KU-825-838

E00387

REFRACTIVE SURGERY

Dimitri T. Azar, MD
Director of Corneal and Refractive Surgery Services
Massachusetts Eye and Ear Infirmary
Associate Professor of Ophthalmology
Harvard Medical School

Associate Scientist
Schepens Eye Research Institute
Department of Ophthalmology
Harvard Medical School
Boston, Massachusetts

Formerly
Associate Professor of Ophthalmology
Director, Keratorefractive Surgery Service
The Wilmer Ophthalmological Institute
The Johns Hopkins University School of Medicine
Baltimore, Maryland

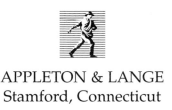

APPLETON & LANGE
Stamford, Connecticut

EAST GLAMORGAN GENERAL HOSPITAL
CHURCH VILLAGE. near PONTYPRIDD

Notice: The authors and the publisher of this volume have taken care to make certain that the doses of drugs and schedules of treatment are correct and compatible with the standards generally accepted at the time of publication. Nevertheless, as new information becomes available, changes in treatment and in the use of drugs become necessary. The reader is advised to carefully consult the instruction and information material included in the package insert of each drug or therapeutic agent before administration. This advice is especially important when using, administering, or recommending new and infrequently used drugs. The authors and publisher disclaim all responsibility for any liability, loss, injury, or damage incurred as a consequence, directly or indirectly, of the use and application of any of the contents of this volume.

Copyright © 1997 by Appleton & Lange
A Simon & Schuster Company

All rights reserved. This book, or any parts thereof, may not be used or reproduced in any manner without written permission. For information, address Appleton & Lange, Four Stamford Plaza, PO Box 120041, Stamford, Connecticut 06912-0041.

97 98 99 00 01 / 10 9 8 7 6 5 4 3 2 1

Prentice Hall International (UK) Limited, *London*
Prentice Hall of Australia Pty. Limited, *Sydney*
Prentice Hall Canada, Inc., *Toronto*
Prentice Hall Hispanoamericana, S.A., *Mexico*
Prentice Hall of India Private Limited, *New Delhi*
Prentice Hall of Japan, Inc., *Tokyo*
Simon and Schuster Asia Pte. Ltd., *Singapore*
Editora Prentice Hall do Brasil Ltda., *Rio de Janeiro*
Prentice Hall, *Upper Saddle River, New Jersey*

Acquisitions Editor: Jane Licht
Production Service: Andover Publishing Services
Designer: Janice Barsevich Bielawa

PRINTED IN THE UNITED STATES OF AMERICA

ISBN 0-8385-8276-1

9 780838 582763

90000

To my parents

To Lara and Nicholas, Welcome!

To Nathalie,
for sharing my profession with dedication and excellence,
my long working hours with patience and assistance,
my leisure time with cheerfulness and laughter,
and my happiest moments with affection and optimism;
and for giving us Nicholas and Lara . . .

And to Ilene Gipson, Claes Dohlman, and all my teachers.

CONTENTS

EAST GLAMORGAN GENERAL HOSPITAL CHURCH VILLAGE. near PONTYPRIDD

CONTRIBUTORS

Indu Arora, MD
Research Fellow, Corneal Service
Department of Ophthalmology
The Wilmer Ophthalmological Institute
The Johns Hopkins University School of Medicine
Baltimore, Maryland

M. Farooq Ashraf, MD
Assistant Professor of Ophthalmology
The Wilmer Ophthalmological Institute
The Johns Hopkins University School of Medicine
Baltimore, Maryland

Kerry K. Assil, MD
Medical Director,
The Sinskey Eye Institute
Santa Monica, California

Dimitri T. Azar, MD
Director of Corneal and Refractive Surgery Services
Massachusetts Eye and Ear Infirmary
Associate Professor of Ophthalmology
Harvard Medical School

Associate Scientist
Schepens Eye Research Institute
Department of Ophthalmology
Harvard Medical School
Boston, Massachusetts

Formerly
Associate Professor of Ophthalmology
Director, Keratorefractive Surgery Service
The Wilmer Ophthalmological Institute
The Johns Hopkins University School of Medicine
Baltimore, Maryland

Nathalie F. Azar, MD
Director of Pediatric Ophthalmology and
    Strabismus Service
Massachusetts Eye and Ear Infirmary
Department of Ophthalmology
Harvard Medical School
Boston, Massachusetts

Georges Baikoff, MD
Professor
Chirurgie Oculaire
Centre d'Ophthalmologie
Clinique Clairval
Marseille, France

Richard E. Braunstein, MD
Assistant Clinical Professor
Department of Ophthalmology
Edward S. Harkness Eye Institute
Columbia-Presbyterian Medical Center
Columbia University College of Physicians
    and Surgeons
New York, New York

Salim I. Butrus, MD
Assistant Clinical Professor
Department of Ophthalmology
George Washington University
Georgetown University
Attending Surgeon
Department of Ophthalmology
Washington Hospital Center
Washington, DC

Jonathan D. Carr, MD
Clinical Associate
Department of Ophthalmology
Emory University School of Medicine
Atlanta, Georgia

Charles Casebeer, MD
Clinical Professor of Ophthalmology
University of Utah
Casebeer Eye Center
Scottsdale, Arizona

Wallace Chamon, MD
Coordinator
Refractive Surgery Sector
Department of Ophthalmology
Paulista School of Medicine
São Paulo, Brazil

Tat Keong Chan, MD, FRCS, FRCOphth
Senior Lecturer
Department of Ophthalmology
National University of Singapore
Singapore, Singapore
Clinical Fellow, Corneal Service
The Wilmer Ophthalmological Institute
The Johns Hopkins University School of Medicine
Baltimore, Maryland

Shu-Wen Chang, MD
Research Fellow, Corneal Service
The Wilmer Ophthalmological Institute
The Johns Hopkins University School of Medicine
Baltimore, Maryland

William W. Culbertson, MD
Professor
Department of Ophthalmology
Bascom Palmer Eye Institute
University of Miami School of Medicine
Miami, Florida

Jan Daniel, MD
Fellow
Department of Ophthalmology
Emory University School of Medicine
Atlanta, Georgia

Thierry David, MD
Chef de Clinique
Université Paris VI
Faculté de Médicine Broussais-Hotel Dieu
Assistant des Hospitaux
Department of Ophthalmology
Hotel Dieu
Paris, France

Martin G. Edwards, MD
Department of Ophthalmology
Walson United States Air Force Hospital
Fort Dix, New Jersey
Department of Ophthalmology
The Wilmer Ophthalmological Institute
The Johns Hopkins University School of Medicine
Baltimore, Maryland

Forrest J. Ellis, MD
Clinical Fellow
Divisions of Pediatric Ophthalmology and
    Oculoplastic Surgery
Department of Ophthalmology
The Wilmer Ophthalmological Institute
The Johns Hopkins University School of Medicine
Baltimore, Maryland

Vadim Filatov, MD
Corneal Fellow
Massachusetts Eye and Ear Infirmary
Harvard Medical School
Greenwich Eye Center
Greenwich, Connecticut

Charles W. Flowers, Jr, MD
Assistant Professor
Director of Refractive Surgery
Division of Ophthalmology
Charles R. Drew University of Medicine and Science
Los Angeles, California

Dasa V. Gangadhar, MD
Corneal Fellow
Massachusetts Eye and Ear Infirmary
Harvard Medical School
Eye Clinic of Wichita
Wichita, Kansas

Claudio Genisi, MD
Department of Ophthalmology
General Hospital
Venice, Italy

Marcela Gomez, MD
Clinical Research Coordinator
Cornea and Refractive Surgery
Cornea Consultants
Boston, Massachusetts

R. Bruce Grene, MD
Assistant Clinical Professor
Department of Ophthalmology
University of Kansas Medical School
Wichita, Kansas

Maged S. Habib, MD
Research Fellow, Cornea Service
The New York Eye and Ear Infirmary
New York, New York

Tae Won Hahn, MD
Research Fellow, Corneal Service
Department of Ophthalmology
The Wilmer Ophthalmological Institute
The Johns Hopkins University School of Medicine
Baltimore, Maryland

Khalil D. Hanna, MD
Assistant Professor
Department of Ophthalmology
Bascom Palmer Eye Institute
University of Miami School of Medicine
Miami, Florida

David R. Hardten, MD
Assistant Clinical Professor
Department of Ophthalmology
University of Minnesota
Attending Surgeon
Department of Ophthalmology
Phillips Eye Institute
Minneapolis, Minnesota

Peter Hersh, MD
Associate Professor
Director, Corneal and Refractive Surgery
Department of Ophthalmology
UMDNJ-New Jersey Medical School
Newark, New Jersey
Director, Cornea and Laser Institute
Hackensack University Medical Center
Teaneck, New Jersey

Jesper Ø. Hjortdal, MD, PhD
Department of Ophthalmology
Århus University Hospital
Århus, Denmark

David G. Hunter, MD, PhD
Assistant Professor
Division of Pediatric Ophthalmology and Strabismus
Departments of Ophthalmology and Biomedical
   Engineering
The Wilmer Ophthalmological Institute
The Johns Hopkins University School of Medicine
Baltimore, Maryland

Sandeep Jain, MD
Research Fellow, Corneal Service
Department of Ophthalmology
The Wilmer Ophthalmological Institute
The Johns Hopkins University School of Medicine
Baltimore, Maryland

W. Todd Johnson
Corneal Service
Massachusetts Eye and Ear Infirmary
Harvard Medical School
Boston, Massachusetts

Carol L. Karp, MD
Assistant Professor of Clinical Ophthalmology
Bascom Palmer Eye Institute
University of Miami School of Medicine
Miami, Florida

Kenneth R. Kenyon, MD
Senior Surgeon
Massachusetts Eye and Ear Infirmary
Associate Clinical Professor, Ophthalmology
Harvard Medical School
Cornea Consultants
Boston, Massachusetts

Johnny M. Khoury, MD
Research Fellow, Corneal Service
Department of Ophthalmology
The Wilmer Ophthalmological Institute
The Johns Hopkins University School of Medicine
Baltimore, Maryland

Douglas D. Koch
Associate Professor
Cullen Eye Institute
Department of Ophthalmology
Baylor College of Medicine
Houston, Texas

Ernest W. Kornmehl, MD
Clinical Instructor
Department of Ophthalmology
Harvard Medical School
Associate Clinical Professor
Department of Ophthalmology
Tufts University School of Medicine
Co-director, Novatec Laser Program
Massachusetts Eye and Ear Infirmary
Boston, Massachusetts

Jeffrey C. Lamkin, MD
Assistant Professor
Department of Ophthalmology
Northeastern Ohio Universities College of Medicine
Kent, Ohio

Thomas M. Leitman, MD
Research Fellow
F. I. Proctor Foundation
University of California, San Francisco
San Francisco, California

Russell L. McCally, PhD
Associate Professor
Department of Ophthalmology
The Wilmer Ophthalmological Institute
The Johns Hopkins University School of Medicine
Principal Staff Physicist
The Johns Hopkins Applied Physics Laboratory
Laurel, Maryland

Peter J. McDonnell, MD
Professor
Department of Ophthalmology
University of Southern California School of Medicine
Doheny Eye Institute
Los Angeles, California

Mariana D. Mead, MD
Clinical Instructor
Department of Ophthalmology
Harvard Medical School
Practicing Ophthalmologist
Ophthalmic Consultants of Boston
Boston, Massachusetts

David Miller, MD
Associate Clinical Professor
Department of Ophthalmology
Harvard Medical School
Cornea Consultants
Boston, Massachusetts

Samuel E. Navon, MD, PhD
Massachusetts Eye and Ear Infirmary
Harvard Medical School
Boston, Massachusetts
Department of Ophthalmology
King Khaled Eye Specialist Hospital
Riyadh, Saudi Arabia

Lee T. Nordan, MD
Assistant Clinical Professor
Jules Stein Eye Institute
University of California
Los Angeles, California

Gregory S. H. Ogawa, MD
Assistant Professor, Ophthalmology
Director, Corneal Service
Department of Surgery, Division of Ophthalmology
University of New Mexico Health Sciences Center
Albuquerque, New Mexico

Joseph Pasternak, MD
Assistant Director
Cornea and External Disease
Division of Surgery
Department of Ophthalmology
National Naval Medical Center
Bethesda, Maryland

K. Scott Proctor
Refractive Surgery Service
The Wilmer Ophthalmological Institute
The Johns Hopkins University School of Medicine
Baltimore, Maryland

Paolo Rama, MD
Department of Ophthalmology
General Hospital
Venice, Italy

Peter A. Rapoza, MD
Assistant Clinical Professor
Department of Ophthalmology
Harvard Medical School
Massachusetts Eye and Ear Infirmary
Cornea Consultants
Boston, Massachusetts

Cynthia J. Roberts, PhD
Assistant Professor
Biomedical Engineering Center and Department
    of Ophthalmology
The Ohio State University
Columbus, Ohio

Michael J. Rogers, MSE
Departments of Biomedical Engineering and Applied
    Physics Laboratory
Johns Hopkins University
Laurel, Maryland

Gary S. Rubin, PhD
Associate Professor
Lions Vision Research Center
The Wilmer Ophthalmological Institute
The Johns Hopkins University School of Medicine
Baltimore, Maryland

Luis Ruiz, MD
Director and Specialist in Refractive Surgery
Centro Ophthalmologico Colombiano
Bogota, Colombia

Ameed Samaha, MD
Department of Ophthalmology
American University of Beirut
Beirut, Lebanon

David J. Schanzlin, MD
Professor
Department of Ophthalmology
Shiley Eye Center
University of California, San Diego
La Jolla, California

Theo Seiler, MD, PhD
Department of Ophthalmology
University Eye Clinic Dresden
Dresden, Germany

Stephen G. Slade, MD
Clinical Faculty
Department of Ophthalmology
University of Texas Medical School
Director, The Laser Center
Houston, Texas

Janine Austin Smith, MD
Medical Officer
Laboratory of Immunology
National Eye Institute
National Institutes of Health
Bethesda, Maryland

Mark G. Speaker, MD, PhD
Associate Clinical Professor
Department of Ophthalmology
New York Medical College
Valhalla, New York
Director, Cornea Service
Department of Ophthalmology
The New York Eye and Ear Infirmary
New York, New York

Walter J. Stark, MD
Professor of Ophthalmology
Director, Corneal Service
The Wilmer Ophthalmological Institute
The Johns Hopkins University School of Medicine
Baltimore, Maryland

J. B. Stevens, MD
Fellow
Cornea Consultants
Boston, Massachusetts

Leon Strauss, MD
Department of Ophthalmology
The Wilmer Ophthalmological Institute
The Johns Hopkins University School of Medicine
Baltimore, Maryland

Jonathan H. Talamo, MD
Assistant Clinical Professor of Ophthalmology
Harvard Medical School
Massachusetts Eye and Ear Infirmary
Cornea Consultants
Boston, Massachusetts

Keith P. Thompson, MD
Department of Ophthalmology
Emory University
Emory Vision Correction Center
Atlanta, Georgia

Vance Michael Thompson, MD
Assistant Professor
Department of Ophthalmology
University of South Dakota School of Medicine
Director of Refractive Surgery
Sioux Valley Hospital
Sioux Falls, South Dakota

Ikuko Toda, MD
Fellow
Schepens Eye Research Institute
Boston, Massachusetts
Assistant Ophthalmologist
Department of Ophthalmology
Tokyo Dental College
Ichikawa-shi, Chiba
Japan

Kazuo Tsubota, MD
Assistant Professor
Department of Ophthalmology
Keio University School of Medicine
Shinjuku, Tokyo
Chairman
Department of Ophthalmology
Tokyo Dental College/Ichikawa General Hospital
Ichikawa, Chiba
Japan

Suhas W. Tuli, MBBS, MD
Research Fellow, Corneal Service
Department of Ophthalmology
The Wilmer Ophthalmological Institute
The Johns Hopkins University School of Medicine
Baltimore, Maryland

Stephen A. Updegraff, MD
Medical Director, L.C.A. Vision
Tampa, Florida
Clinical Instructor
University of South Florida
Tampa, Florida

Steven M. Verity, MD
Assistant Professor
Department of Ophthalmology
St. Louis University School of Medicine
Anheuser-Busch Eye Institute
St. Louis, Missouri

Michael D. Wagoner, MD
Medical Director,
Chair, Department of Ophthalmology
King Khaled Eye Specialist Hospital
Riyadh, Saudi Arabia

PREFACE

This book describes many of the surgical techniques in the rapidly changing field of refractive surgery, their indications, patient selection, complications, and drawbacks. We have reviewed anatomy, wound healing, pharmacology, optics, topography, and instrumentation as they relate to refractive surgery. We highlight the principles of incisional, lamellar, and laser corneal surgery. It is my hope that this book will serve as an introduction to this rapidly evolving field.

It was not until my first face-to-face meeting with Jane Licht, my witty and energetic publisher, that I realized that the idea of a refractive surgery textbook could in fact materialize. My prior skepticism about this project dissipated as the differences between my objectives and those of the publisher became negligible. We originally envisioned a small textbook that would cover topography, RK, PRK, and KM in order to introduce the general ophthalmologist and the corneal specialist to refractive surgery. It was 1994; refractive surgery was experiencing a renaissance. In the ensuing two years, our vision became that of a more comprehensive book covering as many new topics and techniques as possible, torturing Ms. Licht with current developments until the last possible moment before publication.

As I dedicate this book to my family, I would like to express my gratitude to the contributors who were willing to consume their precious time, spending long hours writing and revising manuscripts. I was amazed at their willingness to do so, given that my early refractive surgical learning experience came from attending courses many of the contributors have taught at the American Academy of Ophthalmology, International Society of Refractive Surgery, and the American Society of Cataract and Refractive Surgery. Several were willing to contribute chapters to this book while they were in the process of writing or publishing their own books!

I would like to thank Drs. Leon Strauss, Walter Stark, and Morton Goldberg for their kind assistance in reviewing manuscripts and offering advice throughout the various stages of this project. I would also like to acknowledge the valuable assistance of Scott Proctor and Niels Buessem. Their relentless communication with the publisher and with contributors, and Scott's maintenance of a rigid filing system, were paramount in keeping the project on schedule.

As I write this preface, I open a new page in my academic life, assuming responsibilities at the Massachusetts Eye and Ear Infirmary and the Schepens Eye Research Institute, and I now realize how indebted I am to my loyal friends at the Wilmer Institute for their many efforts towards the production of this book.

Dimitri T. Azar, MD

FOREWORD

Evolution of medical information progresses inexorably, though sometimes unpredictably. The lifetime of a major new clinical concept often lasts no longer than one to three decades; and, then, new or revitalized ideas emerge, and like juggernauts, vigorously plow ahead, casting aside pre-existing beliefs that stand in their way. Their rate of growth, interestingly, is akin to that of a new colony of microorganisms; i.e., an S-shaped curve with an initial slow phase, followed by exponential and sometimes explosive growth, finally terminating in a plateau, or, in some cases, a final steep descent and even extermination. For example, the last quarter of the 20th century may reasonably be considered the golden age of vitreous surgery, at least as we now know it. This is not to say that we have seen the final innovative ideas in this arena; indeed, we are about to enter important derivative activities utilizing vitreoretinal surgical techniques, such as submacular surgery, retinal cell transplants, drug delivery, and hopefully, gene transfer. The age of initial revolutionary ideas, however, occurred in the early 1970s, and many of the later concepts and techniques should be considered important refinements instead of epiphanies.

Now, with the passage of time, the field of refractive surgery rises and glows, piquing our interests and challenging our priorities. These refractive ideas promise to rejuvenate both therapeutic and cosmetic approaches to ocular problems that, according to conventional wisdom, have previously been considered technically, economically, or ethically insurmountable. As in the case of most such innovations involving human health and its associated commercial enterprises, there is a spectrum of opinion, with enthusiastic advocates and their understandable hyperbole recognizable at one end, and died-in-the-wool naysayers at the other

extreme. Of course, the "truth" lies somewhere in the middle. With history in mind, one can predict that ingenious ideas, instruments, and surgical procedures will rather quickly and dramatically proliferate in this emerging field. Darwinian natural selection, influenced, sometimes regrettably but unavoidably, by the marketplace will have its say, and within a decade or so, refractive surgery will evolve more completely. Eventually, the public will become well served by a combination of properly evaluated surgical procedures and superbly trained eye surgeons. This process requires a continual sifting of new concepts and techniques. Through repeated trial and error that are enhanced by ethical, objective, and wise evaluation of scientifically obtained clinical data, a mature discipline will emerge that benefits patients who are carefully selected, informed, treated, and followed up.

In the early stages of its evolution, now about to enter the exponential phase of growth, the field of refractive surgery needs to undergo some periodic respites that allow both the evaluation and the teaching of new ideas and data that have become available to date. Herein lie the value of Dimitri Azar and his welcome book. During his several years at the Wilmer Eye Institute, Dr. Azar displayed the set of attributes required of an editor and author of a compendium whose goals include promulgating new surgical ideas for the therapists of both today and tomorrow; namely, highly developed ethics, communicative skills, intellectual prowess, and technical virtuosity. He is also well endowed with the combination of exuberance and perseverance that are necessary both for proselytizing favorable principles and practices, and simultaneously promoting the caution that is essential whenever patients are subjected to revolutionary interventions that have not yet been wholly vindicated. Indeed, as pointed out by the author:

> We must continue to validate refractive surgical procedures by ensuring their predictability and reproducibility through controlled and well designed scientific investigations.

Dr. Azar's imprimatur is evident throughout this book—his ideas, his original writings and illustrations, and, of course, his selection of outstanding American and international authors. Importantly, the authors represent both younger and older refractive surgeons—gay blades and experienced savants, so to speak. Both groups have much to offer, and, as they themselves would be quick to admit, their valuable offerings represent information which is state-of-the-art, but which, of necessity, is in dramatic flux. Future editions (and one hopes there will be several) will reflect the result of careful clinical scrutiny; some current ideas that are fervently propounded will die, and better ones will evolve.

Perhaps the very vigilant among us would wish to be clairvoyant before embarking on this journey, utilizing a crystal ball to predict what the future of this field foretells; on the other hand, the excitement and much of the value of unpredictable and presently unfathomable new ideas would be lost. We should look to the future, therefore, with pleasure and bated breath, but also with judicious circumspection. There will be many opportunities for appropriate mid-course corrections. For the moment, however, this book is an outstanding contemporary summary of refractive surgery for both the neophyte and the sophisticate. It is the forerunner of an epoch of eye surgery that will occupy our minds and our operating rooms for years to come.

Morton F. Goldberg, MD
Director and Chairman
The Wilmer Ophthalmological Institute
Baltimore, Maryland
September 1996

FOREWORD

Refractive Surgery is a well-written, beautifully illustrated, and compendious review, comprehensively but not exhaustively covering the nascent field of surgically changing the shape of the cornea in order to reach a point where spectacles will be regarded as no longer necessary if not otiose. Notwithstanding the fact that various incisional procedures have been tried over the past 40 years to assuage the problem of ametropia, it is clear that radial keratotomy, and some of the defects that have been perceived in its execution and stability, are what brought the greatest amount of attention to refractive surgery. I personally have always had difficulty with the concept of wounding a crystalline and beautifully regimented tissue simply because of a problem in curvature. There is no doubt, however, that in certain professions, and in certain temperaments, wearing spectacles can create an insufferable and intolerable problem, which cannot be entirely obviated by contact lenses.

I am now persuaded that what once was the "art" of refractive surgery has recently reached the level of early scientific codification. While there is much yet to be learned, there is no question that this type of surgery can be efficacious, safe, and with the recent application of the excimer laser, quite elegant. Further refinements are to be expected. I know of several ophthalmologists who have undergone this form of surgery themselves. Since a great deal of refractive surgery will be performed outside of the ambit of insurance reimbursement, a high degree of ethics will be required of practitioners in order to avoid foisting marginal surgery on the gullible for reasons of one's own remuneration. Textbooks such as this, and the ongoing scientific evaluation of the surgical procedures and their outcomes, will be

tremendous reinforcements for such standards of professional comportment.

If I am not in any sense an expert on corneal refractive surgery, this foreword gives me great pleasure to write because I do regard myself as an expert on Dr. Dimitri Azar. Dimitri has already had three careers: 1) he completed his ophthalmology residency in Lebanon but had to leave that country during the time of its "troubles" in the late 1970's and 1980's; 2) after a Fogarty fellowship he did his second residency in ophthalmology at the Massachusetts Eye and Ear Infirmary, where he also completed a corneal fellowship under Dr. Claes Dohlman and associates, and finally went on to become Chief Resident for one year; 3) and after leaving the Infirmary, he joined the faculty at the Wilmer Ophthalmological Institute, where he founded the first refractive surgical service at that institution. He was an enormous success at the Wilmer, built a thriving practice, obtained National Eye Institute funding for his research program, published many valuable papers on corneal refractive surgery, and was ultimately promoted to Associate Professor at the Johns Hopkins University Medical School.

When the occasion arose to find a new Director of the Cornea Service at the Massachusetts Eye and Ear Infirmary, the Search Committee had the collective epiphany that it would be wonderful if we could interest Dimitri, among other capable candidates, to consider the position. We are delighted that he accepted the position in Boston, where he has also been recently named Associate Chief of Ophthalmology because of his myriad responsibilities. Dimitri is renowned for his equable personality, diplomatic skills, energy, courteousness, intelligence, research inquisitiveness, and surgical and teaching skills. He has been awarded the "Teacher of the Year Prize" both at the Massachusetts Eye and Ear Infirmary when he was Chief Resident, and at the Wilmer Ophthalmological Institute when he was a faculty member. His multivalent talents are amply demonstrated in the design of this textbook as well as in the many chapters of which he is a co-author. I and my colleagues at the Massachusetts Eye and Ear Infirmary are thrilled that he has once again joined us as a clinical and intellectual compatriot. Having witnessed what he has achieved at a comparatively early stage of his career, one enthusiastically contemplates the glories of his productivity and contributions that lie ahead.

Frederick A. Jakobiec, MD, DSc (Med)
Henry Willard Williams Professor of
Ophthalmology, Professor of Pathology, and
Chairman, Department of Ophthalmology
Harvard Medical School
Chief of Ophthalmology
Massachusetts Eye and Ear Infirmary
September 1996

SECTION I

Introduction

CHAPTER 1

Terminology, Classification, and Definitions of Refractive Surgery

Mariana D. Mead ▪ Dimitri T. Azar

WHY PERFORM REFRACTIVE SURGERY?

Most patients with refractive errors obtain excellent visual results with spectacles and contact lenses. Some individuals, however, have jobs and careers that require better uncorrected visual acuity than they are able to obtain with glasses. Others have ocular or medical conditions that make contact lens wear difficult or dangerous. Still others have anisometropia and spectacle-related anisophoria such that corrective spectacle lenses result in prominent eye strain and an unacceptable degree of discomfort. For these patients, refractive surgery may be of benefit.

Still other patients simply wish to dispense with their contact lenses or spectacles, to be able to see without visual aids. Several studies have explored the motivations of patients seeking radial keratotomy (RK). Approximately 75% of patients wished to see well without physical dependence on spectacles or contact lenses.[1,2] Others wanted to have refractive surgery to improve their cosmetic appearance. For many physicians, operating on a normal eye simply to rid a patient of glasses or contact lenses seems aggressive. "Demand-driven rather than disease-driven treatment is new to surgeons who are accustomed to operating to improve or prevent poor corrected vision that is due to disease."[3] However, as well-controlled, multicenter studies show excellent predictability and stability with a variety of refractive surgical procedures, refractive surgery has been accepted by many formerly skeptical physicians. Previous biases will be overcome by progress as we continue to develop increasingly successful and predictable refractive surgical options for our patients. Anyone who has performed refractive surgery knows that these patients generally are delighted and very satisfied. We must continue to validate refractive surgical procedures by ensuring their predictability and reproducibility through controlled and well-designed scientific investigations.

EMMETROPIA AND THE AMETROPIAS

The successful performance of refractive surgery demands a thorough understanding of the optics of the human eye. The refractive power of the eye is predominantly determined by three variables: the power of the cornea, the power of the lens, and the length of the eye. In emmetropia, these three components combine in such a way as to produce no refractive error. When an eye is emmetropic, a pencil of light parallel to the optical axis and limited by the pupil focuses at a point on the retina (ie, the secondary focal point of an emmetropic eye is on the retina) (Fig 1–1). The "far point" in emmetropia (defined as the point conjugate to the retina in the nonaccommodating state) is optical infinity.

Eyes with refractive errors can have abnormalities in one or more of the above variables, or all variables can be in the normal range but incorrectly correlated, resulting in a refractive error. For example, an eye with

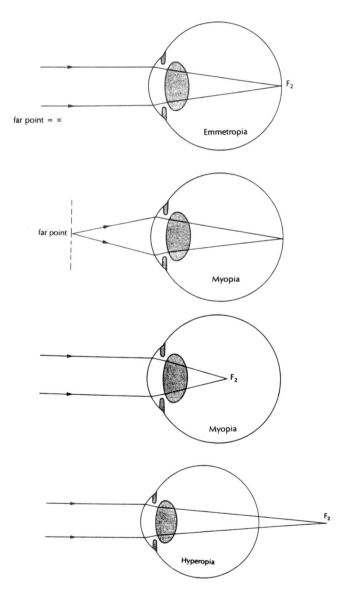

Figure 1–1. Schematic diagrams of emmetropia, myopia, and hyperopia. In emmetropia (top), the far point is at infinity, and the secondary focal point (F2) is at the retina. In myopia, the far point is in front of the eye, and the secondary focal point, F2, is in the vitreous. In hyperopia (bottom), the secondary focal point, F2, is located behind the eye. (Modified with permission from *Azar DT, Strauss L. Principles of applied clinical optics. In: Albert D, Jakobiec F, eds.* Principles and Practice of Ophthalmology. *Philadelphia: WB Saunders; 1994.*)

an axial length in the upper range of normal may be myopic if the corneal variable is also in the steeper range of normal. In a myopic eye, a pencil of parallel rays is brought to focus at a point anterior to the retina. This point, the secondary focal point of the eye, is in the vitreous. Rays diverging from the far point of a myopic eye will be brought to focus on the retina without the aid of accommodation.

The hyperopic eye, on the other hand, brings a pencil of parallel rays of light to focus at a point behind the retina. Accommodation of the eye may produce enough additional plus power to allow the light rays to focus on the retina. Rays converging toward the far point farther behind the eye will be focused on the retina while accommodation is relaxed.

For full correction of myopia and hyperopia, a distance corrective lens placed in front of the eye must have its secondary focal point coinciding with the far point of the eye so that the newly created optical system focuses parallel rays onto the retina. Keratorefractive surgical procedures, instead of using corrective lenses, alter the corneal refractive power, thereby affecting further refraction of light rays reaching the cornea.

Astigmatism may be caused by a toric cornea or, less frequently, by astigmatic effects of the native lens of the eye. Astigmatism is regular when it is correctable with cylindrical or spherocylindrical lenses so that pencils of light from distant objects can be focused on the retina. Otherwise, the astigmatism is irregular.

Presbyopia

Presbyopia is the age-related loss of the ability to sustain comfortably the accommodation necessary for clear vision. The amplitude of accommodation wanes with age. Age of onset of presbyopia will vary with the refractive error and its method of correction. For example, myopes corrected with spectacles can simply remove their glasses for improved reading vision. A latent hyperope, on the other hand, uses his or her accommodative reserve for clear distance vision; and as the amplitude of accommodation wanes with age, reading difficulties emerge.

Presbyopia is an important aspect of the informed consent of keratorefractive patients. Surgically corrected presbyopic myopes will need reading glasses as they age, whereas before surgery they could remove their spectacles to read. Undercorrected myopes may experience less than optimal distance vision, but may retain some of their ability to see clearly at near distances. Patients over 40 considering refractive surgery for myopia must appreciate the extent to which they exchange dependence on distance spectacles for dependence on spectacles for near vision. Patients should be advised of the alternative of attempted undercorrection in one (monovision) or both eyes to offset the problems of presbyopia as well as the possible gradual shift toward hyperopia, which has been reported in as many as 43% of patients 10 years after RK.[4]

REFRACTIVE PROCEDURES: CLASSIFICATION

New keratorefractive techniques are continuously being developed and old techniques refined and simplified, all with the goal of allowing patients to obtain a high level of visual acuity without the use of optical aids. Dr George Waring has provided us with an extensive classification scheme, which allows categorization of keratorefractive procedures based on surgical techniques.[5] Alternatively, grouping keratorefractive procedures by the refractive error being treated provides a framework for understanding the mechanical basis for refractive effect (Table 1–1). With each type of refractive error, it remains useful to divide the procedures into incisional/coagulation, lamellar, and laser techniques. With this classification scheme it can be seen that, depending on the refractive error to be corrected, similar

procedures can be applied to or oriented on the cornea in a variety of ways to correct various refractive errors. For example, lamellar procedures may involve the subtraction or addition of tissue, whereas incisional and coagulation techniques can be radial, circumferential, or localized. Additionally, techniques can be combined, as in laser in situ keratomileusis (LASIK), where lamellar surgery is combined with excimer treatment of the corneal bed.

This discussion will include only currently accepted keratorefractive procedures as well as those with a reasonable chance of being accepted in the near future.

Myopia

Myopia is the most common visually significant refractive error, with a prevalence of nearly 25% for Caucasians and 13% for African Americans.[6] Numerous procedures have been developed to treat myopia by altering the corneal curvature (ie, keratorefractive procedures). The cornea is responsible for 60% of the eye's refractive power, and small changes in curvature can produce significant refractive changes. The long-term safety of intraocular lens placement in phakic myopic eyes and clear lens extraction has not been established, and they are not currently recommended treatments for myopia (see Chapter 42). Similarly, posterior scleral

TABLE 1–1. CLASSIFICATION OF KERATOREFRACTIVE PROCEDURES

	Incisional	Coagulation	Lamellar	Laser
Myopia	Radial keratotomy (1.5–5 D)		Keratomileusis (5–18 D)* • Cryolathe • Nonfreeze planar BKS	Photoretractive keratectomy (excimer PRK) (1–7 D)
	Phakic IOLs and clear lens extraction (>15 D)		Keratomileusis in situ* Intracorneal rings Intracorneal implants	Laser in stiu keratomileusis (LASIK)
			Epikeratophakia (epikeratoplasty, onlay lamellar keratoplasty)	Intrastromal solid state picosecond lasers
Hyperopia	Hexagonal keratotomy	Radial intrastromal thermokeratoplasty (HTK) (up to 3 D)	Hyperopic ALK (4–6 D) Homoplastic ALK (6–20 D) Hyperopic keratophakia Keratophakia Intracorneal implants	Laser thermokeratoplasty (LTK) (up to 4 D) Hyperopic PRK Hyperopic LASIK
Aphakia	Intraocular lenses		Epikeratophakia Keratophakia Intracorneal implants	
Astigmatism	Astigmatic keratotomy Wedge resections/relaxing incisions	Arcuate intrastromal thermokeratoplasty	Astigmatic LASIK	Consecutive spherocylindrical or elliptical photoastigmatic keratectomy (PAK) Erodible-mask excimer Arcuate laser thermokeratoplasty

*May be combined with excimer laser treatment of the lenticules or bed (LASIK).

techniques for severe myopia have been suggested as a means of retarding the progress of high myopia but will not be discussed. Theoretically, corneal procedures can correct myopia by flattening the anterior curvature or changing the index of refraction of the cornea. All procedures to be discussed in this chapter for the treatment of myopia modify the corneal thickness to produce anterior curvature alterations except RK, in which the corneal curvature is flattened by tectonic weakening without changing the central thickness.[7]

Incisional Procedures for Myopia

Radial keratotomy for myopia involves deep and radial corneal stromal incisions, which weaken the paracentral and peripheral cornea and flatten the central cornea. This reduces the refractive power of the central cornea and thereby lessens myopia (Fig 1–2). Radial keratotomy (RK) was performed by ophthalmologists in the Soviet Union including Beliaev,[8] Yenaliev,[9] and Fyodorov and Durnev[10–13] in the early 1970s. In 1978, RK was performed for the first time in the United States.[14,15] Since then, radial keratotomy has been studied thoroughly, most notably by the National Eye Institute (NEI)-funded, multicenter Prospective Evaluation of Radial Keratotomy (PERK) study, a collaborative effort of nine clinical centers. Although the surgical techniques employed in this study have been modified over the past 15 years, the study continues to yield important information about the natural history, safety, predictability, and stability of RK. Newer RK techniques may have better predictability and fewer complications as a result of the adoption of age-related nomograms with fewer incisions, ultrathin diamond knives, better knife calibration, more accurate ultrasonic corneal pachymeters, and improved blade design (see Chapter 16).

Approximately 250,000 RK operations are performed annually in the United States,[4,16] and the American Academy of Ophthalmology considers RK to be a safe and effective procedure in appropriately selected patients.[17] Patients with low and moderate degrees of nonprogressive myopia (up to 5 D) have the best results with RK in achieving the highest levels of uncorrected visual acuity. In patients with higher amounts of myopia (6 to 10 D), the response to surgery is much more variable[18–27] and undercorrection is to be expected. The age of the patient partially determines the upper limit of attainable correction. Older patients achieve a greater correction by approximately 0.75 to 1.00 D per 10 years of age exceeding 35 years.[28] The surgeon currently can manipulate three variables in attempting to achieve accuracy: central optical zone and the number and depth of incisions. Other patient variables are more difficult to quantitate. For example, it is possible that the premenopausal female with a flat cornea, low intraocular pressure, and a small corneal diameter will achieve less correction than would be generally predicted for a paticular RK technique.[29–31]

Despite attention to these factors, predictability of results still can be problematic for the patient seeking perfection.[19–32] Three early studies of predictability have concluded that about 70% of eyes will have a residual refractive error within ±1 D of the predicted result and 90% within ±2 D.[17,29–32] Later studies, with a staged approach, report 80% to 90% of eyes within 1 D of emmetropia.[17,33,34]

Stability of refraction after radial keratotomy is inadequate (see Chapter 21).[4,35] The 10-year PERK results reveal long-term instability of refractive errors; 43% of eyes changed refractive power in the hyperopic direction by 1 D or more (hyperopic shift) between 6 months

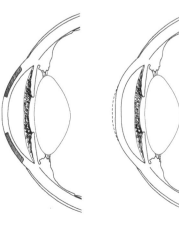
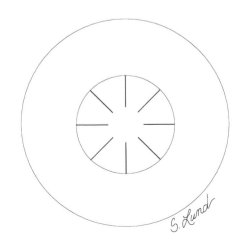

Figure 1–2. In radial keratotomy, radial incisions are placed in the cornea (left), resulting in forward bowing of the "midperipheral" cornea and compensatory flattening of the central cornea (middle). Postoperative appearance of radially symmetric spokes can be appreciated (right). The details of the procedure are described in Chapter 19.

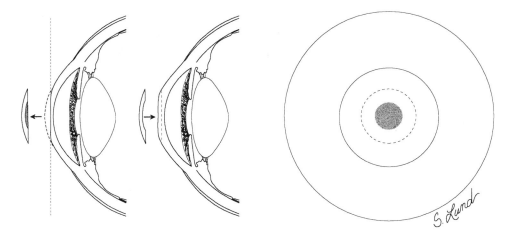

Figure 1–3. Schematic illustration of myopic keratomileusis. The shaded area refers to the location of tissue subtraction. A corneal button is raised using a microkeratome, and is reshaped using a cryolathe (left). When the button is replaced, the central cornea is flattened (middle). Area of central flattening is shown (right, shaded area).

and 10 years.[4] Perhaps technique refinements such as the use of ultrathin gemstone knives and fewer mini-RK incisions will lessen this tendency.

Lamellar Procedures for Myopia

Keratomileusis refers to carving or chiseling the cornea. Although the concept of corneal carving was introduced in 1949, the first reported clinical results were not published until 1964 by Jose Barraquer.[36–37] Keratomileusis was first performed in the United States in 1980 by Swinger.[38]

For myopia, keratomileusis involves excision of a lamellar button (lenticule) of the patient's cornea with a microkeratome, reshaping the lamellar button and replacing it in position with or without sutures (Fig 1–3). The microkeratome applanates the cornea, and slides through a suction ring placed at the limbus. The suction ring height varies to allow the specific diameter of the cornea to be excised to protrude above the mi-

crokeratome track. For myopia, the removed lenticule is treated such that the central corneal curvature is flattened and the overall refractive power of the cornea decreases. The button (lamellar autograft) can be reshaped with a cryolathe, a microkeratome, or an excimer laser. Alternatively, in situ automatic corneal shaping with a second pass of the microkeratome modifies the stromal bed rather than the cap (Fig 1–4). Keratomileusis also can be performed as a homoplastic procedure, in which a central disc of the patient's cornea is removed, and replaced with a lathed disc of donor cornea.

Barraquer's original keratomileusis procedure, called *cryolathe keratomileusis,* involved freezing and reshaping the removed lenticule with a cryolathe (Fig 1–3). Significant advances have improved the predictability of this cryolathe procedure, but the advances in strumentation and surgical skills necessary for the procedure limit its use. Although the procedure enables

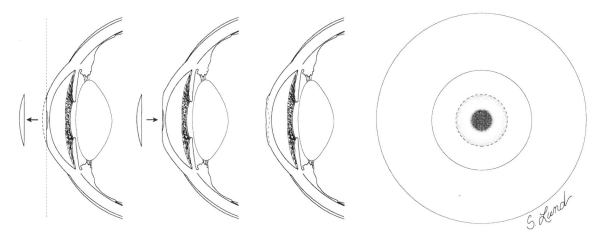

Figure 1–4. Schematic illustration of in situ automatic corneal reshaping of the keratomileusis bed. The shaded area refers to the location of tissue subtraction. A corneal button is raised using a microkeratome (left). A second pass modifies the stromal bed to allow corneal flattening after replacing the cap (middle).

correction of large degrees of myopia, major problems such as irregular astigmatism, unpredictability, and long visual recovery time (freezing damages tissue) may be encountered.[39–43] The nonfreeze planar keratomileusis technique as devised by Barraquer, Krumeich, and Swinger (BKS) in 1983 replaced the cryolathe with a cutting device and a newer microkeratome.[44]

Myopic keratomileusis is able to correct 5 D to 18 D of myopia,[39,40] but is generally considered for patients with 7 to 15 D of myopia, although the upper limit of correction may depend on the initial radius of curvature.[7,38] Corrections beyond 18 D require greater tissue resections, resulting in instability and unpredictability.[38,39]

Automated lamellar keratoplasty (ALK), also called *keratomileusis in situ,* was initially developed for higher myopia (Fig 1–4). ALK uses a mechanized microkeratome secured by a suction apparatus to remove a plano lenticule. This microkeratome, or "automatic corneal shaper," was developed by Luis Ruiz to provide a more consistent thickness and diameter of the corneal lenticule. The second pass of the microkeratome in the stromal bed resects a disc of central corneal stroma. The corneal cap generally is replaced on the stromal bed without sutures. The lenticule, at the time of the first pass, can be secured by a small residual hinge of tissue (flap) to minimize the possibility of losing the cap. Although the initial results of keratomileusis in situ are promising, more studies are necessary to determine predictability and effectiveness in higher myopes (see Chapter 26).

After lenticule removal, the excimer laser can be used to ablate the corneal stromal bed or the button after keratomileusis or keratomileusis in situ. The 193-nm argon fluoride (ArF) laser is currently used to flatten the central corneal curvature.[45,46] The button can then be returned to its treated bed and will often adhere adequately without the need for sutures (Fig 1–4). When the laser treatment is performed on the stromal bed under a flap, the procedure is known as *laser in situ keratomileusis,* or LASIK (see Chapter 34).

Irregular astigmatism is common after ALK, fortunately often decreasing with time. Reports of clinically significant irregular astigmatism after all types of myopic keratomileusis vary but may be as high as 10% to 15%.[40,46,47] Although the automatic microkeratome has improved reproducibility and predictability, ALK remains a technically demanding procedure, with a steep learning curve. For residual refractive errors, incisional refractive techniques can be performed after ALK to increase the degree of central corneal flattening.

The placement of synthetic materials into the cornea can be used to correct myopia. Intracorneal rings can be threaded into a peripheral midstromal tunnel or placed in a peripheral lamellar microkeratome bed to effect flattening of the central cornea.[48,49] Their advantage lies in the avoidance of manipulation of the central cornea and visual axis (Fig 1–5). Alternatively, synthetic intracorneal implants can be placed in a centrally dissected corneal stromal pocket. Although early studies on intracorneal implants dealt with aphakic correction (Fig 1–6), intrastromal lenses are now under study for myopic correction.[50] Intracorneal lenses with high indices of refraction, such as polysulfone, are undergoing refinement in the laboratory, and may prove useful.[51–53]

Epikeratoplasty (also known as *epikeratophakia* and *onlay lamellar keratoplasty*) was introduced by Kaufman, Werblin, and Klyce at the LSU Eye Center in the late 1970s and early 1980s.[54,55] It involves removal of the ep-

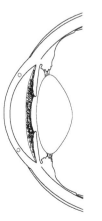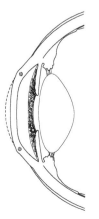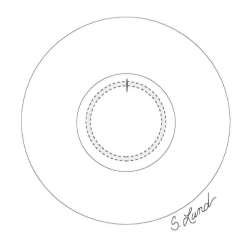

Figure 1–5. Schematic illustration of intrastromal ring. The ring is placed in the stroma (left) resulting in central flattenting (middle). The central cornea is not manipulated (right).

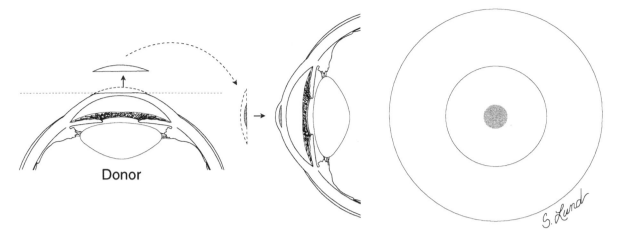

Figure 1–6. Schematic illustration of intracorneal implants. The intrastromal implant can be harvested from a donor eye (left) or made of synthetic material (right). The shaded area refers to the location of the donor lenticule.

ithelium from the patient's central cornea and preparation of a peripheral annular keratotomy. No microkeratome is used. A lyophilized donor lenticule (consisting of Bowman's layer and anterior stroma) is reconstituted and sewn into the annular keratotomy site (Fig 1–7).[56] Theoretical advantages of epikeratophakia are its simplicity and reversibility.[57] Although this procedure is capable of correcting greater degrees of myopia than keratomileusis, the complications of irregular astigmatism, delayed visual recovery, and prolonged epithelial defects are common.[39,58] Although possibly useful in unilateral high myopia in children at high risk for amblyopia, its general use in the treatment of myopia has been abandoned largely owing to the potential for loss of best corrected visual acuity. Synthetic mate-

rials for epikeratoplasty and improved means of attaching the lenticule to the cornea may allow epikeratoplasty to become a potentially useful technique in the treatment of myopia in the future.

Laser Procedure for Myopia

Excimer laser corneal surgery was introduced in 1983 by Trokel and Srinivasan for linear keratectomy.[59] Progress was slowed by unpredictable wound healing, but large-area ablation laser technology or *photorefractive keratectomy* (PRK), proven to be a valuable tool in refractive surgery, has been progressing at a very rapid rate (Fig 1–8). Two basic properties are the foundation of excimer laser refractive surgical techniques.[60] First, there is a potential for minimal or no residual refractive

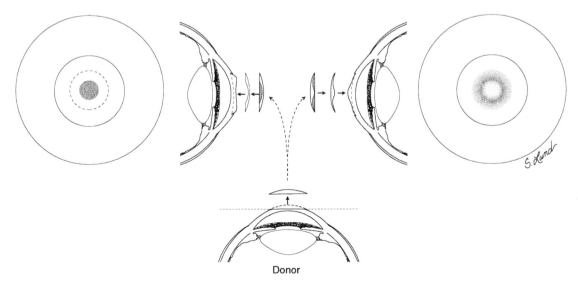

Figure 1–7. Schematic illustration of epikeratoplasty. A preshaped donor lenticule (bottom) is sutured to the recipient stromal bed to correct myopia (left) and hyperopia (right). The shaded areas refer to the locations of tissue subtraction. This procedure is described in detail in Chapter 29.

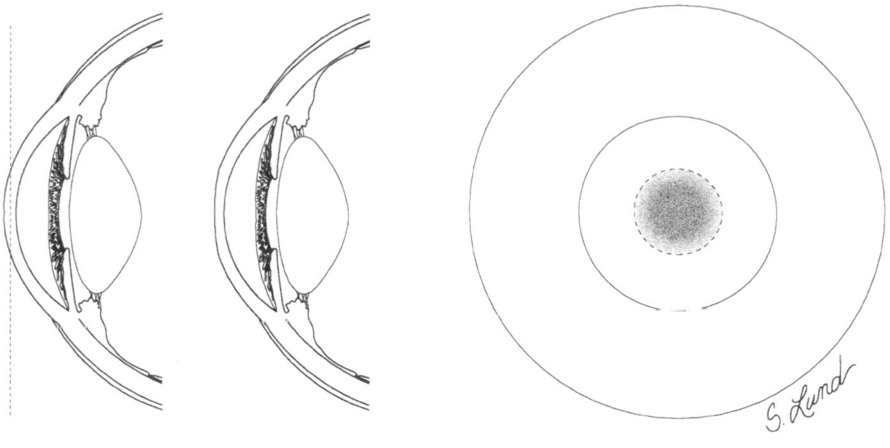

Figure 1–8. Schematic illustration of photorefractive keratectomy showing central subtraction of anterior stroma (left) resulting in corneal flattening (middle). The shaded area refers to the location of tissue subtraction. More tissue is removed from the central as compared to the paracentral region (right).

error after excimer laser surgery. Second, the excimer laser–ablated surface has the potential of being smoother than that obtainable by other surgical techniques because of the submicron accuracy with which the ultraviolet radiation energy ablates the corneal surface.

The 193-nm argon fluoride (ArF) excimer laser is utilized in PRK to maximally ablate corneal tissue centrally, tapering peripherally, with the goal of flattening the corneal surface of myopic individuals. Three types of excimer lasers are currently available: wide-area ablation, scanning slit, and flying spot lasers. The excimer laser wide-area ablation beam is manipulated to achieve corneal flattening through one of two techniques. Most commonly, a diaphragm or a slit changes the size of the ablation aperture over the course of the exposure, allowing maximum laser ablation centrally with less peripherally. Use of an ablatable mask is also being investigated. The mask consists of a plastic polymer (PMMA), which is placed in the laser path and ablated with successive laser pulses. For myopic treatments, the mask is thinnest centrally and progressively thicker toward the edges; the excimer beam penetrates the center first, ablating the central cornea first, and then peripheral ablation occurs with successive pulses. Scanning slit and flying spot lasers are used primarily in Europe, and are currently under clinical investigation in the United States.

The depth of ablation necessary for correction of myopia is highly dependent on the size of the treatment zone. To minimize haloes and edge glare in patients with moderate myopia, most clinical investigations are employing treatment zones of 6 to 6.5 mm, which may require significant ablation of the anterior stroma.

In the United States the use of excimer lasers in humans is under control of the US Food and Drug Admin-

istration (FDA) (Washington, DC), which has to date approved the applications of two companies in the United States: Summit Technology (Waltham, MA) and VisX (Sunnyvale, CA). For myopia of 1 to 7 D, PRK has been shown to result in a high rate of preservation of best corrected visual acuity and minimal complications. In most series, 90% of patients achieve 20/40 or better uncorrected acuity and are within 1 D of emmetropia. In this moderate myopia group, the initial overcorrections generally regress toward emmetropia over several months with stabilization after 6 to 12 months. Long-term follow-up in the United States is needed to assess stability over multiple years. Dense subepithelial haze occurs rarely, but may reduce the best corrected visual acuity (see Chapter 33).

Highly myopic patients often regress 6 to 12 months after surface PRK, presumably because of stromal regeneration and/or epithelial hyperplasia, which cause resteepening of the ablated zone.[61] The incidence of subepithelial haze is also greater in PRK treatments exceeding 6 D. Aspheric ablations and multipass/multizone strategies may minimize wound-healing corneal responses and may improve the predictability in the treatment of higher degrees of myopia.

Intrastromal solid state picosecond lasers are more compact and portable than excimer lasers, but their development is in its early stages.[62] By removing tissue from the stroma or making intrastromal ablation to flatten the central cornea, the epithelium and Bowman's layer are spared and thus smoother surfaces with less keratocyte fibroblastic responses are possible with intrastromal lasers.[63] The intelligent surgical laser (ISL) system is focused in the corneal stroma, creating small cavities and gas bubbles that disappear within 60 minutes. The anterior cornea of experimental animals collapses and flattens (see Chapter 35). Early human studies have failed to demonstrate similar collapses in the space created by the ablated tissue. Numerous questions remain to be answered before intrastromal ablation becomes an acceptable keratorefractive procedure.[63,64]

Hyperopia

Although hyperopia affects approximately 40% of the adult population,[65,66] it is much less visually significant than myopia. The great majority of young hyperopes regard their eyes to be optically "normal." They may experience early presbyopia and manifest hyperopia in their mid to late 30s. Overcorrections after radial keratotomy may require surgical intervention, but a waiting period of approximately 1 year may be necessary.[67]

Many of the keratorefractive procedures used for hyperopia are similar in design to those used to treat myopia but act to increase the cornea's refractive power. Keratorefractive procedures to treat aphakia often are similar to those for high hyperopia.

Incisional/Coagulation Procedures for Hyperopia

Mendez devised the "hexagonal keratotomy" procedure in 1985 to treat hyperopia, which was the first incisional treatment for hyperopia in humans.[68–70] Hexagonal keratotomy consisted of circumferential connecting hexagonal peripheral cuts around a clear 4.5- to 6.0-mm optical zone, which allowed the central cornea to steepen, thereby decreasing hyperopia (Fig 1–9).[68] Wound healing was a major problem with this continuous cut, leading to anterior displacement of the central cornea, excessive scarring at the incisions, and induced astigmatism. In 1989, nonintersecting hexagonal incisions were described by Jensen and Men-

dez.[71] Corneal scarring, optical aberrations, and irregular astigmatism, however, remained a significant problem even after placement of nonintersecting hexagonal keratotomy incisions. Modifications have been suggested, such as T cuts just posterior to the point where the tangential cuts meet, with a reported decreased incidence of astigmatism (T hexagonal keratotomy).[71,72] Until recently, only isolated reports of serious complications had been described with this evolving technique for the correction of low to moderate amounts of hyperopia.[67,73] In 1994, complications in 15 eyes of 10 patients who had undergone hexagonal keratotomy were reported. Complications included problems with glare, photophobia, polyopia, fluctuation in vision, overcorrection, irregular astigmatism, corneal edema, corneal perforation, bacterial keratitis, and endophthalmitis.[74] These authors concluded that "hexagonal keratotomy appears to be an unpredictable, unsafe surgical procedure with a high complication rate, and it should be abandoned until well controlled experimental trials establish its safety and efficacy."[74]

Radial intrastromal thermokeratoplasty shrinks the peripheral and paracentral stromal collagen, producing a peripheral flattening and a central steepening of the cornea to treat hyperopia (Fig 1–10). Radial thermokeratoplasty (hyperopic thermokeratoplasty, or HTK) for the correction of hyperopia was developed in Russia in 1981 by Fyodorov. A retractable cautery probe tip produces a series of preset depth (approximately 95%) stromal burns in a radial pattern similar to that used in RK (see Chapter 37).[75–78] Although an initial reduction in hyperopia was observed, lack of predictability and significant regression are problems.[75–78] However, there may be less induced astigmatism with radial thermokeratoplasty than with hyperopic ALK or hexagonal keratotomy.[79]

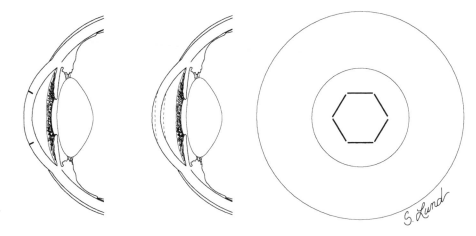

Figure 1–9. Schematic illustration of hexagonal keratotomy.

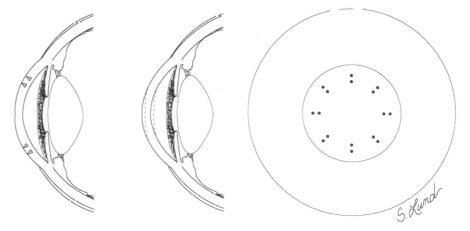

Figure 1–10. Schematic illustration of radial intrastromal thermokeratoplasty and laser thermokeratoplasty.

Lamellar Procedures for Hyperopia

In hyperopic keratomileusis (automated lamellar keratectomy or hyperopic ALK), a deep lamellar keratectomy is performed with a microkeratome, elevating a corneal flap. The stromal bed subsequently develops ectasia under the flap, which is replaced without additional surgery (Fig 1–11). Alternatively, the stromal side of the resected disc is remodeled into a convex hyperopic lenticule that, when placed in the original stromal bed, results in steepening of the central cornea (Fig 1–12).

Hyperopic ALK works best for low levels of hyperopia, but predictability is low and the risk of progressive ectasia limits its usefulness to 4 to 6 D of hyperopia. For larger degrees of hyperopia, homoplastic ALK has been performed. In this procedure, the microkeratome removes a small disc (80 to 100 μm in thickness, 5 to 7 mm in diameter) which is discarded and replaced by a 350- to 400-μm thick donor lenticule (generated using the microkeratome). Although hyperopia between 4 and 10 D has been treated successfully,[80] the safety and efficacy of hyperopic and homoplastic ALK have not been fully established and long-term follow-up is lacking.

Hyperopic epikeratophakia uses a prepared donor lenticule without microkeratome removal of tissue (Fig 1–7). Although theoretically safer than keratomileusis, it lacks predictability and may induce irregular astigmatism.[81]

Keratophakia is the technique of creating a corneal lens for the purpose of reshaping the cornea to create a steeper anterior cornea and increased refractive power. Keratophakia, developed by José Barraquer, can be used to correct high hyperopia, as well as aphakia. Like keratomileusis, the surgery is technically complex and difficult to perform. A lamellar keratectomy is first performed with a microkeratome on the recipient's cornea. A fresh or preserved donor cornea also undergoes a la-

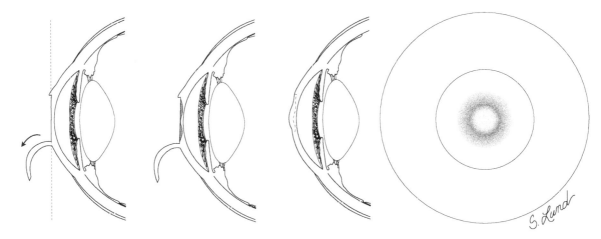

Figure 1–11. Schematic illustration of flap keratomileusis (left). Myopic and hyperopic corrections are possible under the flap. Hyperopic correction results from either spontaneous ectasia of the posterior stroma (not shown) or from combining the flap technique with hyperopic laser treatment as illustrated (central left). The flap is then replaced (central right). The shaded area refers to the location of tissue subtraction (right).

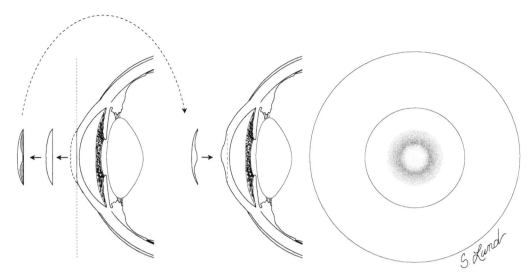

Figure 1–12. Schematic illustration of hyperopic keratomeleusis using a cryolathe to reshape the stromal lenticule and increase central corneal curvature. The shaded area refers to the location of tissue subtraction (right).

mellar keratectomy. From this donor specimen, epithelium, Bowman's layer, and anterior stroma are removed to create a stromal lens, which is then shaped into a meniscus lens of desired specifications after preservation by a variety of means (refrigeration in tissue culture medium, freezing, or freeze-drying). This stromal lens is placed intrastromally within the recipient and the anterior lamellar cap is sutured in place (Fig 1–6).

Because of the complexity of keratophakia, synthetic intracorneal lenses were developed. Hydrogel intrastromal implants for hyperopic correction are biocompatible, but still require preparation of a lamellar bed with a microkeratome.

Laser Procedures for Hyperopia

Solid-state infrared lasers, like the holmium:YAG (Ho:YAG) laser, have been used in a peripheral intrastromal radial pattern (laser thermokeratoplasty, or LTK) to treat hyperopia of 4 D and less.[82] LTK works by causing thermal shrinkage of stromal collagen in the paracentral cornea with a resultant steepening of the central corneal curvature, thereby reducing hyperopia (Fig 1–10). Recent work on human eyes has demonstrated appropriate topographic changes with at least short-term stability.[83] This laser energy can be delivered by a handheld probe or slit beam system and appears most useful for limited amounts of hyperopia and hyperopic astigmatism. However, the long-term effects and refractive stability of Ho:YAG laser thermokeratoplasty are unknown.

The excimer delivery system can deliver a specific ablation pattern with or without an erodible mask, which allows for maximum ablation in the midperiphery for an overall steepening of the optical zone (hyperopic PRK; Fig 1–13). This contour created for hyperopic correction is prone to regression because of epithelial hyperplasia and new collagen formation. Early clinical experience with hyperopic PRK under a keratomileusis flap (hyperopic LASIK), however, is promising.

Aphakia

Refractive techniques for the correction of aphakia include intraocular lens implantation, keratophakia, and epikeratoplasty. Keratophakia has been previously discussed as a treatment for hyperopia. Epikeratophakia has been described previously for myopia and hyperopia. In aphakic keratoplasty, the donor tissue lens is thicker in the center than in the periphery. Widespread use of epikeratophakia is limited because of problems with epithelial healing and graft clarity. However, epikeratophakia has a role in the aphakic contact lens–intolerant patient at high risk for intraocular procedures. Its main use is in the correction of aphakic children aged 1 to 8 who are spectacle- and contact lens–intolerant in order to avoid amblyopia. The highest success rates in epikeratophakia have been reported in the treatment of 8- to 18-year-old patients with aphakia.[84]

Intracorneal lenses also may prove to be of benefit in treating aphakia. Hydrogel,[85] as well as materials with a high index of refraction, like fenestrated polysulfone,[86] may prove to be safe for use in patients who

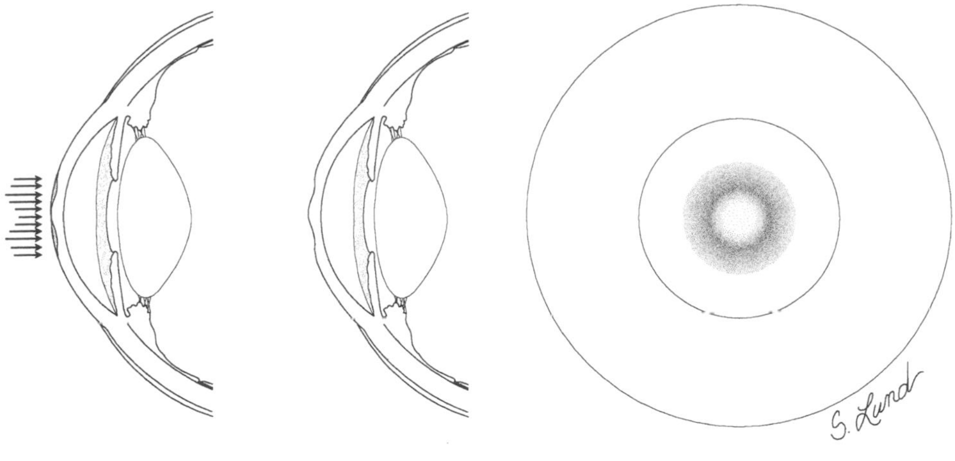

Figure 1–13. Schematic illustration of hyperopic photorefractive keratectomy. The shaded area refers to the location of tissue subtraction. More stromal tissue is removed in the paracentral as compared to the central region.

are contact lens–intolerant and in whom intraocular lenses are contraindicated.

Astigmatism

Naturally occurring astigmatism is very common, and up to 95% of eyes may have some clinically detectable astigmatism in their refractive error.[87] Between 3% and 15% of the general population has astigmatism greater than 2 D.[88] Although there is some variability, approximately 10% of the population can be expected to have naturally occurring astigmatism greater than 1 D, where the quality of uncorrected visual acuity might be considered unsatisfactory.[89,90] The incidence of astigmatism following extracapsular cataract extraction greater than 2 D is approximately 25% to 30%,[91,92] although it is lower after phacoemulsification.

Visual acuity is expected to decline for the different degrees of astigmatism. Astigmatism of 0.50 to 1.00 D usually requires some form of optical correction. An astigmatic refractive error of 1.00 to 2.00 D decreases uncorrected vision to the 20/30 to 20/50 level, whereas 2.00 to 3.00 D may decrease uncorrected visual acuity to the 20/70 to 20/100 range.[89]

Incisional Procedures for Astigmatism

Although Snellen first published on the surgical correction of astigmatism in 1869,[93] keratotomy procedures to treat astigmatism are still not well standardized, and there is much less published information about them than about radial keratotomy.

Astigmatic keratotomy (AK) involves performing transverse (also called tangential, or T) cuts in an arcuate or straight fashion perpendicular to the steep meridian of astigmatism (see Chapter 22). Although current techniques are certain to be refined in the future, AK

offers the patient a very good chance of significant improvement by correcting astigmatic errors.[94–96] In general, patients with greater than 1.5 D of astigmatism may be candidates for astigmatic keratotomy. Deeper and longer incisions produce greater effect, but cuts beyond 75° are not recommended. Effects of cuts increase dramatically with age. The use of the mechanized arcuate keratome for astigmatism is summarized in Chapter 17.

The Ruiz procedure employs trapezoidal cuts, four transverse cuts inside two radial incisions. Although important in its time, stacking multiple rows of astigmatic incisions is no longer felt to be prudent because of poor predictability. A pair of tangential or arcuate incisions achieve significant correction. Additional incisions have minimal added benefit.

Relaxing incisions in the steep meridian, often with wedge resections, and resuturing in the flat meridian were developed by Troutman.[97,98] Although the procedure is effective in decreasing astigmatism, clinical results are highly unpredictable and the procedures are reserved for the correction of postkeratoplasty astigmatism.[99–101]

Laser Procedures for Astigmatism

Laser transverse linear keratectomy for astigmatism has been replaced by the use of excimer laser keratectomy treatment of astigmatism. The laser beam can be directed though a moving slit aperture, or a scanning laser slit beam can be used to deliver an excimer laser pattern capable of treating astigmatism. The erodible-mask technique involves ablation of a PMMA toric button, mounted on a quartz plate transparent to the 193-nm radiation, held by a plastic eyecup. Using a wide laser aperture, the laser ablates the PMMA and then the cornea, thereby allowing the anterior shape of the mask to be transferred onto the cornea, producing the desired astigmatic correction. Corneal wound healing and remodeling occur at the two truncated ends along the axis of the ablated cylinder, and therefore there is a net hyperopic shift (see Chapter 32). The procedure is therefore suitable for compound myopic astigmatism but inadvisable in patients with hyperopia.

Arcuate applications of thermokeratoplasty (with Ho:YAG laser or deep stromal hot needle) to the flat meridian are in early clinical trials in the United States.[102]

No discussion of astigmatism would be complete without a mention of the endless possibilities we have to address naturally occurring astigmatism during cataract surgery by planning location of wound, length of incision, sutures versus no sutures, and concurrent placement of arcuate keratotomy incisions.

SUMMARY

A multitude of motivations lead patients to consider refractive surgery. Increased predictability and reproducibility of a number of keratorefractive surgical procedures have led to an overall increased acceptance of this rapidly evolving field. Special attention to informed consent is vital for these procedures, as the vast majority of these eyes are normal except for their refractive error.

A classification scheme based on type of refractive error to be corrected permits a logical approach to treatment and provides a framework for the development of new procedures.

The clinician must keep constantly in touch with the literature as more of these keratorefractive techniques are proven to be safe, predictable, effective, reliable, stable, and reproducible.

REFERENCES

1. Bourque LB, Rubenstein R, Cosand B, et al. Psychosocial characteristics of candidates for the Prospective Evaluation of Radial Keratotomy (PERK) study. *Arch Ophthalmol.* 1984;102:1187–1192.
2. Powers M, Meyerowitz BE, Arrowsmith PN, Marks RG. Psychosocial findings in radial keratotomy patients two years after surgery. *Ophthalmology.* 1984;91:1193–1198.
3. Sugar A. Has radial keratotomy finally come of age? *Ophthalmology.* 1993;100:979–980.
4. Waring GO, Lynn MJ, McDonnell PJ, et al. Results of the Prospective Evaluation of Radial Keratotomy (PERK) study 10 years after surgery. *Arch Ophthalmol.* 1994;112:1298–1308.
5. Waring GO. Making sense of Keratospeak IV—classification of refractive surgery 1992. *Arch Ophthalmol.* 1992;110:1385–1391.
6. Sperduto RD, Seigel D, Roberts J, Rowland M. Prevalence of myopia in the United States. *Arch Ophthalmol.* 1983;101:405–407.
7. Swinger CA, Barraquer JI. Keratophakia and keratomileusis—clinical results. *Ophthalmology.* 1981;88:709–715.
8. Beliaev VS, Ilyina TS. Scleroplasty in the treatment of progressive myopia. *Vestn Oftalmol.* 1972;3:60–63.
9. Yenaliev FS. Experience in surgical treatment of myopia. *Vestn Oftalmol.* 1978;3:52.
10. Fyodorov SN. Surgical correction of myopia and astigmatism. In: Schachar RA, et al, eds. *Keratorefraction.* Denison, TX: LAL Publishing; 1980;141–172.
11. Durnev VV, Ermoshin AS. Determination of dependence between the length of anterior radial nonperforating incision of cornea and their effectiveness. In: *Transactions of the Fifth All-Union Conference of Inventors and Rationalizers in Ophthalmology Field.* Moscow: 1976:106–108.
12. Durnev VV. Decrease of corneal refraction by anterior keratotomy method with the purpose of surgical correction of myopia of mild to moderate degree. In: *Proceedings of the First Congress of Ophathalmologists of Transcaucasia.* Thilisi; 1976:129–132.
13. Fyodorov SN, Durnev VV. Operation of dosaged dissection of corneal circular ligament in cases of myopia of a mild degree. *Ann Ophthalmol.* 1979;11:1185–1190.
14. Bores LD, Myers W, Cowden J. Radial keratotomy—an analysis of the American experience. *Ann Ophthalmol.* 1981;13:941–948.
15. Bores LD. Historical review and clinical results of radial keratotomy. In: Binder PS, ed. Refractive Corneal Surgery: The Correction of Aphakia, Hyperopia and Myopia. *Int Ophthalmol Clin.* 1983;23:93–118.
16. Waring GO, Lynn MJ, Nizam A, et al. Results of the evaluation of radial keratotomy (PERK) study five years after surgery. *Ophthalmology.* 1991;98:1164–1176.
17. Waring GO. Ophthalmic procedures assessment—radial keratotomy for myopia. *Ophthalmology.* 1993;100:1103–1115.
18. Sanders DR, ed. *Radial Keratotomy Surgical Techniques.* Thorofare, NJ: Slack; 1986.
19. Waring GO, Lynn MJ, Fielding B, et al. Results of the Prospective Evaluation of Radial Keratotomy (PERK) study four years after surgery for myopia. *JAMA.* 1990;263:1083–1091.
20. Deitz MR, Sanders DR, Marks RG. Radial keratotomy: an overview of the Kansas City Study. *Ophthalmology.* 1984;91:467–477.
21. Arrowsmith PN, Marks RG. Visual, refractive, and keratometric results of radial keratotomy: a five year followup. *Arch Ophthalmol.* 1989;107:506–511.
22. Sawelson H, Marks RG. Five year results of radial keratotomy. *Refract Corneal Surg.* 1989;5:8–20.

23. Arrowsmith PN, Sanders DR, Marks RG. Visual, refractive, and keratometric results of radial keratotomy. *Arch Ophthalmol.* 1983;101:873–881.

24. Rowsey JJ, Balyeat HD, Rabinovitch B, et al. Predicting the results of radial keratotomy. *Ophthalmology.* 1983;90:642–654.

25. Neumann AC, Osher RH, Fenzl RE. Radial keratotomy: a comprehensive evaluation. *Doc Ophthalmol.* 1984;56:275–301.

26. Kremer FB, Marks RB. Radial keratotomy: prospective evaluation of safety and efficacy. *Ophthalmic Surg.* 1983;14:925–930.

27. Waring GO. *Refractive Keratotomy for Myopia and Astigmatism.* St. Louis, MO: CV Mosby; 1991.

28. Waring GO. Radial keratotomy. *Ophthalmol Clin North Am.* 1992;5:695–707.

29. Lynn MJ, Waring GO, Sperduto RD, the PERK Study Group. Factors affecting outcome and predictability of radial keratotomy in the PERK study. *Arch Ophthalmol.* 1987;105:42–51.

30. Arrowsmith PN, Marks RG. Evaluating the predictability of radial keratotomy. *Ophthalmology.* 1985;92:331–338.

31. Sanders DR, Deitz MR, Gallagher D. Factors affecting the predictability of radial keratotomy. *Ophthalmology.* 1985;92:1237–1243.

32. Arrowsmith PN, Marks RG. Four year update on predictability of radial keratotomy. *J Refract Surg.* 1988;4:37–45.

33. Spigelman AV, Williams PA, Lindstrom RL. Further studies of four incision radial keratotomy. *Refract Corneal Surg.* 1989;5:292–295.

34. Salz JJ, Salz JM, Salz M, Jones D. Ten years experience with a conservative approach to radial keratotomy. *Refract Corneal Surg.* 1991;7:12–22.

35. Dietz MR, Sanders DR, Reanan MG, DeLuca M. Long term (5 to 12 year) followup of metal blade radial keratotomy procedures. *Arch Ophthalmol.* 1994;112:614–620.

36. Barraquer JI. Keratomileusis for myopia and aphakia. *Ophthalmology.* 1981;88:701–708.

37. Barraquer JI. Qucratomileusis para la correcion de la miopia. *Arch Soc Am Oftalmol Optom.* 1964;5:27–48.

38. Swinger CA, Barker BA. Prospective evaluation of myopic keratomileusis. *Ophthalmology.* 1984;91:785–792.

39. Binder PS. Refractive surgery—its current status and its future. *CLAO J.* 1985;11:358–375.

40. Price FW. Keratomileusis. *Ophthalmol Clin North Am.* 1992;5:673–681.

41. Baumgartner SD, Binder PS. Refractive keratoplasty. Histopathology of clinical specimens. *Ophthalmology.* 1985;92:1606–1615.

42. Jakobiec FA, Koch P, Iwamoto T, et al. Keratophakia and keratomileusis. Comparison of pathologic features of penetrating keratoplasty specimens. *Ophthalmology.* 1981;88:1251–1259.

43. Binder PS, Beal JP Jr, Zavala EY. The histopathology of a case of keratophakia. *Arch Ophthalmol.* 1982;100:101–105.

44. Krumeich JH, Swinger CA. Non-freeze epikeratophakia for the correction of myopia. *Am J Ophthalmol.* 1987;103:397–403.

45. Buratto L, Ferrari M. Excimer laser intrastromal keratomileusis—case reports. *J Cataract Refract Surg.* 1992;18:37–41.

46. Buratto L, Ferrari M, Rama P. Excimer laser intrastromal keratomileusis. *Am J Ophthalmol.* 1992;113:291–295.

47. Arenas-Archila E, Sanchez-Thorin JC, Navanjo-Vribe JP, Hernandex-Lozano A. Myopic keratomileusis in situ: a preliminary report. *J Cataract Refract Surg.* 1991;17:424–435.

48. Fleming JF, Reynolds AE, Kilmer L, et al. The intrastromal corneal ring: two cases in rabbits. *J Refract Surg.* 1987;3:227–232.

49. Burns TE, Ayer CT, Evensen DA, et al. Effects of intrastromal corneal ring size and thickness on corneal flattening in human eyes. *Refract Corneal Surg.* 1991;7:46–50.

50. Werblin TP, Patel AS, Barraquer JI. Initial human experience with Permalens myopic hydrogel intracorneal lens implants. *Refract Corneal Surg.* 1992:8:2326.

51. Lane SL, Cameron JD, Lindstrom RL, et al. Polysulfone corneal lenses. *J Cataract Refract Surg.* 1986;12:50–60.

52. Choyce P. The correction of refractive errors with polysulfone corneal inlays. *Trans Ophthalmol Soc UK.* 1985;104:332–342.

53. Kirkness CM, Steele ADM, Garner A. Polysulfone corneal inlays. Adverse reactions: a preliminary report. *Trans Ophthalmol Soc UK.* 1985;104:343–350.

54. Kaufman HE. The correction of aphakia. *Am J Ophthalmol.* 1980;89:1–10.

55. Werblin TP, Klyce SD. Epikeratophakia—the surgical correction of aphakia: 1. Lathing of corneal tissue. *Curr Eye Res.* 1981;1:123–129 or 591–597.

56. McDonald MB, Kaufman HE, Aquavella JV, et al. The nationwide study of epikeratophakia for myopia. *Am J Ophthalmol.* 1987;103:375–383.

57. McDonald MB, Klyce SD, Suarez H, Kandarakis A, Friedlander MH, Kaufman HE. Epikeratophakia for myopic correction. *Ophthalmology.* 1985;92:1417–1426.

58. Krumeich JH, Swinger CA. Nonfreeze keratophakia for correction of myopia. *Am J Ophthalmol.* 1987;103:397–403.

59. Trokel SL, Srinivasan R, Braren B. Excimer laser surgery of the cornea. *Am J Ophthalmol.* 1983;96:710–715.

60. Steinert RF. Excimer laser photorefractive keratectomy: theory, case selection and variables. In: Brightbill FS, ed. *Corneal Surgery,* 2nd ed. St. Louis, MO: CV Mosby; 512–528.

61. Thompson KP. Photorefractive keratectomy. *Ophthalmol Clin North Am.* 1992;5:745–751.

62. Moretti M. Refractive laser update: solid state refractive lasers evolve slowly. *Refract Corneal Surg.* 1991;7:273–274. News.

63. Assil KK, Quantock AJ. Wound healing in response to keratorefactive surgery. *Surv Ophthalmol.* 1993;38: 289–302.

64. Brown DB, OBrien WJ, Schultz RO. ND:YLF picosecond laser capabilities and ultrastructure effects in corneal ablations. *Invest Ophthalmol Vis Sci.* 1993;34(suppl):1246.

65. Sorsby A. Biology of the eyes as an optical system. In: Duane TD, Jaeger EA, eds. *Clinical Ophthalmology,* rev ed. Philadelphia: JB Lippincott; 1988;1:1394.

66. Sorsby A, Sheraton M, Leary GA, et al. Vision, visual acuity and ocular refraction of young men. *Br Med J.* 1960;1:1394.

67. Tamura M, Mamalis N, Kreisler KR, Anderson CW, Casebeer JC. Complications of hexagonal keratotomy following radial keratotomy. *Arch Ophthalmol.* 1991;109: 1351. Correspondence.

68. Mendez A. Correcao da hipermetropia pela ceratotomia hexagonal. In: Guimarares, R, ed. *Cirugia Refractive.* Rio de Janiero, Brazil: Piramide Livro Medico Editora Ltda; 1987;267–279.

69. Mendez A. Advances in the hyperopic correction with hexagonal keratotomy. Presented at American Society of Cataract and Refractive Surgery Meeting; April 1986; Los Angeles, CA.

70. Mendez A. Hyperopia correction with hexagonal keratotomy. Presented at the Keratorefractive Society Symposium; September 1985; San Francisco, CA.

71. Casebeer JC, Phillips SG. Hexagonal keratotomy. An historical review and assessment of 46 cases. *Ophthalmol Clin North Am.* 1992;5:727–744.

72. Gilbert ML, Friedlander M, Granet N. Corneal steepening in human eye bank eyes by combined hexagonal and transverse keratotomy. *Refract Corneal Surg.* 1990;6: 126–130.

73. McDonnell PJ, Lean JS, Schanzlin DJ. Globe rupture from blunt trauma after hexagonal keratotomy. *Am J Ophthalmol.* 1987;103:241–242.

74. Basuk WL, Zisman M, Waring GO, et al. Complications of hexagonal keratotomy. *Am J Ophthalmol.* 1994;117: 37–49.

75. Feldman ST, Ellis W, Frucht-Pery J, et al. Regression of effect following radial thermokeratoplasty in humans. *Refract Corneal Surg.* 1989;5:288–291.

76. Neumann AC, Sanders DR, Salz J. Radial thermokeratoplasty for hyperopia: encouraging results from early human trials. *Refract Corneal Surg.* 1989;5:50–54.

77. Neumann AC, Fyodorov SN, Sanders DR. Radial thermokeratoplasty for the correction of hyperopia. *Refract Corneal Surg.* 1990;6:404–412.

78. Neumann AC, Sanders DR, Reanan M, et al. Hyperopic thermokeratoplasty clinical evaluation. *J Cataract Refract Surg.* 1991;17:830–838.

79. Neumann AC. Thermokeratoplasty for hyperopia. *Ophthalmol Clin North Am.* 1992;5:753–772.

80. Krumeich JH, Swinger CA. The planar non-freeze lamellar refractive keratoplasty techniques. In: Boyd BF, ed. *Highlights of Ophthalmology,* 30th anniversary ed.: *Refractive Surgery with the Masters.* Coral Gables, FL; 1987; 2:28.

81. McDonald MB. Epikeratophakia. In: Boyd BF, ed. *Highlights of Ophthalmology,* 30th anniversary ed: *Refractive Surgery with the Masters.* Coral Gables, FL; 1987; 2:143.

82. Seiler TH. YAG laser thermokeratoplasty for hyperopia. *Ophthalmol Clin of North Am.* 1992:5:773–780.

83. Seiler T, Matallana M, Bende T. Laser thermokeratoplasty by means of a pulsed Holmium: YAG laser for hyperopic correction. *Refract Corneal Surg.* 1990;6:335–339.

84. Morgan KS, Marvelli TL, Ellis GS, et al. Epikeratophakia in children with traumatic cataracts. *J Pediatrc Ophthalmol Strabismus.* 1986;23:108–112.

85. Werblin TP, Patel AS, Barraquer JI. Initial human experience with Permalens myopic hydrogel intracorneal lens implant. *Refract Corneal Surg.* 1992;8:2326.

86. Climenhaga H, MacDonald JM, McCarey BE, Waring GO. Effect of diameter and depth on the response to solid polysulfone intracorneal lenses in cats. *Arch Ophthalmol.* 1988;106:818–824.

87. Donders RC, Moore WD, trans. *On the Anomalies of Accommodation and Refraction of the Eye.* London, UK: New Sydenham Society; 1864;415–417.

88. Buzard K, Shearing S, Relyea R. Incidence of astigmatism in a cataract practice. *J Refract Surg.* 1988;4:173–178.

89. Duke ESS, Abrams D. Ophthalmic optics and refraction. In: *System of Ophthalmology.* St. Louis, MO: CV Mosby; 1970;5:274–295.

90. Lindstrom RL. The surgical correction of astigmatism: a clinician's perspective. *Refract Corneal Surg.* 1990;6: 441–454.

91. Axt JC. Longitudinal study of postoperative astigmatism. *J Cataract Refract Surg.* 1987;13:381–388.

92. Jampel HD, Thompson JR, Baker CC, et al. A computerized analysis of astigmatism after cataract surgery. *Ophthalmic Surg.* 1986;17:786–790.

93. Snellen H. Die richtung der Haupt meridiane des astigmatischen Auges. *Archiv fur Ophthalmologie.* 1869;15: 199–207.

94. Lindquist TD, Rubenstein JB, Hofmann RF, et al. Astigmatic keratotomy. In: Sanders DR, ed. *Radial Keratotomy: Surgical Techniques.* Thorofare, NJ: Slack; 1986;119–129.

95. Lindquist TD, Rubenstein JB, Rice SW, et al. Trapezoidal astigmatic keratotomy. *Arch Ophthalmol.* 1986;104:1534–1539.

96. Thornton SP. Graded non-intersecting transverse incisions for correction of idiopathic astigmatism. In: Sanders DR, ed. *Radial Keratotomy: Surgical Techniques.* Thorofare, NJ: Slack, Inc; 1986;91–103.

97. Troutman RC. Microsurgical control of corneal astigmatism in cataract and keratoplasty. *Trans Am Acad Ophthalmol Otolaryngol.* 1973;77:563–572.

98. Troutman RC: Corneal wedge resections and relaxing incisions for postkeratoplasty astigmatism. In: Binder PS, ed. Refractive Corneal Surgery: The Correction of Astigmatism. *Int Ophthalmol Clin.* 1983;23(4):161–168.

99. Krachmer JH, Fenzl RE. Surgical correction of high postkeratoplasty astigmatism. *Arch Ophthalmol.* 1980;98:1400–1402.

100. Krachmer JH, Ching SST: Relaxing corneal incisions for postkeratoplasty astigmatism. In: Binder PS, ed. Refractive Corneal Surgery: The Correction of Astigmatism. *Int Ophthalmol Clin.* 1983;23(4):153–159.

101. Cherry PMH, Rodgers KJ, Arndt J. Corneal wedge resection in rabbits. *Ann Ophthalmol.* 1984;16:632–636.

102. Neumann AC, Sanders DR, Reanan M, DeLuca M. Hyperopic thermokeratoplasty: clinical evaluation. *J Cataract Refract Surg.* 1991;17:830–838.

CHAPTER 2

Corneal Anatomy and Physiology

Dimitri T. Azar ▪ Wallace Chamon ▪ Sandeep Jain

BACKGROUND

The cornea is the avascular outer portion of the eye. According to Gullstrand's schematic eye, the cornea is responsible for more than 70% of the optic power of the eye in relaxed accommodation status. Changing 10% of the optic power of the anterior corneal surface would cause a shift of 4.87 D in the patient's refraction.[1] These characteristics explain why cornea surgeries are the most commonly performed refractive procedures.

Corneal horizontal and vertical diameters average 12.6 and 11.7 mm, respectively, in adults, whereas in premature infants corneal diameter can be as small as 6.2 mm.[2,3] Human corneas continue to grow after birth until the end of the third year.

Central corneal thickness averages 0.58 mm in the first week of life,[4–6] thinning to 0.52 mm in adults.[7–10] Corneal thickness does not change with aging after the fifth year of life,[11,12] but increases on average 0.016 mm during pregnancy.[13] The minimal corneal thickness is localized at the line of sight in 69% of eyes, and at a maximum displacement of 0.4 mm in 5% of eyes.[7] Normal peripheral enlargement of corneal thickness is approximately 22% at 5 mm of the line of sight. The anterior corneal curvature is steeper in infants (47.59 D during the first 6 months of life), declining and stabilizing to 42.69 D in the third year of life.[14] Recently, new technologies showed that the posterior surface of the cornea does not follow the same pattern of the anterior surface, and the toricity of the posterior surface has been shown to influence as much as 14% of corneal astigmatism.[15,16] The distance between the corneal apex and the equator of the lens nucleus averages 5.75 mm.[17]

New methods for studying corneal curvatures and biomechanics have been proposed and will improve even more our understanding of corneal behavior under refractive procedures.[18,19] By assuming a uniform angular distribution of stromal lamellae through the corneal thickness, a mechanical model could be designed employing a mathematical analysis known as finite element formulation for simulating the effects of surgical procedures to improve their predictability.[20]

TEAR FILM ANATOMY

The importance of adequate quantity and quality of tears for maintaining a healthy ocular surface is well recognized. The major component of the tear film is the aqueous portion, which is produced by the main lacrimal glands and, to a lesser degree, by the glands of Krause and Wolfring, the accessory lacrimal glands. The most anterior layer of the tear film is the lipid layer produced by the meibomian glands and the glands of Zeis and Moll. The lipid layer is very thin, 0.1 μm thick, and serves to slow evaporation of the tear film from the air.

Conjunctival goblet cells contribute mucus, which facilitates the formation of a hydrophilic layer to coat the corneal surface and traps foreign particles within the tear film; these are moved toward the medial canthus with each blink. Several additional components of tears, including lactoferrin, lysozyme, and IgA, are important in preventing colonization of the ocular surface by potential pathogens. Lysozyme, an enzyme that cleaves the bacterial cell wall, is produced by the lacrimal gland, as is lactoferrin, which is an iron-containing enzyme with antibacterial properties that also inhibits the complement system.

The rate of aqueous tear production is approximately 1.2 μl/min, and the volume of tear is 7 μl. The average osmolality of the tear film in humans has been determined to be 302 $\pm$ 6 mOsm/L. This value can increase when tear production is decreased, as in aqueous deficiency or neurotrophic corneal disease or with increased tear evaporation, as seen in meibomitis and lid disease. The osmolarity of tear potassium is approximately 23 mmol/L, whereas the osmolarity of aqueous potassium is approximately 5 mmol/L. Because the blink mechanism spreads the tear film over the ocular surface, abnormalities of the eyelids or orbicularis muscles can affect the health of the ocular surface.

EPITHELIUM AND BASEMENT MEMBRANE

Epithelium

The most superficial layer in the cornea is a nonkeratinized, stratified squamous epithelium that measures 50 μm (or approximately 10% of the thickness of the cornea). The refractive effect of the corneal epithelium is relatively unknown, but it can account for 1.03 D of the eye optic power at the central 2-mm diameter optic zone.[21] Corneal epithelium turns over approximately every 7 days and consists of four to six morphologically distinct cell layers resulting in an epithelial thickness of 40 μm. They are commonly divided into three layers: superficial, middle, and basal cell layers (Fig 2–1). Basal cells undergo mitosis and differentiate in middle and superficial cells. Peripheral, and more superficial, limbal basal cells present a higher mitosis activity than do central basal cells.[22,23] Although no evidence of a specific corneal stem cell has been reported, studies of epithelial dynamics indicate that limbal epithelium is crucial in maintaining the cell mass of corneal epithelium under normal conditions and that it plays an important role in corneal epithelial wound healing. Therefore, a fraction of limbal basal cells are the stem cells for cor-

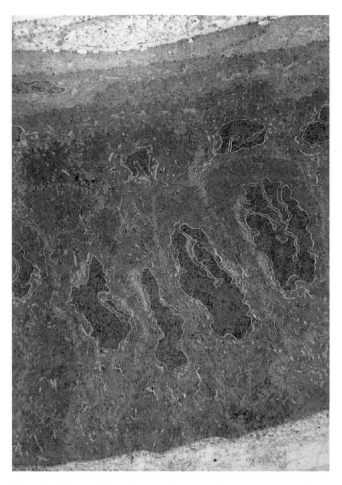

Figure 2–1. Transmission electron micrograph of corneal epithelium showing 6 cell layers. The basal cells are columnar and occupy most of the epithelium. They are attached to the basement membrane and underlying Bowman's layer by adhesion structures including hemidesmosomes and anchoring fibrils.

neal epithelial cell proliferation and differentiation.[23] The factors that contribute to maintaining corneal epithelial thickness are not known. The balance between the pressure exerted by the superficial cell layer under tension and the epithelial growth pressure may determine the thickness of the epithelium at any point in the cornea.[24] This may be important in maintaining corneal curvature after keratorefractive surgery.

Water constitutes 70% of the wet weight of the epithelium.[25] The major epithelial macromolecules include nucleic acids (DNA and RNA), lipids (phospholipids and cholesterol), glycogen, and proteins (glutathione). The epithelium contains high activities of enzymes of glycolysis, Krebs cycle, and Na^+ K^+ ATPase for glucose utilization. Glucose metabolism also occurs through the hexose monophosphate shunt. Under anaerobic conditions the corneal epithelium produces lactic acid. The corneal epithelium has a high concentration of K^+ ions, whereas the stroma is rich in Na^+ ions. The high concentrations of acetylcholine and cholinesterases found in the epithelium may have a role in the cation transport or in trophic nerve function. The epithelium gets much of its oxygen from either the limbal capillaries or from oxygen dissolved in precorneal film. The oxygen consumption of epithelium and endothelium is 5 to 6 μl/mg/h compared with stromal oxygen consumption of 0.23 μl/mg/h.[25]

Basement Membrane

The epithelial layers overlie the basement membrane, which forms a barrier between these layers and the stroma. The sheetlike basement membrane is a specialized extracellular complex of macromolecules that appears early in development and plays a role in cell differentiation and growth, selective permeability, and cell attachment. Adhesion structures (hemidesmosomes and anchoring filaments) attach the basal epithelial cells to the stroma.[26,27]

Extracellular Matrix Macromolecules

The extracellular matrix is composed of fibrous proteins (collagen, laminin, and fibronectin) and polysaccharide glycosaminoglycans (keratan sulfate, chondroitin sulfate, and dermatan sulfate). The major extracellular macromolecules of the basement membrane include type IV collagen and laminins.[28]

Laminins are large multidomain glycoproteins located in the lamina lucida of the basal lamina. Each molecule is composed of three polypeptide chains, which together form the characteristic cross-shaped laminin structure with three short arms and one long arm.[29,30] They promote cell adhesion, growth, migration, and differentiation. Human epithelial cells, in culture, attach to exogenous laminin in a dose-dependent manner.[31] Recent evidence suggests that laminin carbohydrates also participate in these biological responses through their integrin receptors.[32] Laminin plays a significant role in wound healing.[33–35] It is resynthesized within 48 hours following corneal wounding. It first appears under the migrating cells 1 to 2 days after anterior keratectomy and becomes continuous following wound closure.

Fibronectin contains two very similar polypeptide chains linked by disulfide bonds. Each chain has six domains with specific binding sites for integrins, proteoglycans, and collagen.[36] In the unwounded cornea, fibronectin is found in the subepithelial region at the level of epithelial basement membrane and at the

stromal side of Descemet's membrane.[37] Its primary role is to attach cells to extracellular matrix. It does not affect cell proliferation.[38] Rabbit corneal epithelial cells adhere to intact fibronectin, the 75-kD fragment containing the RGDS cell adhesion–promoting sequence, and the 33/66-kD cell adhesion–promoting/heparin-binding fragments of fibronectin.[39–41] The RGD tripeptide (Arg-Gly-Asp) represents an amino acid sequence common to several extracellular matrix components.[42,43] It mediates cell adhesion by interacting with integrins. The αv $\beta 3$ integrin binds to RGD sequences in vitronectin and fibronectin.[44] The $\alpha 5$ $\beta 1$ integrin selectively binds RGD-containing peptides.[45] The synthetic peptides FN-C/H-I, FN-C/H-III, and FN-C/H-V, derived from the amino acid sequence of the 33/66-kD fragment of fibronectin, promote corneal epithelial cell adhesion, spreading, and motility.[46] The classic fibronectin receptor, $\alpha 5$ $\beta 1$ integrin, is expressed in the wounded cornea and in cultured corneal fibroblasts. It plays an essential role in promoting cell adhesion. The $\alpha 5$ $\beta 1$ integrin, not the $\alpha 5$ cytoplasmic domain alone, functions in an early and essential step in fibronectin matrix assembly.[47]

BOWMAN'S LAYER AND STROMA

Bowman's Layer

Bowman's layer is a noncellular layer of randomly oriented collagen fibrils that is located over the corneal stroma and firmly attached to it. Bowman's layer measures approximately 13 μm in thickness; it originates from the mesenchymal cell processes of the superficial stroma at the 14-week gestational age. Bowman's layer does not regenerate, and heals with scar formation.

Bowman's layer was known to stabilize the corneal curvature, but recent studies of biomechanical properties of the cornea, with and without Bowman's membrane, showed that it may not play an important role in the stiffness of the cornea.[48]

Stroma

The corneal stroma is composed of cellular (keratocytes) and extracellular components. Keratocytes are differentiated mesenchymal fibroblasts that produce both the extracellular matrix macromolecules and the enzymes responsible for their remodeling and degradation. Keratocytes occupy 3% to 5% of the stromal volume. The density of keratocytes is highest in the anterior part; it decreases toward the posterior part.

Keratocytes maintain the integrity of both the extracellular fibers and matrix by constant synthetic activity (Fig 2–2). New collagenase synthesis by stromal fibroblasts in and around the repair tissue is the first step in collagen degradation during long-term tissue remodeling. Muller et al have investigated the role of keratocytes in maintaining the highly ordered arrangement of the cornea, reporting that, in contrast to their slender outlook in cross sections, the keratocytes appear as stellate cells with numerous dendritic arborizations in parallel sections.[49] The dendrites are contiguous to large platelike (30- to 50-nm thickness) extensions exhibiting numerous regularly arranged fenestrations and spiny protrusions. Collagen fibers run parallel to the fenestrated planes. Both keratocytes and collagen bundles are mutually organized in a corkscrew fashion. The presence of numerous fenestrations in the platelike extensions, and the mutual corkscrew organization of the keratocytes and collagen bundles, indicate that, in addition to the production of relevant peptides, keratocytes may be involved in the alignment of collagen bundles parallel to the surface.

Extracellular matrix (ECM) occupies a substantial part of the corneal stroma. It is composed of an organized meshwork of macromolecules (collagen, proteoglycans). Stromal thickness averages 450 mm (90% of corneal thickness).

The corneal collagen fibrils form a lattice structure, so arranged that scattering of light is eliminated by mutual interference from individual fibrils.[25] The collagen fibrils are arranged in interlacing bundles (lamellae) which run the full length of the cornea nearly parallel to the surface. The regular arrangement of collagen fibrils separated by less than a wavelength of light is essential for corneal transparency (Fig 2–3). Type I collagen is the primary collagen of the corneal stroma, representing 80% to 90% of the total corneal collagen. Solubility studies have shown that type III collagen (1% to 2%) and type V collagen may also be present, and embryonic tissue may contain type II collagen as well. Scarred corneal collagen is less soluble and less glycosylated and has wider and more variable fiber size than is seen in fetal or normal adult corneal collagen.

The cell-surface proteoglycans are glycosylated proteins linked covalently to highly anionic glycosaminoglycans. The stromal matrix of human cornea contains keratan sulfate proteoglycan (KSPG) and chondroitin and dermatan sulfate proteoglycan (decorin), with KSPG being the major proteoglycan. The heparan sulfate proteoglycan (perlecan) is localized in the basement membranes. The biological functions of proteoglycans are derived from the physiochemical characteristics of the glycosaminoglycan component of the molecule, and from specific interactions through both their glycosaminoglycan and core protein components with the ECM macromolecules. Apart from their hydrodynamic functions, they are involved in many aspects of cell and tissue activities.[50]

KSPG and decorin bind to distinct triple helical sites within each collagen fibril (type I and II) in the

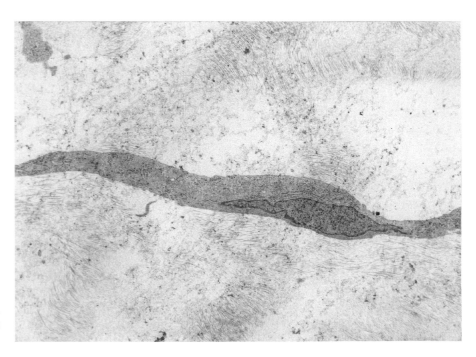

Figure 2–2. Oblique section electron micrograph of a rabbit cornea showing a keratocyte with surrounding collagen fibrils.

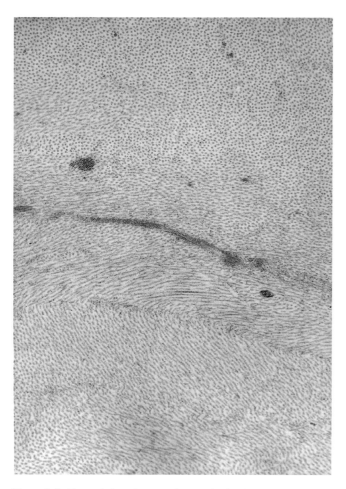

Figure 2–3. Transmission electron micrograph showing regularly spaced collagen fibrils in cross and oblique sections.

adult cornea.[51] Takahashi et al have immunocytochemically confirmed the association of these proteoglycans with type VI collagen in developing (fetal and neonate) rabbit corneas.[52] KSPG plays an important role in corneal transparency. It is absent or reduced in opaque corneal scars and reappears during restoration of transparency. Decorin regulates collagen fibril formation and is a natural regulator of transforming growth factor–β (TGF–β$_1$) activity, which markedly stimulates the synthesis of decorin, mainly as a secreting form.[53] The accumulation of decorin into the matrix is enhanced by L-ascorbate. Fukushima et al have shown that at low concentrations TGF–β binding fragments (decorin and betaglycan ectodomain fragments) enhance the binding of TGF–β to type II receptors and endogenous betaglycan (type III receptor), but at high concentrations they inhibit binding.[54] Decorin may prove to be clinically useful in treating fibrotic diseases caused by overproduction of TGF–β.[55] The modular structure of perlecan harbors multiple domains homologous to the

LDL receptor: laminin, neural crest adhesion molecules, and epidermal growth factor.[56] The strong conservation of these domains, including repetitive sequences and potential alternate splicing, suggests they have vital adhesive and growth regulatory functions. Perlecan binds to growth factors like basic fibroblast growth factor and protease inhibitors.[57] In addition, it acts as a cell-adhesive protein. Matrix cells interact with the core protein of perlecan through β1 and β3 integrins.[58] This interaction is partially RGD independent and is regulated by glycosaminoglycan heparan sulfate.

The synthesis of proteoglycans by human corneal fibroblasts in culture is different from that in vivo.[59] The production of basement membrane–associated proteoglycans (perlecan) increases while corneal stroma–associated proteoglycan synthesis decreases. In the early stages of wound healing following full thickness or anterior keratectomy (manual or excimer) wounds, activated keratocytes produce abnormal glycosaminoglycans and abnormally large proteoglycan filaments.[60–64] The main proteoglycan in the scar tissue is the highly sulfated, dermatan sulfate proteoglycan. The abnormally large proteoglycans are most prominent 2 weeks after wounding, when the corneal scar tissue is maximally hydrated. As healing progresses, the abnormal filaments decrease, but some persist for more than 12 months.

CELL–MATRIX INTERACTIONS

The extracellular matrix (ECM) plays an active and complex role in the regulation of cells, influencing their development, migration, proliferation, shape, and metabolic functions, in addition to providing a scaffolding to stabilize the physical structure of the tissue. Matrix molecules are constantly being remodeled, degraded, and resynthesized during development. During wound healing also there is degradation and resynthesis of matrix components. Regulating the balance of synthesis and degradation of ECM is crucial for both normal embryogenesis and growth and repair and maintenance of proper tissue architecture.

Cellular functions of ECM proteins are largely mediated by integrins, which are present on almost all cells.[65] Integrins are heterodimers having two transmembrane components, a and b subunits. The extracellular domains, in conjunction, bind ECM proteins, and the intracellular domains interact with the actin-based cytoskeleton of the cell, influencing cellular functions. Increasing evidence indicates that integrin receptors can transduce biochemical signals from the extracellular matrix to the cell interior to modulate cell behavior. Upregulation of protein kinase C activity precedes the spread of α 5 β 1 integrin-mediated cell on fibronectin.[66]

Integrins serve as receptors for laminin (α3 β1, α6 β1), vitronectin (αv β3), collagen (α2 β1, α3 β1), and fibronectin (α4 β1, α5 β1, αv β1, αv β3).[67,68] Integrin-based cell-cell and cell-ECM interactions are important in early morphogenesis of the eye. Probes that disrupt integrin-ECM interactions (anti-integrin antibodies and RGD tripeptide) prevent normal eye morphogenesis.[69]

Stepp et al have determined the synthesis, cell surface expression, and localization of integrins in corneal epithelium.[70] The corneal epithelium has a variety of distinct integrin subunits localized in basal and suprabasal cells at sites of cell-cell contact (α2, α3, αv, β1, β5) and basal membrane of the basal cells at the site of cell-substrate interaction (α5, α6, β4). In stationary corneal epithelium, approximately one half of the β1-containing heterodimers are α2 β1; most of the rest are α3 β1. The αv β1, α6 β1, and α5 β1 integrins are present in minor amounts. The α6 β4 integrin is a component of the hemidesmosome. Integrin distribution and production are not dramatically altered during corneal epithelial cell migration over debridement wounds, except at the tip of the leading edge of migrating epithelium. However, at sites of cell-cell interaction and as components of hemidesmosomes in stationary epithelia, integrins are available for rapid recruitment as epithelial cell migration proceeds. Using confocal laser scanning microscopy, Trinkaus-Randall et al have demonstrated age-related changes in the localization of α6 and β4 integrins.[71] The major age-related difference is the loss of continuous α6 and β4 subunits along the basal surface of basal epithelial cells. Integrins aid in the attachment of epithelium to the basement membrane. They participate in maintaining epithelial cell shape, and along with desmosomes, they appear to function as cell-cell adhesion molecules.

Masur et al have identified integrins at the cell surface of noncultured and cultured corneal keratocytes.[72] The presence of α1 β1, α3 β1, and αv-containing integrins in corneal keratocytes facilitates their attachment to collagen, laminin, fibronectin, and vitronectin. When keratocytes are placed in culture, the integrin pattern changes. The classic fibronectin receptor, α5 β1, is then expressed along with additional integrins that bind to fibronectin. Cultured corneal keratocytes prefer fibronectin to collagen, vitronectin, or laminin as the ECM substrate. Similar changes may occur in the wounded

cornea. In regions of scar or fibrous tissue, an upregulated expression of α chains has been reported.

DESCEMET'S MEMBRANE

Descemet's membrane (approximately 10 μm thick) is a product of the secretion of endothelial cells.[25] It is composed of type IV collagen with a high content of glycine, hydroxyglycine, and hydroxyproline. In contrast to the stroma, there are no significant amounts of sulfated glycosaminoglycans. Collagen in Descemet's membrane is insoluble and is more resistant to collagenase than corneal stromal collagen. Although characterized by the usual high hydroxyproline content and peptide helical features of collagen, Descemet's membrane is an unusual collagen in many respects, including a high carbohydrate content, high degree of elasticity, and an amorphous electron microscopic appearance.[25] Descemet's membrane is a barrier to perforation in deep corneal ulcers.

ENDOTHELIUM

The normal corneal endothelium is a single layer of regularly arranged hexagonal cells lining Descemet's membrane. The average endothelial cell count is 2800 cells per square millimeter. Endothelial cell density decreases with age. Cell loss from trauma or inflammation is compensated for by increased cell size and decreased cell density.[25] An active metabolic pump in the endothelium removes fluid that leaks into the stroma and maintains the deturgescent state of the cornea. Endothelial damage results in much more corneal swelling and more rapid swelling than epithelial damage. The endothelium gets most of its required oxygen from the aqueous humor.

EPITHELIAL AND STROMAL WOUND HEALING

Following corneal wounding, the epithelium migrates to cover the defect (Fig 2–4). The cytoskeleton of basal cells in the leading edge of the migrating epithelium is reorganized and the hemidesmosomes disassembled. Focal adhesions of the migrating basal cells replace the adhesion complexes. Vinculin, α-actin, and α5 β1 and α3 β1 integrins, present in the membrane of focal adhesions, serve as provisional adhesion junctions to newly deposited fibronectin in the wound

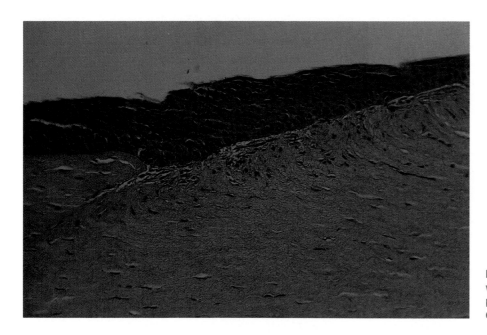

Figure 2–4. Light micrograph showing wedge shaped epithelial hyperplasia accompanied by focal keratocyte activation at the edge of a keratomileusis wound.

bed.[73,74] In penetrating stromal wounds, repair of the anchoring fibril network resumes after re-epithelialization. Patchy reformations of the basement membrane, hemidesmosomes, and anchoring fibrils appear synchronously.[73,74] Segments of the basement membrane become continuous by 1 to 2 months, but small areas of discontinuities and duplications persist for longer periods. Morphometric measurements of the epithelial basement membrane complex in vitamin A–deficient corneas reveal numerous microseparations of the basal epithelial cell membrane with intervening segmental basement membrane duplications and electron dense deposits.[75] Structural abnormalities in the basement membrane correspond with the clinical finding of corneal sloughing.

The role of Bowman's layer in corneal wound healing is not well known. Hsu et al have investigated the mechanism by which anterior stromal puncture reduces the incidence of recurrent erosions.[76] Increased expression of extracellular matrix and immunolocalization of fibronectin, type IV collagen, and laminin at the puncture site suggest that anterior stromal puncture stimulates wound healing by epithelial stromal interactions induced by the breaching of Bowman's layer.

As early as 12 hours following epithelial scrape wounds, fibronectin is deposited over the bare stromal surface in a linear fashion. It provides a temporary scaffold for corneal epithelial migration and adhesion. Epidermal growth factor and interleukin-6 also stimulate cell adhesion and migration by a fibronectin-dependent mechanism, possibly the increased expression of fibronectin receptors.[77,78] Although there have been reports that exogenously applied fibronectin promotes corneal wound healing,[79,80] recent evidence suggests that exogenous fibronectin is not critical for cell adhesion and wound closure. Following anterior keratectomy (mechanical or excimer), fibronectin is deposited inside the stromal lamellae.[81–83] The pattern, time, and distribution of intrastromal fibronectin after excimer keratectomy are not very different from those after mechanical keratectomy.

In the normal cornea tenascin can be detected in the epithelium only. The role of tenascin in ECM interactions is as yet undefined. It has been shown that, following anterior keratectomy, tenascin appears in corneal stroma at the wound area only, particularly at the wound edge. Wounding does not induce any change in epithelial tenascin.[84] Hyaluronic acid (HA) is not normally found in the corneal stroma, but its expression following excimer wounds has been reported.[85] It may represent a nonspecific corneal tissue response to injury. Exogenous HA promotes corneal re-epithelialization.[38] Inoue et al have compared the effect of HA on epithelial cell proliferation in cultured corneas with that of epidermal growth factor (EGF) and fibronectin. HA stimulates epithelial proliferation more than EGF. The results of the study support the possibility of the existence of HA receptors in corneal epithelial cells, by which HA stimulates cell proliferation.

Several recent studies have established a role for polymorphonuclear (PMN) leucocytes and collagenases in corneal healing after alkali burns. PMNs can modulate the biosynthetic functions of corneal cells after alkali burns. They may be responsible for the inhibition of epithelial proliferation. Additionally, alkali-injured corneal cells can modulate the secretion of proteins (18 kD) by PMNs.[86] Metalloproteinases produced by regenerating corneal cells after alkali burns can lead to degradation of laminin in the basement membrane zone.[87] The contribution of PMNs to ECM degradation is not fully known. Ishizaki et al have shown that after alkali burns keratocytes migrate to the injured stroma and transform into myofibroblasts, expressing high levels of collagen I mRNA, smooth muscle α-actin, and vimentin.[88] These myofibroblasts contribute to wound contraction after injury.

REFERENCES

1. Rengstorff RH. Corneal refraction: relative effects of each corneal component. *J Am Optom Assoc.* 1985;56:218–219.

2. Al-Umran KU, Pandolfi MF. Corneal diameter in premature infants. *Br J Ophthalmol.* 1992;76:292–293. Comments.

3. Tucker SM, Enzenauer RW, Levin AV, Morin JD, Hellmann J. Corneal diameter, axial length, and intraocular pressure in premature infants. *Ophthalmology.* 1992;99:1296–1300.

4. Remon L, Cristobal JA, Castillo J, et al. Central and peripheral corneal thickness in full-term newborns by ultrasonic pachymetry. *Invest Ophthalmol Vis Sci.* 1992;33:3080–3083.

6. Autzen T, Bjornstrom L. Central corneal thickness in full-term newborns. *Acta Ophthalmol (Copenh).* 1989;67:719–720.

7. Edmund C. Determination of the corneal thickness profile by optical pachymetry. *Acta Ophthalmol (Copenh).* 1987;65:147–152.

8. Sun FY. Ultrasonic pachymetry of the cornea [in Chinese]. *Chung Hua Yen Ko Tsa Chih.* 1991;27:51–52.

9. Reinstein DZ, Silverman RH, Rondeau MJ, Coleman DJ. Epithelial and corneal thickness measurements by high-frequency ultrasound digital signal processing. *Ophthalmology.* 1994;101:140–146.

10. Rapuano CJ, Fishbaugh JA, Strike DJ. Nine point corneal thickness measurements and keratometry readings in normal corneas using ultrasound pachymetry. *Insight.* 1993;18:16–22.

11. Siu A, Herse P. The effect of age on human corneal thickness. Statistical implications of power analysis. *Acta Ophthalmol (Copenh).* 1993;71:51–56.

12. Herse P, Yao W. Variation of corneal thickness with age in young New Zealanders. *Acta Ophthalmol (Copenh).* 1993;71:360–364.

13. Weinreb RN, Lu A, Beeson C. Maternal corneal thickness during pregnancy. *Am J Ophthalmol.* 1988;105:258–260.

14. Asbell PA, Chiang B, Somers ME, Morgan KS. Keratometry in children. *Clao J.* 1990;16:99–102.

15. Dunne MC, Royston JM, Barnes DA. Posterior corneal surface toricity and total corneal astigmatism. *Optom Vis Sci.* 1991;68:708–710.

16. Patel S, Marshall J, Fitzke FW. Shape and radius of posterior corneal surface. *Refract Corneal Surg.* 1993;9:173–181.

17. Olbert D, Kehrhahn OH. Biometric constancy of the anterior eye segment as demonstrated by slit image photography according to the Scheimpflug principle. *Ophthalmic Res.* 1992;24:27–31.

18. Bachmann W, Jean B, Bende T, et al. Silicon cast method for quantification of photoablation. *Refract Corneal Surg.* 1992;8:363–367.

19. Buzard KA. Introduction to biomechanics of the cornea. *Refract Corneal Surg.* 1992;8:127–138. Comments.

20. Pinsky PM, Datye DV. A microstructurally-based finite element model of the incised human cornea. *J Biomech.* 1991;24:907–922.

21. Simon G, Ren Q, Kervick GN, Parel JM. Optics of the corneal epithelium. *Refract Corneal Surg.* 1993;9:42–50.

22. Ebato B, Friend J, Thoft RA. Comparison of limbal and peripheral human corneal epithelium in tissue culture. *Invest Ophthalmol Vis Sci.* 1988;29:1533–1537.

23. Tseng SC. Concept and application of limbal stem cells. *Eye.* 1989;3:141–157.

24. Dierick HG, Missotten L. Is the corneal contour influenced by a tension in the superficial epithelial cells? A new hypothesis. *Refract Corneal Surg.* 1992;8:54–60. Comments and discussion.

25. Waltman SR, Hart WM. The cornea. In: Moses RA, Hart WM, eds. *Physiology of the Eye.* St. Louis, MO: C.V. Mosby Co; 1987:36–59.

26. Gipson IK: Adhesive mechanisms of the corneal epithelium. *Acta Ophthalmol.* 1992;70(suppl):13–17.

27. Gipson IK, Spurr-Michaud SJ, Tisdale AS, et al. Anchoring fibrils form a complex network in human and rabbit cornea. *Invest Ophthalmol Vis Sci.* 1987;28:212–220.

28. Yurchenco PD, Schittny JC. Molecular architecture of the basement membranes. *FASEB J.* 1990;4:1577–1590.

29. Kleinman HK, Weeks BS, Schnaper HW, Kibbey MC, Yamamura K, Grant DS. The laminins: a family of basement membrane glycoproteins important in cell differentiation and tumor metastasis. *Vitam Horm.* 1993;47:161–186.

30. Engel J. Laminins and other strange proteins. *Biochemistry.* 1992;31:10643–10652.

31. Ohji M, Mandarino L, SundarRaj N, Thoft RA. Corneal epithelial cell attachment with endogenous laminin and fibronectin. *Invest Ophthalmol Vis Sci.* 1993;34:2487–2492.

32. Tanzer ML, Chandrasekaran S, Dean JW, Giniger MS. Role of laminin carbohydrates on cellular interactions. *Kidney Int.* January 1993;43:66–72.

33. Gipson IK, Spurr-Michaud SJ, Tisdale AS, et al. Reassembly of the anchoring structures of the corneal epithelium

during wound repair in the rabbit. *Invest Ophthalmol Vis Sci.* 1989;30:425–434.

34. Stock EL, Kurpakus MA, Sambol B, Jones JC: Adhesion complex formation after small keratectomy wounds in the cornea. *Invest Ophthalmol Vis Sci.* 1992;33:304–313.

35. SundarRaj N, Geiss MJ, Fantes F, et al. Healing of excimer laser ablated monkey corneas. *Arch Ophthalmol.* 1990;108:1604–1610.

36. Gipson IK, Watanabe H, Zieske JD. Corneal wound healing and fibronectin. *Int Ophthalmol Clin.* 1993;33:149–163.

37. Tervo T, Sulonen J, Valtones S, Vannas A, Virtanen I: Distribution of fibronectin in human and rabbit corneas. *Exp Eye Res.* 1986;42:399–406.

38. Inoue M, Katakami C: The effects of hyaluronic acid on corneal epithelial cell proliferation. *Invest Ophthalmol Vis Sci.* 1993;34:2313–2315.

39. Nishida T, Hakagawa S, Watanabe K, Yamada KM, Otari T, Berman MB. A peptide from fibronectin cell-binding domain inhibits attachment of epithelial cells. *Invest Ophthalmol Vis Sci.* 1988;29:1820–1825.

40. Pierschbacher MD, Ruoslahti E. The cell attachment activity of fibronectin can be duplicated by small synthetic fragments of the molecule. *Nature.* 1984;309:30–33.

41. Mooradian DL, McCarthy JB, Skubitz AP, Cameron JD, Furcht LT: Rabbit corneal epithelial cells adhere to two distinct heparin-binding synthetic peptides derived from fibronectin. *Invest Ophthalmol Vis Sci.* 1992;33:3034–3040.

42. Pytela R, Pierschbacher MD, Ruoslahti E. Identification and isolation of a 140 kD cell surface glycoprotein with properties expected of a fibronectin receptor. *Cell.* 1985;40:191 198.

43. Ruoslahti E, Pierschbacher MD: New perspectives in cell adhesion: RGD and integrins. *Science.* 1987;238:492–497.

44. Charo IF, Nannizzi L, Smith JW, Cheresh DA. The vitronectin receptor αvβ3 binds fibronectin and acts in concert with α5β1 in promoting cellular attachment and spreading on fibronectin. *J Cell Biol.* 1990;111:2795–2800.

45. Koivunen E, Gay DA, Ruoslahti E. Selection of peptides binding to the alpha 5 beta 1 integrin from phage display library. *J Biol Chem.* 1993;268:20205–20210.

46. Mooradian DL, McCarthy JB, Skubitz AP, Cameron JD, Furcht LT. Characterization of FN-C/H-V, a novel synthetic peptide from fibronectin that promotes rabbit corneal epithelial cell adhesion, spreading, and motility. *Invest Ophthalmol Vis Sci.* 1993;34:153–164.

47. Wu C, Bauer JS, Juliano RL, McDonald JA. The alpha 5 beta 1 integrin fibronectin receptor, but not the alpha 5 cytoplasmic domain, functions in an early and essential step in fibronectin matrix assembly. *J Biol Chem.* 1993;268:21883–21888.

48. Seiler T, Matallana M, Sendler S, Bende T. Does Bowman's layer determine the biomechanical properties of the cornea? *Refract Corneal Surg.* 1992;8:139–142.

49. Mueller L. IOVS 1995;36(suppl):867. #3974.

50. Yanagishita M. Function of proteoglycans in the extracellular matrix. *Acta Pathol Jpn.* 1993;43:283–293.

51. Hedbom E, Heinegard D. Binding of fibromodulin and decorin to seperate sites on fibrillar collagens. *J Biol Chem.* 1993;268:27307–27312.

52. Takahashi T, Cho HI, Kublin CL, Cintron C. Keratan sulfate and dermatan sulfate proteoglycans associate with type VI collagen in fetal rabbit cornea. *J Histochem Cytochem.* 1993;41:1447–1457.

53. Takeuchi Y, Matsumoto T, Ogata E, Shishiba Y. Effects of transforming growth factor beta 1 and L-ascorbate on synthesis and distribution of proteoglycans in murine osteoblast-like cells. *J Bone Miner Res.* 1993;8:823–830.

54. Fukushima D, Butzow R, Hildebrand A, Ruoslahti E. Localization of transforming growth factor beta binding site in betaglycan. Comparison with small extracellular matrix proteoglycans. *J Biol Chem.* 1993;268:22710–22715.

55. Noble NA, Harper JR, Border WA. In vivo interactions of TGF-beta and extracellular matrix. *Prog Growth Factor Res.* 1992;4:369–382.

56. Noonan DM, Hassell JR. Perlecan, the large low-density proteoglycan of basement membranes: structure and variant forms. *Kidney Int.* January 1993;43:53–60.

57. Timpl R. Proteoglycans of the basement membranes. *Experientia.* 1993;49:417–428.

58. Hayashi K, Madri JA, Yuchenco PD. Endothelial cells interact with the core protein of basement membrane proteoglycan through beta 1 and beta 3 integrins: an adhesion modulated by glycosaminoglycans. *J Cell Biol.* 1992;119:945–959.

59. Hassell JR, Schrecengost PK, Rada JA, SundarRaj N, Sossi G, Thoft RA. Biosynthesis of stromal matrix proteoglycans and basement membrane components by human corneal fibroblasts. *Invest Ophthalmol Vis Sci.* 1992;33:547–557.

60. Cintron C, Covington HI, Kublin CL. Morphological analysis of proteoglycans in rabbit corneal scars. *Invest Ophthalmol Vis Sci.* 1990;31:1789–1798.

61. Cintron C, Gregory JD, Damle SP, Kublin CL. Biochemical analysis of proteoglycans in rabbit corneal scars. *Invest Ophthalmol Vis Sci.* 1990;31:1975–1981.

62. Funderburgh JL, Chandler JW. Proteoglycan of rabbit corneas with nonperforating wounds. *Invest Ophthalmol Vis Sci.* 1989;30:435–442.

63. Rawe IM, Tuft SJ, Meek KM. Proteoglycan and collagen morphology in superficially scarred rabbit cornea. *Histochem J.* 1992;24:311–318.

64. Rawe IM, Zabel RW, Tuft SJ, Chen V, Meek KM. A morphological study of rabbit corneas after laser keratectomy. *Eye.* 1992;6:637–642.

65. Virtanen I, Tervo K, Korhonen M, Paallysaho T, Tervo T. Integrins as receptors for extracellular matrix proteins in human cornea. *Acta Ophthalmol (Copenh).* 1992;70:18–21.

66. Vuori K, Ruoslahti E. Activation of protein kinase C precedes alpha 5 beta 1 integrin-mediated cell spreading on fibronectin. *J Biol Chem.* 1993;268:21459–21462.

67. Lauweryns B, van den Oord JJ, Volpes R, Foets B, Missotten L. Distribution of very late activation integrins in the

human cornea. An immunohistochemical study using monoclonal antibodies. *Invest Ophthalmol Vis Sci.* 1991;32: 2079–2085.

68. Hynes RO. Integrins: versatility, modulation, and signalling in cell adhesion. *Cell.* 1992; 69:11–25.

69. Svennevik E, Linser PJ. The inhibitory effects of integrin antibodies and the RGD tripeptide on early eye development. *Invest Ophthalmol Vis Sci.* 1993;34:1774–1784.

70. Stepp MA, Spurr-Michaud S, Gibson IK. Integrins in the wounded and unwounded stratified squamous epithelium of the cornea. *Invest Ophthalmol Vis Sci.* 1993;34: 1829–1844.

71. Trinkaus-Randall V, Tong M, Thomas P, Cornell-Bell A. Confocal imaging of the α6 and β4 integrin subunits in the human cornea with aging. *Invest Ophthalmol Vis Sci.* 1993;34:3101–3109.

72. Masur SK, Cheung JK, Antohi S. Identification of integrins in cultured corneal fibroblasts and in isolated keratocytes. *Invest Ophthalmol Vis Sci.* 1993;34:2690–2698.

73. Gipson IK, Spurr-Michaud SJ, Tisdale AS, et al. Hemidesmosomes and anchoring fibril collagen appear synchronously during development and wound healing. *Dev Biol.* 1988;126:253–262.

74. Gipson IK, Spurr-Michaud SJ, Tisdale AS, et al. Redistribution of hemidesmosome components during migration of the corneal epithelium. *Invest Ophthalmol Vis Sci.* 1991; 32:1163A.

75. Shams NBK, Hanninen LA, Chaves HV, et al. Effect of vitamin-A deficiency on the adhesion of rat corneal epithelium and the basement membrane complex. *Invest Ophthalmol Vis Sci.* 1993;34:2646–2654.

76. Hsu JKW, Rubinfeld RS, Barry P, Jester JV. Anterior stromal puncture—immunohistochemical studies in human corneas. *Arch Ophthalmol.* 1993;111:1131–1137.

77. Nishida T, Nakamura M, Murkami J, Mishima H, Otori T. Epidermal growth factor stimulates corneal epithelial cell attachment to fibronectin through a fibronectin receptor system. *Invest Ophthalmol Vis Sci.* 1992;33:2464–2469.

78. Nishida T, Nakamura M, Mishima H, Otori T. Interleukin 6 promotes epithelial migration by a fibronectin-dependent mechanism. *J Cell Physiol.* 1992;153:1–5.

79. Kim KS, Oh JS, Kim IS, Jo JS. Clinical efficacy of topical homologus fibronectin in persistent corneal epithelial disorders. *Korean J Ophthalmol.* June 1992;6:12–18.

80. Nishida T, Nakagawa S, Nishibayashi C, Tanaka H, Manabe R. Fibronectin enhancement of corneal epithelial wound healing of rabbits in vivo. *Arch Ophthalmol.* 1984; 102:455–456.

81. Tervo K, van Setten GB, Beuerman RW, Virtanen I, Tarkkanen A, Tervo T. Expression of tenascin and cellular fibronectin in the rabbit cornea after anterior keratectomy. Immunohistochemical study of wound healing dynamics. *Invest Ophthalmol Vis Sci.* 1991;32:2912–2918.

82. Malley DS, Steinert RF, Puliafito CA, Dodi ET. Immunofluorescence study of corneal wound healing after excimer laser anterior keratectomy in the monkey eye. *Arch Ophthalmol.* 1990;108:1316–1322.

83. van Setton GB, Koch JW, Tervo K, et al. Expression of tenascin and fibronectin in the rabbit cornea after excimer laser surgery. *Graefes Arch Clin Exp Ophthalmol.* 1992;230: 178–183.

84. Tervo K, Tervo T, van Setten GB, Tarkkanen A, Virtanen I. Demonstration of tenascin-like immunoreactivity in rabbit corneal wounds. *Acta Ophthalmol (Copenh).* 1989;67: 347–350.

85. Fitzsimmons TD, Fagerholm P, Harfstrand A, Schenholm M. Hyaluronic acid in the rabbit cornea after excimer laser superficial keratectomy. *Invest Ophthalmol Vis Sci.* 1992;33: 3011–3016.

86. Kao WWY, Zhu G, Kao CWC. Effects of polymorphonuclear neutrophils on protein synthesis by alkali-injured rabbit corneas—a preliminary study. *Cornea.* 1993;12: 522–531.

87. Saika S, Kobata S, Hashizume N, Okada Y, Yamanaka O. Epithelial basement membrane in alkali-burned corneas in rats—an immunohistochemical study. *Cornea.* 1993;12: 383–390.

88. Ishizaki M, Zhu G, Haseba T, Shaefer SS, Kao WWY. Expression of collagen-I, smooth muscle alpha-actin, and vimentin during the healing of alkali-burned and lacerated corneas. *Invest Ophthalmol Vis Sci.* 1993;12:3320–3328.

CHAPTER 3

Corneal Wound Healing Following Refractive Keratotomy

W. Todd Johnston ▪ Vadim Filatov ▪ Jonathan H. Talamo

INTRODUCTION

In order to effectively manage patients undergoing incisional keratorefractive surgery it is important to understand corneal wound healing after radial keratotomy (RK). Most histological evaluation of corneal wound healing after RK has been performed in animal models. Human histologic data after incisional keratorefractive surgery are rather limited.

The results summarized in this chapter are organized by layers of corneal tissue (i.e., epithelium, Bowman's layer, stroma, Descemet's membrane and endothelium). Each section starts with human data, followed by relevant animal data. The histologic findings in animals vary significantly according to species. Findings in some animals (nonhuman primates, cats) are more similar to those in humans than those found in other animals (rabbit). Furthermore, significant variations between individuals make it difficult to generalize a particular finding. Nevertheless, general patterns of corneal wound healing following incisional refractive procedures constructed from the varied histological data may explain certain clinical phenomena, such as progressive hyperopia and susceptibility to wound rupture from blunt trauma several years after RK.

EPITHELIUM AND BOWMAN'S MEMBRANE

Human Studies

Histopathologic findings after RK demonstrate that corneal epithelial wound healing following RK differs from normal wound healing patterns. After RK, epithelium slides and proliferates to form an epithelial plug within the wound, which may persist in some incisions 3 to 70 months following RK (Fig 3–1),[1–12] and may be absent in other incision sites sampled at the same time points.[7] The presence of an epithelial plug retards normal stromal apposition in some incisions, preventing complete wound healing for many years after the initial keratotomy. Within epithelial plugs degenerative changes such as nuclear pyknosis, inclusion cysts and intracellular epithelial vacuoles are often present at variable times following RK.[1,3] Inclusion cysts within epithelial plugs may indicate severe epithelial degeneration and have been documented nearly 3 years following RK (Fig 3–2).[1,7,8,10,13]

Most histopathologic studies following RK have demonstrated fractures in Bowman's layer with subsequent misalignment beneath incision sites as long as 70 months following surgery (Fig 3–3).[1–5,7,9,14] Though an epithelial plug may eventually extrude or regress, Bow-

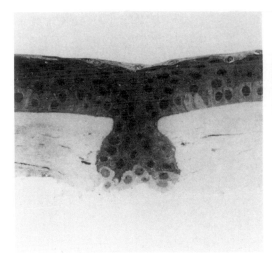
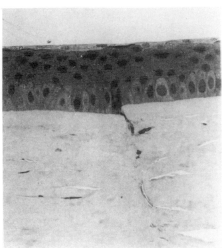

Figure 3–1. Epithelial plug 11 months after repeat RK. *(From Binder et al, Fig 3, p. 436.[5])*

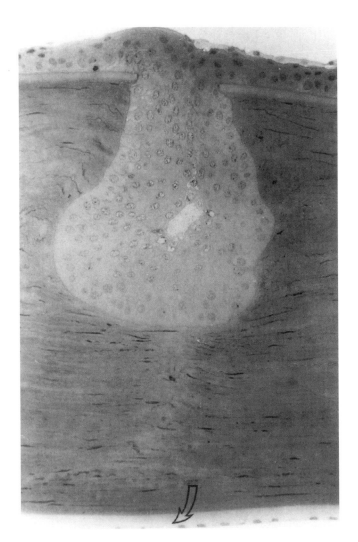

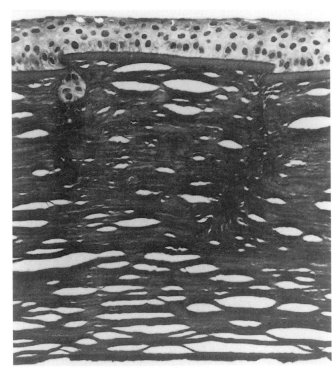

Figure 3–3. Malapposition of Bowman's layer with retained epithelial plug. *(From Deg et al, Fig 7, p. 738.[4])*

Figure 3–2. Epithelial inclusion cyst 26 months after RK. *(From Jester et al, Fig 7, p. 197.[3])*

man's layer never regenerates after RK. In contrast to Bowman's layer, the epithelial basement membrane often reforms, sometimes with duplication, thickening, and hemidesmosome formation reattaching epithelium to the underlying stroma (Fig 3–4).[1–5,7,8] Nevertheless, basement membrane abnormalities, often resembling map-dot-fingerprint changes, may occur even years following RK.[15]

Superficial epithelium also undergoes several changes after RK. Scarring, poor differentiation and absence of microvilli in the overlying corneal epithelium have been reported 6 to 24 months after RK. Hyperplastic epithelium with elevated ridges may be present over corneal incisions up to 70 months postoperatively (Fig 3–5).[4,5,7,11] However, normal epithelium, with dense surface microvilli and prominent cell borders, is more common and has been observed as early as 6 months after surgery.[4,5,7,8] Another change seen in the superficial corneal epithelium following RK may include iron lines, which correlate with increased corneal flattening and irregular astigmatism.[2,16,17]

Animal Studies

Studies of animal corneas demonstrate patterns of epithelial wound healing after RK similar to those of humans. In the owl monkey following RK, epithelium migrates across Bowman's membrane and the stromal bed, extends into the wound, and lines the stroma along the length of the incision.[18] Over time, incisions fill with an epithelial plug, which is replaced over a period of weeks with a marked fibroblastic response (Fig 3–6).[18–20] Other studies using nonhuman primate and canine eyes have found epithelium within the wound site immediately following surgery.[21,20] In the cat, as in the monkey, the epithelial plug is replaced with fibrotic tissue 2 weeks following RK, whereas rabbit corneal incisions have shown continued wound gaping and lack of fibrosis at the same time point.[20] Intraepithelial inflammatory cells may be present at the incision sites intermixed with degenerating epithelial cells after RK. At the same time, the epithelium overlying the incisions often thickens[18,19] and the plasma

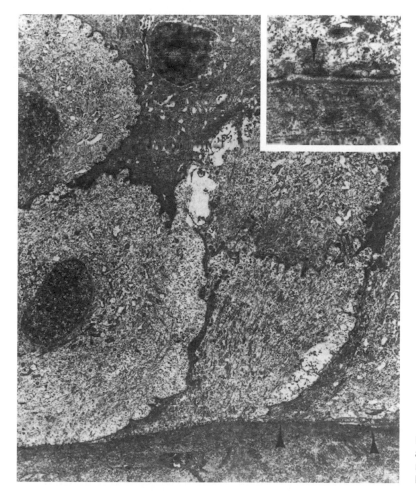

Figure 3–4. Basal lamina associated with retained epithelium and hemidesmosomal attachment to basal cell plasma membrane. Insert shows higher magnification of the epithelial adhesion structures. *(From Jester et al, Fig 3, p. 612.[1])*

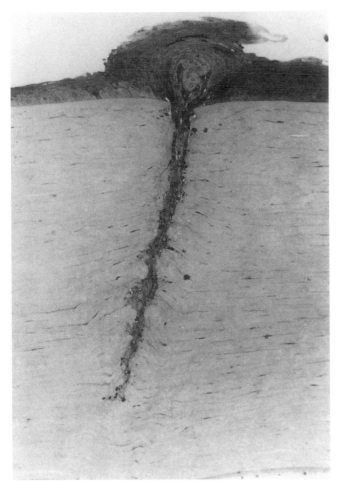

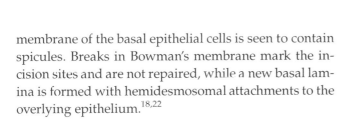

Figure 3–5. Hyperplastic epithelial growth above RK incision site. *(From Binder et al, Fig 8, p. 1589.[7])*

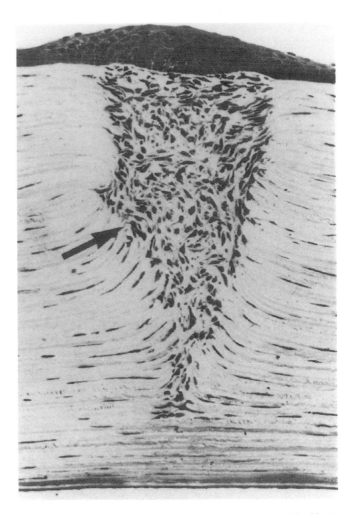

Figure 3–6. Replacement of the epithelial plug with marked fibroblastic response 7 to 14 days after RK. *(From Jester et al, Fig 7, p. 165.[18])*

membrane of the basal epithelial cells is seen to contain spicules. Breaks in Bowman's membrane mark the incision sites and are not repaired, while a new basal lamina is formed with hemidesmosomal attachments to the overlying epithelium.[18,22]

STROMA

Human Studies

Corneal stromal wound healing is the major factor affecting clinical outcome following RK, influencing both the stability and final refractive effect. Immediately following RK, inflammatory cells, damaged keratocytes and edema appear at the incision site.[23] Diffuse edema persists for 1 to 2 weeks around the wound site, de-

creasing significantly by 3 months postoperatively. This may correspond to the initial overcorrection seen 1 to 2 weeks after the procedure, and to the regression of the refractive effect seen at 3 months in the PERK study. Radial incisions often become filled with fine, gray, feathery spicules, which disappear at about 1 year postoperatively from the anterior stroma but may persist for up to 3 years in the posterior stroma (Fig 3–7). These spicules most likely represent disordered collagen fibrils which disappear as the fibrils realign themselves. In these corneas, wound healing is incomplete until the disappearance of the spicules, which usually occurs 2 to 3 years after RK.

Two types of long-term stromal wound healing are described after RK.[24] In the first type, incision scars remain thin and delicate with feathery edges extending laterally from their sides. This type of healing is seen in

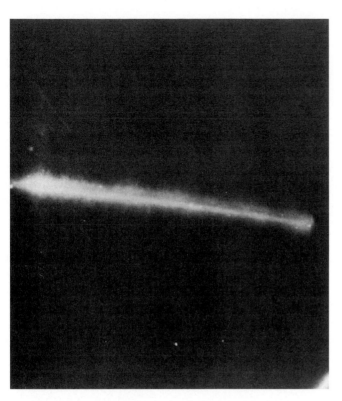

Figure 3–7. Spicules at RK incision site 6 months postoperatively. *(From Waring et al, Fig 4, p. 222.[23])*

patients with a relatively increased refractive effect and is positively correlated with age. The second type of healing forms scars that are rougher and broader, with increased volume and width, and often with multiple epithelial inclusions. Wide variations in wound healing among different individuals may explain some of the variation in refractive outcomes in patients with similar baseline characteristics. Healing may vary not only among individuals, but also among individual incisions.[3–5,7–9] Mild to moderate fibroblastic activity is typically observed within RK wounds, with some fibroblasts containing increased numbers of organelles, such as mitrochondria, ribosomes and endoplasmic reticulum.[2,4,5,7,8] For example, active, normal keratocytes are present in some incisions 10 to 66 months after RK,[4,5] whereas decreased keratocyte density with degenerative changes, such as rough, distended endoplasmic reticulum, may be present in some corneas even 24 months after keratotomy.[1,7] In addition, stromal lamellae underlying RK incisions remain disrupted and randomly apposed many years after RK (Fig 3–8).[2–5,7,8,11] Furthermore, while amorphous collagen and ground substance usually fill in gaps between wound edges,[5,6] they can be absent for more than 1 year after RK.[1–3,7] Although a number of these studies demonstrate that

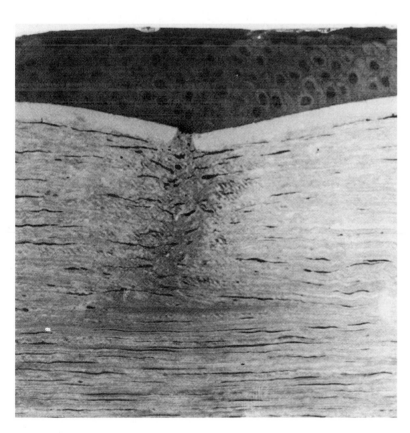

Figure 3–8. Disrupted stromal lamellae with active keratocytes and a break in Bowman's layer 70 months after RK. *(From Binder et al, Fig 3, p. 436 and Fig 6-Left, p. 438.[5])*

stromal wound healing may be delayed for up to 70 months after surgery, others demonstrate wound healing to be more complete as early as 4 months postoperatively (Fig 3–9).

The time course of healing following RK is of the utmost importance, since delayed wound healing may contribute to refractive instability and susceptibility to rupture from blunt trauma.[7,14,25,26] However this is not uniformly the case. In one case, incisions remained intact despite blunt trauma to the face only 2 months after an astigmatic keratotomy reoperation.[27] In the PERK study, blunt trauma severe enough to cause vitreous hemorrhage did not cause splaying of the RK incisions in two eyes 11 and 13 years after RK.[28]

Animal Studies

Studies of stromal wound healing after RK in some animal models show marked differences in healing from humans. Nonhuman primate studies after RK disclose acute stromal inflammation at the incision base within the first 48 hours after RK.[18] Fibroblastic activity at the

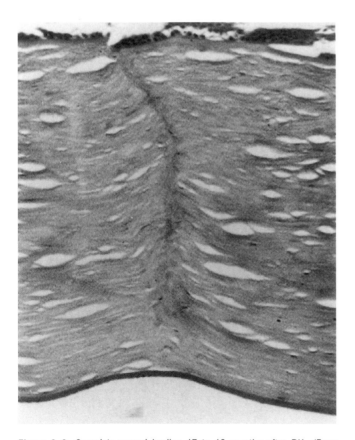

Figure 3–9. Complete wound healing 17 to 18 months after RK. *(From Ingraham et al, Fig 2, p. 684.[2])*

wound site increases by 7 days postoperatively, with very little extracellular matrix present between fibroblasts. One to 2 weeks postoperatively, proliferating fibroblasts begin to replace the epithelial plug within the stroma. By 3 months postoperatively, significant wound contracture occurs with reapproximation of the wound margins. Increased numbers of keratocytes are present, and this newly formed scar contains irregularly spaced, variably sized collagen fibers.

In the rabbit, parallel layers of the incised lamellae are preserved in the deep layers of the wound, but poor reapposition of superficial lamellae remains for many weeks postoperatively.[29] Similar findings are visible with in vivo confocal microscopy, which confirms a remarkable lack of wound healing in a rabbit except in the deepest layers of the incision site. Similar but less dramatic changes are seen in a cat model.[20,30,31] While it is well known that rabbits lack a Bowman's layer, healing disparities are seen mainly in the stromal bed. Unlike rabbits, the epithelial plug in primates and cats is fully replaced with fibroblasts and scar tissue by 2 weeks following RK (Fig 3–10). These studies point out the significant differences in corneal wound healing among humans, rabbits and other animal models used to study RK. These differences in stromal healing response should be kept in mind when interpolating or designing animal studies.

DESCEMET'S MEMBRANE AND ENDOTHELIUM

Human Studies

Endothelial changes after RK are much less pronounced than those observed in the other corneal layers unless a perforation occurs. Endothelial cell loss after RK is of dubious clinical significance,[4,11,32] but has been observed in specimens 3 to 47 months following surgery, with the greatest loss occurring beneath incisions.[3,4,6,32] Endothelial cell loss is greater in perforated corneas and when optical zone size is less than 3.5 mm.[33] Multiple reoperations may also increase the risk of endothelial damage: a 24% endothelial cell loss was noted following five RK procedures.[13] This may be particularly important as staged RK surgery gains in popularity with little limitation to the number of enhancements.

Increases in endothelial cell density after RK have been reported in five eyes 6 to 30 months postoperatively.[33] Changes in endothelial cell morphology such

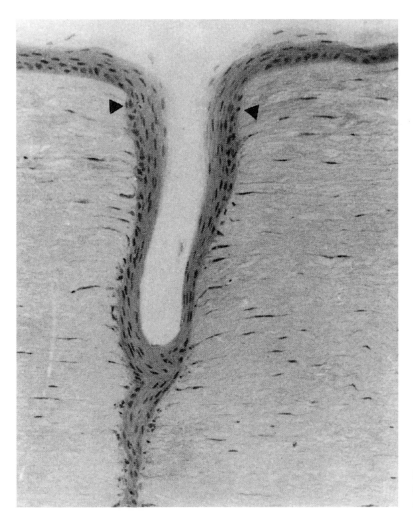

Figure 3–10. Replacement of epithelial plug with fibrotic tissue 3 days after RK in a cat. *(From Garana et al, Fig 1a, p. 3273.*[30]*)*

as pleomorphism, swelling, pitted cell borders, increased mitochondria, vacuoles, cytoplasmic microfilaments and loss of intercellular apposition may also be observed.[2,4,6] One study showed increased pleomorphism when the optical zone was less than 3.5 mm. Another study showed no polymegathism or polymorphism under radial incisions 1 year postoperatively.[32] Overall, endothelial changes in human subjects have been minimal, with significant cell loss occurring only in corneas with very small optical zones and after perforations.

In contrast to animal studies, Descemet's membrane breaks in humans have been noted only after corneal perforation.[6,8,14] In nonperforated corneas Descemet's membrane may increase in thickness following uncomplicated RK, but remains essentially undamaged.[2] Other posterior corneal findings following RK include posterior ridges, retrocorneal membranes, inflammatory cell deposits and epithelial downgrowth

(Fig 3–11).[2,4–7,9,32,34] Like most histological findings following incisional keratorefractive surgery, posterior ridges may be present in most, but not all patients. For example, posterior ridges were absent as early as 6 months after RK in one specimen, while they were observed in another specimen as late as 70 months after RK (Fig 3–12).[2,4–6,32] Inflammatory cell deposits along the retrocorneal surface and stromal necrosis were noted in a cornea complicated by sterile keratitis 4 months after RK, but this is a highly unusual situation.[9]

Animal Studies

In studies of nonhuman primates after RK, no immediate damage is noted in the endothelium after RK (Fig 3–13).[18] Within 1 week of surgery, endothelial cells show only minor mitochondrial changes. Endothelial changes, such as intercellular vacuolation, intracytoplasmic condensation and degenerative changes,

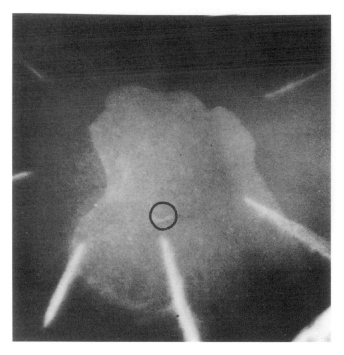

Figure 3–11. Retrocorneal membrane 9 months after RK complicated by microperforation. *(From Binder, Fig 2, p. 249.[34])*

appear 1 to 2 weeks postoperatively. Six months postoperatively, no further changes are seen in the endothelium, and ridges are not observed underlying the incision sites. In another study, linear protrusions are seen below and parallel to incision sites in nonhuman primate corneas 3 months after RK.[35] These posterior ridges correlate positively with the depth of the incision. Other animal studies demonstrate similar ridges below RK wounds.[19,21,22]

Endothelial cells that appear normal are seen in most but not all corneas after RK.[35] Mitochondrial abnormalities, inflammatory cells, thickened endothelium, decreased nuclei counts, vacuoles and intracellular edema are some of the abnormalities seen in the endothelium after RK in animal studies (Fig 3–14a, 3–14b).[18,19,21,22,35] Pleomorphism, loss of cellular organelles, dark spots and ill-defined cellular borders occur in primate corneas up to 3 months after surgery with a statistically significant endothelial cell loss of 8%.[22] In owl monkeys endothelial cell loss was 15% 6 months after RK.[18] In rabbits, endothelium underlying perforated incisions demonstrates more degenerative changes and larger ridges, but endothelial damage in the rabbit model is neither extensive nor permanent.[19]

WOUND HEALING AFTER ASTIGMATIC KERATOTOMY

Astigmatic keratotomy (AK), which utilizes tangential and circumferential incisions to correct astigmatism, exhibits many of the same ultrastructural changes seen after RK. These procedures are frequently performed either in tandem or in short succession.[36,37] AK incisions exhibit a greater tendency to gape postoperatively, perhaps because of the less uniform distribution of tension at the wound edges. Because of this, the epithelial plug may persist for a longer period of time. Fur-

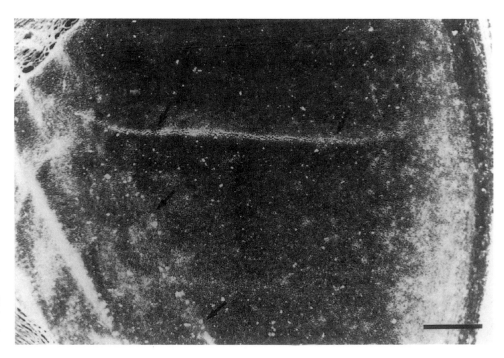

Figure 3–12. Posterior endothelial ridges in endothelium 3 months after RK. *(From Yamaguchi et al, Fig 10, p. 288.[6])*

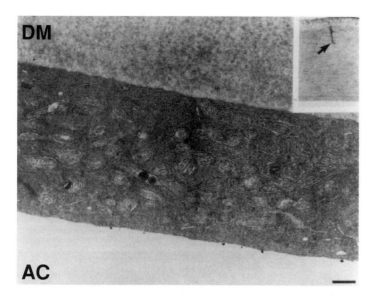

Figure 3–13. Normal endothelium after shallow RK incisions. *(From Yamaguchi et al, Fig 20, p. 326[35])*

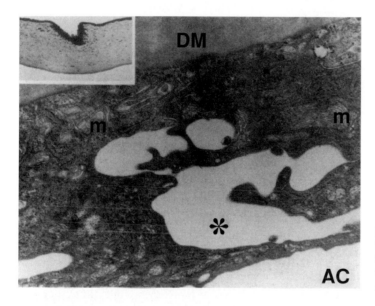

Figure 3–14a. Thickened endothelium with widened intercellular spaces, swollen mitochondria, and endoplasmic reticulum. *(From Yamaguchi et al, Fig 3, p. 2152.[19])*

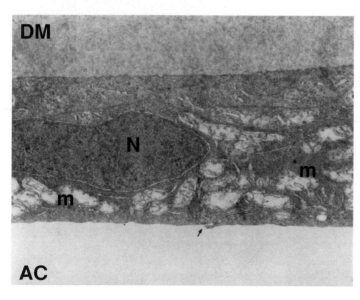

Figure 3–14b. Thickened endothelial cells with swollen mitochondria. *(From Yamaguchi et al, Fig 13, p. 322.[35])*

thermore, delayed wound healing is significantly greater in semiradial incisions than in tangential incisions, with complete healing of semiradial incisions seen in two out of three trapezoidal keratotomies at 9 and 10 months postoperatively.[37]

Intersection of incisions further delays wound healing, with persistence of the epithelial plug and cysts increasing the risks of infection, stromal melting and an irregular topographic result.[1]

SUMMARY

Following RK, epithelium undergoes several changes and forms an intrastromal plug which may last for years after RK prior to its extrusion. Bowman's membrane breaks are permanent, but epithelial basal lamina regenerates and forms a hemidesmosomal attachment to the overlying epithelium, epithelial plug and underlying stroma. Stromal response to RK is varied. Inflammation, keratocyte degeneration and epithelial plugs are eventually replaced with realignment of the collagen fibrils and scar formation. The types of scars and the time course of wound healing varies greatly not only among individuals, but also among incisions. Although smaller optical zones, reoperations and perforations increase the likelihood of endothelial cell loss, it remains clinically insignificant in most cases. Animal studies in nonhuman primates and cats may further delineate corneal wound healing and increase our understanding of refractive outcome after RK.

REFERENCES

1. Jester JV, Villasenor RA, Miyashiro J. Epithelial inclusion cysts following radial keratotomy. *Arch Ophthalmol.* 1983; 101:611–615.
2. Ingraham HJ, Guber D, Green WR. Radial keratotomy: clinicopathologic case report. *Arch Ophthalmol.* 1985;103: 683–688.
3. Jester JV, Villasenor RA, Cavanagh HD, et al. Variations in corneal wound healing after radial keratotomy: possible insights into mechanisms of clinical complications and refractive effects. *Cornea.* 1992;11:191–199.
4. Deg JK, Zavala EY, Binder PS. Delayed corneal wound healing following radial keratotomy. *Ophthalmology.* 1985; 92:734–740.
5. Binder PS, Nayak SK, Sugar J, et al. An ultrastructural and histochemical study of long-term wound healing after radial keratotomy. *Am J Ophthalmol.* 1987;103:432–440.
6. Yamaguchi T, Tamaki K, Shaw EL, et al. Histologic study of a pair of human corneas after anterior radial keratotomy. *Am J Ophthalmol.* 1985;100:281–292.
7. Binder PS, Waring GO, Wang C, et al. Histopathology of traumatic corneal rupture after radial keratotomy. *Arch Ophthalmol.* 1988;106:1584–1590.
8. Durand L, Monnot J-P, Assi A, et al. Complications of radial keratotomy: eyes with keratoconus and late wound dehiscence. *Refract Corneal Surg.* 1992;8:311–314.
9. Karr DJ, Grutzmacher RD, Reeh MJ. Radial keratotomy complicated by sterile keratitis and corneal perforation: histopathologic case report and review of complications. *Ophthalmology.* 1985;92:1244–1248.
10. Vila-Coro AA, Bonafonte S, Del Cotero JN. Epithelial inclusion cysts after radial keratotomy. *Ann Ophthalmol.* 1988;20:367–370.
11. Melles GR, Binder PS, Anderson JA. Variation in healing throughout the depth of long-term, unsutured, corneal wounds in human autopsy specimens and monkeys. *Arch Ophthalmol.* 1994;112:100–109.
12. McNeill JI. Corneal incision dehiscence during penetrating keratoplasty nine years after radial keratotomy. *J Cataract Refract Surg.* 1993;19:542–543.
13. Salz JJ. Progressive endothelial cell loss following repeat radial keratotomy: a case report. *Ophthalmol Surg.* 1982; 13:997–999.
14. Simons KB, Linsalata RP, Zaragosa AM. Ruptured globe secondary to blunt trauma following radial keratotomy. *J Refract Surg.* 1988;4:132–135.
15. Nelson JD, Williams P, Doughman DJ, et al. Map-fingerprint-dot changes in the corneal epithelial basement membrane following radial keratotomy. *Ophthalmology.* 1985;92:199–205.
16. Rashid ER, Waring GO. Complications of radial and transverse keratotomy. *Surv Ophthalmol.* 1989;34:73–106.
17. Steinberg EB, Wilson LA, Coles WH, et al. Stellate iron lines in the corneal epithelium after radial keratotomy. *Am J Ophthalmol.* 1984;98:416–421.
18. Jester JV, Steel D, Smith RE, et al. Radial keratotomy in nonhuman primate eyes. *Am J Ophthalmol.* 1981;92: 153–171.
19. Yamaguchi T, Polack FM, Kaufman HE. Endothelial damage after anterior radial keratotomy. An electron microscopic study of rabbit cornea. *Arch Ophthalmol.* 1981;99: 2151–2158.
20. Jester JV, Petroll WM, Cavanagh HD, et al. Radial keratotomy. I. The wound healing process and measurement of incisional gape in two animal models using in vivo confocal microscopy. *Invest Ophthalmol Vis Sci.* 1992;33:3255–3270.
21. Binder PS, Stainer GA, Akers PH, et al. Acute morphological features of radial keratotomy. *Arch Ophthalmol.* 1983; 101:1113–1116.
22. Yamaguchi T, Asbell PA, Kaufman HE, et al. Endothelial damage in monkeys after radial keratotomy performed

with a diamond blade. *Arch Ophthalmol.* 1984;102: 765–769.

23. Waring GO, Steinberg EB, Wilson LA. Slit-lamp microscopic appearance of corneal wound healing after radial keratotomy. *Am J Ophthalmol.* 1985;100:218–224.

24. Fyodorov SN, Sarkizova MB, Kurasova TP. Corneal bimicroscopy following repeated radial keratotomy. *Ann Ophthalmol.* 1983;15:403–407.

25. McDonnell PJ, Lean JS, Schanzlin DJ. Globe rupture from blunt trauma after hexagonal keratotomy. *Am J Ophthalmol.* 1987;103:241–242.

26. Bloom HR, Sands J, Schneider D. Corneal rupture from blunt trauma 22 months after radial keratotomy. *Refract Corneal Surg.* 1990;6:197–199.

27. Spivack L. Case report: Radial keratotomy incisions remain intact despite facial trauma from plane crash. *J Refract Surg.* 1987;3:59–60.

28. Salz JJ, Villasenor RA, Buchbinder M. Four-incision radial keratotomy for low to moderate myopia. *Ophthalmology.* 1986;93:727–738.

29. Davison PF, Galbavy EJ. Connective tissue remodeling in corneal and scleral wounds. *Ophthalmol Vis Sci.* 1986;27: 1478–1484.

30. Garana RM, Petroll WM, Jester JV, et al. Radial keratotomy. II. Role of the myofibroblast in corneal wound contraction. *Invest Ophthalmol Vis Sci.* 1992;33:3271–3282.

31. Kwitko S, Sinbawy A, McDonnell PJ, et al. Pharmacologic alteration of corneal topography after radial keratotomy. *Ophthal Surg.* 1992;23:738–741.

32. MacRae SM, Matsuda M, Rich LF. The effect of radial keratotomy on the corneal endothelium. *Am J Ophthalmol.* 1985;100:538–542.

33. Chiba K, Oak SS, Hecht S, et al. Morphometric analysis of corneal endothelium following radial keratotomy. *J Cataract Refract Surg.* 1987;13:263–267.

34. Binder PS. Presumed epithelial ingrowth following radial keratotomy. *CLAO.* 1986;12:247–250.

35. Yamaguchi T, Kaufman HE, Asbell PA, et al. Histologic and electron microscopic assessment of endothelial damage produced by anterior radial keratotomy in the monkey cornea. *Am J Ophthalmol.* 1981;92:313–327.

36. Stainer GA, Shaw EL, Akers P, et al. Histopathology of a case of radial keratotomy. *Arch Ophthalmol.* 1982;100: 1473–1477.

37. Deg JK, Binder PS. Wound healing after astigmatic keratotomy in human eyes. *Ophthalmology.* 1987;94:1290–1298.

CHAPTER 4

Corneal Wound Healing Following Laser Surgery

Dimitri T. Azar ▪ Tae Won Hahn ▪ Johnny M. Khoury

The excimer laser allows precise removal of corneal tissue through a photochemical laser-tissue interaction. This interaction results in removal of the most superficial 0.20- to 0.50-mm layer with each pulse.[1–5] The energy of the ultraviolet (UV) photons initially breaks the peptide and carbon-to-carbon molecular bonds. Photon energy in excess of broken chemical bonds excites the fragmented tissue and leads to tissue ablation. This is known as *photoablation*.[7–10] Studies of the argon fluoride (ArF) excimer laser have shown that it produces a 0.2-mm zone of stromal damage with minimal heat transmission beyond this zone.[6,7] The ultrastructure of neighboring corneal zones is preserved. These factors contribute to the excimer laser's ability to make reproducible corneal ablations with sharp demarcation at the edges of treated zones.[8–14]

The optimum UV wavelength for corneal laser ablation was reported to be 193 nm.[8,15] Higher wavelengths (248 or 308 nm) result in undesirable destruction of surrounding tissues due to higher penetration with partial thermal effects; they are also similar to the solar energy UV wavelengths known to be mutagenic or oncogenic.

Photorefractive keratectomy (PRK) with an 193-nm ArF excimer laser was developed to correct refractive errors of the eye predictably and permanently by changing the anterior curvature of the cornea. The initial assumption for PRK was that the excimer laser could remove corneal stroma precisely and gently enough that a wound-healing response would be minimal once the epithelium had covered the ablated corneal surface.

Numerous animal and human studies, however, revealed that corneal wound healing after PRK involves subepithelial fibroplasia and variable degrees of corneal haze. Corneal scarring may contribute to glare, decrease of contrast sensitivity, and loss of best-corrected visual acuity. Scarring may potentially render PRK ineffective and unpredictable and is a major obstacle for widespread clinical application of PRK for high myopia. The excimer laser is also used for the treatment of diseases that affect the anterior one third of the cornea: corneal scars and irregularities, and granular, lattice, and Reis–Buckler's dystrophies.[19–21] Phototherapeutic keratectomy (PTK) is a simple and safe alternative to keratoplasty in patients who have superficial corneal diseases and are poor candidates for corneal graft, but subepithelial haze is also a major problem in PTK, as is postoperative hyperopic shift. Accordingly, corneal wound healing is still an important determinant of the visual outcome of patients undergoing excimer laser keratectomy.[1,15–18]

A pharmacologic approach to modify the corneal wound-healing response has been tried to suppress subepithelial haze and myopic regression after PRK. Corticosteroids are known to reduce the deposition of scar tissue in experimental models of PRK.[22,23] Topical steroids were found to be effective in improving the refractive results and have been commonly used postoperatively, but they have no effect on haze and their effect on the refraction was reported lost after 3 months when steroids were discontinued.[24] Other agents like antimetabolites, growth factors, and interferon are under investigation[23,25,26] (see Chapter 5).

EPITHELIAL WOUND HEALING

After photoablation, the epithelium at the leading edge flattens and migrates over the wound. A thin, electron-dense layer (often called a *pseudomembrane*) develops on the surface of the wound bed and may act as a template or basement membrane substitute to promote smooth, rapid reepithelialization.[27] Once the wound is covered by a single cell layer, mitosis actively occurs and multiple epithelial layers are formed (Fig 4–1).

Following 6-mm excimer ablation of the human cornea, epithelial cells migrate over the wound within 1 to 3 days.[5,6,28] Data from studies of animal and human corneal wound healing following excimer laser keratectomy have shown that there is a tendency for the epithelium to undergo hyperplasia over the ablation bed, which is more pronounced in nontapered ablations.[1,5–7,29–34] Additionally, the epithelial surface does not totally reflect surface irregularities of the stromal ablation bed.[30–33]

In epithelial defects that do not involve the basement membrane, reformation of corneal epithelial adhesion promptly follows epithelial resurfacing.[34–36] Adhesion structure reformation, however, is delayed for up to 2 to 3 months following keratectomy wounds that go below the basement membrane.[35–37] Electron microscopy (EM) and immunolocalization of hemidesmosome, basement membrane, and anchoring fibril components provide evidence of synchronous reappearance of the adhesion structures following keratectomy wounds.[35,37–47] A continuous, reassembled adhesion complex is present 1 to 2 months after the keratectomy in rabbits[38] and 3 months in monkey eyes.[34] Postexcimer EM analyses of corneal epithelial basement membrane zones in monkey eyes have shown discontinuities, duplication, and thickening of the basement membrane as late as 18 months postoperatively.[1,3,5,7,22,48] In corneas with even greater stromal haze, basement membranes were more irregular, focally thickened, and discontinuous.[1,2,16,22] Normaliza-

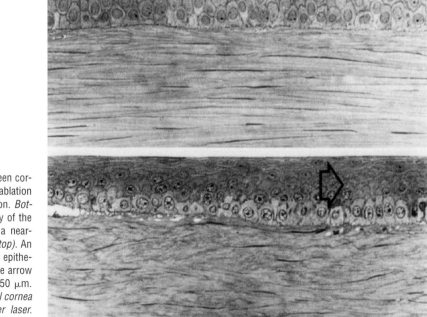

Figure 4–1. Light micrographs of the interface between corneal epithelium and stroma in areas of excimer laser ablation 6 months after exposure. *Top:* central area of ablation. *Bottom:* peripheral area of ablation. Notice the regularity of the basal organization in the central areas as well as a near-normal number of cells in the overlying epithelium *(top)*. An increase in the number of layers of cells within the epithelium is seen at the edge of the ablation *(bottom)*. The arrow indicates the direction of the lesion center. Bars = 50 μm. *(From Marshall et al. Long-term healing of the central cornea after photorefractive keratectomy using an excimer laser.* Ophthalmology. *1988;95:1411–1421.)*

tion of the basement membrane and hemidesmosomal attachments were seen only at 9 months after wounding. Morphometric analysis of the adhesion structures in human eyes after excimer keratectomy has not been reported.

Generally, the corneal epithelium firmly attaches to the stroma throughout the healing process unless there are unexpected problems during and after the procedure; hence, recurrent erosions and persistent epithelial defects are rare. However, evidence from EM studies of human excimer-ablated corneas shows a significant delay in normalization of components of the epithelial basement membrane and of anchoring fibril reformation.[49,50] A failure to reestablish a firm anchoring fibril network contributes to epithelial breakdown,[44] which occurs in 3% of the eyes after PRK[51] and may be the cause of a foreign body sensation, watering, or tenderness in patients who rub the eye.[51-54] Additionally, in experimental excimer ablations, the epithelium can be easily removed as an epithelial sheet 2 to 4 weeks postoperatively, suggesting poor initial epithelial basement membrane adhesion (personal observation).

Human corneas treated with the excimer laser for lattice, macular, and Reis–Buckler's dystrophies that later required corneal transplantation were studied to determine if the time and pattern of reassembly of the corneal epithelial adhesion structures were altered following human excimer laser wounds. These corneal specimens were removed at penetrating keratoplasty 6,

9, 11, and 15 months after initial excimer keratectomy and processed for EM.[49] The basal cell membrane/basement membrane zones of EMs were studied at standardized magnification. Basal epithelial cells from each of three areas of the wound bed were analyzed to determine the reformation of hemidesmosomes, basement membrane, and anchoring fibrils.

The percentage of basal cells with altered parameters of epithelial wound healing was calculated, and morphometric analysis of hemidesmosomes and basement membranes was performed. The results of these studies showed that 29% of cells had normal basement membrane at 6 months, compared with 86% at 15 months. Multilamellar basement membrane was seen in one cornea. Anchoring fibrils were initially decreased but increased gradually after 6 months. Irregular collagen peaked at 9 months, which coincided with the reduction of keratocytes adjacent to the wound (Fig 4–2).[49] These data corroborate the findings of previous studies and suggest that significant alterations of corneal epithelial adhesion and basement membrane persist after 6 months and do not normalize until 1 year. Laminin, present in normal corneas in and below the basement membrane, was immunolocalized to the anterior stroma 1 week after wounding.[5] It concentrated in the basement membrane zone by 3 months, and continued to show discontinuities as late as 18 months after excimer wounding. Type III collagen, ordinarily seen in corneal scars, but not in normal cor-

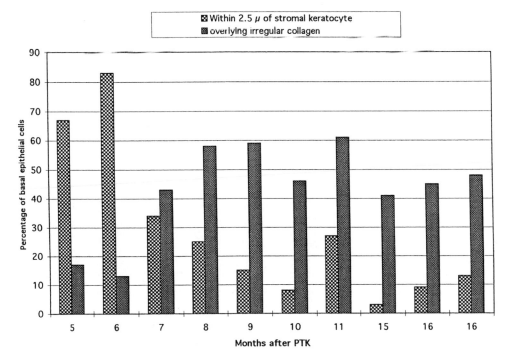

Figure 4–2. The percentage of basal epithelial cells within 2.5 μm of stromal keratocyte and the percentage of cells overlying irregular collagen at different time points after PTK. Results include additional time points, courtesy of Dr. Perry Binder.

neas, began to appear below the epithelium 3 weeks postoperatively and persisted in the anterior stroma.

Bowman's Layer

To achieve clinically acceptable refractive changes with PRK, Bowman's layer is removed in most of the patients. This acellular, fibrotic collagen layer does not regenerate once it is ablated, and its edges retain their tapered appearance after a graded ablation.

The exact physiologic role of Bowman's layer is not clear. A long-standing, but experimentally unproven, hypothesis has been that this layer provides an important contribution to the biomechanical stability of the cornea. Histologically, this point of view was easily accepted because the collagen fibers in Bowman's layer are omnidirectionally oriented and strongly interwoven. However, experiments of uniaxial stress-strain analysis performed on the human cadaver eyes showed that Bowman's layer does not contribute significantly to corneal stability.[57]

Another argument against the mechanical dominance of Bowman's layer is that radial keratotomy (RK) incisions have to be far deeper than the thickness of Bowman's layer to obtain clinically significant refractive results.

The ablation rate of Bowman's layer is slightly different from those of the corneal epithelium and stroma. According to data from enucleated human eyes, the average ablation rates were 0.38, 0.55, and 0.68 μm per pulse in Bowman's layer, stroma, and epithelium, respectively, at a fluence of 205 mJ/cm^2. Predictability of the excimer laser is related to the ablation rate of the corneal layer for a specific radiant exposure and wavelength of the laser.[10]

Ablations confined to Bowman's layer are possible, but in most cases a greater depth of stromal tissue has to be removed than Bowman's layer to obtain the clinically desirable refractive changes. Theoretically refractive change up to 2 D can be induced if ablation is confined to Bowman's layer. Whether ablations confined to Bowman's layer induce subepithelial fibroplasia is not known.[59]

STROMAL WOUND HEALING

Stromal healing following excimer wounds involves migration and proliferation of stromal keratocytes under the area of the wound.[7,16,30] These produce stromal collagen (Fig 4–3). Extracellular matrix (ECM) proteins and glycoproteins are added to the wound bed.[1,3,7,16]

Gradual remodeling of the treatment zone follows, so that by 18 months after excimer wounds the anterior stroma achieves a normal lamellar appearance.

Histologic Findings After Excimer Stromal Scarring

The marked reduction of the keratocytes in the anterior 40 μm of the stroma is the earliest response of the stroma to photoablation in monkey corneas (Fig 4–4).[7,60] The cause for this is not clear, but it is not specific to the excimer laser because the same finding can be observed after scrape injuries.[61] Within the first week keratocytes are converted to fibroblasts that repopulate the anterior stroma.

By approximately 3 to 6 weeks after ablation, the subepithelial zone is filled with fibroblasts showing a marked increase of rough endoplasmic reticulum, cytoplasmic vacuoles, and positive staining for fetal antigen.[60,62] These active fibroblasts are responsible for the production of new ECM components such as type III collagen and fibronectin. Type III collagen, not normally present in the corneal stroma, deposits on the anterior stromal bed. There is also an increased amount of keratan sulfate proteoglycan. During this time, subepithelial haze occurs as a result of the disrupted structure of the anterior stromal lamellae.

Malley and coworkers[5] found in monkeys that subepithelial haze was caused by the production of disorganized layers of type III collagen and the absence of normal keratan sulfate in the subepithelial space for at least 1 month after laser treatment. Subsequent deposition of fibronectin and laminin in the wound bed after reepithelialization suggests a close association between the increased numbers of anterior stromal keratocytes present and the wound-healing response (Figs 4–5 and 4–6).[5,55] Subepithelial haze may also occur because of the larger collagen diameters, increased interfiber spacing, more random orientations, and abnormal glycoproteins. The new material is laid down between the epithelium and the ablated stromal surface, as evidenced by the appearance of type VII collagen-anchoring fibrils throughout the 20- to 40-mm thick zone of new tissue.

Tuft and colleagues[63] have demonstrated this with dichlorotriazinyl aminofluorescein (DTAF) staining in rabbits. The density and distribution of new tissue determine the clinical appearance of the subepithelial haze and the final refractive change. In general, the haze occupies the entire ablated zone and is present in all eyes after ablation.

From approximately 3 months to 1 year after surgery, one of two processes occurs. Most commonly, the

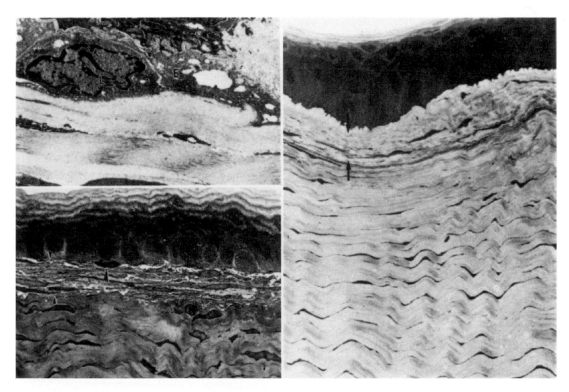

Figure 4–3. Histopathologic findings of anterior stromal scarring *(small arrows)* after excimer laser ablation. *Top left:* four days after ablation, lymphocyte *(L)* is interdigitated between healing vacuolated epithelium *(E)* and residual stroma that contains activated fibrocytes *(F)* (×13,400). *Bottom left:* at 21 days, epithelium is slightly hyperplastic with delayed maturation. Lymphocyte *(large arrow head)* lies between epithelium and underlying connective tissue. A layer of hypercellular, loosely organized scar tissue *(small arrow heads)* lies beneath the epithelium. Remaining stroma shows activated keratocytes with generally compact lamellar architecture (toluidine blue, ×200). *Right:* at 100 days, there is normal stratified epithelium with tall basal cells and a layer of compact subepithelial scar tissue *(between arrows)* approximately 20 μm thick with a transition zone leading to corneal stroma whose architecture is generally normal (toluidine blue, ×200). *(From Hanna et al. Corneal stromal wound healing in rabbits after 193-nm excimer laser surface ablation. Arch Ophthalmol. 1989;107:895–901.)*

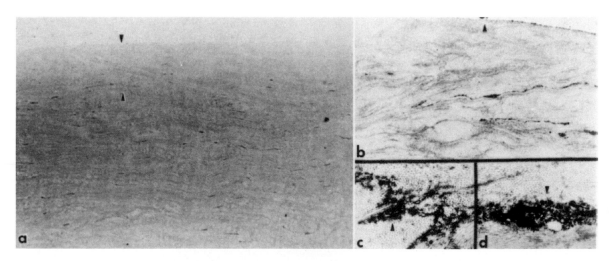

Figure 4–4. Cornea immediately after ablation. A. Light micrograph shows a smooth stromal surface without steps and the ablation of Bowman's layer. The interdigitating anterior stromal lamellae are undisturbed (toluidine blue, ×20). There was a marked decrease in the number of keratocytes in the anterior 40 μm of the stroma *(between arrowheads)*. B. TEM demonstrating small undulations of the surface with a discontinuous, electron-dense condensate and some debris. C, D. Keratocytes in the anterior stroma show disintegration and fragmentation *(arrowheads)* (×25.000). *(From Fantes et al. Wound healing after excimer laser keratomileusis (photorefractive keratectomy) in monkeys. Arch Ophthalmol. 1990;108:665–675.)*

subepithelial zone remodels, the fibroblasts and the type III and type VII collagen disappear, and a reasonably normal lamellar stromal structure emerges that is occupied by keratocytes. This corresponds clinically to a decrease in subepithelial haze. Sometimes, however, the new subepithelial extracellular matrix consolidates into scar tissue, creating a dense layer of apparent type I, irregularly arranged fibrous tissue histologically and a circular corneal scar clinically. Tuft and coworkers[64] demonstrated in rabbits a dramatic decrease in ECM production after the use of topical corticosteroids.

As excimer technology evolves, one of the major obstacles to further clinical application has been the control of subepithelial haze and stromal scarring in the visual axis. This is more pronounced with deeper and larger ablations.[3,4,14,22] The degree of scarring can be lessened with shallower ablations, smaller optical zones, and the use of topical antiinflammatory agents.[4,22] To date, most of the studies evaluating the haze following excimer laser keratectomy have employed only subjective methods. Thus, the natural course of the scar has not yet been fully evaluated, and the effects of drugs that may modulate the scarring process remain difficult to evaluate. Several drugs have

been advocated to minimize stromal scar formation, including mitomycin C. Epithelial defects and recurrent erosions may follow higher concentrations of such topical drugs[22] (see Chapter 5).

Another particular finding of the cornea following excimer wounds is the absence of leukocyte infiltration,[1,3,7,16] which represents a striking difference between these wounds and chemical or inflammatory ulceration. However, epithelial and stromal cells may produce collagenases and cytokines (which are ordinarily leukocyte derived) that may play a role in the pathogenesis of stromal scar formation following excimer keratectomy. Corneal wound healing following excimer keratectomy is different from that following simple debrided wounds, and shows some resemblance to that following mild thermal wounds, where leukocytes are also absent.[65]

Stromal Wound Healing After Excimer: Confocal Microscopy

The pattern of in vivo wound healing following excimer wounds can be determined using confocal microscopy. In collaboration with Dr Rajesh Rajpal at the George-

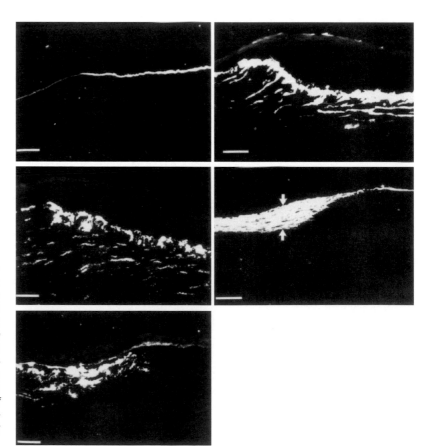

Figure 4–5. Immunofluorescene staining pattern of fibronectin, 1 day *(top left)* and 6 days *(top right)* after laser treatment and 6 days after mechanical keratectomy *(center left)*. The immunofluorescene pattern is similar to that observed for fibrinogen, except at 1 month. One month after laser *(center right)* and mechanical *(bottom left)* treatment, fibronectin fluorescene is observed throughout the newly synthesized connective tissue *(arrows)* *(top left* and *center right,* ×110, bar = 100 μm; *top right, center left,* and *bottom left,* ×220, bar = 50 μm). *(From Malley et al. Immunofluorescene study of corneal wound healing after excimer laser anterior keratectomy in the monkey eye. Arch Ophthalmol. 1990; 108:1316–1322.)*

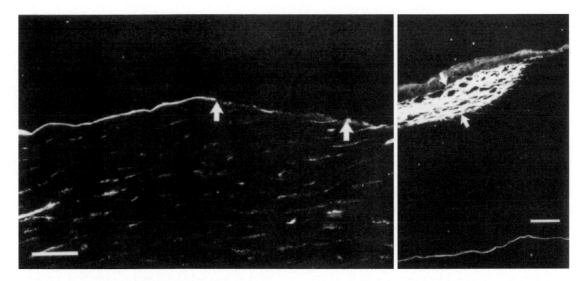

Figure 4–6. Immunofluorescene distribution of laminin. One day after laser treatment *(left)*, no fluorescene is detected over the ablated surface *(arrows)*. Fluorescene is present in adjacent basement membrane. One month after laser treatment *(right)*, positive fluorescene for laminin occurred throughout the newly synthesized connective tissue *(arrows)* (×220, bar = 50 μm). *(From Malley et al. Immunofluorescene study of corneal wound healing after excimer laser anterior keratectomy in the monkey eye.* Arch Ophthalmol. *1990;108:1316–1322.)*

town University Department of Ophthalmology, we have studied the reformation of the epithelium basement membrane, stromal collagen, and keratocytes after excimer laser wounds in rabbit corneas.[66]

Using the 193-nm ArF excimer laser, with a fluence of 160 mJ/cm^2 and an ablation rate of 5 Hz, 100-μm corneal stromal excimer ablations were performed. There was evidence of fibroblastic changes in the anterior stroma, coupled with collagenous stromal scarring in the early stages of wound healing. Anterior stromal keratocytes were elongated and spindle shaped. The degree of keratocyte elongation and the subepithelial collagenous scarring slowly decreased over time, but were not normalized by 6 months postoperatively.[66]

Superficial Concentric PRK

Studies of wound healing following superficial annular keratectomy are consistent with the above observations. We studied epithelial wound healing following Fresnel-like superficial concentric PRK.[67] These corneal excimer ablations stay within the acellular Bowman's layer and, theoretically, would correct greater degrees of myopia with larger optical zones. The results of these experiments (performed in rabbit and monkey eyes) showed epithelial hypertrophy at the edges of the rings, and the epithelial curvature resembled parts of the ablation bed.[67,68] However, when deep annular laser keratectomy was performed, migration and proliferation of ep-

ithelial cells into the central corneal stroma were noted.[69] This phenomenon of intrastromal epithelial migration is excimer specific. The absence of stromal collagen in surrounding areas is suggestive of collagenase activation.

Stromal Wound Healing: Biochemical Aspects

The alterations in epithelial basement membrane reformation and the alterations in subepithelial stromal collagen may be due to collagenase activation in a manner similar to that seen after corneal thermal wounds.[46] Matrix metalloproteinases (MMPs) play an important role in the initial stromal degradation and ultimate matrix regeneration of the cornea following wounding. Modulation of these collagenases may ultimately result in more predictable wound healing and reduction of stromal scarring. The MMPs are active against basement membrane components, and thus may play important roles in remodeling the corneal ECM in normal and pathologic conditions. These MMPs are optimally active at neutral pH, like that of the extracellular space. MMP-2, but not MMP-9, is present in the normal stroma,[46,70] and is more likely to be involved in ECM turnover under normal conditions. Expression of MMP-9 can be induced by stromal cell-culture passaging, organomercurials, and cytochalasin B.[70–72] MMP-9 expression is seen in the initial stages of corneal wound healing after laser ablation. A family of tissue inhibitors of MMPs (TIMPs) exists that includes TIMP-1 and TIMP-2.[73,74] An activated

MMP will fail to cleave its target if TIMPs are present.[74,75] TIMPs are produced in normal tissue and may guard against excessive ECM breakdown.

Studies of collagenase assays following excimer surgery showed that enzymatic activity of a 92-KDa band that was noted in the epithelium of excimer-ablated corneas after 6, 18, and 24 hours was not seen in the epithelium following debrided wounds and untreated controls. A 72-KDa band of enzymatic activity present in the stroma of all treated and control eyes was also seen in the epithelium of excimer-ablated corneas.[65] These short-term studies suggest that, after excimer wounds, MMP-9 (92 KDa) is expressed in corneal epithelium and stroma during wound closure. MMP-2 (72 KDa) activity is present in the stroma prior to wounding and increases following wounding.[65] It is thus possible that these proteolytic enzymes play a role in short-term (MMP-9) and long-term (MMP-2) stromal remodeling in the normal cornea, and in scar formation and clearing postexcimer wounds.

Several human and animal studies suggest that scar formation is more pronounced following deep excimer laser keratectomy.[3,4,22,29] The results of zymographic analysis performed on rabbit stromas obtained following debridement of wounds and superficial (20%) and deep (60%) excimer wounds, 20 and 30 hours after wounding, show increased expression of the 92-KDa MMP with the deeper excimer ablations.[65]

Long-term studies of stromal wound healing following excimer laser keratectomy have shown that stromal scarring and new collagen deposition peak at 1 to 6 months and decrease thereafter.[7,16,30] In addition to the recognized role of collagen matrix remodeling,[73,75–78] several observations indicate that collagenase regulation may be associated with corneal scarring and clearing:

1. Deep stromal excimer ablations are associated with increased stromal scarring and new collagen deposition, compared with superficial ablations.
2. Zymographic analysis of rabbit stromas shows greater MMP-9 expression following deep excimer wounds, compared with superficial wounds.
3. Steroids, known to regulate collagenase expression, result in long-term reduction of collagen deposition in rabbit corneas after excimer wounds and are clinically thought to minimize postexcimer scarring.[16,22]

DESCEMET'S MEMBRANE AND ENDOTHELIUM

The excimer laser is known to be absorbed within a few microns of corneal tissue and not to affect the adjacent structures. Thus, damage to the Descemet's membrane, or endothelium, is not expected. Laboratory and clinical experience have not shown any clinically meaningful changes in the endothelium.

However, experimental studies have revealed a possibility of endothelial damage through shock waves, fluorescence, secondary irradiation, and posterior migration of toxic byproducts.[1,16,79–81] Marshall and colleagues[1] found endothelial damage and loss, possibly caused by shock or acoustic waves after excimer laser incision reaching 40 mm of Descemet's membrane. Dehm et al[79] also showed endothelial alterations with 193-nm excimer laser or diamond incision to 90% of corneal depth. In contrast, 248-nm ablations of similar depth resulted in underlying endothelial cell loss and a surrounding cellular damage. Injury to Descemet's membrane and endothelium is more likely with LASIK than with surface PRK. Intrastromal surgery during LASIK has not been associated with endothelial injury, although the excimer treatment is closer to the endothelium than in surface PRK.[80]

The endothelial wound was healed with the formation of rosettes, multinucleated giant cells, and the production of a fibrillar posterior collagenous layer by 6 months after surgery. Hanna and colleagues[16] observed amorphous fibrillogranular material that appeared in Descemet's membrane in the central zone beneath the 60-mm ablation in rabbits (Fig 4–7). The material migrated forward in Descemet's membrane during the healing period over the next 3 months. The nature of this material is unknown, but immunohistochemical staining of Descemet's membrane and the posterior stroma after ablation in rabbits showed increased amounts of type IV collagen, laminin, fibronectin, and proteoglycans in Descemet's membrane, all suggesting that the ablation activated the endothelium and posterior keratocytes. They have not, however, observed a similar phenomenon in monkey's corneas.[60] At present, evidence of clinically significant postexcimer endothelial damage is lacking.

WOUND HEALING FOLLOWING OTHER EXCIMER LASERS

Excimer lasers can emit UV energy at wavelengths of 193, 248, 308, and 351 nm.[2,85] Each wavelength is pro-

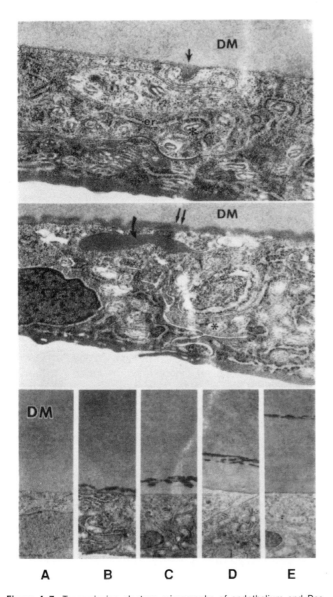

Figure 4–7. Transmission electron micrographs of endothelium and Descemet's membrane *(DM)* after anterior stromal ablation with 193-nm excimer laser. *Top:* 6 hours: Overall structure of cell was preserved with intact plasma membrane, uniform terminal web, and smooth approximation to DM. Mitochondria *(asterisk)* were dilated. Endoplasmic reticulum *(er)* was prominent and contained a fine granular substance. Intercellular space in some areas contained a fibrogranular substance that was also present along the basal aspect of cell adjacent to DM *(arrow)* (×49,250). *Center:* 24 hours: Although endothelial monolayer was preserved, there was cytoplasmic vacuolization and dilatation of mitochondria *(asterisk)* and of endoplasmic reticulum. Apical junctions remained intact. Some basal intracellular spaces were filled with a fibrogranular material *(curved arrow)* that also occupied the outer surface of basal plasma membrane adjacent to DM *(double arrows)* (×38,300). *Bottom:* TEMs of DM and endothelium from 6 hours to 100 days (A through E). Discontinuous layer of fibrillogranular material had moved anteriorly in DM. At 100 days (E) endothelial structure was normal. Discontinuous layer of amorphous fibrillogranular material migrated further forward in DM (×12,500). *(From Hanna et al. Corneal stromal wound healing in rabbits after 193-nm excimer laser surface ablation.* Arch Ophthalmol. *1989;107:895–901.)*

duced by combining a noble gas and a halogen gas in the laser cavity: argon and fluorine (ArF) emit at 193 nm, krypton and fluorine (KrF) emit at 248 nm, xenon and chlorine (XeCl) emit at 308 nm, and xenon and fluorine (XeF) emit at 351 nm. These four wavelengths can be emitted at an irradiance great enough to ablate corneal tissue, a phenomenon termed *ablative photodecomposition.*[2,82]

Kruger et al compared the tissue effects and histologic findings of various excimer laser wavelengths.[2,82] At 193 nm, tissue sections showed smooth uniform walls, without regard to pulse rate or suprathreshold irradiance level (Fig 4–8). In contrast, the stromas treated with the 249-nm laser were irregular and vacuolated with roughly parallel incision edges (Fig 4–9A). Increasing the irradiance caused the incision to bulge (Fig

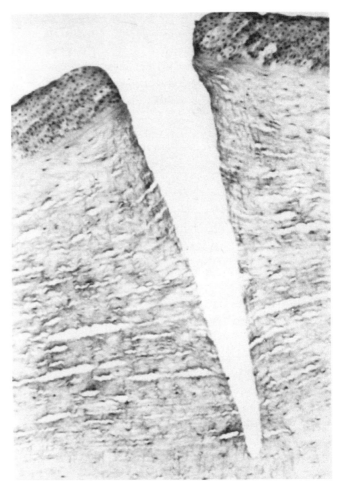

Figure 4–8. Photomicrograph of a 193-nm laser lesion. The lesion produced is similar at all supraablation irradiances and laser firing rates. Note the smooth regular walls with no distortion of the adjacent corneal stroma (×24). *(From Kruger et al. Interaction of ultraviolet light with the cornea.* Invest Ophthalmol Vis Sci. *1985;26[suppl]:1455–1464.)*

4–9B). By further increasing both irradiance and pulse rate, a considerable thermal effect, in which the walls and floor of the ablated stomal tissue melted, was noticed (Fig 4–9C). Photoablation was associated with greater amounts of thermal interaction, as longer wavelengths within the UV spectrum are used. Stromal disorganization and shrinkage were noted with 308-nm excimer lasers. Histopathology of 351-nm corneal laser burns revealed thermal damage. At low pulse rates, tissue removed with a narrow zone of thermal disorganization. The thermal interaction zone surrounding the ablated area broadened when the frequency reached 25 Hz (Fig 4–11).

At low irradiance levels, the cornea remains grossly unaffected by the laser energy. With increased irradiance, coagulation effects are seen at all wavelengths except 193 nm (fine bubbles at 249 nm; large bubbles with charring at 308 nm; shrinkage of adjacent tissues at 351 nm). At 193 nm, tissue ablation occurs with no intervening tissue coagulation, thus suggesting the absence of a thermal component. The threshold for ablation at 193 nm is approximately 50 mJ/cm^2, which is less than that of other excimer laser wavelengths.[2,82] With longer UV wavelengths, the ablation threshold increases logarithmically, as shown in Figure 4–12. The threshold for ablation of 193 nm remains constant as the pulse rate increases. This suggests that 193-nm ablation is purely photochemical.

WOUND HEALING FOLLOWING SOLID-STATE LASERS

Although the excimer laser is currently under clinical investigation for its phototherapeutic and photorefractive uses in treating and reshaping the surface of the cornea, it has several limitations, which include weight and size; safety and maintenance procedures; complicated beam delivery systems; restrictions on the size and shape of ablation zones; and acoustic shock waves resulting from wide area ablations. In an attempt to address some of these limitations, new laser technology has been developed, resulting in second-generation, solid-state corneal lasers. Solid-state technology provides increased reliability, ease of use, and elimination of the need for skilled technical assistance.

Solid-State Lasers for Corneal Surface Ablation

Frequency-quintupled neodymium : YAG (Nd : YAG) laser at 213 nm is capable of ablating corneal tissue with

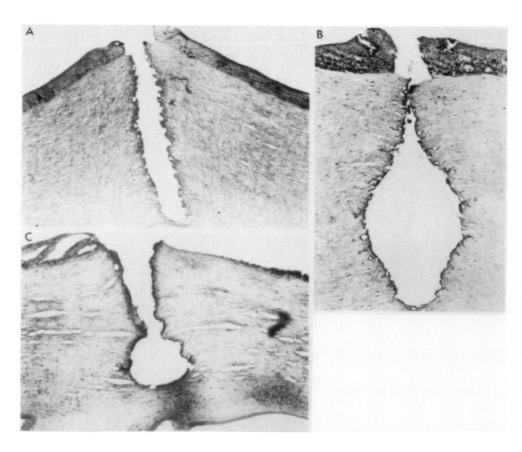

Figure 4–9. The stromal lesions produced with 249-nm laser radiation. A. A linear incision with parallel walls produced at supraablation irradiance. B. The bulging of the walls as the irradiance is increased. C. The lesion produced when both irradiance and firing rate are increased (×24). *(From Kruger et al. Interaction of ultraviolet light with the cornea. Invest Ophthalmol Vis Sci. 1985;26[suppl]:1455–1464.)*

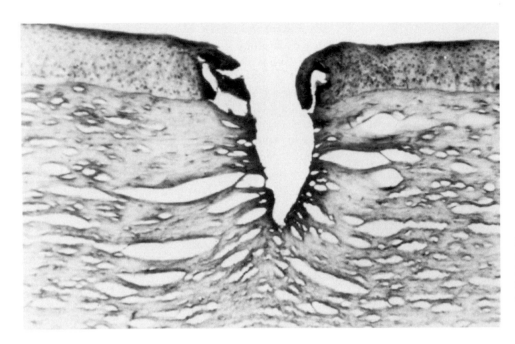

Figure 4–10. Histologic view of a linear excision produced with 308-nm laser radiation. Note the adjacent tissue shrinkage (×24). *(From Kruger et al. Interaction of ultraviolet light with the cornea.* Invest Ophthalmol Vis Sci. *1985;26[suppl]:1455–1464.)*

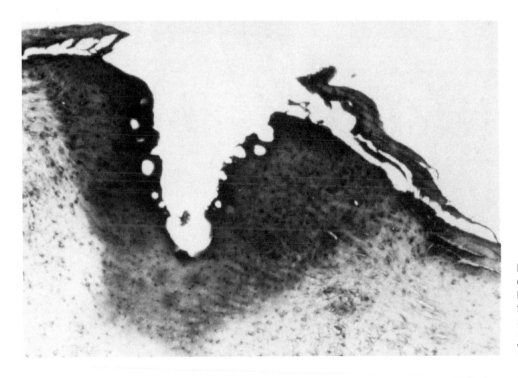

Figure 4–11. Histologic view of a linear excision produced with 351-nm laser radiation. Note the large zone of thermal damage (×24). *(From Kruger et al. Interaction of ultraviolet light with the cornea.* Invest Ophthalmol Vis Sci. *1985;26[suppl]:1455–1464.)*

a degree of precision and tissue damage comparable to the 193-nm ArF excimer laser.[83] Moreover, by coupling the 213-nm laser to a computer-controlled scanning delivery system, microspots (0.5 mm) of far UV laser pulses can be "painted" onto the cornea, facilitating aspheric corneal sculpting. The Q-switched Nd : YAG laser produces a wavelength of 1064 nm, which is modified to emit 213 nm (the Nd :YAG's fifth harmonic). A

fresh, enucleated rabbit eye treated with an ablation zone of 5 mm and an intended correction of 3 D was used for the ultrastructural examination of a 213-nm surface ablation effect.[83] Corneal tissue removed through the use of multiple spiral scanning patterns resulted in unrecognizable laser ablation steps (Fig 4–13). The boundary between ablated corneal stroma and unablated Bowman's layer was similar to that of exci-

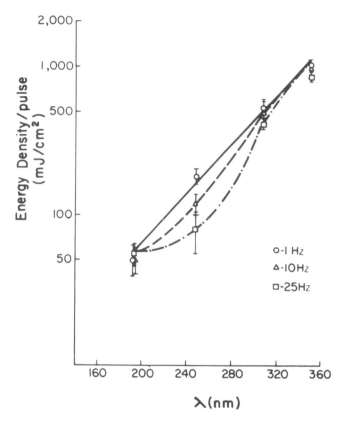

Figure 4–12. Threshold for UV laser corneal ablation, as tested for the four major wavelengths produced by the excimer laser. The departure from the logarithmic relation with lowering of the threshold at 249 nm implies a thermal component of the laser-tissue interaction. *(From Kruger et al. Interaction of ultraviolet light with the cornea.* Invest Ophthalmol Vis Sci. *1985;26:1455–1464.)*

collagen lamellae at the edge of the ablation, with the width of damage zone varying from 0.1 to 0.8 μm—similar to that of excimer laser photoablation.

Solid-state Lasers for Intracorneal Ablation (Intrastromal Lasers)

Lasers capable of removing intrastromal corneal tissue without corneal surface ablation, thus avoiding the disruption of Bowman's membrane and postoperative surface irregularities, are currently being investigated. The purpose of intrastromal ablations is to create an ablated cavity inside the stroma, which, after collapsing, changes the curvature of the anterior corneal surface. The epithelium remains intact; thus, wounding and scarring should be minimal. Intrastromal plasma-

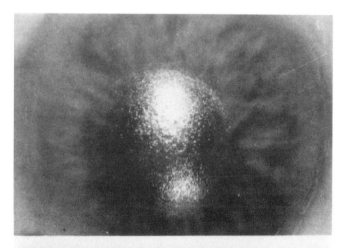

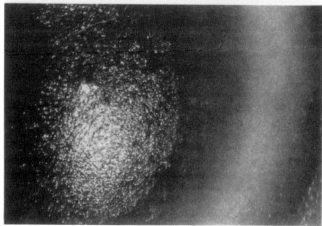

Figure 4–13. Operating microscope appearance of the cornea treated by 213-nm UV solid-state laser PRK. *Top:* the computer-controlled scanning delivery system created a 5-mm ablation zone centered around the pupil. *Bottom:* a magnified ablation zone boundary showed no observable steps. *(From Ren Q, Simon G, Parel JM. Ultraviolet solid-state laser (213-nm) photorefractive keratectomy: in vitro study.* Ophthalmology. *1993;100: 1828–1834.)*

mer-ablated corneas. The endothelial cells of the rabbit cornea beneath the ablation zone were normal. Transmission electron microscopy (TEM) indicated minimal disruption of the collagen fibers (Fig 4–14). Keratocytes, collagen fibers, Descemet's membrane, and endothelial cells beneath the ablation zone appeared normal. Although this laser has been used in experimental studies, it has not yet been approved for clinical use in the United States.

The infrared (1053 nm) picosecond Nd : YLF laser is another solid-state laser that has been modified for UV surface-corneal photoablation by the addition of type I BBO crystals to generate the fifth harmonic (211 nm). This solid-state UV laser is mode locked, thus emitting picosecond pulses that allow the use of a higher pulse rate, resulting in potentially faster ablations.

Utilizing the picosecond Nd : YLF UV pulses at the 211-nm wavelength, Hu et al performed linear incisions on the rabbit cornea.[84] The authors reported neatly cut

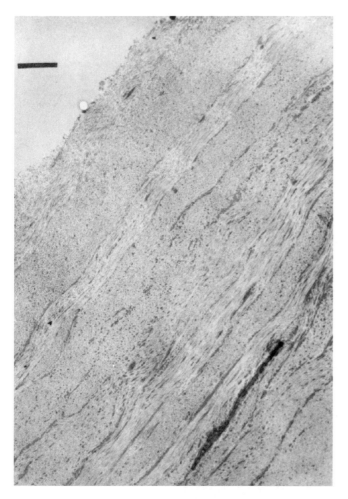

Figure 4–14. Transmission electron micrograph of the cells and collagen fibers subjacent to the ablated surface (bar = 2 μm) shows that the collagen fibers and keratocytes maintained their normal structure immediately after 213-nm PRK. *(From Ren Q, Simon G, Parel JM. Ultraviolet solid-state laser (213-nm) photorefractive keratectomy: in vitro study. Ophthalmology. 1993;100:1828–1834.)*

mediated corneal laser ablation is a potential treatment for myopia, hyperopia, and astigmatism. There are currently two companies manufacturing intrastromal lasers: Phoenix Lasers, Inc, utilizes the Nd : YAG nanosecond laser, and Intelligent Surgical Lasers, Inc, utilizes the Nd : YLF picosecond laser.

Both of these intrastromal lasers are solid-state lasers that allow a wide range of applications but require an excellent aiming mechanism, and are thus equipped with computer-controlled tracking devices. Intrastromal corneal lasers have increased the cone angle to between 22° and 32° to ensure high target irradiance and low posterior irradiance, as compared to a cone angle of approximately 16° for standard YAG capsulotomy. Intrastromal corneal lasers are useful

for the ablation of corneal tissue because they deliver an enormous amount of energy to a small focal spot. This laser–tissue interaction, which is termed photodisruption (or plasma-mediated ablation), is characterized by three major events: (1) plasma formation, (2) shock wave generation, and (3) gas bubble cavitation.[85]

The Q-switched mode-locking Nd : YLf laser is a low-energy and high–repetition-rate picosecond pulse laser with the following parameters: a wavelength of 1053 nm, a repetition rate of 10 to 1000 pulses per second, a pulse energy of 20 to 350 μJ, and a pulse width of 45 picoseconds (Fig 4–15). The double–frequency-pulsed, Q-switched Nd : YAG laser is a high-energy and low–repetition-rate nanosecond pulse laser with the following parameters: a wavelength of 532 nm, a repetition rate of 10 to 200 pulses per second, a pulse energy of 20 to 550 μJ, and a pulse width less than 10 nanoseconds (Fig 4–16).

Niemz et al were the first to investigate intrastromal ablations using the picosecond Nd : YLF laser.[86] The authors reported the appearance of small gas bubbles at the laser's point of focus, with complete resolution within an hour. Figure 4–17 shows the effect of a single picosecond pulse focused underneath Bowman's membrane in a donor human eye. A larger continuous intrastromal cavity of approximately 20 μm in depth is shown in Figure 4–18. Collapse of the smooth cavity walls an hour after laser exposure is shown in Figure 4–19.

Similar results were obtained by Remmel et al.[87] Figure 4–20 shows the formation of microvacuoles by vaporizing the corneal tissue immediately after laser application, with rapid dissemination of these vacuoles after several hours (Fig 4–21).

To determine the efficacy of such intrastromal lasers in the correction of astigmatism, Frueh et al placed intrastromal curved laser patterns 2 mm in length along the horizontal meridians of rabbit eyes using the picosecond Nd : YLF laser.[88] The authors reported corneal flattening in the desired meridian, with a peak of 5.18 ± 2.99 D 24 hours following laser application. There was a complete regression of the effects by 6 weeks postoperatively, and no stromal scarring was observed.

Solid-state Photoablative Decomposition— the Novatec Laser

The Novatec laser system (LightBlade model; Fig 4–22) can be used for surface and intracorneal ablation. It has

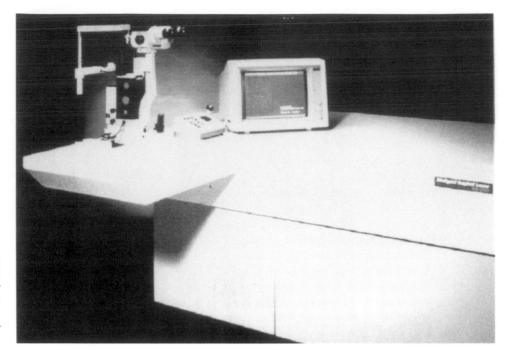

Figure 4–15. The ISL Q-switched, mode-locking Nd : YLF laser with a wavelength of 1053 nm. *(From Rowsey et al.* Alternative Lasers and Strategies for Corneal Modification. *St. Louis: Mosby-Year Book; 1995;269–276.)*

the following approximate parameters when used for surface corneal ablations: a wavelength of 0.2 μm, fluence of 100 mJ/cm^2, spot size varying between 10 to 500 μm, optical zone up to 10 mm in diameter, and computerized scanning delivery system. The use of a scanning beam combined with a low fluence reduces acoustic shock. The eye tracker allows the delivery of laser energy to the appropriate site and improves centration.

Swinger et al performed preliminary preclinical studies on human eye bank eyes using the Novatec LightBlade surgical system.[89] The authors reported that the scanning delivery system is capable of providing a surface quality that is comparable or superior to ones provided by current excimer laser technology. Figure 4–23 demonstrates the fine surface quality produced by such a system, as obtained by scanning electron microscopy (SEM). TEM (Fig 4–24) revealed a very thin pseudomembrane, approximately 1 μm thick, overlying the ablated surface, and the maintenance of the normal corneal structure beneath the ablated area.

Swinger et al also compared the VISX Twenty–Twenty and the Novatec lasers for the myopic correction of 3 D and 6 D on albino rabbit eyes.[89] No differences between the two lasers were identified in the short-term follow-up of 4 to 6 weeks based on clinical appearance, epithelialization, pachymetry, and amount or pattern of haze. An evaluation of the Novatec laser in

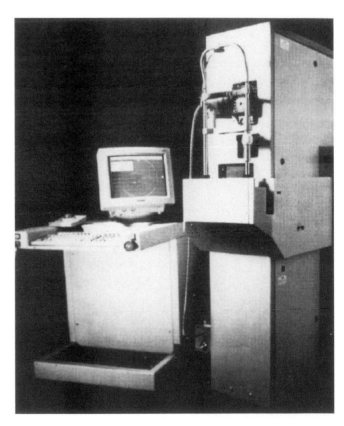

Figure 4–16. The Phoenix double–frequency-pulsed, Q-switched Nd : YAG laser with a wavelength of 532 nm. *(From Rowsey et al.* Alternative Lasers and Strategies for Corneal Modification. *St. Louis: Mosby-Year Book; 1995; 269–276.)*

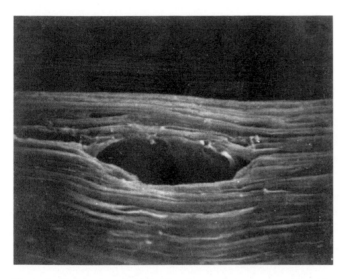

Figure 4–17. Intrastromal ablation in a human donor cornea achieved by a single picosecond pulse. The cavitation has a diameter of approximately 40 μm and a depth of 20 μm. The pulse energy was set at 100 μJ. *(From Niemz et al. Intrastromal ablations for refractive corneal surgery using picosecond infrared laser pulses.* Lasers Light Ophthalmol. *1993;5:149–155.)*

a nonhuman primate model (owl monkey) led Swinger to conclude that the Novatec laser is capable of ablating the primate cornea while producing a clinically regular surface. The primate cornea, following Novatec photorefractive keratectomy treatment, underwent normal epithelialization. Haze developed as it does in human corneas.

OBJECTIVE METHODS OF GRADING LASER-INDUCED STROMAL SCARRING

To date, histologic methods of evaluating laser-induced stromal scarring have been superior to their clinical counterparts. Talamo and associates[22] have used 0.5% DTAF to determine the extent of new collagen formation following excimer corneal wounds. They also demonstrated an inhibitory effect of steroid/mitomycin C combination on this process. Clinical methods of evaluating the haze are mostly subjective in nature. Corneal haze is most commonly graded subjectively as defined by Seiler, Fantes, and colleagues[7]: 0.5, trace haze seen with careful oblique illumination with slit lamp biomicroscopy; 1+, more prominent haze that does not interfere with visibility of fine iris details; 2+, mild obscur-

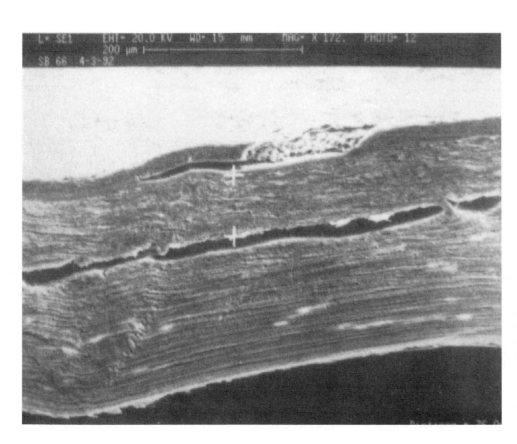

Figure 4–18. Scanning electron micrograph of the periphery of an intrastromal ablation inside a human donor cornea. The pulse energy was set at 140 μJ. Bar = 200 μm. *(From Niemz et al. Intrastromal ablations for refractive corneal surgery using picosecond infrared laser pulses.* Lasers Light Ophthalmol. *1993;5:149–155.)*

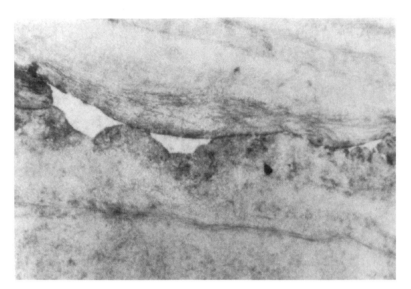

Figure 4–19. Transmission electron micrograph of an intrastromal ablation inside a human cornea. The pulse energy was set at 100 μJ. Fixation took place 1 hour after laser exposure. The beginning of the collapse of the cavity can be seen. The two vacuoles which have not yet collapsed measure about 20 μm. *(From Niemz et al. Intrastromal ablations for refractive corneal surgery using picosecond infrared laser pulses. Lasers Light Ophthalmol. 1993;5:149–155.)*

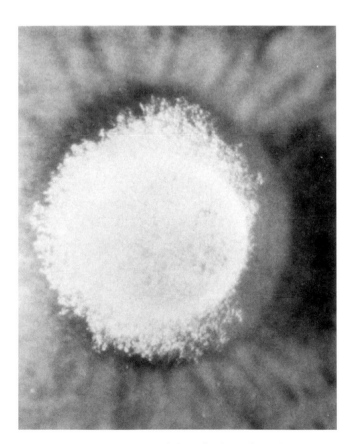

Figure 4–20. Slit lamp photograph immediately postlaser (infrared picosecond Nd : YLF at 1053 nm) application. *(From Remmel et al. Intrastromal tissue removal using an infrared picosecond Nd : YLF ophthalmic laser operating at 1053 nm. Lasers Light Ophthalmol. 1992;4:169–173.)*

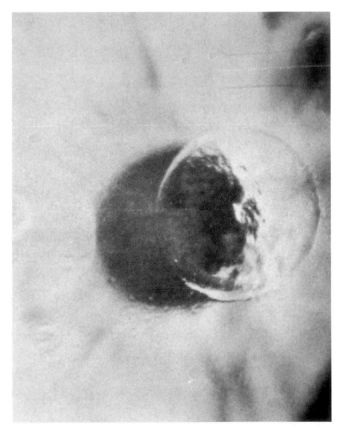

Figure 4–21. Slit lamp photograph 6 hours postlaser (infrared picosecond Nd : YLF at 1053 nm) application. *(From Remmel et al. Intrastromal tissue removal using an infrared picosecond Nd : YLF ophthalmic laser operating at 1053 nm. Lasers Light Ophthalmol. 1992;4:169–173.)*

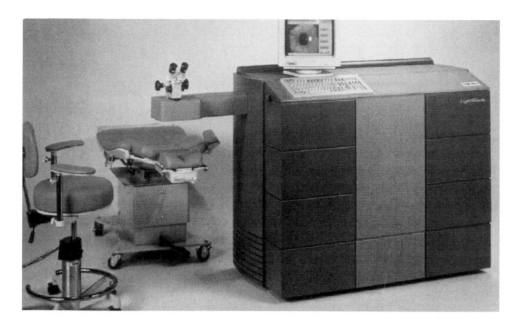

Figure 4–22. Novatec Lightblade solid-state laser system. *(From Swinger CA, Lai ST. Solid-state Photobalative Decomposition—The Novatec Laser. St. Louis: Mosby-Year Book; 1995;261–267.)*

ation of iris details; 3+, moderate obscuration of the iris and lens; and 4+, completely opaque stroma in the area of ablation. Slit lamp photographs may add an element of objectivity, but the haze can be easily exaggerated or eliminated depending on the method of photography.

We have evaluated two new clinical methods of objective measurement of corneal haze. The first method employs a scatterometer (developed at the Johns Hopkins University Applied Physics Laboratory) to measure back-scattered light from a defined region of the corneas under standardized illumination conditions.[90] Briefly, a fiberoptic probe is located at the image plane of the objective lens of a slit lamp. The incident beam (of standardized width) is adjusted to fall at a specified angle (usually 60°) to the surface normal of the cornea at the region of interest. The cornea is viewed and scattered light is collected in the direction of surface normal. Light scattered by the cornea is compared with that scattered from a standard scatterer to standardize the measurements.

This instrument has been tested on rabbits, rats, and humans and found to yield reproducible results.[91] Longitudinal studies on rabbit eyes treated with excimer laser keratectomy shows this method to be sensitive in detecting stromal light scattering over a 1- to 8-week time period following excimer ablations. The data from these experiment show that maximal scatter occurred at, or shortly before, day 18 after excimer laser ablation. In addition, studies comparing corneal haze after LASIK and PRK using the scatterometer have shown significant reduction of corneal light scattering after LASIK[80,92] (Figure 4-25).

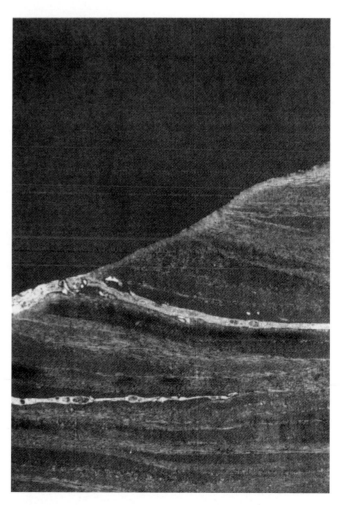

Figure 4–23. Scanning electron micrograph (×30) of the corneal surface of a human eye bank eye following 6 D myopic PRK. *(From Swinger CA, Lai ST. Solid-State Photoablative Decomposition—The Novatec Laser. St. Louis: Mosby-Year Book; 1995;261–267.)*

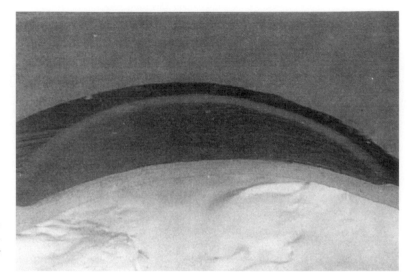

Figure 4–24. Transmission electron micrograph (×10,500) of the anterior cornea of an eye bank eye following 6 D myopic PRK. *(From Swinger CA, Lai ST. Solid-State Photoablative Decomposition—the Novatec Laser. St. Louis: Mosby-Year Book; 1995;261–267.)*

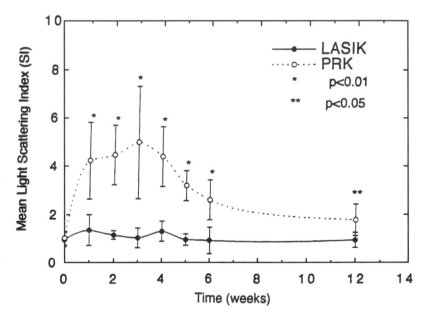

Figure 4–25. Line graphs display the mean light-scattering index as a function of time in rabbit corneas after laser in situ keratomileusis and photorefractive keratectomy. The laser in situ keratomileusis group (closed circles, solid line) has significantly lower mean light-scattering than the photorefractive keratectomy group (open circles, dotted line). Vertical bars represent ±1 S.D. *(From Jain S, Khoury, JM, Chamon W, Azar DT. Corneal light scattering after laser in situ keratomileusis and photorefractive keratectomy. Am J Ophthalmol. 1995;120(4): 532–4.)*

The second method employs high-frequency ultrasound developed at Cornell University Medical College.[93] The results of studies using this method following excimer keratectomy in rabbits showed irregularly distributed echo hyperreflectivity that decreased over 10 weeks. Histopathologic examination showed good correlation between the imaging pattern and increased keratocyte activity. This noninvasive method was also adequate at providing quantitative grading of the excimer-induced stromal scarring.

REFERENCES

1. Marshall J, Trokel S, Rothery S, Schubert H. An ultrastructural study of corneal incisions induced by an excimer laser at 193 nm. *Ophthalmology.* 1985;92:749–758.
2. Kruger RR, Trokel SL, Shubert HD. Interaction of ultraviolet light with the cornea. *Invest Ophthalmol Vis Sci.* 1985;26(suppl):1455–1464.
3. Marshall J, Trokel SL, Rothery S., et al. Long-term healing of the central cornea after photorefractive keratectomy using an excimer laser. *Ophthalmology.* 1988;95: 1411–1421.

4. Seiler T, Kahle G, Kriegerowski M. Excimer laser myopic keratomileusis in sighted and blind human eyes. *Refract Corneal Surg.* 1990;6:165–173.

5. Malley DS, Steinert RF, Pulifito CA, et al. Immunofluorescence study of corneal wound healing after excimer laser anterior keratectomy in the monkey eye. *Arch Ophthalmol.* 1990;108:1316–1322.

6. Kommehl EW, Steinert RF, Puliafito CA, Reidy W. Morphology of an irregular corneal surface following 193 nm ArF excimer laser large area ablation with 0.3% hydroxypropyl methylcellulose 2910 and 0.1% dextran 70, 1% carboxymethyl cellulose sodium or 0.9% saline. *Invest Ophthalmol Vis Sci.* 1990;31:245.

7. Seiler T, Fantes T, Waring GO, Hanna KD. Laser corneal surgery. In: Waring GO III, ed. *Refractive Keratotomy.* St. Louis: Mosby-Year Book; 1992;669–745.

8. Marshall J, Trokel SL, Rothery S, et al. Photoablative reprofiling of the cornea using an excimer laser: photorefractive keratectomy. *Lasers Ophthalmol.* 1986;7:21–48.

9. Goodman GL, Trokel SL, Stark WJ, et al. Corneal healing following laser refractive keratectomy. *Arch Ophthalmol.* 1989;107:1799–1803.

10. Hamilton W, Wood TO. Inlay lamellar keratoplasty. In: Kaufman HE, Barron BA, McDonald MB, et al, eds. *The Cornea.* New York: Churchill-Livingstone; 1988;683–696.

11. McDonald MB, Frantz JM, Klyce SD, et al. Central photorefractive keratectomy for myopia: the blind eye study. *Arch Ophthalmol.* 1990;108:799–808.

12. McDonald T, Borgmann A, Roberts M, et al. Corneal wound healing: I. Inhibition of stromal healing by three dexamethasone derivatives. *Invest Ophthalmol Vis Sci.* 1970;9:703.

13. Munnerlyn CR, Koons SJ, Marshall J. Photorefractive keratectomy: a technique for laser refractive surgery. *J Cataract Refract Surg.* 1988;14:46–52.

14. Trokel SL, Srinivasan R, Barron B. Excimer laser surgery of the cornea. *Am J Ophthalmol.* 1983;96:710–715.

15. Puliafito CA, Steinert RF, Deutch TF, et al. Excimer laser ablation of the cornea and lens; experimental studies. *Ophthalmology.* 1985;92:741–748.

16. Hanna KD, Pouliquen Y, Waring GO, et al. Corneal stromal healing in rabbits after 193 nm excimer laser surface ablation. *Arch Ophthalmol.* 1989;107:895–901.

17. Waring GO. Development of a system for excimer corneal surgery. *Trans Am Ophthalmol Soc.* 1989;87:854–983.

18. McDonald MB, Feantz JM, Klyce SD, et al. One year refractive results of central photorefractive keratectomy in nonhuman primate cornea. *Arch Ophthalmol.* 1990;108:40–47.

19. Stark WJ, Gilbert ML, Goodman GL, et al. Phototherapeutic keratectomy preliminary report. *Invest Ophthalmol Vis Sci.* 1990;31(suppl):243.

20. Stark WJ, Chamon W, Kamp MT, Enger CL, Rencs EV, Gottsh JD. Clinical follow-up of 193-nm ArF excimer laser photokeratectomy. *Ophthalmology.* 1992;99:805–812.

21. Hahn TW, Sah WJ, Kim JH. Phototherapeutic keratectomy in nine eyes with superficial corneal diseases. *Refract Corneal Surg.* 1993;2(suppl):S115–S118.

22. Talamo JH, Gollamudi S, Green WR, De La Cruz Z, Filatov V, Stark WJ. Modulation of corneal wound healing after excimer laser keratomileusis using topical mitomycin C and steroids. *Arch Ophthalmol.* 1991;109:11141–11146.

23. Tuft SJ, Zabel RW, Marshall J. Corneal repair following keratectomy in the rabbit. *Invest Ophthalmol Vis Sci.* 1989;20:1769–1777.

24. Gartry DS, Kerr Muir MG, Lohmann CP, Marshall J. The effect of topical corticosteroids on refractive outcome and corneal haze after photorefractive keratectomy. *Arch Ophthalmol.* 1992;110:944–952.

25. Shah M, Foreman DM, Ferguson MWJ. Control of scarring in adult wounds by neutralising antibody to transforming growth factor b. *Lancet.* 1992;339:213–214.

26. Huang SS, O'Grady P, Huang JS. Human transforming growth factor b-a2 macroglobulin complex is a latent form of TGF-b. *J Biol Chem.* 1988;263:1525–1541.

27. Marshall J, Trokel SL, Rothery S. Photoablative reprofiling of the cornea using an excimer laser. *Br J Ophthalmol.* 1986;70:482–501.

28. DelPero RA, Gistad JE, Roberts AD, et al. A refractive and histopathological study of excimer laser keratectomy in primates. *Am J Ophthalmol.* 1990;109:419–429.

29. Talamo JH, Steinert RF, Puliafito CA. Update on laser corneal surgery. *Int Ophthalmol Clin.* 1990;31:13–23.

30. Tayor DM, L'Esperance FA, DelPero RA, et al. Human lamellar excimer keratectomy: a clinical study. *Ophthalmology.* 1989;96:654–664.

31. L'Esperance FA, Taylor DM, DelPero RA, et al. Human excimer laser corneal surgery: preliminary report. *Trans Am Ophthalmol Soc.* 1988;86:208–275.

32. L'Esperance FA, Warner JW, Telfair WB, et al. Excimer laser instrumentation and technique for human corneal surgery. *Arch Ophthalmol.* 1989;107:131.

33. Hanna KD, Chastang JL, Asfor L, et al. Scanning slit delivery system. *J Cataract Refract Surg.* 1988;15:390–396.

34. Gipson IK, Spurr-Michaud S, Tisdale AS, Keough M. Reassembly of the anchoring structures of the corneal epithelium during wound repair in the rabbit. *Invest Ophthalmol Vis Sci.* 1989;30:425–434.

35. Gipson IK, Spurr-Michaud S, Tisdale AS, Zieske JD. Dynamics of hemidesmosome and focal contact formation during corneal epithelial wound healing. *Invest Ophthalmol Vis Sci.* 1989;30(ARVO suppl):383.

36. Gipson IK. The epithelial basement membrane zone of the limbus. *Eye.* 1989;3:132–140.

37. Gipson IK, Spurr-Michaud SJ, Tisdale AS. Hemidesmosomes and anchoring fibril collagen appear synchronously during development and wound healing. *Dev Biol.* 1988;126:253–262.

38. Gipson IK, Spurr-Michaud SJ, Tisdale AS. Anchoring fibrils form a complex network in human and rabbit cornea. *Invest Ophthalmol Vis Sci.* 1987;28:212–220.

39. Anhalt GJ, Jampel HD, Patel HP, Diaz LA, Jabs DA, Mutasim DF. Bullous pemphigold autoantibodies are markers of corneal epithelial hemidesmosomes. *Invest Ophthalmol Vis Sci.* 1987;28:903–907.

40. Tisdale AS, Spurr-Michaud SJ, Rodriques M, Hackett J, Krachmer J, Gipson IK. Development of the anchoring structures of the epithelium in rabbit and human fetal corneas. *Invest Ophthalmol Vis Sci.* 1988;29:727–736.

41. Azar DT, Spurr-Michaud SJ, Tisdale AS, Moore MB, Gipson IK. Reassembly of the corneal epithelial adhesion structures following human epikeratoplasty. *Arch Ophthalmol.* 1991;109:1250–1255.

42. Azar DT, Gipson IK. Repair of the epithelial adhesion structures following keratectomy wounds in diabetic rabbits. *Acta Ophthalmol.* 1989;67(suppl)102:72–79.

43. Azar DT, Gipson IK. Repair of the epithelial basement membrane adhesion complex of the corneal epithelium following keratectomy wounds in diabetic rabbits. *Invest Ophthalmol Vis Sci.* 1987;28(suppl):53.

44. Azar DT, Spurr-Michaud SJ, Tisdale AS, Gipson IK. Decreased penetration of anchoring fibrils into the diabetic stroma: a morphometric analysis. *Arch Ophthalmol.* 1989; 107:1520–1523.

45. Azar DT, Tisdale AS, Spurr-Michaud SJ, Gipson IK. Altered epithelial-basement membrane interactions in diabetic corneas. *Arch Ophthalmol.* 1992;110:537–540.

46. Matsubara M, Zieske JD, Fini ME. Mechanisms of basement membrane dissolution preceding corneal ulceration. *Invest Ophthalmol Vis Sci.* 1988;29:727–736.

47. Zieske JD, Bukusoglu G, Gipson IK. Enhancement of vinculin synthesis by migrating stratified squamous epithelium. *J Cell Biol.* 1989;109:571–576.

48. Hanna KD, Pouliquen YM, Savoldelli M, et al. Corneal wound healing in monkeys 18 months after excimer laser photorefractive keratectomy. *Refract Corneal Surg.* 1990;6: 340–345.

49. Foutain TR, Azar DT, De la Cruz F, Green WR, Stark WJ. Reassembly of corneal epithelial adhesion structures following human excimer laser keratectomy. *Invest Ophthalmol Vis Sci.* 1992;33:(suppl):345.

50. Ahmad OF, Green R, Stark WJ, Binder PS, Anderson JA, Azar DT. Excimer laser keratectomy: morphometric analysis of epithelial basement membrane and hemidesmosome reformation. *Invest Ophthalmol Vis Sci.* 1993; 34(suppl):703.

51. Gartry DS, Kerr Muir MG, Marshall J. Excimer laser photorefractive keratectomy: 18 month follow-up. *Ophthalmology.* 1992;99:1209–1219.

52. Gartry DS, Kerr Muir MG, Lohmann CP, Marshall J. The effect of topical corticosteroids on refractive outcome and corneal haze after photorefractive keratectomy. *Arch Ophthalmol.* 1992;110:944–952.

53. Tuft SJ, Gartry DS, Rawe IM, Meek KM. Photorefractive keratectomy: implications of corneal wound healing. *British J Ophthalmol.* 1993;77:243–247.

54. Stark WJ, Chamon W, Azar DT, Kamp M. Therapeutic keratectomy: corneal opacities. In: Thompson FB, McDonnell PJ, eds. *Color Atlas/Text of Excimer Laser Surgery.*

55. Fujikawa LS, Foster CS, Gipson IK, Colvin RB. Basement membrane components in healing rabbit epithelial wounds: immunofluorescence and ultrastructural studies. *J Cell Biol.* 1984;98:128–138.

56. Fujikawa LS, Foster CS, Harris TJ, Lanigan JM, Colvin RB. Fibronectin in healing rabbit cornea wounds. *Lab Invest.* 1981;45:120–129.

57. Seiler T, Matallana M, Sendler S, Bende T. Does Bowman's layer determine the biomechanical properties of the cornea? *Refract Corneal Surg.* 1992;8:139–142.

58. Seiler T, Kriegerowski M, Schnoy N, Bende T. Ablation rate of human corneal epithelium and Bowman's layer with the excimer laser (193 nm). *Refract Corneal Surg.* 1990; 6:99–102.

59. Waring GO. *Refractive Keratotomy for Myopia and Astigmatism.* St. Louis: Mosby-Year Book; 1992;721–740.

60. Fantes FE, Hanna KD, Waring GO, et al. Wound healing after excimer laser keratomileusis (photorefractive keratectomy) in monkeys. *Arch Ophthalmol.* 1990;108: 665–675.

61. Crossen CE. Cellular changes following epithelial abrasion. In: Beuerman RW, Crossen CE, Kaufman AG, eds. *Healing Process in the Cornea.* Houston, TX: Gulf Publishing Co; 1989;314.

62. Geiss MJ, Fantes FE, SunderRaj N, et al. Healing of excimer laser ablated monkey corneas: an immunohistochemical evaluation. *Invest Ophthalmol Vis Sci.* 1989;30(suppl): 189.

63. Tuft S, Marshall J, Rothery S. Stromal remodeling following photorefractive keratectomy. *Lasers Ophthalmol.* 1987; 1:177–183.

64. Tuft S, Zabel RW, Marshall JW. Corneal repair following keratectomy: a comparison between conventional surgery and laser photoablation. *Invest Ophthalmol Vis Sci.* 1989;30: 1769–1777.

65. Azar DT, Chamon W, Stark WJ, Stetler-Stevenson W. Matrix metalloproteinase expression in laser-ablated corneas. *Invest Ophthalmol Vis Sci.* 1993;34:(suppl):704.

66. Rajpal RK, Essepian JP, Azar DT, Stark WJ. Confocal microscopy in the study of stromal scar formation post excimer laser keratectomy. *Invest Ophthalmol Vis Sci.* 1993; 34(suppl):802.

67. Azar DT, Chamon W, Green WR, Stark WJ. Time and pattern of epithelial and stromal healing following superficial concentric photorefractive keratectomies. *Invest Ophthalmol Vis Sci.* 1992;33(suppl):766.

68. Rhamsdorf HJ, Smith BJ, Lyons A, et al. Comparison of human stromelysin and collagenase by cloning and sequence analysis. *Biochem J.* 1986;240:913–916.

72. Springman EB, Angleton EL, Birkedahl-Hansen H, Van Wart HE. Multiple modes of activation of latent human fibroblast collagenase: evidence for the role of a Cys-73 active site zinc complex in latency and a cysteine switch mechanism for activation. *Proc Natl Acad Sci USA*. 1990;87: 364–368.

73. Stetler-Stevenson WG, Krutasch HC, Liotta LA. Tissue inhibitor of metalloproteinase-2 (TIMP-2). *J Biol Chem*. 1989; 264:17374–17378.

74. Goldberg GI, Marmer BL, Grant GA, Eisen AZ, Wilhelm S, He C. Human 72-kilodalton type IV collagenase forms a complex with a tissue inhibitor of metalloproteinases designated TIMP-2. *Proc Natl Acad Sci USA*. 1989;86:8207–8210.

75. Liotta LA, Stetler-Stevenson W. Metalloproteinases and malignant conversion. *J Natl Cancer Inst*. 1989;81: 556–557.

76. Stetler-Stevenson WG, Krutzsch HC, Washer MP, Marguiles IMK, Liotta LA. The activation of human type IV collagenase. *J Biol Chem*. 1989;264:1353–1356.

77. Chin JR, Murphy G, Werb Z. Stromelysin, a connective tissue-degrading metalloendopeptidase secreted by stimulated rabbit synovial fibroblasts in parallel with collagenase. *J Biol Chem*. 1989;264:1353–1356. *J Biol Chem*. 1985; 260:12367.

78. Sellers A, Reynolds JJ, Meikie MC. Neutral metalloproteinases of rabbit bone: separation in latent forms of distinct enzymes that when activated degrade collagen, gelatin and proteoglycans. *Biochem J*. 1978;171:493.

79. Dehm EJ, Puliafito CA, Adler CM, Steinert RF. Corneal endothelial injury in rabbits following excimer laser ablation at 193 and 248 nm. *Arch Ophthalmol*. 1986;104: 1364–1368.

80. Koch JW, Lang GK, Naumann GOH. Endothelial reaction to perforating and nonperforating excimer laser excisions in rabbits. *Refract Corneal Surg* (in press).

81. Zabel R, Tuft S, Marshall J. Excimer laser photorefractive keratectomy: endothelial morphology following area ablation of the cornea. *Invest Ophthalmol Vis Sci*. 1988; 29(suppl):309.

82. Krueger RR, Binder PS, McDonnell. *The Effects of Excimer Laser Photoablation on the Cornea*. St. Louis: Mosby-Year Book; 1995;11–44.

83. Ren Q, Simon G, Parel JM. Ultraviolet solid-state laser (213-nm) photorefractive keratectomy: in vitro study. *Ophthalmology*. 1993;100:1828–1834.

84. Hu X, Juhasz T. Corneal ablation with picosecond laser pulses at 211 and 263 nanometers. In: Parel JM, ed. *Ophthalmic Technologies IIII*. Bellingham, WA: SPIE; 1994.

85. Rowsey JJ, Stevens SX, Fouraker BD, et al. *Alternative Lasers and Strategies for Corneal Modification*. St. Louis: Mosby-Year Book; 1995;269–276.

86. Niemz MH, Hoppeler TP, Juhasz T, et al. Intrastromal ablations for refractive corneal surgery using picosecond infrared laser pulses. *Lasers Light Ophthalmol*. 1993;5:149–155.

87. Remmel RM, Dardenne CM, Bille JF. Intrastromal tissue removal using an infrared picosecond Nd : YLF ophthalmic laser operating at 1053 nm. *Lasers Light Ophthalmol*. 1992;4:169–173.

88. Freuh BE, Bille JF, Brown SI. Intrastromal relaxing excisions in rabbits with a picosecond infrared laser. *Lasers Light Ophthalmol*. 1992;4:165–168.

89. Swinger CA, Lai ST. *Solid-State Photoablative Decomposition—The Novatec Laser*. St. Louis: Mosby-Year Book; 1995; 261–267.

90. McCally RL, Hochheimer BF, Chamon W, Azar DT. Objective measurement of haze following excimer laser ablation of the cornea. *Invest Ophthalmol Vis Sci*. 1993; 34(suppl):802.

91. McCally RL, Hochheimer BF, Chamon W, Azar DT. *Simple Device for Objective Measurement of Haze Following Excimer Laser Ablation of the Cornea*. Bellingham WA: SPIE; 1993.

92. Alleman N, Coleman DJ, Chamon W, Azar DT, Stark WJ. High resolution ultrasonographic correlation of corneal haze following excimer laser keratectomy. *Invest Ophthalmol Vis Sci*. 1993;34(suppl):802.

CHAPTER 5

Pharmacologic Modulation of Wound Healing After Keratorefractive Surgery

Sandeep Jain ■ Dimitri T. Azar

Corneal injury evokes an immediate molecular and cellular inflammatory response followed by wound healing. Corneal wound healing involves a complex and well-regulated sequence of events characterized by activation, proliferation, and directed migration of corneal cells toward the wound, and synthesis and subsequent remodeling of the extracellular matrix (ECM). Serine proteases degrade and remodel the ECM. Growth factors (cytokines) coordinate the healing processes.[1] The corneal inflammatory and wound-healing processes are closely intertwined and constitute a mechanism by which corneal defects heal. Following keratorefractive surgery in some patients, these processes may cause unpredictable regression of intended refractive correction and corneal haze. Pharmacologic modulation of the corneal inflammatory and wound-healing response may reduce the adverse effects associated with keratorefractive surgery.

An immediate inflammatory response follows corneal injury, in which arachidonic acid is released through the action of activated phospholipases on cell membrane phospholipids and metabolized to produce prostaglandins (via cyclooxygenase pathway), leukotrienes (via lipoxygenase pathway), and 12(R)-hydroxyeicosatetraenoic (HETE) acid (via cytochrome P-450 monooxygenase pathway).[2,3] Platelet-activating factor (PAF) is another potent inflammatory mediator that is synthesized by the action of phospholipase on membrane phospholipids.[4] The role of arachidonic acid metabolites and PAF as mediators of corneal inflammatory response is well documented. Prostaglandins increase the amount of cyclic adenosine monophosphate and ionic calcium at the nociceptor membrane and decrease the activation threshold. This results in increased central nervous system pain perception. Leukotrienes, HETE acid, and PAF are chemotactic for polymorphonuclear leukocytes. The accumulation of leukocytes is an important feature of the inflammatory reaction. Leukocytes engulf and degrade the debris of necrotic cells and contribute to a tissue defensive response, but they also release enzymes, chemical mediators, and toxic radicals that may prolong inflammation and increase the tissue damage. Keratocytes are differentiated mesenchymal cells that produce both the collagen and ECM macromolecules as well as the enzymes responsible for their remodeling and degradation. Keratocytes form the backbone of the corneal wound-healing response that follows the inflammatory response.

CORTICOSTEROIDS

Corticosteroids inhibit both the inflammatory and the subsequent healing process precipitated by corneal injury. The mechanism of action of corticosteroids has not been fully elucidated, but it has been suggested that steroids interfere with DNA synthesis in keratocytes, producing diminished cellular activity and reduced collagen synthesis. In addition, they inhibit the arachidonic acid cascade by inhibiting phospholipase A2. The mechanism of reversal of regression and improvement in haze following reintroduction of steroid treatment is unclear. An effect on stromal hydration via hyaluronic acid (high molecular weight disaccharide polymer with the capacity to bind large amounts of water) has been postulated. The use of topical steroids after photorefractive keratectomy (PRK) is controversial. Most PRK clinical trials have used corticosteroids postoperatively; however, their study frameworks were not designed to evaluate the therapeutic efficacy of steroids. Potent steroids like dexamethasone and betamethasone have been used under some protocols, while weaker steroids like fluorometholone have been preferred in others. In some studies potent steroids were used for the first postoperative month and then replaced by weaker steroids. The duration of postoperative steroid treatment varied from 5 weeks to 7 months.

There are very few controlled studies in the published literature that have evaluated the efficacy of steroids after excimer keratectomy. In a prospective, double-blind clinical trial conducted by Gartry et al,[5,6] the mean change in refraction following excimer PRK was significantly greater in the steroid-treated group compared with the placebo-treated group at 6 weeks; however, there was no statistically significant difference after the steroids were discontinued. No statistically significant difference in corneal haze was found between the steroid- and placebo-treated groups at any stage. In a prospective, randomized, observer-masked study, O'Brart[7] et al noted a hyperopic shift in the first few weeks after excimer PRK, which regressed toward emmetropia within the first 3 months. Corticosteroid administration caused a greater change in refraction and maintained the hyperopic shift, but the effect was reversed on cessation of treatment. No statistically significant difference in haze between the steroid- and placebo-treated groups was found at any stage. The authors found no justification in routinely administering corticosteroids after excimer PRK. Based on the similarity in clinical outcome following administration of steroids of different potency to identical twins in a double-

blind study, Machat[8] concluded that the need for full-strength topical steroids postoperatively remains questionable (at least for low myopia). These studies suggest a limited role for corticosteroid administration after excimer laser surgery. The role of corticosteroids following radial keratotomy is somewhat better defined. Several studies have shown that corticosteroids do not improve the refractive outcome and do not afford protection against the endothelial cell loss after radial keratotomy.[9,10] Postoperative steroids are not routinely prescribed following radial keratotomy.

In contrast to the above-mentioned studies, in a prospective clinical trial, Fagerholm et al[11] found that only 23% of steroid-treated eyes regressed to myopia of 0.50 diopter at 6 months after PRK, compared with 86% of the steroid-untreated eyes. Corticosteroid administration caused a greater change in refraction and maintained the hyperopic shift. (Steroid-treated eyes had mean refraction in the low hyperopia range.) Subepithelial haze was less in steroid-treated eyes. Fitzsimmons et al[12] found significant refractive and topographical changes following reinstitution of steroids in patients (especially higher myopes) with myopic regression after PRK. The authors favored postponing retreatments in patients with such a response to corticosteroids. Orssaud et al[13] observed early (1 to 3 months postoperatively) and marked (−1.0 to −2.0 D) regressions and significant corneal haze in 22% of eyes in which steroids were not used postoperatively, whereas none of the eyes on a postoperative steroid regimen developed similar regressions or haze. The regression and haze reversed on institution of an intensive steroid regimen. This study highlights the importance of topical steroids, at least in some eyes. Campos et al[14] found significantly less polymorphonuclear leukocytes in the corneal stroma in the steroid-treated rabbit corneas compared with untreated corneas 24 hours after PRK. David et al[15] have reported a reduction in the amount of scar tissue after PRK in rabbit corneas treated with 1% prednisolone acetate. All of these laboratory and clinical studies suggest a beneficial role of corticosteroid administration after excimer laser surgery.

The use of corticosteroids after keratorefractive surgery remains a controversial issue. However, the balance of evidence favors a steroid regimen in which initial intensive therapy is followed by titration of the dosage, and duration of therapy depends on the postoperative effect. In patients with an uneventful postoperative course, steroids are tapered over a period of 3 to 5 months postoperatively. Steroid treatment is restarted or the dosage increased in the event of myopic regression or clinically significant corneal haze. Currently 0.1% fluoromethanolone appears to be the preferred steroid. Potential complications of long-term steroid treatment include increased susceptibility to infections, raised intraocular pressure, reactivation of herpes simplex, cataract formation, and reduced wound strength. The percentage of eyes with raised intraocular pressure ranges from 7% to 23% in different studies. The pressure returns to normal by reducing or discontinuing steroids; in some eyes, however, topical beta-blocker and/or oral carbonic anhydrase inhibitor may be required.

ANTI-INFLAMMATORY DRUGS

Nonsteroidal Anti-inflammatory Drugs (NSAIDs)

Anti-inflammatory drugs can influence the complex interrelation between the molecular and cellular inflammatory mechanism by inhibiting the arachidonic acid metabolism cascade. Nonsteroidal anti-inflammatory drugs (indomethacin, flurbiprofen, diclofenac) inhibit the cyclooxygenase pathway. Diclofenac, in addition, reduces the intracellular levels of free arachidonic acid by enhancing its uptake into the triglyceride pool, thereby inhibiting the lipoxygenase pathway. Phillips et al[2] have demonstrated a sudden and sustained rise in prostaglandin E2 (PGE2) levels, no significant change in leukotrine B4 levels, and significant polymorphonuclear leukocyte infiltration of stroma following excimer laser PRK in rabbit corneas. Diclofenac significantly reduces PGE2 levels but increases leukocyte infiltration in the postexcimer laser-ablated rabbit corneas.

Following excimer laser PRK, patients experience significant ocular pain until corneal re-epithelialization. Despite the use of cold compresses, bandage soft contact lenses, cycloplegics, narcotics, and topical corticosteroids, the pain is not adequately controlled in many patients. Sher et al[16] conducted a randomized, double-masked, parallel-group study of diclofenac sodium 0.1% ophthalmic solution and its placebo vehicle in patients undergoing PRK. Diclofenac was applied topically immediately after surgery and then four times daily until re-epithelialization. Most patients who received placebo experienced pain, starting within 1 hour, peaking at 4 to 6 hours, and lasting from 36 to 48 hours. The diclofenac-treated patients rarely experienced the early peak in pain, had less pain overall until 72 hours postoperatively, and experienced significantly less photophobia and burning or stinging. Significantly

fewer patients on diclofenac required oral narcotics. Postoperative topical use of 0.1% diclofenac (Voltaren Ophthalmic, CIBA Vision Ophthalmics, Atlanta, GA) prior to re-epithelialization may be helpful for the treatment of pain following excimer laser keratectomy. Preoperative treatment does not seem to potentiate the therapeutic effect of postoperative diclofenac therapy.[17] In a retrospective analysis of patients who had undergone PRK, Eiferman et al have reported lower pain scores in 70% of diclofenac-treated eyes.[18]

Loya et al have demonstrated that administration of 0.1% diclofenac qid until wound closure does not delay corneal re-epithelialization following excimer keratectomy.[19] Salz et al[20] have reported two patients who sustained corneal abrasions from blunt trauma to the eye and orbit following PRK. In both patients, the corneal abrasions healed without incident and without recurrent erosions when they were given soft contact lens and treated with diclofenac. Sher et al[16] have also reported no differences in epithelial healing rates between the diclofenac-treated eyes and those not receiving the drug. Following PRK corneal sensitivity decreases to 20% of normal by the second postoperative day, and returns to normal during the first postoperative week. Instillation of diclofenac after PRK does not cause significant long-term reduction of corneal sensitivity and does not delay the recovery of sensitivity.[20] Diclofenac, however, substantially lowers sensitivity in normal corneas.[21]

Nassaralla et al found a significant reduction in corneal haze in rabbits treated with 1% diclofenac for 2 months after −5 diopter PRK.[22] Combination treatment with diclofenac and fluorometholone did not result in a further decrease in haze. Ferrari et al also found the corneal haze and refractive stability to be similar in diclofenac-treated and corticosteroid-treated eyes after PRK for moderate to high myopia.[23]

Other nonsteroidal anti-inflammatory drugs like indomethacin, ketorolac, and flurbiprofen can also be used as topical analgesics. Arshinoff et al reported that pain reduction following treatment with 0.5% ketorolac tromethamine (Acular®, Allergan) in patients undergoing PRK was as effective as with 1% diclofenac sodium.[24] In a multicenter, randomized, double-masked, parallel-group clinical trial, Gwon et al evaluated the local analgesic effect of topically applied 0.03% flurbiprofen sodium in patients undergoing elective unilateral radial keratotomy.[25] Their study suggests that topical 0.03% flurbiprofen safely and effectively relieves ocular pain without affecting corneal sensation in patients undergoing radial keratotomy. David et al have reported a slight reduction in the amount of scar tissue after PRK in rabbit corneas treated with 0.03% flurbiprofen.[15] Arshinoff et al report that flurbiprofen sodium, when administered with topical steroids, significantly reduced post-PRK myopic regression.[24] Diclofenac, used with topical steroids, had much less effect on myopic regression than flurbiprofen. Stoltz et al provide evidence for NADPH-dependent cytochrome P-450 mediated metabolism of arachidonic acid in the corneal epithelium.[3] Flurbiprofen may inhibit both this pathway and the cyclooxygenase and lipoxygenase pathway, thus offering potential advantages over diclofenac.

Platelet-Activating Factor Antagonists

Platelet-activating factor (PAF) antagonists have the potential of inhibiting the corneal inflammatory response.[26,27] Recently PAF has been shown to increase the production of corneal collagenases (MMP-1 and MMP-9).[29] In concert with matrix metalloproteinases, PAF may have a role in the initial ECM breakdown and subsequent remodeling during corneal wound healing. Cohen et al have investigated the role of PAF in corneal transplantation and reported that corneal inflammation, cellular infiltration, vascularization, and edema was inhibited by the PAF antagonist BN-52021.[28] The PAF antagonist BN-50730 blocks the PAF-induced increase in collagenase type I mRNA.[29] Other PAF antagonists include *Ginkgo biloba* derivatives like Egb 761. The use of PAF antagonists after excimer laser surgery has not been evaluated.

ANTIFIBROTIC AGENTS

Fibroblast migration into the area of the wound produces the extracellular structural components of the stromal scar tissue under the area of corneal ablation. Antifibrotic agents inhibit fibroblast function, and thus have the potential of reducing the corneal scarring following excimer keratectomy.

Mitomycins are a group of antitumor antibiotics that covalently bind to DNA upon reductive activation. Mitomycin-C, isolated from *Streptomyces caespitosus*, is a clinically useful member of this group. After intracellular enzymatic reduction it becomes an alkylating agent. Cross-linking of DNA is the major lesion in its cytodestructive action. It inhibits fibroblast function by a dose-dependent inhibition of fibroblast proliferation.[30]

It has the potential of minimizing stromal scar formation following excimer keratectomy by inhibiting fibroblast proliferation. Talamo and colleagues have reported inhibition of subepithelial collagen synthesis in an additive fashion following topical therapy with mitomycin-C drops in conjunction with steroid drops for 14 days following excimer laser keratectomy.[31] Connolly et al have reported significant reduction of corneal light scattering after a single intraoperative annular application of 0.5 mg/ml mitomycin-C in rabbit corneas following excimer keratectomy.[32] The major limitation to the use of mitomycin-C when administered as eyedrops in the postoperative period is the epithelial toxicity that may result in persistent epithelial defects. The local side effects of postoperative topical therapy with mitomycin-C drops include superficial punctate keratopathy, recurrent corneal epithelial defects, crystalline keratopathy, iridocyclitis, and scleral melting.[33,34] Idiosyncratic reactions resulting in serious vision-threatening complications have been reported following administration of a relatively large cumulative dose of mitomycin-C.[35] The potential corneal toxicity is cumulative dose related, which limits the use of mitomycin-C drops for prolonged periods in the postoperative period. In order to minimize these complications, the lowest possible therapeutic concentration should be applied for the shortest effective time period, ensuring minimal corneal contact, particularly when epithelial defects are present.[36] Pery-Frucht et al have reported the use of short-term, low-dose, topical mitomycin-C (0.1 mg/ml twice daily for 5 days) to be an efficient and relatively safe treatment regimen.[37] Chew et al have reported minimal reduction of keratocyte density in the posterior corneal stromal layers after three topical applications of 0.4 mg/ml mitomycin-C.[38] The potential toxicity limits the role of mitomycin-C drops following excimer laser surgery.

5-Fluorouracil is a pyrimidine analog that blocks the enzyme thymidylase synthetase and ultimately inhibits both RNA and DNA synthesis, leading to cell death. Bergman et al found a significantly reduced corneal haze in the 5-fluorouracil treated eyes compared with the untreated controls following excimer PRK; however, the benefit was only transient, as controls cleared to an equivalent haze by 6 weeks.[39] As with mitomycin-C, the potential corneal toxicity limits the role of 5-fluorouracil following excimer keratectomy.

Interferons are a heterogeneous group of proteins produced by the body in response to an antigenic challenge. They can be synthesized using recombinant DNA techniques for clinical use. Interferons can inhibit many aspects of the fibrotic response, such as fibroblast chemotaxis and proliferation and collagen production. Morlet et al have reported a significant reduction of haze in rabbit corneas treated with interferon–α 2 β after PRK and an additive effect when combined with postoperative topical steroids.[40] Mild conjunctival hyperemia was the only side effect noticed.

ANTICOLLAGEN AGENTS

Pharmacologic agents that inhibit cross-linking of collagen enhance the flexibility of scar tissue. Collagen cross-linking is mediated by the copper-dependent enzyme lysyl oxidase. Beta-aminopropionitrile inhibits lysyl oxidase. Moorhead et al have reported that topical application of beta-aminopropionitrile enhances the central corneal flattening by approximately 1.0 D and reduces the refractive regression after radial keratotomy.[41] Treatment with beta-aminopropionitrile enhances the compliance of the peripheral cornea without adversely effecting its structural integrity. Anticollagen agents have not been used after excimer laser surgery.

SERINE PROTEINASES

Corneal Collagenases

To preserve the unique structural and functional properties of the cornea, each of its collagens (types I, II, III, IV, and VII) must be maintained by degradative removal of damaged molecules and replacement with new.[12] Collagen replacement in the wounded cornea is a progressive process of synthesis, degradation, and resynthesis, a process that has been termed *remodeling*. The collagen-degrading enzymes share a common requirement of a metal cofactor for their degradative action, prompting their designation as matrix metalloproteinases (MMPs). Metalloproteinases are divided into three major subclasses: interstitial collagenases, stromelysins, and gelatinases. Interstitial collagenase cleaves native collagens types I, II, and III.[43,44] Stromelysins cleave proteoglycans and are active against laminin, fibronectin, type IV collagen, and a number of globular proteins. Gelatinases are active against denatured interstitial collagens, laminin, fibronectin, and types IV, V, and VII collagens. They include the 72-kDa (MMP-2) and 92-kDa (MMP-9) forms. Azar et al observed gelatinolytic activity of 72-kDa and 92-kDa bands in the migrating epithelium of excimer-ablated

corneas, but not in that of corneas undergoing debridement wounds or in untreated controls.[45] Excimer-treated stromas showed 92-kDa gelatinolytic activity, which was not present in controls. Their results suggest that after excimer ablation 92-kDa type IV collagenase (MMP-9) is expressed in the corneal epithelium and stroma during wound closure, and that the activity of 72-kDa type IV collagenase (MMP-2), present in the stroma prior to wounding, persists after excimer wounding. These proteolytic enzymes may play a role in wound healing and stromal remodeling in the normal cornea, and in scar formation and clearing following excimer wounds. Inhibitors of matrix metalloproteinases like β-mercaptomethyl tripeptide (Peptides International, Louisville, KY) and GM6001 (Galardin®, Glycomed Inc, Alameda, CA) have the potential of modulating corneal wound healing following excimer keratectomy. Although these agents hold promise, their use remains investigational. Currently, none of these agents is used in routine clinical practice.

Plasminogen Activator/Plasmin System

Excimer keratectomy causes minimal damage to tissues adjoining the ablated area; however, the damage may be sufficient to activate the biochemical cascades, leading to the release of inflammatory mediators and proteolytic enzymes into the adjacent tissues.[46] Release of proteolytic enzymes may increase the extent of tissue damage. Plasmin is a normal proteolytic enzyme of the tear fluid. The precursor plasminogen is activated intracellularly by plasminogen activators to become active plasmin. Plasmin activates other enzymes like procollagenase and macrophage elastase and degrades many matrix proteins like fibronectin and laminin. Minimizing tissue degradation by the plasminogen activator/plasmin system may facilitate epithelialization and limit the stromal damage. The concentration of plasmin in the tear fluid of normal, healthy, untreated eyes is very low (< 0.2 μg/ml tear fluid). Lohmann et al have reported higher concentrations of plasmin in tear fluid of all patients following excimer laser PRK.[46] Patients who regressed more than 1.0 D after excimer laser surgery had higher preoperative plasmin levels. This may indicate that high preoperative levels of plasmin may be associated with aggressive wound healers. In their animal studies, Lohmann et al found a strong immunoreactivity for plasminogen activators in the epithelium overlying the excimer-ablated area and a weak staining in the anterior stroma 3 days to 3 months postoperatively. In contrast, Tervo et al found a statistically significant decrease in tear fluid plasmin activity during the first and second postoperative days after PRK.[47] Significant elevation of both tear fluid flow and plasmin flux values occurred during the first 2 postoperative days; however, the proteolytic activity due to plasmin actually decreases because of the acceleration of tear fluid flow.

Aprotinin is a polypeptide that inhibits plasmin. O'Brart et al have reported no beneficial effect on the refractive outcome and visual performance, and a higher degree of corneal haze in patients treated with low-dose topical aprotinin (40 IU/ml) after excimer laser keratectomy.[48] Studies using a combination of aprotinin and corticosteroids after PRK are under way.

GROWTH FACTORS

Growth factors are elements of a complex biologic signaling language that provides the basis for intercellular communication.[1] They are potent peptide regulatory factors that coordinate the proliferation, migration, and differentiation of cells, and control the synthesis and remodeling of the ECM. They play a crucial role in controlling ocular morphogenesis at the cellular and molecular level.[49] In the uninjured cornea, growth factors control the balance between cell production and loss and maintain the normal differentiated architecture. In the injured cornea, they regulate and integrate the complex ocular wound-healing mechanism via both autocrine and paracrine mechanisms. A potential dynamic interaction exists among various growth factors in controlling short-term epithelial and stromal wound healing and long-term remodeling. Therapeutic use of growth factors is currently investigational; however, they have the potential of significantly contributing to ocular therapy in the future.

Epidermal Growth Factor

Epidermal growth factor (EGF) and transforming growth factor-alpha (TGF-α) are members of a family of single-chain polypeptide growth factors that bind to a transmembrane tyrosine kinase receptor to stimulate protein synthesis and cellular proliferation. EGF stimulates corneal epithelial proliferation and migration.[50] It stimulates the proliferation of stromal fibroblasts, increases collagen and fibronectin synthesis, and increases fibronectin receptor activity.[51] The EGF-induced mitogenic effect is characterized by its dose-dependent downregulation.[52] In order to prevent receptor down-

regulation during treatment, Sheardown et al have suggested the use of a controlled-release system to deliver a continuous optimal dose of EGF for a prolonged period, in preference to multiple topical eyedrops of higher concentration.[53] Recently EGF has been used to promote corneal re-epithelialization following alkali burns, epikeratoplasty, traumatic corneal ulcers, and herpetic ulcers.[54–58] It increases the tensile strength of corneal incisions.[59]

TGF-α is a member of the EGF family with approximately 40% homology to EGF, and it binds to the EGF receptor.[60] It is essential for normal ocular morphogenesis.[61] It has been localized in the human corneal epithelium.[62] Autocrine production of TGF-α may control the normal turnover of corneal epithelium. TGF-α bound to *Pseudomonas* exotoxin inhibits fibroblast proliferation and may be used as a fibrosis inhibitor.[63]

Transforming Growth Factor

Transforming growth factor-beta (TGF-β) is a multifunctional growth factor. The three known mammalian TGF-β isoforms (TGF-β 1 to 3) are homo- or heterodimers with overlapping biologic functions mediated by three distinct cell surface receptors (TGF-β receptor types I to III). Type I receptor mediates the cell matrix interactions; type II receptor functions as a transmembrane serine-threonine kinase to mediate the antiproliferative activity; and type III receptor (betaglycan) is a proteoglycan devoid of biological activity.[64–66] Betaglycan cooperates with the type II receptors on TGF-β binding and acts as a dual modulator of TGF-β access to the signaling receptors.[67] TGF-β 2 has been localized in the superficial limbal epithelial cells of the human cornea.[68] This location is consistent with its possible role in the transdifferentiation of conjunctival to corneal epithelium. It has been localized in corneal fibroblasts following epithelial wounding. In vitro studies on human corneal stromal fibroblasts reveal that TGF-β stimulates proliferation and motility of stromal fibroblasts and increases collagen and fibronectin synthesis.[69] In addition to stimulating the synthesis of extracellular matrix, TGF-β suppresses matrix degradation by collagenases. It decreases the synthesis of proteases that degrade matrix proteins (matrix metalloproteinases) and increases the synthesis of protease inhibitors that block the activity of such proteases. In addition, it increases the interaction of cells with the ECM, possibly by increasing the expression of integrin receptors. TGF-β 1 causes a dose-related inhibition of epithelial cell proliferation. By itself it does not affect cell adhesion or migration, but it inhibits the stimulatory effects of EGF, suggesting that it serves as a modulator of EGF.[70] Phillips et al have examined the TGF-β–induced initiation and pattern of corneal angiogenesis.[71,72] TGF-β stimulates angiogenesis indirectly by recruiting inflammatory cells.

Fibroblast Growth Factors

Fibroblast growth factors (FGFs) comprise a family of at least five structurally related proteins, of which acidic and basic FGFs are the prototypes. Both types of FGF affect cell proliferation and differentiation.[73] Acidic FGF has been localized in the corneal epithelium.[74] It is overexpressed during active epithelial migration.[75] Basic FGF is present mainly in the ocular basement membranes, complexed with heparan sulfate proteoglycan.[74,76] In the intact cornea, it has been localized in the epithelial cells, and only small amounts are present in the Bowman's layer.[77] Epithelial cells do not actively secrete basic FGF. Injury-related passive release of intracellular basic FGF is its predominant route of deposit in Bowman's layer.[78] Fibroblast growth factor is endowed with a pleiotropism of biologic activities, the most striking of which are related to wound healing.[79,80] FGF stimulates epithelial cell proliferation and promotes stromal wound healing, stimulating the fibroblasts to proliferate and to synthesize ECM components. Topical application of basic FGF (bFGF) has been shown to promote corneal epithelial and stromal healing without morphologically adverse reactions or intraocular and systemic penetration.[81] FGFs are highly angiogenic and may be responsible for corneal vascularization.[82]

David et al have investigated the influence of topical bFGF on both epithelial and stromal healing after excimer laser keratectomy in rabbits.[83] Basic FGF (10 μg/application) was administered four times daily until complete epithelial healing. A highly significant acceleration in epithelial wound-healing speed and lower mean subepithelial haze scores were seen after bFGF treatment. No significant difference could be seen between steroid-treated and bFGF-treated eyes.

Platelet-Derived Growth Factor

Platelet-derived growth factor (PDGF) is a dimeric molecule composed of A and/or B polypeptide chains (PDGF-AA/AB/BB). It is a major mitogen and chemoattractant. The presence of PDGF receptors in human corneal epithelium, fibroblasts, and endothelium and the mitogenic effects of PDGF on corneal cells suggest that it may play a role in corneal wound healing.[84]

ANTIOXIDANTS

Free radicals are reactive species, capable of independent existence and containing one or more unpaired electrons.[85] Free radical–mediated injury includes DNA damage, enzyme inactivation, and lipid peroxidation. They have been detected during excimer laser ablation of plastics and biologic tissues. The mechanism of free radical production after excimer corneal ablation, and their identification and characterization are currently under investigation. Recent evidence suggests that 193-nm excimer irradiation of collagen in the presence of water may fracture the peptide bonds and produce short-lived free radicals that have a high UV absorbance.[86,87] This may explain the apparent dependence of corneal ablation rate on tissue hydration, despite the transparency of water at 193-nm wavelength. Nakagawa has characterized the free radicals generated during pulsed excimer laser (308 nm) ablation of collagen using electron spin resonance spectroscopy (spin trap technique).[88,89] His findings support the view that free radicals are produced during excimer laser ablation because of specific bond breakage and fragmentation of protein chains (photodisruption) without thermal damage at the target site. Absorption of a UV component of the laser-induced fluorescence may cause photoionization and water radiolysis. Free radical–mediated cellular and extracellular injury may trigger a wound-healing response that results in the production of corneal haze.

Reactive oxygen species is a collective term that includes oxygen-containing radicals like superoxide (O_2—) and hydroxyl (OH—). Hydroxyl radicals are a fearsomely reactive species that can attack all biologic molecules. In contrast, the superoxide radical has limited chemical reactivity. Reactive oxygen species (O_2— and OH—) degrade corneal stromal macromolecules (proteoglycans and collagen) directly by scission of covalent bonds and indirectly by enhancing susceptibility to hydrolytic enzymes.[90,91] They induce collagen aggregation and cross-linking, and alter collagen–fibroblast interactions, collagen solubility, and mechanical strength.[92,93] Jain et al have reported that application of a combination of antioxidants, superoxide dismutase, and dimethyl sulfoxide significantly reduces corneal light scattering after excimer laser keratectomy in rabbit corneas.[94] The authors suggest that development of an assay to determine the preoperative free radical scavenging capacity of individuals may be useful to predict the extent of postoperative corneal haze. Currently, antioxidant use to modulate corneal wound healing remains investigational.

CORNEAL EXTRACELLULAR MATRIX MACROMOLECULES

The ECM plays an active and complex role in the regulation of cells, influencing their development, migration, proliferation, shape, and metabolic functions, in addition to providing a scaffolding that stabilizes the physical structure of the tissue. During wound healing, there is degradation and resynthesis of matrix components. Regulating the balance of synthesis and degradation of ECM is crucial for normal embryogenesis and growth, and for the repair and maintenance of proper tissue architecture.

Fibronectin

Fibronectin is an ECM protein of the corneal stroma. It mediates cellular adhesion via interaction with integrins and provides a temporary scaffold for corneal epithelial migration. In the unwounded cornea, fibronectin is found in the subepithelial region at the level of epithelial basement membrane and at the stromal side of Descemet's membrane.[95] Following excimer keratectomy, fibronectin is deposited under the ablation bed.[96,97] Although there have been reports that exogenously applied fibronectin promotes corneal re-epithelialization,[98,99] recent evidence suggests that exogenous fibronectin is not critical for wound closure.[100] Latvala et al have found cellular fibronectin in the subepithelial scar tissue up to 12 months after excimer keratectomy.[101]

Proteoglycans

The cell surface proteoglycans are glycosylated proteins linked covalently to highly anionic glycosaminoglycans. Apart from their hydrodynamic functions, their involvement in many aspects of cell and tissue activities has been demonstrated.

Keratan sulfate proteoglycan (KSPG) plays an important role in corneal transparency. It is absent or reduced in opaque corneal scars and reappears during restoration of transparency. Chondroitin and dermatan sulfate proteoglycan (decorin) regulate collagen fibril formation and are natural regulators of TGF-β activity.[102,103] Decorin may prove to be clinically useful in treating fibrotic diseases caused by overproduction of TGF-β.[104] Heparan sulfate proteoglycan (perlecan) binds to growth factors like basic fibroblast growth factor and protease inhibitors.[105] In addition, it acts as a cell-adhesive protein.

Proteoglycans have important biologic functions. Pharmacologic agents that can control pysicochemical interactions of proteoglycans may have the potential of favorably influencing corneal wound healing.

REFERENCES

1. Jain S, Azar DT. Extracellular matrix and growth factors in corneal wound healing. *Curr Opin Ophthalmol.* 1994; 5(4):31–34.
2. Phillips AF, Szerenyi K, Campos M, Krueger RR, McDonnell PJ. Arachidonic acid metabolites after excimer laser corneal surgery. *Arch Ophthalmol.* 1993;111: 1273–1278.
3. Stoltz RA, Conners MS, Dunn MW, Schwartzman ML. Effect of metabolic inhibitors on arachidonic acid metabolism: evidence for cytochrome P-450 mediated reactions. *J Ocul Pharmacol.* 1994;10(1):307–317.
4. Bazan HEP, Tao Y, Hurst JS. Platelet-activating factor antagonist and ocular inflammation. *J Ocul Pharmacol.* 1994;10(1):319–327.
5. Gartry DS, Kerr Muir M, Lohmann CP, Marshall J. The effect of topical corticosteroids on refractive outcome and corneal haze after photorefractive keratectomy: a prospective, randomised, double-blind trial. *Arch Ophthalmol.* 1992;110:944–952.
6. Gartry DS, Kerr Muir M, Marshall J. The effect of topical corticosteroids on refraction and corneal haze following excimer laser treatment of myopia: an update. A prospective, randomised, double-masked study. *Eye.* 1993;7: 584–590.
7. O'Brart DPS, Lohmann CP, Klonos G, et al. The effect of topical corticosteroids and plasmin inhibitors on refractive outcome, haze, and visual performance after photorefractive keratectomy. A prospective, randomised, observer-masked study. *Ophthalmology.* 1994;101:1565–1574.
8. Machat JJ. Double-blind corticosteroid trial in identical twins following photorefractive keratectomy. *Refract Corneal Surg.* 1993;9:S105–S107.
9. Haverbeke L. Assessing the efficacy of topical corticosteroids following radial keratotomy. *Refract Corneal Surg.* 1993;9:379–382.
10. Yamaguchi T, Asbell PA, Ostrick M, Kissling GE, Safir A, Kaufman HE. Corticosteroid therapy after anterioir radial keratotomy in primates. *Am J Ophthalmol.* 1984;97: 215–220.
11. Fagerholm P, Hamberg-Nystrom H, Tengroth B, Epstein D. Effect of postoperative steroids on the refractive outcome of photorefractive keratectomy for myopia with the Summit excimer laser. *J Cataract Refract Surg.* 1994; 20(suppl):212–215.
12. Fitzsimmons TD, Fagerholm P, Tengroth B. Steroid treatment of myopic regression: acute refractive and topographic changes in excimer photorefractive keratectomy patients. *Cornea.* 1993;12:358–361.

13. Orssaud C, Ganem S, Binaghi M, et al. Photorefractive keratectomy in 176 eyes: one year follow-up. *J Refract Corneal Surg.* 1994;10(suppl):199–205.

14. Campos M, Abed HM, McDonnell PJ. Topical fluorometholone reduces stromal inflammation after photorefractive keratectomy. *Ophthalmic Surg.* 1993;24:654–657.

15. David T, Serdarevic O, Salvoldelli M, Pouliquen Y. Effects of topical corticosteroids and nonsteroidal anti-inflammatory agents on corneal wound healing after photorefractive keratectomy in rabbits. *J Refract Corneal Surg.* 1994;10(suppl):299.

16. Sher NA, Frantz JM, Talley A, et al. Topical diclofenac in the treatment of ocular pain after excimer photorefractive keratectomy. *Refract Corneal Surg.* 1993;9:425–436.

17. Szerenyi K, Wang XW, Lee M, McDonnell PJ. Topical diclofenac treatment prior to excimer laser photorefractive keratectomy in rabbits. *Refract Corneal Surg.* 1993;9:437–442.

18. Eiferman RA, Hoffman RS, Sher NA. Topical diclofenac reduces pain following photorefractive keratectomy. *Arch Ophthalmol.* 1993;111:1022.

19. Loya N, Bassage S, Vyas S, et al. Topical diclofenac following excimer laser—effect on corneal sensitivity and wound healing in rabbits. *J Refract Corneal Surg.* 1994;10:423–427.

20. Salz JJ, Reader AL, Schwartz LJ, Vanle K. Treatment of corneal abrasions with soft contact lenses and topical diclofenac. *J Refract Corneal Surg.* 1994;10:640–646.

21. Szerenyi K, Sorken K, Garbus JJ, Lee M, McDonnell PJ. Decrease in normal corneal sensitivity with topical diclofenac sodium. *Am J Ophthalmol.* 1994;118:312–315.

22. Nassaralla BA, Szerenyi K, Wang XW, Alreaves T, McDonnell PJ. Effect Of diclofenac on corneal haze after photoreactive keratectomy in rabbits. *Ophthalmology.* 1995;102:469–474.

23. Ferrari M. Use of topical nonsteroidal anti-inflammatory drugs after photorefractive keratectomy. *J Refract Corneal Surg.* 1994;10:287–289.

24. Arshinoff S, D'Addario D, Sadler C, Bilotta R, Johnson TM. Use of topical nonsteroidal anti-inflammatory drugs in excimer laser photorefractive keratectomy. *J Cataract Refract Surg.* 1994;20:216–222.

25. Gwon A, Vaughan ER, Cheetham JK, DeGryse R. Ocufen (flurbiprofen) in the treatment of ocular pain after radial keratotomy. *CLAO J.* 1994;20:131–138.

26. Bazan HEP, Tao Y, Hurst JS. Platelet-activating factors antagonists and ocular inflammation. *J Ocul Pharmacol.* 1994;10:319–327.

27. Bazan HE, Reddy ST, Lin N. Platelet-activating factor (PAF) accumulation correlates with injury in the cornea. *Exp Eye Res.* 1991;52(4):481–491.

28. Cohen RA, Gebhardt BM, Bazan NG. A platelet-activating factor antagonist reduces corneal allograft inflammation and neovascularization. *Curr Eye Res.* 1994;13:139–144.

29. Bazan HE, Tao Y, Bazan NG. Platelet-activating factor induces collagenase expression in corneal epithelial cells. *Proc Natl Acad Sci USA.* 1993;90:8678–8682.

30. Yamamoto T, Varani J, Soong HK, Lichter PR. Effects of 5-flurouracil and mitomycin-C on cultured rabbit subconjunctival fibroblasts. *Ophthalmology.* 1990;97:1204–1210.

31. Talamo JH, Gollamudi S, Green WR, De La Cruz Z, Filatov V, Stark WJ. Modulation of corneal wound healing after excimer laser keratomileusis using topical mitomycin-C and steroids. *Arch Opthalmol.* 1991;109:1141–1146.

32. Connolly PJ, Jain S, Stark WJ, McCally RL, Azar DT. Modulation of corneal wound healing after excimer laser keratectomy using intraoperative mitomycin-C. *Invest Ophthalmol Vis Sci.* 1994;35(suppl):3505.

33. Singh G, Wilson MR, Foster CS. Mitomycin eye drops as treatment for pterygium. *Ophthalmology.* 1988;95:813–821.

34. Singh G, Wilson MR, Foster CS. Effectivity and late complications of mitomycin in treatment of pterygium. *Ophthalmology.* 1989;96(suppl):120.

35. Rubinfield RS, Pfister RR, Stein RM, et al. Serious complications of topical mitomycin-C after pterygium surgery. *Ophthalmology.* 1992;99:1647–1654.

36. Ando H, Ido T, Kawai Y, Yamamoto T, Kitazawa Y. Inhibition of corneal epithelial wound healing. A comparative study of mytomycin-C and 5-flourouracil. *Ophthalmology.* 1992;99:1809–1814.

37. Pery Frucht J, Ilsar M. The use of low-dose mitomycin-C for prevention of recurrent pterygium. *Ophthalmology.* 1994;101:759–762.

38. Chew SJ, Deuerman RW, Kaufman HE. In vivo assessment of corneal stromal toxicity by tandem scanning confocal microscopy. *Lens Eye Tox Res.* 1992;9:275–292.

39. Bergman RH, Spigelman AV. The role of fibroblast inhibitors on corneal healing following photorefractive keratectomy with 193-nanometer excimer laser in rabbits. *Ophthalmic Surg.* 1994;25:170–174.

40. Morlet N, Gillies MC, Crouch R, Maloof A. Effect of topical interferon-alpha 2b on corneal haze after excimer laser photorefractive keratectomy in rabbits. *Refract Corneal Surg.* 1993;9:443–451.

41. Moorhead LC, Carroll J, Constance G, Jenkins DED, Armeniades CD. Effects of topical treatment with beta-aminopropionitrile after radial keratotomy in the rabbit. *Arch Ophthalmol.* 1984;102:304–307.

42. Fini ME, Girard MT, Matsubara M. Collagenolytic/gelatinolytic enzymes in corneal wound healing. *Acta Ophthalmol.* 1992;70(suppl 202):26–33.

43. Matrisian LM. Metalloproteinases and their inhibitors in matrix remodelling. *Trends Genet.* 1990;6:121–125.

44. Welgus HG, Jeffrey JJ, Stricklin GP, Roswit WT, Eisen

AZ. Characteristics of the action of human skin fibroblasts collagenase on fibrillar collagens. *J Biol Chem.* 1980;255:6808–6813.

45. Azar DT, Hahn TW, Jain S, Yeh YC, Stetler-Stevensen WG. Matrix metalloproteinases are expressed during wound healing after excimer laser keratectomy. *Cornea.* 1995 (in press).

46. Lohmann CP, Marshall J. Plasmin- and plasminogen-activator inhibitors after excimer laser photorefractive keratectomy: new concept in prevention of postoperative myopic regression and haze. *Refract Corneal Surg.* 1993;9:300–302. Review.

47. Tervo T, Virtanen T, Honkanen N, Harkonen M, Tarkkanen A. Tear fluid plasmin activity after excimer laser photorefractive keratectomy. *Invest Ophthalmol Vis Sci.* 1994;35:3045–3050.

48. O'Brart DPS, Lohmann CP, Klonos G, et al. The effects of topical corticosteroids and plasmin inhibitors on refractive outcome, haze, and visual performance after photorefractive keratectomy—a prospective, randomized, observer-masked study. *Ophthalmology.* 1994;101:1565–1574.

49. Tripathi BJ, Tripathi RC, Livingston AM, Borisuth NS. The role of growth factors in the embryogenesis and differentiation of the eye. *Am J Anat.* 1991;192(4):442–471.

50. Schultz G, Rotatori DS, Clark W. EGF and TGF-a in wound healing and repair. *J Cell Biochem.* 1991;45:346–352.

51. Ohji M, SundarRaj N, Thoft RA. Transforming growth factor-beta stimulates collagen and fibronectin synthesis by human corneal stromal fibroblasts in vitro. *Curr Eye Res.* 1993;12(8):703–709.

52. Kruse FE, Tseng SC. Growth factors modulate clonal growth and differentiation of cultured rabbit limbal and corneal epithelium. *Invest Ophthalmol Vis Sci.* 1993;34(6):1963–1976.

53. Sheardown H, Wdegw C, Chou L, Apel R, Rootman DS, Cheng YL. Continuous epidermal growth factor delivery in corneal epithelial wound healing. *Invest Ophthalmol Vis Sci.* 1993;34:3593–3600.

54. Chung JH, Fagerholm P. Treatment of rabbit corneal alkali wounds with human epidermal growth factor. *Cornea.* 1989;8:122–128.

55. Caporossi A, Manetti C. Epidermal growth factor in topical treatment following epikeratoplasty. *Ophthalmologica.* 1992;205:121–124.

56. Scardovi C, De Felice GP, Gazzaniga A. Epidermal growth factor in the topical treatment of traumatic corneal ulcers. *Ophthalmologica.* 1993;206:119–124.

57. Cellini M, Baldi A, Caramazza N, DeFelice GP, Gazzaniga A. Epidermal growth factor in the topical treatment of herpetic corneal ulcers. *Ophthalmologica.* 1994;208:37–40.

58. Romano A, Peisich A, Wasserman D, Gamus D. Aggravation of herpetic stromal keratitis after murine epidermal grown factor topical application. *Cornea.* 1994;13(2):167–172.

59. Petroutsos G, Sebag J, Courtois Y. Epidermal growth factor increases tensile strength during wound healing. *Ophthalmic Res.* 1986;18:299.

60. Hommel U, Harvey TS, Driscoll PC, Campbell ID. Human epidermal growth factor. High resolution structure and comparison with human transforming growth factor-a. *J Mol Biol.* 1992;227:271 282.

61. Luetteke NC, Qiu TH, Peiffer RL, Oliver PO, Smithies O, Lee DC. TGFa deficiency results in hair follicle and eye abnormalities in targeted and waved-1 mice. *Cell.* 1993;73:263–278.

62. Khaw PT, Schultz GS, MacKay SL, et al. Detection of transforming growth factor-alpha messenger RNA and protein in human corneal epithelial cells. *Invest Ophthalmol Vis Sci.* 1992;33(12):3302–3306.

63. Smyth RJ, Kitada S, Lee DA. The effects of transferrin receptor antibody, transferrin receptor antibody bound to pseudomonas exotoxin and transforming growth factor-a bound to pseudomonas exotoxin on human tenon's capsule fibroblast proliferation. *J Ocul Pharmacol.* 1992;8:83–90.

64. Chen RH, Ebner R, Derynck R. Inactivation of the type II receptor reveals two receptor pathways for the diverse TGF-β activites. *Science.* 1993;260:1335–1338.

65. Ebner R, Chen RH, Shum L, et al. Cloning of a type I TGF-β receptor and its effect on TGF-β binding to the type II receptor. *Science.* 1993;260:1344–1348.

66. Moustakas A, Lin HY, Henis YL, Plamondon J, O'Conner-McCourt MD, Lodish HF. The transforming growth factor β receptors types I, II, and III form hetero-oligomeric complexes in the presence of ligand. *J Biol Chem.* 1993;268:22215–22218.

67. Lopez-Casillas F, Payne HM, Andres JL, Massague J. Betaglycan can act as a dual modulator of TGF-b access to signaling receptors: mapping of ligand binding and GAG attachment sites. *J Cell Biol.* 1994;124:557–568.

68. Pasquale LR, Dorman-Pease ME, Lutty GA, Quigley HA, Jampel HD. Immunolocalization of TGF-β1, TGF-β2, and TGF-β3 in the anterior segment of the human eye. *Invest Ophthalmol Vis Sci.* 1993;34:23–30.

69. Rao RC, Varani J, Soong HK. FGF promotes corneal stromal fibroblast motility. *J Ocul Pharmacol.* 1992;8(1):77–81.

70. Mishima H, Nakamura M, Murakami J, Nishida T, Otori T. Transforming growth factor-beta modulates effects of epidermal growth factor on corneal epithelial cells. *Curr Eye Res.* 1992;11(7):691–696.

71. Phillips GD, Whitehead RA, Stone AM, Ruebel MW, Goodkin ML, Knighton DR. Transforming growth factor

beta (TGF-β) stimulation of angiogenesis: an electron microscopic study. *J Submicrosc Cytol Pathol.* 1993;25(2):149–155.

72. Phillips GD, Whitehead RA, Knighton DR. Inhibition by methylprednisolone acetate suggests an indirect mechanism for TGF-β induced angiogenesis. *Growth Factors.* 1992;6(1):77–84.

73. Peters K, Ornitz D, Werner S, Williams L. Unique expression pattern of the FGF receptor 3 gene during mouse organogenesis. *Develop Biol.* 1993;155(2):423–430.

74. de Iongh R, McAvoy JW. Distribution of acidic and basic fibroblast growth factor (FGF) in the foetal rat eye: implications for lens development. *Growth Factors.* 1992;6(2):159–177.

75. Dabin I, Courtois Y. Acidic fibroblast growth factor overexpression in corneal epithelial wound healing. *Growth Factors.* 1991;(2):129–139.

76. Vlodavsky I, Fuks Z, Ishai-Michaeli R, et al. Extracellular matrix-resident basic fibroblast growth factor: implication for the control of angiogenesis. *J Cell Biochem.* 1991; 45(2):167–176.

77. Wilson SE, Walker JW, Chwang EL, He YG. Hepatocyte growth factor, keratinocyte growth factor, their receptors, fibroblast growth factor receptor-2 and the cells of the cornea. *Invest Ophthalmol Vis Sci.* 1993;34: 2544–2561.

78. Adamis AP, Meklir B, Joyce NC. Rapid communication. In situ injury-induced release of basic-fibroblast growth factor from corneal epithelial cells. *Am J Pathol.* 1991;139: 961–967.

79. Hecpuct C, Morisset S, Lorans G, Plouet J, Adolphe M. Effects of acidic and basic fibroblast growth factors on the proliferation of rabbit corneal cells. *Curr Eye Res.* 1990;9:429–433.

80. Rieck P, Assouline M, Savoldelli M, et al. Recombinant human basic fibroblast growth factor (Rg-bFGF) in three different wound models in rabbits: corneal wound healing effect and pharmacology. *Exp Eye Res.* 1992;54(6): 987–988.

81. Mazue G, Bertolero F, Jacob C, Sarmientos P, Roncucci R. Preclinical and clinical studies with recombinant human basic fibroblast growth factor. *Ann NY Acad Sci.* 1991; 638:329–340.

82. Grant MB, Mames RN, Fitzgerald C, Ellis EA, Aboufriekha M, Guy J. Insulin-like growth factor I acts an angiogenic agent in rabbit cornea and retina: comparative studies with basic fibroblast growth factor. *Diabetologica.* 1993;36(4):282–291.

83. Hoppenreijs V, Pels E, Vrenson G, Felton P, Treffers WF. Platelet-derived growth factor: receptor expression in corneas and effects on corneal cells. *Invest Ophthalmol Vis Sci.* 1993;34:637–649.

84. David T, Rieck P, Renard G, et al. Corneal wound healing modulation using basic fibroblast growth factor after ex-

cimer laser photorefractive keratectomy. *Cornea.* 1995;14: 227–234.

85. Halliwell B. The chemistry of free radicals. *Toxicol Ind Health.* 1993;9:1–21.

86. Kitai MS, Popkov VL, Semchishen VA, Kharizov AA. The physics of UV laser cornea ablation. *IEEE J Quant Electron.* 1991;27:302–307.

87. Ediger MN, Pettit GH, Weiblinger RP, Chen CH. Transmission of corneal collagen during ArF excimer laser ablation. *Lasers Surg Med.* 1993;13:204–210.

88. Nakagawa K. Direct observation of laser generated free radicals from a myocardium target site. *Free Radic Biol Med.* 1992;12:241–242.

89. Nakagawa K. Pulsed UV laser generated short-lived free radicals from biological samples. *Free Radic Res Commun.* 1993;18:223–227.

90. Monboisse JC, Borel JP. Oxidative damage to collagen. *EXS.* 1992;62:323–327.

91. Rivet AJ. Preferential degradation of the oxidatively modified form of glutamine synthetase by intracellular mammalian proteases. *J Biol Chem.* 1985;260: 300–305.

92. Chace KV, Carubelli R, Nordquist RE, Rowsey JJ. Effect of free radicals on corneal collagen. *Free Radic Res Commun.* 1991;12-13:591–594.

93. Ohshima M, Jung SK, Yasuda T, Sakano Y, Fujimoto D. Active oxygen-induced modification alters properties of collagen as a substratum for fibroblasts. *Matrix.* 1993;13: 187–194.

94. Jain S, Hahn TW, McCally RL, Azar DT. Antioxidants reduce corneal light scattering after excimer keratectomy in rabbits. *Lasers Surg Med.* 1995;17:160–165.

95. Tervo T, Sulonen J, Valtones S, Vannas A, Virtanen I. Distribution of fibronectin in human and rabbit corneas. *Exp Eye Res.* 1986;42(4):396–399.

96. SundarRaj N, Geiss MJ, Fantes F, et al. Healing of excimer laser ablated monkey corneas. *Arch Ophthalmol.* 1990; 108:1604–1610.

97. Van Setton GB, Koch JW, Tervo K, et al. Expression of tenascin and fibronectin in the rabbit cornea after excimer laser surgery. *Graefes Arch Clin Exp Ophthalmol.* 1992;230: 178–183.

98. Kim KS, Oh JS, Kim IS, Jo JS. Clinical efficacy of topical homologus fibronectin in persistent corneal epithelial disorders. *Korean J Ophthalmol.* 1992;6(1):12–18.

99. Nishida T, Nakagawa S, Nishibayashi C, Tanaka H, Manabe R. Fibronectin enhancement of corneal epithelial wound healing of rabbits in vivo. *Arch Ophthalmol.* 1984;102:455–456.

100. Ohji M, Mandarino L, SundarRaj N, Thoft RA. Corneal epithelial cell attachment with endogenous laminin and fibronectin. *Invest Ophthalmol Vis Sci.* 1993;34(8):2487–2492.

101. Latvala T, Tervo K, Mustonen R, Tervo T. Expression of

cellular fibronectin and tenascin in the rabbit cornea after excimer laser photorefractive keratectomy—a 12 month study. *Br J Ophthalmol.* 1995;79:65–69.

102. Takeuchi Y, Matsumoto T, Ogata E, Shishiba Y. Effects of transforming growth factor beta 1 and L-ascorbate on synthesis and distribution of proteoglycans in murine osteoblast-like cells. *J Bone Miner Res.* 1993;8:823–830.

103. Fukushima D, Butzow R, Hildebrand A, Ruoslahti E. Localization of transforming growth factor beta binding site in betaglycan. Comparison with small extracellular matrix proteoglycans. *J Biol Chem.* 1993;268(30):22710–22715.

104. Noble NA, Harper JR, Border WA. In vivo interactions of TGF-beta and extracellular matrix. *Prog Growth Factor Res.* 1992;4(4):369–382.

105. Noonan DM, Hassell JR. Perlecan, the large low-density proteoglycan of basement membranes: structure and variant forms. *Kidney Int.* 1993;43(1):53–60.

CHAPTER 6

Corneal Diseases of Importance
to the Keratorefractive Surgeon

Janine Smith ▪ Dimitri T. Azar

In this chapter we discuss the pathogenesis and management of corneal and external diseases that are frequently encountered in the preoperative evaluation and course of management of the keratorefractive surgery patient. Many of these conditions should be identified and treated preoperatively, while others are contraindications for refractive surgery. This chapter will review these corneal conditions, beginning with inflammatory eyelid disease and followed by conjunctivitis and keratitis, tear film abnormalities, atopic and allergic diseases, peripheral corneal ulceration, keratoconus, and corneal dystrophies and degenerations. The relationship of these conditions to refractive surgical procedures will be emphasized.

BLEPHARITIS AND MEIBOMITIS

An examination of the skin of the eyelid as part of the external ophthalmologic examination should include a search for any signs of active inflammation or infection such as periorbital cellulitis. One should also look for evidence of dermatoblepharitis.[1-4] Included in the category of infectious dermatoblepharitis is herpes simplex virus dermatoblephbaritis, her-

pes zoster dermatoblepharitis, and impetigo, a skin infection caused by *Staphylococcus aureus* or group A *Streptococcus pyogenes*, most commonly seen in children. Although the patient may have no current evidence of these processes, the ophthalmologist must carefully probe for any history of herpetic dermatoblepharitis, specifically because recurrent corneal or conjunctival disease or associated corneal hypesthesia are factors that would impact adversely the suitability of these patients for refractive surgical procedures (Fig 6–1).

McCulley et al have formulated a classification system for blepharitis[3]:

1. Staphylococcal blepharitis
2. Seborrheic blepharitis
3. Seborrheic blepharitis with excess meibomian secretions
4. Seborrheic blepharitis with meibomitis
5. Primary meibomitis with dermal involvement

Although patients rarely fit neatly into these categories, this scheme can be helpful in evaluation and treatment. Careful examination of the eyelid margin and characterization of the signs present are the initial diagnostic tools in evaluating keratorefractive surgery patients.

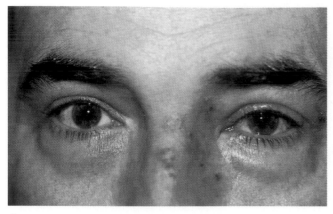

A

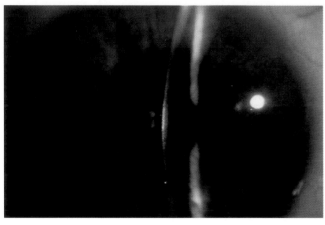

B

Figure 6–1. A. Patient with herpes zoster dermatoblepharitis localized to the left side of the face. **B.** Associated corneal subepithelial scarring is a relative contraindication for laser refractive surgery.

Anterior Blepharitis

Blepharitis is an extremely common condition that requires careful screening in the evaluation of the refractive surgical patient. Staphylococcal blepharitis is the most common nonacute infectious agent of the ocular adnexa, producing the classic sign of the fibrin collarette.[1] Staphylococcal blepharitis can be manifested as acute, ulcerative blepharitis or, more commonly, as chronic blepharitis or blepharoconjunctivitis. In acute, ulcerative blepharitis there is evidence of erythema and ulceration of the anterior lid margin. These findings can be unilateral or bilateral. Generally, conjunctival involvement is not prominent. The entity that general ophthalmologists confront frequently is chronic blepharitis. The patients often report symptoms of burning, foreign body sensation, and crusting of the eyelashes, especially in the morning. On examination, there is ev-

idence of debris adhering to the eyelashes and anterior lid margin, and there may be some thickening of the lid margin itself. Often lashes are missing. There may be evidence of hyperemia of palpebral and bulbar conjunctiva, and papillae involving the limbus. Phlyctenulosis can also accompany this condition. Phlyctenules are sterile, triangular-shaped, predominantly lymphocytic infiltrates characteristically located at the limbal region; their formation is secondary to a type IV hypersensitivity reaction to microbial antigens. Although staphylococcal antigens are the most common inciting factor of this condition, other causes include tuberculosis, coccidioidomycosis, lymphogranuloma venereum, and candidiasis.[2] Chronic staphylococcal blepharitis can involve the cornea with a superficial coarse epitheliopathy and punctate corneal erosions. More serious corneal involvement, such as acute marginal infiltration and ulceration thought to be mediated by type III hypersensitivity reaction to toxins elaborated by the staphylococcal species, is less common. *Demodex folliculorum* infestation of the eyelids results in sleeve formation along the eyelashes and can cause blepharitis as well.

Proper management of staphylococcal blepharitis and associated corneal conditions should increase the likelihood of successful keratorefractive surgery. Antibiotic ointments like erythromycin and bacitracin used for more than 3 weeks are useful in reducing the bacterial load and minimizing symptoms. An eyelid hygiene regimen that includes warm compresses is valuable in the preoperative period, but should be avoided postoperatively. Mild topical corticosteroid preparations are helpful in the perioperative period, especially if marginal corneal infiltrates or phlyctenules are seen. Limited judicious use of topical corticosteroids is advised in patients with associated rosacea blepharitis.

Meibomitis and Meibomian Gland Disease

Dysfunction of the meibomian glands is thought to result in a form of blepharitis that has a wide range of severity. The symptoms are burning, foreign body sensation, and fluctuation of vision that changes with blinking. These patients often give a history of hordeolum and/or recurrent chalazion and its excision. The classic signs of meibomian-gland dysfunction are inspissated meibomian glands, lipid or foam in the tear film, thickening of the lid margin, and hyperemia of the lid margin and conjunctiva. The cornea may be secondarily involved with epithelial erosion, pannus forma-

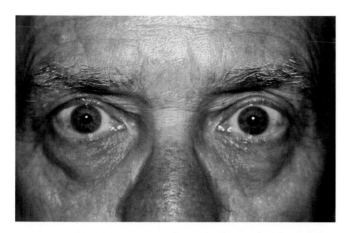

Figure 6–2. Rosacea blepharoconjunctivitis. Note extensive telangectasia of the nose.

tion, marginal infiltration or ulceration, or phlyctenular disease. Sebaceous-gland dysfunction may accompany meibomian-gland dysfunction with associated acne vulgaris, acne rosacea, and seborrheic dermatitis. Examination of the skin of the face will reveal these conditions and direct the ophthalmologist to a detailed examination of the eyelids.

Roscea Blepharitis

Up to 58% of patients with acne rosacea have ocular manifestations of their disease. Acne rosacea is a chronic condition characterized by female predominance, telangiectasias, and pustules along the nose and cheeks.[4] Conjunctival hyperemia and peripheral corneal neovascularization are common; however, the more vision-threatening complications of corneal ulceration, thinning, and perforation are not (Fig 6–2). The etiology of acne rosacea remains unclear. Despite the clear genetic predilection of the condition in persons of Celtic or Northern European ancestry, this condition has been reported in patients of many racial backgrounds. The use of topical corticosteroids in patients with rosacea blepharitis may precipitate corneal ulcerations. A course of preoperative systemic tetracycline, doxycycline, or erythromycin should be considered in keratorefractive surgery patients and continued for 1 to 2 months postoperatively.

BACTERIAL CONJUNCTIVITIS AND KERATITIS

Acute Bacterial Conjunctivitis

The most common organisms colonizing the ocular surface are *Staphylococcus epidermidis* and *Corynebacte-*

rium species.[5] The principal organisms associated with acute bacterial conjunctivitis in the nonimmunocompromised adult are *Staphylococcus aureus, Streptococcus pneumoniae, Neisseria gonorrhoeae,* and *Hemophilus influenzae.* The patient gives a history of redness and tearing, first in one eye and then in the other, which is followed by the mucopurulent discharge and morning crusting that are the hallmarks of this condition. The signs include purulent discharge, conjunctival hyperemia or chemosis, conjunctival membrane formation, subconjunctival hemorrhage, and preauricular lymphadenopathy; the latter is seen only in *Neisseria* conjunctivitis. There may be secondary corneal involvement with superficial epitheliopathy or direct corneal involvement with active keratitis, as in *Neisseria* keratoconjunctivitis. Most mild bacterial conjunctivitis will resolve on its own; however, topical antibiotic therapy has been found to speed recovery and reduce the risks of chronic sequelae.[6] Cultures should be obtained from both eyes and empirical therapy with a broad spectrum antimicrobial begun. If the bacterial conjunctivitis is severe, *Neisseria* species should be ruled out in order to attempt to prevent the consecutive vision-threatening keratitis. Severe signs like marked lid edema, copious purulent discharge, preauricular lymphadenopathy, and membrane formation should provoke the ophthalmologist to act quickly to obtain the appropriate diagnostic cultures and smears to look for intracellular gram-negative diplococci. The Centers for Disease Control and Prevention (CDC) recommend using adjunctive topical therapy and advising sexual partners to obtain evaluation for possible treatment. Unfortunately, this virulent bacteria has the ability to cause rapid suppurative keratitis that results in perforation and has a dismal visual outcome. Keratorefractive surgery should not be performed except after complete resolution of the signs and symptoms of acute conjunctivitis.

Acute Bacterial Keratitis

The majority of cases of bacterial keratitis worldwide are caused by infection with virulent organisms like *Micrococcaceae, Streptococcus spp., Pseudomonus aeruginosa,* and *Enterobacteriaceae.* These infections begin as an epithelial keratitis, and, because of both host and pathogen factors, can erupt with stromal infiltration and edema, possibly progressing to hypopyon formation and stromal suppuration. The major host risk factors for the development of bacterial keratitis are trauma, contact lens wear (Fig 6–3A), history of persistent epithelial defect, which may follow prolonged hypotony (Fig 6–3B), history of herpes simplex keratitis treated with topical corticosteroids, and history of penetrating keratoplasty.[7] Bacterial keratitis may follow refractive surgery procedures. Predisposing factors are similar to those for other corneal surgical procedures. Despite the existence of features that can guide the ophthalmologist in forming an initial impression of the possible pathogen, these are not fail-safe; appropriate diagnostic scrapings and cultures should be obtained. Infectious keratitis resulting from gram-negative rods like *Pseudomonas aeruginosa* tends to produce a fulminant keratitis with stromal abscess formation, generally accompanied by hypopyon formation, and should be suspected in any contact lens wearer whether in the setting of a preoperative evaluation or during contact lens wear after keratorefractive surgery. Some gram-positive organisms like *Staphylococcus* and *Streptococcus* species cause less dramatic infections, but they can nevertheless result in significant corneal scarring and a

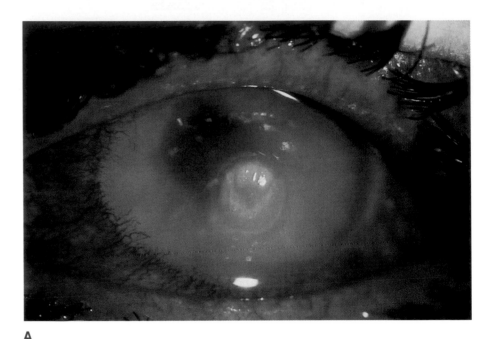

A

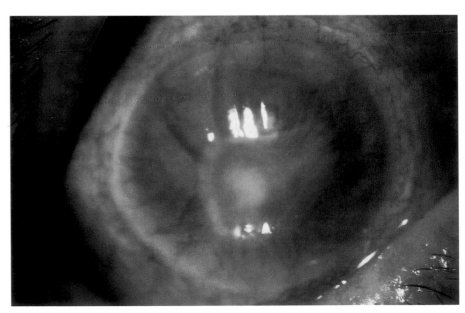

Figure 6–3. A. Bacterial keratoconjunctivitis. The risk factor for the development of bacterial keratitis in this patient is trauma. **B.** Bacterial corneal ulceration following history of persistent epithelial defect because of prolonged hypotony.

B

decrease in visual acuity. *Acanthamoeba* species are increasingly recognized as a cause of infectious keratitis. Although there are scattered case reports of successful treatment of this infectious agent using a variety of agents, definitive treatment of this form of keratitis remains particularly difficult.

Chronic Bacterial Conjunctivitis and Keratitis

Chronic bacterial conjunctivitis is most commonly caused by infection with *Staphylococcus aureus*.[8] The eyelids are often involved as well, a condition thought to be related to the toxins elaborated by this class of bacteria. This entity is discussed in full in the section on blepharitis and meibomitis above. Other causes of chronic bacterial conjunctivitis are the gram-negative bacteria like *Moraxella lacunata, Serratia marcescens, Escherichia coli, Klebsiella pneumoniae,* and *Proteus* species. *Moraxella lacunata* and *Staphylococcus* species can also cause marginal blepharitis. Appropriate cultures should be obtained and directed antimicrobial therapy begun in order to minimize the morbidity of this condition.

Adult inclusion conjunctivitis is secondary to infection with *Chlamydia trachomatis* immunotypes D, E, F, G, H, I, J, and K and is an important cause of chronic conjunctivitis in the adult, an entity distinct from trachoma. Transmission is through contact of the eye with infected secretions. The history is often one of chronic ocular limitation and redness, which may be accompanied by mucopurulent discharge. The most helpful sign in diagnosis is a prominent lymphoid reaction, that is, conjunctival follicles that may involve the bulbar or limbal conjunctiva and preauricular lymphadenopathy. There may be micropannus formation in the cornea, superficial epitheliopathy on the superior cornea, and even subepithelial infiltrate formation. Patients with chronic follicular conjunctivitis seeking keratorefractive surgical procedures complain of chronic redness and ocular irritation with or without contact lenses. Treatment can ameliorate symptoms and increase their contact lens tolerance. It is advisable to treat these patients preoperatively. If untreated, this infection can lead to persistent keratitis and/or conjunctivitis, resulting in corneal and conjunctival scarring. This can be completely avoided, as oral tetracycline 1.0 to 1.5 g daily or oral doxycycline 100 mg bid for 2 weeks is curative.[9]

A form of chronic bacterial keratitis, termed *infectious crystalline keratopathy,* has been described. The etiologic agent is primarily *Streptococcus viridans,* although other causative agents have been implicated. The history often involves previous treatment with topical corticosteroids, which is thought to be important for the development of the characteristic sign of pauci-inflammatory stromal disease. Crystalline opacities are seen within the stroma, and these are accompanied by few signs of active infection or inflammation. Corneal culture must be obtained from the infiltrate, and prolonged therapy with appropriate antibiotics is often required. Corneal infection with nontuberculous mycobacteria can also become chronic. Similarly, patients often have been previously treated with topical corticosteroids and show minimal signs of inflammation. Special media and therapy are required. Crystalline keratopathy is a contraindication for keratorefractive surgery.

VIRAL CONJUNCTIVITIS AND KERATITIS

The major etiologic agents of acute viral conjunctivitis are herpes simplex, adenovirus, and varicella zoster. There are 41 antigenically distinct serotypes of adenovirus, a nonenveloped DNA virus that is probably the most common cause of viral conjunctivitis in the adult. There are three clinical presentations of infection with adenovirus: pharyngoconjunctival fever (PCF), epidemic keratoconjunctivitis (EKC), and acute nonspecific follicular conjunctivitis (NFC). Pharyngoconjunctival fever is most commonly caused by adenovirus serotypes 3, 4, and 7, but it can also be caused by other serotypes. In this instance, the follicular conjunctivitis is accompanied by fever, pharyngitis, and regional lymphadenopathy. Constitutional symptoms frequently are encountered. The conjunctivitis is generally bilateral but not severe, and secondary corneal involvement is usually restricted to mild epithelial keratitis. In contrast, EKC is more serious and can have significant ocular morbidity. Epidemic keratoconjunctivitis is caused most commonly by adenovirus serotypes 8 and 19 and also by types 2, 3, 4, 5, 7, 10, 11, 13, 14, 15, 16, and 29. This highly contagious condition produces symptoms of watery discharge, redness, irritation, and itching. The corneal signs, which occur in 80% of patients, have been classified into five stages.

In stage 1 a fine, diffuse punctate epithelial keratitis is present for 2 to 5 days. In stage 2, fine and coarse epitheliopathy involves the deep epithelium. Stage 3 is characterized by the initial formation of the deep epithelial infiltrates, which have been well described and are equally well recognized clinically. Stage 4 shows the full formation of classic subepithelial infiltrates (Fig 6–4). And in stage 5 there is a coarse granularity to the epithelium late in the clinical course.[10] The conjunctiva shows hyperemia, chemosis, follicle formation, and membrane or pseudomembrane formation, which may result in conjunctival scarring. Judicious use of topical corticosteroids is reserved for severe conjunctival or corneal involvement. Although nonspecific follicular conjunctivitis does not affect the cornea and resolves without sequelae, these patients serve as a reservoir for adenovirus in the community. A history of acute adenoviral infection should not be a contraindication for keratorefractive surgery except when corneal involvement is noted. If there is none, the surgery should be rescheduled for at least 1 month. The presence of chronic subepithelial infiltrates may be a contraindication for refractive surgery.

Herpes simplex conjunctivitis can accompany both primary and recurrent infections and need not be associated with dermatoblepharitis or keratitis. Clinical signs include preauricular adenopathy, a mild follicular or papillary conjunctivitis, and conjunctival hyperemia. Membrane formation does not usually occur. In 30% to 60% of patients, a keratitis will develop that may range in severity from a diffuse punctate epithelial keratitis to typical dendritic keratitis. Recurrent ocular herpes can present as isolated conjunctivitis, epithelial and stromal keratitis, or uveitis. There are virus-related factors and host immune response characteristics that seem to be important in the pathogenesis of recurrent ocular herpetic disease.

Herpes simplex keratitis can take many forms. Most keratorefractive surgeons consider herpetic keratitis to be a contraindication for surgery. Epithelial keratitis is a sign of active viral replication during primary or recurrent infection (Fig 6–5).[4] Punctate keratitis can

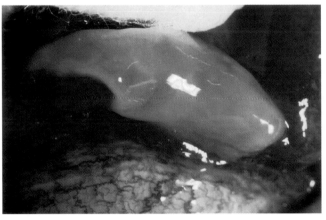

A

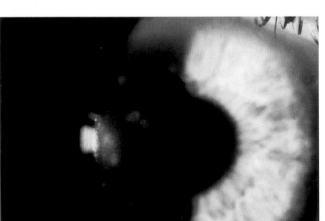

B

Figure 6–4. **A.** Adenoviral membranous conjunctivitis. **B.** Classic subepithelial infiltrates that persist for several months following the initial EKC episode.

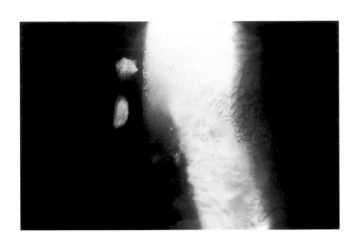

A

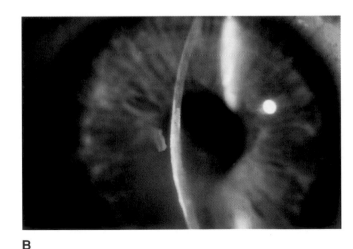

B

Figure 6–5. **A.** Epithelial keratitis, as evidenced by rose bengal staining, is a sign of active herpes simplex viral replication. **B.** Disciform keratitis just below the visual axis results in reduced visual acuity.

accompany the conjunctivitis seen with primary herpes simplex infection, or it can occur without the conjunctivitis before dendrite formation or as a manifestation of drug toxicity. Dendritic epithelial keratitis can be seen during recurrent or primary infection. Keratorefractive surgery may reactivate dormant viral disease. Geographic epithelial keratitis should be distinguished from trophic ulceration caused by chronic disease. The pathogenesis of herpetic stromal disease is not clearly understood and may take the form of disciform keratitis or necrotizing keratitis (Fig 6–5A). Topical corticosteroids for these conditions should be applied based on the degree of inflammation and the likelihood of active viral replication. Herpes zoster stromal keratitis is thought to be related to immunologic mechanisms that are not clearly delineated. The effectiveness of systemic acyclovir in conjunction with corticosteroids is currently being evaluated in the Herpetic Eye Disease Study. Topical corticosteroids are a mainstay of treatment for this difficult disorder. The signs of stromal inflammation and epithelial disease are well recognized and can result in corneal neovascularization, stromal scarring, and corneal irregularities.

The varicella zoster virus causes two clinically distinct entities: chicken pox and herpes zoster, or shingles. If the vesicular eruption of chicken pox involves the skin of the eyelids, or the conjunctiva itself, small lesions resembling phlyctenules may form at the limbus.[11] A keratitis may rarely occur as superficial punctate keratitis, or even as dendritic keratitis. In zoster, conjunctivitis is a common sign often accompanying the painful, vesicular, dermatomal dermatitis. Other conjunctival signs include hyperemia, follicular or papillary hypertrophy, petechial hemorrhages, and membrane formation. The adjacent episclera or sclera may also be involved. Keratitis, discussed above, is a contraindication for keratorefractive surgery (Fig 6–5B).

A chronic follicular conjunctivitis can occur as a toxic response secondary to infection with the poxvirus, molluscum contagiosum. A pearly white, umbilicated lesion may hide among cilia along the lid margin and elaborate toxins onto the conjunctival surface, leading to chronic follicular conjunctivitis. A superficial epitheliopathy may also be seen in addition to micropannus formation. These lesions respond to excision and cryotherapy, which should be performed before surgery. Patients should be educated about the risks of combining keratorefractive surgery with the excision of molluscum lesions.

TEAR ABNORMALITIES AND EXPOSURE KERATITIS

Tear Film Abnormalities

A frequently utilized measure of tear production is the Schirmer test, which measures the volume of tears produced over a 5-minute period using Whatman No. 41 filter paper placed in the inferior fornix under standard conditions: dim illumination, normal blink rate, and no talking or chewing.[12] The amount of wetting of the filter paper is measured with 15 mm of wetting over 5 minutes, which is considered to be the minimum normal time for tear production. Topical anesthetic can be applied before performing the test in an attempt to diminish reflex tear production. In 83% of patients with dry eyes, the Schirmer test will show a value less than 5.5 mm.[13] The marginal tear film strip or tear meniscus present on the lower eyelid can also be an indicator of the amount of tear produced. The height of the tear meniscus should be 0.5 to 1.0 mm. The most specific diagnostic tests for keratoconjunctivitis secca (KCS) are the presence of rose bengal staining of devitalized epithelium and Schirmer's testing with topical anesthetic. The detection of increased tear lactoferrin concentration and tear osmolarity are the most sensitive indicators of dry eye syndrome.[14] The recovery time following refractive surgery is prolonged in patients with dry eyes, generally because of superficial epithelial keratitis and persistent epithelial defects (Fig 6–6).

The most frequently encountered tear abnormality is a deficiency of tear volume. Aqueous tear deficiency may be caused by inadequate tear production or excessive tear evaporation.[15] It is important to determine if

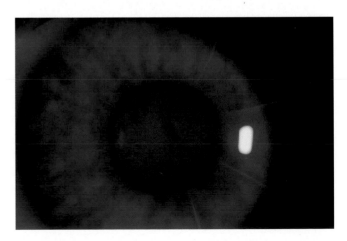

Figure 6–6. Dry eye syndrome. The recovery time following refractive surgery is prolonged in patients with dry eyes generally because of superficial epithelial keratitis.

the etiology of aqueous deficiency is related to ocular or to systemic disease. There are multiple congenital ocular diseases that are associated with aqueous deficiency, including Riley–Day (familial dysautonomia),[16] anhidrotic ectodermal dysplasia, multiple endocrine neoplasia, Adie syndrome,[17] and congenital hypoplasia or aplasia of the lacrimal gland. Idiopathic aqueous deficiency frequently develops in middle-aged women, but it can occur secondary to systemic diseases associated with autoimmune disorders, infiltrative disorders, and neurologic conditions that affect the autonomic nervous system and thereby the lacrimal gland innervation. Conditions that are characterized by infiltration of the lacrimal gland itself, such as lymphoma, amyloidosis, pulmonary fibrosis, graft versus host disease, hemochromatosis, and a host of hematopoietic disorders, can result in replacement of normal gland tissue, thereby causing dry eyes. Disorders more likely to be encountered in the relatively healthy potential refractive surgery patient include autoimmune thyroiditis, sarcoidosis, and systemic lupus erythematosus (SLE). There are several infectious causes of dry eye, including hepatitis B and C, syphilis, trachoma, tuberculosis, and HIV-related diffuse infiltrative lymphadenopathy syndrome, in which CD + cells infiltrate the lacrimal gland and lymphatic tissues.

Keratoconjunctivitis sicca in conjunction with xerostomia comprise primary Sjögren's syndrome. If a known history of both dry eye and dry mouth is obtained, further investigation is warranted to rule out rheumatologic disease, as the key elements of this condition are focal lymphoid infiltrates in the lacrimal and salivary gland and autoantibody formation: ANA > 1:320, rheumatoid factor > 1:320, SS-A or SS-B antibodies.[18] Rheumatoid arthritis is the autoimmune disease most frequently associated with dry eye; however, clear linkage has also been demonstrated for progressive systemic sclerosis, primary biliary cirrhosis, dermatomyositis, and SLE.

Mucus deficiency can result in inadequate wetting of the ocular surface.[19] As a result, dry areas appear within the tear film after the blink, and the degree of tear film stability can be quantified by calculation of the tear break-up time (TBUT) after instillation of 2% fluoroscein solution and examination with oblique illumination using a cobalt blue filter. There should be at least 10 seconds' duration between the blink and the appearance of the first dry area.[20] Inadequate mucus production can occur whenever the conjunctival goblet cells are affected, most frequently with chemical burn, ocular cicatricial pemphigoid, Stevens–Johnson syndrome,

vitamin A deficiency, and administration topical phospholine iodide.[21] Complete lipid deficiency is primarily seen in ectodermal dysplasia secondary to the congenital absence of meibomian glands.[22] This rare condition is characterized by meibomitis and blepharitis, which also cause increased tear lipids, exacerbate the poor wettability of the tear film, and increase evaporation of the aqueous component of the tears.[23] Attention to examination of the eyelids will often reveal inspissation of glands, scurf along the lashes, and debris in the tear film itself; this should alert the ophthalmologist to the presence of significant eyelid disease that may not even be symptomatic.

Many medications can decrease tear production; these often can be obtained over the counter and are not even considered "medicine" by patients. Antihistamines are probably most commonly taken by young patients, and they clearly reduce tear production, as do nasal decongestants, antitussives, and some analgesics that contain antimuscarinic compounds. Any agent with anticholinergic properties, such as antidepressants, antihypertensives, antiulcer medications, and some antiarrhythmics, will inhibit tear production. Some of the beta-adrenergic antagonists, specifically Proctolol and Timolol, have been shown to decrease tear production as measured by Schirmer's test.

A careful history searching specifically for symptoms of dry eye is indicated in the evaluation of the refractive surgery patient. First, the discomfort must be characterized. Is there foreign body sensation, burning, or heaviness of the eyelids? Does itching accompany the symptoms? Is the quality of the irritation sharp or dull? Exacerbating factors should also be explored. Is the discomfort pronounced at a particular time of day or under certain ventilatory conditions? For example, dry eye symptoms are often exacerbated by activities like reading, in which the frequency of blinking is reduced because of the effort required to concentrate. Relieving factors should also be determined. Do artificial tear preparations, closure of the eyelids, or conditions of increased ambient humidity ameliorate the symptoms? The classic symptom of dry eye syndrome is foreign body sensation, which is least noticeable early in the day and increases over the course of the day, punctuated by sharp pain that may be followed by reflex tearing. Severe dryness can be manifest as photophobia, whereas minimal dryness may be asymptomatic. The presence of redundant conjunctiva at the inferior limbus may exacerbate the symptoms of tearing and foreign body sensation in dry eye patients (Fig 6–7).

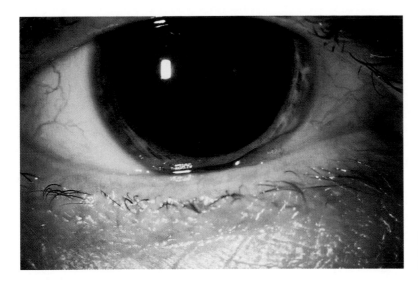

Figure 6–7. Redundant conjunctiva at the inferior limbus in a patient with KCS. This may exacerbate the symptoms of tearing and foreign body sensation in dry eye patients.

Neurotrophic Keratitis

Neurotrophic keratopathy refers to changes that occur in the cornea secondary to disruption of corneal innervation by the fifth cranial nerve. Corneal anesthesia results, leading to decreased tear production. The blink rate can also be decreased while the tear film osmolarity is increased. The trigeminal nerve provides trophic factors that are necessary for the maintenance of healthy corneal epithelium. This process may be related to the transport of specific proteins along the neurons that supply the cornea. In addition, corneal epithelial mitosis appears to be damaged when corneal innervation is disrupted, reportedly secondary to reduction in glycolytic and respiratory cell activity. An epithelial defect with heaped-up edges is a characteristic finding (Fig 6–8A). This can occur either in herpetic viral infections, in which the virus travels via retrograde axoplasmic flow to the trigeminal ganglion where it can become dormant, or in response to space-occupying lesions, like aneurysms or tumors, that compromise trigeminal nerve function. Recurrences of the epithelial defects and prolonged periods required for corneal epithelial wound healing are frequently encountered. Vascularization of the cornea can follow repeated episodes of epithelial defects (Fig 6–8B). Clearly these patients should not undergo keratorefractive surgery.

Neuroparalytic Keratitis

Neuroparalytic keratitis results when the seventh cranial nerve is disrupted. This nerve supplies the orbicularis oculi muscles that allow the eye to blink, so that anything affecting it results in impaired eyelid closure, leading to an abnormal preocular tear film. The blink is

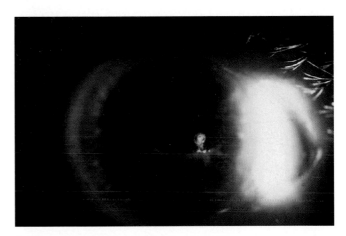

A

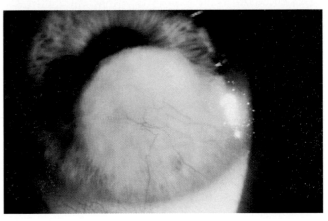

B

Figure 6–8. A. Epithelial defect with heaped-up edges in a patient with neurotrophic keratitis. **B.** Vascularization of the cornea can follow repeated episodes of neurotrophic epithelial defects.

an important mechanism for hydrating the corneal surface, as it serves to spread the tear film over the ocular surface. The lipid layer of the tear film must be maintained in order to minimize evaporation of the tear film. The exposed epithelium becomes dehydrated when the exposed tear film evaporates. The inferior one third of the cornea is typically involved with epithelial breakdown when lagophthalmos is significant. A tarsorrhaphy is frequently required to treat this condition (Fig 6–9A).

Exposure Keratopathy

Exposure keratopathy may result from a variety of causes: thyroid disease, lagophthalmos secondary to neuroparalytic disease, and cicatricial ocular diseases.

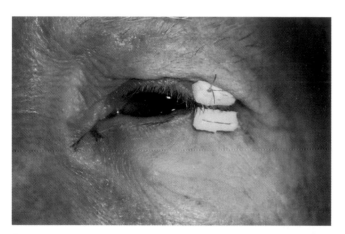

A

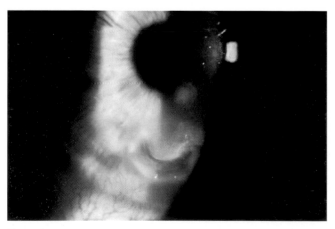

B

Figure 6–9. A. Exposure keratitis. A tarsorrhaphy is frequently required to treat this condition. General thinning is exacerbated by bacterial superinfection. **B.** The inferior one third of the cornea undergoes epithelial breakdown when there is significant lagophthalmos.

Any exposed corneal epithelium quickly becomes desiccated, causing cell membrane damage and death. There is loss of corneal epithelial cells and thinning of the entire corneal epithelium. The thinned cornea is especially susceptible to infectious agents (Fig 6–9B).

IMMUNOLOGIC DISEASE OF THE CONJUNCTIVA AND CORNEA

Introduction

The ocular surface is exposed to a wide range of foreign material, and this antigenic load can result in a variety of immunologic processes within the conjunctiva, cornea, and sclera. Although there are no lymphatic channels within the eye itself, mucous-membrane–associated tissue, termed *conjunctival-associated lymphatic tissue,* or CALT, has been theorized to play a key role in antigen presentation and processing and can be secondarily involved in pathologic processes like lymphoma. All four types of hypersensitivity response have been described as involving the ocular surface. Perhaps the most common ocular manifestation of allergy is allergic conjunctivitis, the result of a type I hypersensitivity response to environmental allergens like pollen and molds, which reach the ocular surface and come into direct contact with the mucous membranes that contain eosinophils, mast cells, and immunoglobulin-E (IgE). The triad of mast cells, IgE, and appropriate allergen results in cross-linking of IgE molecules via activation of a serine esterase, which in turn triggers degranulation of the mast cells and release of vasoactive amines like histamine, eosinophil chemotactic factor (ECF), and platelet-activating factor (PAF); eosinophil granule major basic protein (EMBP) and prostaglandin D2 are also released.[24] Histamine results in conjunctival hyperemia, via H2 receptors,[25] and itching, via H1 receptors,[26] so characteristic of this condition. Other symptoms include tearing and burning; these frequently occur at the time of year that corresponds to the offending allergen's peak production. Patients sensitive to the pollen of trees and grasses suffer exacerbations in the spring and early summer, respectively, whereas ragweed produces its pollen in most abundance early in the fall.

Conjunctival edema is manifest as papillae formation and may be accompanied by edema of the eyelids themselves. A thin, watery discharge is seen acutely, and there is no involvement of the cornea, unless dellen formation has occurred secondary to pronounced localized chemosis. It is not uncommon for the patient to report classical symptoms of hay fever conjunctivitis while showing a paucity of clinical signs suggestive of that condition, so a careful history should be obtained. Itching is the cardinal symptom of allergy, and the pa-

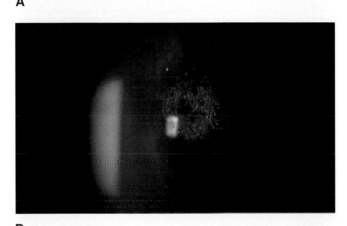

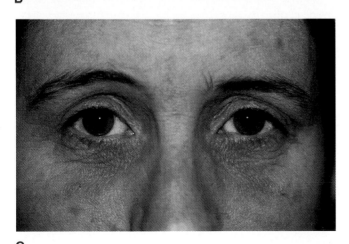

Figure 6–10. A. Atopic keratoconjunctivitis associated with atopic dermatitits of the eyelids. **B.** Steroid cataract may be associated. **C.** Mild atopic disease. Maceration of the canthal skin and excoriation of the periorbital region is exacerbated by scratching.

tient often recognizes well the pattern of exacerbated symptoms during a particular season or among specific environmental factors. If further diagnostic study is warranted, a conjunctival scraping to search for eosinophils can be performed, in addition to skin testing for particular allergens; positive results are 87% predictive of ocular hypersensitivity.[27]

Atopic Keratoconjunctivitis

The term *atopy* refers to type I hypersensitivity reactions of tissue-based IgE antibodies to environmental antigens, which can be confirmed by a positive Prausnitz–Kustner reaction or by a wheal-and-flare response to intradermal injection of the offending allergen. Although atopy is seen in 3% to 15% of the general population,[28] 25% to 40% of affected individuals display ocular manifestations of the syndrome in addition to bronchial asthma, seasonal or perennial rhinitis, hay fever, or urticaria.[29] Atopic dermatitis is manifested during childhood; the scaly, lichenified rash most frequently affects intertrigenous zones and is likely termed *eczema* by pediatricians. The salient features of atopic keratoconjunctivitis include atopic dermatitis of the eyelids (Fig 6–10A), papillary conjunctivitis, and epithelial and stromal corneal disease; these are most likely to become manifest during early adulthood and are generally bilateral. Steroid cataract may be associated (Fig 6 10B). The patient will consistently reveal a history of tearing, burning, watery discharge, and the production of mucous strands, with a strong component of ocular itching and rubbing. This may be one reason to discourage atopic patients from undergoing keratorefractive surgery. Maceration of the canthal skin and excoriation of the periorbital region are not uncommon and are exacerbated by scratching (Fig 6–10C). The eyelids' margins are thickened and scaly while the conjunctiva may appear pale; however, conjunctival hyperemia, papillary hypertrophy, and chemosis are likely to be present during periods of active inflammation. This cycle can become chronic with the development of subepithelial fibrosis and conjunctival cicatrization, which tend to involve the inferior fornix.

Although the initial corneal sign of atopic keratoconjunctivitis (AKC)—a superficial epitheliopathy with intraepithelial microcysts—is not generally vision threatening,[30] more serious corneal manifestations can occur. The epitheliopathy can progress with the formation of infiltrates, the development of corneal neovascularization, and corneal scarring. This is associated with surface irregularities and contact lens intolerance. As a result, many patients with atopic disease may seek refractive surgery procedures. It is important to distinguish AKC from hay fever conjunctivitis because patients with AKC may be poor candidates for surgery. Pannus formation is seen in the majority of patients and may progress to vascularization of the stroma.[31] Indolent, centrally located, oval-shaped ulcers have been reported in severe cases, in addition to pseudogerontotoxon, Horner–Trantas dots, and peripheral corneal ulceration.[32] A strong relation between atopy and keratoconus has been described; 25% of patients with atopic dermatitis[33] and 16% of patients with AKC demonstrate classic signs of keratoconus.[34] Accordingly, atopic patients are not good candidates for refractive surgery, in contrast to patients with seasonal or perennial allergic conjunctivitis. The importance of obtaining a detailed history and physical examination in the evaluation of patients seeking refractive surgery cannot be overemphasized. Unfortunately, these patients are also poor candidates for contact lens wear. Anterior subcapsular "shield" cataracts or posterior polar cataracts are seen in 8% to 10% of patients with atopic dermatitis; these are generally visible during adolescence and are not related to topical corticosteroid therapy because patients who have not been treated for AKC develop them as well.[35]

Vernal Keratoconjunctivitis

Another example of type I hypersensitivity response involving the ocular surface is *vernal keratoconjunctivitis.* This condition affects young men more than women and is reported more frequently in areas of warm climate like that of the Middle East and South America.[36] Classically, this is a bilateral conjunctivitis in which "cobblestone papillae" form in the upper palpebral conjunctiva, variably accompanied by gelatinous hypertrophy of the limbal region and a frequently mild keratopathy. The two forms of disease are limbal and palpebral vernal keratoconjunctivitis; the limbal form is more commonly seen in darker-complected individuals.[37] These limbal papillae may contain Horner–Trantas dots, superficial infiltrates of degenerated eosinophils, lymphocytes, polymorphonuclear cells, and epithelial cells.[38] Corneal involvement is generally mild with an epithelial keratopathy, but in some cases, pannus formation, even epithelial ulceration, can result. A circumscribed, oval-shaped epithelial defect located in

the superior cornea or shield ulcer can be problematic and often requires the administration of topical corticosteroids for resolution. There is a characteristic ropy discharge present in contrast to the thin, watery discharge of acute allergic conjunctivitis. The involved cells appear to be mast cells, goblet cells, which are present in increased numbers, and lymphocytes, which elaborate histamine, mucus, and eosinophilic major basic protein, respectively.

Giant Papillary Conjunctivitis

Because many refractive surgery prospective patients are long-term contact lens wearers, a thorough examination of the palpebral conjunctiva is indicated (Fig 6–11A). Giant papillary conjunctivitis (GPC) has been found in conjunction with contact lens wear, protruding suture material, and the use of prosthe-

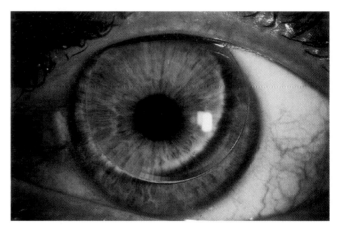

A

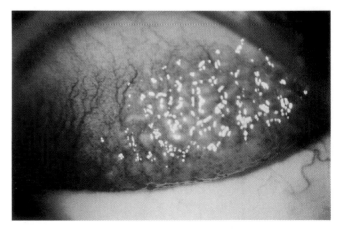

B

Figure 6–11. A. Contact lens wear in a refractive surgery–prospective patient. **B.** Giant papillary conjunctivitis of the upper palpebral conjunctiva.

ses[39] (Fig 6–11B). It has been postulated that protein deposition on the lenses, hypoxia, and bacterial colonization of the lenses are all involved in the pathogenesis of this condition; but this remains unclear. The hypothesis that protein deposits build up on the surface of the contact lens, which may become altered and act as antigens in initiating a type I hypersensitivity response, is supported by the amelioration of symptoms simply by discontinuation of contact lens wear. Keratorefractive surgery is thus a viable alternative for many patients with giant papillary conjunctivitis (Figs 6–12, 6–13). Other factors must be involved as well, as these patients do not have a history of atopy. The features of full-blown GPC are excess mucus production, giant papillae formation on the upper palpebral conjunctiva,

and contact lens intolerance; interestingly, some patients do not have such severe signs. Histopathologic examination of affected conjunctiva reveals plasma cells, lymphocytes, mast cells, eosinophils, and basophils. In addition, tear IgE is elevated in these patients. Therefore, a combination of types I and IV hypersensitivity reactions may be the etiologic basis for this condition. Some patients have a history of GPC, despite a lack of active symptoms; this should be clearly determined and appropriately treated before entertaining a refractive surgery procedure.

Ocular Cicatricial Pemphigoid

The ocular surface may be the site of involvement in chemical burns (Fig 6–14) and in immunologic condi-

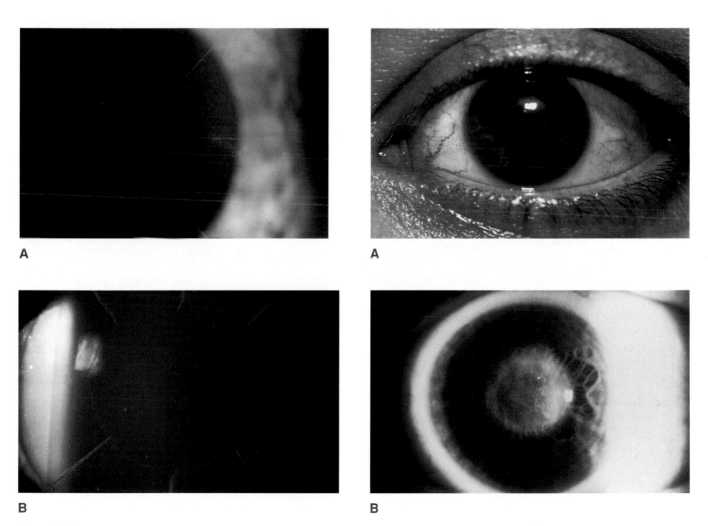

Figure 6–12. A. Appearance of the cornea after radial keratotomy in a patient with giant papillary conjunctivitis. **B.** Retroillumination showing superficial epithelial keratitis in close proximity to the "optical zone" marker.

Figure 6–13. A. External appearance of cornea following PRK. **B.** The extent of light scattering in the area of the scar is extenuated by photographing the same eye with scleral scatter.

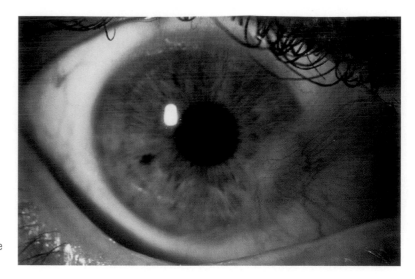

Figure 6–14. Development of superficial pannus at the site of involvement of corneal thermal injury.

tions, including bullous diseases of the skin and mucous membranes; examples of such conditions are ocular cicatricial pemphigoid, bullous pemphigoid, Stevens–Johnson syndrome, and Reiter's syndrome. It is important to diagnose these conditions in order to avoid exacerbation of the disease process following ocular surgery. Perhaps the most commonly seen of these is ocular cicatricial pemphigoid (OCP), a chronic, progressive disease. The early signs of disease of conjunctival hyperemia, papillary response, and chemosis are nonspecific. A key diagnostic feature that indicates chronicity is foreshortening of the inferior fornix. A characteristic subepithelial fibrosis appears as white fibrous tissue readily visible just beneath the superficial conjunctiva; with progression of the disease this can contract, resulting in symblepharon formation. Additionally, the goblet cells are affected and lacrimal gland ducts sclerosed, resulting in both mucus and aqueous tear deficiency.[40] These each can cause devastating effects on the cornea, which may be further compromised by trichiatic lashes, exposure, and secondary conjunctival cicatrization.

The involvement of the cornea in OCP has been well characterized by Foster as follows: Conjunctival inflammation and minimal fibrosis with mucoid discharge comprise stage 1. The development of cicatricial changes in the inferior fornix designates stage 2. Stage 3 is marked by progression of cicatrization, early corneal involvement, trichiasis, and manifestation of tear film disturbance. Finally, stage 4 is represented by severe dry eye with keratinization of the ocular surface and ankyloblepharon formation. The diagnosis is not difficult in advanced cases; however, early manifestations may be nonspecific in middle-aged adults. Subepithelial fibrosis is a reliable sign to screen for this condition.

A variety of other causes of cicatricial changes of the conjunctiva should be determined in the evaluation of the ocular surface of a potential refractive surgery patient. A history of adenoviral or beta-hemolytic streptococcal conjunctivitis or radiation exposure may explain some degree of conjunctival scarring that generally does not progress as does OCP. In addition, any history of Stevens–Johnson syndrome can explain mild to severe conjunctival changes, and some medications have been found to cause a similar appearance. The glaucoma medications are perhaps the most frequent offenders: epinephrine, pilocarpine, and ecothiophate. The antiviral medication, idoxuridine, has been implicated as well.[41]

Connective Tissue Disease

Systemic rheumatologic disease can be manifest initially in the eye, which makes the ophthalmologist very important in the evaluation of these patients. The systemic vasculitis most likely to involve the eye is rheumatoid arthritis. In this condition, the diagnosis is usually made before the ocular manifestations occur, of which keratoconjunctivitis sicca is the most common. Sjögren's syndrome in 24% to 31% of rheumatoid arthritis patients has been demonstrated by lacrimal gland biopsy.[42] This syndrome can cause corneal disease, which may be a mild epitheliopathy or may progress to sterile or infectious infiltration of the peripheral cornea with attendant acute keratitis, sclerosing keratitis, or keratolysis.[43] Fifteen percent of patients with rheumatoid arthritis show corneal involvement, which most frequently takes the form of sterile peripheral stromal infiltration accompanied by episcleritis.[44] Of the severe manifestations, the most common is a sclerosing keratitis, in which peripheral stromal opacification progresses accompanied by stromal vascularization and associated scleritis. Acute stromal keratitis also occurs in the setting of scleritis, whereas furrowing of the cornea may occur without scleritis. Refractive surgery should be avoided in these patients. Melting of the cornea, or keratolysis, the most severe of these corneal manifestations, is an aggressive, destructive process that can result in perforation (Fig 6–15). The proposed etiology of these findings is type III (immune complex) hypersensitivity; circulating immune complexes have been isolated from the serum and synovial fluid of these patients.[45] With appropriate treatment, including

immunosuppressive therapy, the disease process may be halted. Significant astigmatism and surface irregularity may bring the patient to the attention of the refractive surgeon. Keratorefractive surgery may worsen the ocular condition and is contraindicated (Fig 6–15).

Systemic lupus erythematosus can cause a superficial epitheliopathy, keratoconjunctivitis sicca, and, rarely, peripheral ulcerative keratitis. Corneal thinning may rarely occur centrally, requiring patch grafting (Fig 6–16). The corneal manifestations of polyarteritis nodosa tend to be severe, consisting of peripheral ulceration that can accelerate to involve the entire limbal region. There is loss of tissue secondary to the enzymes

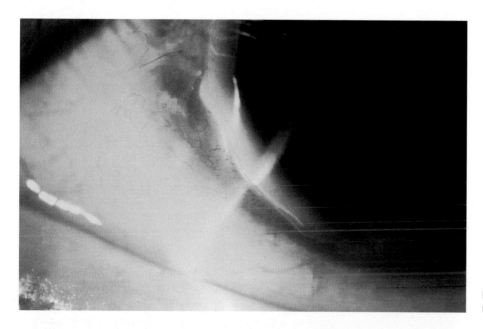

Figure 6–15. Rheumatoid melting of the corneal periphery.

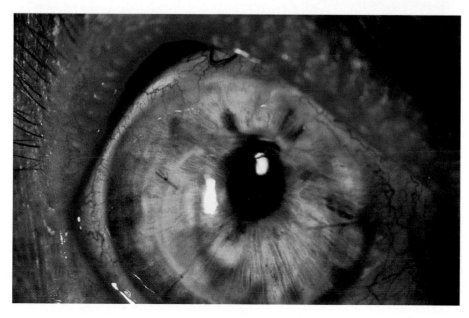

Figure 6–16. Appearance of corneal patch graft for perforated desmatocoele that occurred in the central cornea.

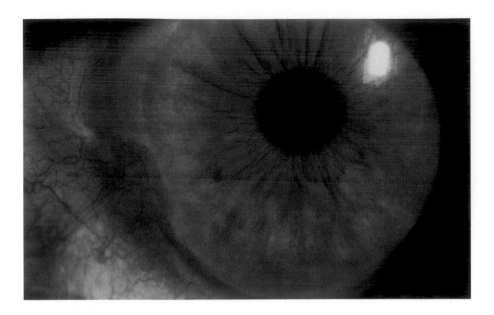

Figure 6–17. Fuchs' marginal keratitis.

produced by the phagocytic white blood cells attracted to the region by immune complex formation. Peripheral ulcerative keratitis can also be seen in Wegener's granulomatosis, even as the presenting sign of disease. The lesion starts at one region of the limbus and can progress to involve the entire limbus, even moving centrally. Fuchs' marginal keratitis may have a similar presentation (Fig 6–17). Relapsing polychondritis is characterized by inflammation of the cartilage of the ears, nose, and trachea. This serious disorder can be accompanied by peripheral ulcerative keratitis thought to be secondary to the formation of antibodies against type II collagen. Progressive systemic sclerosis can have the following ocular manifestations: keratoconjunctivitis sicca, foreshortening of the inferior fornix, and blepharophimosis.

Mooren's Ulcer

Mooren's ulcer was first characterized by Bowman, but it was in 1854 that the name Mooren became associated with this rare entity. This idiopathic peripheral ulcerative keratitis is unaccompanied either by episcleritis or by scleritis and can be unilateral or bilateral. Young men often have the more severe bilateral form of disease. The ulcer begins peripherally and progresses both circumferentially and centrally. There is infiltration of the involved cornea, followed by vascularization and thinning. This process is thought to be related to type III hypersensitivity reaction, with phagocytic cells causing much of the tissue destruction by the elaboration of powerful enzymes. Again, these patients may be re-

ferred for keratorefractive evaluation because of astigmatism, but keratorefractive surgery should be avoided because of the risks of uncontrolled perioperative exacerbations.

KERATOCONUS AND CORNEAL DEGENERATIONS

Keratoconus

Keratoconus was first described In 1854 and termed *conical cornea.*[46] This condition is characterized by progressive corneal ectasia, lack of active inflammation, and the formation of a conical protrusion, which may be round or nipple-shaped. Thinning of the cornea is bilateral and is maximal at the apex of the cone; it can result in high myopia and irregular astigmatism (Fig 6–18); consequently, optical correction achieved with rigid contact lenses is often superior to that with spectacles in the early course of the disease process. Ironically, hard contact lens wear has been associated with keratoconus.[47] However, a cause-and-effect relation has not been clearly elucidated.[48] A condition of corneal warpage secondary to contact lens wear was initially described by Hartstein[49] and has been further characterized by Wilson and others, who, based on computer-assisted analysis of videokeratoscope images of 12 contact lens wearers who had distorted or changing keratometry measurements, described the following corneal topographic patterns: central irregular astigmatism, loss of radial symmetry, and reversal of the normal flatting of the cornea from the

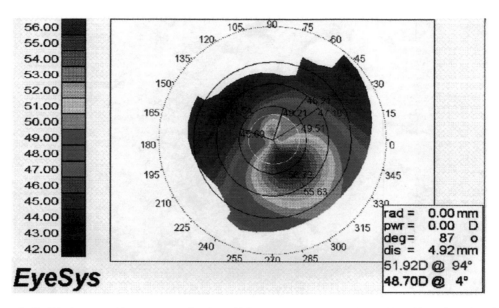

Figure 6–18. Videokeratographic appearance of patient with keratoconus, showing high myopia and irregular astigmatism.

periphery (Fig 6–19).[50] Additionally, the resting position of the contact lens was related to the initial corneal topographic pattern in 9 of 21 eyes and a topographic pattern similar to that seen in keratoconus was found in some patients with superior-riding lenses. They propose the use of a surface asymmetry index, which measures central power disparity between two points 180° apart on the videokeratoscope, to follow central radial corneal symmetry and irregular astigmatism in a qualitative manner. In some cases, 6 months was required to achieve stable topography in patients with contact lens–induced corneal warpage.

Several slit lamp findings are highly characteristic of keratoconus (Fig 6–20). An annulus of corneal epithelial pigment around the base of the cone is termed a *Fleischer ring*. This deposition within the basal epithelium is often best visualized with the cobalt blue filter.[51] Thin, vertical folds within the posterior stroma and Descemet's membrane were first seen by Wischnig and are termed *Vogt's striae*; they are aligned with the steep axis of the cone.[52] Disruption of both Bowman's layer and Descemet's membrane can occur with the development of subsequent anterior stromal scarring and acute corneal hydrops, respectively. The acute development of florid stromal edema and opacification of hydrops will eventually resolve and produce scarring that may actually be associated with improved visual acuity in some patients.[53] Central subepithelial fibrillary structures and prominent corneal nerves have been described in some patients.[53] Munson's sign is a

V-shaped deformation of the lower eyelid upon downgaze; Rizutti's sign is the focused quality of light directed obliquely toward the limbal region. When these classic findings are present, the diagnosis of keratoconus is clear.

Amsler described the angulation of the horizontal axis image of the placido disk in a patient with a form fruste of keratoconus in 1946.[54] Quantitative measurement of corneal curvature was achieved by Rowsey et al in 1981, using a corneascope to detect early inferotemporal steepening with resultant ovalization of the central corneal mire; keratoconus was diagnosed with this instrument before the development of the characteristic slit lamp findings.[55] Computer-assisted analysis of the complex corneal topographic findings of keratoconus was first reported by Klyce in 1984.[56] Several authors further characterized two corneal topographic patterns typical of keratoconus: inferotemporal steepening and central steepening with an associated asymmetric astigmatic pattern.[57,58] In addition, there was a statistically significant difference in the following parameters in eyes with keratoconus, compared with normal eyes:

1. Central corneal power
2. Difference in corneal power between fellow eyes
3. Steepening of the inferior compared with the superior cornea

It has been clearly shown that radial keratotomy performed on patients with keratoconus can result in an unstable cornea, which is at risk for delayed corneal perforation.[59] Computed corneal topographic analysis

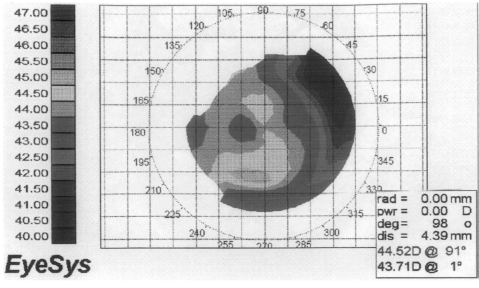

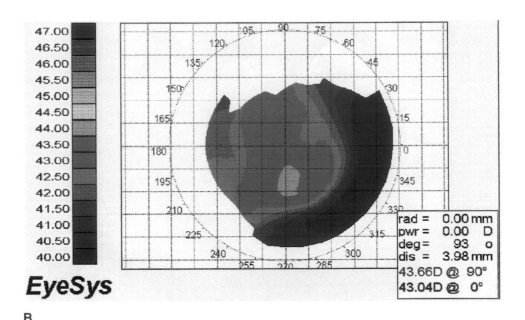

Figure 6–19. A. Corneal warpage secondary to contact lens wear showing central irregular astigmatism and loss of radial symmetry 10 minutes after contact lens discontinuation. **B.** Videokeratographic appearance of cornea 3 weeks after discontinuation of contact lens wear showing partial reversal of corneal warpage.

has improved dramatically over the past few years and can presently serve to detect subtle corneal findings that could impact the outcome of refractive surgery. The earliest findings of keratoconus, which are not discernible by any other diagnostic modality presently available, constitute one example. Wilson and others have described their experience with the use of corneal topography in the process of screening patients for refractive surgical procedures. Thirty-three percent of

these eyes were found to have abnormal topography: 38% of eyes with contact lens–induced warpage and 5.7% of eyes with keratoconus.[60] Potential refractive surgery patients should be thoroughly examined with the benefit of this useful technology in order to detect and appropriately manage corneal topographic abnormalities and to prevent surgical misadventures.

Keratoconus has been found to be clearly associated with atopy, trisomy 21, or Down's syndrome,

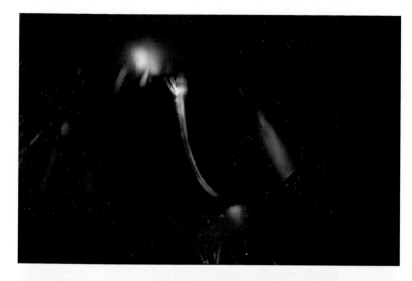

Figure 6–20. Slit lamp appearance of cornea in keratoconus showing apical thinning and scarring as well as forward bulging of the lower lid (Munson's sign).

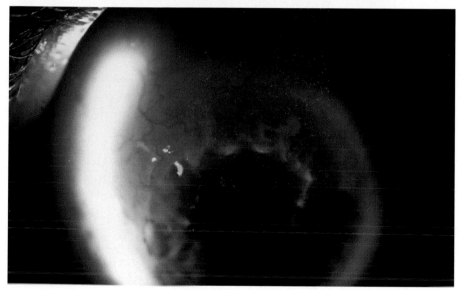

Figure 6–21. Vascularized thin cornea with lipid deposition at the junction of normal and diseased cornea in a patient with Terrien's degeneration following superior patch grafting.

Ehlers–Danlos syndrome, and osteogenesis imperfecta. There are many other connective tissue diseases that have been linked to keratoconus including neurofibromatosis, pseudoxanthoma elasticum, icthyosis, and Marfan's syndrome.[61] The incidence of keratoconus has also been found to be increased in retinitis pigmentosa, Leber's congenital amaurosis, retinal aplasia and coloboma, aniridia, and vernal keratoconjunctivitis.[62]

Noninflammatory Corneal Thinning Disorders

Other noninflammatory corneal thinning disorders include keratoglobus, Terrien's and pellucid marginal degenerations, and posterior keratoconus. Patients with these conditions are not good candidates for refractive surgery. A nonprogressive, diffuse corneal thinning and resultant globular corneal ectasia occurs in kerato-globus, in which there is no evidence of the iron deposition or corneal scarring of keratoconus. The thinning is maximal at the corneal periphery; in this condition the cornea is more prone to perforation from minimal trauma.[63] Treatment is similar to that of keratoconus. In pellucid marginal degeneration the corneal thinning is inferior and peripherally located and the resultant corneal protrusion is above the zone of thinning. Again the slit lamp findings of keratoconus are absent except for Descemet's folds, which are abolished with gentle digital pressure. There are no corneal blood vessels associated with the thinning, which helps to distinguish this condition from Terrien's marginal degeneration. In the latter, the thinned cornea is vascularized and frequently lipid is deposited at the junction of normal and diseased cornea (Fig 6–21). Posterior keratoconus, also known as keratoconus posticus circumscriptus, is an uncommon disorder in which a focal indentation of the central posterior corneal surface can be associated with stromal scarring. In contrast to other conditions in this group, it is usually unilateral and congenital, although rare bilateral cases have been reported in the literature.[64] Mannis et al have described the corneal topography of one patient who had a central area of steepening and paracentral flattening, suggesting that the anterior corneal surface may be involved in this condition.[65] High myopia or astigmatism is commonly noted, but the response of these conditions to keratorefractive procedures is not known. It is believed that conventional keratorefractive procedures are unpredictable, risky, and unstable in patients with corneal thinning disorders. Corneal reinforcement surgery has been advocated for several of these conditions whenever impending perforation, as sometimes occurs in Terrien's marginal degeneration and in keratoglobus, is encountered.

CORNEAL DYSTROPHIES

Epithelial Dystrophies

A corneal dystrophy is a hereditary, bilateral corneal disease that is only rarely associated with systemic disease. The most useful way to classify these conditions is by location of the site of primary pathology. Beginning with the anterior cornea, epithelial dystrophies have in common a predisposition for the development of recurrent erosions and persistent epithelial defects. Both Cogan and Guerry described a syndrome of visible, aberrant epithelial formations, later termed *map–dot–fingerprint* dystrophy. Thickened multilaminar, subepithelial basement membrane material forms areas of thin lines and thicker irregular geographic areas. Intraepithelial microcysts of epithelial-cell debris form dots. These lesions are best visualized with sclerotic scatter or retroillumination. There are data to support the proposal of an autosomal dominant mode of transmission that becomes manifest in middle age. Symptoms are worst in the early morning and visual acuity often improves during the day; there is some resolution of the epithelial edema with evaporation. The etiology of this common dystrophy appears to be related to abnormal basement membrane production, which fails to adhere properly to the overlying epithelium and predisposes to the development of recurrent erosions (Fig 6–22). The cycle of abnormal basement membrane adhesion and impaired epithelial maturation can be broken in some patients with a variety of treatment modalities like anterior stromal micropuncture and epithelial debride-

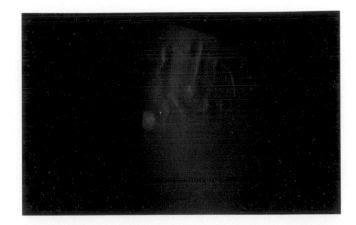

A

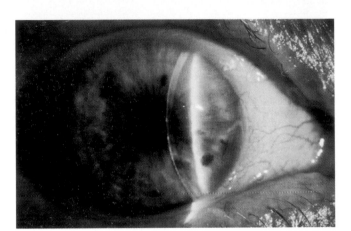

B

Figure 6–22. A. Basement membrane dystrophy. **B.** Abnormal basement membrane production prevents proper adhesion of the overlying epithelium and predisposes to the development of recurrent erosions.

ment. Epithelial debridement with or without excimer laser surgery may be beneficial in recalcitrant cases. Excimer laser surgery may be the procedure of choice for lower myopes suffering from recalcitrant dystrophic recurrent erosions.[66]

Meesmann's dystrophy is characterized by the presence of diffuse, uniform intraepithelial cysts throughout both corneas manifest early in life. Histopathology of these lesions shows a PAS-positive material termed *peculiar substance*, which is as yet unidentified. This autosomal dominant condition was also described by Stocker and Holt in 1955, and histopathologic examination further revealed a thickened basement membrane that was also PAS positive.[67] Symptoms are generally mild and related to mild ocular irritation and foreign body sensation.

In Reis–Bucklers' dystrophy, diffuse, irregular opacities at the level of Bowman's membrane take on a characteristic reticular appearance. The gradual development of intervening anterior stromal haze between these lesions causes decreased visual acuity. This condition also shows autosomal dominant inheritance. Histopathology reveals destruction of Bowman's layer and the accumulation of an indistinct fibrillar material in its place. Although the etiology of this dystrophy remains unclear, the histopathologic features are characteristic and unfortunately result in frequent, recurrent erosions as well as reduction in visual acuity. Anterior membrane dystrophy of Grayson and Wilbrandt and honeycomb dystrophy of Thiel and Behnke may be variants of Reis–Bucklers' dystrophy (Fig 6–23). The anterior location of the lesions in these conditions causes them to respond well to excimer laser keratectomy.

Vortex dystrophy is a term that describes the finding of whorl-like lines within the corneal epithelium (Fig 6–24). These can actually be seen in a variety of settings, with Fabry's disease or its asymptomatic female carriers being the most widely cited. Chloroquine, amiodarone, and indomethacin administration can all result in a similar picture. Band keratopathy can be inherited as a primary disorder whose characteristic histopathologic finding of calcium deposition within the epithelium and Bowman's layer is identical to that seen in the more common condition resulting from chronic ocular irritation or systemic disease (Fig 6–25). Anterior mosaic dystrophy is characterized by polygonal white to gray lesions found in the deep epithelium and Bowman's layer. The intervening clear zones give the crocodile shade of green appearance to the anterior cornea.

Stromal Dystrophies

There are three major stromal dystrophies, which are well characterized. Granular dystrophy, also termed

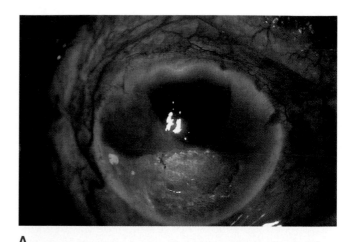

A

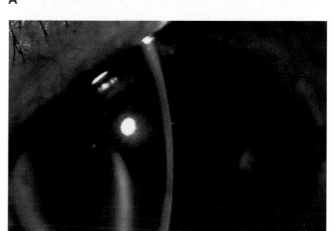

B

Figure 6–24. A. Band keratopathy showing calcium deposition within the epithelium and Bowman's layer in the inferior cornea. **B.** Following EDTA treatment, the cornea is re-epithelialized and shows complete resolution.

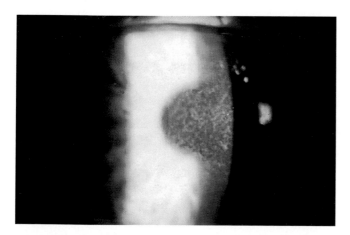

Figure 6–23. Reis-Bucklers' dystrophy with "honeycomb" appearance at the level of Bowman's layer. *(Courtesy of Walter J. Stark, MD.)*

Groenouw's dystrophy type I, is inherited as an autosomal dominant disorder and is manifest early in life with the presence of discrete, gray-white deposits within the central anterior stroma (Fig 6–26). These deposits consist of hyaline degeneration and stain prominently with Masson's trichrome stain.

Lattice dystrophy is an autosomal dominant condition that is readily discernible upon slit lamp examination secondary to the highly characteristic linear opacities that are most prominent in the central corneal stroma. In addition, a haze may be present in the anterior stroma and basal epithelium because of deposition of amyloid, the causative agent of this condition. The amyloid stains with Congo red, is birefringent, exhibits dichroism, and stains with thioflavin-T when viewed under epifluorescent microscopy. In typical lattice dystrophy there is no systemic disease, but lattice dystrophy can be a part of systemic amyloidosis, that is, Meretoja's syndrome or lattice dystrophy type II. In Avellino dystrophy, findings of granular dystrophy are combined with those of lattice dystrophy, as seen in a well-documented family.[68] In each the corneal stroma between the granular deposits is clear in the early course of the disease, but can develop a subtle coarse, ground-glass appearance with time that can profoundly affect visual acuity (Fig 6–27).

Macular dystrophy is inherited as an autosomal recessive disorder and typically involves the entire cornea. It applies early in life in conjunction with reduced vision owing to the indistinct stromal lesions surrounded by milder opacification of the intervening stroma and involvement of the limbus. The endothelium may be involved and the cornea may be thinned. Histopathology of this condition reveals abnormal keratan sulfate-like deposits within the stroma secondary to deficient sulfotransferase, a hydrolytic enzyme, within the cornea. These lesions stain with PAS stain, colloidal iron, and Alcian blue. The profound reduction in visual acuity in these patients generally necessitates penetrating keratoplasty by adulthood.

The other stromal dystrophies are less common and include polymorphic stromal dystrophy, gelatinous droplike dystrophy, central crystalline dystrophy, central cloudy dystrophy, posterior amorphous stromal dystrophy, and congenital hereditary stromal dystrophy. With the exception of gelatinous droplike dystrophy of François, these conditions do not significantly interfere with vision. The response of the cornea in these dystrophies to refractive surgery procedures is not known. In polymorphic stromal dystrophy, irregular, white, axial opacities are seen in the deep stroma and do not affect visual acuity. They represent amyloid deposits, which appear late in life and are not related to lattice dystrophy. Another manifestation of primary amyloidosis is gelatinous droplike dystrophy. This condition may show autosomal recessive inheritance and is characterized by lobular, elevated, accumulated material within the stroma and epithelium of the cornea. Central crystalline dystrophy, or Schnyder's crystalline dystrophy, results in yellow to white linear opacities within the stroma that are found to be composed of neutral fats and cholesterol on histopathologic examination. Prominent corneal arcus and Vogt's limbal girdle may be associated with this condition. Systemic lipid abnormality may or may not be seen in these patients. Central cloudy dystrophy of François rarely affects vision and is characterized by subtle, gray opacities within the deep stroma, which are indistinct and faintly visible under oblique illumination. Patients with posterior amorphous stromal dystrophy exhibit deep stromal, sheetlike opacities that may be combined with iris anomalies like correctopia or pseudopolycoria. In addition, several forms exist and are classified according to predominant site of stromal involvement: central, peripheral, and diffuse. The central cornea may be thinned. Because this disorder is stable and has been seen in conjunction with a variety of iris malformations, it may represent a mesenchymal dysgenesis disorder. Congenital hereditary stromal dystrophy is manifest as flaky opacification of the central and peripheral cornea. Histopathologic examination has revealed abnormal, small collagen fibrils.

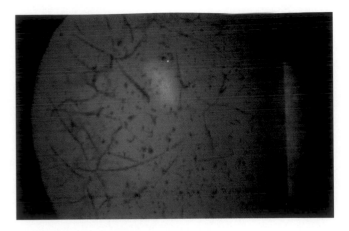

Figure 6–26. Lattice dystrophy.

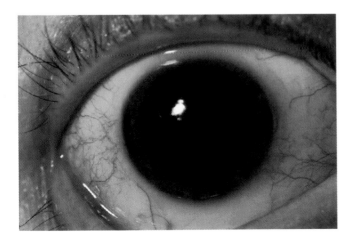

Figure 6–25. Granular dystrophy. An autosomal dominant disorder showing evidence of discrete, gray–white deposits within the central anterior stroma. *(Courtesy of Walter J. Stark, MD.)*

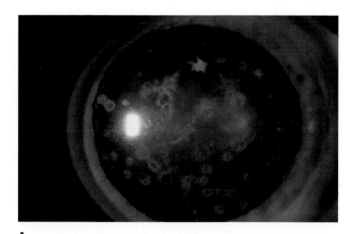

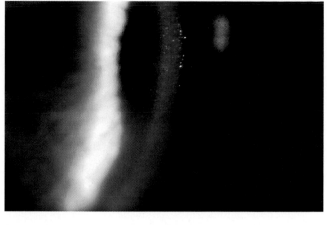

Figure 6–28. Fuchs' late hereditary endothelial dystrophy showing evidence of stromal edema and endothelial irregularities.

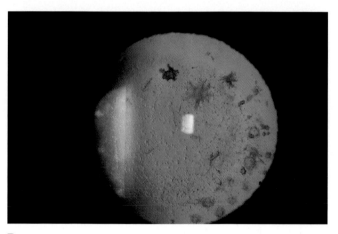

Figure 6–27. A. Avellino dystrophy. Clinical appearance prior to PTK. **B.** The corneal stroma between the granular deposits shows evidence of both subtle linear branching deposits and a ground-glass appearance following PTK. *(Courtesy of Walter J. Stark, MD.)*

edema. Histopathologic examination reveals reduced numbers of endothelial cells and irregular basement membrane material deposited in focal areas. Refractive surgery is generally contraindicated in patients with endothelial dystrophies because of the risks of exacerbating endothelial dysfunction. These patients are good candidates for penetrating keratoplasty.

Endothelial Dystrophies

Congenital hereditary endothelial dystrophy was first described in 1960 by Maumenee.[69] This devastating condition is present at birth, and profound stromal and epithelial edema are evident. It can be inherited as autosomal dominant or recessive. There are no associated systemic or ocular findings. The endothelium and, in some cases, portions of Descemet's membrane are profoundly affected. The etiology is unclear. At the other end of the spectrum lies Fuchs' dystrophy, or late hereditary endothelial dystrophy, a common condition affecting middle-aged women predominantly (Fig 6–28). Gradual deterioration of adequate endothelial-cell functioning results in guttae formation, thickening of Descemet's membrane, and stromal and epithelial

REFERENCES

1. Groden LR, Murphy B, Rodnite J, et al. Lid flora in blepharitis. *Cornea.* 1991;10:50.
2. Belin MW, ed. *External Disease and Cornea in the Basic and Clinical Science Course.* Philadelphia: American Academy of Ophthalmology; 1990.
3. McCulley JP, Sciallis GF. Meibomian keratoconjunctivitis. *Am J Ophthalmol.* 1977;84:788.
4. Browning DJ, Proia AD. Ocular rosacea. *Surv Ophthalmol.* 1986;31:145.
5. Perkins R, Kundsin RB, Pratt M, et al. Bacteriology of normal and infected conjunctiva. *J Clin Microbiol.* 1975;1:147.
6. Gigliotti F, Hendley JO, Morgan J, et al. Efficacy of topical antibiotic therapy in acute conjunctivitis in children. *J Pediatr.* 1984;104:623.
7. O'Brien TP, et al. *Update on Ocular Infectious Diseases.* Baltimore: 1994.
8. Thygeson P, Kimura S. Chronic conjunctivitis. *Trans Am Acad Ophthalmol Otolaryngol.* 1963;67:494.
9. Oriel JD. Chemotherapy. In: Oriel G, Redgeway G, Schachter J, et al, eds. *Chlamydial Infections.* Cambridge, UK: Cambridge University Press; 1986.
10. Dawson C, Hanna W, Wood T, et al. Adenovirus type 8 keratoconjunctivitis in the United States. III. Epidemiologic, clinical and microbiologic features. *Am J Ophthalmol.* 1970;69:473.

11. Pavan-Langston D. Major ocular viral infections. In: Galasso G, Whitely R, Merrigan T, eds. *Antiviral Agents and Viral Diseases of Man*, 3rd ed. New York: Raven Press, 1990.

12. Schrimer O. Studien zur Physiologie und Pathologie der Tranenabsonderung und Tranenabfuhr. *Arch Klin Exp Ophthatmol.* 1903;56:197.

13. van Bijsterveld OP: Diagnostic tests in sicca syndrome. *Arch Ophthalmol.* 1962;82:10.

14. Galen SR. *Beyond Normality.* New York: John Wiley and Sons; 1975.

15. Holly FJ, Lemp MA. Tear physiology and dry eye. *Surv Ophthalmol.* 1977;22:69.

16. Liebman SD. Riley-Day syndrome: long-term ophthalmologic observations. *Trans Am Ophthalmol Soc.* 1968;66:95.

17. Esterly NB, et al. Pupillotonia, hyporeflexia and segmental hypohidrosis: autonomic dysfunction in a child. *J Pediatr.* 1968;73:852.

18. Fox R. Pathogenesis of Sjögren's syndrome. *Rheum Dis Clin North Am.* 1993;18:517.

19. Lemp MA, Dohlman CH, Kuwabara T, et al. Dry eye secondary to mucus deficiency. *Trans Am Acad Ophthalmol Otolaryngol.* 1971;75:1223.

20. Vauley GT, Leopold IH, Gregg TH. Interpretation of tear film breakup. *Arch Ophthalmol.* 1977;95:445.

21. Perkins R, Kundsin RB, Pratt M, et al. Bacteriology of normal and infected conjunctiva. *J Clin Microbiol.* 1975;1:147.

22. Mishima S, Maurice DM. Oily layer of tear film and evaporation from corneal surface. *Exp Eye Res.* 1961; 1:39.

23. Holly FJ. Tear film physiology. *Am J Optom Physiol Opt.* 1980;57:252.

24. Abelson MB, Madiwale N, Weston JH. Conjunctival eosinophils in allergic ocular disease. *Am J Ophthalmol.* 1975; 80:123.

25. Abelson MB, Udell IJ. H2 receptors in the human ocular surface. *Arch Ophthalmol.* 1981;99:302.

26. Weston JH, Udell IJ, Abelson MB. H1 receptors in the human ocular surface. *Invest Ophthalmol Vis Sci.* 1990; 20(suppl):65.

27. Abelson MB, Smith LM, Chambers W. Conjunctival allergen challenge: a clinical approach to studying allergic conjunctivitis. *Arch Ophthalmol.* 1990;108:84.

28. Allansmith MR, Abelson MB. Immunologic diseases. In Smolin G, Thoft RA, eds. *The Cornea,* 1st ed. Boston: Little, Brown; 1983.

29. Rich LF, Hanifin JM. Ocular complications of atopic dermatitis and other eczemas. *Int Ophthalmol Clin.* 1985;25:61.

30. Friedman SJ, Schroeter AL, Hamburger HA. IgE antibodies to *Staphylococcus aureus.* Prevalence in patients with atopic dermatitis. *Arch Dermatol.* 1985;121:869.

31. Hogan MJ. Atopic keratoconjunctivitis. *Am J Ophthalmol.* 1953;36:937.

32. Smolin G, O'Connor GR. *Ocular Immunology.* Philadelphia: Lea & Febiger; 1981.

33. Friedlaender MH. *Allergy and Immunology of the Eye,* 1st ed. San Francisco: Harper & Row; 1970.

34. Tuft SJ, Kemeny DM, Dart JK, et al. Clinical features of atopic keratoconjunctivitis. *Ophthalmology.* 1991;98:150.

35. Hogan. Atopic keratoconjunctivitis. *Am J Ophthalmol.* 1953;36:937.

36. Biegelman MN. *Vernal Conjunctivitis* Los Angeles: University of Southern California Press; 1950.

37. Smolin G, O'Connor GR: *Ocular Immunology.* Philadelphia: Lea & Febiger; 1981.

38. Trantas: Sur le catarrge printaniet. *Arch Ophthalmol (Paris).* 1910;30:593.

39. Allansmith MR, Korb DR, Griener JV, et al. Giant papillary conjunctivitis in contact lens wearers. *Am J Ophthalmol.* 1977;83:697.

40. Leonard JN, Wright P, Haffenden GP, et al. Skin diseases and the dry eye. *Trans Ophthalmol Soc UK.* 1985;104:467.

41. Patten JT, Cavanaugh HD, Allansmith MR. Induced ocular pseudopemphigoid. *Am J Ophthalmol.* 1977;83:443.

42. Ericson S, Sundmark E. Studies on the sicca syndrome in patients with rheumatoid arthritis. *Acta Rheum Scand.* 1970;16:60.

43. Watson PG, Hayreth SS. Scleritis and episcleritis. *Br J Ophthalmol.* 1976;60:163.

44. See 12 Watson

45. Jayson MIV, Easty DL. Ulceration of the cornea in rheumatoid arthritis. *Ann Rheum Dis.* 1977;36:428.

46. Nottingham, G. *Practical Observations on Conical Cornea.* London: 1854.

47. Brightbill FS, Stainer GA. Previous hard contact lens wear in keratoconus. *Contact Intraocul Lens Med J.* 1979;5:43.

48. Gasset AR, Houde WL, Garcia-Bongochea M. Hard contact lens wear as an environmental risk in keratoconus. *Am J Ophthalmol.* 1978;85:339.

49. Hartstein J. Corneal warping due to wearing of corneal contact lenses: a report of 12 cases. *Am J Ophthalmol.* 1964; 71:348.

50. Wilson SE, et al. Topographic changes in contact lens-induced corneal warpage. *Ophthalmology.* 1990;97:737.

51. Glass JD. The iron lines of the superficial cornea: Hudson-Stahle line, Stocker's line and Fleischer's ring. *Arch Ophthalmol.* 1964;71:348.

52. Vogt A. Reflexlinien durch Faltung spiegein der Grenzflachen im Bereiche von Corneo, Linsenkapsel und Netzhaut. *von Graefes Arch Ophthalmol.* 1919;99:296.

53. Bron AJ, et al. Fibrillary lines of the cornea. A clinical sign in keratoconus. *Br J Ophthalmol.* 1975;59:136.

54. Amsler M. Keratocone classique at keratocone fruste: arguments unitaires. *Ophthalmologica.* 1946;111:96.

55. Rowsey JJ, et al. Corneal topography: corneoscope. *Arch Ophthalmol.* 1981;99:1093.

56. Klyce SD. Computer assisted corneal topography high resolution graphic presentation and analysis of keratoscopy. *Invest Ophthalmol Vis Sci.* 1992;25:1426.

57. Wilson SE, et al. Corneal topography of keratoconus. *Cornea.* 1992;10:2.

58. Rabinowitz YS, et al. Computer assisted corneal topography of keratoconus. *Refract Corneal Surg.* 1989;5:400.
59. Durand L. Complications of radial keratotomy: eyes with keratoconus and late wound dehiscence. *Refract Corneal Surg.* 1992;8:311.
60. Wilson SE, Klyce SD. Screening of corneal topographic abnormalities before refractive surgery. *Ophthalmology.* 1992;101:147.
61. Krachmer JH, et al. Keratoconus and related noninflammatory corneal thinning disorders. *Surv Ophthalmol.* 1984; 28:293.
62. Duke-Eider S, Leigh AG. *System of Ophthalmology: Diseases of the Outer Eye.* London: Henry Klimpton; 1985;8:964.
63. Gregoratos N, et al. Blue sclerae with keratoglobus and brittle cornea. *Br J Ophthalmol.* 1971;55:42.
64. Goldsmith AJB. Bilateral circumscribed posterior conical cornea. *Trans Ophthalmol Soc UK.* 1943;63:180.
65. Mannis W, et al: Corneal topography of posterior keratoconus. *Cornea.* 1992;11:351.
66. Azar DT, Jain S, Woods K, et al. Phototherapeutic keratectomy. In Salz JJ, McDonnell PJ, McDonald MB, eds. *Corneal Laser Surgery.* St. Louis, MO: Mosby-Year Book; 1995:213–226.
67. Stocker FW, Holt LB. Rare form of hereditary epithelial dystrophy. *Arch Ophthalmol.* 1955;53:536.
68. Folberg R, Alfonso E, Croxatto O, et al. Clinically atypical granular dystrophy with pathologic features of lattice-like amyloid deposits. *Ophthalmology.* 1988;95:47.
69. Maumenee AE. Congenital hereditary corneal dystrophy. *Am J Ophthalmol.* 1960;50:1114.

CHAPTER 7

Patient Evaluation for Refractive Surgery

Jonathan Carr ■ Peter Hersh

Two aspects of refractive surgery make it a unique surgical procedure necessitating a novel approach to patient selection and preoperative evaluation. First, the eye to be operated upon is generally healthy. Second, success is ultimately defined by patient satisfaction, an outcome comprising both objective and subjective patient perceptions.

PHILOSOPHICAL ISSUES

Increased patient interest and evolving attitudes toward refractive surgery within the profession now make it important that all ophthalmologists be conversant with the complete menu of surgical and nonsurgical options for the ametropic patient so that they can properly counsel their patients regarding the advisability and the risks and benefits of each of these procedures. Although some surgeons may philosophically advise against any type of surgical intervention in an otherwise healthy eye, it remains the ophthalmologist's responsibility to afford considered information and advice to potential refractive surgical patients.

The most common reason for a patient requesting refractive surgery is the desire for independence from spectacle or contact lens correction. Whereas the former goal may derive from the difficulty that patients may incur wearing spectacles for a number of lifestyle activities (for example, sporting and outdoor pursuits), the latter may be related to various perceived or actual problems with contact lens wear. Patients often find contact lens wear inconvenient. Moreover, actual discomfort or more severe difficulties with contact lenses may drive the patient toward refractive surgical options.

Although all forms of refractive surgery have inherent risks to the healthy eye, other forms of optical correction are not without potential problems. Patients who perceive difficulty with their spectacles may simply not wear their corrective lenses, living instead day-to-day with uncorrected, relatively poor vision that may place them in a suboptimal circumstance or, during some activities, at actual risk. For example, some patients with 20/20 vision may choose to live with vision of 20/80 because of a perceived difficulty with spectacles. Moreover, contact lenses may have actual morbidities, ranging from minimal discomfort to sight-threatening infections. Giant papillary conjunctivitis, sequelae of corneal hypoxia, sterile infiltration, and microbial keratitis may all complicate contact lens wear, precluding successful use in many patients. In one well-controlled study, users of extended-wear lenses had a 10- to 15-fold risk of ulcerative keratitis compared with daily-wear soft lens users.[1] In a related article, the annual incidence of ulcerative keratitis was described as 20.9 per 10,000 when using extended-wear soft contact lenses, and 4.1 per 10,000 when using daily-wear soft contact lenses.[2] Although refractive surgical procedures are not without risk, patients who are using contact lenses are also ultimately accepting a degree of risk to their sight.

Thus, the philosophical decision whether to undertake refractive surgery is not simply one of whether it is appropriate to operate on an otherwise healthy eye. Rather, specific patient circumstances must be carefully considered in order for both the ophthalmologist and the patient to arrive at an appropriate, informed decision.

GUIDELINES FOR PATIENT SELECTION

As experience with refractive surgery has improved, insight has been gained into the absolute and relative contraindications associated with these procedures (Table 7–1). Ideally, a prospective patient should have an entirely normal eye with an appropriate refractive error. However, patients often request treatment of eyes that have problems for which surgery might be contraindicated.

Absolute Contraindications

Although advice regarding the propriety of refractive surgery must always be individualized to each patient's risk–benefit ratio, the following situations suggest that refractive surgery be avoided. Patients with systemic immunologic disorders like rheumatoid arthritis, systemic lupus erythematosus, polyarteritis nodosa, and other collagen vascular diseases are at risk of inflammatory and wound-healing sequelae that may cause severe corneal complications. Refrac-

tive surgery in such patients should be avoided. Contraindications may also derive from the health of the eye itself. Patients with severe dry eye syndromes, including those with conjunctival cicatrizing disorders like Stevens–Johnson syndrome, ocular cicatricial pemphigoid, and the chemically burned ocular surface, are poor candidates because of wound-healing problems that may supervene following surgery (see Chapter 4). Patients with keratoconus and other ectatic corneal dystrophies should be identified preoperatively. Such patients may frequently present to the refractive surgical practice because of their poor vision with optical correction. Because the optical and physical effects of refractive procedures and the long-term prognosis are unclear in these patients, refractive surgery is contraindicated in such situations. Similarly, patients with irregular astigmatism should be advised against refractive procedures, although future research and developments may address this patient subset.

Relative Contraindications

Immunodeficiency of any cause is a relative contraindication to refractive surgical procedures on the basis both of possible aberrant wound healing and of predisposition to infection in such patients. One might be less likely to perform photorefractive keratectomy on a diabetic patient, for instance, for fear of a persistent epithelial defect following surgery. Preexisting corneal disease may lead to advice against any form of refractive surgery. Patients with a history of herpetic keratitis, for example, may be at risk for recrudescence of the disease following surgery. The response of patients with corneal dystrophies, degenerations, and dysgeneses is unclear. A patient with a mild degree of dry eye may be intolerant of contact lens wear and may reasonably be considered for a refractive procedure, although the added risk should be considered in deciding to perform such a procedure rather than correcting with spectacles.

Patients with glaucoma, too, should be treated with caution, especially if postoperative corticosteroid use may exacerbate the patients' intraocular pressure problems. Patients with incipient cataract should also be avoided because refractive errors can be corrected during subsequent cataract surgery. Monocularity is generally a contraindication for refractive surgery in the good eye. However, surgery in the amblyopic eye may be undertaken in selected cases. Finally, prospective patients under the age of 18 to 21 years proba-

TABLE 7–1. REFRACTIVE SURGERY CONTRAINDICATIONS

Contraindication	Specificity	Conditions
Absolute	General	Systemic collagen vascular disease
	Eye specific	Keratoconus, other ectatic corneal dystrophies
		Irregular astigmatism
		Ocular surface disease: (chemical injury, conjunctival cicatricial disease)
Relative	General	Immunodeficiency
		Diabetes mellitus
	Eye specific	Monocularity
		Dry eye
		Other preexisting corneal diseases

bly should not be considered as their refraction may not be stable.[3,4]

THE PREOPERATIVE CONSULTATION VISIT

The goals of the preoperative consultation visit are two-fold. First, it is important to assess prospective patients carefully in order to assure that only those considered appropriate actually undergo surgery (Table 7–2). Moreover, it is critically important to assess patient expectations before embarking on irreversible surgical procedures. It must always be stressed that the goal of refractive surgery is to reduce the patient's *dependency* on glasses and contact lenses—not to make all patients free from all optical appliances for all tasks at all times. Patients with such expectations will often be disappointed.

The patient often has contemplated at great length the risks and benefits of refractive surgery and has already made the decision to undergo it. Nevertheless, a thorough discussion of the data on the various available refractive procedures is important to inform the patient fully. Other patients simply present to the office for information regarding refractive surgery in general as well for advice about their specific circumstance. In all cases, the risk and benefits of the different procedures should be explored in addition to the patient's desires and expectations.

Assessment of Contraindications and Appropriateness for Surgery

A patient history should be taken to assess any absolute or relative contraindications to surgery. In addition to the contraindications cited above, there are a number of

TABLE 7– 2. GUIDELINES FOR PREOPERATIVE EXAMINATION

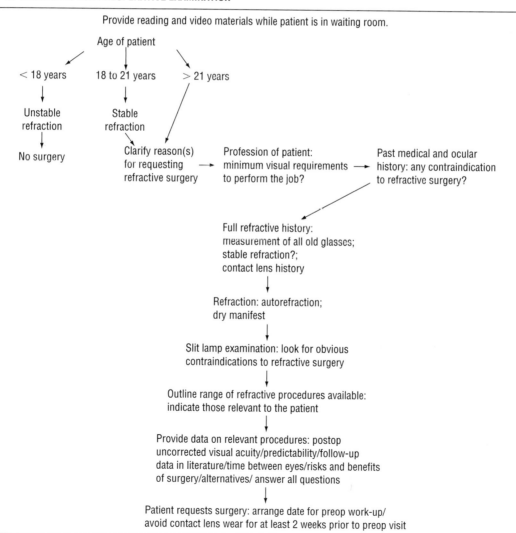

situations where the surgeon will advise the patient against refractive surgery. Stability of the patient's refraction over time should be ascertained. Review of old spectacles, prescriptions, or patient charts may give the appropriate assurance of refractive stability. Refractive surgery rarely should be undertaken on the basis of a single day's refraction. If corroborating data are not available, the patient should be scheduled on another day to verify the refraction measurements.

The patient who presents from another refractive surgeon requesting fellow eye surgery when dissatisfied with the procedure of the first eye requires close scrutiny. Such patients often have unrealistic expectations and will probably not be satisfied with the outcome of a second procedure. If there is any doubt, it is wise to advise against further procedures.

Assessment of Patient Needs and Expectations

One priority of the initial consultation visit is careful documentation of the patient's reason for wanting refractive surgery. The most commonly offered is the desire to be independent of glasses or contact lenses, a wish commonly voiced by patients who are physically intolerant of contact lenses. In such cases, it is important to elicit the actual reason for the patient's inability to wear contact lenses—for example, a dry eye or severe ocular allergy—because this may have a bearing on whether or not to proceed with surgery.

The other main group of factors compelling patients to consider refractive surgery relates to professional or specific leisure activities. Visual requirements of certain occupations, such as in law enforcement, the armed forces, and the aviation industries, and the acceptability of the various refractive surgical procedures by the authorities in these professions should be ascertained. The patient with 20/20 postoperative vision will be dissatisfied if rules of their chosen profession preclude refractive surgery. Specific visual tasks should also be explored. For instance, patients with certain professions should be advised against surgery when uncorrected near acuity is as important as distance acuity.

Investigators have explored the demographic characteristics of prospective radial keratotomy patients and have analyzed their particular motivations for requesting surgery.[5,6] Of radial keratotomy patients in the Prospective Evaluation of Radial Keratotomy (PERK) study, 73% of women and 58% of men wanted surgery in order to avoid being dependent on glasses. This included a fear of being without corrective lenses in an emergency. Thirteen percent of all PERK patients had

previously worn glasses but not contact lenses, 34% of patients wore both glasses and contact lenses, and 53% had tried contact lenses and reverted to wearing glasses alone. Interestingly, only one third of patients who had stopped wearing contact lenses did so because of physical or physiologic problems. Other reasons for desiring RK included occupational reasons (6% of cases), participation in sports (5%), and cosmesis (3%).

A recent study of patients undergoing excimer laser photorefractive keratectomy (PRK) similarly has shown approximately half of patients citing independence from glasses or contact lenses as their primary reason for undergoing PRK. Only 5% cite sports or occupational endeavors as their primary motivation (Hersh P, 1996, unpublished data).

Review of Risks and Benefits

Those procedures relevant to the patient's particular refractive error should be clearly explained. This includes the usual indices of success, such as uncorrected visual acuity of 20/20 or 20/40 and estimations of the predictability and stability of the refractive correction. Well-informed patients will often want a review of published studies of the various procedures. The surgeon thus should have knowledge of such information (see Chapters 21 and 33).

When outlining the risks of the procedure, it is helpful to stratify them into the optical side effects and the medical–physical risks. Optical risks should include discussion of undercorrection and overcorrection. It is helpful for most patients to have this demonstrated by over- and undercorrecting their myopia using lenses in a trial frame, even though this is only an approximate example. Presbyopia and the immediate or ultimate need for near correction should be addressed in addition to possible refractive changes as the patient ages. Subjective optical problems should also be explained in detail, particularly glare, halos, and the starburst phenomenon. The extent to which these various optical side effects play a role in the different refractive procedures under consideration should also be reviewed. For example, starbursts might be more likely to occur after an eight-incision radial keratotomy with a small optical zone (and a large pupil size) than after PRK. Diurnal fluctuation of vision following radial keratotomy and long-term expectations of refractive stability should also be discussed.

When discussing ultimate visual acuity, it is perhaps best to inform patients of their relative chances of obtaining both 20/20 and 20/40 vision after a specific procedure for their refractive error. However, because there is a chance that the patient may fall into the categories of over- and undercorrection, this risk must be acceptable to the patient before proceeding with surgery. The ability to perform reoperations in the event of suboptimal correction and the expectations of such enhancement procedures should be reviewed.

Patients who have reached the age of presbyopia should understand that obtaining emmetropia will necessitate the use of reading glasses postoperatively. Many patients will not find this a problem because they prefer to have unaided distance acuity rather than reading acuity. However, some older patients may not understand this point, and, after hearing it explained, will elect to defer the procedure. Some patients may be candidates for monovision, with refractive surgical correction of only the dominant eye, leaving the nondominant eye myopic for near vision (see Chapter 10). Preoperative trial of monovision contact lens correction may predict which patients will be satisfied with this option.

More general ocular risks include corneal scarring or infection, which potentially could limit the best-corrected visual acuity and ultimately require penetrating keratoplasty. Micro- and macroperforations of the cornea are a real risk in both RK and automated lamellar keratoplasty (ALK), whereas this is somewhat less of a risk in excimer PRK. One point to discuss in preoperative RK cases is the anticipated strategy in the case of perforation—perhaps discontinuing the procedure before completion and continuing at a later date if advisable. This will allay the patient's fears should perforation occur (see Chapter 25).

Finally, there is a theoretical risk of a patient suffering from vision-threatening complications like corneal melting, cataract, and endophthalmitis after the procedure. The patient should be apprised of these risks and the incidence of their occurrence. Moreover, in cases where preoperative visual acuity is less than 20/20 secondary to other pathologies, it must be understood that the refractive procedure will not improve this baseline best-corrected vision.

Discussion of the potential benefits of the planned refractive procedure requires that the surgeon impart honest, realistic information to the patient so that he or she can decide in an informed manner. Unfortunately, the many advertisements testifying to the fact that you will *throw away your glasses* encourage the patient to think that these are risk-free procedures. If the surgeon does nothing to correct this misimpression, there is a real risk that, in the event of a legitimate complication, a

fully informed consent might not have been obtained. Often, giving the patient time to review the consultation and develop further questions will be rewarded by a more knowledgeable patient who has appropriate expectations of the procedure's outcomes.

Reading Materials

The majority of patients will wish to think about their options after the initial meeting, which is often a screening-type visit. It is helpful to offer appropriate reading materials for further patient education. This can even involve giving certain motivated patients copies of actual journal articles in which the salient information is highlighted. Videotapes may be helpful as well.

Patient education materials have developed in recent years as a response to legal and patient-related issues. Such materials should address the main issues and go some way to impart enough information for the patient to be able to give an informed consent. The educational materials may contain the following:

- review of ocular anatomy and a discussion of refractive error and astigmatism
- outline of the preoperative visit and what should be expected by the patient before, during, and after surgery
- outline of the particular surgical procedures available and their indications
- outline of the likely postoperative course
- list of benefits to expect as a result of the procedure, including the published success of the procedure(s)
- description of the risks and complications of the procedure(s) and perhaps a sample of the informed consent form
- suggestions for treatment alternatives, including glasses and contact lenses

Questionnaire

Preoperative patient questionnaires are an easy way for the surgeon to obtain information about his or her refractive surgery population. Questionnaires to assess the level of patient education and patient awareness can be used before surgery, which can lead the surgeon to present a more or less complex explanation during the preoperative visits. Questionnaires given during the postoperative course can help alter the surgeon's usual postoperative management.

Time Interval Between Eyes

The time period between surgery on the first and second eye varies for the different types of procedure. It is important to apprise the patient of this interval because of the optical consequences of uniocular treatment. It may also influence which procedure a patient elects to undergo. Currently most surgeons performing RK are comfortable offering their patients fellow eye surgery within a few weeks. In contrast, patients having PRK must currently wait 3 months between eyes to comply with the recommendations of the US Food and Drug Administration in the current clinical trials. Similarly, patients undergoing ALK on both eyes are likely to wait approximately 2 to 3 months between eyes, as the surgeon will want to evaluate the effect of surgery on the first eye in order to predict more accurately predict the outcome for the second eye.

GUIDELINES FOR PREOPERATIVE EXAMINATION

Following the initial information consultation visit, the complete preoperative examination should take place (Table 7–3).

Eye Examination

The preoperative visit is usually the patient's second visit. During this visit, it is important to provide an entirely normal ocular exam, including dilated fundus examination. One needs to be particularly careful in examining the anterior segment to look for preexisting corneal diseases that might contraindicate a refractive procedure.

Refraction

Refraction is the most important part of the examination and is best carried out by two separate observers to assure accurate measurements. A cycloplegic refraction should also be obtained to confirm that the patient is not accommodating during the dry refraction. All refractions should be compared and any discrepancies resolved. If refractions are not consistent and reproducible, the patient must be reexamined on another occasion (see Chapter 8).

Keratometry

Keratometry readings and refractive astigmatism should agree, and any irregularities of keratometer mires evaluated to expose ocular surface disorders or incipient keratoconus.

Computer-Assisted Videokeratography

Corneal topography has become a standard for assessment of prospective refractive surgery patients. Investigators have demonstrated situations where a topographic map of the cornea may change a decision about a refractive procedure.[7] For example, computerized topography may reveal a heretofore undiagnosed case of keratoconus, a contraindication for refractive surgery.[8,9] Topography has also been used to assess the severity of other ectatic corneal diseases.[10,11] Even though these diseases should be revealed with a good clinical examination, routine preoperative corneal topography can aid in identifying mild cases of such pathologies.

The corneal topographic map may used in the surgical planning of the patient's treatment. For astigmatic and other procedures, it is useful to have a map available in the operating room for reference during the procedure. The map can subsequently be used in the postoperative period to generate a differential topography map that illustrates exactly what the particular procedure has achieved. This facilitates decisions in subsequent management of the patient.

Contrast Sensitivity and Glare Testing

A baseline contrast sensitivity test may be helpful when there are postoperative complaints of *foggy* vision, *dull* vision, and glare, cases in which an abnormal contrast sensitivity or glare test may be found.

Perioperative Contact Lens Wear

It is common practice for prospective refractive surgery patients to discontinue lens wear prior to assessment in order to ensure that refractive measurements are taken of a cornea whose topography has not been perturbed by the contact lens—soft lenses about 1 week and rigid lenses 3 weeks, preoperatively.

A proportion of contact lens wearers are going to have abnormal corneal topographies preoperatively, and some of these will be considered to have contact lens–induced corneal warpage.[12] A patient with a topographic pattern suggestive of keratoconus who also wears contact lenses should be invited back for repeat topography after a period without contact lens wear. This would also apply to patients who have irregular astigmatism in the presence of contact lens wear. How long should we routinely expect contact lens wearers who have these problems with corneal warpage to discontinue their use of contact lenses preoperatively? Wil-

TABLE 7–3. GUIDELINES FOR PREOPERATIVE EXAMINATION

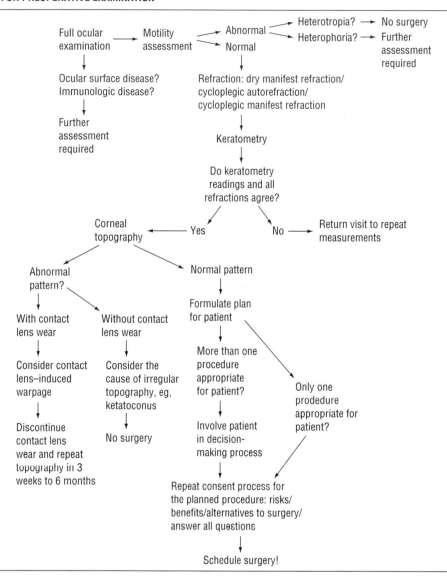

son suggests that for persons wearing soft contact lenses whose topographies suggest corneal warpage, a period of 1 to 1.5 months would probably be sufficient, although if such patients still have an abnormal topographic pattern after that period, further time without the lenses should be allowed before any decisions are made.[12]

An additional contact lens–related issue to consider is their use during the time interval before treatment of the second eye. During this time there will be a problem with anisometropia and aniseikonia. The patient who has less than a 3 D difference between the two eyes may not require any correction in the fellow eye between surgeries. For some patients, this

monovision is the endpoint in their management, and they will not want surgery to correct their error in the second eye. Significant anisometropia requires contact lens correction, and for motivated patients who have been contact lens intolerant, further contact lens wear can usually be tolerated in the short term. Other patients in this situation will simply leave their second eye uncorrected while waiting for surgery. The patient who wears a contact lens in the second eye is usually asked to stop using the lens at least 1 week prior to surgery. Clearly for a patient in whom one has suspected contact lens–induced corneal warpage, no contact lens wear should be allowed between surgery on the two eyes.

Pupil Size

Measurement of the diameter of the entrance pupil in both light and dark conditions may identify patients who have very large pupils, which may exacerbate edge effects of the optical zone following refractive procedures (for example, glare, halo, and the starburst phenomenon).

Ocular Dominance

Ocular dominance should be ascertained preoperatively. Asking the patient to look through a hole in a card and observing the eye used is one clue to the preferred eye. In addition, the patient may be instructed to hold a finger in front of the two eyes and gaze at a distant object. The patient should see two images of the finger, with the denser image contralateral to the dominant eye. Assessment of ocular dominance is important as it is preferable to recommend surgery on the nondominant eye initially, in order to bring any information learned from surgery on the first eye to the operation on the second. If only uniocular surgery is recommended in anticipation of monovision, however, surgery on the dominant eye should be considered.

Ocular Motility Issues

Accurate examination of the patient for heterophoria and heterotropia is required. Patients with a heterotropia may suffer from either diplopia or amblyopia, which will probably contraindicate refractive surgery. The patient with a phoria may well have problems after refractive surgery if not recognized and appropriately counseled. For example, consider the young myopic patient who has worn spectacles that are slightly decentered so that the patient is looking through that part of the lens nasal to the optical center. This patient will have spent considerable time looking through base-in prism. Any coexisting exophoria at near will therefore become much more difficult to control following refractive surgery, especially as the patient approaches the age of presbyopia.

Specular Microscopy and Pachymetry

If there is a question about possible corneal edema or endothelial cell dysfunction, specular microscopy should be formed to document the endothelial cell density and morphology. Corneal thickness measurements will indicate the functional capacity of the endothelium. Patients with compromised endothelial cell function should not undergo refractive surgery.

Informed Consent

Appropriate and complete informed consent is essential in the refractive surgery practice. The main points that should be covered during the consent process are as follows:

- The nature of the proposed treatment.
- Outline of the risks and benefits of the proposed treatment. These may be divided into the optical and physical risks for easier understanding. One must inform the patient of all risks (even rare risks) associated with the procedure in question because only then will the patient be able to decide in an informed manner whether to have surgery performed on the normal eye.
- Explanation of alternatives to the proposed treatment. In the context of refractive surgery, this must include a comment about the option of doing nothing, an important option in these elective procedures.

The appropriate selection, education, and evaluation of the prospective patient for refractive surgery is essential to obtaining satisfactory outcomes. Attention to the details of patient expectations, preoperative examination, and appropriate surgical strategies will likely reap the reward of patients who are satisfied with their preoperative and postoperative treatment and their ultimate visual outcome.

REFERENCES

1. Schein OD. The Microbial Keratitis Study Group. The relative risk of ulcerative keratitis among users of daily wear and extended wear soft contact lenses. A case control study. *N Engl J Med.* 1989;321:773.
2. Poggio EC, Glynn RJ, Schein OD, et al. The incidence of ulcerative keratitis among users of daily-wear and extended-wear soft contact lenses. *N Engl J Med.* 1989;321: 779–783.
3. Deitz MR. Patient selection and counseling. In: Sanders DR, Hofmann RF, Salz JJ, eds. *Refractive Corneal Surgery.* Thorofare, NJ: Slack, Inc; 1986:43.
4. Smith RS. Radial keratotomy in teenagers: a dubious idea. *Refract Corneal Surg.* 1989;5:315–320.
5. Bourque LB, Rubenstein R, Cosand B, Waring III GO. Psychosocial characteristics of candidates for the Prospective Evaluation of Radial Keratotomy (PERK) study. *Arch Ophthalmol.* 1984;102:1187–1192.
6. Brook RH, Ware JEJ, Davies-Avery A, et al. *Conceptualization and Measurement of Health for Adults in the Health Insurance Study: Overview.* Santa Monica, CA: Rand Corporation; 1976;8.

7. Wilson WE, Klyce SD. Advances in the analysis of corneal topography. *Surv Ophthalmol.* 1991;35(4):269–277.

8. Maguire LJ, Bourne WM. Corneal topography of early keratoconus. *Am J Ophthalmol.* 1989;108:107–112.

9. Rabinowitz YS, McDonnell PJ. Computer-assisted corneal topography in keratoconus. *Refract Corneal Surg.* 1989;5: 400–408.

10. Maguire LJ, Klyce SD, McDonald MB, Kaufman HE. Cor-neal topography of pellucid marginal degeneration. *Refract Corneal Surg.* 1987;5:394–399.

11. Wilson SE, Lin DTC, Klyce SJ, Insler MS. The corneal topography of Terrien's marginal degeneration. *Refract Corneal Surg.* 1990;6:15–20.

12. Wilson SE, Lin DTC, Klyce SD, et al. Topographic changes in contact lens–induced corneal warpage. *Ophthalmology.* 1990;97:734–744.

SECTION II

Optics and Topography

CHAPTER 8

Optics Rediscovered
for the Keratorefractive Surgeon

Leon Strauss ▪ Dimitri T. Azar

Clinicians are accustomed to thinking in terms of spherocylindrical spectacle correction of naturally occurring refractive errors. We shall review traditional clinical optics and add to this framework current thoughts on the optics of keratorefractive procedures.[1–14]

GEOMETRIC OPTICS

The ray of geometric optics is a line drawn perpendicular to each of a train of light wave fronts. When such a ray passes obliquely from a medium of lower index of refraction to a medium of higher index of refraction, the velocity of the associated waves is reduced and the ray is bent toward the normal (perpendicular) to the refracting interface. The change of direction is governed by Snell's law: the quotient of the angle of incidence and the angle of refraction equals the quotient of the indices of refraction of the second and the first media (Figs 8–1 and 8–2).

$$n_i \sin i = n_r \sin r$$

where n_i is the index of refraction of the first medium, i is the angle of incidence, n_r is the index of refraction of the second medium, and r is the angle of refraction.

Prisms and Lenses

Upon entering and again when exiting a prism, light is refracted following Snell's law. This results in deviation of the light rays toward the base of the prism. If one imagines a lens to be a continuous array of prisms of various strengths, Snell's law describes the passage of rays through each part of the lens.

Images and Vergence

In order to analyze the behavior of light passing through lenses, one begins with a simplifying assumption, imagining a lens to be spherical and infinitely thin. An *optical axis* passes perpendicularly through the center of the lens. This central part of the lens has no prismatic power; hence rays striking it from any direction pass undeviated. Suppose that an extended object stands some distance away from the lens; rays emanating from points on this object strike the lens. In order to understand the behavior of these rays, and thus the formation of images of points on the object, it is helpful to consider two focal points and three cardinal rays. (We consider the case of a convex lens and a real image; analysis of other cases is similar.) (see Fig 8–3.) All rays passing through the primary focal point on the optical

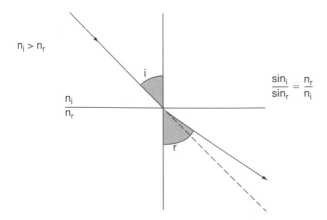

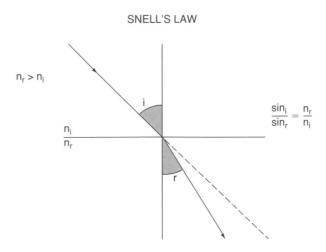

SNELL'S LAW

Figure 8–1. When rays strike a surface, they may be refracted, as shown, or reflected. The relation between the angle of incidence *(i)* and the angle of refraction *(r)* is governed by Snell's law. When light travels from one medium to another with a higher index of refraction, the rays are bent toward the normal to the surface. *(Reprinted with permission from: Azar DT, Strauss L. Principles of applied clinical optics. In: Albert D, Jakobiec F, eds. Principles and Practice of Ophthalmology: The Harvard System. Philadelphia: WB Saunders; 1994.)*

Figure 8–2. When light travels from one medium to another with a lower index of refraction, the rays are bent away from the normal to the surface. A critical angle of incidence *(i)* may be reached if the angle of refraction *(r)* reaches 90°. Light rays striking the surface with an angle of incidence greater than the critical angle will be completely reflected. *(Reprinted with permission from: Azar DT, Strauss L. Principles of applied clinical optics. In: Albert D, Jakobiec F, eds. Principles and Practice of Ophthalmology: The Harvard System. Philadelphia: WB Saunders; 1994.)*

axis emerge from the lens parallel to the optical axis. Rays parallel to the optical axis come to focus, after refraction by the lens, at the secondary focal point. These facts are consequences of Snell's law. To reveal the formation of an image of a point source of light, rays are drawn from that point: (1) through the center of the lens; (2) parallel to the optical axis and, after passing through the lens, to the secondary focal point; and (3) from the point source, through the primary focal point, continuing to the lens, and exiting the lens parallel to the optical axis. Construction of these "cardinal" rays enables us to understand and calculate the locations of images. Another helpful construct is that of "vergence." The inverse of the distance, *u*, from object point to lens (diopters of divergence) plus the power of the lens, *D*

(diopters), equals the inverse of the distance, *v*, to the image point (diopters of convergence).

$$U + D = V$$

where *U* is the vergence of object rays entering the lens = $1/u$, *D* is the power of the lens in diopters, and *V* is the vergence of image rays leaving the lens = $1/v$.

The validity of this vergence analysis is also derived from Snell's law. When the simplifying assumption of "thin" lenses is relaxed, so that lenses are allowed to have significant thickness, nodal points and principal planes replace the conceptual center of the infinitely thin lens (Fig 8–4).

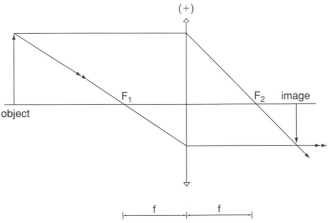

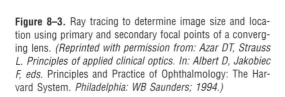

Figure 8–3. Ray tracing to determine image size and location using primary and secondary focal points of a converging lens. *(Reprinted with permission from: Azar DT, Strauss L. Principles of applied clinical optics. In: Albert D, Jakobiec F, eds. Principles and Practice of Ophthalmology: The Harvard System. Philadelphia: WB Saunders; 1994.)*

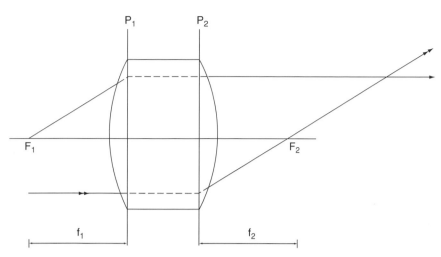

The focal lengths f1 and f2 are measured
from the principal planes P1 and P2, respectively

A

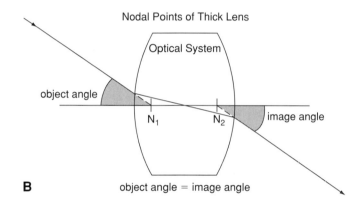

Nodal Points of Thick Lens

B

object angle = image angle

Figure 8–4. A. Principal planes and focal points of an optical system. Note that the focal lengths are measured from the respective principal planes. As shown in the diagram, when the index of refraction is the same on both sides of the optical system, $f_1 = f_2$. If the index of refraction is greater on the side of f_2, then f_2 is greater than f_1. **B.** A ray directed at the primary nodal point, N_1, forming a certain angle with the optical axis, leaves the secondary nodal point, N_2, forming the same angle with the optical axis. In other words, rays incident to one nodal point emerge from the second nodal point parallel to the original direction of the entering ray. When the index of refraction is the same on both sides of the optical system, the nodal points lie at the intersection of the principal planes with the optical axis. *(Reprinted with permission from: Azar DT, Strauss L. Principles of applied clinical optics. In: Albert D, Jakobiec F, eds.* Principles and Practice of Ophthalmology: The Harvard System. *Philadelphia: WB Saunders; 1994.)*

Magnification

Magnification characteristics of optical systems may be defined in several ways. Where an image is formed of an object, linear magnification may be defined to be the quotient of the sizes, measuring perpendicular to the optical axis, of image and object. Measuring along the optical axis, the quotient of image and object sizes is called *axial magnification,* and is found to be the square of the above-described linear magnification. Considering the eye's view through optical systems, it is useful to speak of angular magnification, the quotient of the angles subtended by the image and object as viewed with and without the optical system, respectively.

REFRACTIVE ERRORS OF THE HUMAN EYE

Emmetropia

The nonaccommodating emmetropic eye brings any pencil of parallel rays (eg, from a point on an object at

optical infinity) to focus at some point on the retina. The secondary focal point of such an eye is located on the retina, and the *far point* (defined as the point conjugate to the retina in the nonaccommodating state) is optical infinity (Fig 1–1).

Myopia

The myopic eye brings pencils of parallel rays to focus at points anterior to the retina. The secondary focal point of the eye is in the vitreous. Rays diverging from a point on the far-point plane of the eye will be brought to focus on the retina without the aid of accommodation. The spectacle correction of myopia involves placing a diverging lens in front of the eye so that the secondary focal point of the lens coincides with the far point of the eye. Pencils of parallel rays striking the lens will be diverging when they leave as though they originated from the far point of the eye; hence they will be brought to focus on the retina. Refractive surgical correction of myopia is achieved by flattening the front surface of the eye. When the myopic error is fully corrected, pencils of parallel rays are brought to focus on the retina.

Hyperopia

The hyperopic eye brings pencils of parallel rays of light to focus at points behind the retina. Accommodation of the eye may produce enough additional plus power to bring a parallel (or even a diverging) pencil of rays to focus on the retina.

Astigmatism

Astigmatism of the eye's optical system may be caused by asymmetry of the cornea or, less frequently, of the lens. Astigmatism is *regular* when it is correctable with a spherocylindrical lens, so that pencils of light from distant objects can be focused on the retina. Otherwise, the astigmatism of the eye is called *irregular*. Fortunately, naturally occurring refractive error of the eye tends to be the result of toricity of the cornea, and therefore regular, so that spherocylindrical corrective lenses allow acuity similar to that found in emmetropic eyes. Regular astigmatism is *with the rule* when the steepest (most refracting) meridian lies near 90°. It is correctable by a spherocylindrical lens with plus-cylinder, whose axis lies near 90°, or minus-cylinder, with axis near 180°. When the steepest meridian is near the 180° meridian, the eye's astigmatism is termed *against the rule,* and is correctable by plus-cylinder, with axis at 180°, or minus-cylinder, with axis at 90°. When astigmatism is regular, but the principal meridians do not lie close to 90° and 180°, the astigmatism is termed *oblique.*

Correction of Refractive Errors and Visual Distortions

A distance "corrective" lens placed in front of the eye must have its secondary focal point coinciding with the far point of the eye, so that the resulting optical system focuses parallel pencils onto the retina. Eyes with myopia, hyperopia, and largely regular astigmatism are commonly corrected to approximately 20/20 acuity with spectacles. Aside from the cosmetic and practical inconveniences, what are the drawbacks of spectacle correction? Minus lenses minify the perceived image by roughly 2% per diopter. To the extent that the minus power is astigmatic, the minification is meridionally unequal, thereby distorting the image. Minification is somewhat beneficial because the periphery is brought into view. Plus lenses, on the other hand, magnify the image but create a peripheral scotoma between what is

viewed inside and what is viewed outside the spectacle frame. The farther away from the optical center the line of sight deviates, the more prism is encountered; hence the well-known pincushion and barrel distortions of hyperopic and myopic spectacles, respectively. Off-axis viewing and lens tilt produce changes of the effective sphere and cylinder. These effects are of course greater with higher-power lenses and may be particularly disturbing when the two eyes have markedly different refractive errors.

Binocular spectacle correction of oblique astigmatism distorts each eye's view and, when the axes are not the same, tilts the perceived three-dimensional field. The perceived tilt occurs when both eyes are corrected and disappears when either eye is occluded. Differential meridional minification can be reduced at the expense of clarity by decreasing the cylinder power and by rotating the axis of the correcting cylinder toward 90° or 180° degrees (Fig 8–5).

One might wonder how to tailor refractive surgery for a patient whose spectacle adaptation has required such compromises. Should the surgery aim at less than full correction of astigmatism and rectification of axes towards 90° or 180°? We would not think so, as full correction at the cornea minimizes, rather than creates, these effects. Considering vision with spectacles after refractive surgery, we may expect that changes of astigmatism toward with or against the rule will reduce perceived spectacle-corrected spatial distortion (tilt). On the other hand, a patient who begins without oblique astigmatism, but later obtains glasses to correct significant postsurgical oblique residual astigmatism, may encounter such distortion for the first time and find it disturbing (Fig 8–6). In practice, a number of undercorrected patients complain of distortions that seem not to result from meridional magnification. They describe double images, which are not eliminated by monocular patching.

It may be that some patients, who have long-standing adaptation to spectacle-induced distortion and tilt, experience discomfort for some time when they have these distortions removed through surgery or contact lens wear. Until readaptation occurs, absence of optical distortion is perceived by the patient as a disturbing change in binocular spatial sense.

Anisometropic patients may seek refractive surgery because spectacles may produce symptoms related to aniseikonia and anisophoria. By reducing the anisometropia, surgery may give long-term relief.

Regarding myopic spectacle minification, when optical correction is moved from the spectacle plane to

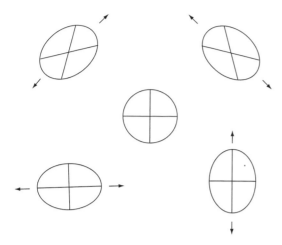

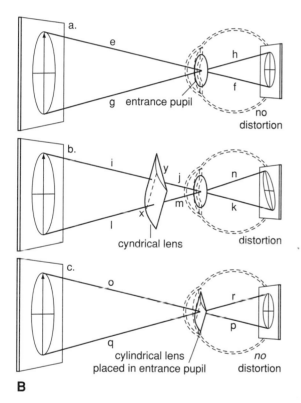

Figure 8–5. A. Monocular distortion caused by meridional magnification. If the retinal image is magnified more in one direction than the other (as indicated by the arrows) vertical lines may become slanted, horizontal lines may become tilted, and objects may appear taller or shorter. **B.** The relation between the position of a cylindrical lens relative to the entrance pupil of a nonastigmatic eye and the distortion of the retinal image produced. **a.** No distortion in the absence of the cylindrical lens. **b.** Distortion produced by the cylindrical lens located in the usual spectacle plane. **c.** No distortion when the cylindrical lens is placed hypothetically in the entrance pupil of the eye. *(Reprinted with permission from: Guyton DL: Prescribing cylinders: the problem of distortion.* Surv Ophthalmol. *1977; 22:177–188.)*

the cornea by contact lenses or surgery, a larger retinal image of the Snellen chart is formed on the retina, so that if the optical resolving power, ie, clarity of image, is preserved, there should be an artifactual improvement of Snellen acuity. One may therefore reason that postoperative acuity should be compared with preoperative rigid contact lens correction in order to judge the effect of the surgery on the optical quality of the eye. This is not a new idea; we may recall that the pre-implant cataract surgeon could hold a plus lens several inches in front of an aphakic eye, so that the patient could read hugely magnified 20/20 letters, viewed one at a time, through the resulting telescope.

Lens Effectivity

Two lenses of unequal power at unequal distances from the eye may each give exact distance correction of that eye, so long as each focuses parallel pencils of rays at the eye's far point. When a newer object is viewed through the same two lenses, vergence calculations show that the amount of accommodation required to focus the diverging rays on the retina is quite different. For instance, a spectacle-corrected myope accommodates less to read a book at 25 cm than the same myope corrected with contact lenses. This notion, that the near effectivity of distance-corrective lenses depends on vertex distance, is, of course, of great interest to the practitioner considering the advisability of contact lenses or refractive surgery for the incipiently presbyopic myope, who has been enjoying the near effectivity of minus spectacles.

OPTICAL ASPECTS OF PREOPERATIVE EVALUATION FOR KERATOREFRACTIVE SURGERY

Contact Lens Wear

In order for the cornea to return to its natural shape, soft contact lens wear should be discontinued for 3 days and rigid lens wear for 3 weeks.

Vertex Distance

For refractive error over 5 D, vertex distance should be measured from the rear surface of a corrective lens in order to calculate the refractive power at the cornea.

Anisometropia

Knapp's rule tells us that with purely axial anisometropia, which may occur in cases of unilaterally high

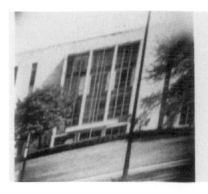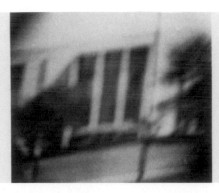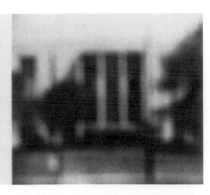

Figure 8–6. Photographic simulation of altering the astigmatic correction to reduce distortion. *Left:* distorted image resulting from full spectacle correction of oblique astigmatism. *Center:* decreased *amount* of distortion obtained by reducing the cylinder power. *Right:* improved *direction* of distortion (vertical) as well as decreased amount of distortion obtained by rotating the plus cylinder axis to 180° and reducing the cylinder power. *(Reprinted with permission from: Guyton DL. Prescribing cylinders: the problem of distortion.* Surv Ophthalmol. *1977;22:177–188.)*

myopia, equal image sizes on the two retinas are achieved when each refractive error is corrected with a spectacle lens placed at the anterior focal point of the eye, which is about 16 mm in front of the cornea. The geometric-optics argument for this does not consider the possibility that the highly myopic eye may have stretched-apart spacing of photoreceptors, which would tend to minify the view. If these anisometropes do not have disturbing aniseikonia with spectacles, might they after keratorefractive surgery? Placement of a corrective contact lens should allow preoperative investigation of this possibility and adequate counseling to the unilaterally high myopic patient about possible postoperative discomfort and adaptation.

Aniseikonia may be unavoidable in refractive surgery of the preoperatively iseikonic bilateral high myope. After surgery of one eye, the other eye may require contact lens wear as the only remedy for aniseikonia until the second eye has similar surgery. Thus, when discussing the risks of surgery preoperatively, contact lens–intolerant patients with high myopia should be apprised of the difficulties they may face should the outcome of surgery on the first eye be unsatisfactory.

Cycloplegic Refraction

Refraction is repeated after cycloplegia in order to discover whether accommodation has been active during the previous "dry" refraction, in which case the cyclopleged eye will show less myopia. For example, a young person with spasm of accommodation would in this manner be identified before surgery, so the surgical plan would be based on the true refractive error. On the other hand, there may be a shift with cycloplegia toward greater myopia, which is caused by *spherical aberration* as the peripheral optics of the eye are exposed by dilation (Fig 8–7).

Hyperopia

When cyclopleged, the hyperopic eye has insufficient plus power to focus the image of a distant object on the retina. Gazing at distance without cycloplegia, the least plus required for clear distance vision is termed *absolute hyperopia*. The most plus the eye can accept without

Figure 8–7. Spherical aberration. Rays of light striking the periphery of a spherical lens are bent more than the central rays. *(Reprinted with permission from: Azar DT, Strauss L. Principles of applied clinical optics. In: Albert D, Jakobiec F, eds. Principles and Practice of Ophthalmology: The Harvard System. Philadelphia: WB Saunders, 1994.)*

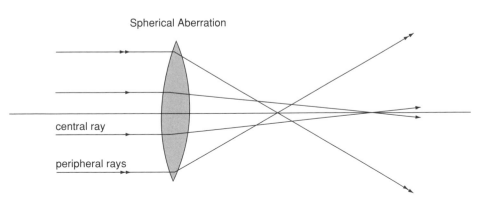

Spherical Aberration

central ray

peripheral rays

blurring of the image is the *manifest hyperopia*. The diopters between the least and most accepted plus constitute the amount of hyperopia that is *facultative*. If accommodation is not as relaxed after fogged refraction as it is with cycloplegia, the difference between the manifest and cycloplegic refractions is considered the amount of hyperopia that is *latent*. As a hyperopic patient advances in age, absolute hyperopia approaches manifest hyperopia (which in turn increases to approach the cycloplegic hyperopia). Under ideal circumstances, surgery for hyperopia should aim at correcting the cycloplegic refractive error, the difficult point here being the assessment of the tenacity of the accommodative tone that constitutes the latent portion of the hyperopia.

Diabetes

The diabetic lens may fluctuate in size and curvature with changes in blood sugar. Diabetic candidates for keratorefractive surgery need to be identified in order to assess the stability of refractive error. Diabetes is a relative contraindication for elective corneal surgery, given that a duplicated basement membrane, recurrent erosions, and persistent epithelial defects occur more frequently in the diabetic corneal epithelium than in the nondiabetic one.

Pupil Size

Size of the entrance pupil (the image transmitted through the cornea) should be estimated in brightly and dimly lit conditions. If the entrance pupil is larger than the optical zone in dim but photopic conditions, then an annulus of cornea surrounding the optical zone will transmit rays to the fovea. We may then be concerned that focus through this annulus is significant and is not the same as it is through the central cornea, or that its scars and irregularity may degrade the foveal image. The Styles–Crawford effect, ie, the notion that the orientation of photoreceptors favors reception of light passing through the central cornea, would encourage hope that the noncentral cornea will cause little image degradation even when the entrance pupil is large enough to allow these photons to reach the fovea.

Extraocular Motility Examination

Extraocular muscle examination and measurements of the amplitude of convergence and divergence can prove helpful prior to keratorefractive surgery. Distance and near cover and alternate cover tests reveal tropias and phorias. Polarized lens stereopsis tests and tests such as red–green Worth lights, which give less stimulus to fusion, may be used to evaluate the degree and stability of fusion and presence of suppression. Keratorefractive surgery may result in reduction or increase in accommodative demands in various circumstances. The spectacle-corrected myope brought to emmetropia by surgery will experience increased demand at near because of the loss of near effectivity of distance-corrective minus lenses. To the extent that myopia is undercorrected, accommodative demand at near will be reduced, giving relief to the presbyope but possibly constituting a cause of concern for someone less presbyopic who has convergence insufficiency. A young esophore with a low reserve of fusional divergence might become symptomatic if overcorrection of myopia, resulting in hyperopia, creates an increased demand for accommodation with its associated accommodative convergence. Measuring with prisms the amplitudes of convergence and divergence (far and near, with or without accommodation) helps to predict whether a change of accommodative demand is likely to stress a weakness of convergence or divergence. If the patient is to function without glasses after surgery, there will be no spectacles in which to grind ameliorating prisms.

Accommodation

Assessment of the amplitude of accommodation before surgery allows the refractive surgeon to formulate a plan for near vision, eg, full correction versus partial, equal correction versus monovision. In general, the difference in diopters between least and most spheres accepted with clear vision while gazing at a distant target is the amplitude of accommodation. Measuring the near point while wearing myopic spectacles will tend to overestimate the amplitude of accommodation because of the near effectivity we have discussed above. Unequal or unusually small amplitudes suggest traumatic injury, drug effects, third cranial nerve paresis, lack of effort, spasm of accommodation, or erroneous distance refraction. One may expect a myope or anisometrope with natural monovision who has not bothered to wear glasses to have developed lower amplitude of accommodation than usual, whereas a long-time uncorrected hyperope will probably have built up greater amplitude than usual.

Spectacle Overcorrection of Myopia

The spectacle overminused myope with presbyopic symptoms may become nonpresbyopic when the unnecessary minus is removed. Discovery of the over-minused state may require cycloplegia (which should be part of every preoperative evaluation), or at least prolonged fogging with plus lenses during refraction, as the patient may have sustained the extra accommodative tone for years. The patient should be given a new pair of lenses, and surgery should be delayed if the accommodation is 1 D or greater. Patients will find that the correct glasses are not as functionally impairing as the overminused lenses were, but they may still desire surgical correction. The surgery should be based on the cycloplegic refraction if the cycloplegic manifest is accepted. This situation requires great care in choosing amount of correction; even after surgery some of these patients will be unable to relax accommodative tone, so that correction based on the cycloplegic preoperative refraction may persistently be felt to be insufficient. The surgeon may then be faced with the patient's demand for further surgery based on this residual accommodative tone, leading to the patient being deliberately converted from an overcorrected myope to a latent hyperope! The overminused bifocal wearer similarly will complain at a younger age of blur in the middle distance and will regain use of the amplitude of accommodation with a corrected distance prescription.

OPTICAL CONSIDERATIONS AFTER REFRACTIVE SURGERY

Pupil Size

According to the geometric-optical reasoning discussed above, when the entrance pupil is larger, the less central cornea becomes relevant for foveal vision; the "Styles–Crawford effect" argument states that these rays of oblique incidence are less visually significant on the retina. Night myopia, however, is a well-recognized entity dependent on noncentral rays, with the more myopic refractive error of the eye attributed to the greater plus power of the peripheral lens, which is exposed as the pupil dilates. If the peripheral lens is optically important in dim light, is not the peripheral cornea as well? Modifying the cornea from prolate to oblate shape, ie, making the cornea flatter in the center and steeper in the periphery, should contribute to the myopic shift occurring with pupil dilation and the peripheral zones of both the lens and the cornea curving more than the central regions. The optical importance of peripheral corneal irregularity and scars and of central corneal haze are subjects of investigation. Should

the surgery produce irregular astigmatism of the central cornea, the effect on uncorrected and spherocylindrical-spectacle–corrected vision is uncertain. To date, attempts to classify these cases have not identified factors that would accurately predict whether or not good spectacle correction can be achieved. The consequences of decentration of surgery are also a matter of interest, as this may bring irregularity, scattering, or diffraction into the more fovea-relevant zone. Occasionally after a long period, there is a diurnal fluctuation of refractive error after radial keratotomy, leading to increased myopia in the morning. Glasses may be prescribed as the patient's needs dictate.

Oval Topographic Zones After Astigmatic Surgery

Successful surgery for astigmatism creates a spherical central corneal zone. The outline of this spherical region has oval isopters, the narrower aspect being the meridian where the difference in curvature between central and peripheral cornea is greatest. In conditions where the pupil is large enough for the peripheral cornea to become relevant, the resulting second image or blur may be noticeable, particularly as sharp and blurred details vary with tortion of the eye or object being observed. Unlike the patient with uncorrected astigmatism whose vision is blurred, these patients have a clearer image created by the central zone, so that the blurred effects may be readily perceived in contrast to the sharper aspect of the image. The combination of relatively sharp focus and a second image may be more disturbing than more diffuse blur.

Streak Retinoscopy

Streak retinoscopy is performed in the customary manner with attention to the central reflex. The "straddling" method of axis refinement is often helpful. Subjective refinement with Jackson cross-cylinder technique is performed as usual. Corneal topography, the astigmatic dial, and the stenopeic slit may be useful when retinoscopy is difficult.

During streak retinoscopy the other eye is fogged with plus sphere lenses, while an *against* motion is observed to confirm that the eye is indeed fogged. Most clinicians customarily approach neutrality through the observation of *with* motion in unoperated corneas, finding this to be easier even after keratorefractive surgery. There is reason, however, to favor minus cylinder technique, using *against* motions after refractive surgery. Influence of the peripheral steeper cornea is minimized if the endpoint of retinoscopy is the onset of neutralization of any part of the *against* motion in the cornea (usually seen in the flattest central cornea). It is common for postoperative patients with slight undercorrection to report that their vision is still sharp with their old spectacles; similarly, a naive refractionist depending on complete neutralization of *against* motion as an endpoint may overcorrect some patients by as much as the full amount of the surgical correction. Furthermore, when against motion is observed, the patient is fogged and therefore less likely to accommodate during the retinoscopy.

The following phenomena may be observed with the retinoscope and utilized to refine the axis of the corrective cylinder after refractive surgery:

Break

The retinoscopic reflex is not perfectly aligned so that the streak falls on the adjacent iris.

Skew

The perceived movement of the streak does not exactly parallel the movement of the retinoscope. This is often helpful in the presence of irregular postoperative astigmatism, where break is not as easily observed.

Straddling

With the supposedly corrective cylinder in place and a *with* motion observable, the reflexes observed 45° on either side of the supposed axis are compared. When using plus cylinders, the correct axis is approached by turning toward the thinner, brighter of the two. When using minus cylinders, the axis is rotated away from the thinner, brighter reflex. (Adding some minus sphere or moving closer to the eye creates the *with* motion reflex necessary to observe this phenomenon.)

The reflex obtained when the pupil is dilated may appear confusing after keratorefractive surgery (eg, scissoring). In this situation, the retinoscopist should concentrate on the central three millimeters. Retinoscopy should not be inadvertently performed off-axis, as the patient gazes askance, giving the retinoscopist a false impression of astigmatism.

Automated Refractors

The use of automated refractors after refractive surgery is of little value, given the variability of the results. More consistent results appear to occur with some automated refractors if the patient is cyclopleged. Cycloplegia reduces false myopia resulting from accommo-

dation, but this may be opposed by the accompanying dilation of the pupil, which may expose the steep peripheral portions of the cornea.

Topographic Maps

Frequently, the axis of astigmatism obtained after retinoscopy and subjective refraction (including refinement using a Jackson cross-cylinder) may be different from that obtained by topographic maps. In such situations, it is helpful to repeat the subjective refraction, beginning with the axis and power suggested by the topographic maps. Lenticular astigmatism should be suspected if there are significant disparities between the topography and subjective findings.

Astigmatic Dial

The astigmatic dial provides an indication of axis and power of cylinder. The test is used when retinoscopy and the Jackson cross-cylinder fail to reveal astigmatism or seem to give untrustworthy results as occurs in some patients with irregular postoperative astigmatism. The patient is asked, while fogged to about 20/40 acuity, to identify the lines that appear blackest and sharpest. The minus cylinder axis is determined by multiplying the smaller ''hour'' number by 30. Minus cylinder is added until the lines appear equally blurred. (The plus cylinder axis is 90° from the minus cylinder axis described above. Each step of plus cylinder must be accompanied by a step of minus sphere.)

Stenopeic Slit

This device is useful for subjective refraction of eyes with irregular astigmatism and uninformative retinoscopy. The stenopeic slit may be considered an elongated pinhole, which corrects in the meridian perpendicular to the slit. The sphere that gives best acuity is selected. The stenopeic slit is introduced before the eye and rotated to the position providing greatest clarity. Sphere is again adjusted to improve acuity further, indicating the power necessary at the meridian parallel to the slit. The slit is then rotated 90°. The change of sphere (plus or minus) required to improve image clarity when the stenopeic slit is rotated 90° is determined. This corresponds to the approximate axis and power of cylinder correction. With the indicated spherocylindrical combination before the eye, the result can be further refined with a ±1.00 D Jackson cross-cylinder. For instance, −3 D when the slit is oriented at 180° and −5 D when the slit is oriented at 90° would suggest a corrective lens to be −3.00 −2.00 × 180.

PRESCRIBING SPECTACLES AFTER REFRACTIVE SURGERY

Because many patients may still need occasional spectacle correction after surgery, the spectacle prescription of a young postoperative patient may be deliberately allowed 0.25 to 0.50 D more minus than is needed for emmetropia at infinity, so that sharpest vision may be achieved with a small amount of accommodative tone. This is most helpful for blunting postoperative diurnal fluctuation and aiding the patient to achieve better acuity for those tasks requiring sharpest distance vision.

In the event that cyclopegia is required to confirm a daytime distance refraction, Halliday has suggested placing an aperture before the eye to simulate an undilated pupil by blocking the peripheral rays.

Regarding near vision, on the one hand a large pupil in dim light gives increased myopia, requiring less add through involvement of the steeper peripheral cornea; on the other hand, in bright light the pupil may be small enough for a pinhole-effect improvement of the range of accommodation.

Anisometropia

At 10 years, 14.7% of patients in the PERK study had not had their second eye operated on. Presumably, many such one-surgery patients are then adult-onset anisometropes. Unless a contact lens is worn in the contralateral eye, one must expect the usual problems of anisometropic spectacle correction, ie, aniseikonia and unequal vertical prism when the gaze goes up and down, particularly with bifocal use. Novis and Rubin observe that vertical anisophoria seems to be much more significant than aniseikonia in the etiology of asthenopia in spectacle-corrected anisometropia.

In general, care for the patient with anisometropia requires identification of sensory and motor adaptations that have already been formed or that will be required with the lenses prescribed. Partial correction or a balance lens is often prescribed when amblyopia is deep or symptoms due to anisophoria or aniseikonia are found to be too disturbing with bilateral full correction. When evaluating hyperopic anisometropes for refractive surgery, one should be aware that such patients are especially likely to have developed amblyopia. Refractive correction is then neither helpful nor disturbing; a "balance" lens similar to that of the other eye is usually prescribed. Significantly undercorrected keratorefractive surgical results may be accepted well by these patients.

With postoperative anisometropia and good acuity of one eye and some amblyopia of the other, there may be some degree of stereopsis and central suppression of the nondominant eye. Suboptimal keratorefractive surgical correction of the dominant eye may be readily apparent. If the dominant eye becomes approximately emmetropic after refractive surgery, one may nevertheless prescribe spectacles in order to protect an essentially monocular patient.

Monovision surgical correction—one eye for distance and one eye for near—may be attempted for some anisometropes, particularly when there is good vision in each eye and demonstrable inability to fuse or appreciate stereopsis. Anisophoria and aniseikonia, which may be experienced with spectacle lens monovision, may or may not be apparent with monovision created by contact lenses or refractive surgery. Trial with contact lenses or formal aniseikonia testing may help to predict this aspect of the surgical result.

High myopes undergoing refractive surgery may have preexisting suppression and strabismus. Surgical undercorrection of the nondominant eye is unlikely to produce discomfort. Surgical overcorrection may, however, lead to accommodative spasm and perhaps an esodeviation. Relief here may be provided with contact lenses or surgical reduction of the hyperopia. Advances in keratorefractive procedures for hyperopia may lead to reliable surgical reduction of consecutive hyperopia.

Spasm of Accommodation

The inability to relax the ciliary muscle suitably is termed *spasm of accommodation*. This may cause blurred vision, asthenopia, headache, or seeming increase in myopia. As in cases of uncorrected hyperopia or astigmatism, spasm of accommodation may develop in overcorrected myopes. With prolonged reading, the prepresbyopic adult may develop spasm of accommodation with consequent blurred distance vision and discomfort. Iridocyclitis, anticholinesterase drugs used for glaucoma, and psychogenic stress may also cause spasm of accommodation. Exophoria may elicit convergence that is neurologically tied to accommodation. To treat accommodative spasm, one may correct astigmatism with glasses, give as much plus as acceptable in a dry refraction, prescribe reading glasses, or occasionally use chronic cycloplegia or bifocals.

Convergence Insufficiency

Suppose that a young myope has borderline convergence insufficiency and that surgical undercorrection of myopia produces discomfort with near vision because accommodation, and hence accommodative convergence, are decreased so that the inadequate fusional convergence is stressed. In this case, correcting the residual myopia with glasses or further surgery will remove the cause of the discomfort.

Presbyopia

Having worn spectacles that undercorrect myopia, a presbyope may first encounter difficulty with near focus when the spectacles are changed to give full correction. The increase in demand for accommodation is even greater if the new full correction is accomplished at the cornea by contact lenses or corneal surgery, so thereby losing the near-effectivity benefit of myopic spectacles; moreover, the option of removing the glasses for near vision is lost as well. The bifocal wearer who has been under-minused has been seeing the middle distance rather than distant objects clearly through the top of the bifocals. If fully corrected with keratorefractive surgery, the middle distance, which was clear, may be blurred with and without reading glasses. The patient may decide either to get used to this or to obtain task appropriate spectacles.

PRESCRIBING FOR PRESBYOPIA AFTER REFRACTIVE SURGERY

General considerations are as follows: beginning with an add typical for the patient's age, the resulting range of accommodation is measured and the add is adjusted to bring the patient's near tasks within the zone of clarity and comfort. The standard tables of adds typical for various ages may suggest adds larger than necessary for these patients, whose corneas may give a multifocal effect. Usually the patient is best served by placing most of the range of clarity farther away than the chosen working distance, choosing a lesser add. This avoids blur of the middle distance and gives a larger range of accommodation.

Fluctuating Vision

When fluctuating refractive error is found after surgery, like the diurnal change seen after radial keratotomy, a high-riding progressive add may provide useful adaptability for near vision, the appropriate add being found as needed.

Unequal Amplitude of Accommodation

Eyes with unequal visual acuities, but equal amplitudes of accommodation, should be given equal adds. On the other hand, when the amplitudes of accommodation are unequal, adds are prescribed so that each eye is using half of its respective amplitude of accommodation for clarity at the desired reading distance. The presumption here is that this amount of accommodation will be produced by equal accommodative innervation of the two eyes.

The very anisometropic patient whose eyes have different ranges of accommodation may require unequal adds; the more myopic eye will need less plus in its bifocal segment. Patients with horizontal phorias require special consideration because more or less reading add may aggravate their phorias; adding or taking away increments of add in a trial frame may enable such a patient to judge a comfortable balance of focusing requirements and fusional amplitudes. If the presbyope has an esophoria, a stronger add will minimize accommodative convergence. On the other hand, the patient with exophoria may benefit from a slightly weaker add so that accommodative convergence will be stimulated. Patients with large cylindrical errors may require cross-cylinder subjective near refraction, as tortion of the globe may occur with convergence and down gaze.

Bifocal Type

Bifocal segments may be either round-top or flat-top. *Image jump* occurs with the abrupt change of prism power encountered as the line of sight crosses into a round-top segment. Flat-top segments minimize image jump on myopic and hyperopic spectacles. *Image displacement* increases as the object is viewed through the peripheral parts of a lens in the manner governed by Prentice's rule. Flat-top segments minimize image displacement on myopic spectacles but accentuate it on hyperopic spectacles.

The surgically undercorrected myope benefits from a flat-top segment with minimal jump (because the optical center of the add is near the top of the segment) and minimized prismatic displacement effect of the add (counterbalanced by the opposite effect of the underlying minus lens). The overcorrected myope, now hyperopic, must choose between the two problems; a flat-top segment gives minimal jump and more displacement, and a round-top segment causes image jump with less displacement.

In general, the top of the segment is usually approximately at the lower limbus. The segment height may be placed farther down for a first pair of bifocals in order to minimize the obstruction of distance vision. The segment may be placed higher in bifocals used primarily for reading as well as in pediatric cases of eso-deviation. As the patient looks downward, the two eyes should enter the top of the segments simultaneously, which may require the optician to place segment heights so as to match facial asymmetry. Horizontal decentration of segments may be adjusted to assist the patient who has a horizontal phoria.

Meridional anisometropia at the 180° axis (vertical power meridian) of the underlying distance correction gives the eyes increasingly unequal amounts of vertical prism as gaze turns down far enough to use the bifocal or trifocal. The difference in prism encountered may induce a symptomatic phoria or diplopia. Prentice's rules states that the inequality of power in the vertical meridian multiplied by the distance below the optical center (in centimeters) is the induced vertical prism. One may expect that a new, induced phoria of 1.5 to 2 prism diopters is likely to cause problems. This may be minimized by slabbing off prism from the more myopic lens, compromising the underlying distance refraction, occluding one segment with translucent tape, lowering the optical centers of the distance correction, or using differing segment types for the two eyes.

Of course, many of the potential problems of bifocal use may be avoided with single-vision reading glasses.

When the amplitude of accommodation is small enough so that a useful near-vision bifocal segment cannot give clarity in the intermediate range, an intermediate correction may be desirable, given as trifocals (usually one-half the full add), progressive-add bifocals, or separate intermediate-zone glasses. The patient who alternates tropia with suppression may be given a stronger add for one eye and a weaker add for the other eye, choosing at will to view the clearer image. The range of accommodation may appear larger after keratorefractive surgery, where the cornea has multifocal effect.

CONCLUSION

The combination of physical and psychophysical aspects of refractive surgery promises to be fertile ground for many optical adventures; we have enjoyed the chance to think about these matters and hope that reviewing them in this way has been helpful.

ACKNOWLEDGMENT

L.S. wishes to thank Dr. Carl Rosen for imparting to his students his love of optics and insistance that patients' comfort and clarity receive the attention they deserve.

REFERENCES

1. American Academy of Ophthalmology: Ophthalmology, Optics, Refraction, and Contact Lenses: Basic and clinical science course, section 3. San Francisco; 1991.
2. Azar DT, Strauss L. Principles of applied clinical optics. In: Albert D, Jakobiec F, eds. *Principles and Practice of Ophthalmology: The Harvard System.* Philadelphia: WB Saunders; 1994.
3. Bennett AG, Rabbetts RB. *Clinical Visual Optics.* London: Butterworths; 1985.
4. Duane TD, Jaeger EA, eds. *Clinical Ophthalmology.* Philadelphia: Harper & Row; 1988.
5. Garcia GE. *Handbook of Refraction.* 4th ed. Boston: Little, Brown; 1989.
6. Guyton DL. *Continuing Ophthalmic Education: Retinoscopy: Minus Cylinder Technique.* Philadelphia: American Academy of Ophthalmology; 1986.
7. Guyton DL. *Continuing Ophthalmic Video Education: Retinoscopy: Plus Cylinder Technique.* Philadelphia: American Academy of Ophthalmology; 1986.
8. Guyton DL. *Continuing Ophthalmic Video Education: Subjective Refraction: Cross-Cylinder Technique.* Philadelphia: American Academy of Ophthalmology; 1987.
9. Michaels DD. *Visual Optics and Refraction: A Clinical Approach.* 3rd ed. St. Louis: CV Mosby; 1985.
10. Milder B, Rubin M. *The Fine Art of Prescribing Glasses Without Making a Spectacle of Yourself.* 2nd ed. Gainesville, FL: Triad Scientific Publishers; 1991.
11. Moses RA, Hart WM, eds. *Adler's Physiology of the Eye.* 8th ed. St. Louis: CV Mosby; 1987.
12. Rubin ML. The sliding lens paradox or the unexpected effect of longitudinal ("to-and-fro") motion of plus spectacle lenses. A treatise on lens effectivity. *Surv Ophthalmol.* 1974;17:180–195.
13. Rubin ML. *Optics for Clinicians.* 3rd ed. Gainesville, FL: Triad Scientific Publishers; 1978.
14. Sloane AE, Garcia GE. *Manual of Refraction.* 3rd ed. Boston: Little, Brown; 1979.

CHAPTER 9

Centering Refractive Corneal Surgical Procedures

Forrest J. Ellis ▪ David G. Hunter

An improperly centered refractive surgical procedure can cause glare, irregular astigmatism, monocular diplopia, ghost images, poor contrast sensitivity, and unpredictable refractive outcomes.[1,2] Despite its importance, the proper centration of corneal procedures is not well studied clinically, and it remains the subject of considerable debate. In the early 1980s, several authors proposed centering techniques that were based on the incorrect assumption that the refraction of light entering the eye is centered on the visual axis.[3–5] However, the visual axis, while useful for theoretical calculations of image sizes in a model eye, has little to do with the refractive elements encountered by rays of light traveling through the eye. In fact, the "visual axis" of an eye with a markedly eccentric pupil may not pass through the pupil at all—instead, it may pass through the iris!

Walsh and Guyton[6] and Uozato and Guyton[7] noted that rays of light passing through the optical elements of the eye must pass through the entrance pupil of the eye. They proposed that corneal surgical procedures should concentrate on the center of the entrance pupil. Uozato, Guyton, and Waring[8] reviewed in detail all other methods of centering corneal procedures and concluded that each was based on erroneous assumptions. Maloney,[2] Mandell,[9] Cavanaugh et al,[10] Klyce and Smolek,[11] and Roberts and Koester[12] all agreed that refractive surgical procedures should be centered on the center of the entrance pupil of the eye. Recently, Lin et al[13] implied that the location of the corneal light reflex should be considered when centering corneal surgical procedures, whereas Pande and Hillman[14] stated that the corneal intercept of the visual axis is the preferred point of centration; thus, the debate continues.

In this chapter, we will summarize the optical principles supporting selection of the center of the entrance pupil as the proper point of centration for refractive corneal procedures. We will discuss the theoretical errors that have led others to recommend that corneal surgical procedures be centered on the corneal light reflex or the visual axis. We will also review the limited clinical studies investigating the consequences of poor centration and present a practical approach to identifying the center of the entrance pupil at the time of surgery.

DEFINITIONS

Much of the confusion surrounding proper centration of refractive surgical procedures results from a misunderstanding of the terms describing the refraction of light by the optical system of the eye. The key misconception is the assumption that familiar terms like *optical axis* and *visual axis* can describe the behavior of a decentered optical system. The following section briefly reviews relevant definitions in the context of their relation to corneal refractive surgery.

Optical Axis, Nodal Points, and Visual Axis

The *optical axis* of any optical system is the line passing through the center of curvature of each optical element comprising the system.[15] The human eye is not an aligned optical system; thus, there is no straight line that can describe the optical axis. A ray striking the primary *nodal point* leaves the secondary nodal point with an identical inclination to the optical axis (Fig 9–1).[16] Because the human eye has no true optical axis, it also has no true nodal points.

The *Gullstrand schematic eye* attempts to work around the nonideal behavior of the human eye by treating it as a centered optical system. Thus, a conjugate pair of nodal points exist in Gullstrand's model. The *reduced schematic eye* is further simplified, assuming only one nodal point. The *visual axis* is a broken line that connects the fixation point with the fovea, passing through the nodal point(s) (Fig 9–1).[15] These assumptions allow the refraction and magnification of objects and images to be calculated for the human eye using Gaussian optics. Considering that these schematic models treat the eye as a centered optical system, it should be clear that they will be of little use in explaining or predicting the behavior of a significantly decentered system—for example, the optical system of a patient with a markedly eccentric pupil or an abnormally large angle lambda.

Pupil, Optical Zones, and the Chief Ray

The *true pupil* is an aperture that limits the amount of light passing through an optical system. The *entrance pupil* is the virtual image of the true pupil formed by the refractive properties of the aqueous and the cornea, whereas the *exit pupil* is the image of the true pupil formed by the refractive properties of the crystalline lens and the vitreous humor. When we look at a person's eye, we see the entrance pupil. Clinical measurements of the pupil actually measure the entrance pupil. The entrance pupil is approximately 14% larger than, and 0.3 mm anterior to, the true pupil (Fig 9–2).[17] The exit pupil can be viewed from the posterior pole of the eye.

The *optical zone* is the area of the cornea overlying the entrance pupil (Fig 9–3).[2] The optical zone is the only part of the cornea that refracts the light rays forming the foveal image. The *chief ray* is a ray emanating from an object point that passes through the center of the entrance pupil (Fig 9–2).[18] The *limiting rays* are the bundle of rays emanating from an object point that pass just inside the edge of the entrance pupil. The limiting rays are the same throughout the optical system; that is, the same light rays are limiting rays as they pass through the entrance pupil, the true pupil, and the exit pupil. When the retinal image is blurred, the chief ray defines the center of the blur circle (assuming a round

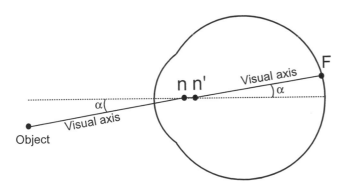

Figure 9–1. Gullstrand schematic eye demonstrating conjugate pair of nodal points *(n, n')*. A ray of light with an angle α to the optical axis and passing through the primary nodal point *(n)* will leave the secondary nodal point *(n')* at the same angle α. The *visual axis* is the line connecting the point of fixation *(object)* through the nodal points of the eye to the fovea *(F)*.

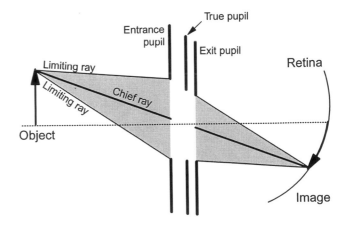

Figure 9–2. Schematic representation of the three pupils of the eye *(entrance pupil, true pupil,* and *exit pupil)*. The *chief ray* and *limiting rays* for a single object point are also indicated.

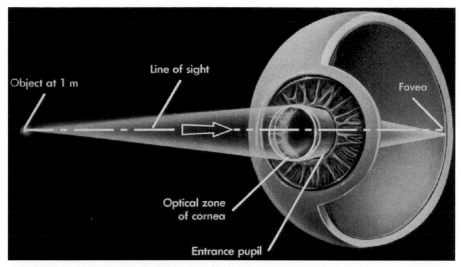

A

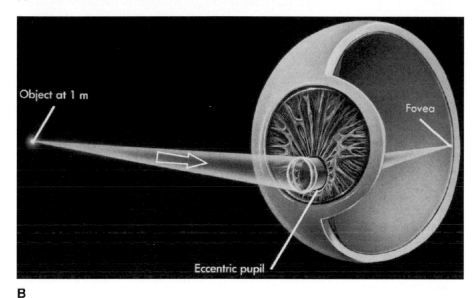

B

Figure 9–3. Location of the *optical zone* and *line of sight* in the eye. **A.** Normal pupil. **B.** Eccentric pupil. Note that in (B), the optical zone and line of sight are displaced far from the location of the corneal light reflex. *(Reproduced with permission from Uozato H, Guyton DL, Waring GO III. Centering corneal surgical procedures. In: Waring GO III, ed. Refractive Keratotomy for Myopia and Astigmatism. St. Louis: Mosby-Year Book, 1992; 493.)*

pupil with a spherical refractive error), and the limiting rays define the edge of the blur circle for each object point.

Line of Sight and Pupillary Axis

The *line of sight* is the line connecting the fixation point with the center of the entrance pupil (Figs 9–3 and 9–4).[17] The line of sight corresponds to the chief ray of the light emanating from the fixation point. In an aligned optical system with a round pupil centered on the optical axis, the line of sight is equivalent to the optical and visual axes. In the eye, with its noncentered optics, the line of sight is not equivalent to the visual or optical axes, which are not determinable.

The *pupillary axis* is the line perpendicular to the cornea that passes through the center of the entrance pupil (Fig 9–4). This line will pass through the center of curvature of the anterior corneal surface. The pupillary axis can be located by centering the corneal light reflex in the center of the patient's pupil while the examiner sights monocularly from directly behind the light source.

Angles Kappa and Lambda

Clinicians often refer to the angle between a coaxially sighted corneal light reflex and the pupillary center as the angle kappa. In fact, the angle kappa is the angle between the nonexistent visual axis and the pupillary

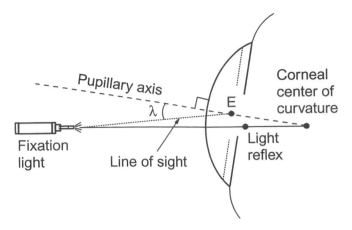

Figure 9–4. Schematic diagram of the anterior segment of the eye, viewed from the top, to demonstrate *pupillary axis* and *angle lambda* (λ). *(E)* is the center of the entrance pupil. The true pupil is closer to the center of curvature than the entrance pupil. *Light reflex* is the corneal light reflex.

axis; thus, it is not possible to measure such an angle in the eye. The angle between the line of sight and the pupillary axis, which can be measured clinically (Fig 9–4), is referred to as the angle lambda.[15] In normal subjects, the angle lambda is typically 3° to 6°.[15]

PREVIOUSLY DESCRIBED CENTERING TECHNIQUES

The *corneal light reflex* (also referred to as the first Purkinje–Sanson image) is the basis of several techniques for centering corneal surgical procedures. The light reflex is formed when a light source is reflected by the convex surface of the cornea, producing a virtual image behind the cornea (Fig 9–4). Gullstrand's schematic eye can be used to calculate the location of the corneal light reflex. When a point source of light is located at infinity and the corneal radius of curvature is 7.8 mm, the corneal light reflex is 3.9 mm behind the surface of the cornea or 0.85 mm posterior to the plane of the entrance pupil.[7]

The location of the corneal light reflex is not a constant. When a point source of light is moved from infinity toward the eye, the corneal light reflex moves a few hundredths of a millimeter closer to the cornea. As the eye moves from side to side, a previously centered corneal light reflex is displaced with respect to the center of the pupil and the cornea. This variability in the location of the corneal light reflex limits its use as a guide for centering corneal surgical procedures.

Other techniques for centering corneal surgical procedures have been developed and promoted. Osher's optical centering device is used to identify and

mark the corneal light reflex (although it can be modified to help the surgeon locate the center of the entrance pupil). The Weck and Zeiss fixation lights and Thornton's fixation target utilize binocular (noncoaxial) sighting through a microscope. The error induced when these techniques are used, which has been extensively detailed,[7,8] makes them inappropriate for centering corneal refractive procedures.

CENTERING CORNEAL SURGICAL PROCEDURES

Importance of Proper Centration

An improperly centered procedure will produce unwanted glare and unpredictable refractive outcomes. Light reaching the fovea must pass through the optical zone of the cornea; thus, the optical zone must be clear of any scarring or irregularity. A small error in centration can place a radial keratotomy (RK) incision scar or the edge of a photorefractive ablation zone in the optical zone.

Light reaching the fovea is refracted within the optical zone; thus, corneal power is relevant only in this location. An error in centration can produce unpredictable corneal curvature in the optical zone, leading to poor refractive outcomes in patients with markedly decentered optical systems. Maloney[2] calculated that if a 4-mm optical zone (overlying a 4-mm entrance pupil) is decentered 1 mm, only 70% of the light rays falling on the retina will have passed through the optical zone.

The optical zone must be larger than the entrance pupil to provide glare-free vision. The minimum optical zone diameter increases with increasing pupil size, desired glare-free visual field angle, and anterior chamber depth.[12] In order for a patient with a 4-mm pupil to have a 15° glare-free visual field, the diameter of the clear optical zone must be at least 5.38 mm.[7] O'Brart et al[19] performed 4-mm photorefractive keratectomy (PRK) ablations in one eye and 5-mm ablations in the other eye of 33 patients. The patients were more likely to complain of glare or decreased night vision in the eye with the 4-mm ablation zone. The authors did not attempt to determine whether errors in centration contributed to the glare.

Centration of Corneal Procedures in a Reduced Schematic Eye

Imagine for a moment that the eye is an aligned optical system represented by a reduced schematic eye with a coaxial cornea, pupil, lens, fovea, and fixation point. Where should a refractive corneal procedure be centered in such an eye? Under these circumstances, most of the currently available methods of centering corneal surgical procedures will mark the same central spot: the geometric center of the cornea (Fig 9–5A). These methods include those based on the coaxially sighted corneal light reflex, on the center of the entrance pupil, and on the corneal intercept of the visual axis.

Several commercially available centering targets may not mark the correct corneal location even in an aligned, coaxial, reduced schematic eye. As mentioned above, the Weck, Zeiss, and Thornton targets provide a fixation target that is not coaxial with the viewing eye of the surgeon. Many ophthalmic surgeons sight monocularly, or strongly favor one eye, making proper centration with these fixation devices less predictable.[8]

Pupil Eccentricity

How does the eye create an image on the fovea when the pupil is eccentric? To answer this question, decenter the pupil in the optical system described above (Fig 9–5B). Even if the rays traveling along the visual axis are

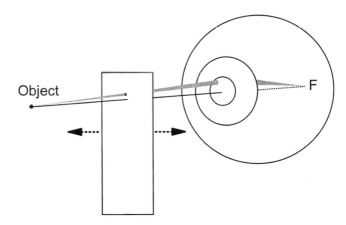

Figure 9–6. Demonstration of consequences of an eccentric pupil. *F* is the fovea. *Shaded area* indicates the path of light through the pinhole aperture and pupil. *Solid line* indicates straight line from object to fovea. *Dotted arrows* indicate movement of the pinhole occluder.

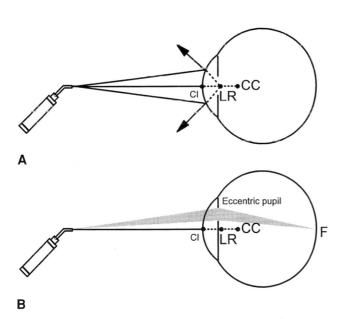

A

B

Figure 9–5. Locating the center of a corneal procedure in a reduced schematic eye. **A.** centered optical system (all optical elements are aligned). *CI* is the corneal intercept of the line connecting the fixation target with *LR*, the corneal light reflex, which in this case coincides with the corneal intercept of the visual axis and the geometric center of the cornea. *CC* is the center of curvature of the cornea. **B.** All optical elements are aligned except for an eccentric pupil. The shaded area indicates the path of light from the fixation target to *F*, the fovea. Note that *CI* is not included within the shaded area and therefore does not participate in the refraction of the light reaching the fovea.

blocked, the eye will still form a focused foveal image of the object. The bundle of rays from the object must pass through, and be refracted by, the optical zone of the cornea. The same bundle of rays must pass through the entrance pupil to reach the fovea. In a living eye, the photoreceptors will reorient their long axis toward the center of an eccentric pupil, not toward the visual axis.[20,21] The image of the object does not move as the pupil is decentered because the optical system of the eye forms an image on the fovea regardless of pupil location.

To demonstrate that an eccentric pupil does not move the image and necessitate a compensatory eye movement to maintain fixation, perform the following simulation (Fig 9–6): Cut a strip of paper 1 cm wide and 3 cm long and place a pinhole opening near one end of the strip. Close one eye and fixate on a target across the room. Place the pinhole before the open eye and move it from side to side and up and down, simulating different degrees of pupil eccentricity. As long as the pinhole aperture stays within the entrance pupil of the viewing eye, the image remains stationary regardless of aperture movement. (The simulation does not exactly match the situation in the eye, as the extra "pupil" is in front of, rather than behind, the cornea. When the pinhole is moved beyond the edge of the entrance pupil of the viewing eye, the image disappears. In addition, a subject with an uncorrected refractive error may note slight movement.)

Variations in Corneal Curvature and Clarity

Imagine again a model eye with aligned optical elements, but with a central power of 60 diopters (D) and a peripheral power of 55 D. Assume no refractive error is present when the pupil is centered in this model eye system. However, when the pupil is eccentric, the refractive power encountered by the bundle of light rays passing through the entrance pupil is 55 D, making the eye approximately 5 D more hyperopic. In this case the refractive power along the visual axis is irrelevant.

What if the model eye has a central corneal scar causing glare and irregular astigmatism? With a centered pupil (Fig 9–7A), the corneal irregularities overlie the entrance pupil. This light will be scattered, and no spherocylindrical lens will sharply focus the light onto the fovea. If the pupil is eccentric (Fig 9–7B), the rays of light encountering the central scar do not participate in the formation of a foveal image. The image will be in sharp focus on the fovea without glare or irregular astigmatism. In this situation, the scar on the visual axis of the model eye is irrelevant.

Foveal Eccentricity

Now consider a different scenario: a model eye with centered optical elements and a centered pupil, but with an eccentric fovea. For foveal fixation, the optical axis will not be aligned with the fixation point. In the model eye, this misalignment of the optical and visual axes is referred to as a positive- or negative-angle

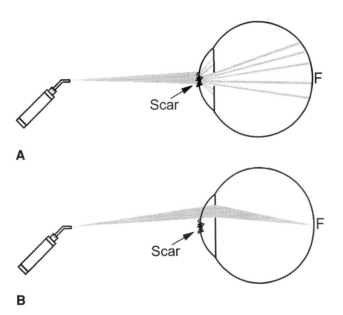

A

B

Figure 9–7. A model eye with centered optical elements and a central corneal scar. **A.** Central pupil. The light striking the scar is scattered as it passes through the entrance pupil. *F* is the fovea. **B.** Eccentric pupil. The light striking the scar is scattered, but the scattered rays of light do not participate in forming a foveal image. The light that forms the foveal image does not pass through the scar, and a sharp foveal image is formed by the clear optical zone over the eccentric entrance pupil.

kappa. (For the reasons stated earlier, the term *angle lambda* is more appropriate when this occurs clinically.) When the optical axis is misaligned in this way, light rays emanating from the fixation point pass through the entrance pupil of the eye and are brought into focus on the fovea. Once again, it is the optical zone over the entrance pupil of the eye, and not the area of cornea overlying the visual axis, that is acting upon the light rays of interest.

Summary of the Role of the Visual Axis and the Optical Zone

It is apparent from the situations described above that the visual axis is of no use in locating the bundles of light refracted by the eye. Thus, even if the human eye were a perfectly aligned optical system, and even if one could determine exactly the intercept of the visual axis with the cornea, this would not matter to the surgeon planning a corneal refractive procedure. The only part of the cornea that matters is the optical zone: the area of the cornea overlying the entrance pupil of the eye. We therefore agree with the conclusion of others[2,7,9–12] that the center of the entrance pupil is the proper centration point for corneal refractive surgical procedures.

RECENTLY DESCRIBED CENTERING TECHNIQUES

Lin et al[13] recently used corneal topographic analysis to evaluate centration of the ablated zone in 97 eyes following excimer laser photorefractive therapy for myopia. The authors centered their treatments halfway between the corneal light reflex and the center of the entrance pupil when the two did not coincide (11% of patients). They did not provide any data or theoretical evidence supporting such a selection. They concluded that the pupillary center was slightly more difficult to identify than the corneal light reflex, and that decentration of the ablation zone from the pupillary center did not cause significant increases in irregular astigmatism, as measured by the surface regularity index (SRI). Based on their results, the authors proposed that centering excimer laser refractive procedures on the "visual axis" (corneal light reflex) rather than the center of the entrance pupil "could be tolerated by the patient."

There were several potential problems with the study, which may have led to erroneous conclusions. The authors incorrectly equated the corneal light reflex with the "visual axis." Pilocarpine was used to decrease the size of the pupil before estimating the location of the center of the entrance pupil, which may have placed the center of the entrance pupil in an unnatural position (see below). In their data analysis, they measured decentration of the ablation zone from the center of the entrance pupil rather than from the intended center of the ablation zone. The ablation zone was decentered greater than 1 mm in only two of the 97 eyes studied (maximum 1.5 mm), and no patients with eccentric pupils were studied, making it difficult to generalize the results to the most difficult patients—those with markedly eccentric pupils or large-angle lambdas. Since publication of that article, Lin[22] has stated that "centration of the excimer laser beam relative to the center of the entrance pupil is a basic requirement to reduce glare and edge effects from PRK."

Pande and Hillman[14] have recently modified an autokeratometer to mark the geometric corneal center, the corneal light reflex, the entrance pupil center, and a "visual axis." They incorrectly defined "visual axis" as a line connecting the fovea to the object of interest, without regard to the nodal points of the eye. They concluded that the corneal light reflex most closely estimates the location of the corneal intercept of the "visual axis." They assumed that the visual axis is the optimal centration point for corneal surgery, and therefore concluded that the coaxially sighted corneal light reflex should be used to best identify the optimal centration point for corneal surgical procedures.

Several authors have disputed the conclusions of Pande and Hillman.[14] Mandell[23] noted that Pande and Hillman's method did not locate the visual axis—it simply marked a line joining the fixation point to the corneal center of curvature, which by definition is the line passing through the coaxially sighted corneal light reflex. A similar method for marking this location was previously described by Uozato,[3] who later discounted this technique.[7] Guyton[24] pointed out that the authors' method simply aligned the optical axis of the measuring instrument with the fovea of the eye, without regard to the path of light rays through the optical system of the eye. He also stated that the paper provided no evidence supporting the theoretical assumption that the visual axis is the optimal centration point.

RECENT STUDIES OF REFRACTIVE CORNEAL SURGERY CENTRATION

The increased interest in centration of corneal refractive surgery has led several surgeons to attempt to measure accurately the centration of their corneal procedures and to identify some of the consequences of poor cen-

tration. In several of these studies,[25,26,27] decentration was measured only from the corneal vertex, or "visual axis," making the results difficult to interpret with respect to the center of the entrance pupil. Cavanaugh et al retrospectively analyzed the centration of their PRK procedures.[10,25] In one study, in which decentration was measured only from the corneal vertex, the authors concluded that decentration of greater than 1 mm may have decreased postoperative uncorrected and best-corrected acuities.[25] In the second study,[10] the distance from the center of the entrance pupil to the center of the post-PRK flat zone was measured in 49 patients. The average decentration was 0.4 mm (range, 0.1 to 1.1 mm). There was no correlation between the amount of decentration and visual acuity (uncorrected or best corrected) in these patients. However, since the maximum decentration was small compared with the first study, there were not sufficient data to detect such a correlation. The authors did not attempt to identify any correlation between decentration and glare, decreased contrast sensitivity, or irregular corneal topography in the optical zone.

Klyce and Smolek[11] studied decentration error from the center of the pupil in two groups. In the first group (18 eyes), average decentration was 0.79 mm (range, 0 to 2.2 mm). The amount of decentration did not correlate with best-corrected visual acuity. Other parameters of visual acuity (uncorrected acuity, glare, contrast sensitivity, corneal irregularity) were not studied. In the second group (19 eyes), average decentration was 0.47 mm, and no attempt was made to evaluate the visual consequences of decentration.

Lin[22] reviewed the decentration from the center of the exit pupil in 502 eyes, and reported a mean decentration of 0.34 mm, with a range of 0 to 1.50 mm. He also performed corneal topographic analysis, including calculation of the SRI, a measurement of irregular astigmatism and "optical performance." He did not attempt to correlate decentration with SRI in this study, but in an earlier study of a subset of these patients, Lin et al[13] found that SRI did not correlate with decentration. Lin[22] concluded that the pattern of ablation was more important than the location of the center of the ablation. However, not enough of the procedures were decentered to allow a correlation to be detected, and other parameters (glare, contrast sensitivity, and visual acuity) were not studied.

Marking the Center of the Ablation Zone

The authors of the studies of centration accuracy claim that they are now able to keep errors in centration (that is, the distance from the center of the entrance pupil to the center of the ablated area) down to 0.29 to 0.47 mm.[11,22] Unfortunately, they provide few specifics as to how they accomplished these improvements. Cavanaugh et al[25] attributed their improved results over time to "improved technique and enhanced attention to detail." Lin[22] stated that "centration results improved with experience as surgeons were better able to recognize . . . [loss of fixation during treatment]." Klyce and Smolek[11] improved their alignment technique "solely through careful attention to centration by both the surgeon and the assistants." They advised having assistants with a different perspective provide feedback to the surgeon regarding the centration of the procedure. They recommended using a corneal ring marker with cross hairs, followed by a hand-held vacuum suction ring to unequivocally mark the desired area of ablation. Other surgeons do not use a fixation ring, allowing the patient to maintain his or her own fixation throughout the procedure.

Postoperative Measurement of Centration

Schwartz-Goldstein et al[28] measured optical zone centration from the center of the entrance pupil and compared decentration with a variety of clinical outcomes. They found that 3 of 6 patients with 1.00 mm or greater decentration had a high glare/halo score. There was a weak statistical association of centration with patient satisfaction, attempted refractive correction, and change in keratometric cylinder

Sun et al[29] found that the methods used to mark the center of the ablation zone in the studies above are subject to interobserver variability of 50%, even with a well-defined flattened zone. They also noted that epithelial hyperplasia and collagen production will conceal portions of the flattened zone, further increasing measurement errors. They recommended performing corneal mapping 1 to 2 weeks after surgery to identify optimally the flat zone, and they proposed using a compass to identify accurately the center of the ablation zone.

PUPILLARY DILATION

Only the rays passing through the entrance pupil of the eye centered about the chief ray contribute to the formation of a foveal image. For this reason, a refraction can vary depending on the amount of pupillary dilation, without regard to the state of accommodation. The natural pupil center shifts nasally and superiorly with miosis.[30] Schwartz-Goldstein et al[28] noted a systematic decentration of PRK inferonasally and attributed this to the preoperative use of pilocarpine. A careful manifest refraction in an examination room with modest lighting to produce 3- to 4-mm natural pupils may be the best to compare with the cycloplegic refraction. Therefore, both a manifest refraction and a dilated refraction should be performed, especially in patients with eccentric or irregular pupils or in patients whose pupils dilate eccentrically. This extra step can help the surgeon identify patients who may develop problems postoperatively when different lighting levels cause variability in the postoperative refraction.

RECOMMENDED TECHNIQUE FOR OPTIMAL CENTRATION IN CORNEAL REFRACTIVE SURGICAL PROCEDURES

Based on the optical principles and experimental results described above, we recommend the following procedure for optimal centration of corneal surgical procedures. The surgeon must keep in mind that although this recommended procedure is most consistent with modern understanding of the optics of the eye, experimental evidence and published clinical data are lacking in this area, especially in patients with markedly decentered optical systems.

The patient should fixate a light or target that is coaxial with the examiner's sighting eye. This can easily be accomplished by placing a fixation spot in the exact center of one of the viewing tubes of the microscope. A 1- or 2-mm mark will not interfere significantly with the microscope optics. Errors from any potential decentration of the surgeon's pupil are negligible.[2] If already available, Osher's optical centering device may also be used as a coaxial fixation target (but the instructions that describe how to mark the corneal light reflex should be disregarded).

Marked miosis displaces the entrance pupil center,[30] which may increase unwanted optical aberrations when the pupil redilates after surgery. Therefore, the pupil should be in a natural state, not under the influence of any pharmacologic agents. Adjust the intensity of the light in the operating microscope until the pupil diameter is 3 to 4 mm. Klyce and Smolek[11] advise marking the center of the entrance pupil at three different pupil sizes (using different light intensities) to increase precision; however, if the three marks do not coincide, we recommend using the mark placed at a pupil diameter of 3 to 4 mm.

Occlude the patient's nonoperative eye and ask the patient to fixate on the target. The surgeon must sight monocularly through the tube containing the fixation spot. The surgeon should then mark the cornea overlying the center of the pupil as seen through the operating microscope, ignoring the corneal light reflex. Centration errors are less likely to be symptomatic if a larger ablation zone is used.

Examples

To demonstrate potential sources of error in centration of corneal refractive procedures, consider the following hypothetical case examples:

Case 1

A patient with a 3-mm pupil decentered 3 mm temporally presents for radial keratotomy. Where should the procedure be centered?

If the corneal light reflex method is used, the temporal horizontal RK incision will pass through the optical zone. The patient will complain of glare, and the incision within the optical zone will lead to unpredictable corneal curvature in this area, with unpredictable refractive results.

If the recommended entrance pupil method is used, no incision will go through the optical zone, so glare will be no more of a problem than usual. The temporal horizontal incision will be placed closer to the limbus than usual, while the nasal horizontal incision will be placed closer to the geometric center of the cornea than is customary. It is not known whether such a peripheral displacement of corneal incisions will change the effectiveness of the procedure in the optical zone when compared with a more central procedure. Planned undercorrection may minimize this potential problem.

Case 2

A pseudophakic patient with a peaked pupil and anterior corneal scarring from previous keratitis presents for phototherapeutic keratectomy. Where should the procedure be centered?

If the corneal light reflex method is used, the ablated zone may only partially cover the cornea overlying the entrance pupil. Peripheral portions of the scar overlying the pupil may not be ablated, leaving residual glare. The edge of the ablated zone will cross the entrance pupil, creating irregular astigmatism and producing less predictable refractive results.

If the recommended entrance pupil method is used, scar will be removed from the entire optical zone,

and the cornea overlying the entrance pupil will be evenly ablated, minimizing irregular astigmatism. It is not known whether the proximity of the limbal epithelium to one edge of the ablated zone will alter the pattern of remodeling and subepithelial scarring normally observed following photoablation.

FUTURE DIRECTIONS

Whereas optical considerations point to the center of the entrance pupil as the best center for refractive surgical procedures, experimental and clinical evidence is needed to confirm these theoretical analyses. The outcome of various centration techniques must be investigated to determine the importance of nonoptical factors, such as wound healing or the topography of asymmetric procedures. These analyses should investigate postoperative function in more detail and in more patients with markedly decentered optical systems than has been studied to date.[10,22] Postoperative function should be studied in terms of glare, contrast sensitivity, refractive outcomes, and long-term stability in this special group of patients. Centration of the procedure should be measured postoperatively using timing and technique similar to that advocated by Sun et al.[29] Other studies should investigate changes in corneal shape that occur with decentered RK incisions, perhaps including mathematical models predicting the tectonic consequences of such procedures. The contribution of asymmetric remodeling to the maturation of eccentrically placed PRK procedures must also be investigated systematically. Until such studies are performed, the selection of the optimal point of centration of corneal refractive procedures must be guided primarily by our understanding of optical principles.

SUMMARY

In the human eye, light passing from an object of interest to the fovea passes through the optical zone of the cornea, which overlies the entrance pupil of the eye. The visual axis, corneal vertex, and geometric center of the cornea are irrelevant to the path taken by these light rays. We therefore recommend that the proper centration point for corneal refractive procedures is the center of the entrance pupil. Other described techniques may induce errors in centration, especially when used in patients with eccentric pupils or large-angle lambdas. Centration errors may result in irregular astigmatism, scarring overlying the entrance pupil, or unpredictable changes in corneal shape in the optical zone, which may cause glare, monocular diplopia, ghost images, poor contrast sensitivity, or unpredictable refractive outcomes. Future studies should attempt to describe in detailed quantitative terms the consequences of proper and improper centration in a group of patients with markedly decentered optical systems (eg, eccentric pupils) and in a group of patients who have experienced inadvertently decentered refractive surgical procedures, comparing these results with the outcomes in a group of patients with normal eyes who have undergone well-centered procedures.

REFERENCES

1. Binder PS. Optical problems following refractive surgery. *Ophthalmology.* 1986;93:739–745.

2. Maloney RK. Corneal topography and optical zone location in photorefractive keratectomy. *Refract Corneal Surg.* 1990;6:363–371.

3. Uozato H, Makino H, Saishin M, Nakao S. Measurement of visual axis using a laser beam. In: Breinin GM, Siegel IM, eds. *Advances in Diagnostic Visual Optics.* Berlin: Springer-Verlag; 1983;22.

4. Steinberg EB, Waring GO III. Comparison of two methods of marking the visual axis on the cornea during radial keratotomy. *Am J Ophthalmol.* 1983;96:605.

5. Thornton SP. Surgical armamentarium. In: Sanders DR, Hofman RF, Salz JJ, eds. *Refractive Corneal Surgery.* Thorofare, NJ: Slack, Inc; 1986;134–135.

6. Walsh PM, Guyton DL. Comparison of two methods of marking the visual axis on the cornea during radial keratotomy. *Am J Ophthalmol.* 1984;97:660–661. Letter.

7. Uozato H, Guyton DL. Centering corneal surgical procedures. *Am J Ophthalmol.* 1987;103:264–275.

8. Uozato H, Guyton DL, Waring GO III. Centering corneal surgical procedures. In: Waring GO III, ed. *Refractive Keratotomy for Myopia and Astigmatism.* St Louis: Mosby-Year Book; 1992;491–505.

9. Mandell RB. The enigma of corneal contour. *CLAO J.* 1992;18:267–273.

10. Cavanaugh TB, Durrie DS, Riedel SM, Hunkeler JD, Lesher MP. Centration of excimer laser photorefractive keratectomy relative to the pupil. *J Cataract Refract Surg.* 1993;19(suppl):144–148.

11. Klyce SD, Smolek MK. Corneal topography of excimer laser photorefractive keratectmomy. *J Cataract Refract Surg.* 1993;19(suppl):122–130.

12. Roberts CW, Koester CJ. Optical zone diameters for photorefractive corneal surgery. *Invest Ophthalmol Vis Sci.* 1993;34:2275–2281.

13. Lin DTC, Sutton HF, Berman M. Corneal topography following excimer photorefractive keratectomy for myopia. *J Cataract Refract Surg.* 1993;19(suppl):149–154.

14. Pande M, Hillman JS. Optical zone centration in keratorefractive surgery. *Ophthalmology.* 1993;100:1230–1237.

15. Lancaster WB. Terminology in ocular motility and allied subjects. *Am J Ophthalmol.* 1943;26:122.

16. Ogle KN. *Optics,* 2nd ed. Springfield, IL: Charles C Thomas; 1968;149.

17. Bennett AG, Francis JL. The eye as an optical system. In: Davson H, ed. *The Eye.* New York: Academic Press; 1962; 4:101.

18. Fry GA. *Geometrical Optics.* Philadelphia: Chilton; 1969;110.

19. O'Brart DPS, Gartry DS, Lohmann CP, Kerr-Muir MG, Marshall J. Excimer laser photorefractive keratectomy for myopia: comparison of 4.00- and 5.00-millimeter ablation zones. *J Refract Corneal Surg.* 1994;10:87–94.

20. Bonds AB, Macleod DIA. A displaced Stiles–Crawford effect associated with an eccentric pupil. *Invest Ophthalmol Vis Sci.* 1978;17:754.

21. Enoch JM, Laties AM: An analysis of retinal receptor orientation. II. Prediction for physiologic tests. *Invest Ophthalmol Vis Sci.* 1971;10:959.

22. Lin DTC. Corneal topographic analysis after eximer photorefractive keratectomy. *Ophthalmology.* 1994;101:1432–1439.

23. Mandell RB. Optical zone centration for keratorefractive surgery. *Ophthalmology.* 1994;101:216–217. Letter.

24. Guyton, DL. More on optical zone centration. *Ophthalmology.* 1994;101:793–794. Letter.

25. Cavanaugh TB, Durrie DS, Riedel SM, Hunkeler JH, Lesher MP. Topographical analysis of the centration of excimer laser photorefractive keratectomy. *J Cataract Refract Surg.* 1993;19(suppl):136–143.

26. Cantera E, Cantera I, Olivieri L. Corneal topographic analysis of photorefractive keratectomy in 175 myopic eyes. *Refract Corneal Surg.* 1993;9(suppl):19–22.

27. Spadea L, Sabetti L, Balestrazzi E. Effect of centering excimer laser PRK on refractive results: a corneal topography study. *Refract Corneal Surg.* 1993;9(suppl):22–25.

28. Schwartz-Goldstein BH, Hersh PS et al. Corneal topography of phase III excimer laser photorefractive keratectomy: Optical zone centration analysis. *Ophthalmology.* 1995;102:951–62.

29. Sun R, Gimbel HV, DeBroff BM. Recommendation for correctly analyzing photorefractive keratectomy centration data. *J Cataract Refract Surg.* 1995;21:4–5. Letter.

30. Fay AM, Trokel SL, Myers JA. Pupil diameter and the principal ray. *J Cataract Refract Surg.* 1992;18:348–351.

CHAPTER 10

Monovision Refractive Surgery

Sandeep Jain ▪ Indu Arora ▪ Dimitri T. Azar

The presbyopic population in the United States is expected to double every 5 years until the year 2010. Increasing numbers of young contact lens wearers are moving into the presbyopic age, and many are also becoming intolerant to contact lens wear. A promising alternative treatment for presbyopia, known as monovision, can be refractive surgical correction of one eye for distance and the other eye for near. Several surgeons target refractive surgery patients for monovision; however, the indication, success rate, and limitations of monovision in refractive surgery remain unclear in current ophthalmic literature.

Ideally, the monovision patient should see clearly at all distances. The binocular clear vision range should be continuous and equal to the sum of the monocular clear ranges, without interference from the blurred image of the other eye. The patients should not have problems in functioning at home, while driving, or at work. Monovision success rates for contact lens wearers vary, depending on study design and population; average rates of 60% and 80% are typical. The variability in reported success rates stems from the differing criteria used to define success, variations in study duration, ambiguous definitions of base population, and lack of

This chapter is reproduced with modifications from *Survey of Ophthalmol.* 1996; 40:491–499.

criteria for minimum contact lens wearing times. Some of the failures may also be related to contact lens intolerance that is not attributable to monovision.

In this chapter, we attempt to clarify the factors predictive of clinical success and visual performance in monovision refractive surgical patients. Preoperative use of monovision contact lenses may identify patients who have the potential of successfully adapting to monovision refractive surgery. We have reviewed the published literature to correlate successful monovision with the following factors: ability to suppress monocular blur, ocular dominance, high contrast and low contrast visual acuity, stereopsis, fusional ranges, phorias, and task performance ability.

Our MEDLINE search strategy identified 2887 unique citations, of which 42 articles satisfied our initial inclusion criteria. The bibliographic search yielded another 19 articles. Forty-two articles[1–42] were original papers, and 19 were reviews or correspondence.[43–61] The articles were abstracted and summarized in a review article in *Survey of Ophthalmology.*

MONOVISION SUCCESS

Monovision success was defined as adequate adaptation to 1 to 2 diopters of monocular blur after 3 weeks or more; it was calculated from articles whose criteria include age of more than 40 years, astigmatism of less than 1 D, no previous monovision experience, and no previous contact lens intolerance.

Monovision success was calculated from 19 articles.[1-19] (See Table 10-1.) Other articles reported success rates, but they did not meet our definition of monovision success, nor did they match our inclusion criteria. The duration of follow-up period ranged from 3 weeks to 5 years. The mean success rate was 76% (434 successful monovision patients out of a total of 573). Monovision failure resulted either from contact lens intolerance or from poor visual adaptation to monovision. The success rate of monovision in patients who can tolerate contact lenses is important because of its applicability to the success rate after refractive surgery. The success rate increased from 69% (100/144) to 86% (124/144) when we excluded the contact-lens–related failures.[6,17]

FACTORS INFLUENCING MONOVISION SUCCESS

Ocular Dominance and Sighting Preference

Ocular dominance plays an important role in the overall success of monovision. Fifteen studies[4-17,19] specified the blurred eye (and followed patients for more than 3 weeks). In 95% of patients (407/427), the dominant eye was corrected for distance[4-6,8-11,13-17,19] (Table 10-1). When the dominant eye was corrected for distance viewing, the overall monovision success rate was 75%.

The majority of patients demonstrated sighting dominance at both distance (90%) and near (80%) with sighting dominance tests (hole-in-the-card and mirror test).[20,21] The sensory dominance test (anisometropic blur test) identified 20% of patients with no sighting preferences at distance. Correcting the dominant sighting eye for distance improved visual locomotor tasks that require directional prediction[22] (walking, driving) and produced lesser esophoric shifts at distance.[23]

For successful monovision, constant interocular suppression of blur is advantageous. Patients with alternating dominance (no sighting preferences) have constant interocular blur suppression.[21] Patients with strong sighting preferences have reduced interocular blur suppression, decreased binocular depth of focus, and higher monovision failure rates.

Interocular Suppression of Blur

In successful monovision wearers (greater than 1 year of monovision correction wear) the interocular sup-

pression of blur was approximately two orders of magnitude greater than unsuccessful monovision wearers (3 to 4 vs 2 log% contrast).[16] Blur suppression was the same irrespective of which eye was blurred and was unaffected by test spot diameter.[13,24,25]

Age

The mean age for studies that reported monovision success (Table 10-1) ranged from 47.7 to 55 years.[1,2,5-16,18] No available articles compared the success rate in younger versus older presbyopes. Two articles[7,10] (63 patients) examined differences between the average age of successful and unsuccessful monovision patients. These differences (48.3 vs 50.5 years, respectively) were not statistically significant.[23,26,27]

Stereoacuity

Stereoacuities of 100 seconds of arc or better are generally considered normal in presbyopes. Twelve articles[3,9-11,15-17,26,28-31] measured stereopsis in monovision (Table 10-2). Stereopsis in monovision ranged from 23 to 73 arc sec for distance and from 50 to 113 arc sec for near. Unsuccessful monovision patients had 50 to 62 arc sec reduction in stereopsis compared with successful monovision patients.

Phorias

An average of 0.6 to 0.9 prism diopter esophoric shift at distance was seen with monovision.[23,30] The esophoric shift in successful monovision patients was less than the shift in unsuccessful monovision patients. No differences in fusional vergence ranges were noted between successful and unsuccessful monovision patients.[27]

VISUAL PERFORMANCE IN MONOVISION

Binocular Visual Acuity

Table 10-3 summarizes the effect of monovision on binocular visual acuity.[15,16,20,26,28,33] Each logMAR line corresponds to 0.1 logMAR unit. Monovision lenses produce a small reduction in high- and low-contrast visual acuity compared with the binocular vision condition at standard (40 to 75 candelas per square meter) room illumination.

The reduction of binocular visual acuity in monovision, compared with binocular vision, was greater in low illumination (5 cd/m^2) than in high illumination

TABLE 10–1. SUCCESS LEVEL IN MONOVISION

Study	Patient Characteristics				Eye Corrected for Distance	Monovision		Reason for MV Failure
	No.	Age	M	F		Duration	Success	
Williams[1]	38	50–60	—	—	—	3 wk	84%	Conact lens related Inability to adapt to MV
Gauthier[2]	72	50–54	—	—	—	1 mth	64%	Occupational visual demand Contact lens related
Beddow[3]	6	—	—	—	—	1 mth	100%	
Josephson[4]	20	—	4	16	Dominant	1 mth	70%	
Kuhl[5]	22	53	8	14	Dominant	1 mth	55%	
Back[6]	117	42–77	—	—	Dominant	3 mth	67%	Distance blur and ghosting Near blur and ghosting Contact lens related
Fonda[7]	13	49	1	12	More myopic	2.7 yr	85%	
Fleischman[8]	28	45–57	—	—	Dominant	4–18 mth	71%	
Kastl[9]	6	55	0	6	Dominant	2.7 yr	100%	
Koetting[10]	50	50.3	—	—	Dominant	2 mth	82%	
Sevigny[11]	2	48	—	—	Dominant	3 mth	0%	Loss of depth perception Impaired ability to drive
London[12]	7	47.7	1	6	Less mobile	—	100%	
Schor[13]	18	52	6	12	Dominant	2 mth	100%	
Sheedy[14]	18	52.3	—	—	Dominant	2 mth	94%	
Papas[15]	23	51.3	—	—	Dominant	1 mth	43%	Impaired ability to judge distances Night driving difficulties
Harris[16]	20	51.7	—	—	Dominant	3 wk	90%	
Hersh[17]	29	—	—	—	Dominant	5 yr	81%	Contact lens related
Molinari[18]	30	46–50	—	—	—	2.5 mth	88%	Poor fusional comfort
Scarborough[19]	54	—	—	—	Dominant	—	90%	Loss of visual effectiveness and/or depth perception

Abbreviation: MV, monovision.

(250 cd/m²).[28] The low-contrast binocular distance visual acuity in monovision decreased by 0.05 ± 0.02 logMAR unit with +1 D ocular blur of the nondominant eye.[33] Thereafter, with each additional diopter of ocular blur, visual acuity decreased by 0.02 logMAR unit. The decrease in high-contrast binocular visual acuity showed considerable variability. The mean binocular visual acuity reduction in monovision with the dominant eye corrected for distance was 0.04 logMAR unit with a fixed 3.5-mm pupil and 0.07 logMAR unit with a fixed 7.0-mm pupil.[33] Residual astigmatic errors, particularly in the dominant, distance-corrected eye at oblique axis, cause greater binocular visual acuity loss in monovision (greater than 1 Snellen line with +0.5 D of astigmatic defocus).[33]

Peripheral Vision and Visual Fields

Monovision causes no significant effect on binocular peripheral visual acuity. Peripheral visual field width is marginally better (1° to 3°) in the nondominant eye (corrected for near) than in the dominant eye.[32] The average decrease in size of the visual field through the far-point lens and the near-point lens are within the variation in measurements expected when taking fields.[3] Static visual fields are not adversely affected by monovision correction.

Contrast Sensitivity

The contrast sensitivity function increases by a factor of $\sqrt{2}$ when the stimulus is viewed binocularly rather than monocularly (binocular summation).[34,62,63] Thus, in the absence of monocular defocus, the binocular contrast sensitivity is approximately 42% greater than monocular contrast sensitivity. With increasing monocular defocus, the binocular contrast sensitivity decreases steadily and then falls below the monocular contrast sensitivity, showing binocular inhibition.[35] If the defocus is further increased (beyond + 2.5 D defocus), the

TABLE 10–2. STEREOPSIS IN MONOVISION

Study	Age (mean)	Stereopsis in MV[a] Distance	Stereopsis in MV[a] Near	Change from BV Distance	Change from BV Near	MV Success	Stereopsis in MV Success	Stereopsis in MV Failure
Beddow[3]	—	—	38%[c]	—	3%	100% (5/5) at 2 mth	38%	
Kastl[9]	55	—	50	—	—	100% (6/6) at 2.6 yr	50	—
Koetting[10]	50.3	—	96[d]	—	—	82% (41/50) at 2 mth	88	150
Sevigny[11]	48	—	25%	—	20%	0% (0/2) at 3 mth	—	25%
Papas[15]	51.3	73[b]	—	—	—	43% (10/23) at 1 mth	—	—
Harris[16]	51.7	—	90[e]		43	90% (18/20)at 3 wk	—	90
Erickson(1)[26]	50.6	—	72[e]	—	36	37% (7/19) of study	40	90
			91[d]	—	41	patients were past MV	94	88
Erickson(2)	—		95[e]	—	59	wearers for at least	69	110
			117[d]	—	68	3 mths	84.3	137
Back[28]	57.0	24[b]	113[e]	15	67	Short study	—	—
McGill[29]	54.7	—	>80 in 60%	—	42	Short study	—	—
McLendon[30]	—	—	34%[c]	—	36%	67% (4/6) at 1 mth	44%	14%
Lebow[31]	—	—	106[d] (0.37–1.5D blur) 445[d] (1.75–2.75D blur)	—	—	All 10 were past MV wearers		
Hersh[17]	—	Gross Stereopsis[c]	—	—	—	81% (22/27 at 5 yr)	—	—

[a]Dominant eye was corrected for distance in all except Erickson(2), where nondominant eye was corrected for distance. Howard Dolman, Randot, and Titmus Stereotest values are mean stereopsis rounded to nearest decimal in arc seconds. Keystone Airplane Series values represent percent stereopsis.
[b]Howard Dolman test.
[c]Keystone Airplane Series with Telebinocular.
[d]Wirt Titmus Stereotest.
[e]Randot Stereotest.
Abbreviations: BV, binocular vision; MV, monovision.
(From Jain S, Arora I, Azar DT. Success of monovision in presbyopes. Surv Ophthalmol. 1996;40:491–499. With permission.)

binocular contrast sensitivity reverts to the monocular level, indicating suppression of the defocused eye. In successful monovision patients, ocular blur reduces binocular summation of middle to high spatial frequencies (greater than 4 cycles per degree).[34] With increasing ocular blur, the binocular summation at lower frequencies is also reduced; in addition, the peak contrast sensitivity shifts toward higher spatial frequencies. When ocular blur is greater than +2 D, binocular summation is essentially lost. Because binocular summation is affected at higher spatial frequencies, monovision is not suited for occupations requiring fine, detailed work.[34] The contrast sensitivity function at low photopic levels (10 cd/m^2) shows no significant differences between monovision and other forms of presbyopic corrections.[36] At this low luminance, the suppression of interocular blur in monovision is poor.

Task Performance

Reduction of task performance in *monovision*, compared with binocular vision (≤6%) is much lower than reductions in *monocular vision*, compared with *binocular vision* (30%), for activities that require high stereopsis (point-

ers and straws).[14,16] For activities that require minimal stereopsis but good visual acuity (letter editing), task performance decreases minimally in monovision and monocular vision (≤6%). For activities that require moderate stereopsis (card filing), performance decrease in monovision is less than that in monocular vision. With increased adaptation, there is some improvement in task performance.[37]

Anisometropic Blur Suppression

Successful monovision patients see clearly by virtue of an interocular suppression of blur.[13,24,25] The anisometropic blur suppression test measures the suppression of monocular blur of fused contours that is essential for clear binocular vision under monovision conditions. The test target is a back-illuminated circular aperture in a white card with rheostat-controlled front illumination. At zero front illumination, a clear image from the distance-corrected eye and a blurred image from the near-corrected eye can be perceived. The front illumination is increased until only the clear image is perceived. The anisometropic blur suppression is proportional to the luminance contrast threshold (log%

TABLE 10–3. LOGMAR VISUAL ACUITY IN MONOVISION[a]

Study	High-Contrast Charts[b]				Low-Contrast Charts				Successful MV patients
	MV Mean	ΔBV Mean	Monovision		MV Mean	ΔBV Mean	Monovision		
			Success	Failure			Success	Failure	
At standard room illumination (75 cd/m²)									
Papas[15]	0.02	0.08	—	—	0.26	0.04	—	—	43.5% (10/23)
Harris[16]	0.02	0.05	—	—	0.36	0.08	—	—	90% (18/20)
Robboy[20]	0.05	—	—	—	0.24	—	—	—	Short study
	0.06[b]	—	—	—	0.22	—	—	—	
Erickson[26]	0.07	0.04	0.03	0.10	0.28	0.09	0.23	0.32	37% (7/19)
	0.09[b]	0.06	0.03	0.13	0.26	0.07	0.25	0.27	
Collins[33]	—	0.07	—	—	—	0.07	—	—	Short study
At high illumination (250 cd/m²)									
Back[28]	−0.05	0.04	—	—	0.11	0.06	—	—	Short study
At low illumination (5 cd/m²)									
Back[28]	0.20	0.10	—	—	0.51	0.10	—	—	Short study

[a]All values are in LogMAR units.
[b]With near correction on dominant sighting eye.
Abbreviations: MV, monovision; ΔBV, change from binocular vision.
(From Jain S, Arora I, Azar DT. Success of monovision in presbyopes. Surv Ophthalmol. *1996;46:491-499. With permission.)*

contrast) at which the clear image, not the blurred image, is perceived. Log numbers 1 to 5 correspond to background luminance of 563, 320, 56, 6, and 0.6 cd/m², respectively.

Anisometropic blur suppression increased by approximately an order of magnitude for small spot sizes following short-term (1 day) adaptation to anisometropia. In marked contrast to the preadapted stage, blur suppression was greater when the blurring lens (near correction) was placed over the nondominant eye. In contrast to the anisometropic blur suppression test, the AO vectographic test measures ocular dominance characteristics with nonfused diplopiclike images. It reveals that suppression of the blurred eye in monovision was enhanced by increasing the amount of anisometropia, and that a 0.50 to 1 D greater add was required to induce 100% suppression at near than at distance.[25] The mean blur suppression in 18 successful monovision wearers was 3.1 to 3.2 log% contrast.[13] Blur suppression increased in 50% of patients at 2 months by 0.5 ± 0.5 log% contrast when the dominant eye was corrected for distance while increasing in only 28% of patients when the nondominant eye was corrected for distance.

Binocular Depth of Focus

In patients with alternating dominance (no sighting preference), the binocular depth of focus is approximately equal to the sum of monocular depths of focus.[21] Although the monocular depths of focus does not vary with differences in sighting preferences, the binocular image becomes blurred in patients with strong sighting preference as the object moves from the dominant-eye monocular clear range to the nondominant-eye monocular clear range. In patients with strong sighting preferences, the depth of focus under monovision condition is considerably less than the sum of the monocular depths of focus.[21]

Stereopsis

A significant increase ($P < .05$) in stereopsis is seen after 3 weeks of monovision adaptation.[16] The reduction in stereoacuity is greater for unsuccessful monovision patients, and smaller for successful monovision patients.[26] In young subjects (23 to 28 years), stereoacuity was reduced to worse than 50 arc sec (from initial values of 20 arc sec) with 2 to 2.5 D of monocular blur.[25] Increasing the ocular blur caused a concurrent increase in stereoscopic threshold.[38]

In presbyopes, the stereoacuity decreased considerably when the ocular blur was greater than +1.75D.[31] Monovision reduced secondary fusion in 10% to 20% of patients, indicating some binocular stress, but simultaneous perception and gross stereopsis were not affected.[31]

Horizontal Phorias and Vergence

Esophoric shifts are speculated to indicate the binocular visual stress created by monovision. The magnitude of esophoric shift was greater with the nondominant eye corrected for distance. Divergence and convergence ranges at distance were smaller with monovision. The reduction in fusional vergence ranges was significant when the nondominant eye was corrected for distance.

Presbyopes generally demonstrate a moderate to large exophoria at near. This was reduced by 2.5 to 5.2 prism diopters with monovision.[27,30,31] The divergence ranges at near (base-in break at 21.2 Δ, recovery at 15.2 Δ) were significantly smaller ($P < .05$) in monovision, but the convergence ranges showed no changes.

Conclusions

Presbyopes with strong sighting preference, with significant reductions of stereoacuity with monocular correction, and with minimal interocular suppression may not be good candidates for monovision refractive surgery. Because the contrast sensitivity function is reduced at higher frequencies with monovision, patients engaged in occupations requiring fine work may experience difficulties with monovision. Large esophoric shifts with monovision correction or visual symptoms associated with esophoria are potential contraindications for monovision.

Refractive surgery has been utilized to provide monovision in presbyopes. In myopic presbyopes, the dominant eye may be fully corrected for distance vision while the nondominant eye is undercorrected, thus producing monovision. However, reversing this surgery will be at best difficult and at worst impossible. Refractive surgery should not be viewed as a solution for presbyopia, but rather as an option available to carefully selected patients who demonstrate a potential for adapting to the visual compromises inherent in monovision.

Demonstration of the visual effects of monovision may be used to determine the adaptability of patients to monovision. Trial of monovision contact lenses preoperatively may be the best method of identifying patients who might do well with monovision refractive surgery. The adaptation period should be greater than 3 weeks. During the adaptation period, patients may experience blurring of vision, difficulty in driving at night, and loss of stereopsis. Many patients do not learn to ignore or suppress these effects. The absence of significant changes in blur suppression and task performance after successful adaptation may suggest that early success is predictive of long-term patient satisfaction. However, preadaptation with optical lenses may not actually mimic the true effects of refractive surgery combined with those of monovision. Many of the modest vision decreases seen with monovision achieved in contact lens wear can be expected to be exacerbated when combined with the potential side-effects of refractive surgery.

In addition to the occasional serious, vision-threatening complications, patients undergoing monovision refractive surgical correction must be informed of the risks of reduced visual acuity and stereopsis. A spectacle lens corrected for distance must be prescribed for the near-vision eye to perform tasks requiring good distance vision. The potential effects of refractive surgical monovision correction during driving are of major concern. Deficits of visual acuity and contrast sensitivity during monovision have some finite effect on target identification. Distance and near ghosting that occasionally present in monovision patients are attributable to incomplete suppression of interocular blur. When present, these secondary images can be distracting. The ability to suppress blur may improve with adaptation, but performance equivalent to binocular vision may never be achieved. Monovision patients may experience hazy vision and occasional loss of balance during the adaptation period.

In spite of its limitations, with properly exercised professional judgment and appropriate clinical screening, surgically created monovision may prove to be effective for correcting presbyopia in many patients.

REFERENCES

1. Williams CE. An evaluation of the CSI plus series with emphasis on monovision fitting. *Int Contact Lens Clin.* 1983;10:172–180
2. Gauthier CA, Holden BA, Grant T, Chong MS. Interest of presbyopes in contact lens correction and their success with monovision. *Optom Vis Sci.* 1992;69:858–862.
3. Beddow DR, Martin SJ, Pheiffer CH. Presbyopic patients and single vision contact lenses. *South J Optom.* 1966;8:9–11.
4. Josephson JE, Caffery BE. Monovision vs. aspheric bifocal contact lenses: a crossover study. *J Am Optom Assoc.* 1987;58:652–654.
5. Kuhl SA, Henry VA, Bennett ES. Clinical evaluation of fitting presbyopic patients with contact lenses. *J Am Optom Assoc.* 1992;63:182–186.
6. Back AP, Holden BA, Hine NA. Correction of presbyopia with contact lenses: comparative success rates with three systems [see comments]. *Optom Vis Sci.* 1989;66:518–525.

7. Fonda G. Presbyopia corrected with single vision spectacles or corneal lenses in preference to bifocal corneal lenses. *Trans Ophthalmol Soc Aust.* 1966;25:78–80.

8. Fleischman WE. The single vision reading contact lens. *Am J Optom Arch Am Acad Optom.* 1968;45:408–409.

9. Kastl PR. Stereopsis in anisometropically fit presbyopic contact lens wearers. *CLAO J.* 1983;9:322–323.

10. Koetting RA. Stereopsis in presbyopes fitted with single vision contact lenses. *Am J Optom Arch Am Acad Optom.* 1970;47:557–561.

11. Sevigny J. The binocular status of two mono-vision patients—case report. *Can J Optom.* 1982;44:137–141.

12. London R. Monovision correction for diplopia. *J Am Optom Assoc.* 1987;58:568–570.

13. Schor C, Carson M, Peterson G, Suzuki J, Erickson P. Effects of interocular blur suppression ability on monovision task performance. *J Am Optom Assoc.* 1989;60:188–192.

14. Sheedy JE, Harris MG, Busby L, Chan E, Koga I. Monovision contact lens wear and occupational task performance. *Am J Optom Physiol Opt.* 1988;65:14–18.

15. Papas E, Young G, Hearn K. Monovision vs. soft diffractive bifocal contact lenses: a crossover study. *Int Contact Lens Clin.* 1990;17:181–186.

16. Harris MG, Sheedy JE, Gan CM. Vision and task performance with monovision and diffractive bifocal contact lenses. *Optom Vis Sci.* 1992;69:609–614.

17. Hersh D. A novel modality for management of presbyopic contact lens patients. *Opt J Rev Optom.* 1969;106:35–40.

18. Molinari JF. A clinical comparison of subjective effectiveness of monovision, aperture-dependent and independent bifocal hydrogel lens fittings. *Optom Weekly.* 1973;64:28–29.

19. Scarborough ST, Lopnaik RW. A two-eyed look at the presbyopic patient. *Contact Lens Forum.* 1976;1:48–57.

20. Robboy MW, Cox IG, Erickson P. Effects of sighting and sensory dominance on monovision high and low contrast visual acuity. *CLAO J.* 1990;16:299–301.

21. Schor C, Erickson P. Patterns of binocular suppression and accommodation in monovision. *Am J Optom Physiol Opt.* 1988;65:853–861.

22. Trevarthen CB. Two mechanisms of vision in primates. *Psychol Fortsch.* 1968;31:299–350.

23. McGill EC, Erickson P. Sighting dominance and monovision distance binocular fusional ranges. *J Am Optom Assoc.* 1991;62:738–742.

24. Schor C, Landsman L, Erickson P. Ocular dominance and the interocular suppression of blur in monovision. *Am J Optom Physiol Opt.* 1987;64:723–730.

25. Heath DA, Hines C, Schwartz F. Suppression behavior analyzed as a function of monovision addition power. *Am J Optom Physiol Opt.* 1986;63:198–201.

26. Erickson P, McGill EC. Role of visual acuity, stereoacuity, and ocular dominance in monovision patient success. *Optom Vis Sci.* 1992;69:761–764.

27. McGill EC, Erickson P. The effect of monovision lenses on the near-point range of single binocular vision. *J Am Optom Assoc.* 1991;62:828–831.

28. Back A, Grant T, Hine N. Comparative visual performance of three presbyopic contact lens corrections. *Optom Vis Sci.* 1992;69:474–480.

29. McGill E, Erickson P. Stereopsis in presbyopes wearing monovision and simultaneous vision bifocal contact lenses. *Am J Optom Physiol Opt.* 1988;65:619–626.

30. McLendon JH, Burcham JL, Pheiffer CH. Presbyopic patterns and single vision contact lenses II. *South J Optom.* 1968;10:7–10,31,36.

31. Lebow KA, Goldberg JB. Characteristic of binocular vision found for presbyopic patients wearing single vision contact lenses. *J Am Optom Assoc.* 1975;46:1116–1123. Review.

32. Collins MJ, Brown B, Verney SJ, Makras M, Bowman KJ. Peripheral visual acuity with monovision and other contact lens corrections for presbyopia. *Optom Vis Sci.* 1989;66:370–374.

33. Collins M, Goode A, Brown B. Distance visual acuity and monovision. *Optom Vis Sci.* 1993;70:723–728.

34. Loshin DS, Loshin MS, Cornear G. Binocular summation with monovision contact lens correction for presbyopia. *Int Contact Lens Clin.* 1982;9:161–165.

35. Pradhan S, Gilchrist J. The effect of monocular defocus on binocular contrast sensitivity. *Ophthal Physiol Opt.* 1990;10:33–36.

36. Collins MJ, Brown B, Bowman KJ. Contrast sensitivity with contact lens corrections for presbyopia. *Ophthalmic Physiol Opt.* 1989;9:133–138.

37. Sheedy JE, Harris MG, Gan CM. Does the presbyopic visual system adapt to contact lenses? *Optom Vis Sci.* 1993;70:482–486.

38. Westheimer G, McKee SP. Stereoscopic acuity with defocussed and spatially filtered retinal images. *J Opt Soc Am.* 1980;70:772–778.

39. Peters HB. The influence of anisometropia on stereosensitivity. *Am J Optom Arch Am Acad Optom.* 1969;46:120–123.

40. Wyzinski P. Why are refractive surgeons still wearing glasses? *Ophthalmic Surg.* 1987;18:349–351.

41. Back AP, Woods R, Holden BA. The comparative visual performance of monovision and various concentric bifocals. *Trans Br Contact Lens Assoc Conf.* 1987:46–47.

42. Boerner CF, Thrasher BH. Results of monovision correction in bilateral pseudophakes. *J Am Intraocul Implant Soc.* 1984;10:49–50.

43. Koetting R. Monocular fitting: a viable alternative for the presbyope. *J Am Optom Assoc.* 1982;53:134–135.

44. Kastl PR. Is the quality of vision with contact lenses adequate? Not in all instances. *Cornea.* 1990.

45. Bier N. Prescribing for presbyopia with contact lenses. *Am J Optom Arch Am Acad Optom.* 1967;44:687–710.

46. Erickson P. Potential range of clear vision in monovision. *J Am Optom Assoc.* 1988;59:203–205.

47. Wesley NK. The control of presbyopia without bifocals. *J Am Optom Assoc.* 1976;47.

48. Josephson JE, Erickson P, Back A, et al. Monovision [see comments]. *J Am Optom Assoc.* 1990;61:820–826. Review.

49. Josephson JE, Caffery B. Bifocal hydrogel lenses: an overview. *J Am Optom Assoc.* 1986;57:190–195.

50. Harris MG. Informed consent for presbyopic contact lens patients. *J Am Optom Assoc.* 1990;61:717–722.

51. Erickson P, Schor C. Visual function with presbyopic contact lens correction. *Optom Vis Sci.* 1990;67:22–28. Review.

52. McMonnies CW. Monocular fogging in contact lens practice. *Aust J Optom.* 1974;57:29–32.

53. Beier CG. A review of the literature pertaining to monovision contact lens fitting of presbyopic patients: clinical considerations. *Int Contact Lens Clin.* 1977;4:49–56.

54. Rothman SM. Monovision fitting of contact lenses for presbyopia: review and personal comments. *J Optom Vis Dev.* 1985;16:19–21.

55. Weidt AR, Cunin BM. The bifocal alternative. *Contact Intraocular Lens Med J.* 1981;7:250–251.

56. Wood WW. Monovision does work. *Optom Management.* 1985;21:49–50.

57. Garland MA. Monovision and related techniques in the management of presbyopia. *CLAO J.* 1987;13:179–181.

58. Weidt AR, Cunin BM. The bifocal alternative. *Contact Intraocul Lens Med J.* 1981;7:250–251.

59. Koetting R. Monocular fitting: a viable alternative for the presbyope. *J Am Optom Assoc.* 1982;53:134–135.

60. Rosenwasser HM. Monovision. *J Am Optom Assoc.* 1991; 62:892–893. Letter; comment.

61. Harris MG, Classe JG. Clinicolegal considerations of monovision. *J Am Optom Assoc.* 1988;59:491–495.

62. Jain S, Arora I, Azar DT. Success of monovision in presbyopes: Review of the literature and potential applications to refractive surgery. *Surv Ophthalmol.* 1996;40: 491–499.

63. Rose D. Monocular versus binocular contrast thresholds for movement and pattern. *Perception.* 1978;7:195–200.

64. Blake R, Fox R. The psychophysical inquiry into binocular summation. *Perception Psychophys.* 1973;14:161–185.

65. Mann CC. Can meta-analysis make policy? *Science.* 1994; 266:960–962.

CHAPTER 11

Contrast Sensitivity and Glare Testing in Keratorefractive Surgery

Gary S. Rubin

More than 200,000 refractive surgery procedures are performed in the United States each year[1] and their safety and efficacy have been evaluated in numerous large and small clinical trials. Despite this careful scrutiny, several outstanding and controversial issues remain concerning the effect of keratorefractive surgery on visual function. One reason for the lingering concern is that evaluation of visual function after surgery has largely been confined to measurement of visual acuity. Acuity tells us about the eye's ability to resolve fine detail at high contrast, but it may not adequately describe the ability to see large, low-contrast patterns like faces or nearby objects. In addition, acuity tests are usually conducted in a darkened examination lane with moderately bright test targets. The results may not generalize to other situations, such as high, ambient lighting (eg, out-of-doors in bright sunlight) or dim illumination (eg, night driving). For these reasons, many people now argue that visual acuity testing should be supplemented by other tests of visual function. In the evaluation of refractive surgery, the two most frequently discussed alternatives are *contrast sensitivity* and *glare sensitivity* tests.

CONTRAST SENSITIVITY TESTING

In recent years, contrast sensitivity testing has been widely promoted as an important adjunct to, or even a replacement for, visual acuity testing. Whereas visual acuity tests measure how large an object must be for the patient to discern the critical details, contrast sensitivity measures how much a pattern must vary in luminance for it to be seen.

In the normal, healthy human eye, contrast sensitivity and visual acuity typically vary in the same fashion. For example, reduced visual acuity due to ametropia causes a predictable reduction of contrast sensitivity.[2,3] But various types of visual dysfunction, including cerebral lesions, optic neuritis, glaucoma, diabetic retinopathy, and amblyopia, may cause a reduction in contrast sensitivity despite near normal Snellen acuity. Similarly, in patients with mild to moderate cataracts, it has been shown that visual acuity does not correlate well with contrast sensitivity, particularly at low spatial frequencies.[4-6]

Although it is clear that contrast sensitivity and visual acuity need not go hand in hand, what does contrast sensitivity loss tell us about a patient's visual disability? Photographic simulations of the world as seen though a cataract suggest that the loss of contrast sensitivity makes the world appear hazy or washed out.[5] Loss of contrast sensitivity at low spatial frequencies makes it difficult to recognize faces and to navigate safely and efficiently through unfamiliar environments.[7,8] Patients with normal contrast sensitivity can tolerate substantial reductions in the contrast of printed text with little effect on reading speed. But patients with reduced contrast sensitivity require high-contrast text in order to read well, and may be severely handicapped by low-contrast text that is found, for example, when colored letters are printed on colored paper.[9] Finally, older adults with low contrast sensitivity are more likely to report difficulty with everyday visual tasks like reading and recognizing faces.[10]

Contrast sensitivity was originally developed as a research tool, and for theoretical reasons most investigators use sinewave grating patterns: alternating light and dark bars that have a sinusoidal luminance profile. Sinewave gratings vary in spatial frequency (bar width) and contrast. A contrast sensitivity function is derived by measuring the lowest detectable contrast across a wide range of spatial frequencies, as illustrated by the curves in Figure 11–1.

Traditional methods for measuring contrast sensitivity require relatively expensive and sophisticated equipment—typically, a computer-controlled video display—and employ time-consuming psychophysical procedures. More recently, several contrast sensitivity tests have been developed for clinical use. These include plate tests with photographically reproduced sinewave gratings and various low-contrast optotype tests. There is considerable controversy about whether it is necessary to measure contrast sensitivity at several spatial frequencies using sinewave gratings or whether a single global measure of contrast sensitivity is adequate for clinical purposes. Patients with anterior segment disorders may experience either a general loss of contrast sensitivity across a wide range of spatial frequencies or a more restricted loss in the middle to high spatial frequencies. We have shown that overall changes in contrast sensitivity and changes near the peak of the function are more important than subtle bumps and wiggles in the curve.[9] Thus, global tests of contrast sensitivity provide about as much useful information as tests that measure multiple points along function.

The Pelli–Robson Letter Sensitivity Chart is a commercially available test that provides a single, global measure of contrast sensitivity (Fig 11–2).[11] Letters of constant size are arrayed in triplets of decreasing contrast. When viewed at the recommended test distance, the letters subtend 3° of visual angle, equivalent to a 20/720 Snellen letter. These large letters have been shown to provide a reliable measure of contrast sensitivity, even for patients with visual acuities down to 20/400.[12]

Contrast Sensitivity in Radial Keratotomy

Contrast sensitivity functions have been measured in several groups of radial keratotomy (RK) patients with conflicting results. Several studies have reported no

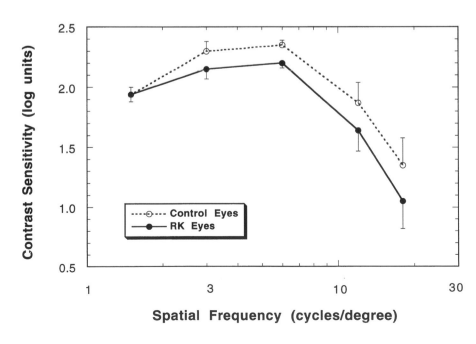

Figure 11–1. Contrast sensitivity function shows significant reduction at middle and high spatial frequencies after RK surgery.

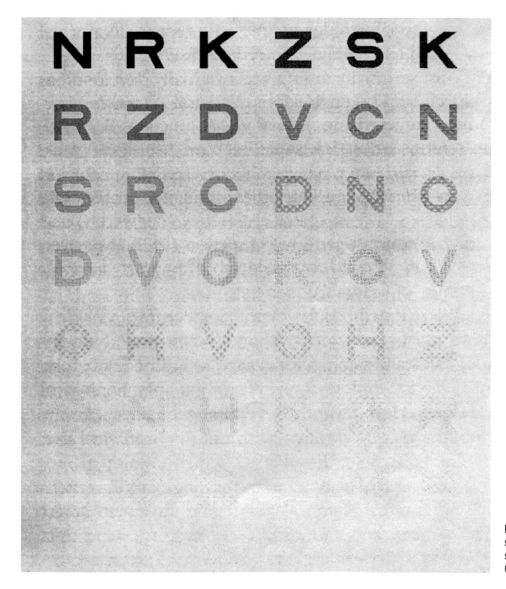

Figure 11–2. Pelli–Robson letter sensitivity chart. The letters are of constant size with decreasing contrast. Copyright 1996 Metropia Ltd.

loss of contrast sensitivity for RK eyes compared with eyes of normal control subjects,[13] the unoperated eyes of RK patients,[14] or the preop contrast sensitivity of eyes that later underwent RK.[14,15] All of these studies were small, as they used fewer than 15 subjects. Four other studies have reported significant declines in contrast sensitivity following RK surgery. A study of six RK patients found reductions at middle spatial frequencies (3 to 6 cycles/degree) at 1 year postop testing.[16] A second study of 30 patients reported decreases at low to middle spatial frequencies (2 to 8 cycles/degree) up to 4 months after surgery, which resolved by 1 year postop.[17] The third study compared the RK eye to the unoperated eye of 69 individuals enrolled in the Prospective Evaluation of Radial Keratotomy (PERK) study. There was a significant loss of contrast sensitivity at middle to high spatial frequencies (6 to 18 cycles/degree) up to 2 years after surgery.[18]

In a preliminary study of 20 RK eyes,[19] we found reductions in contrast sensitivity at spatial frequencies at or above 3 cycles/degree. The differences between RK eyes and contralateral control eyes are illustrated in Figure 11–1.

Contrast Sensitivity in Photorefractive Keratectomy

Contrast sensitivity tests have not been used extensively in studies of photorefractive keratectomy (PRK). Two studies[20,21] of 6 eyes and 31 eyes, respectively, reported no loss of contrast sensitivity at 3 or 6 months postop, but few details were provided. A more comprehensive study of 81 PRK patients tested contrast sensitivity with the Pelli–Robson chart at various intervals from 1 week to 1 year after treatment. There was an initial, significant drop of contrast sensitivity by a factor of two (.3 log units) at 1 week postop. Sensitivity gradually improved over the course of 1 year, but average test scores were still reduced by 50% (.2 log unit) at the last follow-up visit.

One group of investigators has used low-contrast visual acuity to evaluate PRK.[22,23] Low-contrast acuity measures the *smallest* contrast object rather than the *lowest contrast* object that can be recognized at a given size. Strictly speaking, such tests do not measure contrast sensitivity; however, the results are similar for the two types of measures. The low-contrast acuity results from three studies show little acuity loss for conventional high (90%)-contrast letters, but they indicate a marked reduction of visual acuity for letters of 5% contrast. The acuity loss reaches a maximum of as much as five lines at about 1 to 3 months postop. The loss subsides over the period of 4 months to 1 year postop.

Functional Significance of Contrast Sensitivity Loss

The size of the contrast sensitivity loss varies considerably across the studies reporting losses. One of the four RK studies reported losses of less than .1 log unit of contrast sensitivity,[18] whereas another reported losses up to .4 log unit.[17] A .1 log unit loss translates into a change of less than 15% in the amount of contrast required to identify an object. Although statistically significant, such a small change in contrast sensitivity would be of doubtful functional significance. On the other hand, a .4 log unit loss translates into a 250% change in the contrast required to recognize objects (ie, objects that could be recognized at 10% contrast before RK have to be 25% contrast after RK). We have shown that contrast sensitivity changes of this magnitude are functionally significant, at least in older individuals.[10] A contrast sensitivity loss of .3 log unit was associated with a 2.5- to 3.5-fold increase in the likelihood of reporting difficulty with a wide variety of daily vision tasks, such as reading a menu, identifying faces, seeing the edges of steps or curbs, and driving at night.

There have been few attempts to correlate contrast sensitivity loss with visual symptoms following RK or PRK, but one study reported that contrast loss was greatest in subjects who expressed subjective visual complaints. However, the contrast loss was generally small and did not correlate with the severity of the symptoms.[18]

GLARE SENSITIVITY TESTS

The most common visual side effects of refractive surgery are problems related to glare. Glare can refer to a variety of phenomena. *Discomfort glare* describes the sensation experienced when the overall illumination is too bright—for example, when the midday sun is reflected from sand or snow. In extreme cases, discomfort glare may result in pain or photophobia. In milder cases, it is sometimes referred to as photoaversion. *Glare recovery* is a measure of the speed with which the visual system regains function following exposure to a bright light. Any disorder that alters the dynamics of light and dark adaptation may affect glare recovery. Photostress tests are designed to measure glare recovery. *Disability glare* refers to the reduced visibility of a target owing to the presence of a light source elsewhere in the visual field. A common example is the reduced visibility of road signs in the presence of oncoming headlights.

Disability glare occurs when light from the glare source is scattered by the ocular media. This scattered light forms a veiling luminance that reduces the contrast and thus the visibility of the target. This effect is simulated in Figure 11–3. The contrast of the pattern can be defined in several ways. Here we use a definition that is common in the psychophysical literature:

$$\text{Contrast} = \frac{L_{max} - L_{min}}{L_{max} + L_{min}}$$

where L_{max} is the maximum luminance and L_{min} is the minimum luminance in the pattern. According to this definition, contrast can range from 0%, when the minimum and maximum luminances are the same, to 100% when the minimum luminance is 0 (regardless of the maximum luminance). The bar pattern on the left of Figure 11–3 has a contrast of 68%. On the right, scattered light raises the luminance of the target and background by 18 units each. This reduces the contrast to 43%.

Glare symptoms following refractive surgery are presumed to be caused by excessive light scatter; hence, the interest in disability glare tests. Most disability glare tests are simple in concept. A conventional visual function test, usually acuity or contrast sensitivity, is administered in the presence of a glare source. The glare source can be a spot, bar, or ring of light, or an extended bright background. The disability glare score can be obtained either from performance on the glare test alone, or by comparing performance with and without the glare source. The latter method is favored when there is concern about potential retinal or neurologic factors that would depress performance on the basic vision test without the glare. However, the former method provides more reliable data when retinal/neural factors are not an issue.[24]

The most popular clinical glare tests are those employing the Brightness Acuity Tester (BAT).[25] The BAT

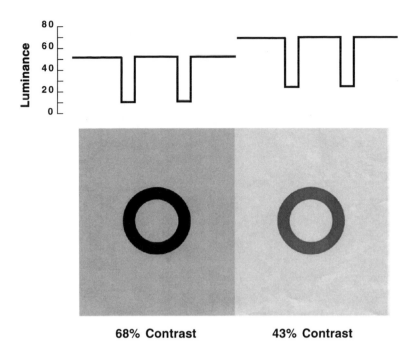

Figure 11–3. Simulation of disability glare. The patterns on the left have greater contrast than those on the right. The difference in luminance shown in the bar pattern on the left is similar to that on the right, but the contrast is greater. Above the letter "O" is its luminance profile.

is a brightly illuminated hemispherical cup held in front of the eye through which a conventional eye chart is viewed. When used with a contrast sensitivity test like the Pelli–Robson Chart, or with a low-contrast acuity test like the Regan Chart,[26] the BAT produces a reliable and valid measurement of intraocular light scatter.[24] However, the BAT is most often used with a conventional high-contrast acuity chart, which reduces the sensitivity and validity of measurement. Although several commercial nighttime glare tests have been introduced, none has been shown to give reliable (ie, repeatable) measurements.

Like contrast sensitivity, disability glare tests provide information about visual function that cannot be found in visual acuity tests alone. Studies of disability glare and cataracts have shown that glare problems cannot be simply explained by changes in visual acuity.[27,28] The dissociation between visual acuity and glare sensitivity is particularly evident in cases of posterior subcapsular cataract,[4,29] capsular opacification,[30] and corneal edema.[5]

Disability Glare in RK

It has been reported that the majority of RK patients see starburst or haloes at night but that these symptoms are not disabling, except for the few patients who have given up nighttime driving.[31] In the PERK study, 17% of participants reported trouble with glare at 1 year after treatment.[32] However, none of the 435 participants in the 1-year follow-up study failed the Miller–Nadler glare test that was part of the PERK study. The Miller–

Nadler test has been shown to have poor reliability and low sensitivity to moderate amounts of light scatter.[24] Other studies using more sensitive instruments have been inconclusive. One study of 15 patients drawn from the PERK study reported significant glare disability for flickering targets, but not for static ones.[33] A preliminary study of four RK patients showed dramatic glare effects under low luminance conditions that simulated nighttime driving.[34] But a study of disability glare at low and high luminance found no difference between preop and 1 month postop for either light level.[15]

Disability Glare in PRK

As in RK, reports of glare, starburst, and haloes are common side effects of PRK. In a study of 202 PRK patients, subjective complaints of glare or decreased vision at night were reported by 59% of patients at 6 months and 21% of patients at 1 year following treatment.[35] Objective measures of disability glare have produced inconsistent results. One study of six PRK eyes reported no loss of acuity under glare conditions at 6 months after treatment, but no details of the methodology or results were provided.[20] Others have found significant loss of acuity with glare using the glare test that is part of the Humphrey Auto Refractor. This test uses a low-contrast acuity chart bounded by an extended glare source above and below the line of acuity letters. No published reliability data are available for this instrument, but, its low-contrast optotypes would be likely to provide a more sensitive measure of disability glare than high-contrast optotypes. Results with the Humphrey instrument showed a loss of three acuity lines with glare for 12% of PRK patients in one study.[36] The magnitude of the glare effect is strongly dependent on the size of the attempted refractive error correction. None of the patients with 3 D or less of refractive error experienced significant glare disability, whereas 43% of those with 9 D or more lost at least three acuity lines with glare.[37] A recent study employing a 6-mm ablation zone instead of the previous 4 to 5 mm reported no difference in preop versus postop disability glare using a nighttime glare test that had proven to be very sensitive to glare in patients with RK.

Functional Significance of Increased Glare Disability

The natural assumption that disability glare measurements would be correlated with difficulty in performing everyday tasks under glare conditions, such as driving at night in the face of oncoming headlights, has been surprisingly difficult to corroborate. One study looked at the subjective reports of cataract patients, using a standardized questionnaire, but was unable to find an association between glare test results and glare symptoms.[38] We also found little relation between disability glare measurements and subjective difficulty with daily tasks under glare conditions.[10] One potential reason for the lack of correlation between glare tests and glare symptoms is that patients do not always distinguish between the various types of glare phenomena. Discomfort glare or glare recovery problems may be confused with disability glare. Because the glare tests used in the refractive surgery studies only measured disability glare, any confusion in the subjective reports of glare symptoms would weaken the statistical relation between objective and subjective glare assessment. In any event, neither the psychophysical measurement of disability glare nor the subjective assessment of glare symptoms leads to a clear understanding of the frequency and seriousness of this potential side effect of refractive surgery.

Mechanism of Contrast Sensitivity Loss and Glare in RK and PRK

There are at least two distinct mechanisms for glare and contrast sensitivity changes following refractive surgery. The most familiar is increased intraocular light scatter, caused by the corneal scars in the case of RK, or associated with corneal haze in the case of PRK. Although light scatter is usually discussed in the context of glare, it will also cause a reduction in the contrast sensitivity. At a qualitative level, the concept is simple:

light from the bright regions of a visual stimulus is scattered over the entire image, including the contrasting dark parts of the stimulus. This reduces the light:dark ratio, which is stimulus contrast. The addition of a glare source provides more light to scatter and further reduces contrast.

Several studies have measured the increase in intraocular light scatter following refractive surgery. One study used a newly developed instrument, the Straylightmeter,[39] to evaluate light scatter in 19 RK eyes that were tested 2 or more years after surgery. Compared with unoperated control eyes, there was a 40% increase in light scatter for undilated RK eyes and a 200% increase for pharmacologically dilated RK eyes.[40]

A theoretical analysis of the effects of wide-angle light scatter on disability glare demonstrates that light scatter has little effect on high-contrast acuity with glare, but a much larger effect on low-contrast acuity with glare.[41] This prediction is verified by the glare data for both RK and PRK.

For PRK, numerous studies have attempted to correlate corneal haze observed at the slit lamp with visual outcome, including contrast sensitivity and disability glare. However, haze seen in the slit lamp is the result of backscatter, or light scattered out of the eye toward the observer. Backscatter has a negligible effect on the quality of the retinal image. Forward light scatter is responsible for the image degradation but is much harder to quantify by observation. Fortunately, the Straylightmeter measures forward light scatter and is insensitive to backscatter.[22] Straylight meter measurements with PRK patients have yielded conflicting results. One study of 10 PRK eyes showed an association between reduced low-contrast acuity and increased light scatter.[22] A subsequent study, however, reported no increase in light scatter for 12 PRK eyes.[42] The second study suggests that the discrepancy may be caused by the larger ablation zone used (6 mm versus 4 mm).

The second cause of glare and contrast sensitivity loss is the introduction of higher-order aberrations at the cornea. RK and PRK differentially change the curvature of the central and peripheral regions of the cornea. For RK, this change is commonly modeled as an induced spherical aberration. Calculations of spherical aberration based on photokeratoscopic data were in rough agreement with predicted changes in the contrast sensitivity functions for four RK eyes. However, there was close quantitative agreement for only one of the four eyes.[43]

PRK produces a duplex optical system with a central in-focus zone and an annular out-of-focus zone. An optical model of this duplex system predicts little change in high-contrast acuity, but a more noticeable effect on contrast sensitivity.[44] Interestingly, the optical model predicts that contrast sensitivity loss should decrease as the amount of refractive error increases. This is because the contribution of the out-of-focus annulus decreases as the ametropia increases.

Spherical aberration is seldom discussed in the context of disability glare. However, a theoretical model of the duplex optical system in PRK eyes predicts the appearance of haloes and ghost images often associated with glare disability.[44] This prediction is supported by data from a PRK study, in which spherical aberration computed from corneal topography data was highly correlated with glare disability.[45] One study has attempted to look at light scatter and refractive changes in the same group of PRK patients.[46] Refractive errors seemed to be associated with the appearance of haloes around bright objects, whereas light scatter was associated with starburst phenomena.

SOURCES OF VARIATION IN GLARE AND CONTRAST SENSITIVITY STUDIES

From this review of glare disability and contrast sensitivity loss following refractive surgery, it is apparent that there is considerable variability and inconsistency in the reported findings. Some studies report dramatic and clinically significant visual side effects, while others report none, even for similar types of vision tests. There are several possible explanations for this variability. First, the tests themselves may be subject to large amounts of measurement error. Although this may be a contributing factor, especially for early studies based on tests that were subsequently shown to have poor reliability, most recent studies have used tests that have been shown to be reliable and valid.[24] A second factor may be the inherent variability of the patients. Several of the reviewed studies have used small numbers of patients, perhaps a dozen or less, and they have neither the statistical power to detect subtle changes nor the means for setting reasonable confidence intervals on the size of measured effects. A third factor, or group of factors, should not be neglected: the differences in surgical procedures or measurement conditions that may influence the visual outcome.

An important surgical factor that has been identified in studies of refractive surgery is the size of the clear zone for RK or the size of the ablation zone for PRK. A smaller clear zone was associated with more subjective glare complaints in a subset of PERK patients.[18] Theoretical models suggest that a larger ablation zone will result in fewer visual side effects, and a recent PRK study using 6-mm ablation instead of the former 4 to 5 mm found fewer light-scatter problems.[42] Unfortunately, the size of clear zone or ablation zone is often confounded with the amount of refractive error to be corrected, and higher refractive errors have been associated with more frequent visual complaints. Closely related to the size of the optical zone is the potential role of pupil size. Pupillary dilation results in a much larger increase in light scatter for RK eyes, compared with unoperated eyes,[40] and the largest glare effects are measured under nighttime viewing conditions.[34] Pupil size also interacts with spherical aberration in determining the quality of the retinal image.[47,48] Clinical studies of RK and PRK frequently do not measure or control pupil size, so this may add considerable variability to the results.

The healing process following refractive surgery has a well-known time course. Studies of visual function in RK and PRK differ in time after surgery when the tests are performed. One group of investigators has carefully monitored corneal haze (backscatter), forward light scatter, and disability glare at fixed intervals over a 1-year period following PRK. They reported that the time course of disability glare was not closely related to corneal haze[49] but, rather, was associated with forward light-scatter measurements.[22]

CONCLUSIONS

Despite numerous studies of visual function following refractive surgery, it is difficult to draw firm conclusions about the potential for contrast sensitivity loss or glare disability. Clinically significant reduction of contrast sensitivity and increase in glare disability has been reported for some groups of patients. This, combined with the frequent though seldom severe complaints of visual side effects from the procedures, argues strongly for additional research in this area. We now possess the tools to assess light scatter, contrast sensitivity, and glare with practical, reliable, and valid instruments. Future studies will need to identify and control potentially important variables, such as pupil size, follow-up time, and details of the surgical procedure that may account for the variability in previous studies. It is hoped that a better understanding of the factors that contribute to visual changes following refractive surgery will enable us to predict more accurately who will benefit from current procedures and new innovations for the treatment of refractive error.

REFERENCES

1. Kraff MC, Sanders DR, Karcher D, Raanan M, DeLuca M, Neumann G. Changing practice patterns in refractive surgery: results of a survey of the American Society of Cataract and Refractive Surgery. *J Cataract Refract Surg.* 1994; 20(2):172–178.

2. Marmor MF, Gawande A. Effect of visual blur on contrast sensitivity. *Ophthalmology.* 1988;95:139–143.

3. Campbell FW, Green DG. Optical and retinal factors affecting visual resolution. *J Physiol.* 1965;181:576–593.

4. Elliott DB, Gilchrist J, Whitaker D. Contrast sensitivity and glare sensitivity changes with three types of cataract morphology: are these techniques necessary in a clinical evaluation of cataract? *Ophthalmic Physiol Opt.* 1989;9: 25–30.

5. Hess RF, Carney LG. Vision through an abnormal cornea: a pilot study of the relationship between visual loss from corneal distortion, corneal edema, keratoconus and some allied corneal pathology. *Vision Res.* 1979;18:476–483.

6. Adamsons IA, Rubin GS, Vitale S, Taylor HR, Stark WJ. The effect of early cataracts on glare and contrast sensitivity: a pilot study. *Arch Ophthalmol.* 1992;110:1081–1086.

7. Lennerstrand G, Ahlström CO. Contrast sensitivity in macular degeneration and the relation to subjective visual impairment. *Acta Ophthalmol (Copenh).* 1989;67(3):225–233.

8. Marron JA, Bailey IL. Visual factors and orientation-mobility performance. *Am J Optom Physiol Opt.* 1982;59:413–426.

9. Rubin GS, Legge GE. Psychophysics of reading. VI—The role of contrast in low vision. *Vision Res.* 1989;29(1):79–91.

10. Rubin GS, Bandeen-Roche K, Prasada-Rao P, Fried LP. Visual impairment and disability in older adults. *Optom Vis Sci* (in press).

11. Pelli DG, Robson JG, Wilkins AJ. The design of a new letter chart for measuring contrast sensitivity. *Clin Vision Sci.* 1988;2:187–199.

12. Rubin GS. Reliability and sensitivity of clinical contrast sensitivity tests. *Clin Vision Sci.* 1988;2:169–177.

13. Carney LG, Kelley CG. Visual losses after myopic epikeratoplasty. *Arch Ophthalmol.* 1991;109:499–502.

14. Trick L, Hartstein J. Investigation of contrast sensitivity following radial keratotomy. *Ann Ophthalmol.* 1987;19: 251–254.

15. Olsen H, Andersen J. Contrast sensitivity in radial keratotomy. *Acta Ophthalmol.* 1991;69:654–658.

16. Tomlinson A, Caroline P. Effect of radial keratotomy on the contrast senstivity function. *Am J Optom Physiol Opt.* 1988;65:803–808.

17. Krasnov M, Avetisov S, Makashova N, Mamikonian V. The effect of radial keratotomy on contrast sensitivity. *Am J Ophthalmol.* 1988;105:651–654.

18. Ginsburg AP, Waring GO, Steinberg EB, et al. Contrast sensitivity under photopic conditions in the prospective evaluation of radial keratotomy (PERK) study. *Refract Corneal Surg.* 1990;6:82–91.

19. Hamburg T, Azar D, Rubin G, Blair S. Comparison of acuity, contrast sensitivity, and disability glare with contact lenses before and after radial keratotomy (RK) surgery. *Invest Ophthalmol Vis Sci.* 1994;35(4 suppl):1637.

20. Eiferman RA, O'Neill KP, Forgey DR, Cook YD. Excimer laser photorefractive keratectomy for myopia: six-month results. *Refract Corneal Surg.* 1991;7(5):344–347.

21. Sher NA, Chen V, Bowers RA, et al. The use of the 193-nm excimer laser for myopic photorefractive keratectomy in sighted eyes. A multicenter study. *Arch Ophthalmol.* 1991; 109(11):1525–1530. Comments.

22. Lohmann CP, Fitzke F, O'Brart D, Muir MK, Timberlake G, Marshall J. Corneal light scattering and visual performance in myopic individuals with spectacles, contact lenses, or excimer laser photorefractive keratectomy. *Am J Ophthalmol.* 1993;115(4):444–453.

23. Lohmann CP, Gartry DS, Muir MK, Timberlake GT, Fitzke FW, Marshall J. Corneal haze after excimer laser refractive surgery: objective measurements and functional implications. *Eur J Ophthalmol.* 1991;1(4):173–180.

24. Elliott DB, Bullimore MA. Assessing the reliability, discriminative ability, and validity of disability glare tests. *Invest Ophthalmol Vis Sci.* 1993;34:108–119.

25. Holladay JT, Prager TC, Trujillo J, Ruiz RS. Brightness acuity test and outdoor visual acuity in cataract patients. *J Cataract Refract Surg.* 1987;13:67–69.

26. Regan D, Neima D. Low-contrast letter charts as a test of visual function. *Ophthalmology.* 1982;90:1192–1120.

27. Hirsch RP, Nadler MP, Miller D. Glare measurement as a predictor of outdoor vision among cataract patients. *Ann Ophthalmol.* 1984;16:965–968.

28. Rubin GS, Adamsons IA, Stark WJ. Comparison of acuity, glare, and contrast sensitivity before and after cataract surgery. *Arch Ophthalmol.* 1993;111:56–61.

29. Abrahamsson M, Sjostrand J. Impairment of contrast sensitivity function (csf) as a measure of disability glare. *Invest Ophthalmol Vis Sci.* 1986;27:1131–1136.

30. Knighton RW, Slomovic AR, Parrish RK. Glare measurements before and after neodymium-YAG laser posterior capsulotomy. *Am J Ophthalmol.* 1985;100:708–713.

31. Rashid ER, Waring GO. Complications of radial and transverse keratotomy. *Surv Ophthalmol.* 1989;34: 73–106.

32. Cartwright CS, Bourque LB, Lynn M, Waring GO. The PERK Study Group. Relationship of glare to uncorrected visual acuity and cycloplegic refraction 1 year after radial keratotomy in the prospective evaluation of radial keratotomy (PERK) study. *J Am Optom Assoc.* 1988;59:36–39.

33. Atkin A, Asbell P, Justin N, Smith H, Wayne R, Winterkorn J. Radial keratotomy and glare effects on contrast sensitivity. *Doc Ophthalmol.* 1986;62:129–148.

34. Applegate RA, Trick LR, Meade DL, Hartstein J. Radial keratotomy increases the effects of disability glare: initial results. *Ophthalmology.* 1987;19:293–297.

35. Kim JH, Hahn TW, Lee YC, Joo CK, Sah WJ. Photorefractive keratectomy in 202 myopic eyes: one year results. *Refract Corneal Surg.* 1993;9(2 suppl):11–16.

36. Seiler T, Wollensak J. Myopic photorefractive keratectomy with the excimer laser. One-year follow-up. *Ophthalmology.* 1991;98(8):1156–1163.

37. Seiler T, Wollensak J. Results of a prospective evaluation of photorefractive keratectomy at 1 year after surgery. *Ger J Ophthalmol.* 1993;2(3):135–142.

38. Elliott DB, Hurst MA, Weatherill J. Comparing clinical tests of visual function in cataract with the patient's perceived visual disability. *Eye.* 1990;4:712–717.

39. van den Berg TJTP. Importance of pathological intraocular light scatter for visual disability. *Doc Ophthalmol.* 1986; 61:327–333.

40. Veraart HG, van den Berg TJ, Ijspeert JK, Cardozo OL. Stray light in radial keratotomy and the influence of pupil size and stray light angle. *Am J Ophthalmol.* 1992;114(4): 424–428.

41. Beckman CME. Letter imaging through light scattering eye media in the absence and presence of glaring light. In: *Vision Science and Its Application, 1994 Technical Digest Series.* Washington, DC: Optical Society of America; 1994;2: 94–97.

42. Harrison JM, Tennant TB, Gwin MC, Applegate RA, Tennant JL, van den Berg TJ, Lohmann CP. Forward light scatter at one month after photorefractive keratectomy. *J Refract Surg.* 1995;11(2):83–88.

43. Hemenger R, Tomlinson A, Caroline P. Role of spherical aberration in contrast sensitivity loss with radial keratotomy. *Invest Ophthalmol Vis Sci.* 1989;30:1997–2001.

44. Baron W, Munnerlyn C. Predicting visual performance following excimer photorefractive keratectomy. *Refract Corneal Surg.* 1992;8:355–362.

45. Seiler T, Reckmann W, Maloney RK. Effective spherical aberration of the cornea as a quantitative descriptor in corneal topography. *J Cataract Refract Surg.* 1993;19:155–165.

46. O'Brart DP, Lohmann CP, Fitzke FW, et al. Disturbances in night vision after excimer laser photorefractive keratectomy. *Eye.* 1994;8(pt 1):46–51.

47. Holladay JT, Lynn MJ, Waring GO, Gemmill M, Keehn GC, Fielding B. The relationship of visual acuity, refractive error, and pupil size after radial keratotomy. *Arch Ophthalmol.* 1991;109:70–76.

48. Applegate RA, Gansel KA. The importance of pupil size in optical quality measurements following radial keratotomy. *Refract Corneal Surg.* 1990;6:47–54.

49. Lohmann C, Gartry D, Muir M, Timberlake G, Fitzke F, Marshall J. "Haze" in photorefractive keratectomy: its origins and consequences. *Lasers Light Ophthalmol.* 1991;4: 15–34.

CHAPTER 12

Corneal Topography: Basic Principles

Michael J. Rogers ▪ Russell L. McCally ▪ Cynthia J. Roberts ▪ Dimitri T. Azar

Corneal topography refers to a description of the anterior corneal surface shape. It is used to gain insight about the optical performance of the eye in general and the cornea in particular. Topographic measurements are currently used to plan and to evaluate the outcome of refractive surgery and to diagnose corneal pathology. In this chapter the basic concepts and current issues in corneal topography are reviewed.

TERMINOLOGY

Some important landmarks on the cornea can be described, using the dimensions of Gullstrand's schematic eye.[1] These features are illustrated in Figure 12–1. The tear film of the anterior corneal surface acts like a convex mirror to form a virtual, erect image of reflected light. This image is called "the first Purkinje image" or the "corneal light reflex," and is the basis of many topographic measurement methods. If the central corneal radius of curvature is 7.80 mm, then when the eye is fixating a light source, the corneal light reflex is located approximately 3.90 mm posterior to the surface of the cornea.[1] As indicated in Figure 12–1, this image lies along a normal to the corneal surface.

The entrance pupil is the virtual image formed by refracted light from the real pupil, and it is located about 3.05 mm posterior to the corneal surface.[1] Thus,

the corneal light reflex is about 0.85 mm posterior to the entrance pupil. In general, the center of the entrance pupil (E in the figure) and the corneal light reflex are *not* coaxial.

The line of sight is a line connecting a fixation point at optical infinity with the center of the entrance pupil.[1] The pupillary axis is a line normal to the corneal surface passing through the center of the entrance pupil. It is usually temporal to the line of sight, and the angle between them is in the range of 3° to 6°. The pupillary axis and the line of sight both pass through the center of corneal curvature.

Historically, the cornea was considered to have a central optical zone with nearly constant curvature, outside of which the cornea became increasingly aspheric.[2] More recently, Waring described four surface zones on the cornea.[3] The central zone generally refers to the central 3 to 4 mm of the cornea, although sometimes a more specific definition is needed. Probably the most important definition of the central zone is that area of the cornea contributing to formation of the foveal image. The paracentral zone is an annulus with inner and outer diameters of 4 mm and 7 mm, respectively. The peripheral zone is an annular region with inner and outer diameters of 7 mm and 11 mm, respectively. The limbal zone is the border, about 0.5 mm wide, between the cornea and sclera. Of course, discrete divisions like these simplify the true situation

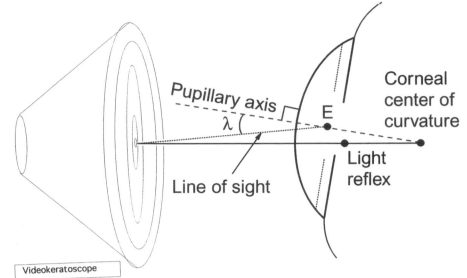

Figure 12–1. Location of the corneal light reflex, the line of sight, and the pupillary axis for a schematic eye fixating on the light. The pupillary axis and line of sight both pass through the center of the entrance pupil *(E)*. Angle lambda is usually 3° to 6°, with the pupillary axis directed temporal to the line of sight. *(Adapted from Uozato H, Guyton DL. Am J Ophthalmol. 1987;103:264–275.)*

because the corneal curvature varies continuously, but the terminology is widely accepted for clinical purposes.[2,3]

A meridian is defined as a great circle passing through the center of the cornea. (A great circle is a circle formed on the surface of a sphere by the intersection of a plane passing through the center of the sphere.[4] Although the cornea is not spherical, the concept of a great circle is the best way to visualize a meridian.) Meridians are located by their angular position, increasing counterclockwise from 0° at the 3 o'clock position to 180° at the 9 o'clock position.[3] A semimeridian is a direction on the corneal surface from its center, and it is located by its angular position from 0° at the 3 o'clock position, increasing counterclockwise around the full 360°. An axis refers to the direction in a cylindrical lens along which there is no power.

There is some confusion over the terms *apex* and *vertex* as applied to the cornea. According to Webster, both terms refer to a point on a shape furthest from its base.[4] A vertex can also refer to the point where the axis of a curve intersects the curve itself.[4,5] Maloney suggested denoting the high point of the cornea as the corneal vertex and the apex as the region of greatest curvature.[5] However, Waring defined the apex as the high spot of the cornea.[3] We will use Webster's definition of apex, and will not differentiate between apex and vertex. Still, it is very important to understand that the high point and the region of greatest curvature do not necessarily coincide.

Corneal topography is frequently described in terms of radius of curvature. The definition of radius of curvature at a point on a smooth plane curve is as follows[6]:

$$\rho = \frac{\left[1 + \left(\dfrac{dy}{dx}\right)^2\right]^{\frac{3}{2}}}{\left|\dfrac{d^2y}{dx^2}\right|} \tag{1}$$

An *apical* radius of curvature is simply the radius of curvature at the apex of a curve, and it may be determined by applying Equation 1 to such a point. In practice, instruments that measure corneal curvature cannot determine the apical radius of curvature at a point; rather, they determine the average central radius of curvature in a small area around the apex.

In order to determine a radius of curvature at a point on a three-dimensional surface, a two-dimensional curve must be defined by intersecting the surface with a plane. This is so because, according to Equation 1, radius of curvature is defined at a point on a two-dimensional plane curve. Such a defining curve and the radius of curvature associated with it are uniquely defined by the orientation of the intersecting plane (except in the special case of a perfect sphere). In describing the optical performance or shape of an aspheric optical element, two perpendicular planes are conventionally defined.[7,8] These are the tangential (also called meridional) and sagittal (also called transverse) planes, which are illustrated in Figure 12–2. A tangential plane is a plane containing both an off-axis object point and the optical axis. The sagittal plane is perpendicular to the tangential plane, and it also contains the object point and the surface normal to that object point. An infinite

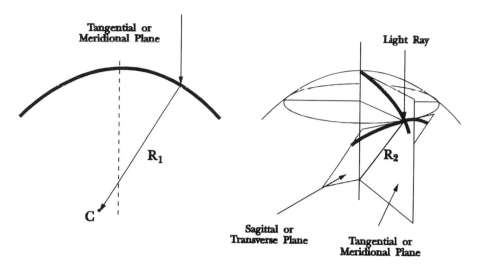

Figure 12–2. Schematic illustration of the tangential and sagittal planes of an optical surface. *(Adapted from Gao Y.* Polynomial Modeling of the Corneal Surface to Improve the Measurements of Topography. *Columbus: Ohio State University; 1994. Dissertation.)*

number of such planes correspond to all of the object points in space.

The tangential radius of curvature at a point on a surface is determined as the radius of curvature at that point along a curve defined by the intersection of the tangential plane with the surface; the sagittal radius of curvature is similarly defined. Both radii of curvature lie along the surface normal. For a spherical surface, the tangential and sagittal radii of curvature are identical everywhere, and their centers of curvature are both on the optical axis. However, for an aspherical surface, the tangential and sagittal radii of curvature are independent of one another, they may vary from point to point on the surface, and their centers may both be off of the optical axis. The intersection of the normal to the curve with the optical axis has been referred to as the *axial distance* and has been used to approximate radius of curvature in corneal topography.[9] For a spherical surface, the axial distance is equivalent to the radius of curvature. However, for an aspherical surface, the axial distance may be quite different from any true radius of curvature, whether in the tangential or the sagittal direction.[9]

Radius of curvature, which is an indicator of shape, has been described in terms of dioptric power, which is an indicator of optical performance, a practice that has led to some confusion.[9] Although paraxial equations, by definition, are only valid near the optical axis, they are frequently used in geometric optics to estimate optical performance. The paraxial refractive power *P,* of a single refracting surface with apical radius of curvature *r,* for light traveling from a medium with refractive index *n* to a medium with refractive index *n'*, is shown in Equation 2.

$$P = \frac{n' - n}{r} \qquad (2)$$

This equation predicts that refractive power is inversely proportional to the radius of curvature. Thus, in the central paraxial region, a surface with a small radius of curvature has more refractive power than one with a larger radius of curvature. However, it is important to note that Equation 2 is only valid in the central 1 to 2 mm of the corneal surface. Outside that region, refractive power is not necessarily inversely proportional to radius of curvature.[9] The region of interest for corneal topography covers an area of the corneal surface over 8 mm in diameter, well outside the paraxial region, but corneal topography instruments commonly apply the same Equation 2 over the entire region. To be precise, we will use the term *dioptric power* to describe the values displayed by corneal topography "power" maps, which are based on corneal shape, and our use of the term *refractive power* will refer strictly to optical performance. Dioptric power maps should not be interpreted, even qualitatively, as refractive power maps.

DESCRIPTIONS OF CORNEAL SHAPE

The cornea is aspherical in shape.[10,11] The average central radius of curvature of the normal human cornea is about 7.8 mm, but there is variation about this value. The radius of curvature becomes larger peripherally.[11]

Mandell studied the corneal shapes of eight subjects using photokeratoscopy and found that apical radii of curvature ranged from 7.3 to 8.2 mm.[10] He examined several simple mathematical curves as descriptors of corneal shape and found that the best fit for any single semimeridian of the cornea was an ellipse. The best-fitting ellipses had eccentricities ranging from 0.2 to 0.85, with an average value of 0.48. He also found that the apex was decentered from the line of sight in every case.

Because ellipses are useful for describing corneal surface shape and have recently been applied in the assessment of corneal topography devices,[9,12,13] we will consider their characteristics in some detail. Figure 12–3 illustrates an ellipse, which is a type of conic section. A conic section is a shape that can be obtained by intersecting a double-napped right circular cone with a plane,[6] and is defined as follows:

> ... the locus of a point P that moves in the plane of a fixed point F, called a focus, and a fixed line d, called a directrix, such that the ratio of the distance of P from F to its perpendicular distance from d is a constant, e, called the eccentricity.[14]

The definition of an ellipse is "the set of all points in a plane, the sum of whose distances from two fixed points in the plane (the foci) is constant."[6]

In mathematical texts, the equation for an ellipse is frequently formulated in terms of the lengths of the major and minor axes, $2a$ and $2b$, respectively.[6] The ellipse shown in Figure 12–3 has its major axis parallel to the y axis and its center at $(0, -a)$, so that an apex of the ellipse is located at the origin; the general equation for such an ellipse is

$$\frac{x^2}{b^2} + \frac{(y + a)^2}{a^2} = 1 \tag{3}$$

For any ellipse, the eccentricity is

$$e = \frac{\sqrt{a^2 - b^2}}{a} < 1 \tag{4}$$

The apical radius of curvature, R_0, can be determined by taking the appropriate derivatives of Equation 3 at the origin and substituting these into Equation 1. The result is

$$R_0 = a(1 - e^2) \tag{5}$$

(Note that for a circle, which is a special case of an ellipse with $a = b$, Equation 5 gives the radius as $R_0 = a$, as expected.)

Bennett described another formulation of a conic section for use in aspheric contact lens design.[7] For a

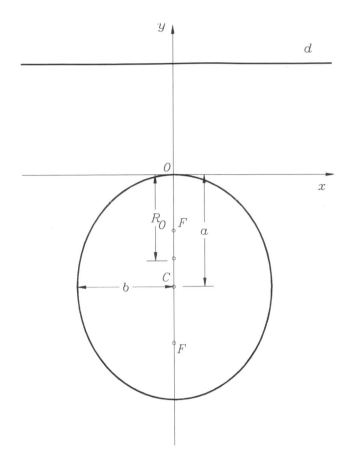

Figure 12–3. Geometry of an ellipse with its major axis parallel to y axis and origin at $(0, -a)$. One apex of the ellipse is located at the origin. In the figure, C is the center of the ellipse, F are the foci, d is the directrix, and a and b are the major and minor axes, respectively. Note that for this ellipse the apical radius of curvature, R_0, is shorter than a. *(From Rogers MJ.* Topography-Based Excimer Laser Ablation of an Irregularly Astigmatic Surface. *Baltimore: Johns Hopkins University; 1994. Master's thesis.)*

conic section located in the x–y plane with its apex at the origin and its major axis parallel to the y axis, the curve is defined in terms of the apical radius of curvature, R_0, and the index of peripheral flattening, or shape factor, p, as

$$x^2 = -2R_0y - py^2 \tag{6}$$

in which the shape factor is related to the eccentricity by $p = 1 - e^2$. The shape factor describes the degree and type of asphericity. For example: $p < 0$ describes a hyperbola, $p = 0$ describes a parabola, $0 < p < 1$ describes a *prolate* ellipse (an ellipse in which the radius of curvature increases with distance from the apex), $p = 1$ describes a circle, and $p > 1$ describes an *oblate* ellipse (radius of curvature decreases with distance from the apex). Thus, the central cornea is approximated by a prolate ellipsoid.

Another method to describe the shape of the cornea mathematically is by a series of orthogonal polynomials. Zernike polynomials are a complete set of orthogonal polynomials used to describe surface shapes that are nearly spherical. Webb demonstrated the application of Zernike polynomials to surfaces occurring in ophthalmology and suggested that they may be the best descriptor of the cornea.[15]

In another approach, Howland and colleagues fitted fourth-order Taylor polynomials to corneal surface files obtained from a computer-assisted videokeratoscope.[16] After fitting the surface data, they could calculate the mean corneal curvature at any point on the surface. After comparing plots of calculated and measured radius of curvature data, they found that the polynomial description captured gross curvature features but lost some of the fine detail portrayed by the original curvature data. They also noted that the polynomial description demonstrated greater overall curvature than the measured data, but they did not determine the source of this inconsistency. With refinement, they suggested that this method could provide a classification scheme for normal and pathologic corneas.

Raach analyzed the meridional variations in corneal dioptric power due to astigmatism using Fourier techniques.[17] He condensed dioptric power data from a computer-assisted videokeratoscope into a weighted average for each meridian and plotted it as a function of the meridional orientation. This average profile was decomposed into a sum of sinusoids. The amplitude of the two-cycle sinusoid represented the magnitude of regular astigmatism. Higher- and lower-frequency sinusoidal components represented the irregular astigmatic components.

Corneal shape can also be summarized with statistical indices. Dingeldein, Klyce, and Wilson designed the surface asymmetry index (SAI) and studied its correlation with best spectacle-corrected visual acuity.[18] The SAI is a measure of the difference in corneal dioptric power along opposing semimeridians. A theoretically perfect sphere or spherocylinder would have an SAI of zero. Similarly, Wilson and Klyce designed the surface regularity index (SRI) and studied its relation to visual acuity.[19] The SRI measures the variation in corneal dioptric powers at adjacent keratoscope points in the central cornea; like the SAI, it would be zero for an ideal sphere. In their study, Wilson and Klyce found that the SRI was a better predictor of visual acuity than the SAI.[19]

EARLY CORNEAL MEASUREMENTS

The first Purkinje image provides a measure of corneal shape and is the basis for most methods of measuring the corneal surface. The earliest known attempt to measure the curvature of the anterior corneal surface was in 1619 by Father Christopher Scheiner (1573–1650).[20,21] Scheiner compared images reflected from the surface of the cornea with those reflected by glass balls of various diameters.

The independent discoveries of astigmatism by Thomas Young (1773–1829) and George Biddell Airy (1801–1892) in 1800 and 1825, respectively, stimulated further interest in examining corneal shape.[21] In 1808, David Brewster (1781–1868) used the Purkinje image from a candle flame to observe the shape of a conical cornea.[21,22] In 1847, Henry Goode described the first keratoscope.[21] It was a small, luminous square, which he held a few inches in front of the eye, allowing him to detect abnormal corneal shape by observing the corneal reflex. This early keratoscope provided a qualitative measure of corneal deformity.

Hermann Ludwig Ferdinand von Helmholtz (1821–1894) is generally credited with invention of the ophthalmometer, or keratometer, in 1854,[23] although it has also been attributed to Jesse Ramsden (1735–1800).[24] The keratometer made possible the first quantitative measurement of the corneal radius of curvature. Louis Emile Javal (1839–1907) and Hjalmar August Schiøtz (1850–1927) improved Helmholtz's design by about 1880.[20]

Working independently of Goode, in 1880 a Portuguese oculist named Antonio Plácido (1840–1916) developed his own handheld keratoscope for detecting corneal irregularities.[21] Plácido's disc, as it came to be called, consisted of a flat disc 23 cm in diameter, with alternating light and dark bands drawn on its surface and a central aperture for viewing the corneal reflex of the rings. In that same year, Plácido went on to develop the first photokeratoscope by using a camera in conjunction with his disc to record the corneal reflex. At about the same time, Javal reported that he had developed his own keratoscope and photokeratoscope, apparently independently of Plácido.[20,21] Javal went on to present the first known application of photokeratoscopy to the observation of a pathologic corneal irregularity.[21] In his review of keratoscopy, Clark attributed the invention of *quantitative* photokeratoscopy to Gullstrand,[25] and he described the major developments from Gullstrand's work up to the end of the 1960s. (Also noteworthy is Clark's review of keratometry.[26])

KERATOMETRY

The keratometer measures the average radius of curvature of the central cornea along a single meridian. Today's clinical keratometer is based on the same design as that developed by Helmholtz and by Javal and Schiøtz.[27] The principle of keratometry, which is fundamental to many quantitative keratoscopy techniques, is illustrated in Figure 12–4. Because the anterior corneal surface acts like a convex mirror in reflecting light, the size of the reflected image is related to the corneal radius of curvature. The keratometer makes quantitative measurements of this reflected image. If the cornea is illuminated with an object whose size and distance from the corneal surface are known, the radius of curvature can be determined by measuring the size of the reflected image. In practice, the distance from the object to the reflected image is fixed by placing the object in a mount with a fixed-focus eyepiece. This arrangement requires the object–image distance to be equal to the working distance of the eyepiece in order to bring the image to sharp focus. Measurement of the image height is facilitated by an optical doubler. (For a description of optical doubling, see Bennett.[27])

In Figure 12–4, we have adopted the following conventions: incident light travels from left to right, distances to the left of the optical surface are negative, and those to the right are positive. An object of height h is located a distance o from the vertex, V, of a convex mirror with radius r. A ray from point Y of the object is directed toward the center of curvature, C, and is reflected back along itself. Another ray from Y' directed toward the focal point, F, of the mirror becomes parallel to the axis after reflection. Thus, a virtual image of point Y is formed at point Y'. If h' is the height of Y' above the axis, then by similar geometry

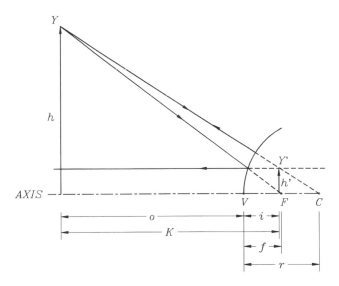

Figure 12–4. The principle of keratometry (see text).

$$\frac{h'}{h} \approx \frac{f}{f - o} \tag{7}$$

Because of the fixed-focus eyepiece, the distance from object to image under proper focus conditions is a constant, $K = i - o$. If o is very large, i will be very close to f, and we can write $(f - o) = (i - o) = K$. The focal point of the mirror is located at $f = r/2$ from the vertex. Substituting for f and $(f - o)$ and solving for r, we have

$$r \approx 2K\frac{h'}{h} \tag{8}$$

Three approximations made by the keratometer should be noted:

1. The cornea is a spherical convex mirror with the center of curvature on the optical axis.
2. Paraxial equations are sufficiently accurate to determine the path of light rays.
3. The dioptric power, P (on most keratometers), is determined from the radius of curvature by the paraxial Equation 2, where the refractive index of the cornea is assumed to be 1.3375. This so-called keratometer index, which differs from the true refractive index of the cornea (1.375, according to Maurice[11]), is a factor that gives approximately correct total corneal power measurements by compensating for the negative power of the posterior corneal surface.[28]

In most keratometers, the object projected onto the cornea, called a *mire,* consists of two illuminated crosses separated by about 3 mm. Thus, the keratometer measures the *average* radius of curvature in one meridian within the central area of the cornea. The curvature can be measured along any meridian by rotating the eyepiece-target assembly. For example, if a cornea is astigmatic, the principal radii are determined by making two measurements.

CORNEAL TOPOGRAPHY SYSTEMS

Although several other methods for measuring corneal topography have been reported, some of which are now commercially available, Plácido disc–based topography systems still dominate in clinical practice. Consequently, this discussion of specific topography methods will emphasize videokeratoscopy.

Videokeratoscopy

The need for accurate corneal measurements in order to plan refractive surgery stimulated increased interest in measuring the corneal surface in the late 1970s.[29] New techniques were sought to obtain more detailed information about the shape of the cornea. Most of these techniques were enhancements of keratoscopes and photokeratoscopes. Functionally, the principal difference between a keratometer and a keratoscope is in the coverage provided; a keratometer typically uses a simple mire with only two reference points, but a keratoscope usually projects a pattern over a large area of the cornea. Both instruments rely on measuring the reflected image of a target, and they calculate the radius of curvature based on the size or location of the image.

In 1981, Rowsey and colleagues described a modified photokeratoscope, called the Corneascope, that utilized a comparator to determine the corneal radius of curvature at a point on any of the rings.[30] The comparator allowed the keratoscope photo to be variably enlarged until a point of interest on one of the rings in the photo matched the corresponding point on a standard set of rings. The required magnification was used to determine the radius of curvature at that point.

Also in 1981, Doss and colleagues introduced mathematical techniques for analyzing keratoscope photographs to determine radius of curvature.[31] They used a computer program to calculate the radius from the measured radial distance to each ring in the photo. Their algorithm assumed that the radius of curvature of the cornea at its apex was 7.8 mm, and they calculated the radius of curvature at each ring by constructing a series of arcs tangentially connected at the ring locations. In 1983, Rowsey and Isaac described a technique in which they manually digitized keratoscope photos of calibration spheres and used regression to develop a relation between the ring locations and the radius of curvature.[32] They incorporated the regression results in a computer program that could be used to analyze digitized keratoscope photos of patient corneas.

Klyce refined the algorithms developed by Doss and used statistical methods to reduce errors from manual digitization.[33] Klyce's algorithm eliminated the assumption of a 7.8-mm apical radius of curvature by estimating the central radius of curvature from the average radius of the image of the innermost keratoscope ring. His computer program presented results in the form of a three-dimensional representation of the corneal shape. Corneas were also displayed as "distortion plots," or spherical difference plots, showing how the corneal shape differed from a sphere. Further refinements to the algorithms developed by Doss were published by van Saarloos and Constable.[34] Maguire and Singer worked with Klyce to add a color-coded display

showing contours of constant dioptric power.[35] This *isodioptric* display is one of the standard displays in computer-assisted videokeratoscopes now commercially available, and is probably the most widely used. Examples of isodioptric displays of test surfaces are shown in Figures 12-5 and 12-6. The first integrated computer-assisted videokeratoscope system was described by Gormley and colleagues in 1988.[36] Typical of the systems now available, it included a lighted target, a CCD video camera to capture the keratoscope image, and computer digitization of the ring locations using an edge detection algorithm.

A number of studies have examined the accuracy and reproducibility of different videokeratoscope systems,[37–44] but most of these studies used spherical test objects and thus did not address fundamental limitations of the technique.[12]

Surface Reconstruction Methods and Limitations

Like the keratometer, most videokeratoscopes attempt to measure the radius of curvature at points on the corneal surface and then to convert the measurement to paraxial dioptric power. As we pointed out earlier, the paraxial description of refractive power is an approximation valid only near the optical axis (recall Equation 2). However, videokeratoscopes are used to measure a region that is approximately 8 mm in diameter. Roberts showed that videokeratoscopes do not display refractive power accurately over this entire region, and thus they may produce incorrect qualitative patterns.[9] Thus, dioptric power data produced by videokeratoscopes should be considered a description of shape only, *not* refractive power. Both corneal shape and refractive power are meaningful quantities for understanding optical performance, but the distinction is essential for correct interpretation of corneal measurements.

Commercially available computer-assisted videokeratoscope systems use different proprietary algorithms to compute the radius of curvature. All suffer from the fact that there is insufficient information in the two-dimensional image of the corneal reflex to uniquely determine the three-dimensional shape of the cornea.[45] The situation is illustrated in Figure 12-7. A virtual image of an object point is created by reflection at the corneal surface. The virtual image is focused at the film plane when it is at the working distance of the camera. However, there is more than one reflecting surface, each with different radii of curvature, that can produce the same virtual image. In order to construct a unique three-dimensional solution to the problem, as-

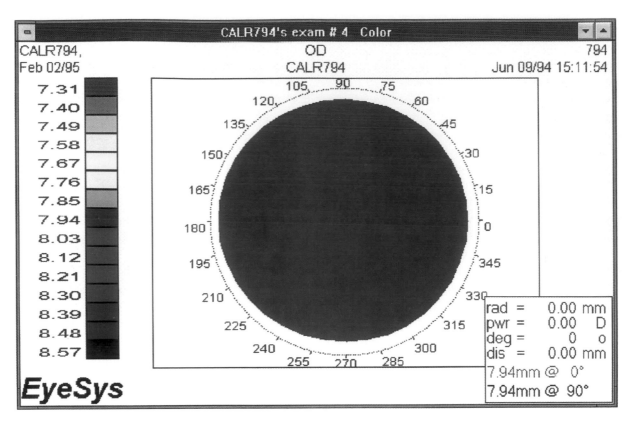

Figure 12–5. Isodioptric videokeratoscope map of a 7.94-mm radius calibration sphere. The videokeratoscope measures radius of curvature, but the scale at left is in diopters, calculated from $P = 0.3375/r$. For a sphere with a constant radius of curvature, the color map is relatively uniform (within the limits of measurement accuracy). *(From the EyeSys Corneal Analysis System, EyeSys Laboratories, Houston, TX.)*

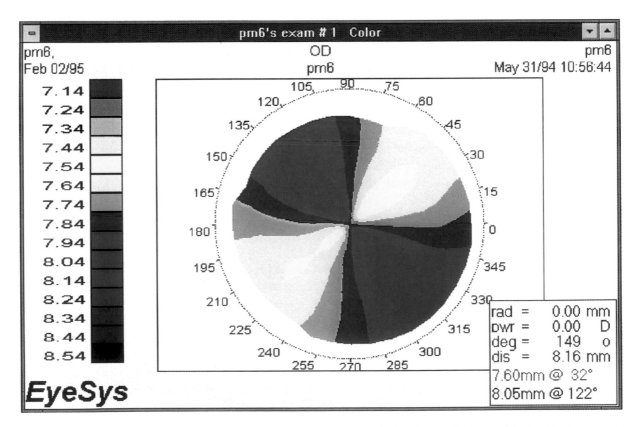

Figure 12–6. Isodioptric videokeratoscope map of a toric contact lens. Because the lens has maximal and minimal radii of curvature in meridians that are orthogonal to one another, it illustrates regular astigmatism. The radius of curvature of the front surface of the lens ranges from 7.9 to 7.3 mm. *(From the EyeSys Corneal Analysis System, EyeSys Laboratories, Houston, TX.)*

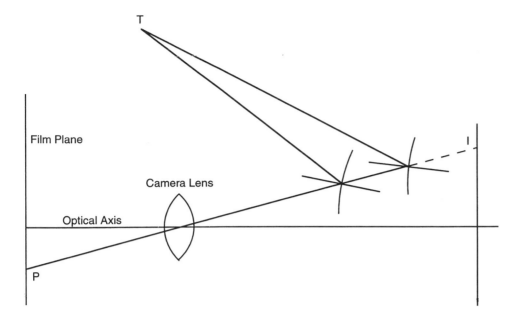

Figure 12–7. The difficulty in uniquely reconstructing a surface from keratoscopy data. An object point reflected by the corneal surface creates a virtual image, which is focused at the film plane. Because more than one surface can produce the same virtual image, assumptions must be made in order to construct a solution. *(From Wang J, Rice DA, Klyce SD.* Refract Corneal Surg. *1989; 5:379–387.)*

sumptions about the geometry of the cornea are necessary. Fundamentally, the keratometer encounters the same problem and, as discussed earlier, makes assumptions to overcome it.

Many videokeratoscopes overcome the ambiguity of surface reconstruction by calibrating the mire images on a series of standard spherical surfaces with known radii of curvature.[12,46] An internal table of the mire locations for the calibration surfaces is created. When a measurement is made of a cornea, the measured locations of the mire images are compared with those obtained during calibration in order to determine the radius of curvature at each point. This technique is essentially an adaptation of the method proposed by Rowsey et al.[30] Measurements of aspherical surfaces using this method are subject to error caused by the spherical bias of the calibration procedure.[12,45]

Several consequences of spherical bias merit further discussion. When a light ray is reflected by a surface, it lies in the same plane as the incident ray and the surface normal. All of the surface normals of a spherical optical surface pass through the optical axis, and the center of curvature at each surface point is also located on the optical axis. For such a surface, a reflected ray and the center of curvature are contained in the same plane. However, a spherical surface is a special case; for the more general case of an aspheric surface, the center of curvature and the radius of curvature must be defined in terms of planes intersecting the surface at the point of interest, and they will vary with the orientation of such planes (conventionally, the tangential and sagittal planes). In any case, for an aspheric surface the plane defined by the reflected ray and the surface nor-

mal may not contain the optical axis. A spherically biased videokeratoscope cannot resolve this type of optical performance, so that some information about an irregular surface is lost. To characterize completely the surface normal, which ultimately defines optical performance, both the sagittal and the tangential radii of curvature are necessary.

Spherically biased systems do not determine the tangential or instantaneous radius of curvature because they assume that the center of curvature lies on the optical axis.[12] Roberts quantified the error in the dioptric power determinations of the EyeSys Corneal Analysis System (EyeSys Laboratories, Houston, TX) by comparing measured and theoretically calculated curvature for a sphere and an ellipsoid with known dimensions.[12] In that study, the EyeSys videokeratoscope was characterized as spherically biased because it calculates radius of curvature by comparing the keratoscope image dimensions with a look-up table. The videokeratoscope measured the sphere under conditions of perfect alignment to within 0.10 D of the "true" paraxial power. Comparison of measured and theoretical paraxial dioptric power for the ellipse showed that at the inner four rings the measurement error was less than 0.25 D, but it increased peripherally to a maximum of 3.22 D at the outermost ring. Comparisons between aligned and misaligned measurements indicated that the misalignment error was small compared to the inherent error of the algorithm itself. However, comparison of the measured results to calculations using a formula based on axial distance showed that the instrument accurately reproduced the axial distance rather than the radius of curvature. Similar results were obtained for the Topographic Modeling System (Computed Anatomy, New York, NY).[13]

Currently available Plácido disc–based topography systems also are incapable of measuring the sagittal radius of curvature because, with a target consisting of a series of concentric rings, it is not possible to measure distortion of the virtual image in the sagittal direction.[12] A rectilinear keratoscope target like that proposed by Shimmick and Munnerlyn may be able to overcome this shortcoming because it would be able to resolve image displacement in two orthogonal directions.[47] In a new product under development by EyeSys Laboratories, a pattern of spokes is superimposed on the Plácido disc target to produce a "checkerboard" Plácido. Measurement of the sagittal radius of curvature would be possible by analyzing the distortion of the reflected checkerboard pattern in the sagittal direction.

An algorithm for computing corneal curvature that avoids the assumption of corneal sphericity and allows the instantaneous center of curvature to lie off the optical axis (but still in the tangential plane) was introduced by Wang, Rice, and Klyce in 1989.[45] They found that the maximum error for measurement of an ellipsoid was reduced from 8% for a spherically biased algorithm to 2% for the new method. Increased computation time and sensitivity to noise have prevented its implementation so far. Several manufacturers of corneal topography devices have developed, or are in the process of developing, algorithms based on tangential or instantaneous radius of curvature, rather than axial distance. Systems in which the tangential or instantaneous radius of curvature is currently available as an output include the EyeSys Corneal Analysis System, the Keratron Corneal Imaging Analyzer (Optikon 2000, Italy), and the Alcon EyeMap EH290 Corneal Topographer (Irvine, CA). A similar algorithm is currently being developed for the Topographic Modeling System. However, no data have yet been published examining the accuracy of any of these algorithms in measuring radius of curvature. These algorithms will potentially determine the tangential radius of curvature more accurately than a spherically biased algorithm, but they still neglect the sagittal radius of curvature.

Videokeratoscope Measurements of Corneal Elevations

Although most topography systems describe the corneal surface in terms of radius of curvature, an alternate characterization is to describe the surface in terms of elevation with respect to a reference plane, a quantity sometimes called *sag* or *surface height*. Several commercially available videokeratoscopes are capable of deriv-

ing sag from radius of curvature data, and in some of the newer non-Plácido disc–based systems, sag is the fundamental measurement quantity.

As noted previously, corneal height elevations were used for analyzing corneal surface shape in a system developed by Klyce.[33] This system produced wireframe models of corneal surface shape and plots of spherical difference, which Klyce called distortion plots. Young and Siegel described a technique that they called "isomorphic corneal modeling," which used existing tools to produce wire-frame representations of corneal shape from videokeratoscope measurements.[48,49] They used a Visioptics EH-270 videokeratography system to obtain their data because it produces data in the form both of sag values and of radius of curvature. The data were imported into a commercially available software program that permitted wire frame displays, subtraction of one curve from another, free rotation of the wire frame, and scalable axes.

The accuracy of videokeratoscope sag values has not been thoroughly assessed. However, some systems that use sag values as the fundamental measurement quantity allow differentiation between a "hill" and a "valley" on the corneal surface, an ability that current Plácido disc–based systems do not have.

Rogers, McCally, and Azar investigated the accuracy of sag values derived from Plácido disc–based topography measurements (unpublished data). A proprietary algorithm provided by EyeSys Laboratories was used to derive sag values for an ellipsoid with known dimensions, based on published topographic data obtained with the EyeSys Corneal Analysis System.[12] Comparison of the derived and theoretically calculated sag values showed that the maximum error was less than 0.1%. Further investigation is needed to assess the accuracy of sag values for the more important case of a generally irregular surface.

Centering Corneal Topography

Corneal topography is increasingly used for planning surgical procedures. For this purpose, topography data should be centered on a useful and easily determined reference point. Uozato and Guyton discussed centering procedures for corneal surgery, and their discussion applies to corneal topography as well.[1] They recommended centering on the entrance pupil while the patient fixates on a target that is made to be coaxial with the observer's line of sight. They also illustrated the centration error that arises from centering on the corneal light reflex instead of the entrance pupil (Fig 12–1). Topography should be referenced to the center of the entrance pupil, but the concentric rings of a videokeratoscope target center on the corneal light reflex, and the two locations do not generally coincide. The offset can be significant for an irregular cornea and must be taken into account when using videokeratoscope data.[5] Some videokeratoscope systems have incorporated an algorithm that searches the captured image for the edge of the entrance pupil. This is a step in the right direction, but we have not seen any data regarding how well the pupil is located. The Keratron Corneal Imaging Analyzer has the ability to move the center of the topographic data display at the user's discretion. Therefore, if the user observes that the map is not centered on the pupil, he or she can move the map to that location and recalculate it with reference to the newly identified center. Because calculations are referenced to a new central axis that remains normal to the corneal surface, the movement requires rotation of this reference axis, as

well as translation. This is illustrated in Figures 12–8 and 12–9 for a photorefractive keratectomy (PRK) patient. The radius of curvature–based dioptric map (labeled *true* in the figures) is given on the left, and the axial distance–based dioptric map (labeled *axial* in the figures) is on the right. The pupil center is shown by the small white cross, and the reference axis on which the map is centered is shown by the large white cross. Figure 12–8 represents the original set of maps obtained at the time of the patient exam. Figure 12–9 represents the recalculated maps after the reference axis has been moved to the pupil center. The axial map is dramatically altered by moving the reference axis, while the radius of curvature map is only minimally affected. Because axial distance is defined relative to a specific axis, it is therefore sensitive to changes in axis location. Radius of curvature, on the other hand, is axis independent.

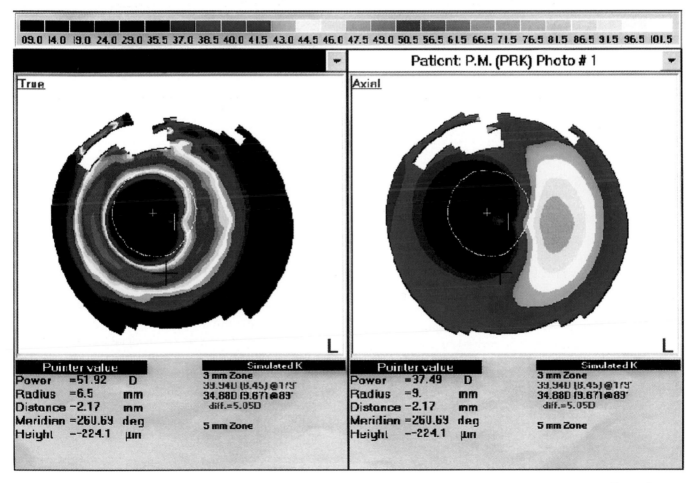

Figure 12–8. Original maps obtained with a Keratron Corneal Image Analyzer (Optikon 2000, Italy) after photorefractive keratectomy. The pupil center is shown by the small white cross. *Left:* Radius of curvature–based dioptric map. *Right:* Axial distance–based dioptric map. *(Courtesy of Alliance Medical Marketing, Inc., Jacksonville Beach, Florida.)*

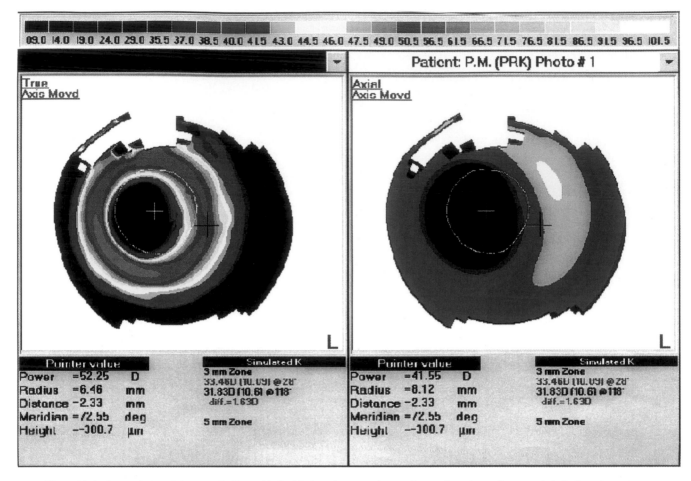

Figure 12–9. Recalculation of the maps in Figure 12–8 with the reference axis superimposed on the pupil center. *Left:* Radius of curvature–based dioptric map. *Right:* Axial distance–based dioptric map. *(Courtesy of Alliance Medical Marketing, Inc., Jacksonville Beach, Florida.)*

Other Topography Systems

Raster Photogrammetry

Rasterstereography, or raster photogrammetry, was described by Frobin as a method for measuring body surfaces.[50] Warnicki and colleagues introduced a corneal topography system that relies on raster photogrammetry.[51] A version of this system that is now commercially available was described by Belin and colleagues.[52] The system projects a grid onto the corneal surface, and the camera captures an image of the grid. Both the projector and the camera are set up so that their axes make known offset angles with the optical axis of the eye. Topical fluorescein is used to stain the corneal tear film to enhance the grid projection. Elevations are computed at each grid intersection based on the distortion in the grid and the known projection and camera angles. From these elevations, radius of curvature or dioptric power information is calculated. Accuracy of dioptric power determinations on spherical test objects was reported to be within 0.21 D[53]; however, we are not aware of any data regarding the accuracy of the system on general aspherical test objects.

One advantage of the raster photogrammetry system is that, because it relies on fluorescein rather than the tear film to reflect the projected grid, it can be used intraoperatively. However, it does not work with standard fluorescein in balanced salt solution; instead, the fluorescein requires a viscous artificial tear vehicle. This leads to a *disadvantage:* because artificial tear preparations have been found to alter videokeratoscope measurements of corneal topography,[54,55] it is likely that application of such a viscous fluid on the corneal surface may disguise the true corneal shape.

Moiré Topography

Moiré topography has been used in medicine to depict the three-dimensional shape of various parts of the hu-

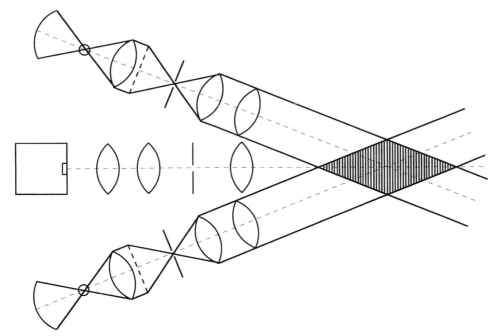

Figure 12–10. Additive moiré projection. *(From Jongsma FHM, Laan FC, Stultiens BATh. In: Parel J-M, Ren Q, eds.* Ophthalmic Technologies IV, Proc SPIE; *1994;2126:3–10.)*

man body.[56,57] Briefly, the technique relies on creating an interference pattern of alternating light and dark bands, using two grid projectors. The principle is illustrated in Figure 12–10. The bands are projected onto the object being measured, and they reveal contours of constant distance from the grid. Jongsma and colleagues applied the Moiré technique to obtain high-resolution measurements of the corneal surface using discrete Fourier analysis.[58] They reported an axial resolution of 3 μm and a lateral resolution of 40 × 30 μm. Like the raster photogrammetry method, application of a fluorescein solution was required in order to make the cornea a diffusely radiating surface. Thus, this implementation of the Moiré technique also measures a distorted surface.

Pancorneal Slit Topography

Another approach to corneal topography uses a series of captured slit images to determine corneal surface height with respect to a reference plane (RK Snook: True Topography and Pachymetry, unpublished). The technique sequentially projects a slit of light (similar to a conventional slit lamp) onto the cornea from 45 angles to the left and to the right of the camera axis. An image is captured at 10 slit positions each for the left and right projections. Analysis of the digitized images yields the surface height of the anterior corneal surface. A commercial system with this configuration recently became available (Orbscan, Orbtek, Salt Lake City, UT). It has

shown excellent potential in providing topographical (height) maps of the anterior and posterior surfaces of the cornea as well as corneal thickness (pachymetry) measurements, which will prove helpful in increasing our understanding of the corneal response to various refractive surgical procedures.

REFERENCES

1. Uozato H, Guyton DL. Centering corneal surgical procedures. *Am J Ophthalmol.* 1987;103:264–275.
2. Mandell RB. The enigma of the corneal contour. *CLAO J.* 1992;18:267–273.
3. Waring GO. Making sense of keratospeak II: proposed conventional terminology for corneal topography. *Refract Corneal Surg.* 1989;5:362–367.
4. Mish FC, ed. *Webster's Ninth New Collegiate Dictionary.* Springfield, MA: Merriam-Webster; 1984.
5. Maloney RK. Corneal topography and optical zone location in photorefractive keratectomy. *Refract Corneal Surg.* 1990;6:363–371.
6. Swokowski EW. *Calculus with Analytic Geometry.* Alternate ed. Boston: Prindle, Weber & Schmidt; 1983.
7. Bennett AG. Aspheric contact lens surfaces. *Ophthal Opt.* 1968;8:1037–1040, 1297–1300, 1311;9:222–230.
8. Jenkins FA, White HE. *Fundamentals of Optics.* 3rd ed. New York: McGraw-Hill; 1957.
9. Roberts C. The accuracy of "power" maps to display curvature data in corneal topography systems. *Invest Ophthalmol Vis Sci.* 1994;35:3525–3532.

10. Mandell RB, St. Helen R. Mathematical model of the corneal contour. *Br J Physiol Opt.* 1971;26(3).183–197.

11. Maurice DM. The cornea and sclera. In: Davson H, ed. *The Eye.* New York: Academic Press; 1984.

12. Roberts C. Characterization of the inherent error in a spherically-biased corneal topography system in mapping a radially aspheric surface. *J Refract Corneal Surg.* 1994;10:103–116.

13. Roberts C. Analysis of the inherent error of the TMS-1 Topographic Modeling System in mapping a radially aspheric surface. *Cornea.* 1995;14:258–265.

14. Beyer WH. *CRC Standard Mathematical Tables and Formulae.* 29th ed. Boca Raton, FL: CRC Press; 1991.

15. Webb RH. Zernike polynomial description of ophthalmic surfaces. In: *Ophthalmic and Visual Optics Technical Digest.* Washington, DC: Optical Society of America; 1992: 38–41.

16. Howland HC, Glasser A, Applegate R. Polynomial approximations of corneal surfaces and corneal curvature topography. In: *Ophthalmic and Visual Optics Technical Digest.* Washington, DC: Optical Society of America; 1992: 34–37.

17. Raach TW. Quantitative model of corneal astigmatism from topographic data. In: *Ophthalmic and Visual Optics Technical Digest.* Washington, DC: Optical Society of America; 1992:24–27.

18. Dingeldein SA, Klyce SD, Wilson SE. Quantitative descriptors of corneal shape derived from computer-assisted analysis of photokeratographs. *Refract Corneal Surg.* 1989;5:372–378.

19. Wilson SE, Klyce SD. Quantitative descriptors of corneal topography: a clinical study. *Arch Ophthalmol.* 1991;109: 349–353.

20. Gorin G. *History of Ophthalmology.* Wilmington, DE: Publish or Perish; 1982.

21. Levene JR. The true inventors of the keratoscope and photo-keratoscope. *Br J Hist Sci.* 1965;2:324–342.

22. Levene JR. Sir David Brewster (1781–1868) and the clinical detection of corneal abnormalities. In: *12th International Congress on the History of Sciences.* Paris; 1968;8: 105–109.

23. Southall JPC. *Introduction to Physiological Optics.* New York: Dover Publications; 1937.

24. Mandell RB. Jesse Ramsden: Inventor of the ophthalmometer. *Am J Optom.* 1960;37:633.

25. Clark BAJ. Conventional keratoscopy—a critical review. *Aust J Optom.* 1973;56:145–155.

26. Clark BAJ. Keratometry: a review. *Aust J Optom.* 1973;56: 94–100.

27. Bennett AG, Francis JL. The eye as an optical system. In: Davson H, ed. *The Eye.* New York: Academic Press; 1965.

28. Mandell RB. Corneal power correction factor for photorefractive keratectomy. *J Refract Corneal Surg.* 1994;10:125–128.

29. Klyce SD, Dingeldein SA. Corneal topography. In: Masters BR, ed. *Noninvasive Diagnostic Techniques in Ophthalmology.* New York: Springer-Verlag; 1990.

30. Rowsey JJ, Reynolds AE, Brown R. Corneal topography. *Arch Ophthalmol.* 1981;99:1093–1100.

31. Doss JD, Hutson RL, Rowsey JJ, Brown DR. Method for calculation of corneal profile and power distribution. *Arch Ophthalmol.* 1981;99:1261–1265.

32. Rowsey JJ, Isaac MS. Corneoscopy in keratorefractive surgery. *Cornea.* 1983;2:133–142.

33. Klyce SD. Computer assisted corneal topography: High resolution graphic presentation and analysis of keratoscopy. *Invest Ophthalmol Vis Sci.* 1984;25:1426–1435.

34. van Saarloos PP, Constable IJ. Improved method for calculation of corneal topography for any photokeratoscope geometry. *Optom Vis Sci.* 1991;68:960–965.

35. Maguire LJ, Singer DE, Klyce SD. Graphic presentation of computer-analyzed keratoscope photographs. *Arch Ophthalmol.* 1987;105:223–230.

36. Gormley DJ, Gersten M, Koplin RS, Lubkin V. Corneal modeling. *Cornea.* 1988;7:30–35.

37. Antalis JJ, Lembach RG, Carney LG. A comparison of the TMS-1 and the corneal analysis system for the evaluation of abnormal corneas. *CLAO J.* 1993;19:58–63.

38. Hannush SB, Crawford SL, Waring GO, et al. Accuracy and precision of keratometry, photokeratoscopy, and corneal modeling on calibrated steel balls. *Arch Ophthalmol.* 1989;107:1235–1239.

39. Hannush SB, Crawford SL, Waring GO, et al. Reproducibility of normal corneal power measurements with a keratometer, photokeratoscope, and video imaging system. *Arch Ophthalmol.* 1990;108:539–544.

40. Koch DD, Foulks GN, Moran CT, Wakil JS. The Corneal Eyesys System: accuracy analysis and reproducibility of first-generation prototype. *Refract Corneal Surg.* 1989;5: 424–429.

41. Koch DD, Wakil JS, Samuelson SW, Haft EA. Comparison of the accuracy and reproducibility of the keratometer and the Eyesys Corneal Analysis System Model I. *J Cataract Refract Surg.* 1992;18:342–347.

42. Legeais J-M, Ren Q, Simon G, Parel J-M. Computer-assisted corneal topography: accuracy and reproducibility of the topographic modeling system. *Refract Corneal Surg.* 1993;9:347–357.

43. Tsilimbaris MK, Vlachonikolis IG, Siganos D, et al. Comparison of keratometric readings as obtained by Javal ophthalmometer and Corneal Analysis System (Eyesys). *Refract Corneal Surg.* 1991;7:368–373.

44. Wilson SE, Verity SM, Conger SL. Accuracy and precision of the Corneal Analysis System and the Topographic Modeling System. *Cornea.* 1992;11:28–35.

45. Wang J, Rice DA, Klyce SD. A new reconstruction algorithm for improvement of corneal topographical analysis. *Refract Corneal Surg.* 1989;5:379–387.

46. McCarey BE, Zurawski CA, O'Shea DS. Practical aspects of a corneal topography system. *CLAO J.* 1992;18:248–254.

47. Shimmick J, Munnerlyn C. Corneal analysis with a rectilinear photokeratoscope. In: *Ophthalmic and Visual Optics Technical Digest.* Washington, DC: Optical Society of America; 1992:2–3.

48. Young JA, Siegel IM. Corneal contour mapping: an isomorphic approach. *CLAO J.* 1993;19:182–185.

49. Young JA, Siegel IM. Isomorphic corneal topography: a clinical approach to 3-D representation of the corneal surface. *Refract Corneal Surg.* 1993;9:74–78.

50. Frobin W, Hierholzer E. Rasterstereography: a photogrammetric method for measurement of body surfaces. *J Biol Photogr.* 1983;51:11–17.

51. Warnicki JW, Rehkopf PG, Curtin DY, et al. Corneal topography using computer analyzed rasterstereographic images. *Appl Optom.* 1988;27:1135–1140.

52. Belin MW, Litoff D, Strods SJ, et al. The PAR technology corneal topography system. *Refract Corneal Surg.* 1992;8:88–96.

53. Belin MW, Zloty P. Accuracy of the PAR corneal topography system with spatial misalignment. *CLAO J.* 1993;19:64–68.

54. Novak KD, Koch DD, Soper B, Padrick T. Changes in computerized videokeratographic measurements induced by artificial tears. *Invest Ophthalmol Vis Sci.* 1994;35(suppl):2062.

55. Yu JS, Wu M, Crosser VA, Tauber J. Changes in corneal topography after instillation of artificial tear lubricants. *Invest Ophthalmol Vis Sci.* 1994;35(suppl):2194.

56. Koepfler JW. Moiré topography in medicine. *J Biol Photogr.* 1983;51:3–10.

57. Takasaki H. Moiré topography. *Appl Optom.* 1970;9:1467–1472.

58. Jongsma FHM, Laan FC, Th. Stultiens BA. A moiré based corneal topographer suitable for discrete fourier analysis. In: Parel J-M, Ren Q, eds. *Ophthalmic Technologies IV. Society of PhotoOptical Instrumentation Engineers;* 1994;185–192.

CHAPTER 13

Corneal Topography: Adjunctive Use in Keratorefractive Surgery

Dasa V. Gangadhar ▪ Jonathan H. Talamo

Interest in refractive surgery has grown explosively over the past several years. Accordingly, detailed analysis of the corneal contour has assumed greater importance for preoperative planning and postoperative analysis. Conventional keratometry has historically been used to evaluate corneal topography. Keratometry, however, evaluates only four individual points on the central 3 mm of the corneal surface, and as such does not adequately represent the optical effects of the central corneal topography. Corneal topographic analysis has evolved from the keratometer to photokeratoscopy to the present-day use of computer-assisted corneal topographic analysis, whereby the majority of the corneal surface can be quantitatively and qualitatively analyzed.

The study of corneal surface topography has been driven by the need to understand the complex changes that may occur after refractive surgical procedures. A better understanding of these changes may help to refine surgical techniques and improve visual results.

This chapter will consider the importance of computer-assisted topographic analysis (computerized videokeratography or CVK) of the cornea for patient screening, preoperative surgical planning, and for monitoring as well as explaining surgical results after refractive surgery. Topographic changes that occur after radial keratotomy (RK), excimer laser photorefractive keratectomy and keratomileusis (LASIK or ALK) will be discussed.

PATIENT SCREENING

Proper patient screening and selection for refractive surgery is as important as the meticulous surgical execution itself. Patients may be deemed poor candidates for refractive surgery based on unrealistic expectations, excessive occupational/recreational risk for ocular trauma, or anatomic abnormalities of the cornea. Careful preoperative study of corneal topography is vital for dealing with the latter difficulty.

Occult Keratoconus

Preoperative screening of candidates for refractive surgery can be greatly facilitated by CVK. Identifying topographic abnormalities that may potentially disqualify a patient from refractive surgical procedures, or at the very least expand the level of informed consent, is a primary role for preoperative CVK.

Occult corneal ectatic disorders, such as keratoconus, can be discovered on routine preoperative screening topography, but they may not be apparent by clinical examination and keratometry alone (Fig 13–1). Qualitatively, the most common topographic pattern seen in early keratoconus is that of a concentric steep area surrounded by concentric bands of progressively decreasing corneal power located at the apex or inferior to the apex of the cornea. Because the topography of keratoconus may be heterogeneous, and interpretation may be subjective, reliable quantitative descriptors have been proposed by Rabinowitz and associates[1] to eliminate interobserver variability and provide a more objective and sensitive tool for the diagnosis of keratoconus. The three most useful quantitative parameters for the diagnosis of keratoconus are as follows:

1. Increased dioptric power at the center of the cornea (> 46.0 D).
2. Positive I–S value, indicating a relatively steeper inferior cornea (calculated by subtracting the average superior corneal power, S, from the average inferior corneal power, I, 3 mm from the center of the cornea).
3. Large differences in the central dioptric power (greater than 1 D) between the two eyes of the same patient.

Historical details of progressive myopia, a family history of keratoconus, clinical findings of compound my-

opic astigmatism, and/or the topographic abnormalities described above should permit accurate diagnosis of occult or early keratoconus in the majority of patients.

Many refractive surgeons feel that patients with subclinical keratoconus should be advised against having refractive surgery. Such patients may experience natural progression of their disease, and anecdotal case reports suggest that the cornea may behave in an unpredictable manner after surgery, resulting in irregular astigmatism and/or unpredictable refractive results.[2,3] However, the degree of corneal steepening/ectasia that is clinically significant remains unknown. As clinical experience expands, refractive surgeons will undoubtedly develop better answers to these questions. Longitudinal studies will be necessary to understand the importance of these subtle subclinical findings with CVK, and to decide if such findings are relative or absolute contraindications to refractive surgery. Until better information is available, extreme caution should be exercised when contemplating keratorefractive procedures in this subgroup of patients.

Contact Lens–Induced Corneal Warpage

Corneal warpage is defined as a contact lens–induced change in corneal curvature. Topographic changes commonly caused by corneal warpage include irregular astigmatism, loss of radial symmetry, and reversal of the normal topographic pattern of progressive flat-

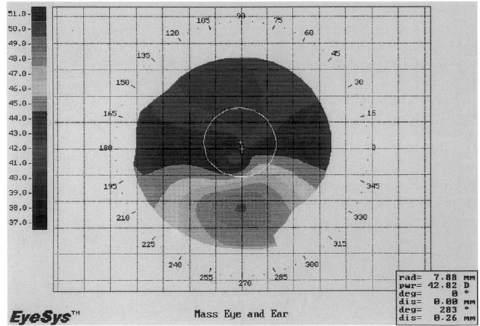

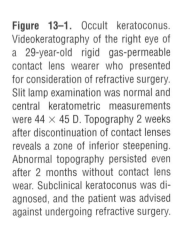

Figure 13–1. Occult keratoconus. Videokeratography of the right eye of a 29-year-old rigid gas-permeable contact lens wearer who presented for consideration of refractive surgery. Slit lamp examination was normal and central keratometric measurements were 44 × 45 D. Topography 2 weeks after discontinuation of contact lenses reveals a zone of inferior steepening. Abnormal topography persisted even after 2 months without contact lens wear. Subclinical keratoconus was diagnosed, and the patient was advised against undergoing refractive surgery.

tening of the corneal contour from the center to the periphery.[4]

Clinically significant changes in corneal topography are more commonly seen with rigid plastic polymer (PMMA) contact lenses, but they may also occur with gas-permeable, or even soft, contact lenses. Decentration of contact lenses can induce topographic changes that may simulate early keratoconus, often causing reduction in best corrected visual acuity (BCVA) (Fig 13–2).

Several months may be required for corneal topography to normalize and/or achieve a stable pattern after discontinuation of contact lenses. Because keratometry and keratoscopy are less sensitive, the topography may appear to normalize sooner using these techniques than after assessment by CVK. Therefore, CVK should be considered the most reliable parameter for initially diagnosing and then following patients with contact lens–induced corneal warpage. Serial refractions and CVK should be performed every few weeks, until the corneal contour and refractive status are stable, before proceeding with a keratorefractive surgical procedure.

Some patients may not achieve a normal topography (ie, persistence of irregular astigmatism, central corneal flattening) and may have permanent alterations in the corneal shape and reductions in best spectacle-corrected visual acuity.[4] Such patients, although in the minority, are not ideal candidates for refractive surgery and perhaps should be discouraged from seeking keratorefractive procedures.

PREOPERATIVE PLANNING

Astigmatism can be either treated by astigmatic keratotomy (AK) alone or combined with radial keratotomy to treat myopia and astigmatism simultaneously. Because the surgical correction of astigmatism has not enjoyed the same level of predictability and reproducibility as the surgical correction of myopia, it is hoped that careful attention to preoperative CVK data will improve results.

Analysis of preoperative topography can be valuable in formulating an individualized surgical "game plan" for treating astigmatism. It can also be useful for detecting conditions that may not be suitable for incisional astigmatic keratotomy. For example, CVK can identify cases of irregular astigmatism that may not be amenable to standard astigmatic keratotomy but may actually benefit from mechanical superficial keratectomy or excimer phototherapeutic keratectomy (PTK) to smooth the corneal surface.

The surgeon can also use CVK to reconcile the meridian, symmetry, and magnitude of corneal and refractive astigmatism. When CVK demonstrates orthogonal astigmatism that corresponds to the refractive axis of astigmatism, the surgeon can be confident in the surgical axis for astigmatic incision placement. In contrast, with orthogonal astigmatism, where the topographic astigmatic axis is significantly different from the refractive axis, underlying lenticular astigmatism has most likely been uncovered. In this scenario, the surgeon should operate on the refractive axis of astigmatism. To

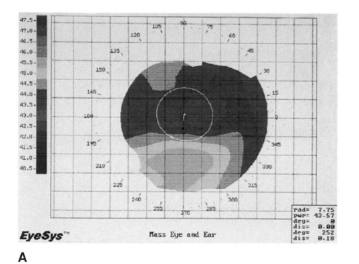
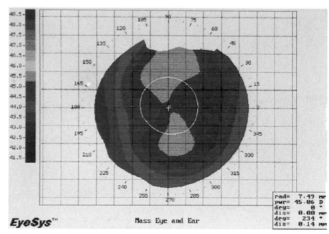

A **B**

Figure 13–2. Contact lens–induced corneal warpage. **A.** Videokeratography of the left eye of a 43-year-old rigid gas-permeable contact lens wearer reveals inferior steepening, simulating keratoconus. Findings in the right eye were similar. **B.** Repeat videokeratography 3 weeks after discontinuing contact lenses reveals normalization of topography, indicating reversible contact lens–induced corneal warpage.

Figure 13–3. Nonorthogonal corneal astigmatism. Videokeratography reveals nonorthogonal astigmatism with the steep hemimeridia located at 90° and 315°. Orthogonal reconstruction of the steep axis most closely approximating the true corneal curvature (averaging of the two steep meridians) would be 112° and 292°. If the axis and magnitude of refractive astigmatism identifies 112° as the steep axis, one can be confident that lenticular astigmatism is minimal and that the astigmatism is primarily corneal. Astigmatic incisions could then be placed at the actual steep hemimeridia as identified by CVK (90° and 315°). This strategy may better address the situation than would incisions at 112° and 292° based on refraction alone.

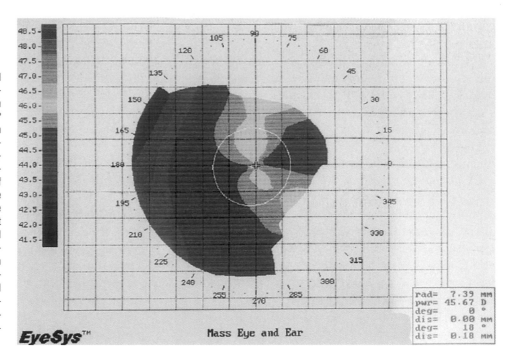

treat corneal astigmatism based on topography alone would simply uncover the lenticular component, yielding an unsatisfactory result.

In cases of nonorthogonal corneal astigmatism, CVK may depict the actual corneal shape more accurately than does the refraction, which artificially assumes the presence of an orthogonal shape. To formulate a proper treatment plan, the surgeon must decide if an orthogonal reconstruction of the topographic axis corresponds to the refractive axis. If this is the case, the surgeon should then place the astigmatic incision at the steep hemimeridia as determined by CVK (Fig 13–3).

The formulation of a treatment plan is more problematic in cases of nonorthogonal astigmatism, where the orthogonal reconstruction of the topography does not correspond to the refractive axis of astigmatism. In such cases, the surgeon should proceed with great caution because the results can be unpredictable. More clinical data are necessary to guide surgical planning for this unusual clinical setting.

Finally, CVK can graphically identify asymmetrical astigmatism (ie, different magnitudes of astigmatism in the two hemimeridia). Astigmatism nomograms guide the surgeon in choosing the length of incisions and optical zone parameters, but they do not currently address asymmetrical astigmatism. CVK may allow the surgeon to modify treatment parameters by guiding him or her in the symmetry of such incisions. For ex-

ample, topography may suggest altering the surgical plan so that a longer incision is placed in the meridian with greater astigmatism and a shorter incision in the opposite meridian (Fig 13–4). In the past, keratometry and refraction have provided insufficient information to guide these decisions. More experience is needed in this arena, but such adjustments in surgical technique may ultimately improve surgical predictability.

CORNEAL TOPOGRAPHIC CHANGES FOLLOWING RADIAL KERATOTOMY

Normal Corneal Shape

A thorough appreciation of the shape variations of the normal cornea is necessary to understand fully the changes that occur after refractive surgery. Both quantitative photokeratoscopy[5,6] and CVK[7] have revealed that normal corneas display a gradually increasing radius of curvature from the center to the periphery. In other words, there is a gradual flattening of the cornea from the center to the periphery, called *normal corneal asphericity* or a *prolate corneal configuration.*

Bogan and associates[8] have extensively studied the topography of normal eyes and have classified corneas into five different qualitative topographic patterns: round, oval, symmetric bow tie, asymmetric bow tie, and irregular. The bow-tie patterns were found to have

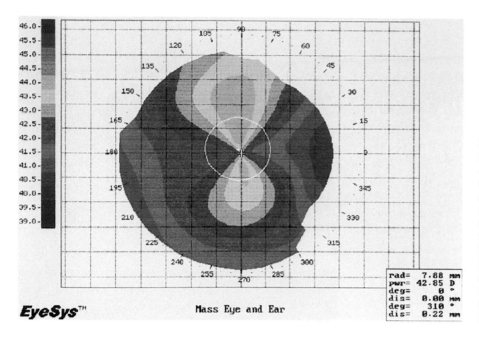

Figure 13–4. Asymmetric astigmatism. Videokeratography of the right eye of a 47-year-old patient reveals asymmetric astigmatism with a greater astigmatic component in the superior versus the inferior cornea. Preoperative refraction showed 3.25 D of with-the-rule astigmatism. Such patients may benefit from asymmetric surgery (ie, longer T-cuts in the region of greater astigmatism). In this patient, a 3-mm T-cut was placed superiorly and a 2-mm T-cut inferiorly. Six weeks postoperatively, refractive astigmatism had been reduced to 0.75 D. Uncorrected visual acuity improved from 20/100 to 20/20.

a statistically significant greater amount of refractive and keratometric astigmatism than the round or oval patterns.

Evolution of Topography Following Radial Keratotomy

After RK, the majority of the corneal surface flattens and the central cornea assumes a disproportionate amount of flattening compared with the periphery. This results in both an augmentation and a reversal of normal corneal asphericity, with the peripheral cornea assuming a steeper topography than the central cornea

(oblate corneal configuration).[5–7] In the majority of instances after RK, evaluation of the midperipheral cornea discloses not only relative steepening compared with the central cornea, but also absolute steepening (increase in dioptric power) in relation to preoperative topography.[9]

Ideally RK creates a relatively homogenous, flat central optical zone centered over the entrance pupil (Fig 13–5). These topographic changes are concurrent with rapid visual recovery and excellent unaided visual acuity. Occasionally, the immediate postoperative central topography may be irregular, resulting in delayed

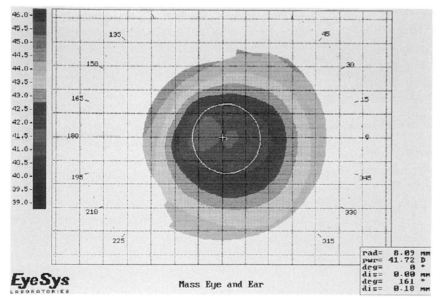

Figure 13–5. Postoperative radial keratotomy. Videokeratography of the left eye of a 36-year-old patient 4 weeks after eight-incision RK for −5 D of myopia. A large, homogenous central optical zone (COZ) can be seen despite the use of a 3.5-mm optical zone for incision placement. Uncorrected visual acuity was 20/20. Concentric rings of progressively higher power can be seen outside the COZ. If the COZ is decentered or if the pupil is dilated, a multifocal lens–type effect could be created.

visual recovery. In a subset of patients, the greatest amount of flattening occurs in the paracentral cornea at the edge of the optical zone defined by the origin of the radial incisions, while the central cornea assumes a relatively steeper topography. These changes create a nipple-shaped central optical zone (COZ) in the immediate postoperative period, resulting in irregular astigmatism and decreased visual function. In most cases, visual function improves as the central cornea flattens over the first several months, thus eliminating the "nipple architecture."[10]

Progressive flattening of the central cornea may continue to evolve for many years after RK. A "hyperopic drift" of >1 D has been reported in 43% of patients in the Prospective Evaluation of Radial Keratotomy (PERK) study.[11] Deitz and associates[12] have reported a similar hyperopic drift in their series. Whether progressive hyperopia will continue to be an issue with the modern thinner diamond knives, improved titratable techniques, and reduced length of radial incisions (ie, mini-RK) remains to be seen.

Optical Side Effects Following Radial Keratotomy

As noted above, corneal asphericity after RK is significantly greater than in the normal unoperated eye. The rate of change in dioptric power from central to peripheral cornea is relatively constant in normal eyes. After RK, there is an increased rate of change in dioptric power between a zone located roughly 2.5 to 3.5 mm from the corneal center. This inflection zone has been called the "paracentral knee" (Fig 13–6). Many refractive surgeons believe that the halo and glare symptoms patients experience after RK are an optical sequelae of this paracentral knee of rapid power change. Many patients also experience "spoking" when viewing point sources of light following RK, particularly in dim illumination. This complaint is usually transient and is most likely caused by meridional variations in paracentral dioptric power stemming from an enhanced flattening effect overlying the radial incisions, rather than by light scattering from the incisions themselves. Interestingly, this side effect appears to be less pronounced following eight-incision RK than when four incisions are placed, presumably because incisions that are 45° instead of 90° apart create a more uniform paracentral topography.

In the normal cornea, dioptric power fluctuates approximately 2 D within the central area of the cornea overlying a standard 4-mm entrance pupil. In a small number of patients, this range nearly doubles after RK,

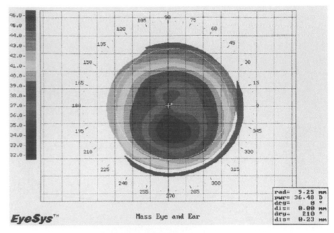

A

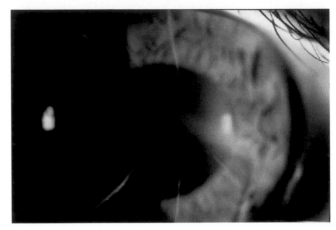

B

Figure 13–6. Prominent paracentral knee after RK. **A.** Videokeratography of the left eye of a 46-year-old patient 4 years after eight-incision RK. Preoperative refraction was −5.50 D sph. The patient experienced progressive hyperopia postoperatively and is presently significantly overcorrected (+3.00 sph. with 20/25 vision). Uncorrected vision is 20/60, but with significant asthenopic symptoms. The topographic map reveals marked central corneal flattening (32 D) with a midperipheral zone of rapid and substantial increase in power to 46 D (exaggerated paracentral knee). **B.** Slit lamp photograph of the same eye. By observing the incision contour, the profound central corneal flattening and rapid midperipheral steepening can be appreciated.

creating a multifocal central optical zone (COZ) with increased likelihood of visual disturbances.[9] (See the discussion of COZ dioptric distribution below.)

Optical Zone Shapes Following Radial Keratotomy

RK results in a central zone of flattening that can vary in configuration and size. Optical zone configurations can be round, oval, bandlike, split, or dumbbell shaped (Fig 13–7). Dumbbell or split optical-zone configurations may result in greater degrees of refractive and keratometric astigmatism than occur with the round

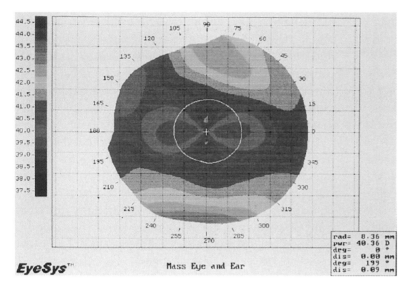

Figure 13–7. Dumbbell-shaped optical zone after RK. Videokeratography of left eye of a 52-year-old patient 3 months after four-incision RK. Uncorrected visual acuity was 20/40, but the patient had fluctuating visual acuity and unstable refractions over the first 3 postoperative months. Dumbbell or split optical zones are far more often associated with diurnal fluctuations of vision than are round or bandlike optical zones.

or bandlike optical zones; these configurations may be more commonly associated with a suboptimal visual outcome (see below). The explanation for this multiplicity of optical-zone shapes is not readily apparent, but it may relate to variability in the depth and/or centration of incisions as well as individual variability in wound healing.[7,13]

Central Optical-Zone Dioptric Power Distribution

Refractive measurements following RK often correlate poorly with uncorrected visual acuity and keratometry, as patients often have better uncorrected visual acuity than would be predicted. This phenomenon can be explained by increased corneal asphericity and the multifocal COZs that can result after RK. Multifocality can be demonstrated clinically by the mainte-

nance of best spectacle-corrected visual acuity at a set distance over a wide dioptric range during cycloplegic refraction.

Multifocal optical zones can exist in two principal patterns. One pattern consists of a large central optical zone of fairly uniform power that encompasses smaller "islands" of differing power. Refraction through the larger optical zone may reveal the presence of residual myopia, but the patient may be able to utilize these small zones (islands) of greater flattening to obtain better vision than may have been predicted (Fig 13–8).[14–16] Alternatively, one may see a small, flat central zone surrounded by concentric rings of higher power (Fig 13–5). If these rings are located over the entrance pupil, a multifocal effect can occur. This phenomenon explains how some presbyopic individuals may obtain excellent uncorrected distance and near visual acuity after RK.

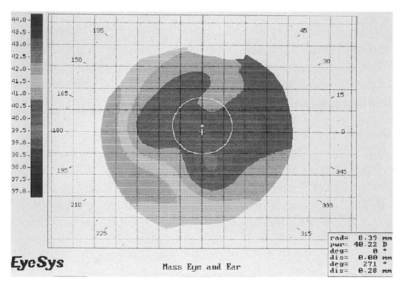

Figure 13–8. Multifocal optical zones after RK. Videokeratography of the left eye of a 62-year-old patient 10 weeks after four-incision RK. Uncorrected visual acuity was 20/70. Although manifest refraction of −1.25 −0.75 × 89° yielded a vision of 20/20, the patient still complained of nocturnal glare and "spoking" around lights. The multifocal optical zone caused degradation of the visual image, even though "normal" corrected Snellen visual acuity was obtainable.

Although discrete optical zones of differing power may appear to be present based on the topographic map produced by CVK (see Fig 13–8), this effect is most likely a function of the arbitrary dioptric intervals of the color-coded power scale used in the analysis of keratoscopic ring images. In reality, there is most likely a progressive blending of powers between multiple optical zones, analogous to a progressive bifocal segment.[17]

Although multifocality may result in some unexpected benefits for the patient, it may also have detrimental effects. In spite of good Snellen visual acuity, some patients with multifocal corneas may have sufficient irregularity of the corneal surface to result in significant degradation in visual image quality. Monocular diplopia or polyopia, ghosting of images, and glare are unwanted detrimental effects that may result, especially in dim illumination as the pupil dilates.[18] Careful correlation of topography with visual indices like contrast sensitivity may more accurately reflect the quality of vision in these patients than Snellen acuity measurements alone.

Diurnal Fluctuations of Visual Acuity after Radial Keratotomy

Diurnal fluctuations of visual acuity after RK have been reported in 1.9% to 60% of patients.[11,19,20] Most complaints of visual fluctuations occur early in the postoperative period (2 to 6 weeks), but some patients may continue to be symptomatic for months or even years after the surgery. McDonnell and associates have found that patients with dumbbell-shaped or split optical zones were more likely than patients with round or bandlike zones to complain of diurnal fluctuations (Fig 13–7). While still anecdotal, this information suggests that different degrees of corneal stability are present with different optical-zone configurations.

Diurnal fluctuations are related to steepening of the cornea in the evening and flattening in the morning following prolonged eyelid closure during sleep. Not all meridians of the cornea change uniformly, and studies have shown that the greatest degree of diurnal steepening occurs in the nasal and inferonasal quadrants. Keratometric changes do not always correlate with the diurnal changes in refraction and CVK. This discrepancy is not unexpected, as keratometry is not a sufficiently sensitive tool to detect the complex changes in corneal topography that occur in these postoperative eyes.

Possible explanations for diurnal fluctuations in vision and topography after RK include fluctuations in intraocular pressure, changes in corneal thickness, and alterations in lid position (closed during sleep and resting at the limbus during waking hours). Additionally, tension exerted by the extraocular muscles during accommodative convergence or orbicularis tension from the lid may further explain the regional variations in topography that occur from morning to evening.[21] Most likely, the etiology of these changes is multifactorial.

Diurnal fluctuations are a reminder that the structural integrity of the cornea is weakened after RK, as the continuity of incised stromal collagen fibers may not be restored for many years.[22] A comparative incidence of postoperative diurnal fluctuations in visual function following the various modern RK techniques (ie, Russian vs American vs combined technique) that have evolved over the past several years has not been reported.

Guiding Enhancements Following Radial Keratotomy

One of the cardinal rules of refractive surgery is to avoid overcorrection. Owing to the inherent biologic variability among individuals, RK has in many ways evolved into a staged procedure, where the surgeon often chooses to err on the side of undercorrection. If the initial surgical correction falls short of the intended or desired result, enhancement surgery can usually be performed. CVK serves as a valuable adjunct to guide the surgeon in this second phase of the surgical procedure. If the topographic map reveals a homogenous optical zone and refraction reveals only residual myopia, the surgeon may simply choose one of several modalities to enhance the initial procedure: reducing the size of the initial optical zone, adding additional incisions in previously uncut cornea, and/or redeepening the original incisions. Alternatively, if CVK clearly identifies induced astigmatism or a localized area of cornea that has responded suboptimally, the surgeon may be able to correlate this with clinical findings of a shallow incision and selectively enhance or redeepen that particular incision. CVK is invaluable in planning enhancement surgery where there is residual or induced astigmatism, but such information must always be used in conjunction with manifest and cycloplegic refraction data.

Refractive surgeons have in their armementarium multiple refractive surgical procedures: RK, excimer laser photorefractive keratectomy (PRK), laser in situ keratomileusis (LASIK), and automated lamellar keratoplasty (ALK). These procedures are not mutually exclusive, in that one procedure may be used to enhance or fine-tune another (see chapter 45). For example, RK or AK can be used to correct residual myopia

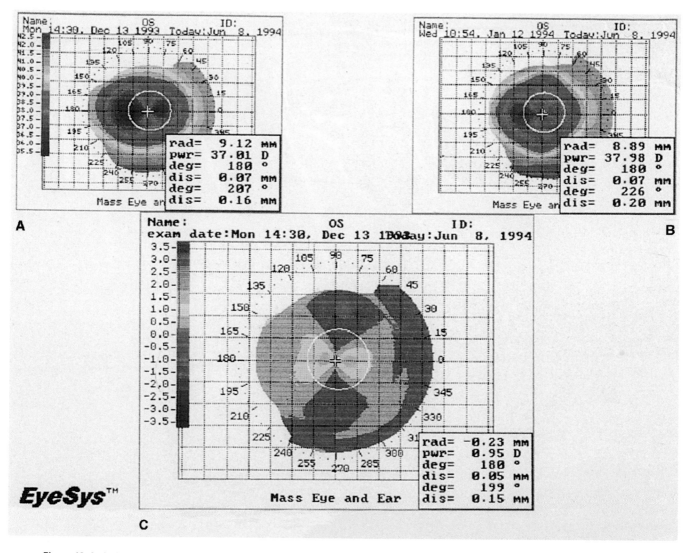

Figure 13–9. Astigmatic keratotomy (AK) after PRK. A 44-year-old patient with a refraction of −6.00 −0.50 × 180° underwent uncomplicated PRK in the left eye. **A.** Eighteen months postoperatively, uncorrected visual acuity was 20/50. Refraction of +1.00 − 2.50 × 12° yielded 20/20 acuity with 2 D of iatrogenically induced cylinder evident on videokeratography. **B.** Six weeks' status postastigmatic keratotomy with paired 3-mm T-cuts in the steep (vertical) meridian, videokeratography, and refraction demonstrate 1 D of residual astigmatism. Uncorrected visual acuity had improved to 20/25. **C.** Difference map showing flattening effect of T-cuts in vertical meridian with steepening in orthogonal meridian.

and/or astigmatism after PRK (Fig 13–9). Similarly, PRK can be used to treat residual refractive errors after RK. In the future, sequential application of these procedures may broaden the range of refractive errors that can be treated safely and predictably.

CORNEAL TOPOGRAPHIC CHANGES FOLLOWING EXCIMER LASER PHOTOREFRACTIVE KERATECTOMY AND KERATOMILEUSIS FOR MYOPIA

CVK has provided invaluable insights into the changes that occur following excimer PRK and laser in situ keratomileusis (LASIK). Information can be obtained re-

garding the uniformity of the ablation, centration relative to the entrance pupil, diameter of the ablated zone, and stability of topographic alterations over time.

Optical-Zone Quality

The precision and uniformity of tissue ablation is a major asset of excimer PRK. An area of relatively uniform surface power is created centrally. Outside this area, a smooth transition in dioptric power is seen until the ablation edge is reached (Fig 13–10). However, not all ablations have a homogenous pattern, and up to 50% of all ablations may have regional internal variations in dioptric power.[23]

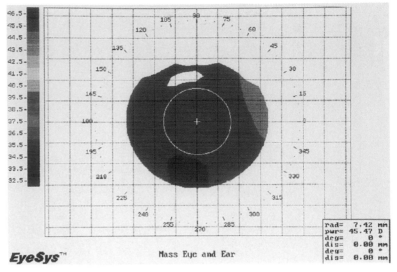

A

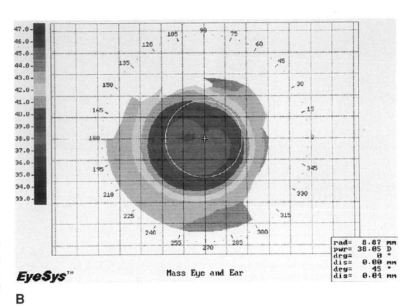

B

Figure 13–10. Topography after excimer PRK. **A.** Preoperative videokeratography of the right eye of a 34-year-old patient awaiting excimer PRK. (Preoperative refraction of −6.50 D sph.) **B.** Six months after PRK, a COZ of fairly uniform flattening is apparent. Uncorrected visual acuity was 20/40. Refraction revealed −1.25 D sph of residual refractive error.

The size of the central area of uniform dioptric power created by PRK can be calculated. This region is called the central optical zone, or COZ. We have examined this parameter in our patients treated for moderate myopia (6 to 8 D) with the VISX 2020 excimer laser system (VISX, Inc, Santa Clara, CA). The distance from the pupil center to where the power changed more than 1 D was defined as the edge of the COZ. The average diameter of the COZ was found to be 3.4 mm in our series of 17 highly myopic patients, despite an ablation diameter of 6 mm. Given the contoured nature of these ablations, this is not unexpected. Theoretically, if the pupil diameter exceeds the confines of the COZ, nocturnal glare symptoms could be expected. These data further emphasize the importance of proper centration of excimer laser ablations.

Topographic Stability

Topographic assessment 1 month after PRK reveals a central area of maximal flattening with mild refractive overcorrection. The initial overcorrection may be the consequence of early variations in epithelial thickness, with the epithelium being thicker peripherally than centrally. Nonuniform stromal swelling (greatest in the periphery of the ablation) may also contribute to the mild overcorrection often seen in the early postoperative period. This is less pronounced after keratomileusis, automated lamellar keratectomy (ALK), or laser in situ keratomileusis (LASIK).

Sequential topography reveals steepening of the central cornea from progressive central epithelial thickening and stromal remodeling over the first 4 to 6 months. The regression of refractive effect is greatest during this period, with stability of central corneal power being achieved in the majority of patients treated for low myopia (2 to 6 D) by 6 to 8 months. Some patients, particularly those with higher attempted corrections, may have continued stromal remodeling for up to 1 year, or longer.[24,25]

The most important factor affecting postoperative refractive stability after PRK is individual variation in wound healing. In approximately 2% to 12% of patients, a "central island" (a localized area of increased power) may develop within the ablation zone (Fig 13–11). This was initially thought to occur only when gases were blown across the cornea during PRK, but it has subsequently been noted even with "no blow" techniques.[26–28] This area of increased power can sometimes be correlated clinically with a localized area of exuberant stromal scarring or haze. The central island phenomenon is most likely a result of local variability in intraoperative stromal hydration (with regional variations in stromal ablation rates), but may also be due to a masking effect from material ejected from the cornea during the treatment process, inhomogeneity in the delivery of laser energy, and/or variability in wound healing.

Greater regression of effect is seen with higher attempted dioptric corrections. The reasons for this response have not been precisely defined, but it may be that the greater stromal excision depth and/or the greater acoustic shock wave effect delivered by large numbers of pulses needed for higher corrections incites a more exuberant healing response than is seen after lower degrees of correction. Following deeper PRK ablations (ie, ≥ 50 μm), some studies suggest that stromal remodeling and refractive regression can be modulated by individual tailoring of steroid regimens. The stability of corneal topography after ALK and LASIK seems to be greater than that after PRK, presumably due to the limited wound healing, and reduced epithelial-stromal interactions (see Chapter 4). Whether this modulation of wound healing is permanent in these situations (moderate to high myopia) or is possible following PRK for lower degrees of myopia remains controversial.[18,29,30]

In a subset of patients refractive regression can rapidly be reversed by topical steroid therapy. Steroid treatment has been shown to alter the corneal hyaluronic acid (extracellular matrix) content,[31,32] and may be a potential explanation for the rapid refractive shifts that can occur. The permanency of such effects is unknown.

Centration

Centration is perhaps the most important technical factor the surgeon controls during excimer PRK. CVK has proven essential for assessment of ablation centration and in guiding technical alterations to improve this vitally important step of the procedure.

Uozato and Guyton have recommended centering refractive procedures on the entrance pupil (see Chap-

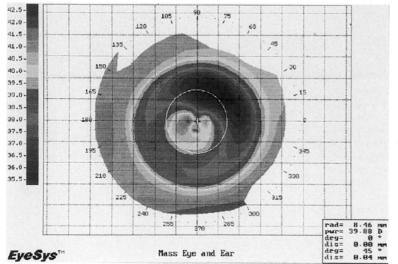

rad=	8.46	mm
pwr=	39.88	D
deg=	0	°
dis=	0.00	mm
deg=	45	°
dis=	0.04	mm

EyeSys™   Mass Eye and Ear

Figure 13–11. Central island after excimer PRK. Videokeratography of the right eye of a 53-year-old patient 6 weeks after excimer PRK. (Attempted correction of −8 sph.) A central island of steepening can be seen within an otherwise uniform ablation. An area of subepithelial and anterior stromal haze was evident biomicroscopically, which corresponded to the topographic findings. Best-corrected visual acuity (BCVA) 6 weeks postoperatively was 20/80, but with significant visual degradation. The refraction appeared undercorrected (−2.50 D spherical equivalent), and intensive topical steroid therapy was begun. Within 2 weeks of increasing steroids, BCVA improved to 20/40 and a hyperopic shift of +3.75 D occurred (refraction of +1.25 sph). The central island persisted, although it was beginning to flatten with respect to the surrounding ablated surface. The mechanisms for such rapid shifts in refraction are unclear, but changes in hyaluronic acid content or stromal hydration shifts of the cornea may be responsible.

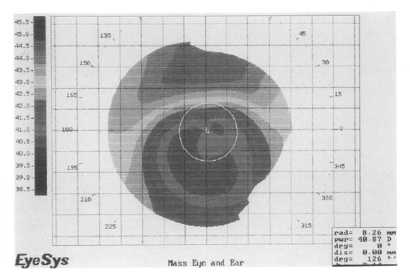

Figure 13–12. Decentered excimer PRK ablation. Videokeratography of the right eye of a 53-year-old patient 7 months after PRK. (Attempted correction of −7.25 D sph.) Ablation is inferotemporally decentered by 1.5 mm. Uncorrected visual acuity is 20/70. Although BCVA was 20/25 with −1.75 D sph, the patient experiences significant nocturnal glare from the ablation edge being within the entrance pupil.

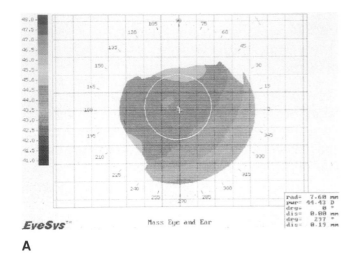

A

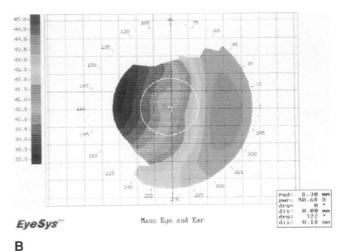

B

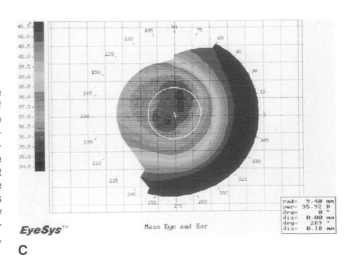

C

Figure 13–13. PRK retreatment for decentered ablation. **A.** Preoperative videokeratography of the left eye of a 23-year-old patient with −8 D of myopia. **B.** Sixteen months postoperatively, refraction had regressed to −1.50 sph. Although BCVA was 20/20, the patient reported glare symptoms. Slit lamp examination revealed moderate anterior stromal haze temporal to the visual axis, and videokeratography showed the ablation to be nasally decentered. **C.** Excimer PRK retreatment was undertaken to correct the residual myopia and to better center the ablation. Intraoperatively, the nasal aspect of the treatment zone was partly shielded with artificial tears so as to ablate selectively the raised temporal scar. Videokeratography 2 months postoperatively shows a well-centered ablation. The elevated temporal crescent has been selectively ablated. Uncorrected vision was 20/30, and the patient reported improved quality of vision.

ter 9).[33] The location of the actual visual axis can be elusive, and the pupil center is thought to approximate closely the center of the optical system for incident light entering the eye. The amount of decentration that will produce clinically significant visual degradation of image quality is unknown. Some studies suggest that decentrations less than 1 mm do not affect uncorrected or best corrected visual acuity while decentrations of greater than 1 mm have an untoward effect on both.[34] Even with preservation of Snellen visual acuity, decentration may result in degradation of the visual image, decreased contrast sensitivity, monocular diplopia, or ghost images.[35] Decentration may also result in some element of multifocality within the COZ and all its attendant problems (Figs 13–12 and 13–13).[36]

Prior studies evaluating centration of excimer ablations have been empiric in nature, identifying the ablation zone center by visual estimation rather than by using quantitative indices.[37–39] We have recently developed a weighted, vector-based differential equation to identify quantitatively the center of the topographic changes induced by PRK or other keratorefractive procedures.[40] When applied to a series of 17 moderate- and high-myopia patients, we have found the central ablation zone to be decentered 0.20 ± 0.16 mm relative to the pupil center. Given the mean COZ size of 3.4 mm in these patients, it is clear that, even with large ablation diameters, precise centration is crucial to ensure a favorable outcome.

Decentrations after LASIK or ALK for high myopia can be of greater clinical importance. Jabbur and Azar have studied the corneal changes after ALK and defined corneal double asphericity parameters that

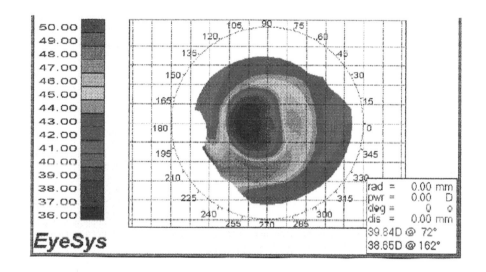

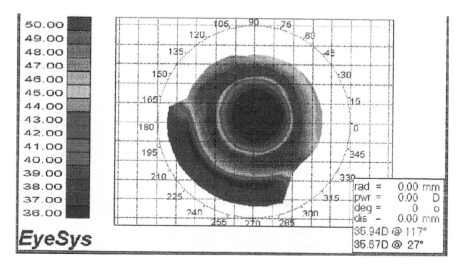

Figure 13–14. Topographical tangential maps following keratomileusis (ALK) in a patient with well-centered treatment (top) and a patient with temporal decentration (bottom). The central cornea is flattened and is surrounded by an annulus of "maximal steepening" creating an edge effect (shown in red). The zone of zero-change from baseline is shown in green, and is located between the central flat zone and the peripheral steep annulus. These landmarks can be used to determine the extent of decentration.[41]

may aid in measuring treatment decentration.[41] They measured decentration of the annulus of maximal steepening using tangential corneal maps, as well as the zone of zero change from baseline, in patients with high myopia of -8 D to -22 D (Fig 13–14). Decentrations of > 0.3 mm were seen in 40% of the patients, most commonly in the inferotemporal quadrants, and occurring in patients with higher degrees of original refractive errors.[41]

Guiding Phototherapeutic Keratectomy and Retreatments Following Photorefractive and Phototherapeutic Keratotomy

CVK is useful for phototherapeutic keratectomy (PTK) and for retreatments after PRK. In PTK, for example, localized areas of elevations and depressions can elegantly be demonstrated on the topographic color map. By selectively shielding the depressions in the cornea using either the epithelium or a masking fluid, a more uniform surface can be created. Similarly, decentrations, central islands, and aberrant healing patterns after PRK can result in localized elevations and depressions. CVK can once again guide the surgeon in selectively masking certain regions of the cornea while leaving other areas exposed. The end result is a more regular corneal surface and improved optical performance (Fig 13–13). These techniques are more challenging when the treatment of LASIK or ALK decentrations are contemplated.

SUMMARY

Modern methods for analyzing corneal topography contribute greatly to the growing field of keratorefractive surgery, providing new insights into the consequences of surgical alteration of the corneal surface. The information provided by CVK permits more exacting patient selection and greater sophistication in surgical planning, as well as providing valuable feedback that should ultimately improve the predictability and visual outcomes of such procedures. As refractive surgical techniques continue to evolve, current and future technologies for corneal contour analysis will undoubtedly play an integral role. In the future, the advent of real-time corneal topographic analysis will allow for continuous "on-line" intraoperative monitoring, providing even greater precision with which to guide surgeons in their quest for surgical correction of myopia, hyperopia, and astigmatism.

REFERENCES

1. Rabinowitz YS, Nesburn AB, McDonnell PJ. Videokeratography of the fellow eye in unilateral keratoconus. *Ophthalmology.* 1993;100:181–186.
2. Mamalis N, Montgomery S, Anderson C, et al. Radial keratotomy in a patient with keratoconus. *Refract Corneal Surg.* 1991;7:374–376.
3. Rabinowitz YS. Keratoconus, videokeratography, and refractive surgery. *Refract Corneal Surg.* 1992;8:403–407.
4. Wilson SE, Lin DTC, Klyce SD, et al. Topographic changes in contact lens-induced corneal warpage. *Ophthalmology.* 1990;97:734–744.
5. Rowsey JJ, Balyeat HD, Monlux R, et al. Prospective evaluation of radial keratotomy: photokeratoscope corneal topography. *Ophthalmology.* 1988;95:322–334.
6. Rowsey JJ, Waring GO, Monlux RD, et al. Corneal topography as a predictor of refractive change in the prospective evaluation of radial keratotomy (PERK) study. *Ophthalmic Surg.* 1991;22:370–380.
7. McDonnell PJ, Garbus J. Corneal topographic changes after radial keratotomy. *Ophthalmology.* 1989;96:45–49.
8. Bogan SJ, Waring GO, Ibrahim O, et al. Classification of normal corneal topography based on computer-assisted videokeratography. *Arch Ophthalmol.* 1990;108:945–949.
9. Bogan SJ, Maloney RK, Drews CD, et al. Computer-assisted videokeratography of corneal topography after radial keratotomy. *Arch Ophthalmol.* 1991;109:834–841.
10. Moreira H, Fasano AP, Garbus JJ, et al. Corneal topographic changes over time after radial keratotomy. *Cornea.* 1992;11:465–470.
11. Waring GO III, Lynn MJ, McDonnell PJ, et al. Results of the Prospective Evaluation of Radial Keratotomy (PERK) Study 10 years after surgery for myopia. *Arch Ophthalmol.* 1994;112:1298–1308.
12. Deitz MR, Sanders DR, Raanan MG. Progressive hyperopia in radial keratotomy; long-term follow-up of diamond-knife and metal-blade series. *Ophthalmology.* 1986;93:1284–1289.
13. Melles GRJ, Binder PS, Anderson JA. Variation in healing throughout the depth of long-term, unsutured, corneal wounds in human autopsy specimens and monkeys. *Arch Ophthalmol.* 1994;112:100–109.
14. McDonnell PJ, Garbus J, Lopez PF. Topographic analysis and visual acuity after radial keratotomy. *Am J Ophthalmol.* 1988;106:692–695.
15. Moreira H, Garbus JJ, Lee M, et al. Multifocal corneal topographic changes after radial keratotomy. *Ophthalmic Surg.* 1992;23:85–89.
16. Lopez PF, Maloney RK, Goodman GG, et al. Subregions of differing refractive power within the clear zone after experimental radial keratotomy. *Refract Corneal Surg.* 1991;7:360–367.

17. Wilson SE, Klyce SD. Topographic analysis and visual acuity after radial keratotomy. *Am J Ophthalmol.* 1989;107:436–438. Letter; comment.

18. Maguire LJ, Bourne WM. A multifocal lens effect as a complication of radial keratotomy. *Refract Corneal Surg.* 1989;5:394–397.

19. McDonnell PJ, McClusky DJ, Garbus JJ. Corneal topography and fluctuating visual acuity after radial keratotomy. *Ophthalmology.* 1989;96:665–670.

20. McDonnell PJ, Fish LA, Garbus J. Persistence of diurnal fluctuation after radial keratotomy. *Refract Corneal Surg.* 1989;5:89–93.

21. Kwitko S, Gritz DC, Garbus JJ, et al. Diurnal variation of corneal topography after radial keratotomy. *Arch Ophthalmol.* 1992;110:351–356.

22. Assil KK, Quantock AJ. Wound healing in response to keratorefractive surgery. *Surv Ophthalmol.* 1993;38:289–302.

23. Lin DTC, Sutton HF, Berman M. Corneal topography following excimer photorefractive keratectomy for myopia. *J Cataract Refract Surg.* 1993;19(suppl.):149–154.

24. Wilson SE, Klyce SD, McDonald MB, et al. Changes in corneal topography after excimer laser photorefractive keratectomy for myopia. *Ophthalmology.* 1991;98:1338–1347.

25. Seiler T, Holschbach A, Derse M, et al. Complications of myopic photorefractive keratectomy with the excimer laser. *Ophthalmology.* 1994;101:153–160.

26. Campos M, Cuevas K, Garbus J, et al. Corneal wound healing after excimer laser ablation. Effects of nitrogen gas blower. *Ophthalmology.* 1992;99:893–897.

27. Parker PJ, Klyce SD, Ryan BL, et al. Central topographic islands following photorefractive keratectomy. *Invest Ophthalmol Vis Sci.* 1993;34(suppl):803.

28. Krueger RR, Campos M, Wang XW, et al. Corneal surface morphology following excimer laser ablation with humidified gases. *Arch Ophthalmol.* 1993;111:1131–1137.

29. Gartry DS, Kerr Muir MG, Lohmann CP, et al. The effect of topical corticosteroids on refractive outcome and corneal haze after photorefractive keratectomy. A prospective, randomized, double-blind trial. *Arch Ophthalmol.* 1992;110:944–952.

30. Tengroth B, Epstein D, Fagerholm P, et al. Excimer laser photorefractive keratectomy for myopia. Clinical results in sighted eyes. *Ophthalmology.* 1993;100:739–745.

31. Fitzsimmons TD, Fagerholm P, Tengroth B. Steroid treatment of myopic regression: acute refractive and topographic changes in excimer photorefractive keratectomy patients. *Cornea.* 1993;12:358–361.

32. Fitzsimmons T, Fagerholm P, Harfstrand A, et al. Steroids after excimer surgery decrease corneal hyaluronic acid content. *Invest Ophthalmol Vis Sci.* 1992;33(suppl):766.

33. Uozato H, Guyton DL. Centering corneal surgical procedures. *Am J Ophthalmol.* 1987;103:264–275.

34. Cavanaugh TB, Durrie DS, Riedel SM, et al. Topographical analysis of the centration of excimer laser photorefractive keratectomy. *J Cataract Refract Surg.* 1993;19(suppl.):136–143.

35. Klyce SD, Smolek MK. Corneal topography of excimer laser photorefractive keratectomy. *J Cataract Refract Surg.* 1993;19(suppl.):122–130.

36. Moreira H, Garbus JJ, Fasano A, et al. Multifocal corneal topographic changes with excimer laser photorefractive keratectomy. *Arch Ophthalmol.* 1992;110:994–999.

37. Cantera E, Cantera I, Olivieri L. Corneal topographic analysis of photorefractive keratectomy in 175 myopic eyes. *Refract Corneal Surg.* 1993;9(2 suppl.):S19–22.

38. Spadea L, Sabetti L, Balestrazzi E. Effect of centering excimer laser PRK on refractive results: a corneal topography study. *Refract Corneal Surg.* 1993;9(2 suppl.):S22–25.

39. Cavanaugh TB, Durrie DS, Riedel SM, et al. Centration of excimer laser photorefractive keratectomy relative to the pupil. *J Cataract Refract Surg.* 1993;19(suppl.):144–148.

40. Almendral DF, Waller SG, Talamo JH. Corneal topography after single and multiple zone excimer photorefractive keratectomy (PRK) for moderate and high myopia. *Ophthalmology.* 1993;100(suppl):108.

41. Jabbur N, Azar DT. Analysis of corneal double asphericity parameters and decentration using axial and tangential maps after A.L.K. *Invest Ophthalmol Vis Sci.* 1996;37(suppl):2565.

CHAPTER 14

Measuring Surgically Induced Astigmatic and Prismatic Corrections

Thomas Leitman ▪ K. Scott Proctor ▪ Nathalie F. Azar ▪ Dimitri T. Azar

Astigmatism is often the vision-limiting factor following cataract, glaucoma, corneal transplant, and refractive surgery. To further refine surgeries like these, and to effectively correct both postsurgical and congenital astigmatism through the use of refractive surgery, the accurate quantification of surgically induced astigmatism is essential.

The term *astigmatism* is used to describe an optical aberration resulting from variation in the refractive power of an optical system across different meridians. An astigmatic cornea is "steep" in one meridian and "flat" in the meridian perpendicular to the "steep" meridian. In stigmatic optical systems, the image of a point source is also a point. Many characteristics of lenses produce images that are not stigmatic; these include astigmatism, spherical aberration, chromatic aberration, and coma.

The degree of surgically-induced astigmatism and spherical correction depends upon the preoperative versus the postoperative refractive power of the eye. A change in astigmatism may be induced by the removal of the lens or a dislocation and/or tilting of an intraocular lens, a phenomenon that can be noted by comparing the results of keratometry with those of manifest refraction. More commonly, an asymmetric change in the curvature of the cornea is responsible for a change in astigmatism. This asymmetric change may be induced by addition or subtraction of tissue, tightening of sutures, wound gape, cauterization, or corneal incisions. This change in curvature may be observed using retinoscopy and refraction measurements, or it can be directly documented by keratometry or corneal topography. In many of the above procedures, a prismatic effect may accompany the spherical or astigmatic correction.

HISTORY

Changes in the cornea following cataract surgery were first noted in 1876 by Mauthner.[1] A flattening of the cornea along a particular meridian after a corneal incision was observed as early as 1900 by Weber, and in 1912 by Schoenbeck,[1] although the authors did not attempt to define the effect of the surgery.

Since its introduction, the vector analysis method has been an accepted technique for the analysis of the effects of cylindrical lenses. Stokes first used this vector analysis technique in a device that measured the amplitude of an astigmatic error.[2] Using his observation that the combination of two thin cylindrical lenses at various angles could approximate the effect of a single cylindrical lens of a different power, Stokes was able to quantify the power of this single lens. He suggested that a positive cylinder could be represented by a vec-

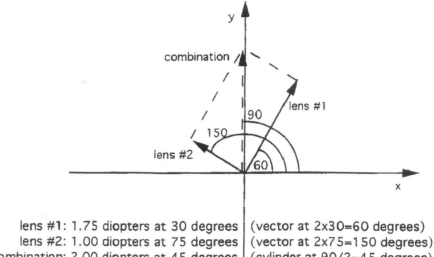

lens #1: 1.75 diopters at 30 degrees | (vector at 2x30=60 degrees)
lens #2: 1.00 diopters at 75 degrees | (vector at 2x75=150 degrees)
combination: 2.00 diopters at 45 degrees | (cylinder at 90/2=45 degrees)

Figure 14–1. A line drawing representing Stokes' method of the analysis of astigmatism.

tor whose magnitude is equal to the optical power of the astigmatism and whose angle is equal to twice the angle of the positive cylinder. The vectors that represented the two cylindrical lenses could then be added to form a new vector that corresponds to a single cylindrical lens (Fig 14–1). Stokes did not provide a proof in his brief presentation to the Royal Society. This method, however, was not intuitive to many scientists, and a proof was provided by other authors. The proof written by Thompson[3] is summarized in Appendix A.

The concept of the vector analysis of astigmatism has been reproduced periodically in the ophthalmic literature (in progressively longer descriptions) and has been adopted for the determination of surgically induced astigmatism, a process in which vectors are sub-

tracted rather than added (Fig 14–2).[4,5] In a comprehensive article, Holladay and colleagues used the trigonometric solutions of the vector analysis method to determine surgically induced astigmatism.[6] A program we have utilized based on a program written by Buzard is presented in Figure 14–3.[7] The program calculates the refractive change following ophthalmic surgery based on the preoperative sphere and cylinder measurements versus the postoperative sphere and cylinder measurements. This computer program is written in the Visual Basic® programming language for Microsoft® Excel 5.0A for the Macintosh; it may also be used in any version of Excel for IBM PC-compatible computers that supports the Visual Basic programming language.

Alpins assigned the term *surgically induced astigmatism* (SIA) to the vector that represented the postop-

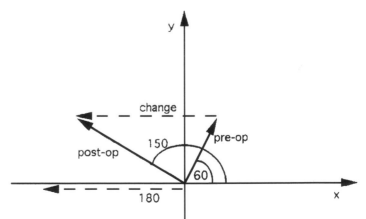

pre-op: 1.00 diopters at 30 degrees | (vector at 2x30=60 degrees)
post-op: 1.75 diopters at 75 degrees | (vector at 2x75=150 degrees)
change: 2.00 diopters at 90 degrees | (astigmatism at 180/2=90 degrees)

Figure 14–2. A schematic illustrating the vector analysis of astigmatism.

```
Function Holladay(preC, preA, postC, postA)
        rpreA = preA * 3.141592 / 180
        rpostA = postA * 3.141592 / 180
        rapostA = rpostA + 3.141592 / 2
        rbpostA = rapostA - 3.14592
        If rapostA > 3.141592 Then
                rmpostA = rbpostA
        Else
                rmpostA = rapostA
        End If
        alpha = Abs(rmpostA - rpreA)
        twobeta = Atn((postC * Sin(2 * alpha)) / (10 ^ -10 + preC +
        postC * Cos(2 * alpha)))
        theta = ((twobeta + 3.141592) / 2)
        SC = (preC * (Sin(theta)) ^ 2) + (postC * (Sin(alpha - theta)) ^ 2)
        finalC = preC + postC - 2 * SC
        If postC = preC And postA = preA Then
                finalC = 0
        Else
                finalCo = finalC
        End If
        Holladay = finalCo
End Function
```

Figure 14–3. A computer program written in Microsoft Visual Basic to calculate the Hollady-derived astigmatic change following ophthalmic surgery.

erative minus the preoperative astigmatism.[8] Alpins also suggested the term *target-induced astigmatism* to determine deviation from intended correction as opposed to preoperative error. Several other authors have suggested methods for the calculation of surgically induced astigmatism, some of which clearly reduce mathematically to Stokes' method. Several of the other suggested methods yield the correct solution when determining with-the-rule and against-the-rule astigmatism, but fail when determining astigmatism at oblique meridians; such methods have a questionable mathematical basis and may lead to inconsistent outcomes.[9–11]

Stokes' method provides clinically useful answers and is mathematically sound. Despite the method's advantages, however, it does have limitations. The algorithm assumes that all corneas exhibiting astigmatism do so only as regular astigmatism, and the algorithm relies on either a refraction or on keratometry readings to determine its result. Refraction measurements are very subjective, and it is unclear how to use the vector method if the keratometer mires are distorted or if the principal meridians found by keratometry are not 90° apart.

CORNEAL TOPOGRAPHY

Several methods that are capable of analyzing irregular astigmatism, a type that is often found when using cor-

neal topography, have been proposed.[12,13] Current modeling systems compute the corneal curvature through a central point along each meridian at several radii. The curvature at any given radius can be viewed as a function of the corneal meridian, and it can be used clinically to help in the management of astigmatism.[14–25]

At a radius of 0.5 mm from the corneal apex, the graph of curvature versus meridian is a sinusoidal function (Fig 14–4). This sinusoidal phenomenon, known since the 18th century as the Equation of Euler, is observed on any given surface, regardless of its irregularity. This principle is mathematically identical to a more elementary equation; the modified Euler equation states that the spherical equivalent is equal to the average curvature, the cylinder is equal to the difference from the minimum to the maximum curvature, and the curvature varies according to a cosine function with a period of 180° (Fig 14–5).

Equation of Euler

$$k = k_1\cos^2\theta + k_2\sin^2\theta$$

Modified Euler Equation

$$k = (se) + \frac{(cyl)}{2} \cdot \cos(2\theta)$$

Through the use of this modified Euler equation, a function for sample preop and postop keratometry

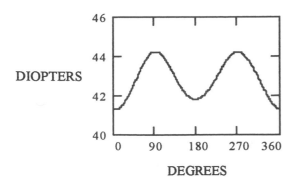

Figure 14–4. Graphic representation of corneal curvature versus corneal meridian. in a patient having with-the-rule astigmatism. The flattest hemimeridian is at zero (360) degrees, while the 90 and 270 hemimeridians are steepest (44.25D).

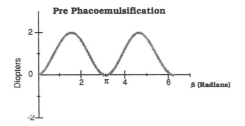

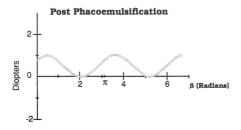

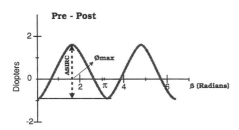

$$SIRC = Spre + Apre \sin^2(ß-øpre-\pi/2) - Spost - Apost \sin^2(ß-øpost-\pi/2)$$
$$= S_{SIRC} + A_{SIRC} \sin^2(ß-øpre-\pi/2)$$

$S_{SIRC} = min$

$SpEq_{SIRC} = (min+max)/2$

$A_{SIRC} = max-min$

$ø_{max} = ø_{SIRC}$

Figure 14–5. Azar's sinusoidal method of calculating surgically-induced astigmatism using the mathematical principle of Euler's equation. It can be utilized to determine astigmatic changes after phacoemulsification or refractive surgical procedures.

readings may be constructed. This function represents the curvature, or the power deduced from the curvature, at a certain radius along various meridians. The subtraction of the preop from the postop functions results in a third function, the surgically induced astigmatic error (SIAE) function, which is also always sinusoidal with a period of 180° (Fig 14–5). It can be shown that this method of subtracting functions will always give a result identical to Stokes' vector method through the use of "rotating vectors," a simple method of subtracting two sine functions of the same period (although not necessarily the same phase or amplitude). Stokes' method is actually a short cut for subtracting these two functions (Appendix A).

The SIAE function can be used in conjunction with corneal topography to analyze accurately a more irregular cornea,[11] as in the case of a patient with keratoconus. The keratometry readings in this case are probably distorted, making both refraction and retinoscopy difficult to measure. It would therefore be difficult to determine preop, as well as surgically induced, astigmatism. The curvature at the central point of the cornea would necessarily obey Euler's equation (ie, in the form of a sine function with a period of 180°). However, if the curvatures at a radius of approximately 1 mm (the image of the second Plácido's disc ring) are plotted, then a different pattern is observed.

This function of corneal curvature versus meridian at a radius of 1 mm from the corneal apex is periodic, and the function can be broken down into harmonics, using Fourier analysis of corneal topography[13]; even a function that appears irregular can be represented as the sum of a series of regular sine functions. The first "prismatic" harmonic has a period of 360°, the second "astigmatic" harmonic has a period of 180°, and other harmonics have progressively higher frequencies or lower periods. The addition of just the first two harmonics gives an excellent approximation of the irregular function of curvature versus meridian at a radius of 1 mm. In fact, the function associated with many corneas can be adequately represented by only the first two harmonics because the amplitudes of the higher frequencies are relatively small.

An example of the corneal topography of a cornea with approximately 1.36 diopters of with-the-rule astigmatism, as determined by Fourier analysis, is shown in Figure 14–6. The steeper, more powerful meridian at approximately 85° can be seen on the graph of meridian versus power in Figure 14–7 and in the yellow areas on the topography map (Fig 14–6).

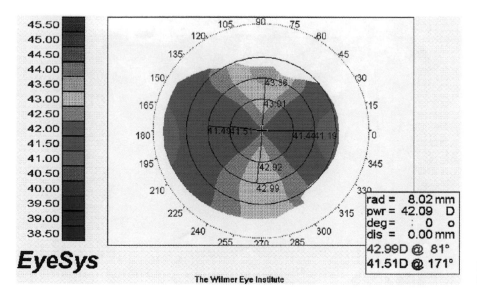

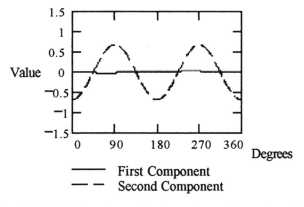

Figure 14–6. Corneal topographic representation of with-the-rule astigmatism.

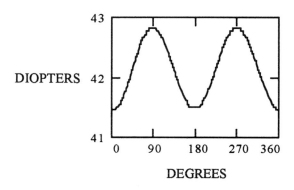

Figure 14–7. Corneal meridian versus corneal power graph corresponding to the corneal topography map in Figure 14–6.

The Fourier transform of the first two harmonics of the fundamental frequency (Fig 14–8) indicates the dominance of the secondary component of the overall astigmatism. It is important to note that the second harmonic, with a periodicity of 180°, is in the same form as Euler's equation, and in a sense this harmonic represents a component of regular astigmatism. The first component, or the first harmonic, has much less of an effect on the overall astigmatism in the Fourier graph. The second Plácido's ring was used for this calculation, but it turns out that any of the Plácido's disc reflections within the image of the pupil give nearly identical results for this patient.

For the patient illustrated in Figure 13–3, Fourier analysis reveals a first "prismatic" component at the 15

degree hemimeridian, accounting for the "nonorthogonal astigmatism." This is compounded to the regular astigmatic (second) component with periodicity of 180 degrees at the 130 degree meridian. Similarly, the patient illustrated in Figure 13–4 with asymmetric astigmatism has a predominant astigmatic (second) component and a smaller prismatic (first) component at the 95 degree hemimeridian.

This method of analysis can also be used to analyze surgically induced astigmatism. The postoperative corneal topography is shown in Figure 14–9. The preop corneal curvature function can be subtracted from the postop corneal curvature function, yielding a third curve. An analysis of the postop result corresponding to the preop cornea is shown in Figure 14–10. It should

Figure 14–8. Fourier transform of the first and second harmonics of the topography map in Figure 14–6; the solid function line represents the first (prismatic) harmonic and the dashed function line represents the second (astigmatic) harmonic.

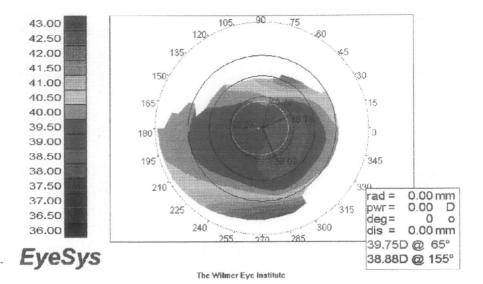

Figure 14–9. Postoperative corneal topography of patient in Figure 14–6.

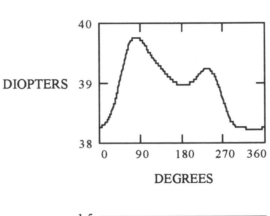

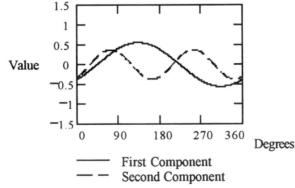

First Component
— — Second Component

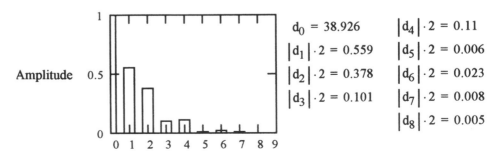

Figure 14–10. Analysis of the postoperative corneal topography corresponding to the preop corneal topography represented in Figure 14–9.

$d_0 = 38.926$ $|d_4| \cdot 2 = 0.11$

$|d_1| \cdot 2 = 0.559$ $|d_5| \cdot 2 = 0.006$

$|d_2| \cdot 2 = 0.378$ $|d_6| \cdot 2 = 0.023$

$|d_3| \cdot 2 = 0.101$ $|d_7| \cdot 2 = 0.008$

$|d_8| \cdot 2 = 0.005$

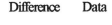

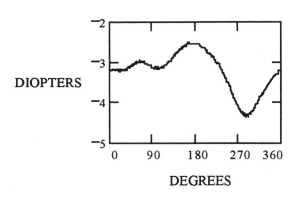

Figure 14–11. Graphic representation of surgically induced corneal topographic change.

be noted that the postop cornea exhibits a greater amplitude of the first harmonic compared with the second harmonic. The curve that represents the surgically induced curvature change at each meridian, shown in Figure 14–11, can be approximated by the sum of a series of sine functions that was calculated using Fourier analysis.

The Fourier analysis of the "difference graph" indicated an overall change of approximately 3.23 D following surgery. There was 1.13 D of the "primary prismatic harmonic" component induced at 131.82°, and 0.81 D of the "second harmonic" component of astigmatism induced at 13.8°. These values were determined using the values that are graphically represented in Figure 14–11. These values are the results of the Fourier analysis of the difference graph. This technique provides a much more accurate, in-depth analysis of surgically induced prismatic and astigmatic changes than an analysis using Stokes' vector analysis method.

CONCLUSION

Using Stokes' vector method is a sound and reliable way to determine surgically induced astigmatism based on keratometry measurements. The only requirement of Stokes' method is the simple subtraction of vectors (or the trigonometric equivalent of vectors). However, the vector method assumes that any astigmatism at all found in pre- and postop corneas is regular, and it permits no consideration for the possible existence of irregular astigmatism or prismatic shifts. It is possible to

represent accurately corneas with some degree of irregular astigmatism using a modified form of the Equation of Euler in conjunction with data acquired from corneal topography. Surgically induced astigmatism can be measured at all corneal meridians by subtracting two such functions. The Fourier analysis of corneal topography has been applied to regular and irregular components of surgically induced astigmatism, and may therefore be used to approximate the curvature of many irregular corneas and the induced prismatic, spherical and astigmatic curvature change of some surgical procedures. This analytical technique may enable a refractive surgeon to better design the appropriate surgical procedure for correcting irregular astigmatism.

REFERENCES

1. Huber C. Myopic astigmatism a substitute for accommodation in pseudophakia. *Doc Ophthalmol.* 1981;52:123–178. Review.
2. Stokes GG. On a mode of measuring the astigmatism of a defective eye; 19th meeting of the British Association for the Advancement of Science, 1849. *Trans Sect.* 1850:10–11.
3. Thompson SP. On obliquely-crossed cylindrical lenses. *Philosophical Mag.* 1900;50(4):317–324.
4. Naylor EJ. Astigmatic difference in refractive errors. *Br J Ophthalmol.* 1968;52:422–425.
5. Jaffe S, Clayman HM. The pathophysiology of corneal astigmatism after cataract extraction. *Trans Am Acad Ophthalmol Otolaryngol.* 1975;79:615.
6. Holladay JT, Cravy TV, Koch DD. Calculating the surgically induced refractive change following ocular surgery. *J Cataract Refract Surg.* 1992;18:429–443. Comments.
7. Buzard K. New formula for vector change in astigmatism. *J Cataract Refract Surg.* 1993;19:815–816. Letter.
8. Alpins NA. A new method of analyzing vectors for changes in astigmatism. *J Cataract Refract Surg.* 1993;19:524–533.
9. Cravy TV. Calculation of the change in corneal astigmatism following cataract extraction. *Ophthalmic Surg.* 1979;10:38–49.
10. Cravy TV. Long-term corneal astigmatism related to selected elastic, monofilament, nonabsorbable sutures. *J Cataract Refract Surg.* 1989;15:61–69.
11. Naeser K. Conversion of keratometer readings to polar values. *J Cataract Refract Surg.* 1990;16:741–745.
12. Raasch T. Quantitative model of corneal astigmatism from topographic data. *Ophthalmic Vis Optics.* 1992;3:24–27.
13. Lietman TM, Azar DT. Analysis of surgically-induced astigmatism. *Invest Ophthalmol Vis Sci.* 1994;35:2195.

14. Axt JC. Longitudinal study of postoperative astigmatism. *J Cataract Refract Surg.* 1987;13:381–388.

15. Jampel HD, Thompson JR, Baker CC, Stark WJ. A computerized analysis of astigmatism after cataract surgery. *Ophthalmic Surg.* 1986;17:786–790.

16. Koch DD, Haft EA, Gay C. Computerized videokeratographic analysis of corneal topographic changes induced by sutured and unsutured 4 mm scleral pocket incisions. *J Cataract Refract Surg.* 1993;19:166–169.

17. Masket S. Keratorefractive aspects of the scleral pocket incision and closure method for cataract surgery. *J Cataract Refract Surg.* 1989;15:70–77. Review.

18. Masket S. Deep versus appositional suturing of the scleral pocket incision for astigmatic control in cataract surgery. *J Cataract Refract Surg.* 1987;13:131–135.

19. Merck MP, Williams PA, Lindstrom RL. Trapezoidal keratotomy. A vector analysis. *Ophthalmology.* 1986;93:719–726.

20. Neumann AC, McCarty GR, Sanders DR, Raanan MG. Small incisions to control astigmatism during cataract surgery. *J Cataract Refract Surg.* 1989;15:78–84.

21. Nordan LT. Quantifiable astigmatism correction: concepts and suggestions, 1986. *J Cataract Refract Surg.* 1986;12:507–518.

22. Richards SC, Brodstein RS, Richards WL, et al. Long-term course of surgically induced astigmatism. *J Cataract Refract Surg.* 1988;14:270–276.

23. Sawusch MR, Guyton DL. Optimal astigmatism to enhance depth of focus after cataract surgery. *Ophthalmology.* 1991;98:1025–1029.

24. Seiler T, Reckmann W, Maloney RK. Effective spherical aberration of the cornea as a quantitative descriptor in corneal topography. *J Cataract Refract Surg.* 1993;19:155–165.

25. Shepherd JR. Induced astigmatism in small incision cataract surgery. *J Cataract Refract Surg.* 1989;15:85–88.

APPENDIX A

Thompson's Proof of the Vector Addition of Obliquely Crossed Cylindrical Lenses

To determine the angle, ϕ, the equation representing the meridian at which the refractive power of a bicylindrical lens system is at its maximum must be evaluated:

$$A \cos^2 \phi + B \cos^2 (\theta - \phi)$$

(1) $$\frac{A}{B} = \frac{\sin2(\theta - \phi)}{\sin2\phi}$$

to which may be given the alternative form

(2) $$\cot2\phi = \frac{\dfrac{A}{B} + \cos2\theta}{\sin2\theta}$$

(3) $$C = A\cos^2\phi + B\cos^2(\theta - \phi) - A\sin^2\phi$$
$$\qquad - B\sin^2(\theta - \phi);$$
$$C = A\cos2\phi + B\cos2(\theta - \phi);$$

(4) $$D = A\sin^2\phi + B\sin^2(\theta - \phi)$$

$$\frac{C}{A} = \cos2\phi + \frac{B}{A}\cos2(\theta - \phi)$$

$$\frac{B}{A} = \frac{\sin2\phi}{\sin2(0 - \phi)}$$

$$\frac{C}{A} = \cos2\phi + \frac{\sin2\phi \cdot \cos2(\theta - \phi)}{\sin2(\theta - \phi)}$$

$$\frac{C}{A} = \frac{\sin2\theta}{\sin2(\theta - \phi)}$$

(5) $$\frac{A}{\sin2(\theta - \phi)} = \frac{B}{\sin2\phi} = \frac{C}{\sin2\theta}$$

(6) $$C^2 = A^2 + B^2 + 2\,AB\cos2\theta$$

(7) $$\sin2\phi = \frac{B}{C}\sin2\theta$$

$$\frac{D}{A} = \sin^2\phi + \frac{B}{A}\sin^2(\theta - \phi)$$

$$= \frac{1}{2}\left\{\frac{\sin2(\theta - \phi) + \sin2\phi - \sin2\theta}{\sin2(\theta - \phi)}\right\}$$

$$= \frac{1}{2}\left\{1 + \frac{B}{A} - \frac{C}{A}\right\}$$

$$= \frac{1}{2}\frac{A + B - C}{A}$$

(8) $$D = \frac{A + B - C}{2}$$

SECTION III

Biomechanics and Instrumentation

CHAPTER 15

Corneal Biomechanics in Refractive Surgery

Jesper Ø. Hjortdal

Corneal biomechanics, the study of mechanics applied to the cornea, explores the normal function of the cornea, predicts changes due to alterations, and proposes methods of artificial intervention.[1] Corneal refractive surgical procedures alter the shape and structure of corneal tissue. The outcome of incisional and laser shrinkage techniques depends on proper alteration of the biomechanical properties of the stroma. Biomechanical effects may confound the direct sculpturing of the corneal stroma in lamellar and laser keratectomy techniques. The purpose of this chapter is to provide an introduction to corneal biomechanics and to discuss the relevance of biomechanics in refractive surgery.

BIOMECHANICS OF THE CORNEA

The term *biomechanics* has been applied to the investigation of a variety of physical and chemical properties. In the present context, elasticity and time-dependent changes will be considered in the relation between deformation and load. The relation between these mechanical properties and the structural components of the cornea, including the collagen fibril, the ground substance, and water, will also be discussed.

Elasticity

The basic elements of elasticity, those of strain and stress, are related through the elastic properties of the material.[2] When a force is applied to a fixed structure, the structure will deform to the point at which the opposing force in the structure balances the applied force. The structure's extent of deformation depends upon both the size and shape of the unloaded structure and the direction of the applied force. Consequently, the relation of absolute deformations to a structure's original undeformed shape is quantified as *strain*, and the applied force is quantified as *stress* (force per unit area). Both deformation and force can be split into tensor components, which are capable of acting parallel or perpendicular to each other. These components eventually give rise to both normal and shear stresses and strains (Fig 15–1).

A *Hookean elastic solid* is a solid that obeys Hooke's law, which states that the stress tensor is linearly proportional to the strain tensor. The *constitutive properties* of a material are determined by the amount the material strains in response to a given stress. A material whose mechanical properties lack symmetry is called *aelotropic* or *anisotropic*. The precise anisotropic level of the cornea is not known. In an *isotropic* material only two

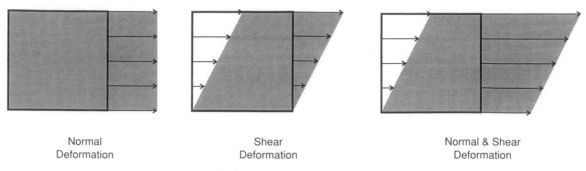

| Normal Deformation | Shear Deformation | Normal & Shear Deformation |

Figure 15–1. Normal, shear, and combined normal and shear deformation.

independent constants, known as the *Lamé constants,* are necessary for connecting stresses and strains because the elastic properties of the specimen and the orientation of the specimen are independent variables. From these two constants the more commonly used *Young's modulus of elasticity, shear modulus,* and *Poisson's ratio* can be calculated.[2] The term *Young's modulus of elasticity* is only valid for linear isotropic materials. For the corneal stroma, a more proper name for the parameter describing the relation between normal stress and normal strain is *elastic stiffness.*[3]

Few biologic materials are linear elastic and isotropic. It is clear that the cornea is not an isotropic material when its microstructure, with ground substance–embedded collagen fibrils running in lamellar sheets parallel to the corneal surface, is considered. Differing elastic properties in the transverse direction across the corneal stroma and in the tangential direction along the corneal membrane are to be expected. The elastic properties of an *ortotropic* material exhibit symmetry in two orthogonal planes; such a model may be a sufficient description of the elastic behavior of the corneal stroma. Nine independent elastic constants are needed to fully characterize an ortotropic material.[2]

The treatment of the corneal stroma as a fibril-reinforced material makes any calculations more objective. The collagen fibrils of the cornea form the fibril part of the material, and the ground substance and water form the "cement" in which the collagen fibrils are embedded. The regular spacing of the collagen fibrils may be promoted by forces of repulsion originating in the ground substance.[4] For stresses in a particular direction, a fiber-reinforced material can be regarded as a homogenous material with the following modulus of elasticity:

$$E_{fm} = E_f bh + E_m(1 - b)$$

The corneal elastic stiffness (E_{fm}) in a particular direction will thus depend upon the *elastic stiffness* of the single fibril (E_f) and the ground substance (E_m), respectively. The *degree of reinforcement* (>b), the volume fraction of fibrils), and the *efficacy factor* (>h), which is a measure of the orientation of the fibrils with respect to the direction investigated, will also affect the corneal elastic stiffness (E_{fm}).[5,6] The elastic stiffness of a collagen fibril has been estimated to be in the order of 0.5 to 1.0 GPa, whereas the elastic stiffness of oak tree and mild steel is in the order of 10 and 200 GPa, respectively.[1,7] The elastic stiffness of the ground substance may be calculated from swelling-pressure experiments of the cornea.[8] The equilibrium stress–strain behavior of the cornea under compression will determine the elastic stiffness of the solid phase, which results from the ground substance alone because the cross-sectional area of the corneal button during compression remains constant.[9,10] At a central corneal thickness of 0.50 mm, the elastic stiffness is approximately 40 kPa. Consequently, the elastic stiffness of the ground substance is a factor of 25,000 less than the elastic stiffness of the fibrils. If all fibrils are oriented along the direction of interest, the efficacy factor is 1; however, if they all are oriented perpendicular to the direction of interest, the efficacy factor is 0. For randomly oriented fibrils in two dimensions, a realistic possibility in the cornea, the efficacy factor is 3/8.[5,11,12] The volume fraction of collagen fibrils in the cornea, otherwise known as the degree of reinforcement, is approximately 0.2.[13,14] If the cited values for the constants in the equation are used and it is assumed that all collagen fibrils are in action, the tangential elastic stiffness of the corneal stroma should be 35 to 70 MPa. In the transverse direction, the elastic *stiffness* should be approximately 30 kPa. Thus, the calculated elastic stiffness of the cornea is approximately 1000 times higher for tangential extension than it is for transverse compression. Regional variability in the orientation of the collagen fibrils, including fibrils crossing between lamellae, may explain the interlamellar adhesive strength increase from center to periphery.[15] Consequently, some regional variability in tangential and transverse corneal elastic stiffness can be expected.

The overall tangential elastic stiffness of the corneal stroma (E_{fm}) has been measured in several in vitro experiments, and the results related to the human cornea are summarized in.[13,16–20] In strip extensiometry experiments, as well as in whole globe experiments, the cornea has been found to behave in a nonlinear elastic fashion, as have other connective tissues; that is, the elastic stiffness increases with increasing stress and strain. The structural reasons for the observed nonlinearity are not completely understood, and it is probable that several factors are involved. In mechanical testing of parallel fibered structures, such as tendons and ligaments, it has been observed that the fibrils are undulated in the relaxed state. The specimen will gradually unfold when it is loaded, whereas the specimen behaves in a linear elastic way when all fibrils are straight.[3] The crimp of collagen fibrils imparts a resilience to the tissue as the fibrils are sequentially straightened and loaded.[21] Furthermore, local reorientation of fibrils under stress may contribute to the nonlinear elastic response of tendons.[6] Finally, structural studies of the conformation of collagen molecules have revealed axial regions of alternating "order" and "disorder."[22] Application of stress to a fibril may result in a preferential unraveling of the regions of disorder, resulting in a nonlinear elasticity of the collagen fibril itself. The fibrils of the normohydrated human cornea have not been found to fold or crimp during unloading, whereas the rabbit cornea has demonstrated such behavior.[23] Stromal striations have, however, been observed in the normal living human cornea, although it is unknown whether these striations correspond to crimped lamellae.[24] The nonlinear elastic behavior of the cornea may be incorporated into the aforementioned fibril-reinforced material model using a parallel spring, variable slack concept.[3] Thus, at a certain strain or stress level, only a fraction of the collagen fibrils will be in action. With increasing strain and stress, more fibrils will be recruited sequentially and will take part in load bearing, while the tissue will behave in a linear elastic manner when all fibrils are active (Fig 15–2).[25]

While the mechanical characteristics of the ground substance do not contribute to the tangential elastic stiffness of the corneal membrane, the ground substance contributes to the membrane's shear strength whereby tension is transferred between neighboring collagen fibrils. The cornea shows very little resistance to shear deformation in the plane tangential to the surface, suggesting that small displacements of a fibril

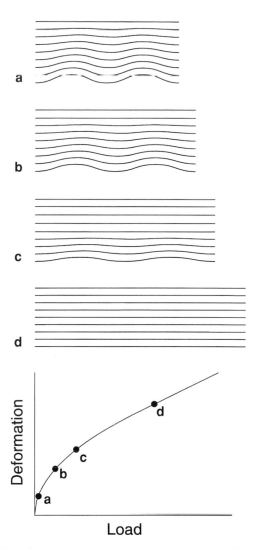

Figure 15–2. Graph showing load versus deformation: more fibrils are recruited with increasing strain and stress, while the tissue behaves in a linear elastic manner when all fibrils are active.

along its length do not result in transmission of significant stress to neighboring fibrils.[26] In preliminary shearing experiments in the rabbit and human cornea, the shear modulae (shear stiffness) have been found to be approximately 1 and 2 kPa, respectively.[26,27] The relation between shear stress and shear strain in the rabbit cornea shows considerable hysteresis and depends on the hydration of the tissue.[26] Although small, the shear stiffness of the human cornea, the major determinant for corneal resistance to bending, is appreciable in applanation tonometry. Similarly, the influence of the shear stiffness may become significant in refractive surgery. After a corneal incision, the shear stiffness will determine the transmission of tensile forces from uncut to cut corneal fibrils, which will influence the curvature change of the corneal surface.

Eliasson and Maurice reported that the distribution of tension across the human cornea in vivo is equal, suggesting that a constant fraction of collagen fibrils across the corneal stroma bears the intraocular pressure load.[26,28] The actual in vivo strain of the human cornea induced by the intraocular pressure remains to be determined; therefore, the elastic stiffness of the human cornea in vivo is also not known. However, observations of the corneal radius of curvature and the subjective refraction in glaucoma patients before and after treatment suggest that the tangential elastic stiffness of the ocular tunics is very high.[29]

Time-Dependent Changes

If a material is suddenly strained to a constant level, the stresses induced in the material may decrease with time, demonstrating a concept known as *stress relaxation*. Similarly, if a material is suddenly stressed by a constant force, the material may continue to deform with time, demonstrating a concept known as *creep*. These phenomena are characteristics of viscoelasticity.[1] The cornea demonstrates viscoelastic changes when tested in vitro. In swelling-pressure experiments, it typically takes 1 to 2 hours before a steady state level is attained.[8,30] Studies of viscoelastic changes along the corneal membrane are not as common. It has recently been found that abrupt pressure loading of the intact human cornea induces an inverse creep phenomenon on the epithelial side and a regular creep phenomenon on the endothelial side of the cornea in vitro. These changes are associated with a decreasing corneal thickness and are probably due to sequential recruitment of active load-bearing collagen fibrils in the posterior part of the cornea during corneal thinning.[20,33]

Corneal hydration has been shown to influence corneal radius of curvature. Associated with an overnight 2.4% increase in cornea thickness, the radius of curvature increases 0.04 mm; with eyelid opening, the cornea thins and steepens slightly.[34] Although the normal cornea shows time-dependent changes, which can possibly be ascribed to changes in corneal hydration, the tissue is remarkably stable and seems insensitive to even prolonged elevated stress levels, as seen in adult patients with chronic glaucoma. The surface contour of the keratoconic cornea, however, changes with time,

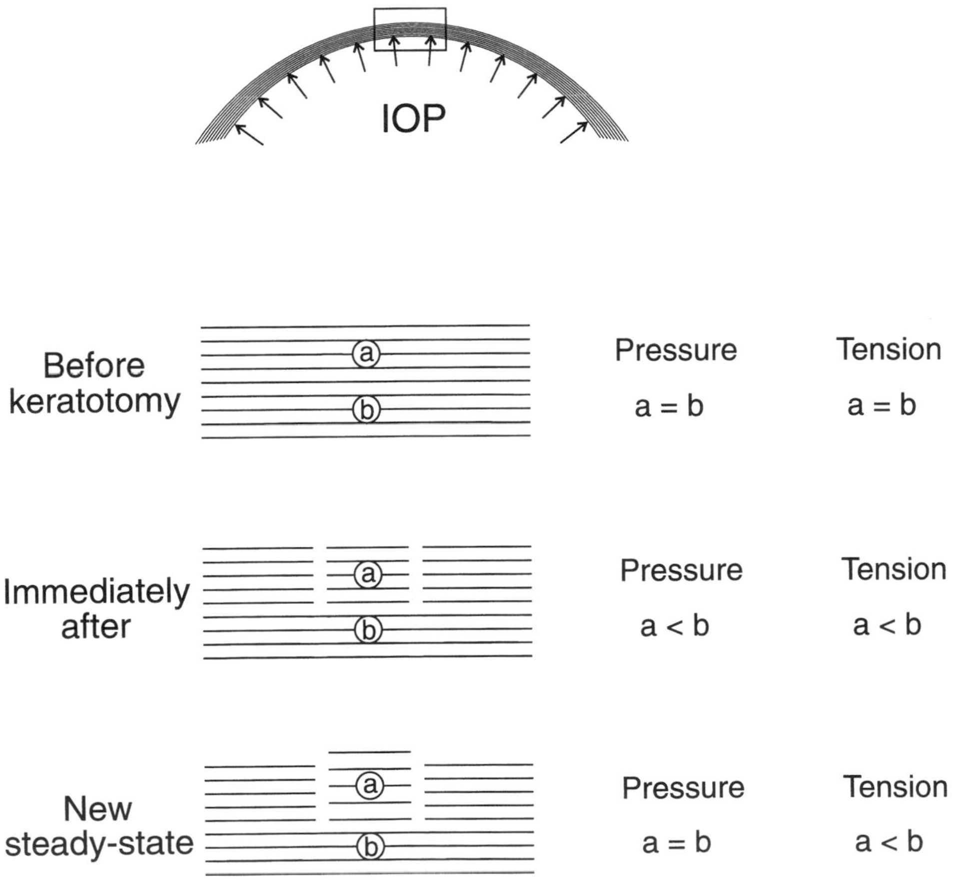

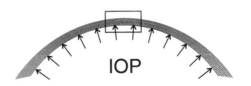

IOP

		Pressure	Tension
Before keratotomy	ⓐ ⓑ	a = b	a = b
Immediately after	ⓐ ⓑ	a < b	a < b
New steady-state	ⓐ ⓑ	a = b	a < b

Figure 15–3. The change in the outer contour of the cornea brought on by shifts in fibril stress and in the distribution of water in the stroma.

principally because of changes in the ground substance.[35,36] It can be hypothesized that the anchorage of the collagen fibrils is gradually compromised in this disease, and that the observed protrusion results from a continuous sliding of the fibrils that causes the tissue to loosen gradually.

In the living eye, the relation between intraocular pressure and corneal thickness is influenced by the permeability of the limiting corneal cell layers and the endothelial fluid pump. Positive as well as negative relations have been described.[37,38] The limiting cell layers are necessary for opposing the expansive force (measured as the swelling pressure) of the corneal stroma, which would otherwise suck water (measured as the imbibition pressure).[39] Thus, even under zero load from the intraocular pressure, the corneal stroma is under a transverse load. The imbibition pressure decreases from the center of the cornea to the corneal periphery, possibly reflecting the pumping capacity of the corneal endothelium and the stroma's resistance to water movement.[30,40,41] Water, the predominant component of the stroma, will move from regions of high pressure to regions of low pressure, thus leveling out any pressure differences. The intraocular pressure, the stress distribution between the corneal fibrils, the swelling pressure of the ground substance, the barrier and pumping functions of the limiting cell layers, and the magnitude of, and resistance to, water flow determine the local corneal hydrostatic pressure.[41] An example may illustrate how changes in fibril stress can influence the distribution of water in the stroma, thereby affecting the outer contour of the cornea (Fig 15–3). If a deep circular trephination is made at the center of the cornea, only the very posterior corneal fibrils can take up tension, whereas the fibrils in the trephined cylinder are relaxed. The local pressure will be smaller in the relaxed cylinder than in the surrounding tissue immediately following the trephination. Water will move from the area of higher pressure to the area of the lower pressure, the cylinder will increase in volume, the local swelling pressure will decrease, and eventually the pressure in the cylinder will be similar to that of the surrounding tissue. If the water resistance and pumping function in the limiting cell layers are constant, the net effect of the trephination will be a small increase in the volume of the cylinder (the low fibril-stress regions) and a small decrease in the arbitrary volume defined by the intact fibrils (the high fibril-stress regions). Experimental support for the influence of membrane stress on local corneal hydration has been provided by McPhee et al.[42]

MECHANICAL ASPECTS OF REFRACTIVE SURGERY TECHNIQUES

Induction of Curvature Changes

The refractive power of the cornea can, in principle, be changed by altering the anterior corneal radius of curvature, the refractive index of the cornea, or the posterior corneal radius of curvature. Until now, only changes in the anterior radius of curvature have been considered feasible, although secondary changes in the posterior corneal surface may occur and slightly modify the total refractive power of the surgically modified cornea. Changes in total refractive index of the cornea have been induced experimentally by implantation of intracorneal lenses with a high refractive index.[43]

Changes in the anterior radius of curvature can be induced by the direct sculpturing of excimer laser ablation, or epikeratophakia.[44,45] Additional sculpturing techniques include intracorneal addition of tissue (keratophakia) and controlled removal of corneal lamellae (keratomileusis), either mechanically or by intrastromal laser ablation.[46–48] Thus, the basis for the direct sculpturing techniques is controlled tissue removal or tissue addition in the central cornea. The developments in controlling the excimer laser beam have led to nearly perfect geometric precision in the ablation pattern when tested on unloaded mechanically stable materials such as plastic polymer (PMMA). The cornea, however, is under load from the intraocular pressure, is not perfectly stiff, and water may redistribute in the tissue if the stress distribution is altered.

The other principle of refractive surgery involves modification of the paracentral and peripheral cornea, whereby the central radius of curvature is passively changed. Some examples of this technique are incisional refractive techniques, thermokeratoplasty, peripheral corneal inlays (intracorneal ring), and gel.[49–52] The operative principles of these peripherally acting methods can be understood, at least qualitatively, based on several biomechanical and surface continuity principles. We will assume that the corneal membrane is fixed at the limbus. The corneal membrane is loaded by the intraocular pressure to a given meridional arc length and has a slightly prolate shape that is steeper at the center (Fig 15–4). The central radius of curvature may then be changed in two ways. First, if the meridional arc length increases, the cornea will become more prolate and the center will steepen, and vice versa. Second, if some peripheral bulging or flattening can be induced, and if the corneal meridional arc length remains

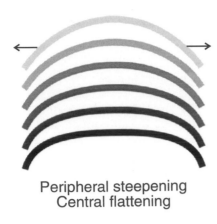

Peripheral steepening
Central flattening

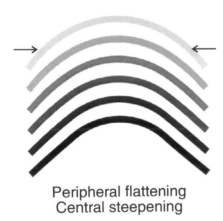

Peripheral flattening
Central steepening

Figure 15–4. Peripheral steepening and central flattening of the cornea, compared with peripheral flattening and central steepening of the cornea.

constant, a varying amount of the arc will be available to cover the central cornea. More arc will be available if peripheral flattening is induced, while less arc will be available if peripheral bulging is induced, thus ensuring the continuity of the central corneal surface. Consequently, in peripheral bulging, the center of the cornea will flatten, whereas in peripheral flattening, the center of the cornea will steepen (Fig 15–4). An increase in the corneal arc length can be induced by increasing the local stress on the corneal membrane, which will strain as a result of its elastic behavior. Peripheral bulging or flattening can be induced by relaxing or shrinking, respectively, a circumferential band of tissue. Alternatively, peripheral bulging may be introduced by an increase in the peripheral volume.

Incisional Operative Techniques

The cutting of stromal lamellae decreases the number of corneal fibrils available to bear the load of the intraocular pressure, thus increasing the mechanical stress on the remaining uncut fibrils. The increased fibril stress will cause the uncut fibrils to elongate. After radial keratotomy (RK), the corneal periphery will bulge outward and, assuming the arc length of the uncut optical zone remains constant, the center of the cornea must flatten in order to preserve surface continuity. In transverse keratotomy, the central corneal flattening observed in the cut meridian may be a consequence of a peripheral local outward bulging. Therefore, the center of the cornea must flatten in the cut meridian in order to preserve surface continuity. Some grading of the effect of incisional operative techniques is possible by varying the size of the central optical zone (COZ) or the number and depth of incisions.[53,54]

The stability of the corneal membrane is decreased after RK. A significant proportion of patients experience continued diurnal fluctuations in visual acuity that are associated with corneal steepening during the day.[55,56] Corneal hydration and intraocular pressure also exhibit diurnal changes. In vitro as well as in vivo increased corneal hydration accentuates the flattening effect of a radial keratotomy, and diurnal variations in corneal hydration correlate with diurnal changes in corneal power.[56–58b] Diurnal variations in intraocular pressure are small, amounting to a few millimeters of mercury. The physiologic range of pressure fluctuations is too small to affect the corneal curvature significantly.[59–60] Long-term clinical studies after RK have shown time-dependent changes in subjective refraction. Some of the initial effect is lost during the first month, while more patients show an increasing, rather than a decreasing, effect of surgery up to 5 years postoperatively.[60b,61] The causes of this phenomena are not known.

Lamellar Refractive Techniques

Epikeratophakia

The epikeratophakia operative technique, in a biomechanical sense, consists of a 360° circumferential partial keratotomy combined with the addition of a tissue lenticule. The partial keratotomy increases the stress on the deeper corneal lamellae, causing the tissue to elongate. If left at this stage, the increased meridional arc length should result in some central corneal steepening of the native cornea. The lenticule is loosely inserted into the pocket and is probably under reduced membrane tension after suture removal. The lack of membrane tension may result in a higher water content in the epilenticule than in the normal cornea, possibly increasing the refractive effect of the procedure.[62]

Keratomileusis and Keratophakia

Keratomileusis involves the removal of a lenticule of the patient's cornea by lamellar dissection. In principle, either the posterior surface of the lenticule or the anterior surface of the nude native cornea may be sculptured by excimer laser ablation or by mechanical lathing or cutting. After intrastromal sculpturing, the lenticule is repositioned on the patient's cornea. By breaking the continuity of the anterior stromal fibrils, only the posterior corneal lamellae can take up tension. They experience higher membrane stresses and exhibit strain. Fibrils in the repositioned lenticule will probably not bear any of the intraocular pressure load. The intrastromal sculpturing procedure's effect on corneal curvature may therefore be modified by hydration changes in the lenticule.

Intrastromal Procedures

The stromal volume can be modified without disturbing the anterior parts of the stromal lamellae, including Bowman's layer, principally using two types of procedures:

1. Increasing the volume of the peripheral cornea either by an intrastromal ring or by injection of gels
2. Intrastromal removal of tissue by laser techniques

Addition of Peripheral Volume

Either insertion of an intrastromal ring in the corneal periphery or injection of gels in a preformed peripheral circumferential channel will induce flattening of the center of the cornea. Qualitatively, the same effect may be induced by a rigid ring and a gel. The addition of matter in the corneal periphery will induce an outward bulging of the corneal surfaces around the implant, thus incorporating excess corneal arc length. Consequently, less of the corneal arc will be available for covering the central cornea, which therefore must flatten.

Intrastromal Ablation

The intrastromal lamellae can be disrupted by the picosecond infrared laser.[48] The procedure results in a net removal of central intrastromal volume, thus displacing the surfaces of the cornea as the stromal cavity is eliminated. With an intended myopic correction, the anterior surface will displace predominantly in the posterior direction, as the cavity is then eliminated by relaxation of fibrils.

Laser Operative Techniques

Excimer Laser

In excimer laser ablation, corneal tissue is removed in order to decrease the corneal thickness. The remaining corneal fibrillae will be exposed to higher levels of membrane stresses, inducing some elongation of the fibrils. A 20% reduction in corneal thickness corresponds to a 25% increase in the corneal stroma's average stress, which is comparable to a 25% increase in the intraocular pressure. However, the induced increase in the corneal meridional arc length will be very small, probably amounting to less than 0.05%. If the edge of the ablation zone is considered fixed, this would induce negligible steepening of the central cornea.

For decades, some ophthalmologists have believed that Bowman's layer serves as a reinforcing structure in the cornea and that damage to this layer is critical to the development of keratoconus. The introduction of the excimer laser caused some to fear that the procedure's ablative properties might eventually induce a keratoconuslike disorder. Recent biomechanical studies of the cornea have not demonstrated any particular mechanically enhancing effect of Bowman's layer.[63,64] Furthermore, clinical follow-up studies of ablated patients did not document excessive corneal steepening after excimer laser ablation. Thus, it seems that Bowman's layer simply serves as the outer layer of the corneal stroma. If the layer is removed, the outer lamellae of the proper corneal stroma take up the mechanical functions of the outer limiting connective tissue layer.

Thermokeratoplasty

Thermokeratoplasty has recently been reintroduced as a surgical procedure. The absorbed light of a Holmium: YAG laser heats a small conic volume of the corneal stroma. The regular straight collagen structure is changed to an irregular recoiled structure when exposed to temperatures above 65°C, and the length of the collagen fibril shrinks to about one third of its original length.[1] However, the elastic stiffness of the heat-denatured collagen molecule is a factor of 1000 less than that of the straight molecule.[1] Therefore, much of the thermal shrinkage can be expected to disappear when the cornea is loaded by the intraocular pressure. Central corneal steepening can be induced by the application of a pattern of paracentral or peripheral burns. The effect of the treatment decreases as the treatment diameter increases.[65] Peripheral shrinkage, which induces a flatter constricting peripheral band through which the central cornea can bulge, accounts for the procedure's effect on corneal curvature.

THE MECHANICS OF THE EYE AFTER REFRACTIVE SURGERY

The biomechanical impact on corneal curvature is founded on immediate elastic effects and on slightly longer-term hydration effects. The cornea, as a living tissue, responds to surgical intervention by wound healing.[66] An important part of the interindividual variability in the effects of radial keratotomy and excimer laser ablation on individuals can probably be attributed to differences in wound healing.[67,68] Wound healing may be interpreted in at least two ways:

1. Healing directly toward re-establishment of the original corneal radius of curvature
2. Healing toward re-establishment of the normal integrity of the cornea

After excimer laser ablation for myopia, a wound-healing response is seen at the site of the ablation. The epithelium thickens and newly formed connective tissue elements are produced.[69] Some of the original flattening effect of the procedure may therefore disappear. It has been speculated that the mechanical attachment between the superficial corneal epithelial cells contributes to the observed epithelial thickening.[70] The other type of wound healing attempts to recover the integrity of the cornea after stromal incisions. Wound healing in the incised cornea may affect biomechanics in one of two ways:

1. The strength of the tissue may be increased.
2. The elastic stiffness of the cornea may be altered.

Corneal Strength

A reduction in corneal strength will make the eye more vulnerable to blunt trauma. The weakest point of the intact, normal eye is located at the equator of the sclera, and the bursting pressure of the intact eye globe is around 5 kg/cm^2, which corresponds to an intraocular pressure of 3700 mm Hg.[26] The maximum tensile strength of corneal tissue strips is around 12.7 MPa, which corresponds to the wall tension developed by an intraocular pressure of 12,000 mm Hg.[17] Our knowledge about human corneal strength after refractive surgery is limited. Some estimates may be made if we assume that the tensile strength of the uncut stromal fibrils is similar to that of the normal cornea, and that

the stress on the uncut fibrils will increase in proportion to the depth of the cut. Such calculations reveal that, at a cutting depth of more than 70% of the corneal thickness, the strength of the incised cornea will be less than that of the equatorial sclera. Procedures in which a fraction less than 70% of the corneal lamellae is cut should not decrease the strength of the eye globe. In radial or circumferential keratotomy deeper incisions are made, and the bursting pressure of the globe will be lower than 3700 mm Hg. These simple calculations are in good agreement with experimental results of corneal integrity.[71] Reinforcement of the strength of corneal incisions occurs with time. The strength of human corneal cataract incisions has been shown to rise slowly over the first month and return to normal after 4 years.[72]

Elastic Stiffness

Wound healing after RK has recently been studied in detail using confocal microscopy.[73–75] In these animal experiments, wound-healing processes in the corneal incisions were found to correlate with wound gape contraction and changes in corneal refractive power. Although a healing response has been observed in human corneal radial incisions, it is not evident either that the tissue involved in the healing processes bears any of the intraocular pressure load or that the wounds eventually contract and modify the refractive power of the human cornea.[73,76] Clinical follow-up studies suggest a biphasic biologic response, with a short-term (months) regression of the effect and a long-term (years) progression of the effect of RK.[61]

TONOMETRY

All types of clinical tonometry involve corneal bending. Factors that alter the bending rigidity of the cornea will therefore affect the readings of tonometry instruments. In normal subjects there is a positive correlation between corneal thickness and intraocular pressure, probably because a thick cornea is more difficult to bend.[77] The change in corneal radius of curvature may also affect tonometry readings. A larger necessary bending force and a larger displaced intraocular volume are required to achieve an equal amount of corneal flattening in an eye with a steep cornea, compared with an eye that has a flat cornea. Both factors tend to falsely increase the intraocular pressure.[78]

Little is known about the errors in tonometry after refractive corneal surgery. Extrapolation from observations in normal corneas suggests that corneal flattening will lead to excessively low pressure measurements in myopic eyes treated with refractive surgery. Corneal thinning, as seen in eyes following excimer laser treatment, also leads to deceptively low pressure measurements. The clinical importance of the small errors possible in tonometry may become clearer when the growing population of corneal refractive individuals ages and develops open-angle glaucoma. The diagnostic criteria for open-angle glaucoma still includes increased intraocular pressure. If the pressure is falsely measured as too low in these patients, the diagnosis may be missed or delayed.

PERSPECTIVES: FINITE ELEMENT MODELING OF THE CORNEA

The present considerations of biomechanics and refractive surgery have all been qualitative. Rational, structural, biomechanically based quantitative models for refractive surgery are necessary to improve the individual clinical outcome, to improve previously known techniques, and to make preliminary evaluations of new techniques. Several quantitative mathematical models for predicting the effect of incisional refractive techniques have been developed. These models include analytical "closed solution" models and finite element models. Although analytical "closed solution" models are more intuitive than finite element models, the latter can handle complex geometries and material properties that are closer to the "real world."[79] A number of analytic and finite element models have been developed for analyzing mechanical deformation in tonometry and refractive surgery.[12,75,80–98] Some of the more recent models are based on the actual corneal microstructure.[12,95,96] However, the models developed for the measurement of corneal deformation can, at their best, only describe elastic changes in the tissue. It should be taken into consideration that stress-induced redistribution of water may bring about viscoelastic changes in the tissue, possibly necessitating additional mathematical procedures to take flow-induced deformation into account.[99,100] Postoperative wound healing may also affect the final structure of the tissue, although it is unclear whether the wound eventually participates in the load bearing of the unsutured, surgically altered corneal stroma at physiologic pressures. Further developments in mathematical modeling are needed; even more critical are experiments to verify the mod-

els and to determine the significance of biomechanics in corneal refractive surgery.

It is necessary to know the shape, thickness, and constitutive properties of the individual cornea in order to make use of experimentally validated mathematical corneal models in individual computer-aided surgery. Approaches to measuring the mechanical properties of individual human corneas in vivo include pressure loading of the eye globe, combined with measurement of the induced deformation.[59b,101] Alternatively, corneal indentation or applanation may be used to deform the tissue.[102] If the deforming load is known or measured, and the induced deformation is measured, it may be possible, by so-called reverse finite element modeling, to infer some mechanical properties of the individual cornea.[103]

CONCLUSION

Corneal refractive surgery is a growing field in anterior segment surgery. In contrast to cataract surgery, the surgeon forms the new biologic lens whose quality is the primary determinant for the success of the operation. The rapid development in the number of techniques, combined with the increasing demand for unaided vision, may help explain why all corneal refractive techniques are empirically based (more or less) and involve various elements to compensate for the variation of biologic responses of the wounded living cornea. It is our hope that increased insight into corneal biomechanics can facilitate the movement of corneal refractive surgery from the genre of medical art to that of medical science.

REFERENCES

1. Fung YC. *Biomechanics. Mechanical Properties of Living Tissues.* New York: Springer-Verlag; 1981.
2. Bisplinghoff RL, Marr JW, Pian THH. *Statics of Deformable Solids.* New York: Dover Publications Inc; 1965.
3. Viidik AA. Functional properties of collagenous tissues. In: Hall DA, Jackson DS, eds. *International Review of Connective Tissue Research.* London: Academic Press; 1973;6: 127–211.
4. Maurice DM. The structure and transparency of the cornea. *J Physiol Lond.* 1957;136:263–286.
5. Krenchel H. *Fibre Reinforcement. Theoretical and Practical Investigations of the Elasticity and Strength of Fibre-Reinforced Materials.* Copenhagen: Akademisk Forlag; 1964.

6. Parry DAD, Craig AS. Collagen fibrils during development and maturation and their contribution to the mechanical attributes of connective tissue. In: Nimni ME, ed. *Collagen: Biochemistry and Biomechanics.* Boca Raton, FL: CRC Press; 1988;2:1–24.

7. Kato YP, Christiansen DL, Hahn RA, et al. Mechanical properties of collagen fibres: a comparison of reconstituted and rat tail tendon fibres. *Biomaterials.* 1989; 10:38–42.

8. Olsen T, Sperling S. The swelling pressure of the human corneal stroma as determined by a new method. *Exp Eye Res.* 1987;44:481–490.

9. Myers ER, Zhu W, Mow VC. Viscoelastic properties of articular cartilage and meniscus. In: Nimni ME, ed. *Collagen: Biochemistry and Biomechanics.* Boca Raton, FL: CRC Press; 1988;2:268–288.

10. Hedbys BO, Dohlman CH. A new method for determination of the swelling pressure of the corneal stroma in vitro. *Exp Eye Res.* 1963;2:122–129.

11. Hukins DWL. Collagen orientation. In: Hukins DWL, ed. *Connective Tissue Matrix: Topics in Molecular and Structural Biology.* London: Macmillan; 1984;5:211–339.

12. Pinsky PM, Datye DV. Numerical modelling of radial, astigmatic, and hexagonal keratotomy. *Refract Corneal Surg.* 1992;8:164–172.

13. Jue B, Maurice DM. The mechanical properties of the rabbit and human cornea. *J Biomech.* 1986;19:847–853.

14. Fatt I, Weissman BA. *Physiology of the Eye. An Introduction to the Vegetative Functions.* 2nd ed. Stoneham, MA: Butterworth-Heinemann; 1992;97–149.

15. Smolek MK, McCarey BE. Interlamellar adhesive strength in human eyebank corneas. *Invest Ophthalmol Vis Sci.* 1990;31:1087–1095.

16. Woo SL-Y, Kobayashi AS, Schlegel WA, Lawrence C. Nonlinear material properties of intact cornea and sclera. *Exp Eye Res.* 1972;14:29–39.

17. Andreassen TT, Hjorth Simonsen A, Oxlund H. Biomechanical properties of keratoconus and normal corneas. *Exp Eye Res.* 1980;31:435–441.

18. Nash IS, Greene PR, Foster CS. Comparison of mechanical properties of keratoconus and normal corneas. *Exp Eye Res.* 1982;35:413–424.

19. Hoeltzel DA, Altman P, Buzard K, Choe K. Strip extensiometry for comparison of the mechanical response of bovine, rabbit, and human corneas. *J Biomech Eng.* 1992; 114:202–215.

20. Hjortdal Jù. Extensibility of the normo-hydrated human cornea. *Acta Ophthalmol (Copenh).* 1995;73:12–15.

21. Baer E, Cassidy JJ, Hiltner A. Hierarchical structure of collagen and its relationship to the physical properties of tendon. In: Nimni ME, ed. *Collagen: Biochemistry and Biomechanics.* Boca Raton, FL: CRC Press; 1988;2:178–199.

22. Fraser RDB, MacRae TP, Miller A, Suzuki E. Molecular conformation and packing in collagen fibrils. *J Mol Biol.* 1983;167:497–521.

23. Gallagher B, Maurice DM. Striations of light scattering in the corneal stroma. *J Ultrastruc Res.* 1977;61:100–114.

24. Bron AJ. Superficial fibrillary lines. A feature of the normal cornea. *Br J Ophthalmol.* 1975;59:133–135.

25. Hjortdal Jù. Regional elastic performance of the human cornea. *J Biomech* 1996. In press.

26. Maurice DM. Mechanics of the cornea. In: Cavanagh HD, ed. *The Cornea: Transactions of the World Congress on the Cornea.* New York: Raven Press; 1988;3: chap 33.

27. Wollensak J, Ihme A, Seiler T. Neue Befunde bei Keratoconus. *Fortschr Ophthalmol.* 1987;84:28–32.

28. Eliasson J, Maurice DM. Stress distribution across the in vivo human cornea. *Invest Ophthalmol Vis Sci.* 1981; 20(suppl):156.

29. Poinoosawmy D, Roth JA. Variations in visual acuity, refraction, and corneal curvature with changes in applanation tension. *Br J Ophthalmol.* 1974;58:523–528.

30. Fatt I. Dynamics of water transport in the corneal stroma. *Exp Eye Res.* 1968;7:402–412.

33. Hjortdal JØ, Jensen PK. In vitro measurement of corneal strain, thickness, and curvature using digital image processing. *Acta Ophthalmol (Copenh).* 1995;73:5–11.

34. Kiely PM, Carney LG, Smith G. Diurnal variations of corneal topography and thickness. *Am J Optom Physiol Opt.* 1982;59:976–982.

35. Maguire LJ, Lowry JC. Identifying progression of subclinical keratoconus by serial topography analysis. *Am J Ophthalmol.* 1991;112:41–45.

36. Fullwood NJ, Tuft SJ, Malik NS, et al. Synchrotron x-ray diffraction studies of keratoconus corneal stroma. *Invest Ophthalmol Vis Sci.* 1992;33:1734–1741.

37. Ytteborg J, Dohlman CH. Corneal edema and intraocular pressure. II. Clinical results. *Arch Ophthalmol.* 1965;74: 477–484.

38. Olson RJ, Kaufman HE. Intraocular pressure and corneal thickness after penetrating keratoplasty. *Am J Ophthalmol.* 1978;86:97–100.

39. Hedbys BO, Mishima S, Maurice DM. The imbibition pressure of the corneal stroma. *Exp Eye Res.* 1963;2: 99–111.

40. Wiig H. Cornea fluid dynamics. I: measurement of hydrostatic and colloid osmotic pressure in rabbits. *Exp Eye Res.* 1989;49:1015–1030.

41. Maurice DM. The cornea and sclera. In: Davson H, ed. *The Eye.* New York: Academic Press; 1984;1B: 303–351.

42. McPhee TJ, Bourne WM, Brubaker RF. Location of the stress-bearing layers of the cornea. *Invest Ophthalmol Vis Sci.* 1985;26:869–872.

43. McCarey BE, Waring GO, Street DA. Refractive keratoplasty in monkeys using intracorneal lenses of various refractive indexes. *Arch Ophthalmol.* 1987;105: 123–126.

44. Trokel SL, Srinivasan R, Braren B. Excimer laser surgery of the cornea. *Am J Ophthalmol.* 1983;96:710–715.

45. Werblin TP. Epikeratophakia: techniques, complications, and clinical results. *Int Ophthalmol Clin.* 1983;23: 45–58.

46. Barraquer JI. Modification of refraction by means of intracorneal inclusions. *Int Ophthalmol Clin.* 1966;6: 53–78.

47. Barraquer JI. Keratomileusis for myopia and aphakia. *Ophthalmology.* 1981;88:701–708.

48. Bille JF, Klancnik EGK, Niemz MH. Principles of operation and first clinical results using the picosecond IR laser. In: Parel J-M, ed. *Ophthalmic Technologies II. Proc SPIE.* 1992;1644:88–95.

49. Fyodorov SN, Durnev VV. Operation of dosaged dissection of corneal circular ligament in cases of myopia of mild degree. *Ann Ophthalmol.* 1979;11:1885–1890.

50. Seiler T, Matallana M, Bende T. Laser thermokeratoplasty by means of a pulsed holmium: YAG laser for hyperopic correction. *Refract Corneal Surg.* 1990;6:335–339.

51. Burris TE, Baker PC, Ayer CT, et al. Flattening of central corneal curvature with intrastromal corneal rings of increasing thickness: an eye-bank eye study. *J Cataract Refract Surg.* 1993;19(suppl):182–187.

52. Simon G, Parel JM, Lee W, Kervick GN. Gel injection adjustable keratoplasty. *Graefes Arch Clin Exp Ophthalmol.* 1991;229:418–424.

53. Jester JV, Venet T, Lee J, Schanzlin DJ, Smith RE. A statistical analysis of radial keratotomy in human cadaver eyes. *Am J Ophthalmol.* 1981;92:172–177.

54. Salz J, Lee JS, Jester JV, et al. Radial keratotomy in fresh human cadaver eyes. *Ophthalmology.* 1981;88:742–746.

55. Santos VR, Waring GO, Lynn MJ, et al. Morning-to-evening change in refraction, corneal curvature, and visual acuity 2 to 4 years after radial keratotomy in the PERK Study. *Ophthalmology.* 1988;95:1487–1493.

56. Schanzlin DJ, Santos VR, Waring GO, et al. Diurnal change in refraction, corneal curvature, visual acuity, and intraocular pressure after radial keratotomy in the PERK Study. *Ophthalmology.* 1986;93:167–175.

57. Maloney RK. Effect of corneal hydration and intraocular pressure on keratometric power after experimental radial keratotomy. *Ophthalmology.* 1990;97:927–933.

58. Simon G, Ren Q. Biomechanical behavior of the cornea and its response to radial keratotomy. *Refract Corneal Surg.* 1994;10:343–356.

58b. MacRae S, Rich L, Phillips D, Bedrossian R. Diurnal variation in vision after radial keratotomy. *Am J Ophthalmol.* 1989;107:262–267.

59. Feldman ST, Frucht-Perry J, Weinreb RN, et al. The effect of increased intraocular pressure on visual acuity and corneal curvature after radial keratotomy. *Am J Ophthalmol.* 1989;108:126–129.

59b. Hjortdal JØ, Böhm A, Kohlhaas M, Olsen H, Lerche R, Ehlers N, Draeger J. Mechanical stability of the cornea after radial keratotomy and photorefractive keratectomy. *Journal of Refractive Surgery* 1996;12:459–466.

60. Hjortdal JØ, Ehlers N. Acute tissue deformation patterns of the human cornea after radial keratotomy. *Journal of Refractive Surgery* 1996;12:391–400.

60b. Deitz MR, Sanders DR, Raanan MG. Progressive hyperopia in radial keratotomy. Long-term follow-up of diamond-knife and metal-blade series. *Ophthalmology.* 1986;93:1284–1289.

61. Waring GO, Lynn MJ, Nizam A, et al. Results of the Prospective Evaluation of Radial Keratotomy (PERK) Study five years after surgery. The Perk Study Group. *Ophthalmology.* 1991;98:1164–1176.

62. Hjortdal JØ, Ehlers N. Epikeratophakia for high myopia. *Acta Ophthalmol (Copenh).* 1991;69:754–760.

63. Seiler T, Matallana M, Sendler S, Bende T. Does Bowman's layer determine the biomechanical properties of the cornea? *J Refract Corneal Surg.* 1992;8:139–142.

64. Hjortdal JØ, Ehlers N. Effect of excimer laser keratectomy on the mechanical performance of the human cornea. *Acta Ophthalmol (Copenh).* 1995;73:18–24.

65. Moreira H, Campos M, Sawusch MR, McDonnell JM, Sand B, McDonnell PJ. Holmium laser thermokeratoplasty. *Ophthalmology.* 1993;100:752–761.

66. Maurice, DM. The biology of wound healing in the cornea. *Cornea.* 1987;6:162–168.

67. American Academy of Ophthalmology. Radial keratotomy for myopia. *Ophthalmology.* 1993;100:1103–1115.

68. Ehlers N, Hjortdal JØ. Excimer laser refractive keratectomy for high myopia. *Acta Ophthalmol (Copenh).* 1992;70: 578–586.

69. Tuft SJ, Zabel RW, Marshall J. Corneal repair following keratectomy. A comparison between conventional surgery and laser photoablation. *Invest Ophthalmol Vis Sci.* 1989;30:1769–1777.

70. Dierick HG, Missotten L. Is the corneal contour influenced by a tension in the superficial epithelial cells? A new hypothesis. *Refract Corneal Surg.* 1992;8:54–59.

71. Luttrull JK, Jester JV, Smith RE. The effect of radial keratotomy on ocular integrity in an animal model. *Arch Ophthalmol.* 1982;100:319–320.

72. Simonsen AH, Andreassen TT, Bendix K. The healing strength of corneal wounds in the human eye. *Exp Eye Res.* 1982;35:287–292.

73. Jester JV, Petroll WM, Feng W, et al. Radial keratotomy. 1. The wound healing process and measurement of incisional gape in two animal models using in vivo confocal microscopy. *Invest Ophthalmol Vis Sci.* 1992;33: 3255–3270.

74. Garana RM, Petroll WM, Chen WT, et al. Radial keratotomy. II. Role of the myofibroblast in corneal wound contraction. *Invest Ophthalmol Vis Sci.* 1992;33: 3271–3282.

75. Petroll WM, New K, Sachdev M, Cavanagh HD, Jester JV. Radial keratotomy. III. Relationship between wound gape and corneal curvature in primate eyes. *Invest Ophthalmol Vis Sci.* 1992;33:3283–3291.

76. Waring GO, Steinberg EB, Wilson LA. Slit-lamp microscopic appearance of corneal wound healing after radial keratotomy. *Am J Ophthalmol.* 1985;100:218–224.

77. Ehlers N, Bramsen T, Sperling S. Applanation tonometry and central corneal thickness. *Acta Ophthalmol (Copenh).* 1975;53:34–43.

78. Whitacre MM, Stein R. Sources of error with use of Goldmann-type tonometers. *Surv Ophthalmol.* 1993; 38:1–30.

79. Buzard KA. Introduction to biomechanics of the cornea. *Refract Corneal Surg.* 1992;8:127 138.

80. Kobayashi AS, Woo S L-Y, Lawrence C, Schlegel WA. Analysis of the corneo-scleral shell by the method of direct stiffness. *J Biomech.* 1971;4:323–330.

81. Schachar RA, Black TD, Huang T. Understanding radial keratotomy. Denison, TX: LAL Publishing; 1981.

82. Sjöntoft, E. In vivo determination of Young's modulus for the human cornea. *Bull Math Biol.* 1987;49:217–232.

83. Arciniegas A, Amaya L. Combined semi-radial and arcuate keratotomy for correction of ametropia: a theoretical bioengineering approach. *J Refract Surg.* 1988;4: 51–59.

84. Vito RP, Shin TJ, McCarey BE. A mechanical model of the cornea: the effects of physiological and surgical factors on radial keratotomy surgery. *Refract Corneal Surg.* 1989; 5:82–88.

85. Rand RH, Lubkin SR, Howland HC. Analytical model of corneal surgery. *J Biomech Eng.* 1991;113:239–241.

86. Hanna KD, Jouve F, Bercovier MH, Waring GO. Computer simulation of lamellar keratectomy and laser myopic keratomileusis. *J Refract Surg.* 1988;4:222–231.

87. Hanna KD, Jouve FE, Waring GO, Ciarlet PG. Computer simulation of arcuate and radial incisions involving the corneoscleral limbus. *Eye.* 1989;3:227–239.

88. Hanna KD, Jouve FE, Waring GO. Preliminary computer simulation of the effects of radial keratotomy. *Arch Ophthalmol.* 1989;107:911–918.

89. Hanna KD, Jouve FE, Waring GO, Ciarlet PG. Computer simulation of arcuate keratotomy for astigmatism. *Refract Corneal Surg.* 1992;8:152–163.

90. Huang T, Bisarnsin T, Schachar RA, Black TD. Corneal curvature change due to structural alternation by radial keratotomy. *J Biomech Eng.* 1988;110:249–253.

91. Bryant MR, Velinsky SA. Design of keratorefractive surgical procedures: radial keratotomy. In: Ravani B, ed. *Advances in Design Automation.* New York: American Society of Mechanical Engineers; 1989;19:383–391.

92. Velinsky SA, Bryant MR. On the computer-aided and optimal design of keratorefractive surgery. *Refract Corneal Surg.* 1992;8:173–182.

93. Sawusch MR, Wan WL, McDonnell PJ. Tissue addition theory of radial keratotomy: a geometric model. *J Cataract Refract Surg.* 17:448–453.

94. Sawusch MR, McDonnell PJ. Computer modeling of wound gape following radial keratotomy. *Refract Corneal Surg.* 1991;8:143–145.

95. Pinsky PM, Datye DV. A microstructurally based finite-element model of the incised human cornea. *J Biomech.* 1991;24:907–922.

96. Pinsky PM, Datye DV. A microstructurally mechanical model of the human cornea with application to keratotomy. *Invest Ophthalmol Vis Sci.* 1994;35(suppl):1296.

97. Howland HC, Rand RH, Lubkin SR. A thin-shell model of the cornea and its application to corneal surgery. *Refract Corneal Surg.* 1992;8:183–186.

98. Jouve F. Modélisation de l'oeil en élasticité non linéaire. In: *Recherches en Mathématiques Appliquées.* Paris: Masson; 1993.

99. Barry SI, Aldis GK. Comparison of models for flow induced deformation of soft biological tissue. *J Biomech.* 1990;23:647–654.

100. Hanna KD, Jouve FE, Kaiss A, Le Tallec P. Viscoelastic model for the human cornea. In: Durand M, El Dabaghi F, eds. *High Performance Computing.* Netherlands: Elsevier Science Publishers BV; 1991;2:632–640.

101. Calkins JL, Hochheimer BF, Stark WJ. Corneal wound healing: holographic stress-test analysis. *Invest Ophthalmol Vis Sci.* 1981;21:322–334.

102. Chang SS, Hjortdal JØ, Maurice DM, Pinsky PM. Corneal deformation by indentation and applanation. *Invest Ophthalmol Vis Sci.* 1993;34(suppl):1241.

103. Chang SS, Maurice DM, Pinsky PM, Datye DV. Determination of mechanical properties of cornea in vivo by indentation. *Invest Ophthalmol Vis Sci.* 1994;35(suppl): 1357.

CHAPTER 16

Radial Keratotomy Instrumentation

Kerry K. Assil

In selecting appropriate instrumentation for incisional keratotomy, the surgeon should pay particular attention to reproducibility, durability, and affordability. Proper instrument selection may facilitate surgical outcome reproducibility and cost-effective care delivery. Furthermore, unnecessary or repeat expenditures may adversely influence delivery of care.

Below, we describe some useful instrumentation and assistive technology for a keratorefractive practice. A survey of the vast variety of available instrumentation is beyond the scope of this text. We will therefore focus instead upon the features that are essential to any system component. We hope that our descriptions will be sufficiently broad to encompass the majority of available systems and to allow for the adaptation of alternative systems.

OPERATING-ROOM EQUIPMENT

Operating-room equipment should be selected according to the room's size limitations. A fully reclining, height-adjustable chair in place of a surgical bed may be more economical of space, possibly permitting space for both slit lamp biomicroscopy and incisional keratotomy. In the event that a reclining chair is selected, it should have prominent side arms (in place of side rails) to assure patient safety. The chair or bed should also accommodate a wrist rest to facilitate surgeon hand position.

The surgeon's chair should be height adjustable and should have a foot bar or pedal control. The chair should also have a back rest and elbow rests, particularly if the surgeon wishes to forgo the wrist rest.

A large array of operating microscopes is now available, specifically designed for delivery of keratorefractive procedures in the office. Microscope selection should be based on the optics quality, including the depth of field. A relatively large depth of field is useful in maintaining focus, as the globe is indented during the procedure. Variable magnification and light source intensity are other valuable features. Secondary procedures (enhancements) often require higher magnification and variable lighting, as these procedures are frequently performed with the pupil dilated for better visualization of previous incisions. Adjustable ocular tilt angle and interpupillary distance are useful as well. Practical foot pedal features include auto focus and x/y control, although these may be compensated for by a lightweight microscope coupled with autoclavable handles. The microscope field illumination light source should consist of either a nearly coaxial focal beam or a concentric illumination ring in order to avoid the bothersome shadows that can accompany corneal surface markings when para-axial light sources are used.

Fixation light systems have evolved to assist with patient cooperation during the procedure, enabling either coaxial visual axis determination (Fig 16–1) and/or automated eccentric gaze globe fixation during the procedure (Fig 16–2).

Improved microscope designs may provide optimal features for in-office delivery of refractive procedures.[1] These proposed microscope designs include a para-axial light source in the form of a ring illumination system of relatively large diameter (concentric to the microscope head), which would enable diffuse surface illumination at high intensity. Thus, the subject would not experience light-induced discomfort because the para-axial light reflex is concentric with, and peripheral to, the entrance pupil. The concentric nature of the light source would eliminate shadows from either corneal markings or the surgeons' hands in the face of para-axial illumination. By placing an infrared filter within the fiber-optic light pathway, the ocular surface would not be desiccated by heat energy, thus enabling the diamond-knife footplates to glide smoothly along the moist epithelial surface in the face of bright surface illumination. Within this system a separate (flashing) fixation light source (red or green) would be coaxial with one of the two ocular objectives within the microscope. Sighting through the complementary eyepiece, the surgeon's view would be coaxial with the patient's line of sight and corneal optical center, which would serve as the closest measurable landmark to the true visual axis.[2] (See Chapter 9 for more details regarding centration of RK and other procedures.)

Coaxial light fixation devices, which are either mounted onto surgical microscopes or aligned within the microscope optical system, make the precise localization of the corneal optical center readily possible (Fig 16–1). Para-axial ocular guidance systems for automated eccentric gaze ocular fixation are now available (Fig 16–2). These enable patients to fixate upon a flashing target light that guides the eye into an eccentric field of gaze opposite to the intended incision site.[3] This eye position maximizes surgical site exposure, facilitating perpendicular orientation to the corneal surface, while minimizing patient discomfort from the bright operating-light source.

A Mayo stand should be large enough to display the instrumentation properly. An autoclave, available within the operating room and capable of rapid instrument sterilization, reduces interoperative time and facilitates quality assurance (with instruments packaged either singly or within an instrument tray). In autoclaving the instrumentation, it is generally important that distilled and deionized water be used to avoid buildup of crystalline precipitates upon the diamond-knife blade and footplates. Modern autoclaves sterilize instruments in less than 10 minutes. Ultrasonic cleansers with plastic fingerlike projections along the chamber base are now available for cleaning the diamond blades

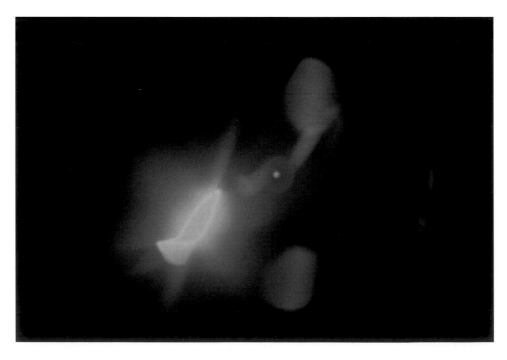

Figure 16–1. Photograph of accessory fixation light source for near-coaxial fixation (red light).

and the corneal markers immediately after they have been rinsed following the procedure. The chamber may be filled with either hydrogen peroxide or distilled deionized water. Cidex should be avoided, as its corrosive action may dislodge the diamond from its base.

While studies of the environment required to minimize sufficiently the risk for airborne contamination during refractive keratotomy are lacking, several simple precautionary measures appear prudent. If the procedures are performed other than in a standard operating-room setting, some consideration may be given to air purification. Simple precautions include the wearing of masks by persons entering the room, the elimination of carpeting or substandard ceiling tiles, and placement of hoods over air vents to redirect the flow of air away from the patient. An air purification system that continuously filters particulate matter from the environment may be considered.

SURGICAL SUPPLIES AND MEDICATIONS

Surgical supplies and medications are listed in typical sequence of use:

1. Surgical mask (antifog)—gown and head cover are often not utilized.
2. Mayo stand cover—sterile field for display of surgical instruments.
3. Anxiolytics—administered prior to the procedure.
4. Analgesics—may include topical nonsteroidal anti-inflammatory medication.
5. Blanket or cover sheet—for patient comfort.
6. Folded towel—placed beneath patient's shoulders to facilitate the chin-up position.
7. Eye patch—occludes patient's nonsurgical eye.
8. Betadine skin prep—taking care to avoid the ocular surface.
9. Sterile open eye surgical drape.
10. Topical antibiotics—broad spectrum.
11. Topical anesthetics—avoiding instillation onto corneal epithelium (to minimize toxicity).
12. Hand-disinfecting solution.
13. Sterile surgical gloves (powderless).
14. Weck cell sponges.
15. 10-0 nylon suture—for intraoperative crossed incisions or perforation.
16. Topical analgesics, steroids, and broad spectrum antibiotics—initiated just prior to the procedure, may be continued for several days thereafter.

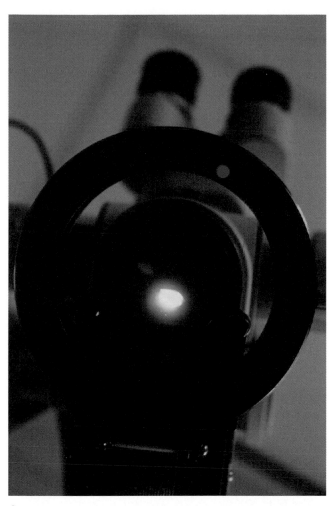

A

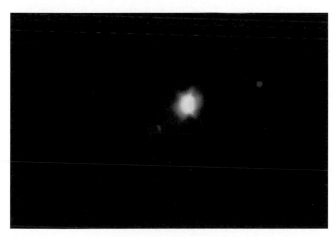

B

Figure 16–2. Accessory eccentric gaze light fixation ring mounted onto operating microscope **(A)** and exaggerated simulation of resultant corneal reflexes, with patient viewing bright illumination source from the operating microscope **(B)**.

EAST GLAMORGAN GENERAL HOSPITAL
CHURCH VILLAGE, near PONTYPRIDD

PRIMARY PROCEDURE INSTRUMENTATION

In selecting surgical instrumentation, the surgeon should concentrate on quality because proper machining will extend the life of the instrument and may improve reproducibility. To contain costs while ensuring instrument quality, the surgeon may wish to avoid such cosmetic packaging features as gold plating, which, because it has a different coefficient of expansion than the underlying steel or titanium, tends to flake off with repeat autoclaving. In general, titanium instruments may be preferable to steel because, in addition to being lighter in weight, they are potentially more durable. When titanium is used, the cross hairs and radial wing extensions may be readily machined from the same sheet of metal as the remainder of the instrument so that the parts are not soldered and the potential for damage caused by repeat autoclaving is minimized. Radial keratotomy instruments are listed in their most common order of use:

Eyelid Speculum

A wire eyelid speculum providing adequate globe exposure is usually sufficient. It is helpful for determining the center of the entrance pupil.

Visual Axis Marker

A blunt-tipped Sinskey hook or jeweler's forceps, for indenting the corneal epithelium, serves as a surgical centration landmark (Fig 16–3).

Central Clear Zone Markers

These are generally provided in two forms, either with a dull contact margin, requiring ink for corneal marking (Fig 16–4), or with a sharper contact margin, obviating the need for surgical dyes. The more refined markers taper to a 4-μm-wide contact margin, providing a precise and prominent surgical landmark. The optical zone marker should be equipped with cross hairs in order to ensure precise concentric placement to the visual axis marking (Fig 16–5). Diameters ranging from 3 to 5 mm in 0.25-mm increments are generally sufficient for these instruments.

Outer Zone Markers

At the time of writing, the ideal outer zone diameter remains to be determined. While recent data suggest that an outer zone diameter of 10 mm may provide a greater range of corneal flattening than one of 8 mm,[4] it may well be that the optimal outer zone size lies somewhere between the 8- and 10-mm diameter range. Furthermore, there are no clinical data presently available to distinguish between the relative value of outer zone marking centered on the limbus versus the central clear zone. Such studies are currently under way, and it is hoped that they will delineate the optimal outer zone diameter and centration site.

Radial Wing Markers

Radial keratotomy (RK) procedures providing greater than eight radial incisions in a single setting are now generally discouraged. Radial wing markers may be obtained for delineating three, four, six, and eight radial

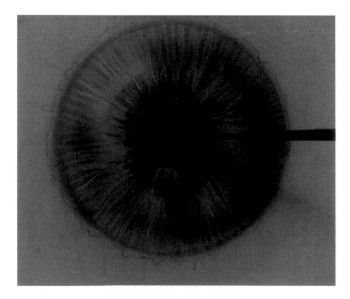

Figure 16–3. Artist's rendition of surgical centration point marking onto the corneal epithelium using a Sinskey hook.

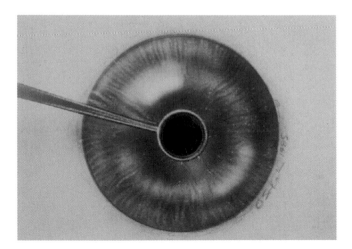

Figure 16–4. Artist's rendition of central clear zone marker without cross hairs.

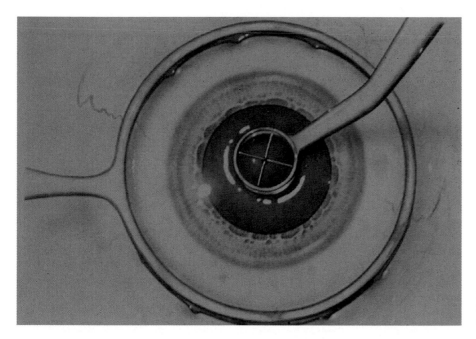

Figure 16–5. Artist's rendition of central clear zone marker with cross hairs. Globe is fixated using a Thornton fixation ring.

incision sites. The markers should be judged for durability, low profile (do not obscure corneal visualization), and sharp contact margins for prominent epithelial indentation. Titanium enables the marker head to be machined from a single sheet of metal, thereby avoiding any durability concerns associated with soldering (Fig 16–6).

Forceps

For globe fixation, proper diamond orientation maintained throughout the incision improves predictability and safety. Globe fixation may also enable more predictable incision depth placement. Typical fixation techniques include the use of 0.3 forceps grasping the conjunctival insertion at the limbus directly across from the radial incision site (Fig 16–7), Kelman 2-point fixation forceps, and Thornton 360° ring forceps (Fig 16–5), each of which also retard globe torsional rotation. Recently, ring fixation forceps with footplate guides for more linear incision placement have been reintroduced.[5]

Radial Keratotomy Knives

The first-generation knives used for the performance of anterior surface RK consisted of steel blades, which were broken and fashioned onto scalpel handles or forceps (Fig 16–8). The introduction of diamond technology for incisional keratotomy coincided with the initiation of the PERK study in the United States (Fig 16–9).[6,7] Traditionally, diamond designs with a cutting edge along the angled margin for performing centrifugally directed incisions (Fig 16–10) were more common than those with a cutting edge along the vertical margin (Fig 16–11) for centripetally directed incisions.[8] Throughout the 1980s, these diamond designs were often modified: changes were made of the angle subtended by the diamond's tip and to the diamond thickness; and a faceted margin was added along the distal portion making it trifaceted.

The combined-technique diamonds were designed in 1991 and became generally available in 1992 (Fig 16–12).[9] These diamonds enable the surgeon to begin the incision at the central clear zone (Fig 16–13), to extend out toward the limbus, and then to reverse direction back toward the central zone (Fig 16–14) without the risk of invading the central clear zone. The angled margin on the front surface, which is the centrifugal cutting component, is sharpened along its entire length. The vertical margin is ground sharp to a cutting edge for a distance of only 250 μm from the blade tip (Fig 16–12).

The blunt superficial portion of the vertical margin prevents undesirable invasion of the central clear zone when the blade tip is initially inserted into the cornea at the clear zone margin. During the next phase, as a centrifugal incision is made toward the limbus (downhill), the diamond produces a linear radial incision groove of variable depth ranging from 55% to 80% of the corneal thickness. Upon arriving at 1 mm of the limbus, the cut-

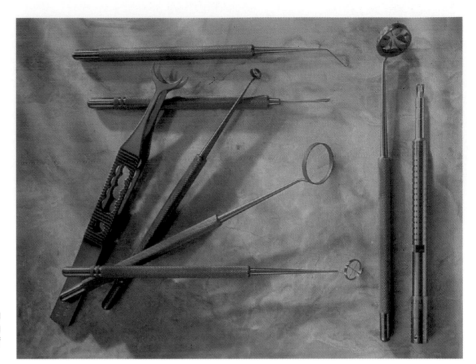

Figure 16–6. Titanium instruments, including central clear zone markers and radial wing markers, machined from a single sheet of metal.

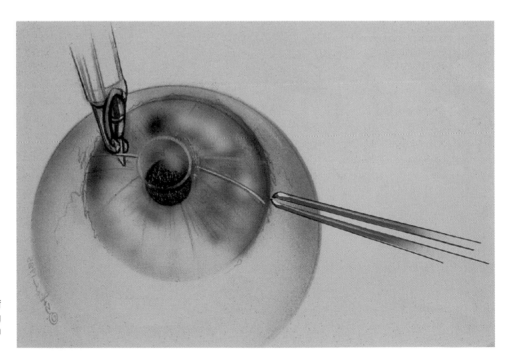

Figure 16–7. Artist's rendition of globe fixation, with forceps grasping the conjunctival insertion across from incision site.

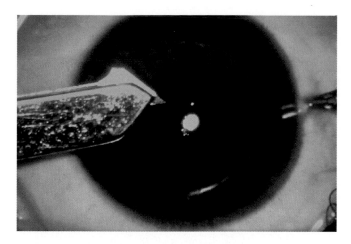

Figure 16–8. Example of early steel blade used for RK.

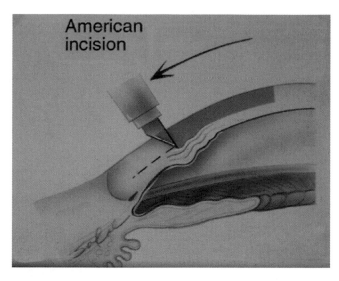

Figure 16–10. Artist's rendition of centrifugal incision.

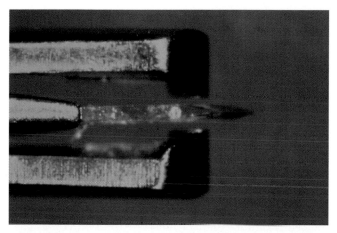

A

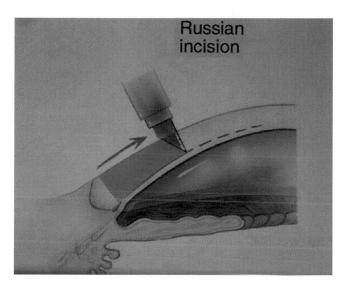

Figure 16–11. Artist's rendition of centripetal incision.

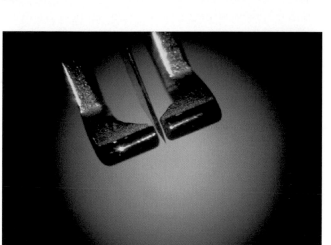

B

Figure 16–9. A. Photograph of early RK diamond, approximating 500 μm in thickness. **B.** Modern thin diamond measuring approximately 100 μm in thickness.

ting motion is reversed centripetally toward the central clear zone within the same groove created by the preceding centrifugal incision. Because the vertical margin of the diamond is sharp only along its distal portion (250 μm), it is difficult for the blade to escape from within the previously incised groove. This centripetally directed motion increases the incision depth uniformly to approximately 80% to 90% of corneal thickness. Once the diamond blade returns to the central clear zone margin, it is unable to advance further. Thus, the ideal features of the centrifugal radial incision method, a linear groove with minimal risk of invading the central clear zone, are combined with the ideal features of the centripetal radial incision method to create a uni-

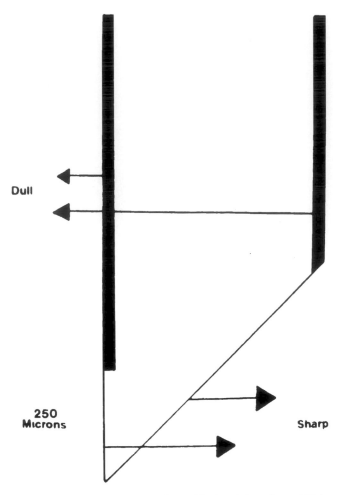

Figure 16–12. Schematic diagram of a combined-technique diamond blade.

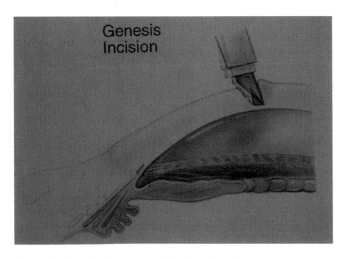

Figure 16–13. Initiation of a combined incision with corneal penetration and undermining of central clear zone margin.

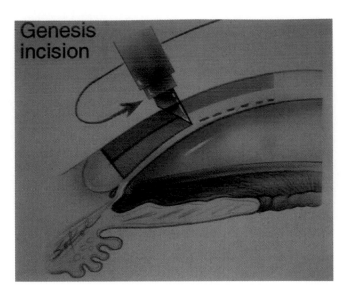

Figure 16–14. Artist's rendition of combined-style incision in progress. Having completed the centrifugal complement of the incision, the surgeon is now retracing centripetally within the original incision groove.

formly deeper incision (for reproducible corneal flattening). By eliminating the need to extend the diamond setting well beyond 100% of corneal thickness, as was routinely done with the centrifugal incision method, the risk of globe perforation may be significantly reduced as well.

In a comparative study using donor eyes, the combined (Genesis) technique for radial incisions demonstrated significantly greater corneal flattening than did the centrifugal (American) method, and outcome variability was reduced compared with the centripetal (Russian) method of incision.[9] Early clinical data appear consistent with these eye-bank studies.[10]

Diamond-Knife Footplates

It is important for the footplate design to be forgiving of undesirable deviations caused by the surgeon's hand by helping to maintain the diamond blade at a uniform stromal depth over a broad range of angular excusions made by the diamond knife on the corneal surface. By designing knife footplates that make minimal radial contact with the corneal surface, the blade will tend to maintain uniform depth within the stroma even if the surgeon's hand rocks (Fig 16–15). The knife footplates should also be relatively broad in order to provide maximal lateral support. In this way, should the surgeon's hand rock from side to side, the footplate's lateral compression upon the cornea maintains perpendicular stromal penetration (Fig 16–16).

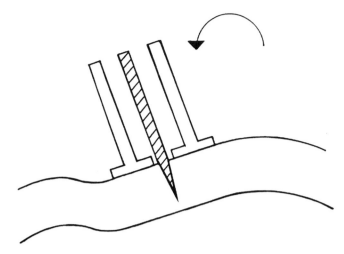

Figure 16–16. Broad lateral contact between the diamond footplates and the corneal epithelium enables the diamond blade to maintain its relative perpendicular orientation on the corneal stroma, despite inadvertent lateral rocking of the diamond knife.

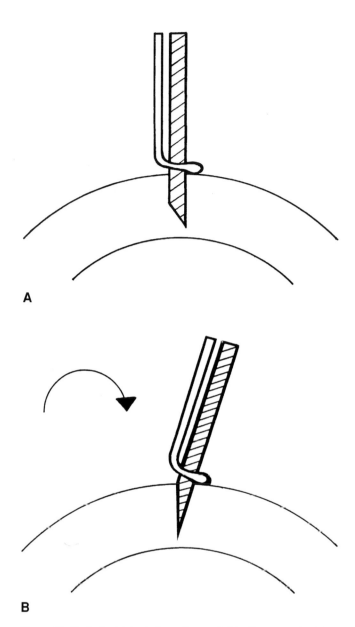

Figure 16–15. A. Footplate design with rounded leading toe and minimal radial epithelial contact. **B.** Minimal footplate radial contact with the epithelium enables the diamond blade to maintain a relatively uniform stromal depth, despite inadvertent rocking motion of the diamond knife.

The knife footplates should additionally be designed to generate minimal resistance against the corneal epithelium over the course of the incision. The leading tips of the footplate should be curved and smoothly polished, thus providing minimal resistance against a dry epithelium. Finally, diamond-knife footplates should be designed to enable easy viewing of both the diamond and the cornea, a feature referred to as having a low profile. We refer to diamond-knife footplates with this combination of features as having a universal design. The recent trend toward globe fixation

rings that contain footplate guidance tracks may facilitate improved incision quality.

Footplate spacing serves as a significant variable affecting incision depth. Widely spaced footplates may cause anterior bowing of the cornea between the footplates, resulting in relatively deeper blade penetration. Conversely, more closely spaced footplates may cause relative posterior corneal displacement, resulting in a shallower incision. It is thus evident that footplate design features are just as important determinants of incision precision and efficiency as are diamond-blade design features. It may therefore be somewhat misleading to suggest that two surgeons, using different diamonds, should achieve identical results.

Other diamond-tip designs currently being utilized include the undercut diamonds designed for maximizing central corneal flattening while affording relatively larger central clear zone diameters, thereby diminishing associated glare and possibly induced astigmatism.[11]

To maximize the shelf life of the diamond tip, it should be readily retractable into a safe housing position when not in use. The diamond knives should be cleaned in distilled deionized water during the autoclave cycle and in balanced salt solution or hydrogen peroxide in the ultrasonic cleanser.

Needle Holder

A standard curved needle holder should be readily available to repair intraoperative crossed incisions or perforations.

Irrigating Cannula

Either an angled 27-gauge or a Rowsey-style irrigating cannula may be used to flush saline solution into the incision groove at the termination of the case. Many surgeons do not routinely irrigate the wounds.

ASTIGMATIC KERATOTOMY INSTRUMENTATION

Several instruments unique to astigmatic keratotomy include central clear zone markers measuring 6, 7, and 8 mm in diameter. To place transverse incisions, 3-mm T-cut markers are generally sufficient, as the anticipated outcome of transverse incisions is titrated by varying the central clear zone size while incision length remains constant. For arcuate keratotomy, the central clear zone size is generally held constant while the arc length is varied. A set of four-, six-, and eight-wing RK markers is sufficient for delineating the desired arc length in most cases. A 6-wing RK marker, for instance, will intersect the central clear zone marker at 60° intervals, whereas an eight-wing marker will do so at 45° intervals.

The design used for performing astigmatic keratotomy may be a standard back-cutting (Russian style), trifaceted (Fig 16–17), or 15° diamond. These blades may be incorporated into a mechanized keratome to improve the surgeon's ability to perform arcuate incisions (see Chapter 17).

SECONDARY PROCEDURE INSTRUMENTATION

Undercorrections may typically be addressed either by adding incisions or by lengthening or deepening the original ones. Instrumentation for adding incisions consists of those used for the primary procedure itself, including corneal topographic analysis to guide in localizing corneal steep zones (Fig 16–18). Incision lengthening is a variable option, particularly during the first several weeks to months following the primary procedure, as minimal cross-linking of stromal collagen has occurred at this stage. For incision lengthening, a Sinskey hook may be used to splay open the superficial (epithelial) portion of the original incisions and a combined-style diamond may be used to elongate the incisions either peripherally or centrally.

Overcorrections may be addressed either pharmacologically, using 4% pilocarpine, or surgically, using selective sutured wound closure of incision sites topographically identified as being excessively flat. A specialized Sinskey hook with a serrated lateral wall may be used to scrape out the epithelial cysts and loose fibrous tissue from within the incision groove (Fig 16–19). Sutured closure using a needle holder and interrupted 10-0 nylon sutures at the 5-, 7-, and 9-mm zone diameters may then be carried out.

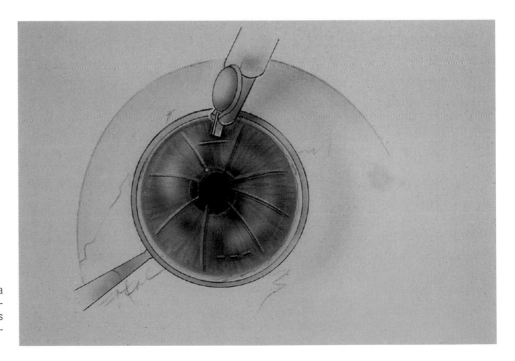

Figure 16–17. Artist's rendition of a trifaceted diamond for performing astigmatic keratotomy. A fixation ring is in position, and the eye has previously undergone eight-incision RK.

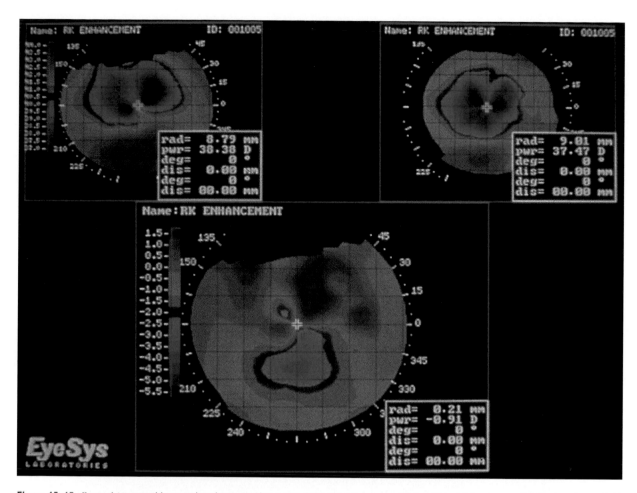

Figure 16–18. Corneal topographic mapping demonstrating postradial keratotomy map with insufficient inferotemporal flattening *(upper left)*. Post second procedure map demonstrates symmetric central flattening, following inferotemporal relaxing incision *(upper right)*. The difference map *(bottom)* demonstrates the change effected by the secondary procedure.

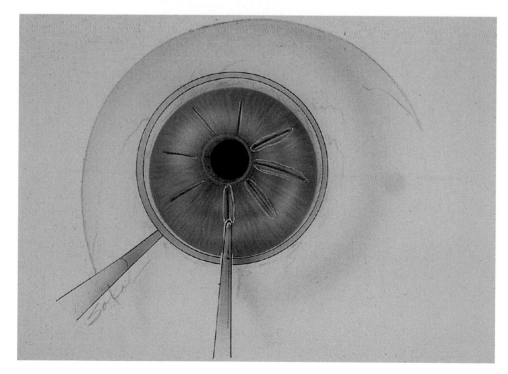

Figure 16–19. Artist's rendition of a modified Sinskey hook used to open a previous keratotomy incision site and to scrape free epithelial inclusion cysts and fibrous debris.

ADDITIONAL ASSISTIVE TECHNOLOGY

Glare Tester

A standard glare tester, including the brightness acuity tester, is a useful ancillary system to screen for subclinical lenticular opacities and also to assist in unmasking subtle, irregular astigmatism, although corneal topography and contrast sensitivity testing may be more accurate in identifying the latter.

Auto Refractor

While there is no substitute for a cycloplegic refraction, automated refraction with the eye in a cycloplegic state may provide a useful starting point in refracting a patient whose baseline error is otherwise unknown.

Computerized Videokeratography (Fig 16–20)

The rapid advances in keratorefractive surgery would not be possible without the aid of sophisti-

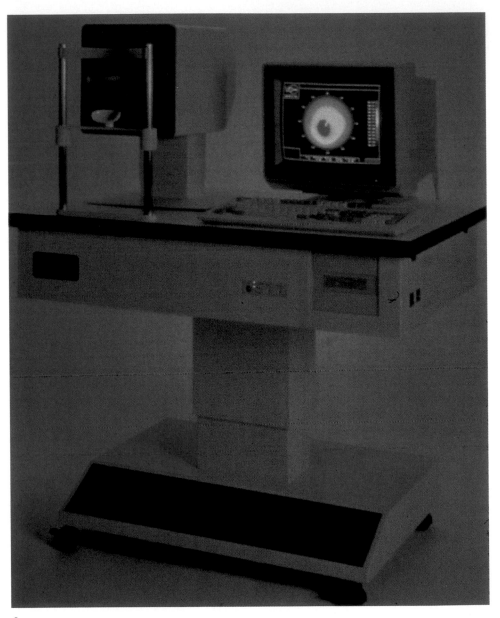

A

Figure 16–20. A. Photograph of a corneal topography system.

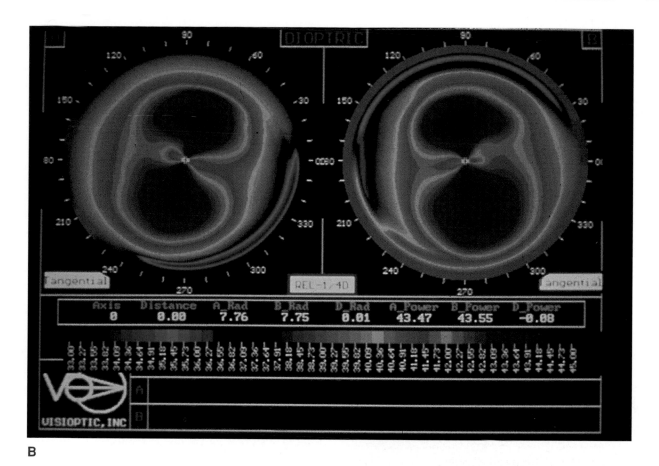

Figure 16–20 (continued). B. A representative topography map provided by a corneal topography system.

cated corneal shape analysis. With the advent of computerized videokeratography, we are now able to explain many of the previously unanswerable questions regarding corneal physiologic optics. Computerized videokeratography in the setting of a kerato-refractive practice facilitates (1) patient screening, (2) surgical planning, (3) documentation of irregular astigmatism, (4) guidance of secondary procedures, and (5) surgeon feedback.

Ultrasonic Pachymeter

The use of intraoperative, real-time solid-state ultrasonography is critical to achieving accurate corneal pachymetry readings (Fig 16–21). It is also advisable to conduct preoperative screening pachymetry to supplement intraoperative measurements (Fig 16–22).

To reduce microperforation risk, intraoperative pachymetry for RK may be conducted within a 3-mm optical zone, that is, 1.5 mm from the visual axis, at the temporal site, and over the thinnest paracentral cornea, as determined by the screening pachymetry. These two

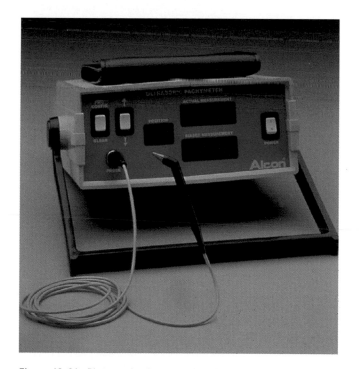

Figure 16–21. Photograph of a corneal pachymeter with digital display monitor, solid-state probe tip, built-in memory, and contact-activated continuous corneal measurements.

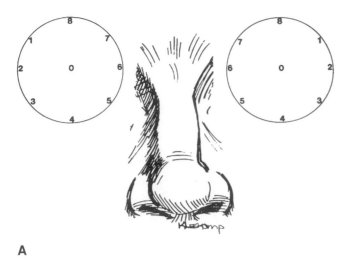

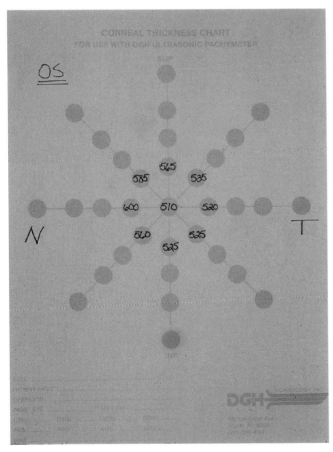

A

B

Figure 16–22.A. Schematic representation of desirable sites for pachymetric corneal measurement, including the apex (position φ) and eight paracentral sites at an approximate 3-mm diameter. **B.** Representative pachymetric measurements at the corneal apex and eight paracentral locations.

loci will often coincide. Optimal design features for an ultrasonic pachymeter should include a solid-state probe tip and contact-activated corneal measurement with consecutive readings; there is no need for a foot pedal, a digital display monitor, or memory for storing sequentially obtained data.

Diamond-Calibration Microscopes

There are multiple optional techniques available for calibrating the length of diamond-tip extension beyond the plane of the footplates. These include the micrometer on the knife itself (Fig 16–23) and several alternative external validation systems. The systems of external validation include plastic blocks (Fig 16–24), coin gauges (Fig 16–25), shadowgrams, and, most recently, diamond-calibrating microscopes (Fig 16–26).

The first diamond-calibrating microscope was developed by Richard Villasenor, and multiple first-generation variants were produced in the late 1980s that offer the benefits of near coaxial magnification to evaluate diamond-tip morphology and calibration of tip extension (Fig 16–27).

There are now a number of coaxial microscope systems designed for precise diamond-tip calibration (Fig. 16–26). Diamond microscopes with the least number of accessory components tend to be accurate and economical. We have found that the ideal calibrating microscopes are those with the following features:

1. High-quality optics that maximize depth of field (Fig 16–28) while minimizing spherical aberration

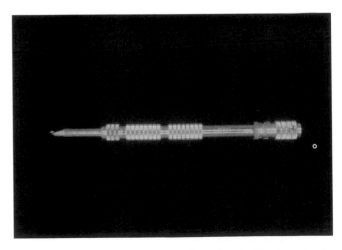

Figure 16–23. Standard RK diamond knife equipped with micrometer for self-contained calibration of diamond-tip extension.

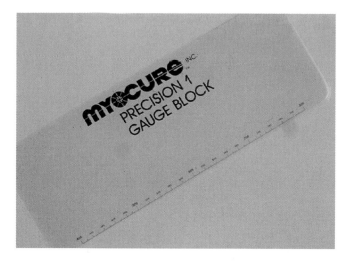

Figure 16–24. Plastic gauge block used for measurement of diamond-tip extension.

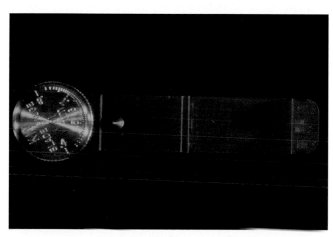

A

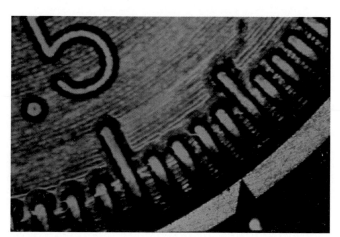

B

Figure 16–25. Standard coin gauge used for diamond-tip calibration **(A)**, in this case suggesting that the diamond tip has been extended approximately 530 μm **(B)**.

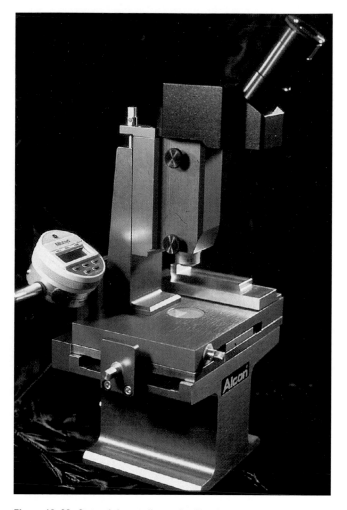

Figure 16–26. State-of-the-art diamond-calibrating microscope.

2. Stages mounted upon cross rollers that minimize vibrational motion
3. Motion detectors (in place of micrometers) capable of reporting diamond-tip excursion relative to the viewing system
4. A rotatable reticule within the eyepiece for precise alignment of both footplates relative to the vertical zero position

The calibrating microscopes also permit the evaluation of diamond defects, including chipping or accumulation of debris (Fig 16–29).

Video Monitor

The surgeon may wish to have a video monitor system attachment to the operating microscope in order to view the procedure in real time to aid the precise centration of the globe within the operative field, and to videotape significant procedures. Although this feature is clearly not mandatory, it may add an incremental benefit in certain clinical settings.

Data-Tracking Software

This may provide the surgeon with outcomes analysis and assist in long-term selection between alternative competing techniques. Such systems can also help in tracking costs and in surgical planning.

INVESTIGATIVE AIDS

Specular Microscopy

Designed for the examination of the corneal endothelial layer, this is of critical value in studies evaluating the impact of keratorefractive procedures on corneal integrity. To date there are no prospective studies demonstrating significant endothelial cell loss in association with anterior surface RK.

Contrast Acuity

Testing will likely become an increasingly important modality in the keratorefractive setting. Because most refractive procedures alter corneal topography and reverse the physiologic positively aspheric shape of the central cornea, they are likely to affect contrast sensitivity adversely. Although any adverse effect of RK on contrast sensitivity appears to be minimal, this assertion may not hold true for extremely small optical zone

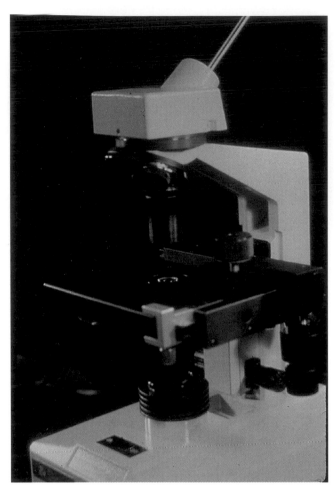

Figure 16–27. Early model diamond-calibrating microscope.

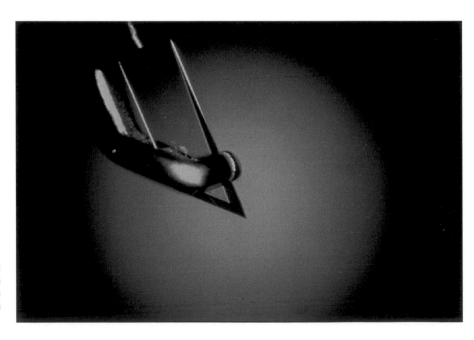

Figure 16–28. Photograph of diamond blade and footplates, demonstrating simultaneous visualization of footplates and diamond blade associated with the large depth of field within the viewing system.

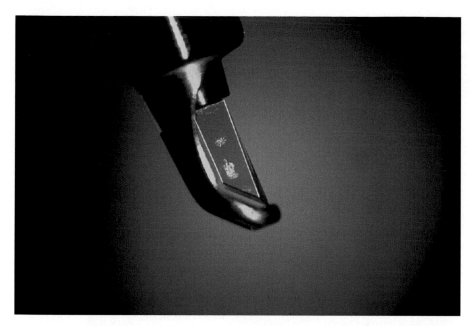

Figure 16–29. Debris accumulated onto diamond blade, readily observable under magnification.

selections. Furthermore, contrast sensitivity data may become more important in selecting between alternative keratorefractive modalities.

Anesthesiometer

This has potential value in assessing postoperative changes in corneal innervation after keratorefractive procedures.

FUTURE ADVANCES

Incisional keratotomy as practiced in 2 to 3 years will most likely differ significantly from our current approach. The technology that is now undergoing clinical investigation includes undercut diamonds, designed for greater range of corneal flattening (Fig 16–30), and computer-assisted diamond knives, whereby real-time pachymeters adjust the diamond-tip extension by optically guided motor drives linked to a computer interface (Fig 16–31).[12] Corneal topographic systems may evolve to permit real-time corneal topographic analysis, further aiding in refinement of technique and diminishing the rate of future enhancements (Figs 16–32 and 16–33). Automated globe fixation systems for controlling intraocular pressure and ocular movement will probably become available as well, adding to outcome predictability and procedural safety.

Perhaps of greatest value will be the advances in understanding corneal wound healing, affording us the capability of pharmacologic corneal shape manipulation.

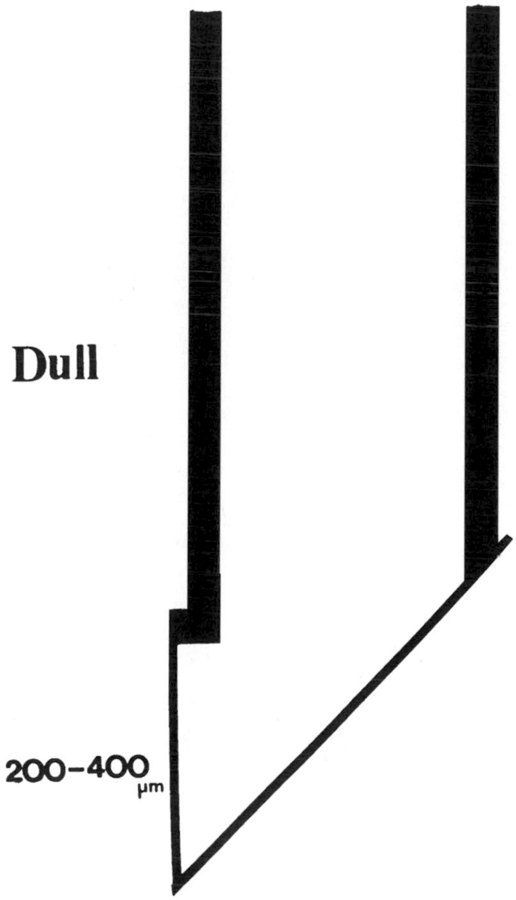

Dull

200–400 μm

Figure 16–30. Schematic representation of a diamond knife blade designed for maximal undermining of the central clear zone.

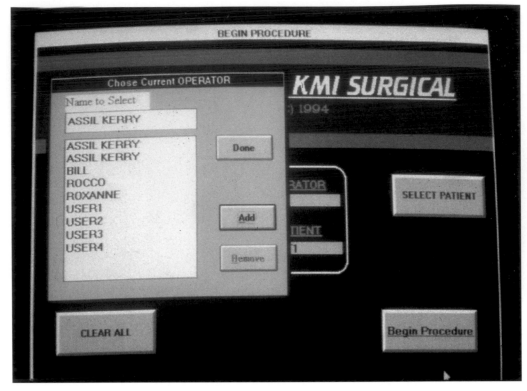

A

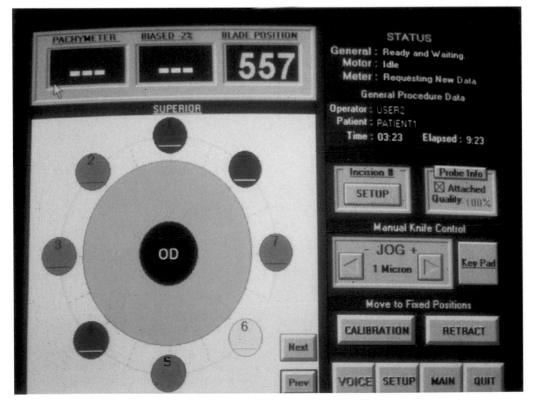

B

Figure 16–31. Sample computer screen displays of programmable diamond system. **A.** Initial setup display. **B.** Incision sequence programming with diamond knife setting.

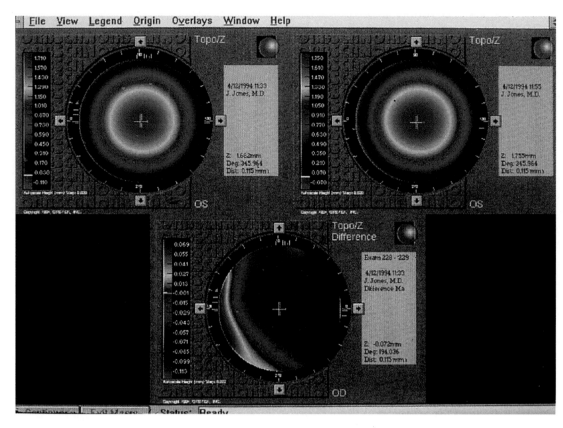

Figure 16–32. Topography map printout provided by the Orbscan slit beam corneal imaging system.

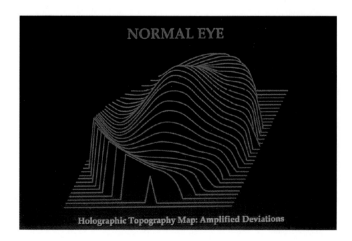

Figure 16–33. Topographic printout of corneal surface shape provided by a holographic-amplified topography mapping system.

REFERENCES

1. Assil KK, Schanzlin JD. Proposed refinements to microscope design. In: *Radial and Astigmatic Keratotomy: A Complete Handbook for Successful Practice of Incisional Keratotomy Using the Combined Technique.* Thorofare, NJ; Slack Inc; 1994;33031.

2. Pande M, Hillman JS. Optical zone centration in keratorefractive surgery. *Ophthalmology.* 1993:100:1230–1237.

3. Assil K, Knepshield W. Light guided eccentric gaze fixation system. Presented at American Society of Cataract and Refractive Surgery Symposium; April 1994; Boston.

4. Chayet A, Assil K, Parks R, Talamo J, and Refractive Keratoplasty Study Group. 8 vs. 10 mm outer zone radial keratotomy. Presented at American Society of Cataract and Refractive Surgery Symposium; April 1994; Boston.

6. Bores LD, Myers W, Cowden J. Radial keratotomy: an analysis of the American experience. *Ann Ophthalmol.* 1981;13:941–948.

7. Waring GO III, Moffitt SD, Gelender H, et al. Rationale for and design of the National Eye Institute Prospective Evaluation of Radial Keratotomy (PERK) Study. *Ophthalmology.* 1983;90:40–58.

8. Melles GRJ, Binder PS. Effect of radial keratotomy incision direction on wound depth. *Refract Corneal Surg.* 1990;6: 394–403.

9. Assil K, Kassof J, Schanzlin DJ, Quantock AJ. A combined incision technique of radial keratotomy: a comparison to centripetal and centrifugal incision techniques in human donor eyes. *Ophthalmology.* 1994;101:746–754.

10. Chayet A, Meyer JC. The combined technique of radial keratotomy. *Semin Ophthalmol.* 1994;9(2):106–109.

11. Assil K, Parks RA, Kratz-Owens K, Quantock AJ. The undercut technique of radial keratotomy: a comparison to the combined technique. Association for Research in Vision and Ophthalmology, Annual Meeting on Investigative Ophthalmology and Visual Science; May 1994; Sarasota, FL.

12. Assil KK, Knepshield W. The sentry programmable diamond for radial keratotomy. Presented at American Society of Cataract and Refractive Surgery, Summer Symposium; September 1993; Los Angeles.

CHAPTER 17

The Mechanized Arcuate Keratome

Khalil D. Hanna ▪ Thierry David ▪ Carol L. Karp ▪ William W. Culbertson

DEVELOPMENT OF KERATOTOMY FOR ASTIGMATISM

Transverse keratotomy for the correction of astigmatism was suggested by Snellen[1] in 1869, studied in laboratory animals by Lans[2] in the 1890s, and used clinically by Bates[3] and others in the late 19th century.[4] Sato used straight transverse incisions to correct astigmatism in the 1940s and 1950s. High astigmatism after penetrating keratoplasty prompted Troutman,[5] Swinger[6] and Krachmer[7] to propose arcuate transverse "relaxing incisions."[8] Interest in radial keratotomy (RK) for myopia and in small-incision cataract surgery led to more emphasis on transverse keratotomy to control naturally occurring astigmatism.[9–12] Many patterns of transverse keratotomy have been proposed, particularly in combination with radial incisions. There is currently a trend to use arcuate transverse keratotomy as the primary means of correcting astigmatism.[13,14] Merlin[13] and others[11,14] have emphasized that arcuate incisions are preferable because the entire incision length is equidistant from the center of the cornea and because the incision is located in an area of equal corneal thickness.

Several factors that may affect the outcome of surgery have been described.[15–17] The excimer laser PRK and AK have been proposed as alternatives to improve the clinical outcomes.[18–20]

Current techniques of making arcuate transverse incisions require the manual use of a micrometric diamond knife. The major problem with this technique is the variability of the depth and the configuration of the incision, depending upon the surgeon's skill. A mechanized keratome designed to make arcuate incisions may increase the reproducibility of the incisions. The instrument has undergone prototype development and has been described in recent publications.[21,22] It is expected that many patients having myopic astigmatism will be eligible for excimer laser PRK if their degree of astigmatism is minimal, or if it has been reduced after astigmatic keratotomy.

DEVELOPMENT OF THE MECHANIZED KERATOME

Description

The arcuate keratome shares many design similarities with the Hanna trephine,[15] substituting a pair of micrometric diamond-bladed knives for the circular trephine blade. Certain features allow the instrument to make reproducible arcuate incisions in the cornea and increase predictability of the results:

1. Double-edged, micrometric diamond knife blades mounted in retractable carriers
2. The ability to fix the arcuate length and excursion of the blades by setting a series of stops according to the instrument markings

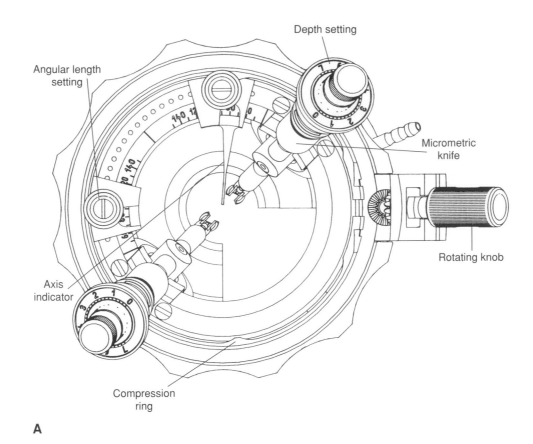

Depth setting

Angular length
setting

Micrometric
knife

Rotating knob

Axis
indicator

Compression
ring

A

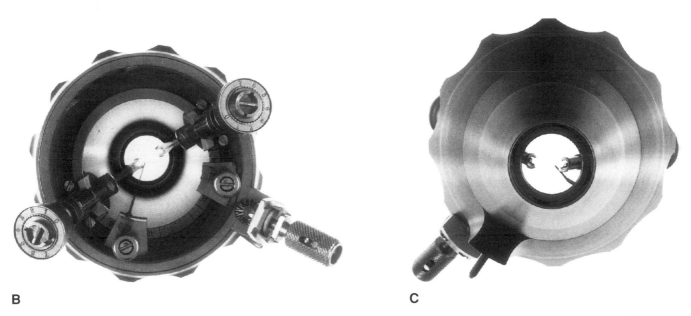

B

C

Figure 17–1. Components of the arcuate keratome. Computer drawing **(A)** and surgeon's view **(B)** show the assembled instrument with a rotation knob, two micrometric diamond knives, and the angular setting. **C.** View of assembled instrument from below demonstrates the centering-axis pointer and the two diamond blades inside the housing cone.

3. A centering guide that is also aligned with the steep meridian to assure proper orientation

4. The ability to set the location of each diamond blade independently at a fixed radius from the center so that symmetric or asymmetric incisions can be made

The keratome (Fig 17–1) has the shape of a truncated cone that is 53 mm in diameter at its upper plane, where the surgeon holds it, and 15.5 mm in diameter at its lower plane, where it attaches to the limbal conjunctiva. It is 41 mm tall and weighs 81 g. The truncated, slightly concave shape results in its being comparatively smaller at its middle and lower planes; it is also smaller in comparison to the Goldmann 3-mirror contact lens at its middle and lower planes. Consequently, it fits well in the orbit, especially in deep-seated eyes.

It consists of two parts: (1) the outer cone that houses the knife carrier and provides fixation and (2) the knife carrier with two micrometric diamond knives.

Housing

The upper rim of the housing has a series of large indentations to ensure steady fixation with finger and thumb (Fig. 17–1). The surface that attaches to the globe has a 15.5-mm outer-wall diameter, an 11-mm inner-wall diameter, and an area in between of 82 mm^2 for suction. The space between the two walls connects to a suction cannula that protrudes from the side of the instrument to which tubing and a syringe can be attached. The inner edge of the suction space contains an 11-mm-diameter removable ring with eight small claws that stabilize the instrument on the limbus and prevent slipping. These also allow use of the instrument without suction. The first clinical cases were done using claws fixation, but then the ring was removed when the instrument proved to be sufficiently stable that incisions could be performed without claws or suction fixation. The effect of suction was studied in the laboratory and was found to affect the reproducibility of the incision depth.[21]

Two parts of the housing—the cone and the upper rim—are joined by a simple spring clip. A gear mechanism turns the knife carrier; it is attached to the upper rim of the housing and is operated by turning a knurled knob that extends obliquely from the upper surface.

Knife Carrier and Micrometric Knives

The two micrometric knives are mounted on a carrier 180° apart. In order to make arcuate incisions of a defined length, a stop mechanism is used. The stop mechanism consists of holes on the blade carrier into which pegs that serve as stops can be inserted. A circular compression ring above the blade carrier has two projections oriented at 180° from each other. When these projections hit the stop pegs, the rotation of the knife carrier ceases. The position of the pegs and the compression-ring projections determine the excursion of the knife blades, and thus the angular length of the incisions. One of the stops has a thin pointer that extends downward in the center of the cone to the corneal surface, where it can be aligned with both the center of the pupil and the steep corneal meridian (Fig 17–2). The compression ring must be rotated to allow placement of the knurled knob that advances the blade carrier in a comfortable position.

The knives are perpendicular to the cornea at 6-mm diameter, and they pivot radially at their attachments to the carrier. A small knob (Fig 17–2) moves each knife radially to determine the zone diameter, which can be altered from 4 mm to 8 mm. Each knife has a double-edged diamond blade oriented parallel to the limbus.

The blades are stored in a safe, retracted position and are exposed by turning the upper knife casing one fourth of a turn so that a spring extends the blade to the preset depth. The depth setting of the blade is adjusted by a calibrated screw mechanism at the top of each knife. Each knife has a semicircular footplate that is open toward the center of the cornea to allow visualization of the blades during cutting. This configuration is different from a standard RK knife, in that the cutting edges of the diamond blade face the closed sides of the footplate. The footplate slides on the surface of the cornea and supports it during the incision.

Maintenance and Sterilization

The blades should be cleaned by the surgeon with hydrogen peroxide or a cleaning soap and distilled water. Alternatively, they may be held in an ultrasound cleaning bath. The entire keratome can be steam autoclaved.

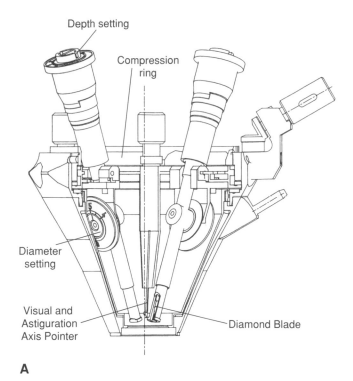

Depth setting

Compression ring

Diameter setting

Visual and Astiguration Axis Pointer

Diamond Blade

A

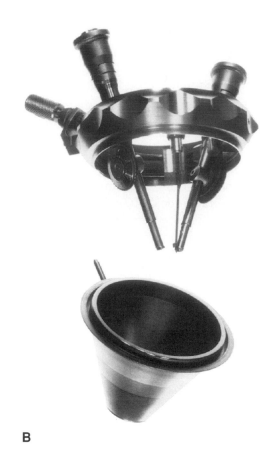

B

Figure 17–2. A. Cross-sectional computer drawing demonstrates the instrument, suction ring, and two diamond knives. The pointer indicates the center of the pupil and aligns with the steep meridian. The diameter-setting knob, when rotated, moves the knife radially, altering the zone diameter. Three variables are set by adjustments on the instrument: zone diameter of the two incisions, angular length of the incisions, and depth of the incisions. **B.** The disassembled instrument shows the double-walled housing cone *(below)* and the diameter setting.

CLINICAL EVALUATION

Correction of Postkeratoplasty Astigmatism

Two prototypes of the keratome were used in 40 patients with postkeratoplasty astigmatism and 16 patients with naturally-occurring astigmatism. Preoperative astigmatism ranged from 4 to 13 diopters.

For patients with postkeratoplasty astigmatism, selection criteria included clear graft by slit lamp microscopy, absent inflammatory reaction and epithelial defects, and readable videokeratograph (Fig. 17–3). All sutures were to have been removed for at least 6 months prior to surgery. No attempt was made to use a rigid nomogram for these cases; each one was planed individually under the guidance of a published nomogram.[21]

Immediately preoperatively, patients were examined using a slit lamp microscope with the beam oriented centrally and vertically over the surface of the cornea and aligned with the vertical 90° meridian. A sterile hypodermic needle or a marking pen was used to make a mark at the 12 o'clock location at the limbus to mark the 90° meridian.

In the operating room, the center of the pupil was marked with a marking pen, and a Mendez protractor was used, first to identify the 90° meridian and then to identify and mark the steep meridian in the upper cornea. In the case of asymmetric astigmatism, when the two steep semimeridians were not 180° apart and had shifted by 10° or more based on the videokeratograph, the two steep semimeridians were marked over the upper sector of the cornea; therefore the incisions were not performed simultaneously, but successively.

Corneal thickness was measured along the diameter of the zone selected for the incisions, using an ultrasonic pachymeter on which the speed of sound was set at 1640 milliseconds. The arcuate keratome was then set to the selected diameter, arcuate length, and blade extension.

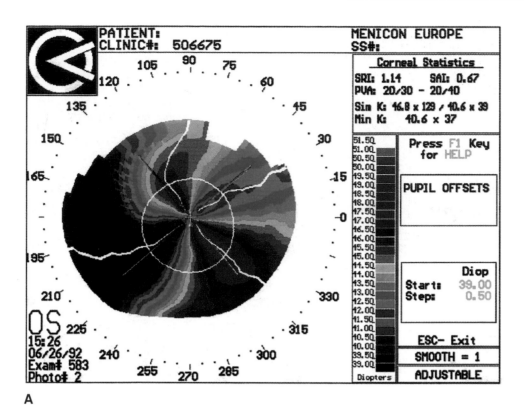

A

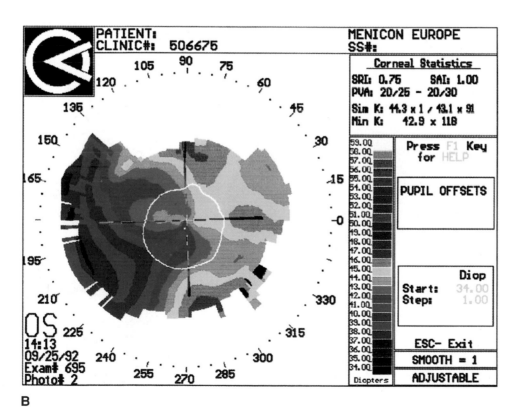

B

Figure 17–3. A. Videokeratograph of a patient with 6.2 D of postkeratoplasty astigmatism. The inferonasal semimeridian is steeper than the superotemporal semimeridian with 10° of axis misalignment. The lower flat semimeridian is 2 D flatter than the upper semimeridian. **B.** Videokeratograph of the same patient 2 weeks after surgery. One pair of incisions of a 60° angular length, a 6.5-mm clear zone, and 80% depth. The videokeratograph shows 1.2 D of astigmatism, but with irregularities that improved over time.

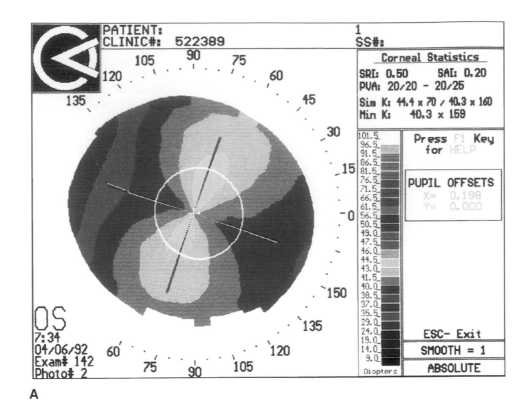

A

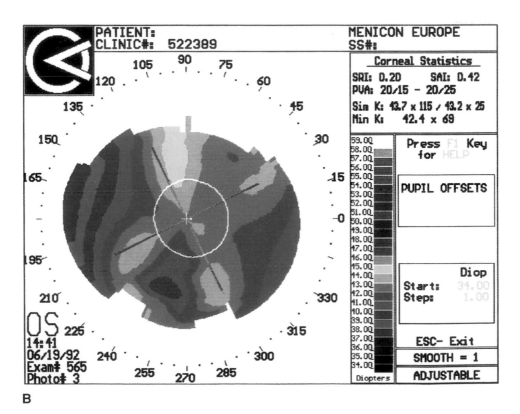

B

Figure 17–4. Videokeratographs of case 6 (Table 17–3), with naturally occurring astigmatism. **A.** Preoperative keratograph shows a bow-tie pattern with approximately 4.2 D of astigmatism; the steep meridian is at 70°. **B.** Videokeratograph 3 months after surgery with the arcuate keratome shows approximately 0.50 D of astigmatism; there is a 35° change in axis toward 90° using the absolute scale with 1 D steps.

TABLE 17–1. NOMOGRAM FOR POSTKERATOPLASTY ASTIGMATISM

Amount of Refractive Astigmatism (D)	Zone Diameter (mm)	Blade Extension (%)	Angular Length (deg)
2.5 to 3.75	6.75	75	60
4.0 to 5.0	6.50	75	60
5.0 to 6.25	6.50	75	70
6.5 to 7.5	6.25	75	70
7.75 to 8.75	6.25	75	80
9 to 15	6.00	75	80

TABLE 17–2. NOMOGRAM FOR ASTIGMATIC KERATOTOMY (NATURALLLY OCCURRING)[a]

Amount of Refractive Astigmatism (D)	Zone Diameter (mm)	Blade Extension (%)	Angular Length (deg)
1.5 to 2.5	7.25	90	60
2.75 to 3.75	7.00	90	70
4.0 to 5.0	7.00	90	80
5.25 to 6.25	6.75	90	80
6.50 to 7.50	6.75	90	90
7.75 to 8.75	6.50	90	90

[a]Over or under age 30: increase or decrease in efficacy by 0.05 D per year.

A small amount of 1.3% methylcellulose (Goniosol) was spread over the end of the footplates to avoid epithelial abrasion. The keratome was lowered to the eye and the indicator aligned with the steep meridian so that its tip was on the center pupil mark. The keratome was then pressed firmly onto the surface of the globe. Each blade was extended into the cornea and advanced at an average angular speed of 10 to 15 degrees per second. Only a single pass was made in early cases. Currently we use two passes to achieve a depth closer to the preset depth. The nomogram now in use is presented in Table 17–1.

Postoperatively, a pressure patch was placed for 1 day in some cases. Thereafter, the eye was not patched, and topical dexamethasone 0.1% and antibiotics were applied tid for 3 weeks and then stopped.

A significant reduction in astigmatism occurred in all cases in which there was an improvement in visual acuity. In many of these cases, some irregular astigmatism persisted after surgery (Fig 17–4). Overcorrection occurred in early cases when an incisional depth setting of 90% was used. In one case, one of the incisions perforated the cornea at the graft–host interface. Two interrupted 10-0 nylon sutures closed the incision at the site of perforation.

Correction of Naturally Occurring Astigmatism

A consecutive series of 16 patients (17 eyes) with naturally occurring astigmatism was treated with the keratome at Bascom Palmer Eye Institute, Miami, Florida,

TABLE 17–3. ASTIGMATISM REDUCTION USING THE ARCUATE KERATOME

Eye No	Preop Astig (D)	Preop Axis (deg)	K1 (D)	K2 (D)	Clear Zone (mm)	Angular Length (deg)	Final Astig (D)	Final Axis (deg)	Final K1 (D)	Final K2 (D)	Flattening (D)	Steepening (D)	Flattening/ Steepening Ratio	Vectoral Change (D)	Change in Spherical Equivalent (D)
1	5.4	95	46.3	40.9	6.5	80	3.2	80	45.4	42.2	0.9	1.3	0.69	3.1	0.2
2	4.2	115	43.0	38.8	7.0	60	2.0	93	42.1	40.1	0.9	1.3	0.69	3.9	0.2
3	2.3	58	44.0	41.7	7.0	60	0.7	96	43.4	42.7	0.6	1.0	0.60	2.2	0.2
4	7.0	86	48.3	41.3	6.5	80	1.8	73	46.2	44.4	2.1	3.1	0.68	5.6	0.5
5	6.3	96	47.7	41.4	6.5	80	1.4	60	45.2	43.8	2.5	2.4	1.04	5.9	−0.05
6	4.1	70	44.4	40.3	7.0	60	1.3	105	43.6	42.3	0.8	2.0	0.40	3.8	0.6
7	5.9	87	44.9	39.0	6.0	80	3.2	59	43.9	40.7	1.0	1.7	0.59	4.7	0.35
8	4.1	86	48.8	44.7	6.5	60	2.1	73	48.0	45.9	0.8	1.2	0.67	1.9	0.2
9	6.0	86	47.7	41.7	6.0	80	2.6	68	46.2	43.6	1.5	1.9	0.79	4.3	0.2
10	5.3	95	46.8	41.5	7.0	80	3.0	73	45.7	42.7	1.1	1.2	0.92	3.0	0.05
11	4.8	79	43.5	38.7	6.5	80	2.5	75	42.1	39.6	1.4	0.9	1.56	2.3	−0.25
12	2.7	87	45.8	43.1	7.5	60	2.0	98	45.2	43.2	0.6	0.1	6*	1.3	−0.25
13	4.6	96	46.6	42.0	7.0	60	3.3	79	45.9	42.6	0.7	0.6	1.17	1.5	−0.05
14	3.0	82	44.6	41.6	7.0	60	1.4	48	43.8	42.4	0.8	0.8	1.00	2.6	0
15	2.3	66	46.2	43.9	7.0	60	1.8	60	45.8	44.0	0.4	0.1	4.00	0.8	−0.15
16	4.8	66	46.3	41.5	6.5	80	2.0	80	44.2	42.2	2.1	0.7	3.00	3.2	−0.7
17	2.6	96	45.7	43.1	7.5	60	1.1	60	45.2	44.1	0.5	1.0	0.50	2.4	0.25

*Incision depths less than 50% of corneal thickness.

and at Hotel-Dieu Hospital, Paris, France, by two surgeons (WWC and KDH, respectively). The criteria for case selection were generally the same as those outlined in the PERK Study.[23] Additional criteria include the presence of 2 D or more of astigmatism and exclusion of eyes with keratoconus or with focal corneal thinning disorders, such as pellucid marginal degeneration. The nomogram used for setting parameters in these cases has been published elsewhere.[21] (A new nomogram was created according to the results of these preliminary cases; Table 17–2.)

The achieved depth was equal to the setting in most cases (Fig 17–5) and shallower than the preset depth up to 30%. Thereafter, the two-sweeps technique was used to improve depth predictability.

Astigmatism reduction varied from 34% to 95%, with a mean vectoral change of 68% (3.12 D) (Table 17–3). Uncorrected visual acuity improved in 80% of eyes (Fig 17–6). Best corrected visual acuity increased two Snellen lines or more in 57% of eyes, and one line in 20% (Fig 17–7). The flattening to steepening ratio varied from 0.40 to 4 (mean 1.09), except in case 12 (Table 17–3) where a 30% depth of incision was used. Change

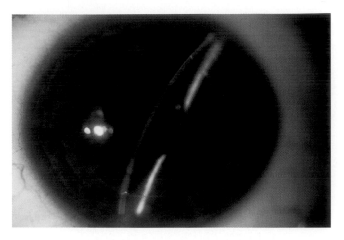

Figure 17–5. Slit lamp photomicrograph shows the smooth arc of a deep incision. *(From* Arch Ophthalmol. *1993; 111(7):998–1004.)*

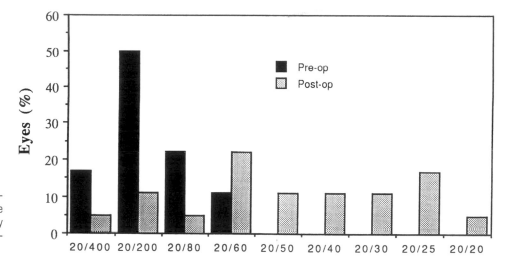

Figure 17–6. Graphic represents visual acuity at 3 months after arcuate keratotomy in 17 cases of naturally occurring astigmatism. Note the improvement of uncorrected vision.

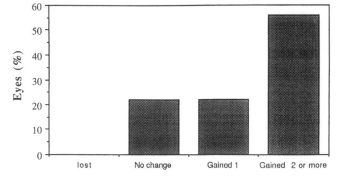

Figure 17–7. Graphic represents the improvement of best uncorrected vision. Uncorrected vision did not improve in 20% of the cases because of associated ametropia.

in spherical equivalent ranged from +0.5 to −0.7 D (mean 0.06 D) (Table 17–3).

COMMENT

Design and Use of the Instrument

The arcuate keratome was designed to fulfill the following goals:

1. Arcuate incisions with accurate and reproducible location, length, configuration, and depth
2. Accurate centering and positioning of the instrument on the steep meridian
3. Steady fixation on the globe during cutting with minimum distortion of the cornea
4. Visualization of the blade while the tissue is being cut
5. Simultaneous production of incisions of the same or differing zone diameters
6. Ergonomic efficiency and ease of use

The design and engineering of this instrument achieved these goals.

The instrument allows the surgeon to alter two different variables for each of the paired incisions because the diameter of the incision zone and the depth of the incision can be different for each incision of the pair. However, the length of the incisions is identical—between 60° and 120°—and the incisions are located 180° apart. If the surgeon wishes to make the two incisions other than 180° apart, as indicated in asymmetric astigmatism and in many cases of postkeratoplasty astigmatism, it is easy simply to use one of the knife blades to make an initial incision and then to lift the keratome and reorient the axis marker along a different meridian to make a second incision. Thus, the instrument is both flexible and capable of assuring considerable uniformity in the execution of the incisions. The arcuate keratome avoids manual wobble and creates a more uniform and accurate incisional depth.

Achieved Depth of the Incisions

Many factors affect the actual depth of the incision in the cornea: the accuracy of the pachymeter, the location of the corneal-thickness readings, the configuration and sharpness of the knife blade,[17] and the speed at which the incision is made. The use of two passes or sweeps increases the incision depth and reduces the difference between the attempted depth and the achieved depth.

Effect of Incision Depth

Better correction was achieved when the incision depth was ≥ 70% of corneal thickness. Undercorrection was observed with shallow incisions.

Effect of Age

The elastic modulus of the cornea changes with age. Keratotomy is more effective in older patients because their elasticity coefficient value is decreased. Better correction was observed in the 30- to 40-year age group (Table 17–3). We think that the relation to age is nonlinear and the curve is not as steep in older persons.

Predictability

There was no overcorrection in the naturally occurring astigmatism cases. Seventeen eyes were within 1 D of the planned correction (Table 17–3). In one case transient overcorrection was present for 2 weeks. Postkeratoplasty cases were less predictable, and overcorrection occurred when 90% deep incisions were made. Interface scarring and original pathology, such as keratoconus, play an important role. The irregularity and the great asymmetry of postkeratoplasty astigmatism decrease the accuracy of nomograms. The insufficiency of nomograms for guiding decisions has propelled the development of an expert system (a computer program that combines patient topography with a finite-element computer model) to help in designating the surgical parameters to be used (KD Hanna et al. Unpublished data).

Stability

All eyes corrected for naturally occurring astigmatism decreased correction during the first 15 days by approximately 10%, except in one where the decrease was 32%. An increased effect with time of about 8% was observed in only one case. Generally the mean correction at 3 months approached 90% of that obtained at the first postoperative day.

Keratotomy versus Laser Keratectomy

The 193-nm excimer laser has been proposed for correcting astigmatism, both by making linear transverse excisions[18] and by making surface ablations.[19] Compared to diamond-knife incisions, the excimer laser creates wider wounds (thereby performing a keratectomy) and increases the risk of endothelial cell damage.[20] Surface ablation requires surgery over the pupil and has a postoperative recovery period of 3 to 12 months.

Whether the arcuate keratome can produce clinical results that are truly superior to manual keratotomy or excimer laser photorefractive keratectomy must await the results of prospective randomized clinical trials.

REFERENCES

1. Snellen H. Die Richtung der Hauptmeridiane des astigmatischen Auges. *Archiv für Ophthalmologie.* 1896;15:199–207.

2. Lans LJ. Experimentelle Untersuchungen über Entstehung von Astigmatismus durch nicht-perforirende Corneawunden. *Archiv für Ophthalmologie.* 1898;45:117–152.

3. Bates WH. A suggestion of an operation to correct astigmatism. *Arch Ophthalmol.* 1894;23:9–13.

4. Schimmelpfennig BH, Waring GO. Development of refractive keratotomy in the nineteenth century. In: Waring GO. *Refractive Keratotomy for Myopia and Astigmatism.* St. Louis: Mosby-Year Book; 1991;171–177.

5. Troutman RC. Microsurgical control of corneal astigmatism in cataract and keratoplasty. *Trans Am Acad Ophthalmol Otolaryngol.* 1973;77:OP563–572.

6. Troutman RC, Swinger CA. Relaxing incisions for control of postoperative astigmatism following keratoplasty. *Ophthalmic Surg.* 1980;11:117–120.

7. Krachmer JH, Fenzl RL. Surgical correction of high postkeratoplasty astigmatism relaxing incisions vs wedge resection. *Arch Ophthalmol.* 1980;98:1400–1402.

8. Swinger CA. Postoperative astigmatism. *Surv Ophthalmol.* 1987;31:219–248.

9. Lindstrom RL, Lindquist TD. Surgical correction of postoperative astigmatism. *Cornea.* 1988;7:138–148.

10. Rowsey JJ. Review: current concepts in astigmatism surgery. *J Refract Surg.* 1986;2:85–94.

11. Binder PS, Waring GO. Keratotomy for astigmatism. In: Waring GO. *Refractive Keratotomy for Myopia and Astigmatism.* St. Louis: Mosby-Year Book; 1991;1085–1198.

12. Thornton SP, Sanders DR. Graded nonintersecting transverse incisions for correction of idiopathic astigmatism. *J Cataract Refract Surg.* 1987;13:27–31.

13. Merlin U. Curved keratotomy procedure for congenital astigmatism. *J Refract Surg.* 1987;3:92–97.

14. Duffey RJ, Jain VN, Tchah H, Hofmann RF, Lindstrom RL. Paired arcuate keratotomy—a surgical approach to mixed and myopic astigmatism. *Arch Ophthalmol.* 1988;106:1130–1135.

15. Waring GO, Hanna KD. The Hanna suction punch block and trephine system for penetrating keratoplasty. *Arch Ophthalmol.* 1989;107:1536–1539.

16. Lowery JA, Parel J-M, Roussel TJ, Simon G, Lee W, Nose I. Artificial orbit system for experimental surgery with enucleated globes. *Ophthalmic Surg.* 1990:21:522–528.

17. Thornton SP, Gardner SK, Waring GO. Surgical instruments used in refractive keratotomy. In: Waring GO. *Refractive Keratotomy for Myopia and Astigmatism.* St. Louis: Mosby-Year Book; 1991:407–489.

18. Seiler T, Bende T, Wollensak J, Trokel S. Excimer laser keratectomy for correction of astigmatism. *Am J Ophthalmol.* 1988;105:177–124.

19. McDonnell PJ, Moreira H, Clapham TN, D'Arcy J, Munnerlyn CR. Photorefractive keratectomy for astigmatism: initial clinical results. *Arch Ophthalmol.* 1991;109:1370–1373.

20. Dehm EF, Puliafito CA, Adler CM, Steinert RF. Corneal endothelial injury in rabbits following excimer laser ablation at 193 nm and 248 nm. *Arch Ophthalmol.* 1986;104:1364–1368.

21. Hanna KD, Hayward M, Hagen KB, Simon G, Parel JM, Waring GO. Keratotomy for astigmatism using an arcuate keratome. *Arch Ophthalmol.* 1993;111:998–1004.

22. Hanna KD, et al. Arcuate keratotomy for astigmatism using a mechanical keratome: early clinical experience. *Invest Ophthalmol Vis Sci.* 1993;34(suppl):1244.

23. Waring GO, Moffitt SD, Gelender H, et al. Rationale for and design of the National Eye Institute Prospective Evaluation of Radial Keratotomy (PERK) Study. *Ophthalmology.* 1983;90:40–58.

CHAPTER 18

Lamellar Refractive Surgery Instrumentation

Shu-Wen Chang ▪ Luis Ruiz ▪ Marcela Gomez

Lamellar refractive surgery, like other keratorefractive surgical techniques, has been performed as an alternative to correction by spectacles or contact lenses for decades. Lamellar refractive surgery for the correction of hyperopia and myopia, better known as *keratomileusis* (KM), was pioneered by J. I. Barraquer, from Bogotá, Colombia, more than 30 years ago. Another lamellar procedure to correct aphakia, termed *keratophakia*, was also introduced by Barraquer. Barraquer's first clinical results for autoplastic myopic keratomileusis (MKM) were published in 1964, and those for keratophakia appeared in 1965.[1] At a time when there was a shortage of donor corneas, he concentrated on the development of autoplastic surgery for the correction of hyperopia and aphakia, and he subsequently developed the technique of *hyperopic keratomileusis* (HKM). His first published results were reported in 1980 (Figures 1–3 and 1–12).[2]

In 1977, Troutman and Swinger introduced the hyperopic procedures in the United States, and Swinger performed the first myopic procedure in 1980. Swinger and Villasenor contributed substantially to the surgical knowledge of keratomileusis in the United States, while Nordan and Maxwell standardized it for consistent and systematic teaching.

On the basis of Barraquer's work, Kaufman and Werblin introduced the onlay lamellar refractive procedure, initially termed *epikeratomileusis* and later *epikeratophakia* (although it is more properly named *epikeratoplasty*) in 1979. A new technique called *nonfreeze planar keratomileusis*, which permitted operations without freezing, was described by Krumeich and Swinger in 1983. More recently, in an effort to avoid the drawbacks of these techniques, keratomileusis in situ has been investigated and performed. At the time of this writing, keratomileusis with intrastromal photoablation using the excimer laser (laser in situ keratomileusis or LASIK) is being refined as a method that effectively and easily combines a surgical procedure and laser technique (see Chapters 26 and 34).

INSTRUMENTS FOR CENTERING AND MARKING THE TREATMENT ZONE

Currently four techniques of keratmileusis are in clinical use: cryolathe, planar with mold, keratomileusis in situ, and excimer laser. Several other methods using newer lasers are being investigated. No matter what corneal surgical procedure is performed, proper centration is required to avoid postoperative complications, like irregular astigmatism and glare, that may interfere with visual function (see Chapters 9 and 16). To obtain optimal corneal centering, the patient fixates on a target or light that is coaxial with the examiner's sighting eye. In other words, the patient fixates on a target and the examiner views the patient's eye from the position of the target before marking a zone concentric with the pupil (Figs 16–3 and 4). There are different views about the precise site where the procedure should be centered. Several investigators argue that the ''visual axis'' is the optimal site of centration, while others have selected the center of the entrance pupil for that purpose.[3,4]

Various techniques have been described for corneal centration using the operating microscope. Steinberg and Waring described the technique used in the PERK study, in which the light reflex was a reference point.[5] The patient fixed on the coiled microscope light filament that emerged from the viewing tubes on the microscope toward 6 o'clock. Viewing is monocular, and when it is through the right microscope ocular the surgeon uses the tip of a hypodermic needle to mark the corneal epithelium at the left end of the rectangular filament reflection and a filament of one half to one width inferiorly toward 6 o'clock. Most surgeons currently center the treatments on the pupil instead of the corneal light reflex (see Chapter 9).

The Osher's centering device (JEDMED, St. Louis) can also be used after it has been attached and removed from the microscope. The screw clamp must be fastened securely to avoid disengagement of the device, although a guard chain is provided to prevent this. One disadvantage of this setup is that the light provided by the fiberoptic tip is dim, so that it is difficult to see its reflection on the cornea and impossible to see it on the pupil. Fortunately, Osher's device is better used to center the treatment on the pupil, ignoring the corneal light reflex (see Chapter 9). Other fixation targets can be attached to the microscope that are centered between the viewing tubes. These are valuable if the surgeon has no ocular dominance while viewing the cornea binocularly. The fixation light in the Zeiss and Weck centering devices and the nonluminous fixation point in Thornton's methods are examples of such devices.[4]

When performing lamellar refractive surgery, specifically automated lamellar keratoplasty (ALK) and laser-assisted in situ keratomileusis (LASIK), after the center has been defined, a mark is made on the eyeball with a specially designed marker (see Fig 26–13).

This marker consists of two concentric circles: an internal one, 3 mm in diameter; and an external one, 10.5 mm in diameter. The two circles are attached by a line that touches the smaller circle tangentially, resulting in a pararadial line. After the marker is soaked in a dye (usually gentian violet or brilliant green), it is placed on the cornea to obtain the marks.[6]

INSTRUMENTATION FOR KERATOMILEUSIS WITH FREEZING

Keratomileusis with freezing allows relatively predictable surgical correction of myopia, to a degree as high as 16 diopters. Major disadvantages of keratomileusis with freezing include the complexity of the technique; the sophisticated technical equipment itself—a microkeratome and a cryolathe; the time required to attain sufficient expertise in handling the two instruments; and the long recovery period due to the changes in the corneal tissue structure after the lenticule is frozen. Surgical instruments necessary for keratomilieusis with freezing are summarized in Table 18–1. Instrumentation includes a microkeratome to perform the lamellar keratectomy, a set of suction rings with which to fix the eye and guide the microkeratome, a microcomputer or calculator for the cryolathe procedure, the cryolathe itself, and the means to prepare the refractive lenticule.

Cryolathe

The Barraquer cryolathe consists of a modified Levin contact lens lathe to which freezing circuits and digital micrometers among other necessary changes have been added. After removal with the microkeratome, the host cornea is placed in a solution designed to protect the keratocytes from freeze damage before cryolathing. The tissue is then turned on the cryolathe (Figs 26–2 and 26–3). During lathing, the corneal tissue, the head stock of the lathe on which the cornea is mounted, and the lathing tool are all brought to approximately −20°C by evaporating carbon dioxide. After reshaping, it is thawed and replaced in the host bed.

The Barraquer-type cryolathe is accurate but technically complex and expensive. Both theoretical and experimental considerations have triggered an effort to simplify this procedure and possibly eliminate the necessity for freezing the tissue. While the process of freezing enables precise shaping of the resected disc, it nonetheless results in keratocyte death and considerable postoperative corneal edema. Both of these factors

TABLE 18–1. SURGICAL INSTRUMENTS FOR REFRACTIVE LAMELLAR KERATOPLASTY

	Keratomileusis with Freezing	Keratomileusis in Situ	Epikeratophakia	Excimer Keratomileusis	LASIK
Colibri eyelid speculum	Yes	Yes	Yes	Yes	Yes
Fixation ring	Yes	Yes	No	Yes	Yes
Applanation lens	Yes	Yes	No	Yes	Yes
Preoperative tonometer	Yes	Yes	No	Yes	Yes
Microkeratome	Yes	Yes	No	Yes	Yes
Cap to protect the denuded cornea	Yes	No	No	Yes	No
Fenestrated lenticule spatula	Yes	Optional[a]	Yes	Yes	Optional[a]
Base for desiccation of the corneal disc	Yes	No	No	Yes	No
Delrin's bases	Yes	No	No	No	No
Base forceps	Yes	No	No	No	No
Cryolathe	Yes	No	No	No	No
Base for BKS planar keratomileusis	Yes	No	No	No	No
Colibri forceps	Yes	No	Yes	Yes	No
Tie forceps	Yes	Optional[b]	Yes	No	Optional[b]
Needleholder	Yes	Optional[b]	Yes	No	Optional[b]
Fine hair brushes	Yes	No	No	No	No
Lenticule container and preservative solutions	Yes	No	No	Yes	No
Heat container for defreezing the lenticule	Yes	No	No	No	No
Computer	Yes	No	No	No	No
Hassburg–Barron trephine	No	No	Yes	No	No
Vannas scissors	No	No	Yes	No	No
Excimer laser	No	No	No	Yes	Yes

[a]Yes if doing a cap technique.
[b]Yes only if the surgeons decide to suture the cap/flap.
Abbreviations: BKS, Barraquer–Krumeich–Swinger; LASIK, laser-assisted in situ keratomileusis.

contribute to a prolonged postoperative recovery period and to delayed epithelialization and epithelial ingrowth.

Microkeratome

Working in situ at the stromal level ensures greater accuracy in the resected thickness than is obtained by the extraocular manipulation of the tissue that occurs in keratomileusis with freezing or planar keratomileusis without freezing. Failure to adjust the thickness of the stromal lenticule to the value given in the table results in a residual defect of under- or overcorrection. Any irregularity in the resected lenticules leads to astigmatism. The microkeratome is associated with high accuracy, predictability, and postoperative stability. Variation in the speed of the passage of the microkeratome and in the pressure exerted by the surgeon's hands on the instrument will result in a different thickness and diameter than was calculated. The higher the speed, the thinner the lenticule, and vice versa.

An applanation tonometer assures adequate pressure for the resection (at least 65 mm Hg). Changeable base plates determine the thickness of the resected disc while various suction rings determine the diameter of the resection. Usually a base plate of 0.30 to 0.35 mm is used for keratophakia, MKM, and HKM, except in the case of high hyperopic corrections, where a 0.40-mm plate is necessary.

An applanation lens is used to verify the diameter of the proposed resection and, if unsatisfactory, the suction ring is changed. The diameter of the resected disc is 8.0 to 8.5 mm for KF or HKM. For MKM, the diameter is typically 7.25 mm when the cryolathe is used. Optical zones should be between 5.75 and 6.00 mm for HKM. Larger optical zones cause poor wound apposition, whereas smaller ones cause subjective symptomatology.

Lenticule Production

In autoplastic refractive procedures, the lenticule is prepared while the patient is on the operating table, whereas in homoplastic procedures the lenticule is usually prepared and stored before surgery.

A number of straightforward programs for calculating lenticule parameters are currently available and are easily modified based on an individual surgeon's results. For keratophaia and homoplastic MKM or HKM, a de-epithelialized donor eye (whole eye or tissue-cultured corneal scleral button) is used. The tissue should be free from scarring or irregularity but need not be of the quality used for transplantation. The tissue is dehydrated in a corneal press to bring it to normal dimensions. If a cornea with a scleral rim is used, it is placed in an artificial anterior chamber and a keratectomy is performed with the microkeratome. The disc obtained by keratectomy, whether from a donor or the patient's eye, is placed in a solution of dye (0.25% light green dye in buffer or McCarey–Kaufman solution) for up to 1 minute, frozen on the cryolathe for up to 2 minutes, and machined to the necessary dimensions. The keratophakia lenticule, which is a positive-meniscus lens, consists of stroma only and measures approximately 0.2 mm thick and 6 mm wide. The KM lenticule has an anterior membrane complex (without epithelium, if homoplastic) besides the stroma. Homoplastic lenticules can be used immediately, stored in the refrigerator for a few days, kept frozen at subzero temperatures, or lyophilized. They may also be ordered from a lens laboratory.

Refractive procedures are most commonly performed on an ambulatory basis under local or topical anesthesia. Reference marks are made on the epithelium over the visual axis to center the keratectomy and in a radial line to realign the anterior cap. A perilimbal suction ring is placed, and the intraocular pressure and proposed diameter of resection are verified. The ring is changed as necessary until the correct diameter is applanated. The circular lamellar disc, resected from the patient by a microkeratome, is replaced, aligned with the reference mark, and attached with a running eight-bite antitorque suture beginning at 12 o'clock. The interface must be cleaned meticulously. The previously prepared keratophakic lenticule is placed into the interface with a spatula and centered over the visual axis. The suture is tied and the tension adjusted under keratometric control so that it is not too tight and a small gap is present for 360°.

Previously, in those rare patients on whom cataract surgery was performed simultaneously, the lens extraction was performed after the keratectomy but before the donor lenticule placement to allow for better visualization.

Hyperopic and Myopic Keratomileusis

The techniques for HKM and MKM are essentially the same. Specialized equipment varies, depending on the technique. In autoplastic, a calculator and Barraquer cryolathe or BKS (Barraquer–Krumeich–Swinger)-1000 refractive set are necessary. Following the keratectomy,[5] the bed is protected with a plastic cap, and the resected disc is placed into a solution of dye and buffer. The thickness of the disc is measured immediately following the keratectomy and after it is removed from the staining solution. A dry run using the estimated computer settings essentially precludes perforation of the disc. The disc is then placed in the Barraquer cryolathe, frozen, and machined to the necessary curvature as determined by the calculator output, from the periphery toward the center in MKM and from the center toward the periphery in HKM. Tissue modification takes approximately 2 minutes. The modified disc, now called the lenticule, is replaced on the bed, aligned with a previously made reference mark, and sutured. Double-running, eight-bite sutures are usually used.

In homoplastic procedures, the resected disc is replaced by the donor lenticule. One needs a Barraquer microkeratome set with suction rings and associated devices to perform the lamellar keratectomy. A resection of a large diameter is preferred in this situation. Following keratectomy in the patient's eye, the resected disc is measured and evaluated for regularity of thickness. Next, the diameter of the bed is measured; its minimal diameter should be larger than the diameter of the precarved corneal lenticule. Then, the precarved lenticule is placed onto the keratectomized bed and the optic zone is centered over the visual axis. The lenticule is then sutured with a running suture of 12 to 16 bites.[7] Further refinements should lead to improved results and more widespread application of the procedure.

INSTRUMENTATION FOR PLANAR LAMELLAR REFRACTIVE KERATOPLASTY

Because freezing corneal tissue results in severe damage to the keratocytes and the lamellar architecture of the cornea, planar lamellar refractive keratoplasty was conceived as an alternative procedure. Two obvious advantages of this technique are a shorter recovery period of the visual function and stability of the correction because of the absence of cryotrauma to the corneal disc. However, this technique is much more unpredictable than keratomileusis with freezing. It also can predispose to corneal ectasia, if the desired correction is very high.

Surgical Technique

The nonfrozen planar keratomileusis technique is performed using the BKS–1000 set (Eye Tech, Balzers, Liechtenstein) (Fig 26–5). The BKS unit is less costly, less complex, and more portable. The technique is basically the same as the one used by Barraquer for keratomileusis, so that only certain steps have to be changed. When performing an MKM, the diameter of the resected disc is 9 mm when the BKS unit is used, and the disc is cut by a single pass with the microkeratome. The latter technique, which employs a newly developed instrument that obviates the need for freezing, requires a button large enough to ensure good fixation in the device.[8] For this reason, a microkeratome that allows a larger resection diameter than the classic Barraquer microkeratome has been newly designed.

When preparing the lenticule with the BKS device, no chemical solutions are used and the disc is modified without freezing.

INSTRUMENTATION FOR KERATOMILEUSIS IN SITU

The instruments necessary for keratomileusis in situ are also summaried in Table 18–1. In keratomileusis with freezing or planar lamellar refractive keratoplasty, the predictability of the surgery relies mostly on the accuracy of the crylathe or the BKS-1000 set, whereas the precision of keratomileusis in situ depends on the accuracy of the keratome. Understanding the microkeratome is vital for evaluating and selecting an ideal surgical instrument.

Microkeratome

The microkeratome has a high-speed oscillating blade that uses the principle of the carpenter's plane to resect corneal discs of different diameters and thickness from either the patient or the donor cornea (Fig 26–1). Keratomes are microprecise machines that can produce parallel-faced lamellar discs with accuracies of 5 to 10 μm. The accuracy of a keratectomy is extremely important for obtaining an ideal result from keratomileusis. Current techniques of keratomileusis, including the excimer laser and mechanical variations, and intracorneal lenses cannot be perfected without predictable, safe, consistent, and minimally traumatic microkeratome sections. The microkeratome looms paradoxically as both a pathway and a barrier to progress in lamellar refractive corneal surgery. Designs of microkeratomes for lamellar refractive surgery have changed significantly in recent years. The main characteristics of the four currently available systems for keratomileusis in situ are shown in Table 18–2. The quality of a keratectomy is assessed by its smoothness, roundness, and the uniformity of its depth and diameter. These qualities depend mostly on the variables of the keratome such as the speed of the pass, the rate of blade oscillation, the sharpness of the blade, the angle of the blade, the gap between the blade and the plate, and the downward force upon the

TABLE 18–2. COMPARISON OF CURRENTLY AVAILABLE MICROKERATOME SYSTEMS

	Steinway	SCMD	MicroPrecision	Draeger
Model name	Automatic Corneal Shaper	SCMD–2000	MicroPrecision™	Draeger Lamellar Keratome
Motor	Electric	Gas-turbine	Gas-turbine	Electric
Control unit	AC powered	DC/AC auto charge	Pneumatic	AC powered
Blade movement	Oscillating	Oscillating	Oscillating	Rotary
Blade cut rate	7500 cuts/min	14,800 cuts/min	20,000 cuts/min	500
Blade angle	25°	22.5°	9°	0°
Torque	Low	High	High	Low
Adjustable suction ring	Yes	No	No	No
Suction source	Electricity	Pneumatic	Pneumatic	Pneumatic
Change of depth plate	Interchangeable plates	Adjustable screw	Adjustable screw	Interchangeable plates
Digital calibrating micrometer	No	No	Yes	—
Reticule applanators	Single	Double	Double	—
Lock between applanator and fixation ring	Yes	No	No	—
Movement across cornea	Mechanical-gear driven	Manual	Manual	Mechanical-screw driven
Diameter of myopic refractive cut	4.2 mm	4.2 mm	4.5 mm	—

keratome. The intraocular pressure (IOP) also affects the result significantly.

The speed of the microkeratome pass is important. Very fast keratectomy results in scraping or plowing of the cornea, whereas slower keratectomies cut by the shearing action of the blade. Excessive speed of the microkeratome causes thinner resections so that very fast kerateceomies should be avoided. A slow and steady keratectomy is ideal. A velocity range of thickness stability exists in the range of 4 to 6 seconds.[9]

There are two major mechanisms of blade movement: oscillating and rotary. The rate of blade movement is another important variable. The speeds of current oscillating keratomes vary from motor-driven devices that reciprocate at 7500 rpm, to gas turbine devices that reciprocate at 20,000 rpm. According to the principle of kinematic reduction of friction, blade movement perpendicular to the cut direction will decrease resistance to cutting. Greater friction causes tissue to "plow up," resulting in an irregular keratectomy. Irregularities in the resected lenticules may lead to significant postoperative astigmatism. Scanning electron microscopic study of a keratectomy performed at 7000 rpm shows multiple ridges, while ridges are absent at 20,000 rpm.[9] There are also significant differences between the 7000- and 20,000-rpm rates in the cuts near Bowman's membrane. The 7000-rpm machine produced a saw-toothed edge that indicates intermittent, almost "pulse" cutting, while the 20,000-rpm machine produced very little of this "chatter." Chatter lines, as observed by Hofman et al,[10] could serve as an intrastromal diffractive optical source, sufficient to produce irregular astigmatism and reduce corrected visual acuity, particularly if the cap is not replaced with perfect alignment.

Another consideration is the sharpness of the cutting blade. Dull blades tend to scrape tissue and cut irregularly. Blades must be remarkably sharp and smooth to increase the depth consistency and smoothness. According to Hofmann's study, no fracture lines, debris, or score lines could be found after 15 repeated practice and experimental procedures with the same round, reusable Draeger circular blade,[10] whereas the blade of the two Barraquer style systems manifested rough, scored, or fractured cutting edges.

In keratome design, the relation between the blade and posterior plate is important. The Barraquer design has a blade angle set to approximately 25°, while other units have blade angles lower than 9°. Blades approaching tissue closer to the 0° plane may theoretically provide smoother resections and less bias or change in depth of cut from surgeon to surgeon. In designing the relation between the blade and posterior plate, it is important to consider how easily the cut cornea will feed through the gap between blade and plate after the cut has been performed. Bottlenecks can cause ripples on the cornea, and must be avoided, particularly when using keratomes with steep blade angles.

The gap is the distance between the blade and the plate. Some manufacturers use a series of plates of varying thicknesses to vary the gap. Plate thickness generally increases in 5-μm steps in this interchangeable system. Others use adjustable screws or differential micrometers to fine tune this distance. These differential micrometer systems use a Mitutoyo stand and measure the distance between the plate and blade to check the keratome gap. Once the gap is checked, changing it is simply a matter of rotating the micrometer screw. To test the gap on plate systems, a keratome holder stands the keratome vertically under the objective of a radial keratotomy microscope. Through the microscope, the surgeon can see the blade and its reflection from the plate. The distance from the blade to its reflection is then measured. When divided by two, this distance correlates with the thickness of the keratectomy. The differential micrometer seems to measure the gap more precisely. Not only can it move exact increments, but it also requires only one plate, thereby removing a variable in keratome construction.

Variation in the speed of the microkeratome passage will also result in a different thickness and diameter than was calculated. Ruiz automated the Barraquer-designed keratome, making the speed of the pass constant (Fig 26–8). One additional interesting feature of the automated keratome is the reverse position. Using this, the surgeon can accomplish a flap or hinged keratectomy by advancing, then reversing, the keratome head to a prescribed point (Fig 26–14). However, flaps can also be constructed using manual keratomes. After completing the partial keratectomy, the surgeon needs only to break the suction and the flap will pass gently through the gap. While manual keratomes do not produce ridges, the automation gears of automated keratomes may give rise to some ridges. The pressure exerted by the surgeon's hands on the instrument during surgery will affect the result as well. The weight of the apparatus upon the eye during the keratectomy is standardized by the Ruiz automated design, while the weight of the surgeon's hand may affect the depth and roundness of the keratectomy when a manual keratome is used.[11–14]

Maintaining IOP is critical, as lower pressures result in shallower keratectomies. Intraocular pressure at the beginning of the keratectomy is always greater than at its termination. If the keratome is sensitive to IOP, the keratectomy thickness may change as IOP changes. It is thus important to study the IOP dependence of a keratome. Strong suction that maintains high IOP requires good exposure of the ocular surface and minimal conjunctival chemosis and edema. Some systems have one adjustable ring that allows for an infinite number of keratectomy sizes. Others have multiple rings that must be placed and removed manually until the right applanation is met. Both systems have their drawbacks. The excessive manipulation needed for the multiring system may lead to greater chemosis and conjunctival edema, which can lower the IOP for a shallow keratectomy, while the adjustable rings are often larger and difficult to place on the eye. A suitable small, adjustable ring is, however, not available now. It would be ideal for a keratome to have a control mechanism that would permit variable suction power to maintain a constant vacuum setting in the suction ring, thereby sustaining the eye at a stable pressure throughout the keratectomy.

AUTOMATED LAMELLAR KERATOPLASTY (ALK)

Keratomileusis in situ is a highly effective surgical technique. However, the microkeratome speed and pressure have been mentioned as factors that lead to a diverging outcome in the desired lenticules. After a search for a technique that excluded these factors, the Automatic Corneal Shaper was developed. It is used to perform ALK and ensures accurate, regular, and predictable resections by making the procedure independent of the human factor. Success depends on close attention to detail in the assembly, operation, and maintenance of the instrument. The device is a precisely manufactured instrument designed to cut corneal lenticules of preselected thickness and diameter automatically. This feature allows the ALK to be more accurate and predictable (see Fig 34–9).

Automated lamellar keratoplasty was reviewed by the American Academy of Ophthalmology (Committee on Ophthalmic Procedures Assessments) to evaluate its safety, efficacy, clinical effectiveness, and appropriate uses.[14] The Academy found in its preliminary review reason for more rigorous evaluation. There were no peer-reviewed articles in the literature as of October 1995 that answered the questions of safety, efficacy and

optical quality of the cuts in a scientifically sound manner.[14] The following is a description of the components of the instruments used in ALK.

The Shaper Head

The shaper head has two parts, upper and lower, joined by a hinge that facilitates its assembly. After a blade is placed between the two parts, the head is closed and fastened by a nut. A motor is connected to the upper body of the shaper head. There are also three pinions that are the core of the automation mechanism of the microkeratome. The movement of the head is uniform and stops automatically. This solves one of the main problems of the original manual technique, namely, the lack of continuous movement of the head at a constant speed, which may result in irregular resections.

The blade is critically important for a successful operation and must meet a number of requirements. The sharp edge has to be of highest quality, and the length, thickness, and type of bevel must be carefully checked. Each blade is individually marked with a dot that has to be visible when the blade is placed in the blade holder. If it is inverted, the resection thickness will differ completely from the desired one. The plates are essential for defining the thickness of the tissue to be resected. The varying thickness of the plates permits varying distances between the plate itself and the sharp edge of the blade. This allows prior adjustment of the resection thickness within a variation range as small as 5 μm. The thickness of each plate is indicated by a number marked on its front side.

The Shaper Motor

The motor used to transmit motive force to the corneal shaper is a 12-V micromotor rotating at 7500 rpm.

The Pneumatic Fixation Ring

The ring basically consists of two parts: one fixates the patient eye and the other raises or lowers the level of the corneal passage, thus varying the diameter of the resection. It also has an adjustable height. It fulfills three basic functions:

1. To fix the ocular globe
2. To increase the IOP up to more than 65 mm Hg so that the resection is uniform and regular as low pressure usually results in an irregular cut and unpredictable resection thickness
3. To serve as a guide for the passage of the shaper head

The Applanation Lens

This lens is a plastic element enabling the surgeon to assess the diameter of the resection to be done; it must be directly related to the height of the fixation ring. The ring on the applanation lens can also be used to verify centration during the procedure.

The Control Unit

The control unit contains the power source for the motor and the connection for the pedal that controls the passage of the shaper head. The pedal has two positions: one for forward and the other for backward movement.

Surgical Technique for Automated Lamellar Keratoplasty

This technique is basically used for myopic, hyperopic, and homoplastic ALK. The setup and execution until removal of the corneal disc are virtually identical; in these techniques they then vary slightly in the use and calibration of the corneal shaper, the manipulation of the stromal bed, and the reattachment of the corneal disc. After the blepharostat has been placed and the cornea has been marked (Fig 26–13), the pneumatic fixation ring has to be placed so that the eyeball is as exposed as possible. It allows slight manual adjustment of the position of the eyeball and helps to raise the IOP in a uniform manner to 65 mm of Hg or more. The tonometer is a conic lens that works by applanation. When adequate IOP has been obtained, the resection diameter is graded with the aid of the applanation lens. The lens is slowly lowered until it rests horizontally. If necessary, the applanation may be centered by slightly shifting the lens. The cornea must be perfectly dry before the lens is placed to avoid a false applanation. A 7.2 applanation lens should be used for the first resection. As soon as the applanation lens is placed on the ring, its height must be adjusted, using the regulating wrench of the ring, to make the applanation coincide with the inner circle marked on the surface of the lens. The wrench is first placed in the corresponding hole and fixed by clockwise rotation. Next, with the wrench fixed, the height of the ring is adjusted using the micrometer located on the upper end of the wrench. When a given height of the ring has produced the applanation needed for the operation, the resection diameter will be equal to the applanation diameter. The applanation lens and the adjustment wrench are removed. The spring butt on the ring handle must be rotated 180° to allow the shaper to pass freely.

The next stage of the surgical procedure is the use of the corneal shaper. It should be stressed that using the shaper without a plate may cause the most severe complication of the procedure, namely, penetration of the blade into the anterior chamber. The shaper should be placed tilted on the fixation ring, then lowered to the horizontal position and inserted into the notch on the side of the handle. The shaper is gently pushed forward until a tooth of the largest pinion engages the first tooth of the dented rack. In that position the shaper is ready to slide and perform the resection (Fig 26–11). When the pedal is pressed, the shaper starts sliding and cutting the disk. It stops automatically when the large pinion reaches the end of the rack. The shaper is then removed inversely to its insertion. There are then two options for the fixation ring: The first is to remove the ring simultaneously with the resected disk. The second is to continue the suction with the ring placed while an assistant removes the resected disk from the corneal shaper and changes the plate for the second resection, using a previously selected applanation lens and the regulating wrench of the ring. The thickness of the disc is measured, and, when the disc is dry, it is placed in a closed container to avoid contamination and extreme changes in its thickness. Recently, the shaper has been changed to obtain a flap instead of the disc, so that all these steps for removing and storing it are no longer necessary. The corneal bed should be inspected, which is more easily done if the surface is dry. The centering for the resection has to be done in both the corneal bed and the disc. The margins of the bed should be equidistant from the outer marked circle, and the inner landmark should be concentric with the circumference of the disc.

Myopic Automated Lamellar Keratoplasty

If the fixation ring was removed, it has to be replaced to perform the second resection; if the fixation ring was not removed, only the applanation lens is placed. The lens has to be selected before the surgery, according to the calculation table, and must be placed on a dry corneal bed. The height-regulating wrench is gyrated until the applanation touches the inner margin of the circle that is marked on the lens. Afterward it is removed and the shaper is positioned as before. When the resection is completed, both the shaper and the ring are removed and the lenticule is examined for the accuracy of its measure. The interface and the disc must be washed with a brush and saline solution, which will prevent cells from proliferating on the interface and produce a much clearer cornea postoperatively. All excess fluid has to be removed by aspiration, and the corneal bed air-dried. As soon as the disc is placed back, the anterior curvature of the cornea will show an applanation equivalent to the said correction.

Hyperopic Automated Lamellar Keratoplasty

No refractive resection is necessary for the correction of hyperopia (Fig 26–17). Once the corneal disc has been checked, the surgeon should wash the corneal bed, air-dry it, and replace the disc in the bed.

For proper replacement of the disc, the surgeon should check the epithelial and stromal sides. They should be identified throughout the surgery, starting as soon as the disc is removed from the microkeratome, and afterward, when it is measured, stored, and cleaned.

To prevent the disc from folding, it is advisable to place it on a fenestrated spatula. Rotate the spatula and lower the disc toward the eye. With a Weck sponge in each hand, quickly rotate the disc to align it with the pararadial reference line. When placed back in the eye, the disc should be in its original position. If, instead of forming a straight line, the segments form an angulation, then the epithelial side is against the stroma. If this occurs, the disc must be removed, both the disk and the corneal surface should be rewashed, and then the disc can be repositioned. Air-dry the edge of the disc and check for centration. Any air trapped under the disc should be gently pushed out with a forceps. Once alignment and centration are verified, there is no need for further manipulation of the disc. Air may be used to enhance the cohesion of the disc to the corneal–stromal surface. Do not overdry the cornea with the air as this may cause corneal irregularities. After carefully removing the eyelid speculum, allow the lids to close and make sure that the disc is not displaced by the lid margins.

Homoplastic Automated Lamellar Keratoplasty

After the corneal disk is obtained by the method described above, it is discarded and a new one is created from donor tissue. The primary procedure must be repeated, using either a whole donor eye or an artificial anterior chamber for anterior donor sections. It is necessary to suture the donor disc to the recipient cornea because the alignment of the donor tissue cannot be precisely duplicated.

Suturing the Corneal Disc

Sutures can be placed only after the position of the corneal disk is rectified. Usually the material used is 10-0 nylon. An eight-bite antitorque running suture is placed. The needle should take 0.75 mm from the disc and 1.0 mm from the periphery. The knot should be buried peripherally.

MICROLAMELLAR KERATOPLASTY

The SCMD system has similar features as the Automatic Corneal Shaper.[14] Some of the different features are addressed here.

Power Console

The control console contains the vacuum pump, the battery, and the vacuum-release solenoid. A multipin connector on the front panel connects the foot pedals. A similar connector on the back connects the rechargeable pump battery. A tubulature connector on the left front panel connects the suction tubing and a "quick-connect" fitting on the right is for the keratome handle. The motor speed is preset at 14,000 rpm (35 to 40 on the pressure dial). Two labeled foot pedals, one for the vacuum and the other for the turbine motor, connect to the console via a single plug. The foot switch does not activate a forward and reverse motion of the microkeratome head. Keratectomy in this system is controlled by the surgeon. The high speed of the turbine may allow for consistent cuts with varying speed of translation across the cornea. However, excessive changes in speed of translation should be avoided. The surgeon should make cuts that feel smooth and natural.

Adjustable Microkeratome Head

The plate in the SCMD microkeratome is continuously adjustable and is not fixed, as it is in changeable plate units. This plate is set by inserting the microkeratome head upside down into the gauging ring attached to the stand. After centering the keratome head within the gauging ring, lift the gauge anvil with the lever on the thickness gauge and slide the head into position. For more accurate reading of the gauge, set the plate from the highest setting to the lowest.

The Pneumatic Fixation Ring

The SCMD system provides typical vacuum fixation rings. Rings are used with applanator lenses to establish disc diameter. A ring with a thin shoulder allows more cornea to be exposed in the aperture and a larger corneal area will be applanated, while a ring with a thick shoulder allows less cornea to be exposed in the aperture and a smaller corneal area will be applanated. In the correct ring, the applanated area should lie just inside the inner edge of the reticule. In a human, a number 8 ring typically yields a disc of 7.25 mm in diameter. However, a number 3 or 4 ring may occasionally be needed. Unlike the larger adjustable ring, the pneumatic fixation rings are smaller and easier to place on the eye. However, excessive manipulation of the multiring system should be avoided to prevent chemosis and conjunctival edema, which can lower the IOP for a shallow keratectomy. Upward and downward motion of the vacuum fixation ring during tissue resection will cause depth variability and should be avoided.

MICROLAMELLAR KERATOMILEUSIS SYSTEM

The MicroPrecision™ microlamellar keratomileusis system has been available since 1991. Most of its features are summarized in Table 18–2.

Microkeratome Head

The microkeratome head in the MicroPrecision™ system also has an adjustable plate system with finite adjustments from 0 to 500 μm in 1-μm increments, allowing for greater accuracy and less built-in error. This may result in better postoperative refractive predictability. The microkeratome head has a micrometer attached to the adjustable plate, which allows for accurate adjustment of the plate under the microscope within the sterile field. The blade angle is set at 9° so that the blade approaches the tissue closer to the 0° plane. It may provide smoother resections and less bias or change in depth of cut from surgeon to surgeon. The open-blade window and its gradual slope allow a direct view of the cutting action during surgery. The tissue does not need to work its way up a 25° slope so that the rippling effect that can cause bottlenecking of the resected tissue is prevented. It may also be easier to remove the corneal button from the keratome.

Digital-Calibrating Micrometer Stand

The digital-calibrating micrometer stand measures the gap between the blade and the adjustable plate. It allows the surgeon to set the depth of the resection to within 1 μm so that there is a greater degree of accuracy, a more precise depth of cut, and, presumably, better postoperative results.

Turbine-Driven Motor

The blade has an oscillation rate of 20,000 rpm with a high torque force, which may provide smoother and more consistent resection with less chatter. The turbine

system avoids inconsistent AC or DC current fluctuations.

ROTATING MICROKERATOME (THE DRAEGER ROTOR KERATOME SYSTEM)

This system was developed for lamellar surgical procedures. It can be used safely in either the patient or the donor cornea.

Micromotors

Two electric micromotors are used to provide well-coordinated speed in the blade rotation and in the transverse movement during the lamellar cutting process. This gives a clean and even tissue interface. The handled keratome and the integrated keratome of the system block are operated through the foot switch of the PowerPac console.

In contrast to the oscillating movements in other systems, the cut is carried out in a continuous and unidirectional rotating motion. To avoid vibrating the tissue during the cutting, a fast-running blade, which always rotates in the same direction, is used. The blade advances through the tissue in an automatic and steady slow speed. The feed rate of the blade in relation to its circumferential speed has been established in a way that minimizes the insult to the tissue. The wound bed remains free of edges and grooves.

The Draeger microkeratome has a pressure plate moving ahead of the rotor blade to ensure that the applanated corneal surface is always parallel to the plane of the cutting blade throughout the entire lamellar dissection. A suction ring attaches to the limbus firmly and in a circular manner, thus ensuring the position and direction of the pressure plate and blade path throughout the entire cut. The vacuum is produced and adjusted by the microsurgical operation units available in hospitals.

The standard setting of the lamellar thickness is 0.25 mm. However, the respective spacer may be exchanged to obtain thicknesses of 0.15 mm or 0.35 mm. Components of the refractive system include:

1. A base plate with system block, integrated rotor keratome, and receptacle ring
2. A die holder
3. Exchangeable dies of 9.5-mm diameter, each with curvatures mathematically equivalent to +8, +12, +15, +18, +21, +24, −8, −12, −15, −18, and −21 D
4. An external ring of 9.5-mm internal diameter

5. A fixation clamp
6. A micron gauge

Refractive Correction Techniques

In the keratomileusis procedure, a lamella of 9.5-mm diameter and a thickness of approximately 0.35 mm is used as dissected from the patient's eye with the hand-held keratome. In both cases the epithelium has to be removed thoroughly.

In preparation for the refractive correction cut, the die holder is inserted into the receptacle. A die with the desired refractive correction effect is inserted into the die holder and held firmly by the fixation clamp. The external ring to be placed around the refractive die has a prominence of 0.10 mm encircling the corneal disc. The corneal disc to be reshaped (either the donor lenticule or the patient's lamella) is placed onto the die upside down (epithelial side down, stroma up). A vacuum is connected and the 9.5-mm corneal disk is sucked firmly to the die. The integrated keratome of the system block is moved on its slide into the operating start position, and the height adjustment knob is turned down to the zero-position stop, bringing the circular blade level with the external ring of the refractive die. Now the height adjustment knob is turned upward to lift the keratome blade to the level of remaining lenticule thickness desired after the refractive cut. The additional thickness to the initial 0.10 mm of the external ring will be indicated by the integrated micron gauge.

Now irrigation is started and the electrically driven refractive correction cut is made across the die, leaving a final lenticule on the die with myopic or hyperopic correction according to the type of the die used. Dies with convex centers render the lenticule thinner in the center (for myopic correction), and dies with concave centers render the lenticule thicker in the center (for hyperopic correction). Sufficient rinsing is particularly important during the refractive cut to avoid friction. Experience has shown that the use of a solution of 0.05% healon in BSS may be very helpful in this condition.

PHOENIX LAMELLAR LENTICULAR KERATOPLASTY SYSTEM

The Universal Keratome (UK) manufactured by Phoenix Keratek offers potential advantages over existing machines. Unlike other machines which require multiple suction rings, applanation lenses and plates, it is a narrow unit with built-in suction ring. The vacuum settings on the machine can be raised or lowered to stan-

dardize the pressure in the eye prior to initiating the incision. The handpiece consists of a removable optical PMMA insert which is ordered for each patient and a smooth blade with a zero degree angle of attack. The machine is designed to compress the cornea into the optical insert which can have a lamellar (planar) shape to create LASIK flaps or remove myopic (plano-convex) or hyperopic (plano-concave) shaped sections on a second pass technique termed lamellar lenticular keratoplasty (Fig 18–1A). Scanning electron microscopic (SEM) studies have confirmed that a lenticular shaped tissue resection is possible unlike other microkeratomes which remove planar (parallel-faced) resections. The oscillating blade (14,000 revolutions per minute) moves across the cornea at a constant speed of 1 mm/second via a linear actuator. The zero degree angle of attack creates no blade chatter marks. Since the corneal tissue is not bent during the resection of the flap, there will be a reduction in the incidence of breaks in Bowman's

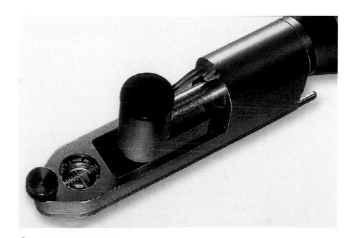

A

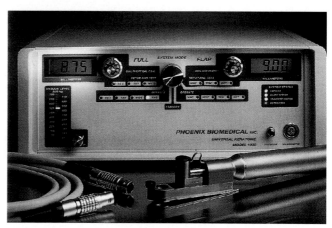

B

Figure 18–1. Universal Keratome. **A.** Handpiece. **B.** Console.

layer. The console itself controls the flap diameter electronically without the need for a mechanical stop mechanism to create a hinge (Fig 18–1B). The surgeon is able to visualize the entire procedure through the optically clear PMMA insert and can center the keratome easily by viewing preplaced corneal marks through the optical insert.

This machine should be ideal for performing the primary cut during LASIK. Further clinical work will need to be done to see if the second pass technique (lamellar lenticular keratoplasty) can reproducibly correct refractive errors.

INSTRUMENTATION IN EPIKERATOPLASTY

Epikeratoplasty (EKP) is a procedure that eliminates the need for a keratectomy on the central cornea. This is a simpler technique than keratomileusis with freezing, but it demands a normal corneal surface for its maintenance. It is less predictable and requires a long time for total visual rehabilitation. It uses a donor cornea instead of the host cornea to achieve the correction of a refractive error.

After removing the corneal epithelium, a precarved lenticule of appropriate refractive power is placed on top of the Bowman's membrane of the patient's cornea; it is then anchored into a circumferential keratectomy (Figs 26–4 and 29–1). The final central corneal thickness may be increased by 0.35 mm or more, depending on the refractive correction. The donor cornea is treated the same as a keratophakia and keratomileusis lenticule, but two steps are added: dehydrating the donor cornea through a corneal press[11] and freeze-drying the tissue after it has been reshaped on the cryolathe.[12]

Myopic EKP was introduced invoking as the main benefit of its capacity to correct severe myopia of up to 30 D. Nevertheless, its use has declined sharply because of associated problems like its extended recovery period, unpredictability, instability of the correction, and epithelial changes that often mandate removal of the lenticule.

The current refractive procedure of choice for pediatric patients is EKP for several reasons. First, it may be more reversible than keratophakia or MKM in youngsters. Thus, should an inaccurate result be obtained or should the refraction change, the lenticule can be replaced. More important, the classic Barraquer microkeratome cannot be used in children younger than four years of age, as the suction rings are too large to adapt to such small globes and narrow palpebral fissures. Therefore, because manual keratectomy is necessary EPI is the only alternative in this age range.

Surgical Technique

Instruments necessary for EKP are summarized in Table 18–1. Myopic EKP begins by marking the visual axis and removing most of the corneal epithelium except for a small central area that contains the visual axis mark and a small peripheral cuff.[13] Removal is initiated by rubbing the epithelium with a blunted cellulose sponge soaked in 4% cocaine solution and completed by rubbing with a Paton spatula. Vigorous aspiration and irrigation are necessary to remove any remnants of the epithelium. Next, a Hessburg–Barron trephine (7 mm) is appropriately set and placed, and a keratotomy is performed to approximately 0.30 mm in depth. Following the keratotomy, the central epithelium is removed, and a 360° wedge resection is made with Vannas scissors central to and continuous with the keratotomy (see Chapter 29). This allows for fixation of the lenticule and migration of the host keratocytes into the acellular lenticule. Following the keratectomy, a spatula is passed peripherally at the level of the base of the keratectomy to crate a 360° potential space approximately 1 mm peripheral to the initial keratotomy. The precarved lenticule, which has been hydrated, is then placed on top of Bowman's membrane and sutured with eight interrupted nylon sutures. The sutures are passed to bisect the thickness of the wing of the lenticule and are then inserted at the base of the keratectomy into the groove of the potential space created by the spatula. This allows for the peripheral wing to be adequately fixed and prevent sliding postoperatively.[7]

LASER IN SITU KERATOMILEUSIS (LASIK)

Experience with planar keratomileusis and the excimer laser in treating mild and moderate myopia led to the idea of joining these two techniques and instruments to take advantage of the high corrective capacity of keratomileusis and the excimer laser's precision in tissue removal. The aim was to overcome the technical difficulties associated with the refractive incision of both the cryolathe and the nonfrozen keratomileusis technique, and thus to achieve an accurate, reproducible, and predictable surgical result (see Chapter 34).

In theory, the combination of surgical procedures and laser photoablation complicates statistical control and the predictability of results because a considerable number of technical variables are involved.[14] In practice, however, the predictability of refractive correction is excellent, surpassing that obtained with purely surgical techniques. The excimer laser can be used to ablate corneal tissue from the resected corneal cap or on the corneal bed. The latter is termed *laser-assisted in situ keratomileusis* (LASIK). The instruments necessary for both procedures are summarized in Table 18–1. Details of these surgical techniques are described in Chapters 26 and 34. The refractive results indicate that this technique may be a valuable tool for treating moderate and mild myopia (Figs 26–22, 23, 24). As laser software improves, this operation should become a promising choice for higher degrees of myopia.

REFERENCES

1. Barraquer JI. Special methods in corneal surgery. In: King JHJ, McTigue JW, eds. *The Cornea.* Washington, DC: Butterworths; 1965.
2. Barraquer JI. Keratomileusis for myopia and aphakia. *Ophthalmology.* 1981;88:701–708.
3. Walsh PM, Guyton DL. Comparison of two methods of marking the visual axis on the cornea during radial keratotomy. *Am J Ophthalmol.* 1984;97:660–661. Letter.
4. Waring GO III. *Refractive Keratotomy for Myopia and Astigmatism.* St. Louis: Mosby-Year Book; 1992;721–774.
5. Steinberg EB, Waring G III. Comparison of two methods of marking the visual axis on the cornea during radial keratotomy. *Am J Ophthalmol.* 1983;96:605–608.
6. Ruiz L. *A Manual on Automated Lamellar Keratoplasty.* Chiron Intra Optics Educational Series.
7. Binder PS. Pathologic findings in cases of refractive corneal surgery. In: *Cornea, Refractive Surgery, and Contact Lenses. Transactions of the New Orleans Academy of Ophthalmology.* New York: Raven Press; 1986:143–159.
8. Binder PS, Akers PH, Deg JK, Zavala EY. Refractive keratoplasty: microkeratome evaluation. *Arch Ophthalmol.* 1982;100:802–806.
9. Rozakis GW. *Refractive Lamellar Keratoplasty.* Thorofare, NJ: Slack, Inc; 1994.
10. Hofmann RF, Bechara SJ. An independent evaluation of second generation suction microkeratomes. *Refract Corneal Surg.* 1992;8:348–354.
11. Safir A, McDonald MB, Klyce SD, Werblin TP, Kaufman HE. The cornea press: restoring donor corneas to normal dimensions and hydration before cryolathing. *Ophthalmic Surg.* 1983;14:327–331.
12. Maguen E, Nesburn AB. A new technique for lathing lyophilized cornea for refractive keratoplasty. *Arch Ophthalmol.* 1982;100:119–121.
13. Swinger CA. Surgical correction of myopia. In: *Cornea, Refractive Surgery, and Contact Lenses. Transactions of the New Orleans Academy of Ophthalmology.* New York: Raven Press; 1986.
14. American Academy of Ophthalmology. Automated lamellar keratoplasty. *Ophthalmology.* 1996;103:852–861.

SECTION IV

Incisional Refractive Surgery

CHAPTER 19

Radial Keratotomy: Operative Techniques

Ernest W. Kornmehl

HISTORY AND BACKGROUND

Donder's treatise *On the Anomalies of Accommodation and Refraction of the Eye*[1] clearly described the clinical and optical principles of refractive errors. This information allowed future clinicians to develop surgical techniques for correcting astigmatism and myopia. Schiotz[2] of Norway was the first ophthalmic surgeon to use an incision to treat astigmatism in 1885. He used a limbal incision 4 months postoperatively to reduce 19.50 diopters of with-the-rule postcataract astigmatism to 7.00 D. In 1894 Bates of New York City suggested an operation for astigmatism after observing six patients with peripheral traumatic and surgical corneal scars who developed corneal flattening in the meridian that intersected the scar with no change in the meridian 90° away.[3] Faber of the Netherlands was the first to use anterior transverse keratotomy to address the occupational needs of his patients.[4] In 1895 a 19-year-old man was rejected from the Royal Military Academy because his uncorrected vision was 20/60 and his refraction was +0.75 −1.50 × 30. Three weeks following a 6-mm-long full-thickness incision at the corneoscleral limbus at axis 120, his uncorrected vision was 20/25 and his refraction was +0.75 −0.75 × 120. Lucciola of Italy reported 10 cases of nonperforating corneal incisions to flatten the steep meridian in 1896.[5]

Lans's doctoral thesis, "Experimental Studies of the Treatment of Astigmatism with Non-perforating Corneal Incisions," was the first published description of systematic experiments describing the effects of nonperforating corneal incisions in rabbits.[6] The results of Lans's studies defined the following basic principles of radial keratotomy[7]:

- Deeper incisions have a greater effect.
- Peripheral bulging and central flattening is induced by nonperforating corneal incisions parallel to the limbus (Fig 19–1A).
- Scarring of keratotomy wounds cause further flattening of the central cornea (Fig 19–1B).
- Arcuate incisions parallel to the limbus cause flattening in the axis perpendicular to them (Fig 19–1C).
- Radial wounds flatten the central cornea and produce peripheral steepening in the meridian parallel to the wounds (Fig 19–1D).

Modern surgery for myopia was initiated by Sato. He observed that patients with keratoconus who experienced breaks in Descemet's membrane and hydrops eventually developed corneal flattening. He subsequently designed the "Sato knife," which was a modified de Lapersonne's knife with an angled sharp tip that could enter the anterior chamber through the limbus

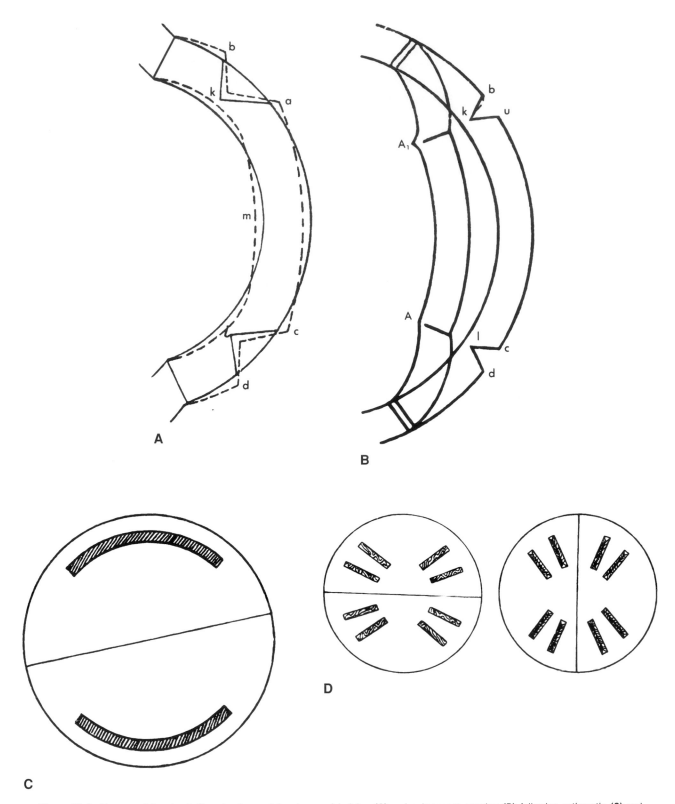

Figure 19–1. Diagram of Lans's studies showing peripheral corneal bulging **(A)** and subsequent scarring **(B)** following astigmatic **(C)** and radial **(D)** keratotomy.

(Fig 19–2A). Sato performed posterior keratotomy in 10 eyes of eight keratoconus patients in 1939[8] and documented corneal flattening. Shortly thereafter, Okamura designed a thin blade with a guard to limit the depth of the anterior corneal incisions (Fig 19–2B). Between 1940 and 1950 Sato performed numerous experiments in rabbits to evaluate the effect of posterior and anterior radial and tangential incisions on corneal curvature. In the early 1950s hundreds of patients underwent anterior and posterior keratotomy for myopia. Patients were lined up on tables adjacent to one another while the surgeon moved from table to table. If an aqueous leak was noted the surgeon would stop, operate on the next patient on the adjoining table, and then return to the first patient to complete the operation. In 1953 Sato, with his colleagues, published his experience with anterior and posterior half incisions in 32 eyes[9] and concluded "this new surgical approach is a proven, safe method which definitely cures or adequately alleviates over 95% of all cases of myopia in Japan."

Unfortunately, the role of the corneal endothelium was not understood when Sato was performing his rabbit experiments and clinical studies. The first case of corneal decompensation in a patient that underwent the "Sato operation" was not documented until 15 years af-ter Sato's death. Of the 681 eyes that were operated on at Juntendo University, 170 eyes in 103 patients were followed up to March 1986, with no information on the other 511 eyes.[10] Of the 170 eyes, 121 (71%) developed bullous keratopathy, and 49 eyes (21%) retained clear corneas. The average time between surgery and the onset of edema was 20 years (range: 15 to 25 years). The results of penetrating keratoplasty in these eyes were much worse than noted in eyes with bullous keratopathy for other reasons. This might be attributed to the incised peripheral host cornea having a reduced number of endothelial cells causing the donor endothelium to spread in order to cover this area, depleting its reserve to the point of edema. Despite the tragic consequences of Sato's work, his rabbit data and clinical results reinforced the findings of Lans and established the following: the effect of the keratotomy increases with greater depth, number, and length of incision; radial incisions placed in one meridian flatten that meridian and slightly flatten the perpendicular meridian; and crossed incisions create more pronounced scarring and should be avoided. Sato's rabbit experiments did not provide insight into the importance of the endothelium because the rabbit endothelium has a regenerative capacity. Sato found anterior incisions alone to be ineffective because

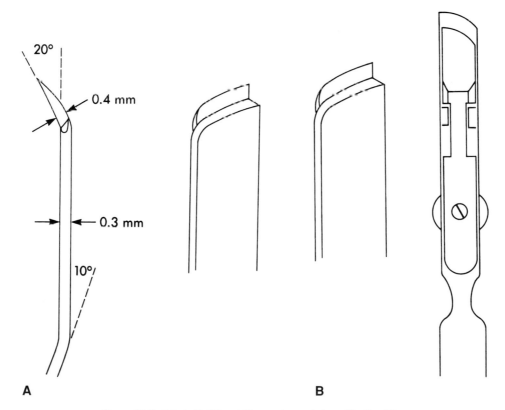

Figure 19–2. Sato knife **(A)** and Okamura's guarded modification **(B)**.

the eye was softened by the limbal stab wounds made prior to the anterior cuts. In addition, the Okamura knife was not sharp enough to cut to 80% depth of the cornea.

Fyodorov visited Japan in 1960 shortly after Professor Sato's death and met with Akiyama to learn Sato's technique of radial keratotomy. On returning to the Soviet Union, he performed Sato's operation with poor results. In 1969 Yanaleyev performed four to twenty-four anterior radial incisions in 426 eyes of 231 patients. The razor blade was set to 0.5 mm in all cases and 80% of the patients (342 eyes) were followed for at least 6 months. He found an average correction of 3 to 4 D, with 73% remaining stable and 27% regressing.[11] Impressed with Yanaleyev's results, Fyodorov and colleagues set out to remove the art from radial keratotomy (RK) and devise mathematical formulas based on anatomic and mechanical parameters of the cornea to calculate the results accurately in each individual case. Using a rabbit model, Durnev observed the change in corneal power was the same with 16 incisions as with 32[12] and documented increased effect with smaller optical zones. He found that optical zones less than 3 mm reduced visual acuity.[13] Fyodorov stressed the importance of each surgeon computing an individual coefficient to allow for variations in surgical technique, especially incision depth. In 1974 Fyodorov began performing anterior RK on patients, using freehand razor-blade fragments in a blade holder. The depth of the incision was checked with a depth gauge. Crystal blades were used in 1978 and guarded knives were made in 1979. Using photokeratoscopy, Fyodorov observed that the central cornea flattened and the peripheral cornea steepened following surgery. He attributed this to intraocular pressure (IOP) pushing the cornea forward after the circular deep ligament was severed.[14] Fyodorov reported exceptionally good results: All 230 eyes with baseline refractions of −1 to −6 D achieved a final refraction within 0.50 D of emmetropia 1.5 years after surgery.[15] These exceptional results have never been replicated.

Bores performed the first RK in the United States at the Kresge Eye Institute in November 1978 with extensive coverage in the popular press. Shortly thereafter a small number of US ophthalmologists began performing the procedure, also with considerable media coverage. The majority of US ophthalmologists remained skeptical and chose not to perform the procedure until further controlled animal and human clinical trials were completed.[16] In early 1981 the Prospective Evaluation of Radial Keratotomy (PERK) was funded. The study protocol called for centrifugal-eight incisions with the diameter of the optical zone based on the spherical equivalent of the refractive error. The effect of age on the final outcome was not appreciated at this time. The PERK investigators employed diamond-bladed knives, ultrasonic pachymeters, and a ridge-style gauge block with a knife cradle. A small group of ophthalmologists opposed implementation of the PERK study and considered it restraint of trade. They felt the procedure had already been proved to be safe and effective, although there was only one report in the American literature.[14] Subsequently separate lawsuits were filed against members of the PERK study[17] and the American Academy of Ophthalmology and three members of its Board of Directors.[18] The case against the members of the PERK study was settled in May 1985 for $250,000 to avoid continued payment of expensive legal fees and the inordinate time commitment that would have been necessary to go to trial. The United States Court of Appeals for the Seventh Circuit found in favor of the Academy on March 3, 1989.

The debate over RK was calmed, and its popularity was reduced in the mid-1980's by the publication of the PERK results and other studies, by the reluctance of insurance companies to cover the procedure, and the higher malpractice premiums demanded by some carriers. Publication of the PERK data and other well-performed studies statistically defined the safety, efficacy, predictability, and stability of the RK procedure.

Renewed interest in RK developed in 1990. This is attributed to both a reduction in fees by third-party payers for nonelectve ophthalmic procedures and by the RK "system" devised by Casebeer. Casebeer performed over 6000 procedures and developed a nomogram using a standardized technique. This enabled novice surgeons to begin performing RK safely and with satisfactory results using his "cookbook" method.

PATIENT SELECTION

Careful patient selection is the key to a successful refractive surgery practice. A good surgical and visual result will not satisfy every patient. It is the surgeon's responsibility to avoid operating on patients with unrealistic expectations, especially when radial keratotomy is being considered. The procedure is successful only if the patient's expectations are met (see Chapter 7).

Borque and colleagues[19] found the typical patient seeking RK was Caucasian, with an equal chance of being male or female, ranging in age from 18 to 44 years, and of a higher socioeconomic status, with 85% of the PERK patients having some post–high school education and 36% reporting annual incomes of $20,000 or more. Studies of the psychologic profiles of PERK patients, compared to a similar group of myopes from Rand Health Insurance, found that the PERK patients were less likely to be depressed, anxious, or to function poorly in their jobs or social lives than the Rand patients.[19] Powers found moderate levels of self-esteem, with 97% of patients reporting stable marriages and occupations over the previous year.[20] This information disproved the theory that the typical patient seeking RK was an unbalanced, chronically dissatisfied risk taker who responded to media hype for the latest health fad. Bourque[19] documented the single, most important reason PERK patients had RK was to be dependent no longer on eyeglasses or contact lenses (65%). Other reasons included occupation (6%) and cosmesis (3%). These data suggest that the overwhelming majority of patients are interested in RK for functional reasons.

Patient selection begins when the patient walks into the room. It is advisable to have a member of the patient's family or a close friend present during the initial ophthalmic examination and discussion of the procedure. This enables the patient to review what was discussed with a trusted confidant and could prove to be essential in clarifying points of discussion if necessary.

History

It is important to inquire about the motivation for considering radial keratotomy. Patients who want to have radial keratotomy to satisfy a loved one should not be considered acceptable candidates. These patients should be given written information describing the procedure to review at home and told to return only if they wish to satisfy their own needs and desires. Patients who demand a "perfect" result or who have unrealistic expectations are not good candidates for surgery.

Pregnancy, collagen-vascular disease, severe atopy, ocular inflammatory disease, and herpes simplex or herpes zoster are contraindications for RK. Patients with a family history of glaucoma must be warned that IOP above 21 mm Hg can alter the final refraction.

Age

Patients less than 21 years of age are generally not offered RK because their refraction may not be stable and because they cannot give independent informed consent in most states. Dietz[21] considers it inappropriate to operate on patients in their teens and early twenties because younger individuals do not achieve as much surgical correction with the same amount of surgery as older individuals and therefore require either a smaller optical zone or more incisions. They are also less likely to have realistic expectations from the surgery. O'Dell and Wyzinski reported a series of bilateral RK in 27 teenagers. Sixty-four percent of eyes were within 1 D of emmetropia an average of 22 months after surgery (range: 3 to 54 months). Although patient satisfaction was high, the report emphasized the problems of overcorrection-induced astigmatism, the need to wear glasses after surgery, and the repeated reoperations to deal with the increases in myopia as the patients got older. Radial keratotomy in patients less than 21 years of age therefore should be discouraged. There is no upper age limit for RK.

Stability of Refraction

Methods to document a stable refraction include obtaining previous clinical records, ascertaining the refractions from old glasses, and determining the age of onset of wearing of glasses. An earlier age of onset suggests a longer time of progression. Also, larger refractive errors are more likely to progress for a longer time.

Contact lenses can change corneal curvature by inducing mild hypoxia and subsequent edema and by remolding the cornea. Corneal warpage is most common in PMMA contact lens wearers although it does occur with gas-permeable and soft contact lenses.[23] The time required for a warped cornea to return to its natural state can vary from hours to months, with some corneas suffering permanant high amounts of astigmatism.[24] Operating on these eyes can alter the surgical plan by 1 to 4 D for the sphere and 1 to 3 D in the cylinder.[30] Contact lenses should be discontinued for at least 1 week prior to surgical evaluation and for longer periods if computerized topography suggests corneal warpage. One should inquire about the prescence of spectacle blur.

Visual Acuity

Both uncorrected and best corrected Snellen visual acuity should be documented during the preop evaluation. Patients who cannot be corrected better than 20/40 are rarely considered for surgery. Patients who are informed of their uncorrected acuity can more easily appreciate their postop result. Patients like to tell their friends they went from 20/400 to 20/25 or 20/20. The Snellan chart is an acceptable tool in clinical practice but is not adequate for clinical studies. The National Eye Institute Visual Acuity Chart described by Ferris should be used in clinical trials.[26]

Refraction

Both the manifest and cycloplegic refraction should be measured, but only the cycloplegic refraction should be used in the surgical plan and for comparing preop and postop surgical results. Using the manifest refraction significantly increases the risk of overcorrection. The PERK study documented one in four eyes having 0.50 D or more of myopia than the cycloplegic refraction, with the baseline refraction measuring an average of 0.25 D more myopia (range: −1.88 to +1.00).[32] Patients with 1.50 to 6.00 D of myopia will likely have the best surgical outcome, although the amount of myopia on which a surgeon will perform RK varies greatly. Patients with greater than 4.00 D of myopia can be acceptable candidates if they are older or willing to accept a decreased probability of achieving 20/40 vision (see Chapter 21).

It is important to document refractive astigmatism during the cycloplegic refraction and compare it to the keratometric astigmatism. The difference between the two is the amount of astigmatism induced by the lens. It may be helpful to demonstrate various clinical results to patients using lenses in a trial frame. If a patient finds 20/25 or 20/30 vision unacceptable, that patient may not be a good candidate for RK. This technique is also helpful in patients that are presbyopic and who insist on emmetropia. Demonstrating an inability to read often convinces these patients to have their nondominant eye undercorrected.

Central Keratometry

It is possible that corneal curvature may influence the refractive effect,[33–35] but there does not appear to be a significant correlation between preop central keratometric power and the effect of RK. It is important to document keratometric power outside the normal range (39.00 to 48.00) because these patients may have an abnormal response to surgery. Very flat corneas may suggest contact lens warpage, while very steep corneas may have keratoconus. Checking keratometric readings in upgaze to look for inferior steepening may help in screening for subclinical keratoconus (see Chapter 12).

Computerized Topography

Computer-assisted corneal topography generates thousands of data points on the anterior corneal surface, and color-coded maps can aid evaluation of the corneal topography. This technology is a sensitive means of detecting subtle regional differences of the cornea as seen in subclinical keratoconus[31–33] and corneal warpage.[34] Photokeratoscopy alone is not sensitive enough to screen for subclinical keratoconus,[35] although photokeratoscopy, retinoscopy, and keratometry in upgaze used together form a sensitive method of screening for subclinical keratoconus. "Radical retinoscopy" as described by Copeland is performed at a working distance of 4 inches from the patient's face. Narrowing of the inferior side of the retina's myopic image proves the inferior cornea is steepening more rapidly than the superior cornea. In most cases, surgery should not be considered in the presence of topographic abnormalities.

Ocular Dominance

The dominant eye is not always the same as the dominant hand and is determined by having patients hold a cardboard sheet with a central hole in front of them with both arms outstretched looking at a distant object binocularly. Patients pull the paper toward them while maintaining fixation on the object. The hole centers on the dominant eye. Although patients will sight a camera or gun with their dominant eye, it is best to test for ocular dominance in the office rather than rely on the recollection of the patient. Most surgeons prefer to operate on the patient's nondominant eye first, so that if the eye overresponds the surgical plan for the dominant eye can be changed.

Slit Lamp Microscopy

Preoperative evaluation of patients undergoing radial keratotomy should include careful examination for anterior basement membrane abnormalities, preexisting corneal scars, Fleiscer ring and Vogt's striae, pigment dispersion, iris transillumination and Krukenberg's spindles, lens opacities, and lens dislocation (see Chapter 6).

Intraocular Pressure

Patients with an IOP above 21 mm Hg are likely to be overresponders while those with an IOP below 10 mm Hg may be underresponders. IOP measurement obtained using applanation tonometry is not likely to be affected by the decrease in scleral rigidity that occurs in myopia.

Dilated Fundus Examination

Every patient should undergo a dilated fundus exam with indirect ophthalmoscopy before having RK. Myopes, particularly pathologic myopes, have an increased risk of developing lattice degeneration, retinal tears, retinal holes, and retinal detachments, and this pathology must be documented and managed preoperatively. Although an atrophic retinal hole would not necessarily be an absolute contraindication for surgery, it is important to inform patients of the presence and potential treatments of preexisting pathology.

Preoperative Pachymetry

Corneal thickness does not seem to affect surgical outcome and thus is not a variable in case selection. Some surgeons elect to perform preoperative pachymetry in patients with borderline topographical maps to screen for keratoconus. Preop pachymetry is not a substitute for intraoperative pachymetry.

PREOP SURGICAL PLANNING

The refractive correction after RK is dependent on the patient's age, the diameter of the central clear zone (optical zone) selected, the number of incisions, and incision depth. The surgeon must use these variables to tailor the desired refractive surgical effect for each patient. The predictability of RK is −1.5 to −2.0 D for 80% to 90% of eyes.[36–39] Patients interested in RK may not be willing to accept this less-than-desirable predictability to eliminate the drawbacks of contact lenses and glasses. The predictability of RK is better in lower myopes, making it a viable alternative to excimer laser PRK and intrastromal rings.

Age

Patient age was not recognized to have a significant effect on surgical outcome until the early 1980s. Using regression analysis, the PERK study documented 0.60 D greater effect per decade[37]; Arrowsmith, 0.48 D greater effect per decade[38]; and Sanders, 0.40 D greater effect per decade.[36] In addition there was greater variability of refractive effect as the optical zone became smaller.[37] Surgeons must be cautious when performing RK on patients over 50 and err on the side of undercorrection regardless of the nomogram being used.

Optical Zone Diameter

Fyodorov and Durnev[14] were the first to suggest that reducing the diameter of the optical zone would produce a greater decrease in myopia. Subsequently Salz and colleagues have shown a statistically significant effect of decreasing the diameter of the optical zone for both four and eight incisions in human cadaver eyes.[40] Mathematical models of RK have supported this conclusion.[41] The PERK study documented a 0.5-mm reduction in the diameter of the optical zone, 4.0 to 3.5 mm, resulting in an increase in refractive change of 0.68 D, and a reduction in the diameter of the optical zone from 3.5 to 3.0 mm resulting in an increase in refractive change of 1.08 D.[37] Based on these data some have suggested that using 0.25-mm steps may be an unnecessary refinement.[42] We routinely use 0.25-mm steps and attribute the large variability of refractive effect achieved between patients within each optical zone group of the PERK study to age not being a variable in the surgical plan. No studies have compared results of 0.25-mm and 0.50-mm steps.

Fyodorov initially advocated optical zones as small as 2.4 mm in diameter but later used a minimum size of 3 mm.[43] Optical zones smaller than 3.0 mm will increase the effect of the surgery but are likely to be associated with increased glare.[44] Although some experienced surgeons recommend optical zone diameters as small as 2.5 mm, most surgeons currently utilize optical zone diameters between 3.0 to 5.0 mm for most of their patients undergoing RK (Fig 19–3).

Incision Number

The number of incisions used for RK has decreased over the past 50 years. Sato made 80 incisions (40 anterior and 40 posterior), Yenaliev started with 32 incisions but eventually recommended 12 incisions, and Fyodorov began with 32 incisions and found that 16 produced an equal effect. Sixteen-incision surgery was recommended when RK was introduced into the United States in 1979.[14] In 1980 Schacher developed a theoretical model of the cornea indicating that eight incisions to the limbus produced most of the corneal flattening.[45] His work was substantiated by a clinical study comparing eight and sixteen incisions using a 3-mm optical zone that yielded a reduction in myopia of 5.21 D and 5.18 D, respectively.[46] These experimental and clinical data, the surgical experience that the final eight incisions were difficult to make because of the weakened cornea, and the availability of surgical alternatives led the majority of surgeons to abandon sixteen-incision RK[47] (Fig 19–4).

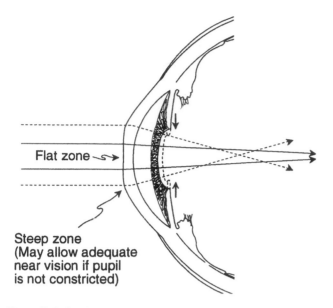

Figure 19–3. Relationship of optical clear zone to pupillary size. The central flat zone is surrounded by a steep zone that may cause significant discomfort if not concentric with the pupil or if the pupil is larger than the optical zone.

In a cadaver eye study using a 3-mm optical zone, four incisions and eight incisions up to the limbus produced 67% and 89%, respectively, of the final flattening.[48] Clinical studies have demonstrated four-incision RK to be effective in correcting low to moderate myopia,[49,50] with few patients being overcorrected. Salz[49] and Spiegleman[50] reported that 86% and 93% of patients with low myopia (−2.00 to −3.12 D) had an uncorrected visual acuity (UCVA) of 20/40 or better after four-incision surgery, with 4% and 0% overcorrected by more than 1 D. The PERK study,[51] employing eight-incision surgery, reported 94% of patients with low myopia (−2.00 to −3.12) had a UCVA of 20/40 or better and 21% were overcorrected by more than 1 D. Salz[49] and Spiegleman[50] report 68% and 84% of patients with moderate myopia (−3.25 to −4.37) had UCVAs of 20/40 or better, and no patients were overcorrected by more than 1 D. In Salz's series,[49] 93% of patients had 20/40 or better uncorrected vision, and 96% were within 1 D of emmetropia following the addition of four more incisions. In the PERK study,[51] 79% of patients with moderate myopia (−3.25 to −4.37) had 20/40 or better uncorrected vision, and 20% were overcorrected by more than 1 D.

Four-incision RK allows the surgeon to evaluate the cornea's initial response to the first four incisions and reduce overcorrections. Patients who are significantly undercorrected may benefit from four additional incisions.[52] Disadvantages of four-incision surgery include a higher risk of irregular astigmatism and

the need for a smaller optical clear zone for any given refractive error, potentially increasing the risk of glare.

Incision Direction

Radial keratotomy incisions can be made from the optical zone to the limbus (centrifugal), from the limbus to the optical zone (centripetal), or from the optical zone to the limbus and limbus to optical zone (two-pass surgery) (see Chapter 16). Up until recently most surgeons in the United States performed centrifugal incisions to decrease the risk of entering the optical zone, which can cause disabling glare, irregular astigmatism, central

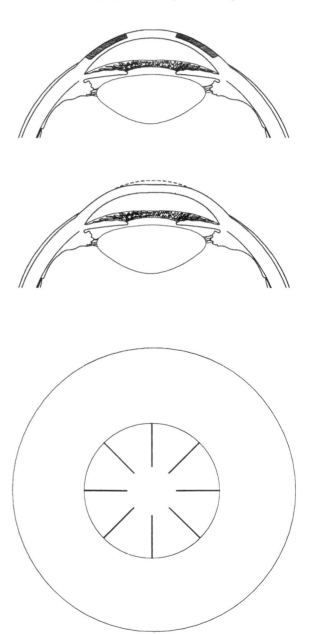

Figure 19–4. Eight-incision RK showing the central flattening (middle). In lower myopes the four oblique incisions may be sufficient to achieve the desired result.

corneal scarring, and loss of best corrected visual acuity (BCVA). Proponents of centripetal incisions suggest this incision is more likely to approach a 90° angle at the optical zone edge and allows continuous visualization of the cutting edge throughout the entire incisional excursion in any meridian.[14,54,55] Melles and Binder compared the efficacy of these techniques in monkeys using light microscopy.[56] Centrifugal incision depth averaged 46% (range: 38% to 61%), whereas centripetal depth measured 74% (range: 53% to 87%). These differences may be explained by the posterior tilt of the front-cutting blade during the centripetal incision, producing a smaller optical zone in the posterior stroma than intended.[57] A clinical series supports these experimental data.[58] A consecutive series of 81 eyes had RK performed by the same surgeon. Fifty-nine eyes had centrifugal surgery and 22 had centripetal surgery. At 3 months 58.9% of the centifugal surgery group and 86.7% (19 of 22 eyes) of the centripetal surgery group had a UCVA of 20/40 or better. Sixty-three percent of the centrifugal surgery group and 91.6% of the centripetal surgery group were within ±2 D of emmetropia at 3 months. Incision depth was estimated with slit lamp microscopy 24 hours postoperatively. The centrifugal incisions were estimated to have depths from 60% to 90%, with significant incision depth variability in individual eyes. Centripetal incision depths ranged from 85% to 100%, with very good consistency in individual eyes as well as in the group. Although these data are useful in comparing the two surgical techniques, it should be emphasized that this study was not randomized, and a uniform technique was not employed in patients having centrifugal surgery.

Two-pass surgery allows the surgeon the advantages of centripetal surgery with the safety of the centrifugal technique. Studies in human cadaver eyes have demonstrated 4.16 D of flattening using the centrifugal technique, 7.71 D for centripetal incisions, and 9.26 D of corneal flattening using the two-pass technique.[59] Other investigators have demonstrated that the second (centripetal) pass in the two-pass technique results in 20% to 30% redeepening of the first (centrifugal) pass at the optical zone.[60] Potential disadvantages of the two-pass technique include the increased risk of forming two tracks that may result in increased scarring and glare.

SURGICAL TECHNIQUES

Centration

Proper centration on the cornea during RK is critical. Poor centration can result in glare and irregular astigmatism, reducing BCVA. An understanding of basic geometric optics is necessary to determine where the optical zone of RK procedures should be centered (see Chapters 8 and 9).

The center of the entrance pupil should be used for centering RK procedures[61,62] The entrance pupil of the eye is the virtual image of the pupil and iris formed by the cornea and is approximately 0.5 mm closer to us and about 14% larger than the real pupil. The line of sight corresponds to the chief ray of the bundle of rays passing through the pupil and reaching the fovea (Fig 9–5). The pupillary axis is the line perpendicular to the cornea that passes through the center of the entrance pupil. The point where the line of sight intersects the cornea is the desired center for the RK optical zone. This point is just temporal to the corneal light reflex and nasal to the intersection of the pupillary axis and the geometric center of the cornea.

The centering technique used in the PERK study[63] consisted of having the patient fixate on the coiled microscope light filament that emerged from the microscope toward 6 o'clock from the viewing tubes, displacing the reflection of the microscope filament from the cornea toward 12 o'clock. The corneal light reflex was also displaced to the right when viewed monocularly through the right ocular. The surgeon compensated for this by marking the corneal epithelium at the left end of the rectangular filament reflection and one half to one complete width of the filament inferiorly with the tip of a hypodermic needle. This technique is prone to error if the patient does not fixate on the center of the light source, and error from the offset estimation by the surgeon. Even though the centering mark in the PERK study was decentered nasally from the entrance pupil by approximately 0.2 to 0.4 mm, glare was minimal.

Optimal corneal centering requires the patient to have a natural undilated pupil and to fixate on a light that is coaxial with the examiner's sighting eye (Fig 9–3). The center of the pupil is marked with a blunt cannula. The position of the corneal light reflex is ignored because it may be misleading[64] and may result in decentered treatments (Fig 19–5).

Intraoperative Pachymetry

The ultrasonic pachymeter is an electronic pulsar that provides short voltage pulses. A piezoelectric crystal changes its shape with each electronic pulse and generates an ultrasonic pulse that is propagated through the cornea, reflected off Descemet's membrane, and received back by the piezoelectric crystal. The impact of the ultrasonic waves on the crystal deforms it once

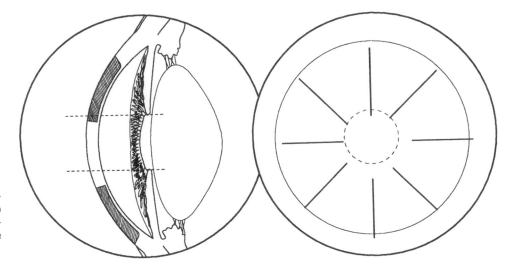

Figure 19–5. Inferotemporal decentration of RK incisions in relation to the pupillary margin. This often occurs when the surgeon centers the treatment on the corneal light reflex.

again, generating an electronic pulse that is sent to a receiver, where it is detected, amplified, and then displayed on an oscilloscope screen or registered on a digital display.[65] Kremer's original calibration for the speed of sound in the cornea of 1640 m/sec is still used by most manufacturers today.[66]

All pachymeters average approximately 30 to 500 measurements in a fraction of a second by either the pulse-locked method or the averaging method. The pulse-locked method records all readings that are within 5 to 10 μm of each other, rejecting those outside that range. The averaging method uses a fixed number of consecutive measurements that must be within 5 to 10 μm of each other to be averaged. The series of measurements is rejected if the readings are too disparate or if the probe is not perpendicular (Fig 16–22) to the corneal surface. Studies comparing ultrasonic pachymeters[67,68] have demonstrated that thickness readings among instruments varied significantly. Values had a range of 49 μm centrally and 59 μm paracentrally among the instruments.

The location of corneal thickness measurements varies among surgeons. Measurements based on 48 consecutive eyes in the PERK study[69] have documented that the cornea became thinner when proceeding superior to nasal to inferior to temporal locations. Using these data and his own experience, Casebeer recommended taking one reading 1.5 mm temporal to the marked central cornea. Other surgeons recommend taking multiple readings at 3, 6, 9, and 12 o'clock since some patients have corneas that are thinnest in locations other than temporally. This may avoid having shallow incisions in areas of increased corneal thickness (Fig 19–6).

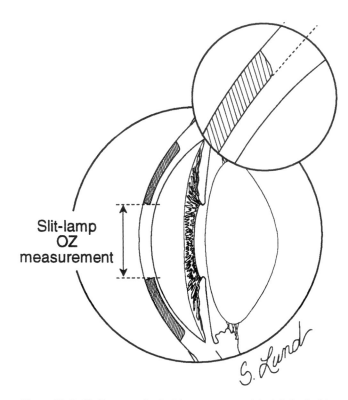

Slit-lamp OZ measurement

S. Lund

Figure 19–6. Shallow superior incision as compared to inferior incision resulting from greater superior pachymetry in comparison with inferior pachymetry.

Blade Calibration

Achieving an incision depth of 80% to 90% corneal thickness is critical to obtaining a satisfactory surgical result. Verifying the extension of the knife blade beyond the footplate using a gauge block has served as the best method of calibrating the depth of the incisions. In the late 1970s and early 1980s a ruler-style gauge block with a calibrated line along the edge was used to calibrate the metal blade fragments in the blade holders. This was a time-consuming procedure, and resetting the blade during surgery to replace a dull one or to extend it for deepening incisions was tedious. The development of the micrometer knife handle theoretically obviated gauge blocks, but experience with inaccurate micrometers, the lack of industry standards for ophthalmic micrometer knives, and the inconsistency in the quality of manufacturing led to the development of a gauge block in which the knife was mounted in a cradle on a platform and and the blade extended over an elevated ridge of calibrated width (Fig 16–25).

Although the coin-gauge blocks used in the PERK study were found to be accurate, Neumann et al[70] found numerous inconsistencies when testing commercial gauge blocks. In general, the errors showed an actual reading higher than what was stated, so that the knife would be set longer than desired, increasing the chance of corneal perforation.

Another significant problem with gauge blocks is the surgeon's inability to align the tip of the blade exactly along the edge of the gauge mark. The farther the knife blade is from the surface of the gauge block and the more the gauge block is tilted from an exact orthogonal orientation to the microscope, the more parallax is induced (Fig 16–25).

Gauges with a micrometer stage and a 100 to 150× magnified calibrated reticle (Fig 16–26) obviate the problems of parallax and inaccurate micrometers. In addition to measuring the extension of the blade, the surgeon can check the alignment of the blade and the foot plates, and for damage to the blade. Au and colleagues[71] found the Magnum optical micrometer to have the smallest measurement error in their study comparing the KOI micrometer (3%), the KOI coin-gauge block (0.07%), and the Magnum optical micrometer (0.04%).

Globe Fixation

Prior to performing incisional keratotomy, the surgeon must decide if he will fixate the globe during the procedure (Fig 16–7). Many surgeons who fixate the globe prefer two-point fixation 180° away from the incision, while others prefer a 360° fixation ring or a Mastel guide. The surgeon should avoid applying pressure to the globe with the fixation instrument when performing centripetal or two-pass surgery. Applying pressure with the fixation instrument during centrifugal surgery may be more acceptable. Although some experienced surgeons have recommended no fixation of the globe during centripetal surgery with a front cutting blade, we do not recommend this, regardless of the surgeon's level of experience. Passing the diamond knife in the Mastel guide may be the best method of fixating the globe and obtaining linear incisions. The surgeon should avoid chipping the tip of the diamond blade as it is introduced or removed from the Mastel guide.

Incision Direction

Center to Periphery (Centrifugal)

Centrifugal incisions are made with either a single-edged 45° angled blade or a double-edged angled blade. With a single-edged angled blade the angle exerts vector forces in both the lateral and posterior directions, displacing some tissue posteriorly without cutting it. The blade has minimal momentum in the area adjacent to the optical zone since this is where the incision originates, further displacing rather than cutting the tissue. As the blade begins to move more of the deeper layers are cut because of the lateral force of the blade, yielding a curved incision that is more shallow adjacent to the edge of the optical zone and deepest near the middle of the incision.

With a double-edged angled blade there is a cutting force in both directions as the knife penetrates the stroma, allowing a deeper cut adjacent to the optical zone and throughout the incision than with a single-edged knife. Also the cut adjacent to the optical zone is more squared.

The knife blade is entered into the cornea with a vigorous, short stab, slightly indenting the cornea adjacent to the optical zone mark. The knife is held vertically for approximately 4 seconds to allow the knife to cut some of the posteriorly displaced stroma. The knife is now pushed across the cornea in a single, smooth motion at a slow, deliberate rate perpendicular to the surface of the cornea without tilting the blade. If the blade is tilted to one side or another the incision is undercut and a wider incision is created. Gentle downward pressure on the knife is applied during the incision to ensure that the blade remains deeply seated in the tissue (Fig 16–10).

The cutting edge of the blade is difficult to visualize as the knife approaches the limbus. The knife is stopped short of the limbal vessels and lifted out of the wound perpendicular to the surface. Care must be taken to avoid letting the momentum of the knife carry the incision into the limbus, which would create excess bleeding without enhancing the effect of the surgery.

Periphery to Center (Centripetal)

Centripetal incisions are usually made with a single-edged, front-cutting vertical blade that creates a smaller vector force posteriorly and therefore displaces less tissue. The incisions begin peripherally, just anterior to the superficial limbal vessels. The blade gains momentum as it travels centrally toward the optical zone and is more likely to cut rather than displace tissue, creating deeper incisions with a squarer configuration adjacent to the optical zone (Fig 16-11).

As with the centrifugal incision, the knife is held vertically, perpendicular to the corneal surface, and pushed across the cornea in a single, smooth motion at a slow, deliberate rate without tilting the blade.

Natural deceleration occurs as the blade approaches the edge of the optical zone. Care should be taken to maintain a uniform rate to avoid staggering at the paracentral part of the wound. Upon completing the incision, the blade should be pulled out perpendicular to the surface and away from the central cornea. The effect of the operation can be enhanced by tilting the handle back toward the limbus and placing the tip of the blade under the edge of the optical zone, creating a smaller optical zone. The knife blade should never be tilted toward the center of the cornea and dragged across the edge of the optical zone. This maneuver extends only the superficial part of the wound, does not enhance the effect of the procedure, and may increase light scattering over the pupil causing glare.

Center to Periphery and Periphery to Center (Two-Pass)

Two-pass incisions are made with a double-edged blade. The back surface of the blade is angled, and the anterior surface is vertical with a cutting edge that varies from 200 to 250 μm (Fig 16-12). During the centrifugal pass the blade exerts vector forces in both the lateral and posterior directions, displacing some tissue posteriorly. During the centripetal pass the blades gains momentum as it travels centrally and cuts tissue that was displaced posteriorly on the initial pass (Fig 19-7). The centripetal cut leaves a square configuration adjacent to the optical cone. The blade cannot enter the optical zone during the centripetal pass because the vertical front-cutting edge is 200 to 250 μm and will only pass through tissue that has already been cut. Gentle downward pressure is applied during the centrifugal incision, with less pressure applied during the centripetal incision to avoid perforation.

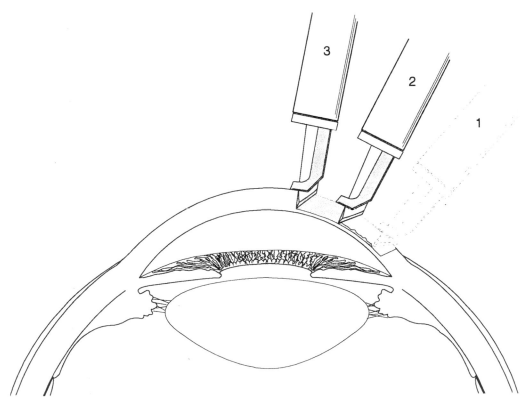

Figure 19-7. Two-pass surgery. After the centrifugal incision the blade is brought from position 1 to 3. Note the redeepening of the base of the incision between positions 1 and 2.

Two-pass surgery provides the deep incisions of centripetal surgery with the safety of centrifugal surgery. A potential disadvantage of two-pass surgery is the increased risk of forming two tracks that may result in increased scarring and glare.

POSTOPERATIVE CARE

Prior to surgery patients receive 10 to 20 mg of Valium, leaving the patient sedated postoperatively. The patient leaves the operative suite with 30 mg of Dalmane, ofloxacin, mild prednisolone, and diclofenac sodium. The Dalmane is taken when the patient arrives at home. Diclofenac sodium is given immediately postoperatively every 5 minutes ×4 and every 2 hours as needed for the first 8 hours and discontinued thereafter. Diclofenac sodium has been shown to decrease corneal sensitivity for 36 hours[72] and significantly to reduce postop pain, possibly by reducing prostaglandin-E2 levels.[73] The use of postop steroids remains controversial. We prescribe prednisolone QID for 1 week to reduce any inflammation that may have resulted from the procedure. Postop steroids will not likely have any effect on the postop refraction[74] unless there is a secondary increase in IOP. Ofloxacin is our antibiotic of choice because it is a solution and has broad antibacterial coverage. It is taken QID for 1 week.

Patients are evaluated 1 day, 1 week, 1 month, 3 months, and 1 year postoperatively, and once a year thereafter.

INTRAOPERATIVE COMPLICATIONS

Radial keratotomy is an elective procedure, and thus the standards for safety and predictability of outcome must be higher than for operations that correct potentially blinding disorders. It is the surgeon's responsibility to inform the patient of the potential complications and to take extreme precautions to prevent them.

Most surgeons currently perform RK under topical anesthesia. Excess topical proparacaine, tetracaine, or lidocaine will roughen and soften the epithelium, increasing the likelihood of a corneal abrasion during the procedure. Toxic reactions to topical anesthetics can occur within 30 minutes of application and include pain, epithelial clouding, corneal edema, and Descemet's striae.[75] Less acute reactions include lid edema, conjunctival hyperemia, and punctate epithelial keratopathy.

Although a regional intraorbital block provides a prolonged anesthetic effect and allows the surgeon better control of the position of the eye, it should not be routinely employed for RK. Complications of retrobulbar injections can produce severe visual loss and include retrobulbar hemorrhage,[76] optic atrophy,[77] and perforation of the globe.[78]

Corneal perforations during surgery can be subdivided into microperforations and macroperforations. Microperforations produce the loss of one or two drops of aqueous that stops spontaneously. There is no shallowing of the anterior chamber, and the procedure may continue at the discretion of the surgeon. A macroperforation is large enough to produce shallowing of the anterior chamber, reqiring suture placement and termination of the procedure.

Microperforations

The incidence of microperforations varies fom 0.006% to 35%,[79] with more recent reports using ultrasonic pachymetry and improved surgical knives reporting rates of 2% to 10%.[80] This rate is likely to be reduced further with the use of the micronscope.

Microperforations occur more frequently in the inferior and temporal cornea[81] because these areas are usually the thinnest; however, they may appear in any location. Factors that increase the chance of corneal perforation include elevation of IOP from fixation during the procedure, using an unfamiliar blade, prolonged dehydration and thinning of the cornea intraoperatively, an inaccurate corneal thickness measurement, and recutting incisions to make them deeper. The management of microperforations includes stopping the incision, checking anterior chamber depth, drying the knife and corneal surface, and retracting the blade before proceeding.

Macroperforations

The incidence of macroperforations varies from 0 to 0.45%.[82] They are best avoided by prompt recognition of a drop of aqueous around the knife blade and foot plates, suggesting a small perforation. This emphasizes the importance of a dry surgical field and knife before beginning the incision. If the anterior chamber shallows and if aqueous continues to leak, a suture should be placed and the procedure terminated. The suture can be removed 2 to 3 weeks later and the procedure completed. It is not uncommon for there to be significant corneal flattening following a macroperforation, with the patient achieving excellent visual acuity even if only two or three incisions were placed. It is important to inform the patient that the corneal flattening will regress and further surgery will be necessary.

Complications of micro- and macroperforations include endothelial damage, scarring of Descemet's membrane, iridocorneal adhesions if the anterior chamber remains flat,[83] laceration of the lens if the blade is carried deeply into the perforation, endophthalmitis, and epithelial downgrowth.[95–97]

Decentered Clear Zone

Unfortunately, the frequency of a decentered clear zone is not reported in the literature. The smaller the clear zone, the greater the effect of decentration, with increased glare and irregular astigmatism (Figs 19–3 and 19–5).

Other potential intraoperative complications include incisions across the visual axis, an incorrect number of incisions, and incisions crossing the limbus, which increases the risk of corneal neovascularization, especially if the patient wears a soft contact lens.

Endothelial Cell Loss

Endothelial cell loss following RK does not appear to be visually threatening. This was a major concern early in the American experience because of the delayed corneal decompensation following the Sato operation. Endothelial cell loss in the first several years following RK has varied from 3% to 10%.[81,90–94] The cell loss is most significant in the first few months after surgery and is not progressive. Using morphometric analysis, McRae and colleagues,[93] demonstrated a 3.3% decrease in endothelial cell density, but no statistically significant change in cell size or shape in either the central or peripheral cornea up to 2 years after surgery.

Eyes that suffered microperforations had more endothelial cell loss than those that did not.[92] Also eyes with central clear zones of 3.0 to 3.5 mm showed a statistically significant change in mean cell density, mean cell perimeter, and mean side length. Eyes with central clear zones of 3.75 to 4.50 mm showed no changes in these parameters.

More long-term studies evaluating the effect of RK on the corneal endothelium are needed to determine if corneal weakning causes increased bending of the cornea and increased endothelial cell loss with blinking and rubbing of the eyes. Also it is not known if the minimal endothelial damage from RK would make the cornea more susceptible to edema following future intra-

ocular surgery or to primary disease such as Fuch's endothelial dystrophy.

Traumatic Rupture of Keratotomy Scars

Following a partial or full thickness corneal incision the collagen fibers do not heal end to end spanning the entire cornea but deposit a new extracellular matrix that cements the two sides of the incision.[98] Thus a corneal scar does not have as much tensile strength and is permanently weaker than the original cornea.

Several laboratory studies evaluating wound strength after RK have been published.[99–101] Larson and colleagues[99] observed that the blunt force required to rupture the globe of rabbits 90 days after eight-incision RK was approximately 50% of that needed to rupture the control eyes not operated on. Ninety-eight percent of the wound ruptures occurred in one or more of the incisions, with patterns that connected one incision to the other and that extended to the sclera, forming stellate wounds. Using a porcine model, Rylander and colleagues[100] demonstrated that ruptures most frequently occurred at the equator in normal eyes and through the cornea in eyes after RK. McKnight and colleagues[101] observed that cat eyes that had undergone eight-incision RK ruptured more readily following BB-gun injuries than the unoperated eye.

Based on these experimental data, it should not be unexpected that patients who have undergone RK are at increased risk for traumatic rupture of the globe following blunt trauma. Binder has reported three eyes with corneal rupture after motor vehicle accidents up to 2 years after surgery.[102] Simmons and Linsalata reported a case of blunt trauma caused by an elbow, resulting in corneal rupture followed by primary repair and subsequent enucleation.[103]

There have been reports of severe blunt trauma to eyes following RK that did not rupture. In one case there was no rupture of the keratotomy scar following severe blunt trauma to an eye 6 months after an eight-incision RK that produced a 75% hyphema and corneal abrasion.[104] in a similar case a patient experienced bilateral facial fractures in a plane crash 4 months after a 16-incision RK, no rupture occurred and the patient recovered 20/20 visual acuity.

To reduce the incidence of traumatic rupture following RK, it is wise to inform patients of this potential complication and insist they wear protective goggle during vigorous athletic and recreational activities such as football, basketball, karate, and racquet sports.

Other potential corneal and intraocular complications include hypertrophic corneal scars, epithelial inclusions, debris and deposits in the corneal scar, herpes simplex keratitis, stellate epithelial iron lines, epithelial basement membrane changes and recurrent erosions, cataract, epithelial downgrowth, iridocyclitis, and ptosis.

Postop Complications

Potential refractive and visual complications include infectious keratitis, endophthalmitis, traumatic rupture of keratotomy scars, overcorrection, undercorrection, increased regular astigmatism, irregular astigmatism, diurnal fluctuation, glare, decreased contrast sensitivity, and monocular diplopia. These complications will be discussed in Chapters 24 and 25.

SUMMARY

Although radial keratotomy can safely reduce low to moderate myopia in most patients, the procedure continues to evolve. There is not a standard surgical technique that is optimal for every patient, and technique should be modified depending on the patient's age and refractive error. Refractive surgeons continue to modify surgical technique in the hope of improving predictability and stability of the results. Experimental and clinical investigations should be performed prior to the widespread application of these modifications.

REFERENCES

1. Donders FC. *On the Anomalies of Accommodation and Refraction of the Eye*. London 1864, New Sydenham Society; 1864;415–417.

2. Schiotz HA. Ein Fall von hochgradigem Hornhautastigmatismus nach Starextraction, Besserung auf operativem Wege. *Arch f Augenheilk*. 1885;15:178–181.

3. Bates WH. A suggestion of an operation to correct astigmatism. *Arch Ophthalmol*. 1894;23:9–13.

4. Faber E. Operative Behandeling von astigmaisme. *Nederl Tijdschr v Geneesk*. 1895;31:495–496.

5. Lucciola J. Traitement chirurgical de l'astigmatisme. *Arch d'Ophthalmol*. 1896;16:630.

6. Lans LJ. Experimentelle Untersuchungen uber Entstehung von Astigmatismus durch nicht-perforirende corneawunden. *Arch für Ophthalmologie*. 1898;45:117–152.

7. Schimmelpfennig BH, Waring GO. Development of refractive keratotomy in the nineteenth century. In Waring GO, ed. *Refractive Keratotomy for Myopia and Astigmatism*. St. Louis MO: Mosby-Year Book, Inc, 1992, pp 174.

8. Sato T. Treatment of conical cornea (incision of Descmet's membrane). *Acta Soc Ophthalmol Jpn*. 1939;43:544–555.

9. Sato T, Akiyama K, Shibata H. A new surgical approach to myopia. *Am J Ophthalmol*. 1953;36:823–829.

10. Akiyama K, Shibata H, Kanai A, Akiyama S, Yamaguchi T, Nakajima A, Waring GO. Development of radial keratotomy in Japan, 1939–1960. In Waring GO, ed. *Refractive Keratotomy for Myopia and Astigmatism*. St Louis MO: Mosby-Year Book, Inc, 1992, pp 212.

11. Yenaleyev FS. Experience in surgical treatment of myopia. *Ann Ophthalmol USSR*. 1979;3:52–55.

12. Durnev VV. Characteristics of surgical correction of myopia after 16 and 32 peripheral anterior radial nonperforating incisions. In Fyodorov SN, ed. *Surgery for Anomalies in Ocular Refraction*. Moscow: The Moscow Research Institute for Ocular Microsurgery, 1981, pp 33–35.

13. Durnev VV, Ivashina AI. Possibility of maximal elongation of incisions in radial keratotomy. In Fyodorov SN, editor. *Surgery for Aomalies in Ocular Refraction*. Moscow: The Moscow Research Institute for Ocular Microsurgery, 1981, pp 19–22.

14. Fyodorov SN and Durnev VV. Operation of dosaged dissection of corneal circular ligament in cases of myopia of mid degree. *Ann Ophthalmol*. 1979;11:1185–1190.

15. Fyodorov SN, Agranovsky AA. Long-term results of anterior radial keratotomy. *J Ocular Therapy Surg*. 1982;1:217–223.

16. Announcement. National Advisory Eye Council meetings Refractive keratoplasty. *Invest Ophthalmol Vis Sci*. 1979;18:882.

17. *Vest v Waring*, 565F. Suppl. 674 (ND Ga 1983).

18. *Schacher v American Academy of Ophthalmology, Inc*, F Supp (ND Ill 1984).

19. Bourque LB, Rubenstein R, Cosand B, Waring GO and the PERK Study Group. Psychosocial characteristics of candidates for the Prospective Evaluation of Radial Keratotomy (PERK) Study. *Arch Ophthalmol*. 1984;102:1187–1192.

20. Powers MK, Meyerwitz BE, Arrowsmith PN, Marks G. Psychosocial findings in radial keratotomy patients two years after surgery. *Ophthalmology*. 1984;91:1193–1198.

21. Dietz MR. Patient selection and counseling. In Sanders DR, Hoffman RF, Salz JJ, editors. *Refractive Corneal Surgery*. Thorofare, NJ: Slack, Inc, 1986, p 43.

22. O'Dell LW, Wyzinski P. Radial keratotomy in teenagers: A practical approach. *Refract Corneal Surg*. 1989;5:315–318.

23. Morgan JF. Induced corneal astigmatism with hydrophilic contact lenses. *Can J Ophthalmol*. 1975;10:207–213.

24. Binder PS. Orthokeratology. In Binder et al, editors. *Symposium on the Cornea. Transaction of the New Orleans Academy of Ophthalmology.* St. Louis, MO: CV Mosby Co, 1980, pp 149–166.

25. Waring GO. Examination and selection of patients for radial keratotomy. In Waring GO, editor. *Refractive Keratotomy for Myopia and Astigmatism.* St. Louis, MO: Mosby–Year Book, Inc, 1992, p 321.

26. Ferris FL, Kasoff A, Bresnick GH, Baily I. New visual acuity charts for clinical research. *Am J Ophthalmol.* 1982; 94:91–96.

27. Waring GO. Examination and selection of patients for refractive keratotomy. In Waring GO, editor. *Refractive Keratotomy of Myopia and Astigmatism.* St. Louis, MO: Mosby–Year Book, Inc, 1992, p 317.

28. Sanders DR, Deitz MR, Gallagher D. Factors affecting predictability of radial keratotomy. *Ophthalmology.* 1985; 92:1237–1243.

29. Rowsey JJ, Balyeat HD, Monlux R, et al. Prospective evaluation of radial keratotomy: photokeratoscope corneal topography. *Ophthalmology.* 1988;95:322–334.

30. Arrowsmith PN, Marks RG. Four year update on predictability of radial keratotomy. *J Refract Surg.* 1988;4:37–45.

31. Maguire LJ, Bourne WM. Corneal topography of early keratoconus. *Am J Ophthalmol.* 1989;108:107–112.

32. Rabinowitz YS, McDonnell PJ. Computer-assisted corneal topography in keratoconus. *Refract Corneal Surg.* 1989;5:400–408.

33. Wilson SE, Lin DTC, Klyce SD. Corneal topography of keratoconus. *Cornea.* 1991;10:2–8.

34. Wilson SE, Lin DTC, Klyce SD, et al. Topographic changes in contact lens induced corneal warpage. *Ophthalmology.* 1990;97:734–744.

35. Rabinowitz YS, Nesburn AB, McDonnell PJ. Videokeratography of the fellow eye in unilateral keratoconus. *Ophthalmology.* 1993;100:181–186.

36. Sanders D, Dietz M, Gallagher D. Factors affecting predictability of radial keratotomy. *Ophthalmology.* 1985;92: 1237–1243.

37. Lynn MJ, Waring GO, Sperdutto RD, et al. Factors affecting outcome and predictability of radial keratotomy in the PERK study. *Arch Ophthalmol.* 1987;105:42–51.

38. Arrowsmith PN, Marks RG. Four year update on predictability of radial keratotomy. *J Refract Surg.* 1988;4:37–45.

39. Werblin TP, Stafford GM. The Casebeer System for predictable keratorefractive surgery: one-year evaluation of 205 consecutive eyes. *Ophthalmology.* 1993;100:1095–1102.

40. Salz JJ, Rowsey JJ, Caroline, P, et al. A study of optical zone size and incision redeepening in experimental radial keratotomy. *Arch Ophthalmol.* 1985;103:590–594.

41. Schacher R, Black T, Huang. *Understanding Radial Keratotomy.* Denison, TX: LAL Publishing Co, 1981, pp 12–37.

42. Lynn MJ, Waring GO, Kutner MH. Predictability of refractive keratotomy. In Waring GO, editor. *Refractive Keratotomy for Myopia and Astigmatism.* St. Louis, MO: Mosby-Year Book, Inc, 1992, pp 352.

43. Fyodorov SN. Surgical correction of myopia and astigmatism. In Schachar AR, Levi S, Schacher S, editors. *Keratorefraction.* Dennison, TX: LAL Publishing Co, 1980, pp 141–172.

44. Smith RS, Cutro J. Computer analysis of radial keratotomy. *CLAO J.* 1984;10:241–248.

45. Schacher RA, Black TD, Huang. A physicist's view of radial keratotomy with practical surgical implications. In Schacher RA, Levy NS, Schacher L, editors. *Keratorefraction. Proceedings of the Keratorefractive Society Meeting.* Dennison, TX: LAL Publishing Co, 1980, pp 195–220.

46. Rowsey JJ, Balyeat HD, Rabinovitch, et al. Predicting the results of radial keratotomy. *Ophthalmology.* 1983;90: 642–654.

47. Swinger CA. Variables in radial keratotomy. *Trans New Orleans Acad Ophthalmol.* 1987;89–110.

48. Salz JJ, Lee JS, Jester JV, et al. Radial keratotomy in fresh human cadaver eyes. *Ophthalmology.* 1981;88:742–746.

49. Salz J, Villasenor R, Elander R, et al. Four-incision radial keratotomy for low to moderate myopia. *Ophthalmology.* 1986;93:727–738.

50. Spiegleman AV, Williams PA, Lindstrom RL. Four incision radial keratotomy. *J Cat Refract Surg.* 1988;14: 125–128.

51. Waring GO, Lynn MJ, Fielding B, et al. Results of the prospective evaluation of radial keratotomy (PERK) study 4 years after surgery for myopia. *JAMA.* 1990;263:1083–1091.

52. Kornmehl EW. Radial keratotomy: incision number, incision direction, peripheral redeepening, and multiple-depth incisions. *Int Ophthalmol Clin.* 1991;31:101–107.

53. Fleming JF. Corneal asphericity and visual function after radial keratotomy. *Cornea.* 1993;12:233–240.

54. Neumann AC, Osher RH, Fenzl RE. Radial keratotomy: a comprehensive evaluation. *Doc Ophthalmol.* 1984;56: 275–301.

55. Neuman AC, McCarty GR. Modified Fyodorov technique: limbus to optical zone cutting. In Sanders DR, editor. *Radial Keratotomy: Surgical Techniques.* Thorofare, NJ: Slack, Inc, 1986, pp 69–87.

56. Melles GRJ, Binder PS. Effect of radial keratotomy incision direction on wound depth. *Refract Corneal Surg.* 1990;6:394–403.

57. Melles GRJ, Wijdh RHJ, Cost B, et al. Effect of blade configuration, knife action and intraocular pressure on keratotomy incision depth and shape. *Cornea.* 1993;12: 299–309.

58. Lee CP. Radial keratotomy: in-to-out and out-to-in. Preliminary results in the Singapore General hospital. *Ann Acad Med Singapore.* 1989;18:141–150.

59. Kassoff MP, Quantock AJ, Assil KK. The genesis technique of radial keratotomy compared to the American and Russian techniques in human donor eyes. *Invest Ophthalmol Vis Sci.* 1993;34(suppl.):1242.

60. Updegraff SA, McDonald MB, Heschel MK. Structural analysis in monkeys of American versus Duotrak incisional keratotomy. *Invest Ophthalmol Vis Sci.* 1993; 34(suppl.):1242.

61. Walsh PM, Guyton DL. Comparison of two methods of marking the visual axis on the cornea during radial keratotomy. *Am J Ophthalmol.* 1984;97:660. Correspondence.

62. Pande M, Hillman JS. Optical zone centration in kerato-refractive surgery: entrance pupil, visual axis, coaxially sighted corneal reflex, or geometric corneal center? *Ophthalmology.* 1993;8:1230–1237.

63. Steinberg EB, Waring GO. Comparison of two methods of marking the visual axis on the cornea during radial keratotomy. *Am J Ophthalmol.* 1983;96:605.

64. Uozato H, Guyton DL. Centering corneal surgical procedures. *Am J Ophthalmol.* 1987;103:264–275.

65. Thornton SP, Gardner SK, Waring GO. Surgical instruments used in refractive keratotomy. In Waring GO, editor. *Refractive Keratotomy for Myopia and Astigmatism.* St. Louis, MO: Mosby–Year Book, Inc, 1992, p 411.

66. Kremer FB, Walton P, Genshimer G. Determination of corneal thickness using ultrasonic pachymetry. *Ann Ophthalmol.* 1985;17:506–507.

67. Salz JJ, Azen SP, Bernstein J, et al. Evaluation and comparison of sources of variability in the measurement of corneal thickness with ultrasonic and optical pachymeters. *Ophthalmic Surg.* 1983;14:750–754.

68. Reader AL, Salz JJ. Differences among ultrasonic pachymeters in measuring corneal thickness. *J Refract Surg.* 1987;3:7–11.

69. Waring GO. Atlas of surgical techniques of radial keratotomy. In Waring GO, editor. *Refractive Keratotomy for Myopia and Astigmatism.* St Louis, MO: Mosby–Year Book, Inc, 1992, p 549.

70. Neumann AC, McCarty GR, Copello B, et al. Enhanced accuracy is necessary for refractive surgery instrumentation. *J Cataract Refract Surg.* 1989;15:220–226.

71. Au YK, Reynolds MD, Chadalavada RC. A study of the optical micrometer, the coin gauge, and the diamond knife micrometer in diamond knife calibration. *Refract Corneal Surg.* 1992.

72. Loya N, Vyas S, Bassage S, Aquavella JV. Effect of topical diclofenac sodium on corneal sensitivity in rabbits. *Invest Ophthalmol Vis Sci.* 1993;34(suppl.):1015.

73. Phillips AF, Szerenyi K, Campos M, McDonnell PJ. Effect of topical cyclo-oxygenase inhibitor and steroid on arachidonic acid metabolism in rabbit corneas subjected to 193 nm excimer laser ablation. *Invest Ophthalmol Vis Sci.* 1993;34(suppl.):704.

74. Haverbeke L. Assessing the efficacy of topical corticosteroids following radial keratotomy. *Refract Corneal Surg.* 1993;9:379–382.

75. Theodore FH. Idiosyncratic reactions of the cornea from proparacaine. *Eye Ear Nose Throat Monthly.* 1968;47: 286–291.

76. Cross WD, Head WJ. Complications of radial keratotomy; an overview. In Sanders D, Hoffman RF, Salz J. editors. *Refractive Corneal Surgery.* Thorofare, NJ: Slack, Inc, 1986, pp 347–399.

77. O'Day DM, Feman SS, Elliott JH. Visual impairment following radial keratotomy: a cluster of cases. *Ophthalmology.* 1986;93:319–326.

78. Lewicky A, Salz J. Special report: radial keratotomy survey. *J Refractive Surg.* 1986;2:32–33.

79. Schachar RA. Indications, techniques, and complications of radial keratotomy. *Int Ophthalmol Clin.* 1983;23: 119–128.

80. Marmer RH. Radial keratotomy complications. *Ann Ophthalmol.* 1987;19:409–411.

81. Rowsey JJ, Balyeat HD. Preliminary results and complications of radial keratotomy. *Am J Ophthalmol.* 1982;93: 437–455.

82. Sawelson H, Marks RG. Two-year results of radial keratotomy. *Arch Ophthalmol.* 1985;103:505–510.

83. Grady FJ. Experience with radial keratotomy. *Ophthalmic Surg.* 1982;13:395–399.

84. Wilhelmus KR, Hamburg S. Bacterial keratitis following radial keratotomy. *Cornea.* 1983;2:143–146.

85. Robin JB, Beatty RF, Dunn S, et al. *Mycobacterium chelonei* keratitis after radial keratotomy. *Am J Ophthalmol.* 1986; 102:72–79.

86. Cottingham AJ, Berkeley RG, Nordan LT, et al. Bacterial corneal ulcers following keratorefractive surgery: a retrospective study of 14,163 procedures, read before the Ocular Microbiology and Immunology Group Meeting, San Francisco, September 28, 1986.

87. Mandlebaum S, Waring GO, Forster RK, et al. Late development of ulcerative keratitis in radial keratotomy scars. *Arch Ophthalmol.* 1986;104:1156–1160.

88. Shivitz IA, Arrowsmith PN. Corneal sensitivity following radial keratotomy. *Ophthalmology.* 1987;94 (suppl.):97.

89. Stern GA, Weitzenkorn D, Valenti J. Adherence of *Pseudomonas aeruginosa* to the mouse cornea: epithelial v stromal adherence. *Arch Ophthalmol.* 1982;100:1956–1958.

90. Rowsey JJ, Balyeat HD, Monlux R, et al. Endothelial cell loss after radial keratotomy. *Ophthalmology.* 1987;94 (suppl.):97.

91. Hoffer KJ, Darin JJ, Pettit TH, et al. Three years experience with radial keratotomy: the UCLA study. *Ophthalmology.* 1983;90:627–636.

92. Chiba K, Oak SS, Tsubota K, et al. Morphometric analysis of corneal endothelium following radial keratotomy. *J Cat Refract Surg.* 1987;13:263–267.

93. McRae SM, Matsuda M, Rich LF. The effect of radial keratotomy on the corneal endothelium. *Am J Ophthalmol.* 1985;100:538–542.

94. Asbell PA, Obstbaum S, Justin N. Peripheral corneal endothelial evaluation post radial keratotomy in PERK patients. *Ophthalmology.* 1984;91(suppl.):122.

95. Gelender H, Flynn HW, Mandlebaum SH. Bacterial endophthalmitis resulting from radial keratotomy. *Am J Ophthalmol.* 1982;93:323–326.

96. O'Day DM, Feman SS, Elliott JH. Visual impairment following radial keratotomy: a cluster of cases. *Ophthalmology.* 1986;93:319–326.

97. Manka RL, Gast TJ. Endophthalmitis following a Ruiz procedure. *Arch Ophthalmol.* 1990;108:21. Letter.

98. Maurice DM. The biology of wound healing in the corneal stroma: Castroviejo lecture. *Cornea.* 1987;6:162–168.

99. Larson BC, Kremer FB, Eller AW, et al. Quantitated trauma following radial keratotomy in rabbits. *Ophthalmology.* 1983;90:660–667.

100. Rylander HG, Welch AJ, Fleming B. The effect of radial keratotomy in the rupture strength of pig eyes. *Ophthalmic Surg.* 1983;14:744–749.

101. McKnight SJ, Fitz J, Giangiacoma J. Corneal rupture following radial keratotomy in cats subjected to BB gun injury. *Ophthalmic Surg.* 1988;19:165–167.

102. Binder PS, Waring GO, Arrowsmith PN, Wang CL. Histopathology of traumatic corneal rupture after radial keratotomy. *Arch Ophthalmol.* 1988;106:1584–1590.

103. Simmons RB, Linsalata RP. Ruptured globe following blunt trauma after radial keratotomy. *Ophthalmology.* 1987;94:148.

104. John ME, Schmitt TE. Traumatic hyphema after radial keratotomy. *Ann Ophthalmol.* 1983;15:930–932.

105. Spivak L. Case report: radial keratotomy incisions remain intact despite facial trauma after plane crash. *J Refract Surg.* 1987;3:59–60.

CHAPTER 20

Secondary Radial Keratotomy Procedures

Richard E. Braunstein ▪ Dimitri T. Azar

This chapter discusses the management of patients who have undergone a single incisional refractive surgery procedure. The benefits and problems of staged incisional refractive surgery are highlighted as well. We have tried to relay an understanding of the surgical procedures and concepts in order to help the refractive surgeon determine their applicability in a given clinical situation.

PLANNED STAGING OF RADIAL KERATOTOMY PROCEDURES

As our understanding of radial keratotomy (RK) has advanced, we have modified both our surgical approach and our desired final postoperative result. While emmetropia remains attractive to patients, especially younger myopes, our experience and research suggest that our refractive goal should be slight undercorrection. PERK study data have revealed a 5-year hyperopic shift in 22% of patients and a 10-year shift in 43%.[1,2] Deitz has also reported a hyperopic shift in 38% of patients following RK using metal blade knives.[3] Because it is not possible to identify these patients preoperatively, one approach is to operate with the intention of leaving patients slightly undercorrected. A small amount of residual myopia permits useful vision at all ages, whereas a hyperopic final correction would be

less desirable. As younger patients become presbyopic, the benefits of additional useful near vision gained from a diopter of myopia and the delayed need for reading glasses will be appreciated. Presbyopic candidates for refractive surgery realize the difficulties with near vision and can opt for more or less undercorrection or monovision (one eye distance, one eye near).

From a practical standpoint, the adjustment of surgical goals must influence surgical planning and method. If the goal is to undercorrect and never go beyond emmetropia, then a staged approach to surgery may be most beneficial. It is safer to aim for undercorrection on an initial procedure and perform secondary (enhancement) procedures after the initial outcome is known, so as to bring the refractive result into an acceptable range for both the surgeon and patient (Fig 20–1).[4] The major difficulty with this approach is the selection of a secondary procedure that will achieve the desired final correction.

Although the term *enhancement procedure* has been popularized through RK courses, we will try to refrain from its use. Patients perceive an enhancement as a less significant procedure with smaller risks designed solely to improve the previous refractive result. In fact, we must take care to inform the patients that a secondary procedure not only carries the same risks as the primary one, but also involves greater technical difficulty. A detailed discussion with overanxious patients may

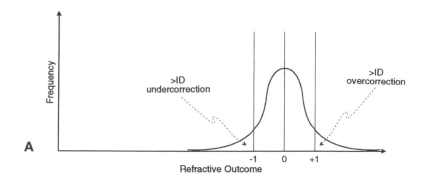

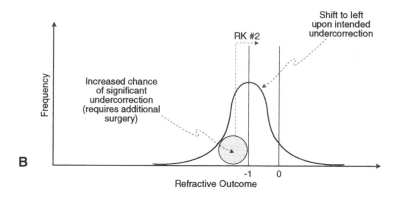

Figure 20–1. Theoretical distribution of refractive outcome. **A.** Aiming at full refraction results in a significant number of patients who are overcorrected. **B.** Aiming at undercorrection results in more undercorrected patients and few overcorrected patients. **C.** Improved distribution around the desired result following reoperation for undercorrection.

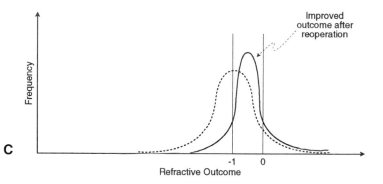

help persuade them to defer additional surgery when their initial refractive procedure has yielded a satisfactory outcome.

The staged approach to refractive surgery has several potential disadvantages as well. Multiple procedures entail extra cost and effort to patients, doctor, and assistants. This includes direct financial costs, time off from work for the patient and escort, and additional time in the office for follow-up examinations. Furthermore, the staged approach seems to raise patients' expectations regarding the final result because of the presumed possibility of refining the refractive outcome through multiple "enhancements."

THE USE OF NOMOGRAMS AND UNEXPECTED RESULTS

Patient Factors

It is evident that different patients will have varying responses to the same refractive surgical procedure. Refractive keratotomy nomograms, which are used to account for different patient variables, have evolved through the experience of many surgeons. A nomogram represents the average response of a large number of patients of the same age and with the same refractive error. In general, younger patients obtain lower surgical benefit than older patients from the same refractive procedure. This phenomenon may be due to the greater wound-healing response in younger patients. However, it is important to note that an individual patient's response may vary significantly from the predicted response based on the results of a nomogram.[5] Although the effect of age on refractive surgery has been quantitated, the influences of gender and intraocular pressure (IOP) on the final refractive result are less well defined.[6,7]

Surgeon Factors

An individual surgeon's nomogram results may also vary greatly, as minute variations in technique may yield significant differences.[6,7] A different brand or style of blade may produce different results. Centripetally (uphill) cut incisions generally produce more of an effect than centrifugally (downhill) cut incisions, and a combination-style incision may be equivalent to a centripetal incision. The amount of pressure used to applanate the blade during the procedure varies among incisions, meridians, and even surgeons. The sharpness of the blade and its overall surface maintenance may yield subtle changes in the incisions, affecting wound healing and refractive outcome (Fig 20–2). Patient cooperation may force the surgeon to modify the procedure intraoperatively. If a combination-style incision is attempted, the surgeon may elect to perform a centrifugal incision rather than attempt to recut back to the central clear zone, or optical zone (OZ). Poor patient fixation may result in a decentered procedure with an unexpected refractive result, such as an induced astigmatism. A surgical complication such as a macro-

perforation may occur that requires suturing or a bandage contact lens, resulting in a variation from the planned surgical outcome.[8] Finally, surgical error while performing the procedure, or use of the incorrect nomogram, may yield an undesired surgical result.

TIMING OF SECONDARY PROCEDURES

Several factors must be taken into account when a second or third refractive procedure on the same eye is considered. Among the most important factors are the patient's uncorrected vision, current refractive correction, and expectation from surgery. Many patients, following RK, will have better uncorrected visual acuities postoperatively than would be expected based on their refractive errors. This may be due to the creation of a multifocal cornea, which allows greater range of correction obtained through slightly off-axis viewing[9,10] (Fig 20–3). The patient's expectations and level of satisfaction need to be reevaluated frequently. Some patients are content with an uncorrected visual acuity of 20/60, whereas others are dissatisfied with 20/20. The surgeon must remind the patient that in most instances refractive surgery is intended to reduce dependence on glasses, and that vision can be enhanced with a spectacle lens in virtually all cases. There is no benefit in rushing to perform a secondary procedure, and it is preferable to wait at least 4 to 6 weeks following the initial procedure. Patients may have a significant change toward myopia or emmetropia in the first few weeks postoperatively. Before additional surgery is considered, adequate time should be allowed for the patients to become accustomed to the new vision and to appreciate better uncorrected distance vision and/or more useful near vision. Patients who were −5.00 D preop may initially be dissatisfied with a −1.50 sph result. Given time, they will have more of a chance to appreciate the significant improvement in their vision. An attempt to simulate monovision by fitting a presbyopic patient with a contact lens on the second eye for a trial period before attempting full correction on the first eye may be useful. Although it is technically easier to operate in the earlier stages of wound healing, there should be no rush to push the eye to emmetropia immediately following the initial procedure. Once the refraction is stable and the patient's needs are appropriately evaluated, a secondary procedure, still aiming toward a final result of slight undercorrection, may be performed.

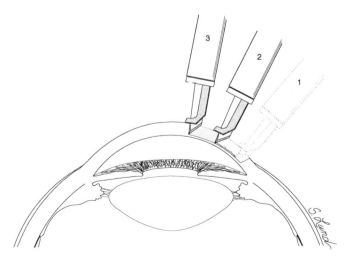

Figure 20–2. Effect of surgical technique on incision depth.

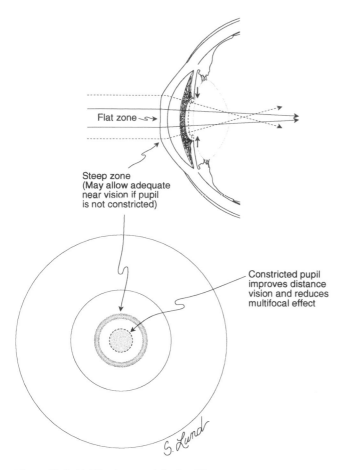

Flat zone →

Steep zone
(May allow adequate
near vision if pupil
is not constricted)

Constricted pupil
improves distance
vision and reduces
multifocal effect

S. Lund

Figure 20–3. Multifocal cornea following RK surgery

CONTRAINDICATIONS TO A SECONDARY PROCEDURE

The refractive surgeon must be aware of the contraindications to performing a secondary procedure. In general, it is preferable not to enhance any eye with less than 0.75 D of residual myopia. The risk for overcorrection in these patients is quite high, and we defer any enhancement procedure even if the patient appears dissatisfied. Patients with clear central zones of 3 mm or less should not be enhanced, regardless of the refraction. These patients are much more likely to suffer from disabling side effects of the surgery. Patients with significant glare or sunbursting following their primary procedure should not be enhanced unless their symptoms subside. If the corneal topography reveals significant induced irregular astigmatism postoperatively, it may not be possible to correct with an incisional technique. The surgeon must carefully follow any change in topography in relation to both the exam and the refraction in order to determine whether the new refractive error is surgically correctable. Although most patients will experience some fluctuation in their vision throughout the course of the day, some patients may have disabling fluctuations of several diopters during the course of the day, requiring multiple pairs of spectacles. These patients should wait for greater stability before additional refractive surgery is considered.

INDICATIONS FOR SECONDARY SURGERY

Secondary incisional surgery should be reserved for patients with residual myopia or astigmatism of greater than 1 D whose uncorrected visual acuity is inadequate for their needs. This secondary procedure, aiming at a slight undercorrection, should only be performed after the patient's needs are carefully assessed. Patients complaining of monocular diplopia postoperatively with induced or residual astigmatism may need a secondary procedure to help alleviate their symptoms.

MANAGEMENT OF UNDERCORRECTION

If a patient is still significantly undercorrected following a primary RK procedure, the initial approach should be to identify any potential error in the surgical planning. Was the initial refraction correct? Was the correct nomogram used and the appropriate optical zone selected? In addition, careful examination of the incisions at the slit lamp may identify incisions that are not of adequate length or depth, resulting in incomplete flattening. The actual OZ can be measured with the slit lamp beam and compared with the OZ selected from the nomogram. Corneal topography can be very helpful in identifying incisions that produce inadequate corneal flattening. Careful slit lamp examination may reveal decentering of the OZ relative to the pupil. This is best visualized in retroillumination so that the edges of the incisions are seen within the pupil (Figs 20–4, 5). If all of these causes are ruled out, it is possible that the patient responds to a lesser extent than would be expected based on his or her age and refractive error. The nomograms represent average values that combine the results of surgery on under- and overresponders. Patients will have varying responses to surgery, and greater wound healing will result in greater regression of the refraction.

MANAGEMENT OPTIONS

Many options and procedures can be utilized following a single refractive surgical procedure with significant

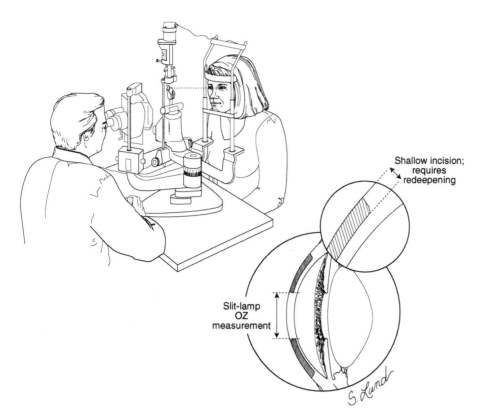

Shallow incision; requires redeepening

Slit-lamp OZ measurement

Figure 20–4. Use of slit lamp to assess radial incisions. In addition to assessing incision depth, the slit lamp is used to measure the achieved OZ.

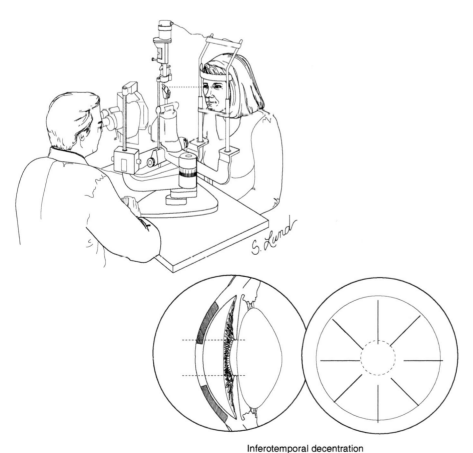

Inferotemporal decentration

Figure 20–5. Use of slit lamp to assess centration of radial incisions. By comparing the central-most extent of incision within the pupil, centration can be evaluated, possibly indicating a need to "decenter" the next surgical procedure.

TABLE 20–1. MANAGEMENT OPTIONS FOR UNDERCORRECTION

Observation
Glasses/contact lenses
Surgery on fellow eye (more than originally planned)
Candidate for monovision
Secondary RK
    Correct identifiable errors in previous surgical plan
    Redeepen/recut original incisions
    Check for different pachymetry result
    Decrease OZ
    Extend mini-RK peripherally
    Increase number of incisions
Use of excimer laser for residual myopia
    OZ already 3 mm or less
    Eight incisions already performed

Abbreviation: OZ, optical zone.

residual undercorrection (Table 20–1). The first step is to determine if there are any obvious identifiable problems. Was the correct nomogram used? Was the pachymetry reasonable? Do the incisions appear of adequate depth and length by slit lamp examination? After obvious problems are ruled out, a patient with significant undercorrection should have a secondary procedure with repeat pachymetry and redeepening of the original incisions. Occasionally the pachymetry reading will be different from the one used for the initial surgical procedure, so that setting the blade at pachymetry for redeepening will have a substantial effect.

If redeepening the incisions does not produce a satisfactory reduction in myopia, then it is possible to decrease the OZ, to extend the incisions more peripherally, or to increase the number of incisions, depending on the previous procedure and the resultant correction (Table 20–2).

Additional surgery, however, is not the only option. Frequently, a patient with residual myopia is best observed for a longer period of time to see if he or she adapts to being less nearsighted and less dependent on glasses without reaching the initial refractive goal. Another alternative is to operate on a smaller OZ in the fellow eye than the nomogram recommends, based on the result from the first eye. This will often give good distance correction in the second eye, and, if appropriate and or desired, the first eye can be left myopic for monovision.

The usefulness of the excimer laser to correct residual myopia following RK has already been established.[11,12] In eyes with high risk of side effects and complications from additional incisional procedures, excimer laser keratectomy (ELK) may allow patients to achieve their desired refractive goal. The predictability of this procedure in eyes that have undergone RK will likely improve as more patients are treated in this manner.

Whatever the situation, the specific options, risks, benefits, and alternatives need to be discussed in detail with the patient to allow for appropriate participation in the decision-making process. After understanding the options, patients will often adjust their expectations and goals.

THE SURGICAL PROCEDURES

A secondary procedure is performed in the same manner as the primary RK procedure. The procedure is done in a microsurgical suite with betadine prep and sterile drape. Oral valium is usually satisfactory for sedation. The eye may be anesthetized with tetracaine, proparacaine, 4% xylocaine, or marcaine, depending on the surgeon's preference. The only important exception is that the pupil should be dilated preoperatively. The red reflex provides better visualization of the previous incisions than does a nondilated pupil.

TABLE 20–2. SURGICAL TECHNIQUES

	Recutting Incisions	Extending Incisions	Adding Incisions
Criteria	Shallow incisions	Existing OZ >3 mm, minimal glare	Existing OZ ≤3.5 mm, ≤4 previous incisions
Optical zone	Same	Smaller, concentric, unless incisions decentered[a]	Same
Additional incisions	None	None	Total ≤8 >8: effect is minimal
Blade	Enhancement/dual cutting	Vertical blade/dual cutting	Dual cutting
Sinskey hook	Yes (recent)	No	No
Incision technique	Redeepening/uphill	Downhill: bridging old incision Uphill: extending incision	Combined technique

[a]Decentered incisions observed at slit lamp preoperatively.
Abbreviation: OZ, optical zone.

Pachymetry is always repeated at the time of surgery in the same locations used in the initial procedure. This result should be compared with the pachymetry result and blade setting used in the primary procedure. The type of blade used depends on the type of procedure to be performed. Specific blade types will be discussed in relation to each of the procedures. The blade should generally be set at pachymetry or according to the nomogram or manufacturer's recommendation. The surgeon should plan to modify the procedure based on the slit lamp examination and corneal topography (Table 20–2). A sketch of the incisions and the corneal topographic map are generally useful in the operating room when performing a secondary procedure.

RECUTTING INCISIONS

Recutting the original incisions is probably the most common secondary procedure performed. An enhancement-style blade or dual cutting blade is easiest and safest for the procedure. The procedure varies in level of difficulty depending on the length of time since the primary procedure. "Fresh" incisions (within the past 6 weeks) are significantly easier to open than year-old wounds. Nevertheless, the procedure can be performed safely and all wounds can be opened with careful surgical technique. We prefer to open the wounds first with a Sinskey hook by gently nudging the tip of the hook through the epithelium and then sliding the hook along the length of the incision to break the epithelial portion of the wound. The wound can then be entered with the diamond knife and recut along its entire length. Great attention should be directed to the paracentral zone to obtain maximum incisional depth in this location.

Alternatively, some surgeons prefer to enter the incisions directly with the diamond knife and not use a Sinskey hook. The blade is tickled into the incision, and the blade tends to drop into the original incisional plane. After recutting the incisions, the wounds may be irrigated with balanced salt solution if significant epithelial plugging was noted preoperatively.

EXTENDING INCISIONS (DECREASING OPTICAL ZONE)

Deciding whether or not to extend incisions centrally depends on several factors. The patient must have residual myopia greater than 1 D with incisions of adequate depth. The OZ should be larger than 3 mm, and

there should be minimal or no complaints of glare. A vertical (Russian style) or dual cutting blade is better to use than an angled blade, as it will produce a deeper incision at the desired OZ.

The patient is asked to fixate on a target and the new OZ marker (usually 0.5 mm smaller than previously) is used to mark the cornea. This should be centered within the original incisions unless preoperatively the incisions were noted to be decentered. The technique differs depending upon the type of blade used. We prefer a dual cutting blade for safety. The blade penetrates the cornea at the new OZ mark directly in line with the original incision, and the blade is then used to cut back to the tip of the original incision and then back to the OZ. If a vertical cutting blade is used, the blade penetrates the cornea at the most central location of the original wound, and a new incision is cut centrally in a centripetal fashion to the new OZ marker. It is probably slightly safer to fixate the globe when extending the incisions into the central OZ, but surgical preferences vary.

ADDING ADDITIONAL INCISIONS

The potential benefit of adding additional incisions depends on the number or incisions already present. Most of the flattening effect occurs from the first four incisions, and after eight incisions have been placed, the additional effect is usually minimal. Patients who have had a four-incision RK with residual myopia are the usual candidates for additional incisions. A centripetal, centrifugal, or dual cutting-style incision can be made, depending on the surgeon's preference. The patient is asked to fixate on a target while the OZ and new incisions are marked. The same OZ used in the primary procedure is normally utilized. The authors do not recommend adding radial incisions to an eight-incision RK, as the additional benefit is usually minimal and adds a significant risk for destabilization of the cornea, producing greater fluctuations in vision and possibly irregular astigmatism.

RESIDUAL OR INDUCED ASTIGMATISM

The management of residual or induced astigmatism is a complex subject (Table 20–3). If residual myopia is still present, the original radial incisions should be recut first before attempting additional astigmatic correction. Careful slit lamp examination and corneal topog-

TABLE 20–3. MANAGEMENT OF RESIDUAL AND INDUCED ASTIGMATISM FOLLOWING RADIAL KERATOTOMY

Condition	Approach	Potential Complication
High residual myopia	Recut/extend original incisions	Increased surface irregularity
Hyperopic spherical equivalent	Avoid further surgery	Increased flattening
Hemimeridional asymmetry by topography	Surgery in steep hemimeridian, asymmetric incisions	Crossing radial incisions, perforation, unpredictability
Previous astigmatic incisions		
Shallow	Recut incisions, pachymetry at astigmatic incision	Macroperforation
Deep, same axis	Extend/add incisions	Crossing radial incisions, unpredictability
Deep, different axis	Suturing if overcorrected, PAK, avoid new incisions	Instability, gaping of neighboring incisions

Abbreviation: PAK, photoastigmatic keratectomy.

raphy are usually helpful in the surgical planning in order to highlight which incisions may be responsible for the residual or induced astigmatism. Additional astigmatic procedures can only be performed if the spherical equivalent is plano or myopic.

If the primary procedure involved the placement of astigmatic incisions, then residual astigmatism present in the same axis can be treated by recutting and/or extending the original astigmatic incisions. The surgical technique is the same used to redeepen radial incisions, described above. A diamond blade designed for astigmatic incisions is usually best suited for this purpose. If no astigmatic cuts are present and the radial incisions have already been recut, astigmatic cuts can be placed in the appropriate axis. An arcuate incision or T-cut technique may be used, but the radial incision must be "jumped" to minimize destabilization of the cornea. If residual astigmatism is present in a different axis from the original astigmatic cuts, following an attempt at recutting, new astigmatic cuts may be placed, or alternatively, excimer laser photoastigmatic keratectomy may be performed.

REFERENCES

1. Waring GO, Lynn MJ, Nizam A, et al. Results of the evaluation of radial keratotomy (PERK) five years after surgery. *Ophthalmology.* 1991;98:1164–1176.

2. Waring GO, Lynn MJ, McDonnell PJ. Results of the prospective evaluation of radial keratotomy (PERK) study 10 years after surgery. *Arch Ophthalmol.* 1994;112:1298–1308.

3. Deitz MR, et al. Long-term (5 to 12 year) follow-up of metal-blade radial keratotomy procedures. *Arch Ophthalmol.* 1994;112:614–620.

4. Werblin TP, Stafford GM. The Casebeer system for predictable keratorefractive surgery. *Ophthalmology.* 1993;100:1095–1102.

5. Jester JV. Variations in corneal wound healing after radial keratotomy: possible insights into mechanisms of clinical complications and refractive effects. *Cornea.* 1992;11:191–199.

6. Melles GR, et al. Effect of blade configuration, knife action, and intraocular pressure on keratotomy incision depth and shape. *Cornea.* 1993;12:299–309.

7. Merlin U, et al. Factors that affect keratotomy depth. *Refract Corneal Surg.* 1991;7:356–359.

8. Leroux les Jardins S, Bertrand I, Massin M. Intraoperative and early postoperative complications in 466 radial keratotomies. *Refract Corneal Surg.* 1992;8:215–216.

9. Moreira H, et al. Multifocal corneal topographic changes after radial keratotomy. *Ophthalmic Surg.* 1992;23:85–89.

10. Lopez PF, et al. Subregions of differing refractive power within the clear zone after experimental radial keratotomy. *Refract Corneal Surg.* 1991;7:360–367.

11. Hahn TW, et al. Excimer laser photorefractive keratotomy to correct residual myopia after radial keratotomy. *Refract Corneal Surg.* 1993;9:S25–29.

12. Seiler T, Jean B. Photorefractive keratectomy as a second attempt to correct myopia after radial keratotomy. *Refract Corneal Surg.* 1992;8:211–214.

CHAPTER 21

Clinical Results of Radial Keratotomy

Vadim Filatov ▪ Jonathan H. Talamo

INTRODUCTION

The goal of this chapter is to give the reader a summary of the results of radial keratotomy (RK). These results can be interpreted based upon analysis of either single or bilateral procedures. In either case, the success of an elective procedure like radial keratotomy is measured by both its objective and its subjective results. The objective variables that are typically assessed after RK include uncorrected visual acuity (UCVA), refraction, and best corrected visual acuity (BCVA). Several other visual factors like contrast sensitivity, glare, diurnal fluctuation, and complications threatening visual loss or distortion have also been examined. These factors are generally measured at various intervals following RK, allowing their stability and predictability to be studied. Subjective evaluations measure the patient's overall satisfaction, perceived need for refractive aids, and the degree to which preoperative expectations were fulfilled. Subjective evaluations also examine whether patients would choose to have RK again.

A number of comprehensive reviews of various aspects of refractive surgical procedures have been published elsewhere.[1-16] The scope of this chapter is limited to the most current analysis of RK. The results of astigmatic keratotomy alone or in combination with RK are covered in other chapters.

RESULTS

The Prospective Evaluation of Radial Keratotomy (PERK) study is an ongoing multicenter clinical trial sponsored by the National Eye Institute to evaluate a standardized technique of radial keratotomy.[1,3,17-27] Four hundred and thirty-five patients who had physiologic myopia between −2.00 and −8.75 diopters underwent RK using eight centripetal incisions made with a diamond micrometer knife. All patients were at least 21 years of age and had stable myopia documented by previous records. Patients were examined at regular intervals, and the results of the procedure at 6 months and at 1,3,4,5,6, and 10 years following RK have been published. Most patients had to wait a mandatory 12 months before having RK performed on the fellow less myopic eye.[22] A recent multicenter study of a combined technique of RK by Verity et al reported better results than those obtained by PERK.[28] The authors have attributed the improvement in the RK results to a number of factors:

1. The improved methodology of a newer incision technique, in which the depth is uniform and the limbus is spared
2. Use of screening and intraoperative pachymetry, in which the incisions are placed in the thinnest corneal quadrant first

3. Use of computer-assisted videokeratography
4. Use of ultrathin diamond knives with improved design and accuracy in tip calibration
5. Incorporation of the patient's age as a variable in the predictive nomograms

The strength of the study was its prospective nature and standardization of the protocol. One shortcoming of the study was the low mean follow-up interval (6.2 months). Fortunately, based on the PERK data, meaningful comparisons of RK results can be made as early as 6 months following RK. Werblin and Stafford reported 3-year follow-up data on 128 patients who have undergone radial/astigmatic keratotomy for the correction of myopia/astigmatism.[2] This study differs from PERK and Verity et al in many ways. Most significantly, it used Casebeer nomograms, which, unlike PERK and like Verity et al, used age to guide the surgical plan. Werblin et al performed RK with a Russian centripetal technique; PERK used the American centrifugal technique; and Verity et al used a combined pass (Genesis) technique. Werblin was one of the first authors to promote a staged approach to RK.

The combined incision technique is thought to combine the safety of the American technique with the efficacy of the Russian technique, achieving deeper incisions than either the American or the Russian techniques while preventing the extension of the incision beyond the optical zone (OZ) toward the visual axis.[28,29] It is important to note that these conclusions were reached without the benefit of a randomized, prospective clinical trial comparing various incision techniques.

Uncorrected Visual Acuity

PERK

Prior to RK, uncorrected visual acuity (UCVA) was worse than 20/40 in 99.7% and less than 20/160 in 66% of operated eyes in the PERK study. Ten years after RK, 579 eyes (85%) had visual acuity of 20/40 or better; 358 eyes (53%) saw 20/20 or better; and only 11 eyes (2%) saw 20/200 (Table 21–1). In the lower myopia group, UCVA of 20/40 or better was attained by 92% of patients 1 year after RK, and this percentage remained stable over 10 years (Table 21–1). UCVA of 20/20 or better was present in 68% of lower myopia patients 10 years after RK, versus 71% 1 year after RK.

In both the moderate and higher myopia groups, the percentage of patients who saw 20/40 or better increased over time. In the moderate myopia group, 86%

of patients saw 20/40 or better, and 60% saw 20/20 or better 10 years after RK, compared with 81% and 49% 1 year after RK (Table 21–2). The increase in the number of eyes that attained UCVA of 20/40 or better 10 years after RK was even greater in the higher myopia group, with 77% and 43% of patients seeing 20/40 and 20/20 or better 10 years after RK (Table 21–3), compared with 63% and 26% 1 year after RK. The increase in the percentage of patients with UCVA of 20/40 and 20/20 or better in the three refractive groups from 1 to 10 years after RK is most likely due to the progressive hyperopic effect of the procedure.

The number of eyes undercorrected by 1 D 1 year after RK differed greatly between the three refractive groups. There was a strong correlation between undercorrection and the degree of preoperative myopia (5%, 26%, and 56% were undercorrected by 1 D or more in the low, moderate, and higher myopia groups, respectively). The percentage of eyes undercorrected by 1 D or more 10 years after RK remained 5% in the lower myopia group; decreased by 12%, from 26% to 14%, in the

TABLE 21–1. PERK RESULTS FOR LOW MYOPIA, IN PERCENT

		Year of Follow-up				
		1	3	4	5[a]	10
UCVA	≥20/40	*92*	*91*	*94*	*95*	*92*
	>20/20	*71*	*74*	*76*	*75*	*68*
Refractive results						
±1.0 D of goal		84	76	73	75	67
±0.5 D of goal		57	46	44	51	47
≥ +1.0 D		11	16	21	18	27
≥ −1.0 D		5	7	6	7	5
≥ +0.5 D		28	38	40	35	43
> −0.5 D		15	17	17	14	8

[a]Five-year data include the results of reoperated eyes, which slightly improves overall visual results.

TABLE 21–2. PERK RESULTS FOR MODERATE MYOPIA, IN PERCENT

		Year of Follow-up				
		1	3	4	5[a]	10
UCVA	≥20/40	*81*	*81*	*79*	*89*	*86*
	>20/20	*49*	*50*	*53*	*63*	*60*
Refractive results						
±1.0 D of goal		62	61	58	67	62
±0.5 D of goal		33	38	49	45	33
≥ +1.0 D		12	19	20	20	25
≥ −1.0 D		26	19	22	13	14
≥ +0.5 D		21	27	29	26	39
> −0.5 D		46	35	36	29	28

[a]Five-year data include the results of reoperated eyes, which slightly improves overall visual results.

TABLE 21–3. PERK RESULTS FOR HIGH MYOPIA, IN PERCENT

		1	3	4	5[a]	10
				Year of Follow-up		
UCVA	≥20/40	*63*	*60*	*58*	*79*	*77*
	>20/20	*26*	*33*	*32*	*43*	*43*
Refractive results						
±1.0 D of goal		38	39	39	49	54
±0.5 D of goal		22	20	23	29	35
≥ +1.0 D		6	13	11	14	18
≥ −1.0 D		56	48	50	37	28
≥ +0.5 D		9	18	16	22	27
> −0.5 D		69	62	61	49	38

[a]Five-year data include the results of reoperated eyes, which slightly improves overall visual results.

moderate myopia group; and by 28%, from 56% to 28%, in the higher myopia group. The percentage of eyes with VA worse than 20/40 in the three refractive groups (8%, 14%, and 23%, respectively) corresponds well with the percentage of eyes in the three groups that were undercorrected by 1 D or more 10 years after RK (5%, 14%, and 28%, respectively). Whether undercorrected eyes represent the majority of eyes with the VA worse than 20/40 is not known.

In summary, UCVA of 20/40 or better is achieved in 92% of patients in the lower myopia group and remains unchanged over the period of 10 years. In the moderate myopia group, UCVA of 20/40 or better is attained by 81% of patients at 1 year, increasing to 86% at 10 years. Similarly, in the high myopia group, UCVA of 20/40 or better increased from 63% of eyes at 1 year to 77% at 10 years after RK.

Finally, although UCVA is the most common measure of the effectiveness of refractive corneal surgery, in some cases UCVA corresponds to what is considered a poor refractive outcome. The reverse also occurs. To reconcile these sometimes conflicting measures, a visual function score combining these two variables (UCVA and refractive error) was devised that classified patients into four categories (excellent, good, fair, and poor). Patients in the excellent category had a refractive error of −1.00 D to + 0.50 D and UCVA of 20/25 or better.[1] Patients in the poor category were either undercorrected by 3 D or overcorrected by 2 D, with UCVA of 20/100 or worse. Patients in the good and fair categories had intermediate values of refractive error and visual acuity. For PERK patients 5 years after RK, 48%, 32%, 13%, and 7% of patients attained visual function scores of excellent, good, fair, and poor, respectively.

Other Studies

Several other studies have been performed in the last decade, although few were prospective.[2,28,30–42] Their results are presented as percentages of patients with UCVA of 20/40 or better, since only a few provided UCVA results of 20/20 or 20/25 or better. It was not known at the time that although UCVA of 20/40 is adequate for driving, it does not predict patients' satisfaction as well as UCVA of 20/25 or better. Another limitation of multistudy comparisons is that subgroup analysis by the degree of baseline myopia often varies between studies and sometimes is not even provided, making direct comparisons between different studies difficult and often inexact.

Despite these limitations, important information about RK can be gleaned from the evaluation and comparison of RK results from a number of different studies. For example, like PERK, best UCVA results have been achieved in patients with the least amount of preoperative myopia. With the exception of Sawelson,[40,43] all studies achieved UCVA of 20/40 or better in 95% to 100% of patients. In the PERK, low myopes achieved UCVA of 20/40 or better in 91% to 95% of eyes, depending on the year of follow-up. Dietz (diamond blade) reported UCVA results of 20/20 or better in 65% of his patients. This compares well to the PERK data, where low myopes achieved UCVA of 20/20 or better in 68% to 76% of eyes, depending on the year of follow-up.

As in PERK, the percentage of patients in these studies with UCVA of 20/40 or better decreased as preoperative myopia increased. Visual results also became more variable as the degree of baseline myopia increased. Moderate myopes achieved UCVA of 20/40 or better in 74% to 90% of patients.[8,30–40] Again this was similar to the PERK data (79% to 89%) depending on the year of follow-up.

Higher myopes (greater than −6 D) faired worst. UCVA of 20/40 or better was achieved in 31% to 77% of patients.[8,30–44] In the PERK data, higher myopes did somewhat better, with 58% to 79% of eyes achieving the same level of VA, depending on the year of follow-up.

Loss of Best Corrected Visual Acuity

PERK

Any elective refractive procedure to reduce myopia in otherwise healthy eyes must not only be efficacious; it must also be safe. Safety can be ascertained by comparing visual function before and after the elective procedure. Best corrected visual acuity is perhaps the most important reflection of visual function and is defined in all studies as best spectacle-corrected visual acuity. Loss of two or more Snellen lines of BCVA is considered visually significant because possible changes of one line (three to five letters) can occur from one examination to another in unoperated eyes, especially with visual acuities of 20/20 or better. In the PERK study, all eyes had a spectacle-corrected visual acuity of 20/25 or better. One year after surgery, BCVA was unchanged in 61%, decreased by one Snellen chart line in 13%, decreased by two to three lines in 0.7%, increased by one line in 24%, and increased by two to three lines in 1.7%, remaining fairly stable over the 10-year period. There was a slight increase in the percentage of patients who lost two to three lines (0.7% at 1 year to 1.4% at 3 years to 3% at 4 years after RK). Loss of BCVA remained unchanged at 3% from 4 to 10 years following RK. BCVA loss was from 20/15 to 20/25 or 20/30. Ten years after RK, BCVA was 20/20 or better in 98%, 20/25 in 1.6%, and 20/30 in 0.4% of eyes in the PERK study. No patient had BCVA worse than 20/30 10 years after RK.

Other Studies

Although many studies describe a variety of visual complications following RK, only two studies with a long follow-up period report the percentage of eyes with the loss of BCVA of two lines or greater.[30,43] These results differ greatly, with only 0.5% of patients in the Dietz study and nearly 10% in the Sawelson study demonstrating this degree of visual loss. The study by Verity et al reports a 0.3% incidence of BCVA loss of two Snellen lines or more, but with only 6 months mean follow-up.[28] The incidence of perforations varies greatly. While Dietz has reported a 36% incidence, PERK and most of the recent studies report a much lower rate of 2% to 3%.

Endothelial cell loss of 5% to 10% has been reported a few weeks following RK. The loss of endothelial cells appears to be self-limiting, but the long-term sequelae are unknown. PERK data indicate that endothelial cell loss does not lead to corneal edema 10 years after RK. Whether corneal decompensation from initial endothelial cell damage may occur 20 or 30 years after RK is still not known.

Fortunately, with recent technical advances and an improved understanding of corneal wound healing after RK, many of these complications can now be minimized. Improved pachymetry, diamond-knife calibration microscopes, and the knowledge that the thinnest area of cornea needs to be incised first reduce the likelihood of perforations, which should decrease the incidence of endothelial cell loss, cataract formation, and endophthalmitis.

Sparing the limbus reduces neovascularization and scarring, making it easier to fit contact lenses following RK. Avoiding intersecting radial and astigmatic incisions reduces scarring, irregular astigmatism, and stromal melting. The reduced number and length of radial incisions may decrease the likelihood of traumatic rupture.

Diurnal Fluctuation

Significant diurnal variation of visual acuity is a nuisance that cannot be easily corrected. In normal corneas, diurnal refractive fluctuation is minimal. Nearly two thirds of patients have stable vision throughout the day. In the remaining third, vision varies by one Snellen line or less.[17] Following RK, diurnal fluctuation is common for the first several months, but appears to be infrequent thereafter.

However, in a small subgroup of PERK patients who complained of any form of visual fluctuation, only 24% had stable vision throughout the day.[19-22] A loss of one line of vision occurred in 37%, of two to three lines in 22%, and of four to six lines in 2% of patients, respectively. A gain of one line of vision was reported in 13%, and two to three lines were lost in the remaining 2% of patients. Despite a poor correlation between manifest refraction and UCVA, diurnal fluctuation of manifest refraction was substantially increased after RK. Whereas 89% of unoperated eyes had less than half a diopter of change in manifest refraction, only 56% of operated eyes were as stable. The major change in refraction occurs within the first hour after awakening and continues for a few hours, after which a small drift persists in some patients.[45] In general, gradual corneal steepening occurred during the day, with a resultant increase in myopia. Diurnal myopic shift of 0.5 to 1.00 D was observed in 33% of operated eyes, compared with 8% of unoperated eyes. Myopic fluctuation did not exceed 1.25 D. The tendency toward diurnal hyperopic shift was low in both groups: 2% in operated and 3% in unoperated eyes. The magnitude of the diurnal change was similar 3 months and 1 year after the RK, reflecting the persistence of wound instability 1 year after RK in this group of patients. The amount of diurnal fluctuation of refractive error did not correlate well with preoperative refractive error, patient age, or change in keratometric power.

It is not known how many patients in the PERK study had objective diurnal variation of vision because only patients who complained of subjective diurnal fluctuation in vision were studied, comprising a very small proportion of PERK patients. Furthermore, of the initial 63 patients who had diurnal symptoms 3 months after RK, only 46 returned for a 1-year follow-up[17]; only 52 patients who were examined at 3 months and 41 patients who were examined at 1 year returned for a 4-year follow-up. Because 83% of these patients had bilateral surgery by this time, only first operated eyes were examined for diurnal fluctuations in this report. Diurnal fluctuation of 0.5 D or more ocurred in 31% of patients between 2.5 and 4 years after RK, compared with 33% at 1 year, reflecting the persistence of diurnal fluctuation 4 years after RK.[4]

The increase in the relative paracentral corneal steepening after RK may contribute to an increased nocturnal myopic shift after RK.[20] Diurnal fluctuation may also be secondary to an increased corneal instability from large numbers or length of RK incisions. Whether decreasing the incision number or length reduces diurnal fluctuation is not known. Diurnal fluctuation may be associated with the degree of endothelial-cell loss. Presumably endothelial cell loss contributes to increased corneal hydration at night, resulting in hyperopic shift upon awakening, with subsequent resolution of edema causing a compensatory myopic shift during the day.

Refractive Outcome

PERK

The median refractive error before surgery in the PERK study was −3.88 D (range, −8.88 to −1.50 D). One year after RK, the mean (SD) decrease in the myopic refractive error was 3.60 D (1.58 D). The mean decrease in the myopia and the width of the standard deviation continued to increase over the 10-year interval period after the surgery. Ten years after the procedure, the mean (SD) decrease in the myopic refractive error reached 4.32 D (1.89 D). The refractive error over the 10-year period shifted from −0.36 D at 6 months to +0.51 at 10 years. The rate of the hyperopic shift of the mean refractive error was smallest in the lower myopia group and largest in the higher myopia group. The mean refractive error 1 to 10 years after the RK changed from +0.14 D to +0.54 D in the lower myopia group, from −0.33 D to +0.30 D in the moderate myopia group, and from −1.19 D to −0.20 D in the higher myopia group.

The percentage of eyes within 0.50 D and 1.00 D of emmetropia varied between the three baseline refraction groups not only in its absolute amount but also by the pattern of change in these numbers over the 10-year period. At the 10-year examination, the refractive error within 0.50 D and 1.00 D of emmetropia was 38% and 60% in all eyes, 47% and 67% in the lower group, 33% and 62% in the moderate group, and 35% and 54% in the higher group. The percentage of eyes within 1 D of the intended correction was greater in the patients with lower preoperative myopia in both the PERK data and in other studies.[1,2,28,30–43] The percentage of patients within 1 D of the intended correction in the three baseline refractive groups was: low myopia (75% to 97%); moderate myopia (50% to 82%); and high myopia (38% to 90%), compared with 67%, 62%, and 54% in the PERK 10-year study (Table 21–4).

Undercorrection

PERK

Undercorrection by more than −1 D 1 year after RK differed greatly among the three baseline refraction groups and correlated well with the degree of preoperative myopia. At 1 year following RK in the PERK study, undercorrection by −1 D or more occurred in 5%, 26%, and 56% of eyes in the lower, moderate, and higher myopia groups, respectively. The percentage of eyes undercorrected by −1 D or more 10 years after RK remained 5% in the lower myopia group, decreased from 26% to 14% in the moderate myopia group, and fell from 56% to 28% in the higher myopia group. Percentages of eyes with undercorrections of more than −0.50 in the three groups were: lower, 8%; moderate, 28%; and higher, 38%.

Other Studies

The PERK result of 17% of undercorrection by 1 D or more at 10 years following RK falls within the spectrum

TABLE 21–4. REFRACTIVE OUTCOME ±1 D OF INTENDED CORRECTION, IN PERCENT

Studies	Low (±1)	Moderate (±1)	High (±1)	All (≥ −1 | ±1 | ≥ +1)		
PERK	67	62	54	17	60	23
Dietz	90	76	90	12	76	13
Arrowsmith	75	50	38	13	53	33
Salz	97	81	45	24	73	3
Shepard	90	82	70	11	76	8
Friedberg	96	81	67		85	

of results from other studies, where 11% to 46% of patients were undercorrected by 1 D or more. Verity et al reported undercorrection by −1 D in 6%, 10%, and 25% of patients in the low (1.00 D to 3.12 D), moderate (3.25 D to 4.25 D), and high (4.50 D to 9.50 D) myopia groups.[28]

Overcorrection

PERK

During the same period, hyperopic shift, which decreased the percentage of undercorrected eyes, correspondingly increased the percentage of overcorrected eyes. Overcorrections in the PERK study were similar in the lower and moderate myopia groups, and occurred least often in the higher myopia group. Percentages of eyes with overcorrections of more than +1 D in the three groups 10 years after the procedure in the PERK study were lower, 27%; moderate, 25%; and higher, 18%.

Other Studies

Like undercorrection, overcorrection by 1 D or more in the PERK study 10 years after RK (23%) fell in between the results of other studies, where the range of patients overcorrected by 1 D or more varied between 3% and 33%.

RK reduced, but did not eliminate, myopia in all baseline refractive groups. The reduction of myopia was directly related to the degree of preoperative myopia. Hyperopic shift that persisted for 10 years after RK resulted in the redistribution of undercorrected patients to overcorrected patients in the PERK and other studies.

Stability of Refractive Error

PERK

Although the average change in refraction for 341 eyes from 6 months to 4 years following RK was only minimally influenced by reoperation (+0.43 ± 0.70 after a single procedure and +0.39 ± 0.87 after reoperation), refractive change from 6 months to 10 years after surgery was examined in eyes that underwent only a primary procedure (n = 330). Between 1 and 10 years, the percentage of eyes undercorrected by more than 1 D decreased from 20% to 11%, while the percentage of eyes overcorrected by more than 1 D increased from 11% to 30%. Between 6 months and 10 years, 43% of 310 eyes

changed in a hyperopic direction by 1 D or more. The percentage of eyes that changed by 1 D or more in the hyperopic direction was relatively constant from 6 months to 10 years, an increase of approximately 5% annually. Overcorrection and undercorrection by more than 1 D occurred in 23% and 17% of patients. In contrast, none of the fellow unoperated eyes of patients 10 years after RK changed by more than 1 D in the hyperopic direction.

The annual rate of hyperopic progression during the first 2 years was 0.21 D/y (95% confidence interval [CI], 0.17 to 0.26 D/y). From 2 to 10 years the rate of hyperopic shift declined to 0.06 D/yr (95% CI, 0.05 to 0.07 D/y). These data are based on eyes that underwent only a primary procedure, but the refractive error for all eyes was not much different.

The degree of hyperopic shift was directly proportional to the degree of preoperative myopia, and hence inversely proportional to the optical zone (OZ) size. The independent effect of these two variables cannot be established, because optical zones were choosen based on the preoperative myopia in the three baseline refraction groups. On average, the refractive change between 6 months and 10 years was +0.50 greater in the eyes with an OZ of 3 mm, compared with eyes in which the optical zones were 3.5 mm or 4 mm. A similar relation was found between incision depth and the degree of hyperopic shift in a separate study.[40] Hyperopic shift, therefore, seems to be more pronounced in eyes that undergo greater surgery to correct higher degrees of myopia.

Qualitative analysis of the PERK data suggests that hyperopic shift was greatest in the eyes that were overcorrected immediately after the operation, supporting the hypothesis that eyes with greater surgery or response to surgery may be more susceptible to a continued hyperopic drift. It is possible that reducing the amount of surgery by decreasing either the number of incisions or their depth or length may decrease the rate of hyperopic shift.

Other Studies

Hyperopic shift that increases gradually after surgery occurred in all studies of RK and was not limited to PERK, indicating that hyperopic shift is an inherent side effect of RK rather than a flaw in the design of the PERK study. A study by Werblin and Stafford presented at the 1994 Academy of Ophthalmology meeting suggests that the degree and the rate of the hyperopic shift may be significantly reduced following RK as it is currently performed compared with the PERK results for low and moderate myopes.[46]

Symmetry of Uncorrected Visual Acuity (Anisometropia)

One year following RK, the difference in UCVA was one line or less in 60% of patients and four to eight lines in 14% of patients, compared with only 1% of patients at baseline.[24] Because most patients who undergo RK have symmetric myopia preoperatively, the success of RK may be gauged in part by its ability to maintain refractive symmetry after surgery. Symmetric postoperative refraction prevents visually significant anisometropia, although it may be desirable in presbyopic patients (monovision). Anisometropia is more symptomatic in presbyopic patients, particularly in patients with myopia in one eye and hyperopia in the other. However, disturbing anisometropia may be present even in patients with excellent and symmetric UCVA because of a greater variation of manifest refraction for a given UCVA after RK. Tolerable anisometropia may be desired if the first eye was overcorrected or monovision was intended. In the PERK study, however, intentional anisometropia was not used to manage presbyopia.

Based on the fact that a 3-D difference in spectacle correction corresponds to a 4-D difference in vertical prism correction and to approximately 5% aniseikonia, anisometropia of 3 D was choosen as the upper limit of what may be tolerated by a patient. It is well known that anisometropia of 2 D is well tolerated by most patients. One year after the surgery on the second eye, 10% of patients had anisometropia greater than 2 D, and only 2% of patients had anisometropia greater than 3 D.

The median difference between the spherical equivalent of the refractive errors of the two eyes was slightly higher 5 years after bilateral RK: 0.62 D (range, 0 to 7) compared with the difference of 0.25 D (range 0 to 2.37) at baseline.

Induced Astigmatism

Radial keratotomy induced 0.50 to 2.75 D of astigmatism in 34% of eyes 3 years after RK.[47] In 10% of eyes the amount of induced astigmatism 3 years after RK exceeded 1 D. A greater increase in astigmatism is associated with a smaller-diameter OZ.

The association of small-diameter OZ and induced astigmatism was also found 6 months after RK in a study utilizing the combined (Genesis) technique.[28] The number of RK incisions did not influence the degree of induced postoperative astigmatism in this study. Because PERK used a standard eight-incisional RK, PERK data cannot assess the influence of incision number on postoperative outcome, including induced astigmatism.

In irregular astigmatism, astigmatic axes are not orthogonal, and corneal curvature change from the center to the periphery exceeds the changes of a normal aspheric cornea. Corneal curvature becomes irregular following RK, and the central cornea flattens accompanied by compensatory peripheral steepening. Fortunately, the degree of induced irregular astigmatism is low, and it rarely affects vision. In some instances, however, irregular astigmatism not only decreases BCVA, but also induces glare.

Need for Glasses/Lenses

One of the most frequently asked questions by the prospective RK patients is what are their chances of being free of glasses and contact lenses after RK. For most patients, this is the major reason for undergoing the procedure. Therefore, the success of the refractive procedure is often judged by whether it obviates the need for optical correction. PERK is one of the studies that has provided us with some data regarding the need for refractive aid wear following RK. Six years after RK, lenswear pattern differed significantly with age, but not with gender. An additional 25% of patients over the age of 40 had to wear lenses for close work, compared with the group below the age of 40. Sixty-four percent of patients under the age of 40 and 40% of patients over the age of 40 did not wear lenses either for near or for distance 6 years after RK. At 10 years, there was almost no change in the freedom from corrective lens wear in patients under the age of 40 (63%), whereas patients over the age of 40 experienced a slight decrease in their freedom from glasses or spectacles for both near and far (33%). The difference between the two age groups can be attributed to the fact that 39% of patients over 40 were presbyopic and required correction at near, compared with only 2% of patients under the age of 40. Whether continued hyperopic shift from 6 to 10 years after RK was the main cause of the increased need for optical correction in the older group remains to be examined. There was no significant difference between the two age groups in the need to wear contact lenses for both distance and near or distance alone. This relation was unchanged at 10 years (35% and 28% were wearing correction for distance ± near at ages below and above 40, respectively). Both groups wore contact lenses 73% of the time for both near and distance. Not surprisingly, the older group wore contact lenses longer for near vision (25% versus 18%), and shorter for distance vision (27% versus 41%). Ten years after RK, 70% of all patients did not wear spectacles or contact lenses for distance vision.

Psychometric Results

From the subjective perspective, patient satisfaction and a retrospective decision to reenroll in the study or to have RK performed again is the ultimate measure of whether RK is a successful procedure. The data from PERK 6-year results suggest that even though only 60% of patients were highly satisfied, 74% felt that their preoperative goals were met, 89% felt that their vision was better after RK, and 94%, given the choice, would have RK performed again. Patient satisfaction and a sentiment that most goals of the procedure were met were greatly influenced by their freedom from glasses and contact lenses, especially at distance, or at both distance and near. Of all RK patients, 96% elected to have the procedure to reduce their dependence on refractive aids, while 6% and 3% of patients elected to have the procedure for professional and cosmetic reasons, respectively.

Reoperation Results

Many consider RK to be a staged procedure. The goal of the initial procedure is slight undercorrection. This is followed by a second procedure, termed *enhancement* by some, which fine-tunes the original refractive result. In the PERK study, the goal of RK was to achieve emmetropia with a single procedure. Nevertheless, a certain subset of PERK patients was left undercorrected. Enhancement was performed on 59 such patients. Reoperations were performed at least 6 months after the initial operation in patients with a cycloplegic, spherical equivalent of at least −1 D of myopia and a UCVA of 20/50 or worse.

Refraction

The average change in refraction from the initial operation was 2.74 D (SD = 1.13), and it ranged from 0.37 to 5.00 D. After enhancement, 77% gained an additional correction of 0.50 D or more, 20% gained less than 0.50 D, and 3% had further regression. The average change in refraction was 1.09 D (SD = 1.05). This was associated with a 1-D flattening of central keratometric power (SD = 0.94). As a result, 51% remained undercorrected

by 1 D, 46% were between +0.12 and −1 D, and 3% were overcorrected by over 1 D.

Surprisingly, despite additional surgery, there was no difference in the refractive stability between the eyes with and without reoperation 4 years following RK.

Visual Acuity

Following reoperations, visual acuity increased by two to nine Snellen lines in 76%, changed one line or less in 22%, and decreased three lines for 2% (one patient). Only 5% of patients had UCVA of 20/40 or better before the enhancement, compared with 64% of patients following reoperation.

Astigmatism

Inadvertent increase in astigmatism of more than 0.50 D was observed in 19% of patients following reoperation. As a result, 15% were left with greater than 1.50 D of astigmatism after the enhancement, compared with 6% after initial RK, and none before any surgery.

Predictability

Refractive outcome following enhancement could not be predicted by the initial response to surgery. In contrast to the primary procedure, the effect of enhancement did not correlate with the depth of incision, OZ size, or age of the patient, and was reduced by neither a proportionate nor a predictable amount of the initial RK response.

SUMMARY

In summary, radial keratotomy is an effective, safe, predictable and stable procedure for the correction of low myopia. Over 90 percent of eyes achieve uncorrected visual acuity of 20/40 or better. The results are slightly less predictable and stable for higher degrees of myopia. Improved UCVA with subsequent freedom from distance correction in a large proportion of eyes resulted in high patient satisfaction with subjective RK results. The loss of BCVA of 2 lines or more occurs in less than 3 percent of patients, but is rarely worse than 20/30.

New techniques, nomograms, and instruments further improved RK results compared with those in the PERK study. Furthermore, limiting RK to low myopia requiring fewer and shorter incisions may reduce and even eliminate hyperopic progression and daily fluctuation of the refractive outcome. A staged approach may also improve predictability with only a slight increase in the potential complication rate.

REFERENCES

1. Waring GO, Lynn MJ, McDonnell PJ. Results of the prospective evaluation of radial keratotomy (PERK) study 10 years after surgery. *Arch Ophthalmol.* 1994;112:1298–1308.

2. Werblin TP, Stafford BS. The Casebeer system for predictable keratorefractive surgery. One-year evaluation of 205 consecutive eyes. *Ophthalmology.* 1993;100:1095–1102.

3. Waring GO, Lynn MJ, the PERK study group, et al. Results of the prospective evaluation of radial keratotomy (PERK) study five years after surgery. *Ophthalmology.* 1991;98: 1164–1176.

4. Rashid ER, Waring GO. Complications of radial and transverse keratotomy. *Surv Ophthalmol.* 1989;34:73–106.

5. Waring GO. Radial keratotomy for myopia. In: Bullock JD, Lindquist TD, eds. Ophthalmic procedures assessment. *Ophthalmology.* 1993;100:1103–1115.

6. Singh D, Grewal SP, Kumar N. Anterior radial keratotomy experience in 600 cases of myopia. *Ann Ophthalmol.* 1984; 16:757–761.

7. Schneider DM, Draghic T, Murthy RK. Combined myopia and astigmatism surgery. Review of 350 cases. *J Cataract Refract Surg.* 1992;18:370–374.

8. Neumann AC, Osher RH, Fenzl RE. Radial keratotomy: a clinical and statistical analysis. In: Troutman RC, ed. Refractive surgery. *Cornea:* 1983;2:47–55.

9. Moreira H, Garbus JJ, McDonnell PJ, et al. Multifocal corneal topographic changes after radial keratotomy. *Ophthalmic Surg.* 1992;23:85–89.

10. Grady FJ. Experience with radial keratotomy. *Ophthalmic Surg.* 1982;13:395–399.

11. Bauerberg J, Sterzovsky M, Brodsky M. Radial keratotomy in myopia of 6 to 12 diopters using full-length deepening incisions. *Refract Corneal Surg.* 1989;5:150–154.

12. Shepard DD. Radial keratotomy: analysis of efficacy and predictability in 1,058 consecutive cases. Part I: efficacy. *J Cataract Refract Surg.* 1986;12:632–643.

13. Shepard DD. Radial keratotomy: analysis of efficacy and predictability in 1,058 consecutive cases. Part II: predictability. *J Cataract Refract Surg.* 1987;13:32–34.

14. Kremer FB, Marks RG. Radial keratotomy: prospective evaluation of safety and efficacy. *Ophthalmic Surg.* 1983;14: 926–930.

15. Powers MK, Meyerowitz BE, Marks RG, et al. Psychosocial findings in radial keratotomy patients two years after surgery. *Ophthalmology.* 1984;91:1193–1198.

16. Kornmehl EW. Radial keratotomy: incision number, incision direction, peripheral redeepening, and multiple-depth incisons. In: Jakobiec FA. *Controversies in Ophthalmology.* Boston: Little, Brown; 1991;31:101–107.

17. Schanzlin DJ, Santos VR, Roszka-Duggan V, et al. Diurnal changes in refraction, corneal curvature, visual acuity, and intraocular pressure after radial keratotomy in the PERK study. *Ophthalmology.* 1986;93: 167–175.

18. Waring GO, Lynn MJ, the PERK study group, et al. Results of the prospective evaluation of radial keratotomy (PERK) study one year after surgery. *Ophthalmology.* 1985;92: 177–198.

19. Lynn MJ, Waring GO, the PERK study group, et al. Factors affecting outcome and predictability of radial keratotomy in the PERK study. *Arch Ophthalmol.* 1987;105:42–51.

20. Santos VR, Waring GO, the PERK study group, et al. Relationship between refractive error and visual acuity in the prospective evaluation of radial keratotomy (PERK) study. *Arch Ophthalmol.* 1987;105:86–92.

21. Holladay JT, Lynn MJ, Fielding B, et al. The relationship of visual acuity, refractive error, and pupil size after radial keratotomy. *Arch Ophthalmol.* 1991;109:70–76.

22. Bourque LB, Cosand BB, PERK study group, et al. Reported satisfaction, fluctuation of vision, and glare among patients one year after surgery in the prospective evaluation of radial keratotomy (PERK) study. *Arch Ophthalmol.* 1986;104:356–363.

23. Binder PS. Four-year postoperative evaluation of radial keratotomy. *Arch Ophthalmol.* 1985;103:779–780.

24. Lynn MJ, Waring GO, the PERK study group, et al. Symmetry of refractive and visual acuity outcome in the prospective evaluation of radial keratotomy (PERK) study. *Refract Corneal Surg.* 1989;5:75–81.

25. Ginsburg AP, Waring GO, Bourque L, et al. Contrast sensitivity under photopic conditions in the prospective evaluation of radial keratotomy (PERK) study. *Refract Corneal Surg.* 1990;6:82–91.

26. Waring GO, Lynn MJ, the PERK study group, et al. Stability of refraction during four years after radial keratotomy in the prospective evaluation of radial keratotomy study. *Am J Ophthalmol.* 1991;111:133–144.

27. Rowsey JJ, Balyeat HD, the PERK study group. Prospective evaluation of radial keratotomy. Photokeratoscope corneal topography. *Ophthalmology.* 1988;95:322–334.

28. Verity SM, Talamo JH, Chayet A, et al. The combined (Genesis) technique of radial keratotomy: a prospective, multi-center study. *Ophthalmology* (in press).

29. Assil KK, Kassoff J, Quantock AJ, et al. A combined incision technique of radial keratotomy. A comparison to centripetal and centrifugal incision techniques in human donor eyes. *Ophthalmology.* 1994;101:746–754.

30. Dietz MR, Sanders DR, Raanan MG. Progressive hyperopia in radial keratotomy. Long-term follow-up of diamond-knife and metal blade series. *Ophthalmology.* 1986; 93:1284–1289.

31. Dietz MR, Sanders DR. Progressive hyperopia with long-term follow-up of radial keratotomy. *Arch Ophthalmol.* 1985;103:782–784.

32. Dietz MR, Sanders DR, Raanan MG. A consecutive series (1982–1985) of radial keratotomies performed with the diamond blade. *Am J Ophthalmol.* 1987;103:417–422.

33. Salz JJ, Salz JM, Jones D. Ten years experience with a conservative approach to radial keratotomy. *Refract Corneal Surg.* 1991;7:12–22.

34. Dietz MR, Sanders DR, Marks RG. Radial keratotomy: an overview of the Kansas City study. *Ophthalmology.* 1984;91:467–478.

35. Salz JJ, Villasenor RA, Buchbinder M. Four-incision radial keratotomy for low to moderate myopia. *Ophthalmology.* 1986;93:727–738.

36. Spigelman AV, Williams PA, Lindstrom RL. Further studies of four incision radial keratotomy. *Refract Corneal Surg.* 1989;5:292–295.

37. Lavery FL. Comparative results of 200 consecutive radial keratotomy cases using three different nomograms. *J Refract Surg.* 1987;3:88–91.

38. Hoffer KJ, Darin JJ, Levenson JE. Three years experience with radial keratotomy. The UCLA study. *Ophthalmology.* 1983;90:627–636.

39. Arrowsmith PN, Marks RG. Visual, refractive, and keratometric results of radial keratotomy. Five-year follow-up. *Arch Ophthalmol.* 1989;107:506–511.

40. Sawelson H, Marks RG. Three-year results of radial keratotomy. *Arch Ophthalmol.* 1987;105:81–85.

41. Arrowsmith PN, Marks RG. Visual, refractive, and keratometric results of radial keratotomy. A two-year follow-up. *Arch Ophthalmol.* 1987;105:76–80.

42. Arrowsmith PN, Marks RG. Evaluating the predictability of radial keratotomy. *Ophthalmology.* 1985;92:331–338.

43. Sawelson H, Marks RG. Five-year results of radial keratotomy. *Refract Corneal Surg.* 1989;5:8–20.

44. Salz JJ, Salz MS. Results of four- and eight-incision radial keratotomy for 6 to 11 diopters of myopia. *J Refract Surg.* 1988;4:46–50.

45. Applegate RA, Howland HC. Magnification and visual acuity in refractive surgery. *Arch Ophthalmol.* 1993;111:1135–1142.

46. Werblin TP, Stafford GM. Should progressive hyperopia be a serious concern after routine refractive keratotomy procedures. *Ophthalmology* (in press).

47. Waring GO, Lynn MJ, Schanzlin DJ, et al. Three-year results of the prospective evaluation of radial keratotomy (PERK) study. *Ophthalmology.* 1987;94:1339–1354.

CHAPTER 22

The Incisional Management of Astigmatism

Lee T. Nordan

Incisional keratotomy continues to be the preferred surgical method of correcting astigmatism. It may be combined with photorefractive keratectomy or with radial keratotomy. This chapter presents the principles and techniques of incisional keratotomy for the management of corneal astigmatism. In 1981, Luis Ruiz, MD, noticed that making five transverse incisions bounded by "pseudoradial" incisions on either side of the optical zone (OZ) resulted in an extremely large effect in rrecting astigmatism, much larger than could be achieved by either transverse or pseudoradial incisions performed separately. He called this procedure the *trapezoidal keratotomy for the correction of astigmatism* (Fig 22–1), which was later renamed the *Ruiz procedure.*

In performing this correction, the meridian perpendicular to the one in which the Ruiz procedure was performed ("the uninvolved meridian") became steeper as the involved meridian became flatter (Fig 22–2). The degree of steepening of the uninvolved meridian was directly proportional to the length of the transverse elements of the Ruiz procedure. In other words, the total correction of astigmatism was equal to the net sum of the flattening of the meridian in which the Ruiz procedure was performed added to the steepening of the flatter ("uninvolved") meridian.

The relation between the transverse length of a Ruiz procedure and the steepening of the "other" meridian of the cornea soon led to a corollary: a Ruiz procedure with a shorter transverse element corrected less astigmatism than a Ruiz procedure with a longer transverse dimension, even though the OZ was the same in both cases. The "involved" meridian did not flatten any differently whether the Ruiz procedure was wide or narrow; it was the "other" meridian that became steeper when the wider transverse incisions were used (Fig 22–3).

This phenomenon meant that an astigmatic cornea could be corrected to numerous spherical corrections by altering the astigmatic keratotomy (AK). An astigmatic procedure could be tailored to an existing spherical ametropia. The profound significance of this phenomenon will be discussed later in the chapter.

Because the spherical equivalent of a patient who undergoes an astigmatic keratotomy becomes more hyperopic while the spherical component of the refraction becomes more myopic, a solid understanding of these terms is essential to comprehend the mechanics of AK. Hoffman coined the descriptive term *coupling* to describe the ratio of the flattening of the principal (steeper) meridian to the steepening of the flatter meridian.[1] This term has stood the test of time and is in widespread use today.

Ruiz procedure patterns were created in which the pseudoradial incisions were perpendicular to the transverse incisions and even "inverted" so that these outer incisions converged toward the limbus. These new

291

styles had no significant effect on the efficacy of the procedure, but one thing was certain: the combination of transverse and radial incisions was far more powerful than either type of incision alone.

At this time, Dr Fyodorov's[2,3] parallel incisions for the correction of astigmatism, which were unpre-dictable in the higher ranges of astigmatism, were giving way to "T-cuts," or flags, that were staggered along the radial incisions on one or either side of the OZ (Fig 22–4). A T-cut was found to have a predictable effect whether it was performed on only one side or on both sides of the visual axis. The Ruiz procedure always had to be performed on both sides of the visual axis.

The presence of a transverse incision made AK much more quantifiable, but the intersection of transverse and radial incisions could lead to delayed corneal healing and epithelial recurrent erosions, especially when metal blades were used. Soon most surgeons tried to avoid joining transverse and radial incisions.

A few other items concerning the Ruiz procedure are noteworthy. Initially, OZs as small as 3 mm were used in the Ruiz procedure. The transverse incisions created very significant glare and irregular astigmatism when placed this close together. The five trans-

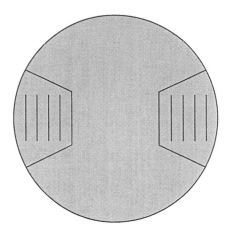

Figure 22–1. The original Ruiz procedure.

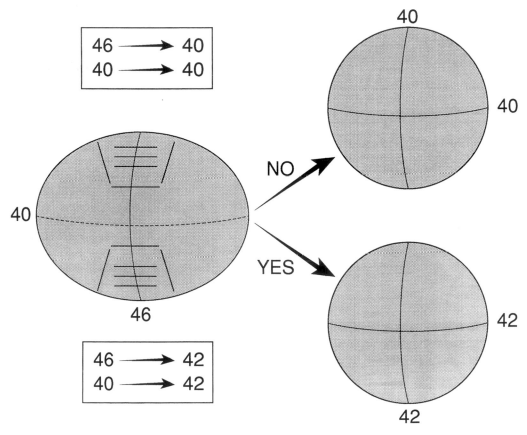

Figure 22–2. Notice that in a Ruiz procedure the flatter meridian steepens from 40 D to 42 D while the steeper meridian flattens from 46 D to 42 D in this example. The *total* change in astigmatism is the sum of the flattening plus the steepening, which in this case equals 4 D + 2 D, for a total of 6 D.

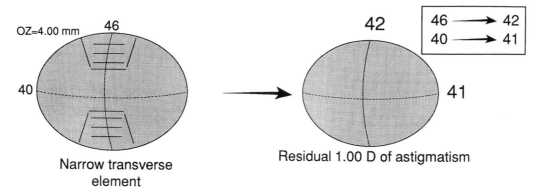

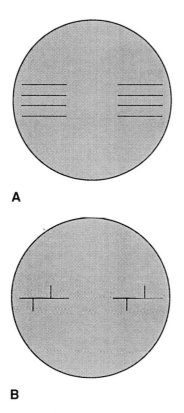

Figure 22–3. This diagram demonstrates that a narrow Ruiz procedure causes less steepening of the flatter meridian. In this case, the narrow Ruiz procedure causes the flatter meridian to steepen from 40 D to 41 D, while the wider Ruiz causes the flatter meridian to steepen from 40 D to 42 D (Fig 22–2).

Figure 22–4. Earlier patterns of astigmatic keratotomy. **A.** Multiple parallel incisions. **B.** "Flags" connected to the radial incision.

verse incisions soon evolved to four. Many surgeons found the predictability of the Ruiz procedure to be poor, no doubt partly because the Ruiz procedure was generally reserved for extremely high astigmatism. The other reason, however, was that most surgeons were not measuring corneal thickness by ultrasound pachymetry at the location of each transverse incision and changing the blade length accordingly. Achieved incision depth,

not blade length, and accurate placement on the involved corneal meridian are crucial to the predictability of a Ruiz procedure.

Some surgeons, even to this day, call any astigmatic incisional procedure a "Ruiz procedure." Actually, the reverse is true; the Ruiz procedure is one form of astigmatic keratotomy, a term that includes all forms of incisional procedures intended to correct astigmatism.

Currently, the most commonly used AK patterns are the arcuate and transverse incisions (T-cut), with or without a peripheral radial incision (Fig 22–5 A–C) and an OZ diameter of 6 to 7 mm. Up to about 4 D of astigmatism can be corrected by a pair of T-cuts, one on either side of the visual axis.

The most common form of Ruiz procedure is the "mini-Ruiz," which involves two transverse elements and an OZ no smaller than 6 mm (Fig 22–6). This approach represents a compromise between the need to correct higher degrees of astigmatism and the preservation of high-quality visual acuity.

The "stepladder" configuration, in which the pseudoradial incisions are perpendicular to the transverse elements, became the preferred form of the Ruiz procedure. This configuration allowed the Ruiz procedure to fit inside a six-incision radial keratotomy (RK) when severe, compound myopic astigmatism was treated. Using the radial incisions as the pseudoradial incisions was not as quantifiable (Fig 22–7).

The correction of astigmatism by means of wedge resection has been investigated for the past 30 years by two of the great corneal surgeons, Jose Barraquer[4–6] and Richard Troutman[7,8] (see Chapter 41). However, the Ruiz procedure has been the subject of only a few limited studies during the past decade.

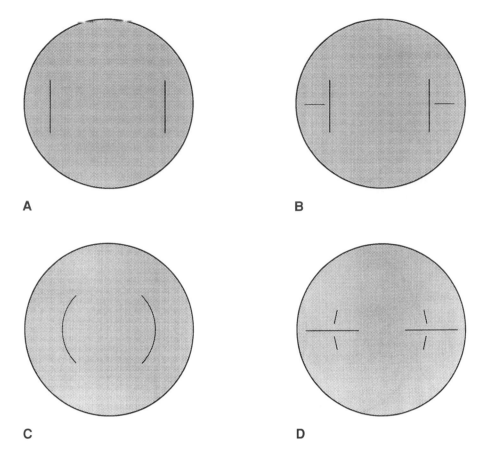

Figure 22–5. The most common astigmatic incisions in 1996. **A.** Transverse (T-cut). **B.** T-cut with radial. **C.** Arcuate. **D.** Chevron.

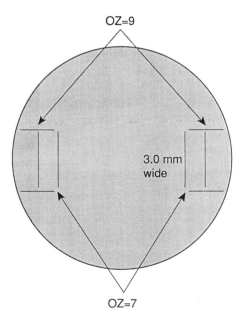

Figure 22–6. The "mini-Ruiz" procedure.

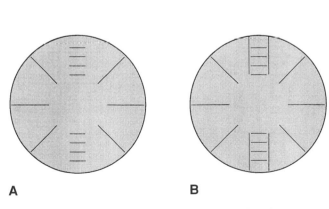

Figure 22–7. The treatment of severe compound myopic astigmatism utilizes one element for treating the astigmatism (Ruiz) and one for the myopia (RK) as in **(B),** rather than combining the radial incisions as part of the Ruiz, as in **(A).**

My experience with 11 penetrating keratoplasty patients who underwent Ruiz procedures was that all except one showed great improvement without complications.

Lindstrom et al[9,10] and Friedlander et al[11,12] have investigated the effect of the Ruiz procedure on cadaver eyes. These studies tended to show a 150% to 200% greater effect than the in vivo procedure (common for cadaver eyes following incisional keratotomy); any generalizations from cadaver eyes to real patients were difficult, at best.

Merlin[13] suggested that better results are possible with arcuate rather than straight astigmatic incisions (Fig 22–5 C). This idea was repopularized by Lindstrom. Arcuate incisions less than 45° tend to act like straight ones, but the excessive gaping and subsequent unpredictability caused by arcuate incisions in the 75° to 90° range is undesirable.

Straight transverse incisions appear rectilinear only when viewed perpendicular to the corneal surface. Using a ping-pong ball as a substitute cornea, it is easy to visualize T-cuts in a three-dimensional view and to understand that these incisions are actually curvilinear because they follow the curved corneal surface (Fig 22–8 A,B). Thus, these "straight" T cuts are really a segment of a great circle around the imaginary corneal sphere, imparting a consistency of action and promoting coupling by gaping less at the end of the incisions. Only when viewed in two dimensions, instead of three, do arcuate incisions appear to be a favorable pattern relative to the center of the cornea, the visual axis. Because all points of an arcuate incision are equidistant from the center of the cornea, an equal amount of wound gape occurs. This equal and large degree of gaping tends to increase irregular astigmatism and makes coupling less predictable.

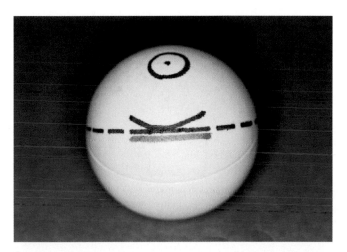

A

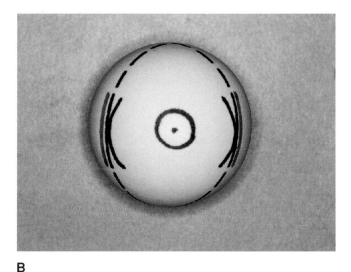

B

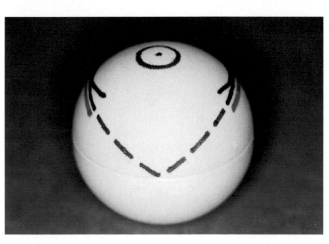

C

Figure 22–8. Demonstrating the curvilinear nature of T-cuts, using a ping-pong ball for a cornea. Notice that the T-cuts (red ink lines) appear straight when viewed perpendicular to the incision **(A)**, but are actually curvilinear **(B)** and a segment of a great circle encompassing the "theoretical corneal sphere" **(C)**, as evidenced when viewed from above the center of the ball (cornea).

MECHANISM OF ACTION

Although the Ruiz procedure was too complicated for routine astigmatic cases, it allowed a great deal to be learned about the mechanics of AK. In order to understand the mechanism of action of an AK, the surgeon should review the basics of refraction and become comfortable correlating the corneal meridian with the appropriate "K", or keratometry, reading and proper component of the refraction. It makes sense, and it is true, that the better refractive surgeons understand refraction better!

To investigate the mechanism of action of an AK, let us consider a mini-Ruiz procedure performed to correct 6 D of astigmatism. The patient's refraction is plano −6 × 180 and the K readings are 40 D @ 180 and 46 D @ 90 (Fig 22–9). Remember, even though the Ruiz procedure is highlighted in this example, the corneal mechanics described are valid for any form of AK.

The surgeon must confirm that the astigmatism is regular, that is, that the patient does not have irregular astigmatism. Astigmatism is a condition in which different meridians of an optical surface have different radii of curvature. Regular astigmatism is an astigmatism

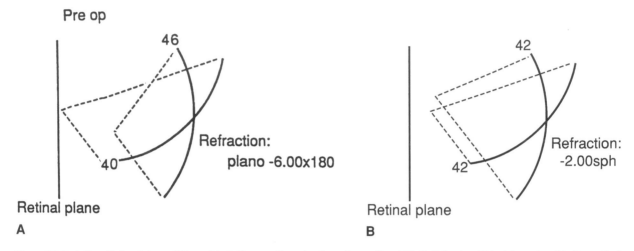

Pre op

46

40

Refraction:
plano -6.00x180

Retinal plane

A

42

42

Refraction:
-2.00sph

Retinal plane

B

Figure 22–9. Astigmatic keratotomy (AK) model. **A.** Preoperative refraction: plano −6 × 180. **B.** Following AK incisions placed in the vertical meridian, the coupling ratio is 2:1. The diagram shows that both meridians following AK now focus light in front of the retinal plane. The spherical equivalent has become more hyperopic (−3 D to −2 D), but the spherical component has become more myopic (plano to −2 D).

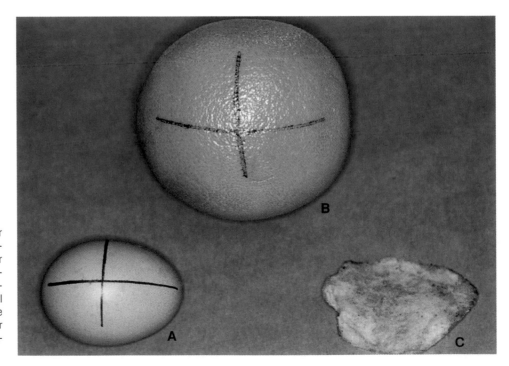

Figure 22–10. Depiction of regular and irregular astigmatism. **A.** In regular astigmatism (egg) the steeper and flatter meridians are perpendicular to each other. **B.** Irregular astigmatism caused by an epithelial (photo) abnormality like punctuate keratopathy (orange). **C.** Irregular astigmatism caused by stromal pathology (potato chip).

that can be corrected by a cylindrical lens, that is, an astigmatism in which the steeper meridian and flatter meridians are perpendicular to each other (Fig 22–10). The cause of irregular astigmatism may be an abnormal epithelium (with normal stroma), as in punctate keratopathy, or an abnormal stroma (with normal epithelium), as in keratoconus or stromal injury and scarring. AK only corrects regular astigmatism.

Because of its high magnification and very thin mire, manual keratometry is the most accurate method of determining even very subtle keratoconus and irregular astigmatism. However, manual keratometry requires an experienced observer. Over the past several years, automated topography has become popular as a screening device for keratoconus because of its ease of use, colorful permanent display, and technician-oriented approach. The accomplished refractive surgeon is urged to study and practice everything that can add to his or her store of useful information about the cornea (Figs 22–11 and 22–12).

In this example, plano −6 × 180°, the steeper (smaller radius of curvature) meridian of the cornea is the vertical one, and the meridian at 180° is the flatter (longer radius of curvature). The astigmatic keratotomy will be performed on the steeper meridian, with its transverse elements perpendicular to the meridian. The primary function of the AK is to cause the flattening of its own meridian, with secondary steepening of the flatter meridian 90° away.

Let us assume a coupling ratio of 2:1. That means, for every 2 D of flattening of the steeper meridian caused by the AK, there will be a simultaneous steepening of the flatter meridian by 1 D. The coupling ratio for a specific AK has been derived empirically through experience (Table 22–1). A surgeon cannot calculate or divine a coupling ratio. Also, the coupling ratio is unpredictable when an AK is performed following a corneal transplant because the encircling scar can change corneal dynamics greatly.

Let us return to our patient with a refraction of plano −6 × 180 (Table 22–2). The flatter meridian of the cornea corresponds to the "plano" term of the refraction and the "6" corresponds to the steeper meridian of the cornea (Fig 22–9). This should seem correct to the surgeon because a steeper meridian creates myopia by focusing light in front of the retina. The plano term of the refraction indicates that light passing through this meridian of the cornea is focused in a line (not a point, because this is an astigmatic cornea) on the retina.

With a refraction of plano −6 × 180, the spherical equivalent (sph + 1/2 cyl) is −3 D and the spherical component of the refraction is plano (Table 22–2).

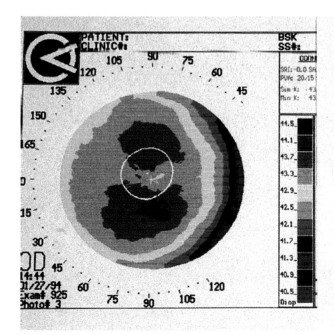 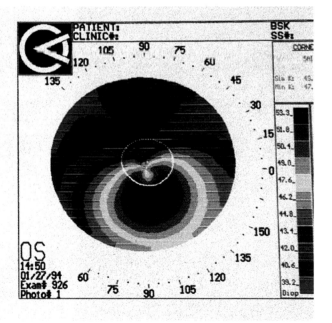

Figure 22–11. A patient with keratoconus that is extremely mild in the right eye and moderate on the left. Manual keratometry and a trained observer are necessary to diagnose keratoconus in the right eye because the automated topography map of the right cornea appears normal in all respects. Automated topography easily alerts the observer to the keratoconus in the left eye that results in severe irregular steepening of the inferior cornea.

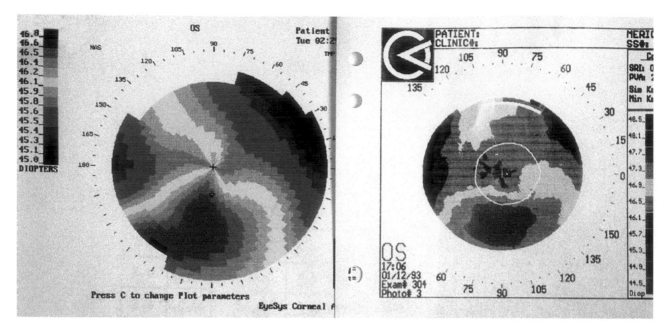

Figure 22–12. Two automated topography maps that may appear similar at first glance are really very different. The patient depicted on the left has keratoconus with a very steep cornea inferiorly, compared to superiorly, and a potential visual acuity (PVA) of from 20/30 to 20/40 as a result of the corneal irregular astigmatism, which was confirmed by manual keratometry. The patient on the right has a difference in corneal curvature between superior and inferior of 1.50 D, a PVA of 20/15 to 20/20, and no irregular astigmatism by manual keratometry.

The spherical equivalent represents the single best representation of the patient's refractive status. A refraction of plano −6 × 180 can be transposed to the plus cylinder form as −6 + 6 × 90. An AK should be performed on the steeper meridian of the cornea, which usually corresponds closely to the plus axis of the refraction. Even though surgeons commonly talk about performing an AK at a certain axis, it should be remembered that the term *meridian* properly refers to the cornea and the term *axis* properly refers to the correcting lens.

For instructional purposes, assume that the perfect AK is performed on this hypothetical patient. All intended incision locations have been measured by ultrasound pachymetry, and the blade length has been changed when more than 5% variation in corneal thickness was encountered.

Achieved corneal depth is crucial to quantifiable AK. A front (Russian)-cutting blade is most commonly used for AK because it affords improved visibility.

What happens to the cornea and the patient's refraction? Because there is a coupling ratio of 2:1, we know that the 6 D of astigmatism will be corrected with two "units" of flattening for every one "unit" of steepening. Therefore, if we consider a total of three units (two units of flattening and one unit of steepening), we can determine the size of one unit by dividing the total

TABLE 22–1. COUPLING RATIOS

Procedure	Size	Coupling Ratio
Long corneoscleral crescentic resection	—	1:1
Arcuate incisions	60°	1:1
T-cuts	3.5–4.5 mm long	2:1
Ruiz procedure	1.5 mm wide	5:1
Ruiz procedure	3 mm wide	3:1
Ruiz procedure	4.5 mm wide	2:1

TABLE 22–2. SUMMARY OF IMPORTANT INFORMATION FOR A HYPOTHETICAL PATIENT

Refraction	plano −6 × 180 −6 + 6 × 90
K readings and/or topography	Verify regular astigmatism
Spherical equivalent	−3 D
Spherical component (− cyl form)	plano
Steeper meridian	90

TABLE 22–3. PREOP/POSTOP TABLE FOR THIS PATIENT

	Preop	Postop
Refraction	plano −6 × 180	−2 sph
Spherical equivalent	−3 D	−2 D
Spherical component	plano	−2 D
K at 90°	46	42
K at 180°	40	42

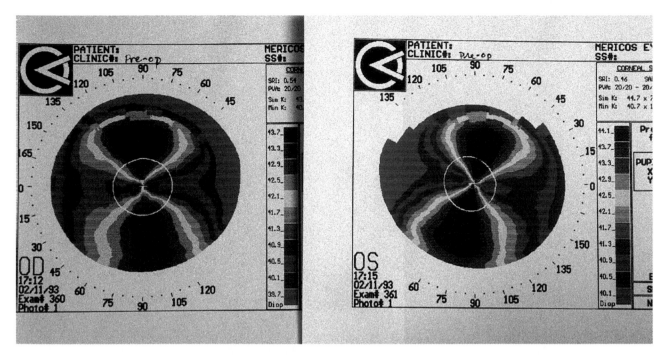

Figure 22–16. An automated topography map highlights the steeper corneal meridian nicely. This information should be correlated with the patient's refraction, keratometry, and slit lamp examination.

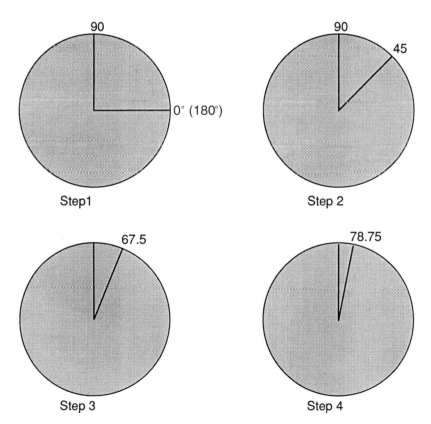

Figure 22–17. A process for estimating the 75th meridian of the cornea, using successive bisection of an angle.

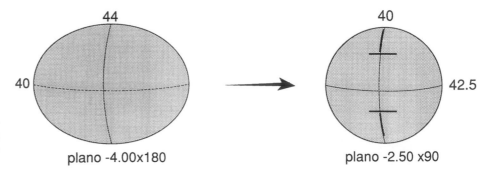

Figure 22–18. Overcorrected astigmatism. This may follow perforations or excessive or unnecessary incisions.

plano -4.00x180

plano -2.50 x90

locations and bisect this sector to find 67.5°. Halfway between 67.5° and 90° is 78.75° (Fig 22–17).

FRONT-CUTTING BLADE

Unlike RK, AK of all patterns is best performed with a front (Russian)-cutting blade. All blades for incisional keratotomy should end in a sharp point, in order to increase consistency of penetration and to avoid macroperforations. This blade configuration allows the surgeon to better visualize the incisions to be made because a back (American)-cutting blade blocks the surgeon's view of where the incision is to be made.

In order to achieve an incision depth of 85% to 90%, the front-cutting blade is set at 95% to 100% of the corneal pachymetry at the point where the incision is to be made. The blade is changed when more than a 5% (0.03 mm) change in pachymetry is noted.

PREOP AND INTRAOP CALCULATIONS

An information resource sheet is used, not only to provide the vital information concerning the patient's refraction, but also to have a convenient place to write down the pachymetry values as they are read out before the surgery. By transposing the patient's refraction into both positive and negative cylinder formats, the surgeon can correlate the patient's steeper meridian with the + cylinder axis and use the − cylinder refraction to predict the refraction following AK. A diagram of the proposed surgery should be drawn *by the surgeon* on a diagram that depicts the surgeon's view.

Performing AK on the improper (flatter) meridian is not uncommon and is usually caused either by clerical mistakes or by a surgeon's unfamiliarity with the principles of refraction that connect corneal meridians and refractive error. It is advantageous for the surgeon

to review the patient's chart and plan these incisional keratotomy cases within a few hours or a day of surgery so that the details of each patient will remain fresh.

The corneal pachymetry is performed with a sterile OZ marker and AK pattern marker before the eye is prepped and the operation commences. The patient is instructed to keep the eyes closed following pachymetry because foreign body sensation (FBS) and corneal drying by evaporation, with subsequent corneal thinning, cannot be appreciated as a result of the topical anesthetic.

SURGICAL TECHNIQUE

The steps of the operative procedure for AK are listed in Table 22–5. A nomogram of T-cuts and arcuate incisions is provided in Table 22–6. Each step is important. The mark of an excellent surgeon is consistency in approach. Note that the blade is set and the speculum is placed in the eye immediately before commencing the procedure. There is a tendency for surgeons who are learning incisional keratotomy to place the speculum in the eye first and then get ready. The cornea thins as a result of evaporation at a rate of about 0.01 mm per minute.

OZ markers are placed concentric with the miotic pupil. In order to obtain a well-placed 7-mm OZ for AK, a 3/5/7-mm OZ marker is more precise than simply a 7-mm OZ marker because the 3-mm portion can be positioned accurately on the miotic pupil.

The eye is patched for 12 to 24 hours, and antibiotic/steroid drops are used every 6 hours for 4 days. Artificial tears are used as desired and the patient is seen the next day after surgery. The patient is examined within every 48-hour period until re-epithelialization is complete.

Nonsteroidal anti-inflammatory (NSAID) medications like Voltaren have a hypesthetic effect on the cor-

TABLE 22–5. ASTIGMATIC KERATOTOMY STEP BY STEP

Preop: patient
1. Proparacaine gtts
   Pilocarpine 1/2% gtts
   Antibiotic gtts
2. Patient's name written on headcover
   Operative eye dot on forehead
3. Valium, 5 mg po

Surgical preparation
1. Microscope coaxial
2. Position patient properly, iris parallel to floor
3. *Verify patient, chart, eye*
4. Proparacaine gtts, OU
5. OZ and astigmatiic axis marked
6. Pachymetry
   Values read aloud and charted
7. Determine bias and blade length
   Chart placed on patient's chest
8. Patient's eye prepped
   If applicable, surgeon moves to second patient and performs pachymetry

Surgery
1. Surgeon dons gloves
2. Sterile handle onto microscope
3. Blade depth set
4. Lancaster speculum in place
5. Copious proparacaine gtts (10–20)
6. Remark OZ and astigmatism axis
7. Fixation forceps or ring applied
8. Instruct patient *not* to follow apparent movement of microscope light
9. RK and AK incisions performed
10. Fixation forceps or ring removed
11. Surgeon retracts diamond blade
12. BSS irrigation only if blood is present in incision
    No irrigation for incision with microperforation
13. Antibiotic gtts/prednisone gtts
14. Lid speculum removed
15. Patient taken to recovery area

TABLE 22–6. TRANSVERSE AND ARCUATE INCISIONS NOMOGRAMS

Nordan Nomogram (Transverse T-cuts) - 85% depth				
Astigmatism	O.Z.	Length	Number Transverse	Number Radial
1.00–1.50 D	7.0 mm	4.5 mm	1 (single)*	1*
1.75–2.25 D	7.0 mm	3.5 mm	2	2
2.50–4.00 D	7.0 mm	4.5 mm	2	2
Composite Nomogram (Arcuate incisions)				
Astigmatism	O.Z.	Length	Degrees	Number Arcuate
1.00–1.50 D	7.0 mm	2.5 mm	40°	2
1.75–2.50 D	7.0 mm	3.0 mm	50°	2
2.75–3.50 D	7.0 mm	3.5 mm	57°	2
3.75–4.50 D	7.0 mm	4.0 mm	65°	2

*Refers to single hemimeridian: combined radial and transverse incision (see Fig 22–5B)

that demonstrates delayed epithelialization for more than a day or two should be patched.

Therapeutic contact lenses should be avoided immediately after incisional keratotomy because they often cause a tight lens syndrome. Such lenses, especially the Ciba-Geigy Focus therapeutic contact lens, have been invaluable following excimer laser procedures that only change the front surface of the cornea rather than its entire thickness.

Because of this gape, AK incisions may present by slit lamp as wider scars than RK incisions. Whereas RK incisions fade noticeably with time, AK incisions do so to a much lesser extent.

COMPLICATIONS

Infection

In AK, topical antibiotics are administered preoperatively, intraoperatively, and postoperatively until epithelialization is complete. As in all eye surgery, these antibiotics are administered prophylactically; it cannot be determined how many corneal ulcers are prevented by such treatment. If complaints progress from only FBS to worsening pain, deep ache, and decreasing vision, the patient should be examined immediately.

If a corneal ulcer does occur, aggressive treatment with fortified antibiotic drops is indicated. Medications are then changed according to the Gram stain and culture reports. The onset of flare and cell in the anterior chamber by slit lamp indicates a more serious corneal ulcer.

nea and can greatly reduce patient discomfort. Such agents may be used every 6 hours for 1 to 2 days, but may tend to reduce epithelial healing if used for an extended length of time. The goal of postoperative care is to accomplish re-epithelialization quickly so that the topical antibiotic and cortisone medications may be stopped.

An AK incision must gape in order to be effective in correcting corneal astigmatism. Therefore, AK patients tend to have FBS for a few days longer than RK patients, especially if the preop astigmatism is in the 3 to 4 D range, necessitating T-cuts of about 4.5 mm in length. Patching such patients for 24 hours initially usually promotes more rapid epithelialization. Any cornea

Perforation

Microperforation during AK is more common than during RK because the transverse incision may be moving toward an area of decreasing corneal thickness. Such microperforations should not be irrigated as this increases the chances of endophthalmitis. The second eye of a proposed bilateral case should not be performed because the potential tragedy of a bilateral endophthalmitis must be avoided.

Macroperforations, defined as any corneal wound that leaks spontaneously, should be sutured with 10-0 nylon at the time of surgery. As in microperforation, the procedure should be completed, so that the patient has a good chance of a successful result following removal of the sutures about 2 to 3 weeks postop. Therefore, the thoughtful AK surgeon must have readily available sterile instrumentation for corneal suturing.

Undercorrection

The patient is monitored until a stable postop result is known. This usually takes about 4 to 8 weeks, depend-

ing upon the severity of the original refraction. There is no known effective medical treatment for an undercorrected AK. Prolonged cortisone drops, patching, and ocular massage are either dangerous or nonproductive. A new pattern of surgical incisions must be planned, requiring considerable ingenuity. The original incisions can be redeepened if they appear to be grossly shallow, but this is often difficult to ascertain accurately by slit lamp. The surgeon must resist the temptation to continually employ merely a smaller OZ, as irregular astigmatism will result.

Overcorrection

Overcorrection following AK means that the preoperative flatter meridian has now become significantly (1.50 D) steeper than the new flatter meridian, and the axis of the correcting cylinder has usually changed by about 90°. After a stable refraction has been recorded, the residual astigmatism can be treated with a second surgical procedure perpendicular to the first (Fig 22–19 A).

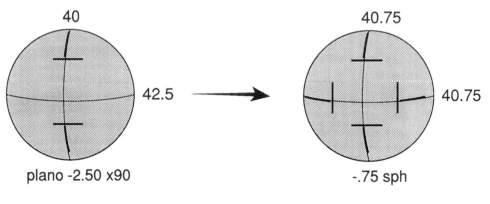

AK for over-corrected AK

A

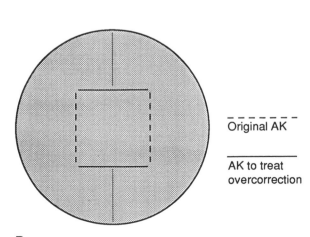

Original AK

AK to treat overcorrection

Figure 22–19. A. one possibility for treating an overcorrected AK patient. **B.** Beware that the AK incisions intended to help an overcorrected AK do not inadvertently join to create a weakened central cornea with irregular astigmatism.

B

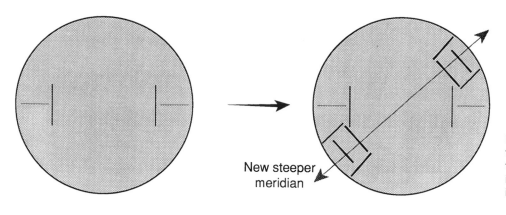

New steeper meridian

Figure 22–20. One possibility for treating an AK that has caused a rotation of the patient's steeper meridian. These cases can demand great imagination by the surgeon.

However, the surgeon must avoid performing the second-procedure incision too close to the first because a hexagonal keratotomy–type incision can be created inadvertently, leading to increased myopia and irregular astigmatism (Fig 22–19 B). The goal of surgery should be reduced by about 1.00 to 1.50 D to avoid another overcorrection.

If the overcorrection has occurred because the OZ used was too small, and irregular astigmatism exists, then suturing the wounds with interrupted 10-0 nylon for 3 to 4 months may be of value. The reduced gaping of the corneal incisions centrally will improve the patient's quality of vision and may permanently reduce the astigmatism. Such suturing does not usually help overcorrected RK procedures long term.

Rotation of Axis with Residual Astigmatism

The same principles apply to this situation as to the undercorrection and overcorrection of astigmatism. This situation is often more difficult, however, because the original incisions may preclude an easy pattern of AK to be oriented on the steeper meridian as a result of the original AK incisions (Fig 22–20).

Irregular Astigmatism

Most irregular astigmatism following AK is created by an OZ of less than 7 mm; OZs less than 6 mm are contraindicated because the amount of glare and reduction in quality of vision in mydriatic situations will be substantial. These problems are increased significantly with long arcuate incisions because arcuate incisions gape more than T-cuts. The suturing of such incisions is a good initial attempt at treatment. A lamellar or penetrating corneal transplant may be necessary, with subsequent phototherapeutic keratectomy (PTK), to achieve the patient's goal of improved, high-quality vision.

Undoubtedly, prevention is a better course to follow by not employing a small OZ initially and making 7 mm the standard OZ for astigmatism of 5 D or less. This covers the vast majority of AK patients. OZs of less than 7 mm require the patient to be well informed about the compromises between effect and reduced quality of vision.

Recurrent Erosions and Superficial Punctate Keratitis

Superficial punctate keratitis occurs frequently after incisional keratotomy (Fig 6–12). Although some short-term recurrent erosions may also bother the patient for up to several months, such long-term problems are very rare following incisional keratotomy using diamond, rather than metal, blades. Classically, the patient complains of FBS and photophobia upon arising in the morning, but the symptoms subside as the day goes on; the epithelial defect has re-epithelialized. Treatment with artificial tears and lubricating ointment before bed and upon arising, plus tincture of time as the epithelium adheres to Bowman's membrane, is usually sufficient to solve the problem. Ongoing use of topical antibiotics is prudent. Even crossed incisions very rarely create long-term recurrent erosion problems. In fact, incisional keratotomy is not contraindicated in patients with anterior basement membrane dystrophy who are plagued by recurrent corneal erosions.

Treatment for a recurrent erosion may range from debridement with a cotton tip applicator and the wearing of a therapeutic contact lens for 6 weeks to focal treatment with a 25-gauge needle tip that perforates Bowman's membrane to promote epithelial adhesion to focal PTK. Although recurrent erosions are classically thought to be caused by a defect of the basement membrane, which is secreted by the epithelium, many patients with severe, recurrent erosions from anterior basement membrane dystrophy have been successfully treated by lamellar corneal transplant. This introduces the possibility that Bowman's membrane may also play an important role in this disease entity, whether it be hereditary or acquired following incisional keratotomy.

SUMMARY

The quantifiable prediction and correction of corneal astigmatism was one of the major advances in anterior segment surgery of the 1980s. Astigmatic keratotomy is now being used by many surgeons to improve the uncorrected vision of patients who are undergoing cataract extraction/IOL implantation, RK, excimer photorefractive keratectomy (PRK), automated lamellar keratoplasty (ALK), laser in situ keratomileusis (LASIK), and penetrating keratoplasty. A knowledge of coupling alerts the surgeon to those cases in which an AK, or a PRK-astigmatism, or a combination of both, may be useful in obtaining the maximum correction of astigmatism, without worsening the patient's spherical refractive status. Judicious use of astigmatic keratotomy remains valuable in providing anterior segment patients with the best possible, appropriate, uncorrected visual acuity.

REFERENCES

1. Hoffmann RF. The surgical correction of idiopathic astigmatism. In: Sanders DR, Hoffmann RF, Salz JJ, eds. *Refractive Corneal Surgery.* Thorofare, NJ: Slack, Inc; 1986:241–290.

2. Fyodorov SN. Surgical correction of myopia and astigmatism. In: Schacher AR, Levi S, Schacher S, ed. *Keratorefraction.* Dennison, TX: LAL Publishing Co; 1980:141–172.

3. Fyodorov SN, Agranovsky AA. Long-term results of anterior radial keratotomy. *J Ocul Ther Surg.* 1982;1:217–223.

4. Barraquer JI. Keratomileusis and keratophakia. In: Rycroft PV, ed. *Corneoplastic Surgery.* New York: Pergamon; 1969. Proceedings of the 2nd International Cornea–Plastic Conference.

5. Barraquer JI. Special methods in corneal surgery. In: King JHJ, McTigue JW, eds. *The Cornea.* Washington, DC: Butterworths; 1965.

6. Barraquer C, Guiterrez A, Espinosa A. Myopic keratomileusis: short term results. *Refract Corn Surg.* 1989;5:307–313.

7. Troutman RC. Microsurgical control of corneal astigmatism in cataract and keratoplasty. *Trans Am Acad Ophthalmol Otolaryngol.* 1973;77:OP563–572.

8. Troutman RC, Swinger CA. Refractive keratoplasty: keratophakia and keratomileusis. *Trans Am Ophthalmol Soc.* 1978;76:329–339.

9. Lindstrom RL, Lindquist TD. Surgical correction of postoperative astigmatism. *Cornea.* 1988;7:138–148.

10. Lindstrom RL. The surgical correction of astigmatism: a clinician's perspective. *Refract Corneal Surg.* 1990;6:441–454. Review.

11. Friedlander MH, Rich LF, Werblin TP, et al. Keratophakia using preserved lenticles. *Ophthalmology.* 1980;87:687–692.

12. Friedlander MH, Safir A, McDonald MB, Kaufman HE, Granet N. Update on keratophakia. *Ophthalmology.* 1983;90:365–368.

13. Merlin U. Curved keratotomy procedure for congenital astigmatism. *J Refract Surg.* 1987;3:92–97.

CHAPTER 23

Incisional Corneal Surgery for the Correction of Hyperopia

Charles Casebeer

INTRODUCTION

Hexagonal keratotomy is a procedure that is rarely used today because of its unacceptably high rate of side effects. This chapter summarizes the history of incisional corneal surgery for the correction of hyperopia, and it reports the evolution, clinical outcomes and complications of hexagonal keratotomy.

HYPEROPIA AS A REFRACTIVE ERROR

Hyperopia is a visual condition in which light rays reach the retina before they come to a focus (Fig 23–1), causing distant objects to appear relatively in focus while closer objects appear relatively blurred. Hyperopia can result because the converging power of the eye is insufficient (refractive hyperopia), the eye is abnormally short (axial hyperopia), or there is a mismatch between the optical power of the eye and its physical length, so that even the most distant rays are not bent enough to focus an image on the retina unless the eye accommodates.

The young person with a small amount of hyperopia may obtain a sharp distance image by increasing the converging power of the eye through accommodation, as the person with normal vision does to read. This same young person may also obtain a sharp near image by accommodating more—much more than a person without hyperopia. The condition may be symptomless for years, even though the accommodating mechanism of the eye is at work for both near and distance vision.

By age 35, however, the power of accommodation may have weakened and the near point receded (Table 23–1) to the point that optical correction for reading is required. By age 37 or a little older, the patient's eyes may have become presbyopic as well, necessitating the addition of more diopters to the already plus correction. This can produce spherical and chromatic aberrations and a more constricted visual field. In terms of vision quality and patient functioning, hyperopia may be more disabling than myopia.

Hyperopia can occur naturally, and is prevalent in 10.4% of a young adult population for the refractive range of +2 to +4 D, or it can occur following radial keratotomy (RK) for myopia.[1] This chapter will focus on the history and surgical techniques of correcting primary hyperopia through incisional keratotomy.

TABLE 23–1. MEAN HUMAN ACCOMMODATION VALUES ACCORDING TO AGE

Age (y)	Mean Accommodation (D)
8	13.8
25	9.9
35	7.3
40	5.8
45	3.6
50	1.9
55	1.3
60+	1.1

SURGICAL CORRECTION OF PRIMARY HYPEROPIA

The goal of surgery for primary hyperopia is visual rehabilitation. This goal is not easily met because steepening of the central cornea is more difficult to achieve surgically than flattening. Various procedures have been used to modify the curvature of the hyperopic cornea, including epikeratoplasty, keratophakia or contact lens implantation, keratomileusis, hot needle or holmium laser thermokeratoplasty, hexagonal or arcuate keratotomy, automated lamellar keratoplasty (ALK), photorefractive keratectomy with or without ALK, clear lens extraction and intraocular lens (IOL) implantation, and contact lens implantation (Table 23–2).[2–36]

THE DEVELOPMENT OF HEXAGONAL KERATOTOMY

Akiyama reported producing central corneal steepening using a hexagonal pattern of intersecting incisions in the posterior cornea of rabbits in 1952.[37] More than 30 years later, Yamashita reported success with incisions in the anterior cornea of rabbits.[38,39] Soon thereafter, Antonio Mendez reported the first results of hexagonal intersecting incisions in humans.

Mendez took pachymetry readings at the selected optical zone (OZ) diameter (5.0, 5.5, or 6.0 mm), and set his blade to 87% of the thinnest pachymetry reading. He connected all incisions at their vortices. While his earlier work predicted 3.5 D of corneal steepening for the 5.0-mm optical zone, 2.5 D for the 5.5-mm zone, and 1.5 D for 6.0-mm zone, he obtained 3.0 ± 0.75 D for the 5.0-mm zone, 2.0 ± 0.75 for the 5.5-mm zone, and 1.5 ± 0.75 for the 6.0-mm zone (zone = diameter of circle made outside of the hexagon; Fig 23–1).[40–42] An increase in corneal thickness of approximately 50 μm as a result of retraction of central corneal collagen was observed in most cases. Overcorrections occurred in 7.8% of the cases, and 20% had induced astigmatism.[43] Poor wound healing was believed to be responsible for the anterior displacement of the central cornea and the excessive scarring at the incision intersection points.

Jensen was also performing this procedure at approximately the same time as Mendez and is credited with having introduced it into the United States.[18] His 1988 report of results with 50 eyes showed mean

TABLE 23–2. REFRACTIVE PROCEDURES FOR THE SURGICAL CORRECTION OF PRIMARY HYPEROPIA

Procedure	Mechanism
Epikeratoplasty	Human donor or synthetic lenticule placed over recipient's cornea denuded of epithelium.
Keratophakia	Recipient's corneal cap removed with the microkeratome. A donor stromal lenticule placed in the bed and covered with the recipient's cap (donor–host "sandwich"). Donor lenticule may be human or synthetic.
Cryolathe keratomileusis	Corneal lenticule removed with the microkeratome, frozen, shaped on the cryolathe, and then replaced. Lenticule may be self or donor tissue.
Hexagonal keratotomy/T-Hex	Six partial thickness incisions placed around the corneal apex, creating a hexagon. In T-Hex, a transverse incision is placed at the vortex of each side of the hexagon.
Thermokeratoplasty (cautery, laser)	Controlled application of heat or laser energy in a radial pattern to shrink peripheral and paracentral stromal collagen to produce a central steepening.
Automated lamellar keratoplasty	Single deep pass of microkeratome, leaving the corneal cap attached by a hinge. Cap assumes steeper central curvature when replaced.
Hyperopic excimer laser photorefractive keratectomy	Laser ablation of tissue from the peripheral cornea.
Automated lamellar keratoplasty in combination with hyperopic excimer laser photorefractive keratectomy	Single deep pass of the microkeratome followed by laser ablation of the corneal cap or stromal bed.
Clear lens extraction and intraocular implantation	Removal of natural lens and implantation of an artificial one that corrects the hyperopia.
Contact lens implantation	Contact lens implanted in posterior chamber on the anterior surface of the natural lens.

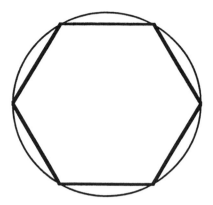

Figure 23–1. The original Mendez hexagonal keratotomy pattern with intersecting incisions. Diameter of the optical zone measured across a circle made to connect the vertices of the hexagon.

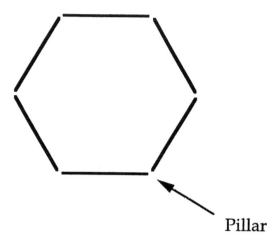

Pillar

Figure 23–2. Hexagonal keratotomy pattern with nonintersecting sides, as modified by Ronald Jensen, MD, in 1989.

changes of 1.00 to 2.65 D, a low level of astigmatism induction, and no complications 1 month postoperatively.[44,45] Also in 1988, Grady reported on successful surgery in 15 of 16 patients, and Neumann and McCarty reported a 2.16 D mean reduction of hyperopia in 15 patients after a mean follow-up of 9.5 months.[15] Uncorrected visual acuity (UCVA) was 20/40 or better in 60% of the eyes, astigmatism was increased a mean of 0.02 D, and no serious complications occurred.[16]

Despite these positive reports, persistent healing defects and astigmatism were frequently associated with intersecting hexagonal incisions. Thus in 1989, Jensen (Fig 23–2) and Mendez (Fig 23–3) independently developed and performed hexagonal keratotomy with nonintersecting hexagonal incisions. In addition, Mendez used an extension or overrun at each incision vortex.

The technique was technically very challenging because the width of the pillars of the hexagon (bridges of

uncut tissue between the vortices) had to be identical. Relatively small differences in pillar width led to asymmetric corneal steepening under the force of intraocular pressure (IOP) (Fig 23–4). The incision extensions (overruns) of the modified Mendez technique did not appear to improve the results of the technique.

To increase corneal stability while retaining the corneal steepening effect, I proposed combined hexagonal and transverse keratotomy incisions, calling it the *T-Hex procedure.* To perform the T-Hex procedure, the sides of the hexagon are constructed first. Care is taken to avoid intersecting the incisions while making the pillars as small as possible (50 to 100 μm). Following creation of the hexagon, a transverse incision, 2.5 to 3.0 mm long, is added approximately 250 μm from each incision vortex (Fig 23–5). This configuration was designed to produce central steepening while avoiding the instability that resulted from intersecting incisions. A group at Tulane University independently proposed a similar hexagonal keratotomy incision technique and studied its effect in cadaver eyes.[14] Later, arcuate keratotomy composed of four nonintersecting arcs that made a circle was tested in human cadaver eyes.[19] Clinical studies, however, were not published.

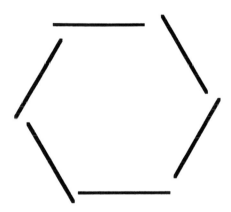

Figure 23–3. Hexagonal keratotomy pattern, with nonintersecting sides and and an extension at each vortex (modified Mendez procedure), 1989.

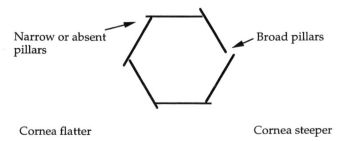

Narrow or absent pillars   Broad pillars

Cornea flatter   Cornea steeper

Figure 23–4. A difference in the amount of uncut tissue (pillars) at the vortices leads to asymmetric anterior bowing and astigmatism.

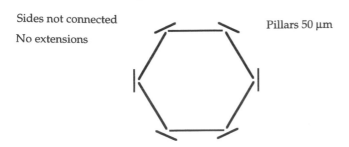

Sides not connected
No extensions
Pillars 50 μm

2.5 mm or 3 mm T cuts

Figure 23–5. The Casebeer T-Hex incision pattern.

Table 23–3 outlines the evolution of the hexagonal keratotomy procedure.

SURGICAL TECHNIQUE: PATIENTS

Clinical Study

In 1991, I performed a clinical study of the T-Hex keratotomy procedure on 110 eyes with hyperopia or hyperopic astigmatism. Of these, 46 eyes of 24 patients were within the limits of the nomogram and were available for follow-up. This follow-up rate of 42% was largely due to the high number of out-of-town referral patients in the practice. Patient characteristics are shown in Table 23–4. The mean age and sex of the group were not unusual considering that hyperopia becomes manifest in middle age and that approximately

equal numbers of women and men seek surgical correction. Patients with astigmatism >1.5 D underwent astigmatism surgery first, followed by T-Hex surgery approximately 6 weeks later.

Patients discontinued rigid contact lenses 3 weeks prior to examination and soft lenses 3 days prior to examination. Each patient underwent a comprehensive ophthalmologic examination, including a cycloplegic refraction, keratometry, tonometry, slit lamp microscopy, and fundus examination.

Patients were fully informed before undergoing a hexagonal keratotomy procedure. This included discussion of available alternatives to surgery, the prognosis for continued spectacle or contact lens wear, and the potential benefits, risks, and complications of this procedure. A questionnaire completed by the patient preoperatively was used to assure that the patient completely understood the surgery.

The visual acuity of each patient was measured in Snellen notation and converted to decimal values, (ie, 20/80 = 0.25).[46] The visual acuity data were also stratified into four groups: 20/10 to 20/20 = good visual acuity; 20/25 to 20/40 = usually functional visual acuity without optical correction; 20/50 to 20/160 = not functional without optical correction; and ≥20/200 = may be considered legally blind in the United States.[47]

Patient Preparation, Pachymetry Measurements, and Blade Setting

Patients were asked to fixate on the light of the operating microscope. The pachymetry measurement was

TABLE 23–3. THE EVOLUTION OF HEXAGONAL KERATOTOMY FOR THE CORRECTION OF HYPEROPIA

Study	Description
First generation: hexagon with connected sides (intersecting incisions)	
Akiyama, 1952	Posterior hexagonal keratotomy in rabbits[37]
Yamashita, 1983	Anterior hexagonal keratotomy in rabbits[38]
Mendez, 1983–1989	Hexagonal keratotomy in sighted humans[40–43]
Jensen, 1987–1989	Introduced hexagonal keratotomy into United States; reported on 190 eyes[44,45]
Grady, 1988	Hexagonal keratotomy in 16 hyperopic eyes[15]
Neumann and McCarty, 1988	Hexagonal keratotomy in 25 hyperopic eyes[16]
Second generation: hexagon with nonconnected sides	
Jensen, 1989	Hexagonal keratotomy with ends of the six incisions not connected
Mendez, 1989	Hexagonal keratotomy with ends of the six incisions not connected and an extension at each vortex (modified Mendez procedure)
Third generation: combined hexagonal and transverse keratotomy and other techniques	
Gilbert, Friedlander, and Granet, 1990	Used combined hexagonal and transverse incisions (Hex-T) to steepen human eye-bank eyes[14]
Casebeer, 1991	Used combined hexagonal and transverse incisions (T-Hex) in humans and reported on 46 surgery cases[18]
Vrabec, Durrie, and Hunkeler, 1993	Studied cadaver eyes and proposed that arcuate keratotomy may be more effective for the correction of hyperopia

TABLE 23–4. T-HEX CLINICAL STUDY: PATIENT CHARACTERISTICS

Number of patients (Eyes)	24 (46)
Age: mean ± SD (range)	55.6 ± 8.31 (35 to 69)
Sex:	
Female	13 (54%)
Male	11 (46%)
Follow-up (months) mean (range)	4.0 (0.25 to 10.25)

TABLE 23–6. CONVERSION TO SPHERICAL EQUIVALENT

Refraction	Spherical Equivalent
+2.00 D + 1.50 D × 90°	+2.75 D
+2.00 D + 2.50 D × 90°	+3.25 D + 2.00 D × 90°
Plano +3.50 D × 90°	1.75 D + 3.50 D × 90°

taken with an ultrasound pachymeter 1.5 mm temporal to the patient's light reflex. The diamond blade was set equal to the pachymetry measurement for all 12 incisions and calibrated with the MicronScope.

The Nomograms

In the Casebeer T-Hex nomogram (Table 23–5), greater reduction of hyperopia is obtained as the OZ decreases and the length of the T-cut increases. Smaller OZs increase the surgical effect. Because pachymetry is taken in the temporal location where it is thinner and the smallest OZ used is 4.5 mm, the incisions are not expected to exceed 80% depth.

For hyperopia up to 4.25 D with astigmatism of 1.5 D or less, no astigmatism incisions were made. With higher amounts of astigmatism (up to 4 D), a staged procedure was used. The refraction was converted to its spherical equivalent (Table 23–6) and the astigmatism-only nomogram (Table 23–7) was to plan the astigmatism surgery, using paired transverse incisions.

The Technique

Patients were usually able to fixate continually on the microscope light. The hexagonal zone marker was used to mark the chosen OZ followed by the T-cut marker, placed approximately 250 μm from the vortices of the hexagon. The hexagon incisions were made first, leaving pillars (uncut tissue) of approximately 50 to 100 μm at the vortices. These were followed by the transverse incisions.

A drop of 0.3% ciprofloxacin was administered. The incisions were not irrigated, inspected, or otherwise disturbed, and a patch was not usually applied. Surgery was not done on both eyes on the same day.

TABLE 23–7. ASTIGMATISM-ONLY NOMOGRAM

**ASTIGMATISM ALONE
T-CUT NOMOGRAM**
DO NOT USE WITH ADDITION OR MODIFICATION OF
RADIAL INCISIONS

PRIMARY & ENHANCEMENT PROCEDURES

SYSTEM EXCEPTION:
Pachymetry at Most Temporal &/or Superior Incision Site

"System" or "Duo Trak" Diamond Blade Set to Pachymetry
Reading A Total of Two Transverse Incisions on the Axis
of the Plus Cylinder. One Transverse Incision
on Each Side of the Cornea

Correction (Diopters)	T-Marker (mm)	Optical Zone (mm)
0.75	2.5	7.00
1.12	3.0	7.00
1.25	2.5	6.00
1.67	3.0	6.00
2.00	2.5	5.00
2.25	3.0	5.00
2.50	2.5	4.75
2.75	3.0	4.75
3.00	2.5	4.50
3.50	3.0	4.50

TABLE 23–5. CASEBEER T-HEX KERATOTOMY NOMOGRAM[a]

Correction (D)	Optical Zone Diameter (mm)	Transverse Cut Length (mm)
1.00	6.00	2.5
1.25	6.00	3.0
1.50	5.75	2.5
1.75	5.75	3.0
2.00	5.50	2.5
2.25	5.50	3.0
2.50	5.25	2.5
2.75	5.25	3.0
3.00	5.00	2.5
3.25	5.00	3.0
3.50	4.75	2.5
3.75	4.75	3.0
4.00	4.50	2.5
4.25	4.50	3.0

[a]Assumes pachometry measurement is taken 1.5 mm temporal to corneal apex and Magnum diamond system blade is set equal to the pachometry measurement.

Postoperative Care

Topical antibiotic–corticosteroid combination was administered QID for 5 days. Application of eye makeup around the eyes or swimming was not permitted for 2 weeks.

Patients were examined 1 to 7 days after the surgery on the first eye, after 3 weeks, and then monthly until the condition was stable. The last visit was usually at 1 year.

Results

The preop UCVA ranged from count fingers to 20/40. Most patients (65.2%) had 20/200 or worse visual acuity (Fig 23–6). Postoperatively, 8.6% had visual acuity in the 20/10 to 20/20 range, 65.2% had 20/25 to 20/40, and 26% had acuity in the range of 20/50 to 20/160, which necessitates optical correction for functioning, and no patient had acuity in the 20/200 or worse range. Thus 74% had 20/40 or better UCVA postoperatively. Seven eyes had a loss of two lines or more of corrected visual acuity, and two eyes had an increase of two lines (Table 23–8). While the best corrected visual acuity (BCVA) of one patient's eye changed from 20/20 to 20/40, no eye lost more than three lines of best corrected vision (Fig 23–7).

The mean preop sphere of +2.04 D was reduced to −0.11 D postoperatively (Table 23–8). Mean cylinder increased from a preop mean of +0.63 D to +1.01 D postop. Mean spherical equivalent changed from +2.35 D preop (range = +0.53 D to +4.38 D) to +0.39 D postop (range = −1.38 D to +3.50 D). The postop mean change in spherical equivalent was 1.96 D. One patient had a microperforation that healed without sequelae.

In this study, we did not observe an increased reduction of hyperopia by virtue of the transverse incisions, as reported by Gilbert and associates.[14]

Mean cylinder increased postoperatively, indicating that the procedure did induce astigmatism, although not to a large degree. Unequal width (asymmetry) of the pillars is the probable cause of induced astigmatism. Enhancement surgery may eliminate some or all of the postop astigmatism.

Like the work of Mendez, our study showed an increase of approximately 50 μm in paracentral corneal thickness resulting from hexagonal keratometry; this was detected during pachymetry measurements before enhancement.[43] The increase does not appear to be related to endothelial cell loss because such loss was not reported by other investigators.[16,17]

TABLE 23–8. T-HEX CLINICAL STUDY: VISUAL RESULTS

	Preop	Postop
Sphere		
Mean	+2.04 D	−0.11 D
Range	+0.03 D to +4.00 D	−1.50 D to +3.00 D
Cylinder		
Mean	+0.63 D	+1.01 D
Range	0.0 D to +3.25 D	0.0 D to +3.5 D
Spherical equivalent		
Mean	+2.35 D	+0.39 D
Range	+0.53 D to +4.38 D	1.38 D to +3.50 D
Mean change		1.96 D
Change in two or more lines of visual acuity		Loss: 7 eyes (15%) Gain: 2 eyes (4%)

SIDE EFFECTS AND COMPLICATIONS OF HEXAGONAL KERATOTOMY

Hexagonal keratotomy has been criticized for inducing an undesirable level of side effects and complications, including irregular astigmatism, glare, and loss of best spectacle-corrected visual acuity.[48–52] However, clinically significant problems with these effects have been infrequent. Werblin believes that patients adjust well to glare and low vision under low light conditions and that most are very happy with their vision, even when there is a loss of one or two lines of best corrected acuity.[51] Irregular astigmatism may occur because of the difficulty in constructing symmetric incisions. A surgeon must be well trained and highly experienced with refractive surgery before attempting hexagonal keratotomy.

As with other kinds of refractive surgery, microperforation or macroperforation can occur. With a macroperforation, the anterior chamber can become shallow or flat, and endophthalmitis is theoretically possible. Recurrent corneal erosion, epithelial cysts, and thickening of the incision have been reported, especially with the older procedure in which the incisions were connected. An increased incidence of retinal detachment, cataracts, significantly decreased endothelial cell count, or glaucoma has not been reported to be associated with hexagonal keratotomy.

NEW DIRECTIONS

The success of RK and PRK for the correction of myopia has drawn attention to the need to provide a surgical modality for the correction of hyperopia. In contrast to the early manifestation of myopia, hyperopia usually

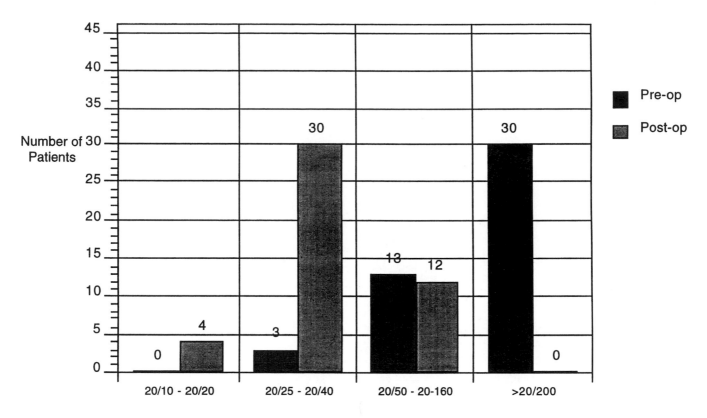

* Visual Acuity Categories:

20/10-20/20   - Good visual acuity

20/25-20/40   - Usually functional visual acuity without optical correction (glasses or contact lenses)

20/50-20/160 - Not functional without optical correction

20/200 or >   - May be considered legally blind in the United States

Figure 23–6. Pre- and postop visual acuity uncorrected.

surfaces in the patient's late thirties and causes significant psychologic distress. The typical patient views the appearance of manifest hyperopia as an unwelcome disability that binds him or her to spectacles for both near and distance vision. Hyperopic patients have often been unaware of the possible surgical resolution of their visual problem, and have shown great interest in this possibility.

Surgeons who were exceptionally skilled in hexagonal keratotomy and were able to offer the procedure to hyperopes obtained good results and found enormous gratification in relieving some patients from their refractive error handicap. However, the procedure was so technically demanding that some surgeons were unable to meet the challenge. Full correction could not be achieved in about 10% of patients.[24] The use of the procedure for RK overcorrections produced some very poor results and led to corneal instability because of the multiple intersecting incisions. An unforseen benefit of these cases, however, was the knowledge that corneal incisions should not intersect.[49]

ALK is another option for the correction of hyperopia. ALK also has a steep learning curve, but it has the major advantage of leaving the anterior cornea uncut while it corrects hyperopic refractive error (see Chapter 26). The mechanism of hyperopic ALK, first observed by Luis Ruiz through aborted keratomileusis cases, is that a deep lamellar incision through the cornea causes corneal steepening and a correction of hyperopia. Ruiz applied these observations to the creation of a nomogram for correcting hyperopia.

The hyperopic ALK procedure can correct up to 5 D of hyperopia with some accuracy, and questionable postoperative stability. Hollis listed the advantages of hyperopic ALK compared with hexagonal keratotomy[24]:

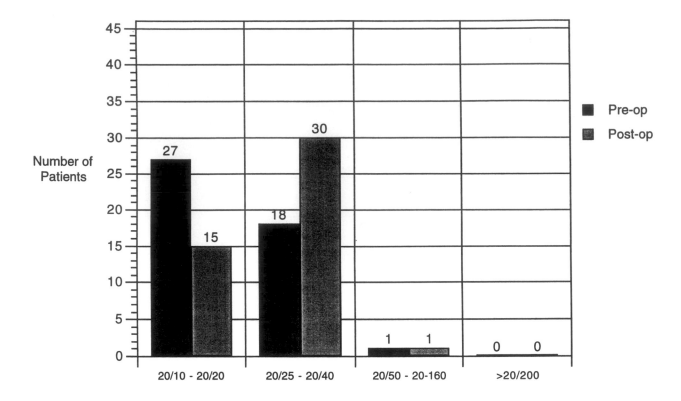

Figure 23–7. Pre- and postop visual acuity with correction.

* There is a much higher success rate.
* There is much less induced astigmatism.
* A better aspherical effect and better near vision may be obtained.
* Results are achieved in about 3 weeks (compared with 6 months for hexagonal keratotomy).
* Delayed healing is eliminated.
* There is much less pain.

Although the precision, predictability, and safety of PRK and hyperopic LASIK have not been established, they seem effective for the surgical correction of hyperopia (see Chapter 37). While hexagonal keratotomy played a role in rehabilitating patients disabled by hyperopia when no other surgical options were available, it has for the most part been superseded by ALK, PRK, and hyperopic LASIK. It is most gratifying to realize that the state of the art of ophthalmic surgery is in constant motion, that refinements continue to be made to already superb surgical equipment, and that

ophthalmic surgeons, never content with what is adequate, continue to search for what is best.

REFERENCES

1. Sorsby A, Sheridan M, Leary GA, Benjamin B. Vision, visual acuity, and ocular refraction of young men. Findings in a sample of 1033 subjects. *Br Med J.* 1960;1:1394–1398.
2. Barraquer JI. Keratophakia. *Trans Ophthalmol Soc UK.* 1972;92:499–516.
3. Erlich MI, Nordan LT. Epikeratophakia for the treatment of hyperopia. *J Cataract Refract Surg.* 1989;15:661–666.
4. Werblin TP, Kaufman HE, Friedlander MH, Granet N. Epikeratophakia, the surgical correction of aphakia III. Preliminary results of a prospective clinical trial. *Arch Ophthalmol.* 1981;99:1957–1960.
5. McCarey BE. Current status of refractive surgery with synthetic intracorneal lenses: Barraquer lecture. *Refract Corneal Surg.* 1990;6:40–46.

6. Lindstrom RL, Lane SS. Polysulfone intracorneal lenses. In: Sanders DR, Hofmann RF, Salz JJ., eds. *Refractive Corneal Surgery.* Thorofare, NJ: Slack Inc; 1986:551–563.

7. Kaufman HE. The correction of aphakia. *Am J Ophthalmol.* 1980;89:1–10.

8. Neumann AC, Fyodorov S, Sanders DR. Radial thermokeratoplasty for the correction of hyperopia. *Refract Corneal Surg.* 1990;6:404–412.

9. Durrie DS, Lesher MP, Cavanaugh TB. Holmium laser thermokeratoplasty for hyperopia and presbyopia: topography and refractive results. Proceedings of International Congress on Cataract, IOL, and Refractive Surgery; 1993; Seattle.

10. Abarca A, Koch DD, Menefee RF, Ebanks TL, Berry MJ. Ho:YAG laser thermal keratoplasty (LTK) for correction of spherical refractive errors. Proceedings of International Congress on Cataract, IOL, and Refractive Surgery; 1993; Seattle.

11. Seiler T, Bende T. Laser coagulation of the cornea with a holmium YAG laser for correction of hyperopia [in German]. *Fortschr Ophthalmol.* 1991;88:121–124.

12. Mendez A. Hexagonal keratotomy for hyperopia. Proceedings of the Keratorefractive Society; 1986; New Orleans.

13. Gilbert ML, Friedlander MH, Aiello JP, Granet N. Hexagonal keratotomy in human cadaver eyes. *J Refract Surg.* 1988;4:12–14.

14. Gilbert ML, Friedlander MH, Granet N. Corneal steepening in human eye bank eyes by combined hexagonal and transverse keratotomy. *Refract Corneal Surg.* 1990;6:126–130.

15. Grady FJ. Hexagonal keratotomy for corneal steepening. *Ophthalmic Surg.* 1988;19:622–623.

16. Neumann AC, McCarty GR. Hexagonal keratotomy for correction of low hyperopia: preliminary results of a prospective study. *J Cataract Refract Surg.* 1988;14:265–269.

17. Jensen RP. Hexagonal keratotomy. Clinical experience with 483 eyes. *Int Ophthalmol Clin.* 1991;31:69.

18. Casebeer JC, Phillips SG. Hexagonal keratotomy: an historical review and assessment of 46 cases. *Ophthalmol Clin N Am.* 1992;5:727–744.

19. Vrabec MP, Durrie DS, Hunkeler JD. Arcuate keratotomy for the correction of spherical hyperopia in human cadaver eyes. *Refract Corneal Surg.* 1993;9:388–391.

20. Grandon SC. Prospective evaluation of hexagonal keratotomy. *Current Research: Refractive and Corneal Surgery Symposium.* Proceedings of International Society of Refractive Keratoplasty; 1993; Chicago.

21. Mendez A. Hyperopia correction with a helicoidal keratotomy. Proceedings of International Congress on Cataract, IOL, and Refractive Surgery; 1993; Seattle.

22. Woodhams JT. Hexagonal keratotomy vs. lamellar keratoplasty in the surgical treatment of hyperopia. Proceedings of Symposium on Cataract, IOL, and Refractive Surgery; 1994; Boston.

23. Casebeer JC, Slade SG, Dybbs A, Mahanti RL. Intraoperative pachometry during automated lamellar keratoplasty. *J Refract Corneal Surg.* 1994;10:41–44.

24. Hollis S. Hyperopic lamellar keratoplasty. In: Rozakis GW, ed. *Refractive Lamellar Keratoplasty.* Thorofare, NJ: Slack, Inc; 1994:79–88.

25. Berkeley RG, Slade SG, Acevedo M. Automated lamellar keratoplasty for hyperopia following RK. Proceedings of Symposium on Cataract, IOL, and Refractive Surgery; 1994; Boston.

26. Dulaney DD. Results of automated lamellar keratoplasty. Proceedings of Symposium on Cataract, IOL, and Refractive Surgery; 1994; Boston.

27. Moore CR. Results of hyperopic lamellar keratoplasty. Proceedings of Symposium on Cataract, IOL, and Refractive Surgery; 1994; Boston.

28. Neumann AC. Automated lamellar keratoplasty: clinical results with myopia and hyperopia. Proceedings of Symposium on Cataract, IOL, and Refractive Surgery; 1994; Boston.

29. Suarez E, Torres F. Hyperopic lamellar keratoplasty. Results in 264 eyes. *Current Research: Refractive and Corneal Surgery Symposium.* Proceedings of International Society of Refractive Keratoplasty; 1993; Chicago.

30. Dausch D, Klein R, Schroder E. Excimer laser photorefractive keratectomy for hyperopia. *Refract Corneal Surg.* 1993; 9:20–28.

31. Ditzen K, Wetzel W. Hyperopic excimer laser PRK combined with automated lamellar keratoplasty. Proceedings of Symposium on Cataract, IOL, and Refractive Surgery; 1994; Boston.

32. Hardten DR, Dougherty PJ, Sher NA, Doughman DJ, Carpel E, Ostrov CS, Lane SS, Lindstrom RL. Hyperopic correction with the 193-nm excimer laser. Proceedings of Symposium on Cataract, IOL, and Refractive Surgery; 1994; Boston.

33. Goes F. Short term results with excimer laser photorefractive keratectomy. *Bull Soc Belge Ophtalmol.* 1992;245: 69–74.

34. McDonald MB, Ahmed S, Pendleton KM. Clinical update on the first cases of hyperopic PRK with a VISX laser. *Current Research: Refractive and Corneal Surgery Symposium.* Proceedings of International Society of Refractive Keratoplasty; 1993; Chicago.

35. Siganos DS, Siganos CS, Pallikaris IG. Clear lens extraction and intraocular lens implantation in normally sighted hyperopic eyes. *J Refract Corneal Surg.* 1994;10: 117–124.

36. Deitz MR, Sanders DR. An implantable contact lens for the posterior chamber for the correction of primary myopia and hyperopia. Proceedings of Symposium on Cataract, IOL, and Refractive Surgery; 1994; Boston.

37. Akiyama K. Study of surgical treatment for myopia. I. Posterior corneal incisions. *Acta Soc Ophthalmol Jpn.* 1952; 56:1142.

38. Yamashita T, Gaster R. Experimental hyperopia correction. Keratorefractive Society Symposium; 1983: Chicago.

39. Yamashita T, Schneider ME, Fuerst DJ, Pierce WJ. Hexagonal keratotomy reduces hyperopia after radial keratotomy in rabbits. *J Refract Surg.* 1986;2:261.

40. Mendez A. Hyperopia reduction with hexagonal keratotomy. Keratorefractive Society Symposium; 1985; San Francisco.

41. Mendez A. Advances in the hyperopia correction with hexagonal keratotomy. American Society for Cataract and Refractive Surgery; 1986; Los Angeles.

42. Mendez A. Correcao da hipermetropia pela ceratotomia hexagonal. In: Guimarares R, ed. *Cirugia Refractive.* Rio de Janeiro, Brasil: Piramide Livro Medico Editora Ltda; 1987: 267–279.

43. Mendez A. Hyperopia reduction with hexagonal keratotomy. Keratorefractive Society Symposium; 1988.

44. Jensen RP. Experience with hexagonal keratotomy. Symposium on Cataract, IOL, and Refractive Surgery; 1988; Los Angeles.

45. Jensen RP. Experience with hexagonal keratotomy. *J Cataract Refract Surg.* 1988;14:580–581.

46. Vila-Coro AA, Vila-Coro AnA. Mean visual acuity. *Am J Ophthalmol.* 1989;107:564–570.

47. Waring GO III.: Standardized data collection and reporting for refractive surgery. *Refract Corneal Surg.* 1992; March/April (suppl).

48. Basuk WL, Zisman M, Waring GO, et al. Complications of hexagonal keratotomy. *Am J Ophthalmol.* 1994;117: 37–49.

49. Tamura M, Mamalis N, Kreisler KR, Casebeer JC. Complications of a hexagonal keratotomy following radial keratotomy (case report). *Arch Ophthalmol.* 1991; 109:1351.

50. Nordan LT, Maxwell WA. Avoid both keratotomy with small optical zones and hexagonal keratotomy. *Refract Corneal Surg.* 1992;8:331.

51. Werblin T. Critique of hexagonal keratotomy raises a ruckus. *Refract Corneal Surg.* 1992;8:408. Letter.

52. Friedlander M. Critique of hexagonal keratotomy raises a ruckus. *Refract Corneal Surg.* 1992;8:408. Letter.

CHAPTER 24

Ocular Infections after Refractive Surgery

Sandeep Jain ▪ Dimitri T. Azar

Several clinical studies have recognized the success and effectiveness of refractive surgery. However, reports of sight threatening ocular infections after refractive keratotomy (RK) and photorefractive keratectomy (PRK) appear periodically in published literature[1–6].

In this chapter, we have systematically compiled[5,6] the reported cases of ocular infections after radial keratotomy to obtain the best available perspective on infections following refractive surgery. We identified pertinent articles through a multistaged, systematic approach. In the first stage, a computerized search of three MEDLINE databases (National Library of Medicine, Bethesda, MD) was performed (1990 to March 1996; 1985 to 1989; and mid-1976 to 1984) to identify all articles describing RK. The term *radial keratotomy* from the Medical Subject Headings (MeSH) supplement to *Index Medicus* (National Library of Medicine, Bethesda, MD) and the text word *keratotomy* were used for a broad and sensitive search. In the second stage, all abstracts were carefully scanned to identify articles, written in English, that described either the complications of refractive keratotomy (RK) or the results of a clinical series. Whole copies of these articles were obtained. Bibliographies of the retrieved articles were manually searched for additional articles. All

identified journals were manually searched up to and including the March 1996 issue, using the same search guidelines. In the third stage, complete articles were reviewed to identify those that reported infections after RK. These articles were grouped as case reports, clinical series, surveys, and reviews. In the last stage, all articles that reported new case(s) of infections were identified and included in the study. Articles reporting previously published cases were excluded. Abstract books of the two major annual ophthalmology meetings, the Association for Research in Vision and Ophthalmology and the American Academy of Ophthalmology, were manually searched to identify unpublished abstracts reporting infections after RK during the study search period (1976 to 1996).

The postop time for onset of infection was determined by calculating the interval between the last surgical intervention (primary procedure or reoperations) and the appearance of initial symptoms. The location of corneal infiltrate with respect to the incisions of a standard, eight-incision radial keratotomy was determined. Infections at each incision included those located within a half-hour clock area on either side of the incision. Each incision was divided into three equal segments to describe infection location within the incision. Cultured microorganisms, associations, and visual outcome after treatment were noted.

A total of 65 infectious episodes (59 keratitis and 6 endophthalmitis) were described in 60 patients. Fifty-one cases followed radial keratotomy.[1,2,7–39] Six of the infections followed PRK, 7 followed PTK, and 1 followed myopic keratomileusis.[38,40–46] There were no reports of infection following ALK. One case of endophthalmitis occurred after PRK, with the other 5 occurring after RK. In 4 patients infections were bilateral, and 1 patient had a repeat episode. Twenty-four (40%) patients were female and 27 (45%) male (data were missing for nine cases). The age of patients ranged from 18 to 80 years, with a median age of 35 years (data were missing for ten cases). Thirty (46%) infections were in right eyes and 18 (28%) in left eyes (data were missing for 17 eyes). Radial keratotomy was performed in 43 (66%) eyes, hexagonal keratotomy in 3, and trapezoidal keratotomy in 3 (data were missing for 3 eyes). The total number of radial incisions was eight or less in 27 (53%) eyes. Fifteen eyes (32%) received more than 8 incisions (range = 10 to 18), with the median number of incisions being 16. Transverse incisions were placed in addition to radial incisions in 15 eyes (23%).

Forty-five percent of infections developed within 2 weeks after the last refractive procedure. The median time of reported early-onset infections was 8.5 days, ranging from 1 to 14 days. Fifty-one percent of infections develop months to years after the last refractive procedure. The median time of reported late-onset infections was 2 years, ranging from 1 month to 5 years. We are aware of one unreported case of acanthamoebae keratitis developing 8 years after RK (EC Alfonso, oral communication, May 1995) and one unreported case of staphylococcal keratitis 9 years after RK (JS Lustgarten, oral communication, May 1995). In the PERK study the frequency of infection was 0.25% (two infections in 793 RK surgeries). Deitz et al reported infection in 0.35% of eyes,[31] and Hoffer et al, in the UCLA study, reported infection in 0.70% of eyes (one infection in 144 RK surgeries).[32] The variability in frequency of infections reported in the three clinical series that reported such cases derives from their small sample size. Most published clinical series do not report any infectious complications. Given that more than 95% of cases in the published literature appear as isolated case reports, the incidence of infections after RK and the cause-and-effect relation of potential associations remain difficult to estimate. Based on a large-scale survey of 63,000 RK cases of over 200 surgeons, Marmer identified infections in only 0.02% of eyes (eight cases of stromal keratitis, two of corneal ulcers, one of microwound abscess, four of endophthalmitis, and one of herpes keratitis).[1] In another survey of the cases of 24 surgeons, Lewicky and Salz identified one case of endophthalmitis, five of bacterial infections, and one of viral keratitis.[39] The total number of surgeries performed by each author was not reported. Such large-scale surveys provide the best estimate of the magnitude of this complication. Two unpublished reports have described infections following RK. Fifty-seven cases of infectious keratitis were noted over a 5-year period of observation in Brazil.[47] The highest incidence of infection was reported to be within the first 2 weeks and between the first and fourth years after surgery. *Staphylococcus aureus* was the most frequently isolated organism. Six cases of delayed keratitis were reported by Cottingham and Berkley.[48] Reoperations were performed in all six cases, and all infections were located inferiorly within the incision sites (Fig 24–1).

Thirty-five eyes of 47 reported eyes (74%) had a single corneal infiltrate, 6 had multiple infiltrates, 3 had central corneal edema, and 3 had no infiltrates (data were missing for 4 eyes). Incisions that cause gaping wounds are more susceptible to infection. The corneal thickness is greatest close to the limbus and thinnest in the central and temporal and inferior paracentral areas. During RK, the depth of corneal incisions is determined by pachymetry and is usually kept constant for all incisions. Constant-depth incisions are likely to produce greater gaping in thinner parts of the cornea, which may explain the preponderance of infections in the inferotemporal quadrant. Sixty-two percent of infections are located in the inferior third of the cornea, as opposed to only 13% in the superior third of the cornea. Incisions (temporal, inferotemporal, inferior, and inferonasal) in the inferotemporal half of the cornea were most susceptible to infection and accounted for 35 (74%) infections (Fig 24–2). Six (13%) infections were located in the temporal incision, thirteen (26%) in the inferotemporal incision, nine (19%) in the inferior incision, and eight (17%) in the inferonasal incision. Of the seven reported perforations, five (71%) were in the temporal quadrant of the cornea (two in the inferotemporal, two in the temporal, and one in the superotemporal incision). One perforation occurred in the inferior incision and one in the inferonasal incision. The tendency for the inferior quadrants to be involved may also be due to factors like proximity of incisions to the lower lid margin, exposure, and surface drying. Transverse incisions, particularly when they cross radial incisions, also produce gaping wounds. In addition, they

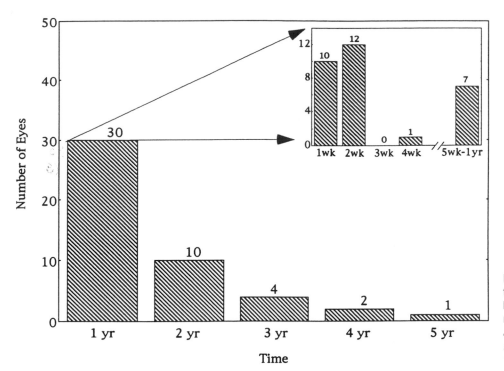

Figure 24–1. Bar diagram showing the onset of infections after refractive keratotomy. *Inset:* Infections occurring within 1 year of surgery. *(From Jain S, Azar DT. Eye infections after refractive keratotomy. J Refract Surg. 1996;12:148–155.)*

may transect corneal nerves and produce anesthesia within the incision.[8,49]

Apart from the three cases of central corneal edema of presumed viral etiology, all infections involved keratotomy incisions. The corneal infiltrates were located in the central third of the incision (optical zone end) in 15 (32%) eyes, in the middle third in 12 (26%), in the peripheral third (limbal end) in 2 (4%), and in the whole length in 3 (6%) eyes (data were missing for 11 eyes). In the 34 eyes for which details were known, the corneal infiltrate was away from the limbus in 85% of eyes.

Associations were identified in 77% of eyes. Eleven percent had multiple associations. Preoperative conditions that were implicated included external ocular pathology in 11% of cases (dry eyes, blepharitis, and chronic vernal conjunctivitis) and systemic infections in 9% of cases (atopy, mycosis, Crohn's disease, and AIDS). Reoperations (additional incisions and enhancements) were the major surgical association. They had been performed in 24%. Cold sterilization of the keratotomy blade was implicated in one case. Intraoperative perforations occurred in 14%. Postop contact lens wear was implicated in 26%. Eight percent suffered postop injury (blunt trauma, extraocular foreign body, and chemical injury), and in 2 eyes postop use of cosmetics (mascara) was implicated.

In our review we observed that 61% of the 15 gram-positive bacterial cultures were isolated from in-

fections occurring within the first 2 weeks (early-onset cases), and that 92% of the gram-negative bacillary cultures were isolated from late-onset infection cases. Gram-positive cocci included *Staphylococcus aureus* in 5 eyes, *Staphylococcus epidermidis* in 5, and *Streptococcus*

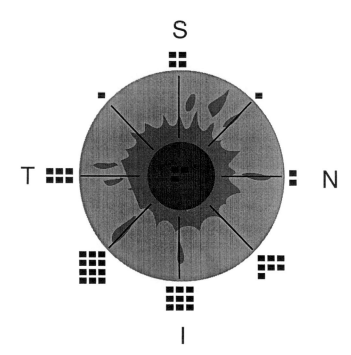

Figure 24–2. Schematic diagram of cornea showing the location of infections with respect to the standard eight radial keratotomy incisions. (*N*, nasal; *T*, temporal; *S*, superior; *I*, inferior). *(From Jain S, Azar DT. Eye infections after refractive keratotomy. J Refract Surg. 1996;12:148–155.)*

pneumoniae in 2. Gram-positive bacilli included diphtheroids in 2 eyes and the anaerobic diphtheroid *Propionobacterium* in 1 eye. Gram-negative bacilli included *Pseudomonas aeruginosa* in 7 eyes, and *Serratia*, *Moraxella*, and *Enterobacter* caused one infection each. Acid-fast bacilli infections were caused by *Mycobacterium chelonei* and fungal infections by *Candida* (Table 24–1).

Refractive keratotomy incisions breach the epithelial integrity. Infections may occur if the antimicrobial and immune defenses are compromised, as in the presence of preexisting ocular, adnexal, and systemic infections. Fibronectin is a stromal extracellular protein that is expressed in the early phase of corneal wound healing.[40] It can bind to a variety of gram-positive cocci, but not to gram-negative bacilli.[51,52] The preponderance of gram-positive coccal infections in early-onset infections may be related to the preferential binding of these bacteria to fibronectin, which is expressed in the early stages of healing after keratectomy wounds. An inadequately sterilized keratotomy knife may, in addition, directly inoculate the microbes deep within the corneal stroma. Intraoperative corneal perforations provide a portal of entry for intraocular infections. Altered corneal microarchitecture along the keratotomy incisions (delayed wound healing, epithelial basement membrane changes, and epithelial plugs and inclusion cysts)[53–55] and tear film redistribution cause epithelial surface irregularities and erosions, facilitating bacterial adherence.[7] Postop mechanical trauma or contact lens–induced hypoxia may erode the epithelial surface or rupture an epithelial plug, predisposing to the development of secondary infection. Spontaneous rupture of an epithelial cyst may incite sterile stromal keratitis. Indiscriminate empirical use of potent topical antibiotics and steroids may encourage infection and decrease the likelihood that organisms can be recovered by standard culture techniques (Fig 24–3).

In 11% of the cases we reviewed, a viral infection (*Herpes simplex*) was presumed, based on the clinical presentation and response to antiviral drugs. Nine (23%) of the 40 cultures were sterile, 6 of which had received empirical topical antibiotic treatment before obtaining cultures. Thirty-seven (88%) of the 42 positive cultures showed bacterial growth and 6 (6%) showed fungal growth. Three cultures showed growth of two or more bacterial colonies. Four cultures were initially negative, but bacteria were isolated in subsequent corneal biopsies (acid-fast bacilli from 2 eyes and gram-positive bacilli from 2 eyes).

Fortified topical cephalosporins were used in 50% of eyes with gram-positive coccal infections. Cefazolin (50 mg/ml) was used in 4 eyes and cephalothin (50 mg/ml) in 1. Vancomycin (50 mg/ml) was used in 2 eyes. In 5 eyes fortified topical aminoglycosides (gentamicin 9.1 to 14 mg/ml, tobramycin 13.5 mg/ml) were used in addition to these antibiotics. Fortified topical aminoglycosides were used in 67% of the 12 eyes with gram-negative infections. Gentamicin (9.1 to 13.6 mg/ml) was used in 6 eyes and tobramycin (13.5 mg/ml) in 1. Fortified topical amikacin (5 mg/ml) was used for the three acid-fast bacilli infections. Ciprofloxacin (3 mg/ml) was used in one case, and was combined with amikacin in another. Topical trifluridine was used for all viral infections. Topical amphotericin-B (5 mg/ml) and oral ketaconazole used for the fungal infections. Topical propamidine (1mg/ml) and polyhexamethylene bijuanide (o · 2 mg/ml) were used to treat the acanthamoeba infection.

TABLE 24–1. MICROBES CAUSING REFRACTIVE SURGICAL INFECTIONS

Microbes	Infection Onset		PRK/PTK	
	Early	*Late*	*Early*	*Late*
Bacterial				
Gram-positive bacilli (diphtheroids)	2	1	0	0
Gram-positive cocci *(Staphylococcus, Streptococcus)*	9	3	0	5
Gram-negative bacilli *(Pseudomonas, Serratia, Moraxella)*	1	11	0	0
Acid-fast bacilli *(Mycobacterium chelonei)*	2	2	0	0
Gram-negative cocci	0	0	0	2
Unknown bacteria	1	1		
Fungal *(Candida)*	3	1	3	0
Viral *(Herpes)*	1	2	0	4
Sterile	5	4		
Protozoa	1	0	0	0
Unknown	1	1		

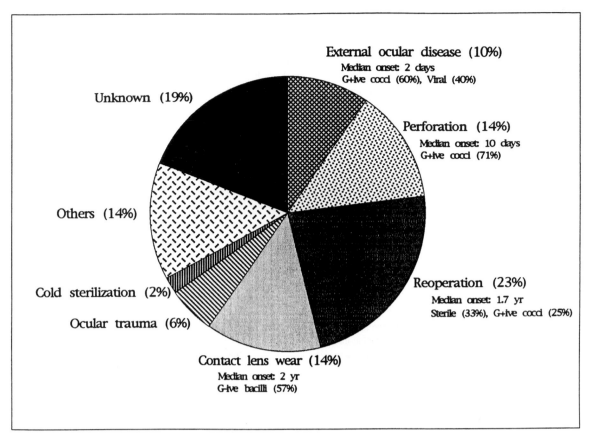

Figure 24–3. Pie diagram showing the relative frequency of factors that may have predisposed to the development of infections after refractive keratotomy. Five eyes had multiple risk factors. *(G–ive,* Gram-negative; *G+ive,* Gram-positive). *(Modified with permission from: Jain S, Azar DT. Eye infections after refractive keratotomy.* J Refract Surg. *1996,12:148–155.)*

Fortified cefazolin and tobramycin were used to treat 45% of the nine sterile keratitis cases. Gentamicin (3 mg/ml) and dexamethasone (1 mg/ml) were used in 1 eye. In one case a thin conjunctival bridge flap was used to cover the inflamed cornea after it failed to respond to all topical treatment. Treatment of endophthalmitis cases was more aggressive and included intravitreal antibiotics and pars plana vitrectomy. Following PTK for HSV-related stromal scarring, 2 of 3 patients were placed on prophylactic trifluoridine and steroids, and one patient was placed on steroids only.

Pre-refractive surgery best corrected visual acuity (BCVA) was better than 20/40 in all cases (Table 24–2). BCVA after complete medical treatment for post-RK infections was 20/40 or better in 63% of eyes and worse than 20/40 in 20%. Nine (13%) eyes required therapeutic keratoplasty, which resulted in a BCVA of 20/40 or better in 4 eyes. The BCVA after the onset of infection was 20/40 or better in 46% of these 28 cases and worse than 20/40 in 53%. After complete medical treatment, BCVA was 20/40 or better in 82% of these 28 cases and worse than 20/40 in 18%. Infections following PRK re-

TABLE 24–2. VISUAL OUTCOME AFTER REFRACTIVE KERATOTOMY INFECTIONS

	BCVA	
Cases[a]	**20/40 or Better**	**Worse than 20/40**
All details known (28)		
At infection onset	13	15
After complete medical treatment	23	5
Partial details known (14)		
At infection onset	—	—
After complete medical treatment	10	5

[a]Data missing for four cases. Following keratoplasty BCVA improved to 20/40 or better in three more eyes.
Abbreviation: BCVA, best corrected visual acuity (see ref. #1).

sulted in final visual acuities of 20/20 in 2 patients, counting fingers in one, and was unknown in 3 patients. The only infection reported with keratomileusis recovered 20/60 spectacle-corrected visual acuity. Following PTK, visual acuity was 20/100 or worse in 4 patients, and better than 20/100 in 3 patients. Data on BCVA after infection onset were missing for 19 eyes (40%). After

TABLE 24–3. ENDOPHTHALMITIS AFTER REFRACTIVE KERATOTOMY

Study	Surgery	Associations	Infection onset	Microbe	Visual Outcome
Gelender[14]	RK (16 incisions)	Perforation	Early (9 d)	*Staphylococcus epidermidis*	20/30
Manka[21]	Trapezoidal keratotomy	Perforation	Early (8 d)	*Staphylococcus epidermidis*	20/25
O'Day[24]	RK (16 incisions)	Perforation Reoperation	Early (10 d)	*Staphylococcus epidermidis*	20/25
Basuk[10]	Hexagonal keratotomy	Perforation Reoperation	Early (12 d)	Sterile	20/40
Durand[12]	RK (16 incisions)	Perforation Reoperation	Late (1.3 y)	—	Keratoplasty

From Jain S, Azar DT. Eye Infections after refractive keratotomy. J Refract Surg. 1996;12:148–155.

TABLE 24–4. CASES REQUIRING KERATOPLASTY AFTER REFRACTIVE KERATOTOMY

Age (y)/Sex	Infection Onset	Associations	Pathogen	Postkeratoplasty Outcome
32/M	1 d	Perforation	*Streptococcus pneumoniae*	20/25 with RGPL
18/F	4 d	—	—	Opaque graft
35/M	14 d	Reoperation Transverse incision	*Mycobacterium chelonei*	VA 20/40
35/M	4 wk	Circumferential incision Topical anesthetic use Therapeutic SCL	Sterile	VA 20/200 Cataract
25/F	1.3 y	Perforation	—	—
35/M	2.8 y	Dry eyes Reoperation Topical steroid use	Sterile	BCVA 20/25

Abbreviations: BCUA, best corrected visual acuity; RGPL, rigid gas-permeable lenses; SCL, soft contact lenses; VA, visual acuity.
From Jain S, Azar DT. Eye Infections after refractive keratotomy. J Refract Surg. 1996;12:148–155.

complete medical treatment, BCVA was 20/40 or better in 53% of these cases and worse than 20/40 in 26%.

Infectious keratitis and endophthalmitis may rarely complicate refractive surgery (Table 24–3). Our study reveals that the risk of infection is greatest within 2 weeks of surgery (early-onset infections); that early-onset infections are mainly caused by Gram-positive bacteria and are associated with intraoperative perforation and preexisting external ocular disease; and that late-onset infections are mainly caused by gram-negative bacteria and are associated with reoperations and postop contact lens wear. Infections are most commonly localized within the paracentral region of the RK incision. Incisions in the inferotemporal third of the cornea harbor the greatest number of infections. The majority of patients recover their preinfection BCVA with conservative management, and few require keratoplasty (Table 24–4).

Our review documents the occurrence of infections after refractive surgery as a relatively rare event. This may be due, in part, to underreporting of this complication. Using proper precautions during surgical planning and postoperative care, and intervening promptly and effectively should infection occur would no doubt lead to further reduction in the frequency of infection and visual compromise.

REFERENCES

1. Jain S, Azar DT. Eye Infections after refractive keratotomy. *J Refract Surg.* 1996;12:148–155.
2. Waring GO, Lynn MJ, Nizam A, et al. Results of the prospective evaluation of radial keratotomy (PERK) study five years after surgery. *Ophthalmology.* 1990;98:1164–1176.
3. Salz JJ, Salz JM, Salz M, Jones D. Ten years' experience with a conservative approach to radial keratotomy. *Refract Corneal Surg.* 1991;7:12–22.
4. Bates AK, Morgan SJ, Steele AD. Radial keratotomy: a review of 300 cases. *Br J Ophthalmol.* 1992;76:586–589.

5. Thacker SB. Meta-analysis: a quantitative approach to research integration. *JAMA.* 1988;259:1685–1689.

6. Dickersin K, Berlin JA. Meta-analysis: state-of-the-science. *Epidemiol Rev.* 1992;14:154–176.

7. Mandelbaum S, Waring GO, Forster RK, et al. Late development of ulcerative keratitis in radial keratotomy scars. *Arch Ophthalmol.* 1986;104:1156–1160.

8. Matoba AY, Torres J, Wilhelmus KR, Hamill MB, Jones DB. Bacterial keratitis after radial keratotomy. *Ophthalmology.* 1989;96:1171–1175.

9. Wilhelmus KR, Hamburg S. Bacterial keratitis following radial keratotomy. *Cornea.* 1983;2:143–146.

10. Basuk WL, Zisman M, Waring GO, et al. Complications of hexagonal keratotomy. *Am J Ophthalmol.* 1994;117:37–49.

11. Beldavs RA, Al-Ghamdi S, Wilson LA, Waring GO. Bilateral microbial keratitis after radial keratotomy. *Arch Ophthalmol.* 1993;111:440.

12. Durand L, Monnot J-P, Burillon C, Assi A. Complications of radial keratotomy: eyes with keratoconus and late wound dehiscence. *Refract Corneal Surg.* 1992;8:311–314.

13. Geggel HS. Delayed sterile keratitis following radial keratotomy requiring corneal transplantation for visual rehabilitation. *Refract Corneal Surg.* 1990;6:55–58.

14. Gelender H, Flynn HW, Mandelbaum SH. Bacterial endophthalmitis from radial keratotomy. *Am J Ophthalmol.* 1982;93:323–326.

15. Holgado S, Luna JD, Juarez CP. Postoperative candida keratitis treated successfully with fluconazole. *Ophthalmology.* 1993;24:132.

16. Hwang DG, Biswell R. Ciprofloxacin therapy of *Mycobacterium chelonae* keratitis. *Am J Ophthalmol.* 1993;115:114–115.

17. Insler MS, Semple HC. Delayed microbial keratitis following radial keratotomy. *CLAOJ.* 1988;14:163–164.

18. Karr DJ, Gruzmacher RD, Reeh MJ. Radial keratotomy complicated by sterile keratitis and corneal perforation: histopathologic case report and review of complications. *Ophthalmology.* 1985;92:1244–1248.

19. Lee CP. Radial keratotomy: in-to-out and out-to-in. Preliminary results in the Singapore General Hospital. *Ann Acad Med Singapore.* 1989;18:141.

20. Mackman G. Delayed sterile keratitis following radial keratotomy successfully treated with conjunctival flap. *Refract Corneal Surg.* 1992;8:122–124.

21. Manka RL, Gast TJ. Endophthalmitis following Ruiz procedure. *Arch Ophthalmol.* 1990;108:21.

22. Maskin SL, Alfonso E. Fungal keratitis after radial keratotomy. *Am J Ophthalmol.* 1992;114:369–370.

23. McClellan KA, Bernard PJ, Gregory-Roberts JC, Billson FA. Suppurative keratitis: a late complication of radial keratotomy. *J Cataract Refract Surg.* 1988;14:317–320.

24. O'Day DM, Feman SS, Elliott JH. Visual impairment following radial keratotomy: a cluster of cases. *Ophthalmology.* 1986;93:319–326.

25. Robin JB, Beatty RF, Dunn S, et al. *Mycobacterium chelonei* keratitis after radial keratotomy. *Am J Ophthalmol.* 1986;102:72–79.

26. Santos CRI. Herpetic corneal ulcer following radial keratotomy. *Ann Ophthalmol.* 1983;15:82–85.

27. Shivitz IA, Arrowsmith PN. Delayed keratitis after radial keratotomy. *Arch Ophthalmol.* 1986;104:1153–1155.

28. Szerenyi K, McDonnell JM, Smith RE, Irvine JA, McDonnell PJ. Keratitis as a complication of bilateral, simultaneous radial keratotomy. *Am J Ophthalmol.* 1994;117:462–467.

29. Dhanda RP, Kalevar V. Radial keratotomy in India: untoward consequences and complications. *Indian J Ophthalmol.* 1990;38:139–144.

30. Grimmett MR, Holland EJ, Krachmer JH. Therapeutic keratoplasty after radial keratotomy. *Am J Ophthalmol.* 1994;118:108–109.

31. Deitz MR, Sanders DR, Marks RG. Radial keratotomy: an overview of the Kansas City study. *Ophthalmology.* 1984;91:467–478.

32. Hoffer KJ, Darin JJ, Pettit TH, et al. Three year experience with radial keratotomy: the UCLA study. *Ophthalmology.* 1983;90:627–636.

33. American Academy of Ophthalmology. Radial keratotomy for myopia. *Ophthalmology.* 1993;100:1103–1115.

34. Kinota S, Wong KW, Biswas J, Rao NA. Changing patterns of infectious keratitis: overview of clinical and histopathologic features of keratitis due to acanthamoeba or atypical mycobacteria, and of infectious crystalline keratopathy. *Indian J Ophthalmol.* 1993;41:3–14.

35. Hersh PS, Kenyon KR. Complications of radial keratotomy: review of the literature and implications for a developing country. *Indian J Ophthalmol.* 1990;38:132–138.

36. Wilson DR, Keeney AH. Corrective measures for myopia. *Surv Ophthalmol.* 1990;34:294–304.

37. Rashid ER, Waring GO. Complications of radial and transverse keratotomy. *Surv Ophthalmol.* 1989;34:73–106.

38. Cooney MJ, Friello PJ, Azar DT. Eye Infections after refractive surgical procedures. *Ophthalmic practice* 1996;14:43–47.

39. Lewicky AO, Salz JJ. Special report: radial keratotomy survey. *J Refract Surg.* 1986;2:32–34.

40. Maguen E, Salz J, Nesburn A, Warren C, Macy J, Papaioannou T, Hofbauer J, Berlin M. Results of excimer laser photorefractive keratectomy for the correction of myopia. *Ophthalmology.* 1994;101:1548–1557.

41. Sampath R, Ridgway AE, Leatherbarrow B. Bacterial keratitis following excimer laser photorefractive keratectomy: a case report (letter). *Eye.* 1994;8:481–482.

42. Faschinger C, Faulborn J, Ganser K. [Infectious corneal ulcers—once with endophthalmitis—after photorefractive keratotomy with disposable contact lens.] [German] *Klinische Monatsblätter für Augenheilkunde.* 1995;206:96–102.

43. Al-Rajhi AA, Wagoner MD, Badr IA, Al-Saif A, Mahmood M. Bacterial keratitis following phototherapeutic keratectomy. *J Refract Surg.* 1996;12:123–127.

44. Vrabec MP, Anderson JA, Rock ME, Binder PS, Steinert RF, Durrie DS, Chase DS. Electron microscopic findings in a cornea with recurrence of *Herpes simplex* keratitis after excimer laser photorefractive keratectomy. *CLAO.* 1994;20: 41–44.

45. Nascimento EG, Carvalho MJ, Defreitas D, Campos M. *Nocardial* keratitis following myopic keratomileusis. *J Refract Corneal Surg.* 1995;11:210–211.

46. Pepose JS, Laycock KA, Miller JK, et al. Reactivation of latent *Herpes simplex* virus by excimer laser photokeratectomy. *Am J Ophthalmol.* 1992;114:45–50.

47. Freitas D, Chaib A, Scarpi M, Guidugli T, Belfort R. Infectious keratitis after radial keratotomy: a Brazilian experience. *Invest Ophthalmol Vis Sci.* 1994;35(suppl):1297.

48. Cottingham AJ, Berkley RP, Nordan LT, et al. Bacterial corneal ulcers following keratorefractive surgery: a retrospective study of 14,163 procedures. Read before the Ocular Microbiology Immunology Group Meeting; September 28, 1985; San Francisco.

49. Shivitz IA, Arrowsmith PN. Corneal sensitivity after radial keratotomy. *Ophthalmology.* 1985;92:734–740.

50. Gipson IK, Watanabe H, Zieske JD. Corneal wound healing and fibronectin. *Int Ophthalmol Clin.* 1993;33:149–163.

51. Woods DE, Straus DC, Johanson WG, Johanson WG. Role of fibronectin in the prevention of adherence of *Pseudomonas aeruginosa* to buccal cells. *J Infect Dis.* 1981;143: 784–790.

52. Kuusela P. Fibronectin binds to *Staphylococcus aureus. Nature.* 1978;276:718–720.

53. Stainer GA, Shaw EL, Binder PS, et al. Histopathology of a case of radial keratotomy. *Arch Ophthalmol.* 1982;100: 1473–1477.

54. Deg JK, Zavala EW, Binder PS. Delayed cornea; wound healing following radial keratotomy. *Ophthalmology.* 1985; 92:734–740.

55. Jester JV, Villasenor RA, Miyashiro J. Epithelial inclusion cysts following radial keratotomy. *Arch Ophthalmol.* 1983; 101:611–615.

CHAPTER 25

Sidestepping the Complications of Incisional Corneal Surgery

Kerry K. Assil ▪ David J. Schanzlin

Over one million Americans have successfully undergone radial keratotomy (RK). Although the serious complications of incisional keratotomy are rare,[1] it is important to become familiar with them, as their prevention requires an awareness and understanding of the potential causes. In the event that a complication occurs, early recognition and prompt therapy will avert a poor outcome in almost every case. The complications associated with incisional keratotomy can be divided into those that are self-limited, occur intraoperatively, occur postoperatively, and are associated with adjunctive therapy.

SELF-LIMITED SIDE EFFECTS

The self-limited side effects include halo effect, starburst effect (Fig 25–1), diurnal visual fluctuation, and early postop regression of effect. In a small subset of patients, these side effects may persist beyond the periop period. They were all evaluated in the PERK study and are discussed in the 5-year analysis of the PERK follow-up results.[2] With the more modern techniques of using shorter-length incisions and thinner diamonds, and the ability to diagnose and treat induced irregular astigmatism using more sophisticated topography systems (Fig 25–2), most surgeons have found side effects to be less severe and of shorter duration than those observed during the period of the PERK study.

Halo and Starburst Effects

By staging the procedure with a variable number of incisions and therefore less frequently producing small optical zone size, the halo and starburst effects may be diminished. These side effects may be less dependent upon direct light scatter from the incisions than upon changes in corneal asphericity ("midperipheral knee"), residual myopia, or induced irregular astigmatism. Corneal topographic analysis may uncover irregular astigmatism, which appears to be more prevalent with four-incision RK carried out to smaller optical zones than with six- or eight-incision RK at slightly larger optical zones. With time, most of these symptoms will resolve. Attempts at early surgical intervention may exacerbate the patient's symptoms.

Diurnal Visual Fluctuation and Early Regression

Diurnal visual fluctuation during the first several postop months is most likely due to immature wound

327

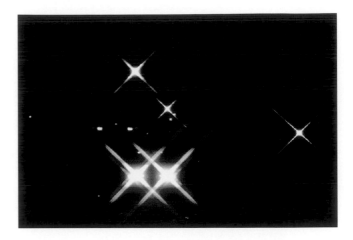

Figure 25–1. Photographic simulation of starburst effect following RK.

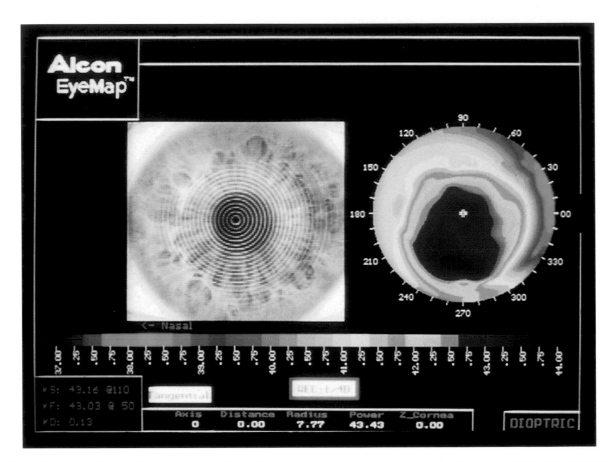

Figure 25–2. Corneal topography map of patient with keratoconus, demonstrating corneal photograph with overlying Plácido ring projections *(left)* and digitized, color-coded topography map *(right)*.

architecture, coupled with stromal corneal edema along the radial incisions.[3–5] Edema develops overnight while the eyelids are closed and results in increased corneal flattening. During the day, as the cornea deturgesces, it tends to resteepen, regressing toward the final refractive outcome upon wound stabilization (4 to 8 weeks postop).[6] The amplitude of the diurnal fluctua-

tion decreases daily as the wounds mature and stabilize.[7–12] During this phase of wound healing, among patients who are adequately corrected, the older population with presbyopia may be aware of hyperopia in the early morning hours with an emmetropic shift by the afternoon. Younger patients will have good vision throughout the course of the day.

Patients with significant residual refractive error appear most bothered by symptoms of visual fluctuation. In patients who are undercorrected, the vision will appear clear in the morning with some gradual increase in myopia by the evening hours. In patients who are overcorrected, the elderly experience hyperopia and presbyopia in the morning with improved hyperopic symptoms in the evening. Overcorrected younger patients (prepresbyopes) may perceive some blurring of vision in the morning and have good acuity in the evening.[11]

It is important to discourage eye rubbing following incisional keratotomy. Such activity may stretch and destabilize the wounds, leading to progressive hyperopia and chronic diurnal fluctuation. Chronic postop contact lens wear (rigid gas-permeable lenses) may also destabilize the wounds. A tincture of time will address most symptoms of diurnal fluctuation.

INTRAOPERATIVE COMPLICATIONS

A number of potential complications may develop intraoperatively as a result of deviations from prescribed surgical protocol or faulty surgical technique. Such potential complications are generally avoided by diligent training, literature review, detailed preparation, and adherence to proper surgical protocols. In the unusual event that a complication does occur, sound judgment can generally remedy the problem.

Topical Medication–Associated Corneal Toxicity

The combination of topical antibiotics, miotics or mydriatics, anesthetics, steroids, and nonsteroidal anti-inflammatory eyedrops may exert significant cumulative toxicity in a subset of patients. The clinical sequelae of such toxic effects include periop exacerbation of dry eye symptoms, or localized intraop or periop sloughing of the corneal epithelium. Residual disinfectant on the tonometer tip may additionally contribute to focal toxicity. Cidex is a particularly corrosive disinfectant and should not be used in a refractive practice. Toxic sequelea may be minimized by instilling eyedrops into the conjunctival fornix (avoiding direct instillation onto the corneal surface) and providing preop punctal occlusion for dry-eyed patients.

Complications Related to Corneal Marking

Inaccurate marking of the visual axis (Fig 25–3) can result in incisions invading the optical zone, leading to a decentered zone of flattening that causes increased

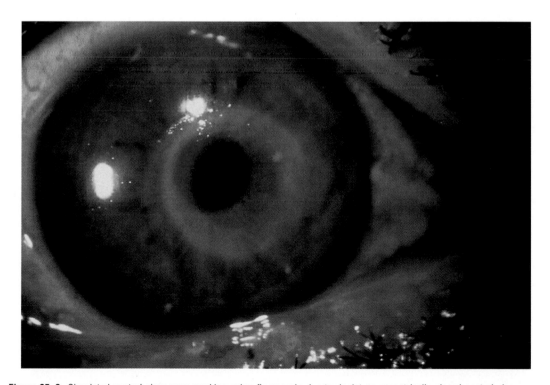

Figure 25–3. Simulated central clear zone marking using fluorescein dye to depict an eccentrically placed central clear zone.

glare and significant irregular astigmatism with monocular diplopia.[13,14] The most common causes of incision decentration are improper estimation of the intraoperative visual axis, arising from inadequate globe centration (inducing errors of parallax) within the operative field and misalignment of the optical zone marker cross-hairs when the epithelial visual axis is marked. Because of the noncoaxial orientation of the microscope light source,[2,6,12,15] the PERK Study Group recommendation for marking the visual axis provides the best approximation.

Coaxial light sources have been designed to reduce the inaccuracies of visual axis determination[16] and to enable the patient to maintain proper fixation during the procedure. When preparing to mark the visual axis, first view the globe under relatively high magnification in order to ensure its proper centration within the operative field, thereby eliminating additional errors of parallax.

Complications Related to Corneal Incising

Incising Beyond Clear Cornea

The extension beyond the clear cornea onto the corneoscleral limbus (Fig 25–4) or the limbal vascular arcades should be avoided in order to prevent subsequent vascular ingrowth.[14,17] Incisions that invade the limbus may eventually render the patient contact lens intolerant owing to associated incision-groove vascularization. Fibrovascular ingrowth may result in corneal destabilization over time, leading to large diurnal fluctuation and progression of refractive effect.

Central Clear Zone Invasion

Central clear zone invasion (Fig 25–5) caused by spontaneous patient eye movement or lack of surgical control represents one of the more worrisome potential complications of centripetal incisions.[18,19] Patient education or globe fixation may reduce, but will not entirely eliminate, the potential for optical zone invasion.[9,14,17]

The combined (Genesis) incision technique was designed in order to address these and other potential complications.[20] The downhill incision provides a relatively shallow linear safety groove; reversing the incision centripetally in the uphill direction adds uniform and reliable depth to the same incision groove up to the optical zone. Because the uphill margin of the blade cuts only along its distal portion, the diamond is incapable of producing deep incisions outside of a previously incised groove, so that it is difficult to incise the visual axis inadvertently when properly employing this technique. Once the central

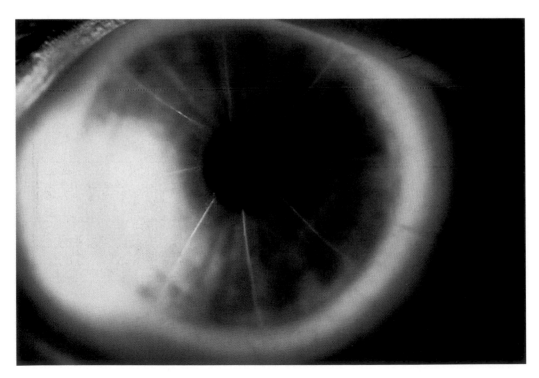

Figure 25–4. RK incisions extending beyond clear cornea onto the corneoscleral limbus.

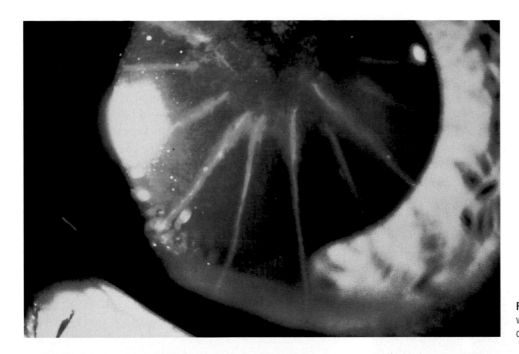

Figure 25–5. RK incisions performed with a metal blade and invading the central clear zone.

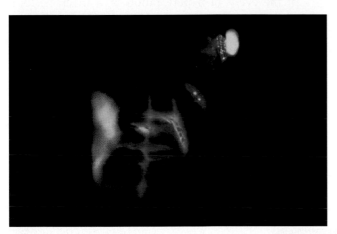

Figure 25–6. Intersecting keratotomy wounds in a patient with keratoconjunctivitis sicca associated with secondary wound melt.

zone has been reached and intentionally slightly undermined, continued pressure should not be applied against the optical zone as the diamond is lifted from the incision groove.

Intersecting Incisions

Intersecting fresh incisions may lead to wound gape and poor healing (Fig 25–6). In the event of such a complication, the surgeon should use interrupted 10-0 or 11-0 nylon sutures to reapproximate the gaped wound margins, burying the knots and leaving the sutures in place for 10 to 12 weeks, or until they loosen. When radial and transverse incisions cross, it is generally best to place a radial suture across the transverse incision margins adjacent to the radial incision.

Unsutured intersecting incisions will often be filled with epithelial plugs. These epithelial plugs develop because severe wound gape does not allow proper wound margin approximation.[21] Epithelial plugs may also become spontaneously extruded, causing transient pain and photophobia and progressive stromal melting.

The first step in treating patients with complications resulting from previously unsutured crossed incisions is to scrape the epithelium from within the wound, using a fine spatula. Next, reapproximate the wound margins with 10-0 nylon. The knots are subsequently buried and the sutures left in place for 4 to 6 months, or until they spontaneously loosen.

Complications Related to Corneal Perforations

The risk of corneal perforation has been reduced with the advent of screening and real-time pachymetry, the availability of microscopes for precise diamond-knife calibration, and the practices of incising the thinnest corneal zones first and of not setting diamonds at substantially greater than 100% of paracentral pachymetry.

A microperforation is one that self-seals and does not continue to leak, even when tested using a Weck cell. Microperforations[22–24] spontaneously seal as the adjacent corneal stroma becomes edematous and tampanades the leak. A perforation will leak upon gentle compression with a Weck cell sponge and, as such, is no longer considered to be a simple microperforation. A macroperforation is one that leaks spontaneously (Fig 25–7).[24,25]

Early recognition of a microperforation, by operating on a relatively dry field (no tear pooling within the cul-de-sac), will prevent its extension into a perforation. Patients with microperforations should be managed with cycloplegia, topical aqueous suppressants such as beta-blockers, a loading dose of broad-spectrum topical antibiotics, and an ocular shield placed over the eye. The eye should not be patched, as this will compress the corneal apex, bow open the incisions, and retard healing. Similarly, collagen shields are not recommended in such cases.

Incising the thinnest quadrant first greatly reduces the risk of a microperforation, as the cornea continues to thin out throughout the procedure.[16,17,26] If a penetration of the diamond into the globe occurs on the very first incision, or on the centrifugally directed component of any incision, the case should be terminated and completed at a later time with repeated pachymetry and diamond calibration because the surgeon cannot determine either the degree to which the diamond has been overextended or the existence of pathologic corneal thinning.

If a microperforation occurs on the second pass of subsequent incisions (directed centripetally), the degree to which the diamond is overextended is probably minimal. In such an event, the surgeon may retract the diamond blade before proceeding.[16] The micrometer on the diamond knife handle should be used to retract the blade 20 μm. Remember, however, that this is an elective procedure, which may be terminated at any time.

In the event of a perforation or a macroperforation, it is prudent to place a single (or multiple) interrupted 10-0 or 11-0 nylon suture to seal the wound and prevent the sequelae of hypotony or of an open wound (Fig 25–8).[27]

The evolution of combined-technique procedures, phasing out centrifugal-style incisions (which set diamonds at up to 120% of the paracentral corneal thickness), and the ability to calibrate diamond knife blades precisely with safety-designed footplates have made macroperforations an uncommon occurrence.

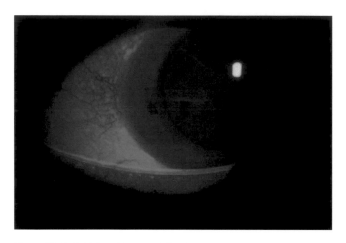

Figure 25–7. Seidel positive test following corneal perforation during RK.

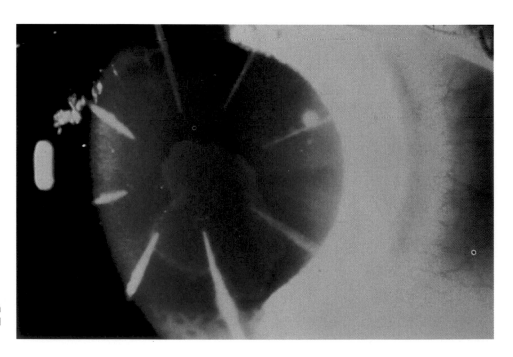

Figure 25–8. Epithelial downgrowth associated with unsutured, perforated keratotomy incision.

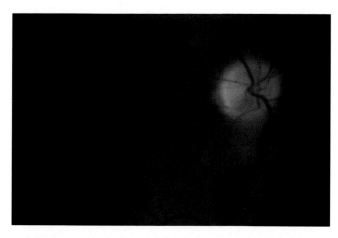

Figure 25-9. Optic nerve atrophy associated with retrobulbar injection.

Miscellaneous Intraoperative Complications

Diamond-Blade Chipping

A diamond fragment serving as an intracorneal foreign body is rare, but possible. The most common cause of a chipped diamond is inadvertent contact against metal instruments, which is easily avoided. Ultrathin diamonds (<80 μm) may also be predisposed to early damage.

Optic Nerve Damage

Optic nerve damage (Fig 25-9)[28] has been reported in association with retrobulbar anesthesia,[29] as has globe penetration[30] with subsequent retinal detachment. Clearly, in highly myopic eyes, the risks of retrobulbar anesthesia outweigh those of the incisional keratotomy procedure itself. Because topical anesthesia is sufficient for performing incisional keratotomy, retrobulbar anesthesia is rarely, if ever indicated.

NON–SIGHT-THREATENING POSTOP COMPLICATIONS

The non–sight-threatening complications related to refractive changes include undercorrection, overcorrection, regression of effect, progression of effect, and induced astigmatism. All of these potential complications are discussed in the PERK 5-year review[12] and in other clinical studies.[9,10,17,25,31,32]

Undercorrection

Undercorrections are not always undesirable and may often be the primary goal of the surgical procedure. Furthermore, in the majority of cases, undercor-

rections can be readily enhanced in secondary procedures.

Overcorrection

Overcorrections,[9,15,25,32] however, may be more difficult to treat and are the basis for a conservative approach to the initial procedure. If moderate overcorrection (+1.50 to +2.50 D) is confirmed early on by cycloplegic refraction, we often treat by using pilocarpine (0.5% to 1.0%) drops QID, for 6 weeks, adding epinephrine or propine drops beginning 2 weeks after the procedure. By stimulating myofibroblast contraction with epinephrine agonists and stimulating wound healing and lowering intraocular pressure with pilocarpine,[4,13] regression of effect may be accelerated and augmented.

The participating surgeons in the PERK Study Group were not aware that age is a variable; consequently, a considerable percentage of older subjects in the PERK study were overcorrected.[15] In the event of mild degrees of long-standing symptomatic overcorrection 4% pilocarpine gel administered each morning is generally sufficient.

The preferred treatment of significant overcorrection is surgical. Four to eight of the incisions should be reopened and any epithelial inclusions or fibrovascular tracks scraped out. The wound margins should be reapproximated with transverse, interrupted 10-0 nylon sutures at 5- and 7-mm optical zones of each incision. The sutures should be relatively long and tight. These sutures may be left in place indefinitely and removed only if needed.

Regression of Effect

Regression of effect is a consequence of the early wound-healing phase and will vary slightly in each patient. Experience with the first eye will generally guide the surgeon in staging the procedure for the second eye. This is one reason why it is recommended to perform the surgical procedure on the nondominant eye first, waiting days, or even weeks, before operating on the other eye. In the great majority of cases, an enhancement procedure can be performed to achieve the desired result.

Progression of Effect

Progression of effect over time appears to have become less common with the use of RK techniques that do not extend incisions out to the limbus. In prior years, many patients who had experienced subsequent significant progression of effect underwent the peripheral redeepening procedures in which incisions radiating from the midperiphery toward the limbus were repeated and the blades were set at the deeper midperipheral measurement.

These redeepened and extended incisions were subsequently prone to ingrowth as fibrovascular tissue advanced centripetally within the groove, providing an increased mass effect with progressive corneal flattening. Because there is no cross-linked stromal collagen within this invading fibrovascular tissue, it renders the wound unstable and creates significant diurnal refractive fluctuation. Such patients are best treated by having the incisions opened, the fibrovascular tissue stripped, and the incisions resutured. The risks of consecutive hyperopia can be minimized by adhering to several guidelines:

1. Performing preop cycloplegic refraction
2. Discontinuing contact lens wear before to surgery (at least 3 days for soft lenses and at least 3 weeks for hard lenses)
3. Stopping incisions approximately 1 mm short of the limbus
4. Recognizing and suturing perforation sites
5. Avoiding peripheral redeepening
6. Discontinuing the use of contact lenses following RK
7. Discouraging eye rubbing

Induced Astigmatism

Another potential complication associated with any keratorefractive procedure is that of induced regular or irregular astigmatism.[12,15] This may occur if fewer incisions are placed, if the incisions are placed asymmetrically about the visual axis, if the incisions are of variable depth, or if the central clear zone is decentered with respect to the visual axis.[5,33,34] The great majority of these refractive aberrations are self-limited and will spontaneously improve within the first 6 postop weeks. Thus, placing additional incisions in the setting of irregular astigmatism is not recommended until the refraction and surface topography have stabilized.

Decreasing best corrected visual acuity (BCVA) is most commonly associated with irregular astigmatism. Corneal topographic analysis is most helpful in determining the extent of persistent irregular astigmatism and tracking its change over time. Furthermore, in the event that subsequent incisions become necessary, topography is useful in determining the optimal location for placing incisions.

Contact Lens Intolerance

Contact lens intolerance is now less common following RK. Newly designed rigid gas-permeable (RGP) lenses with peripheral curves that match the patient's preop parameters are recommended to overcome postop lens fit intolerance (Fig 25–10).[35]

Fibrovascular ingrowth tracks may develop within the incision sites and are most often associated with chronic irritation and hypoxia from subsequent soft contact lens wear.[1,15–17,26] These fibrovascular tracks produce a mass effect that results in corneal flattening. The risk of lens-associated corneal vascularization is greatly reduced by terminating the incision 1 mm shy of the limbus.

Chronic contact lens wear may also provide a direct compressive effect with associated wound stretching and progressive hyperopia. This mechanical effect may be more prominent with rigid lenses.

Epithelial Basement Membrane Disorder

One of the nine clinical research centers participating in the PERK study reported cases of postop recurrent erosion.[12,36] Nonetheless, the ever-present possibility of transient disturbance of the epithelial basement membrane is not surprising because the new epithelial basement membrane adhesion complexes may require 6 weeks, or longer, to mature.

Epithelial Inclusion Cysts

Epithelial inclusion cysts may also appear within the incision grooves and are generally expelled over time without recurrence.[37,38] In the case of crossed, or other-

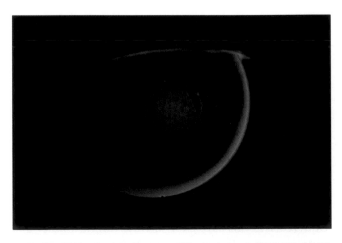

Figure 25–10. Contact lens fit on post-RK eye, demonstrating central pooling of fluorescein dye overlying flattened central zone.

wise gaped, incisions, however, these cysts may become large and problematic, resulting in recurrent erosions as the plug is periodically extruded without subsequent stromal healing. Wounds that have been subjected to multiple repeat incisions may also develop microcysts.

Foreign Particles Within Incision Grooves

Foreign material, including mascara or other cosmetics, powder from the surgical gloves, and even formed crystals from certain antibiotic eyedrops, may also become transiently trapped within the incision grooves. These are generally extruded over time without sequelae. However, it is safer to require patients to discontinue wearing cosmetics for 5 days before surgery. It is also recommended that surgical gloves be meticulously cleaned with moist, sterile gauze or that nonpowdered surgical gloves be worn.

Epithelial Iron Lines

The development of epithelial iron lines tracking parallel to RK incisions has been observed.[39–41] These iron lines do not present any functional consequences, but are most likely due to an alteration in the factors related to tear film distribution and dynamics.[42]

Diminished Corneal Strength

Clearly, in setting unsutured perforations, one would expect long-term compromise in corneal strength.[43–45] There has been much discussion as to whether uncomplicated RK incisions also significantly diminish corneal strength. The controversy centers around anecdotal case reports[45] as well as a number of published clinical animal studies.[46–50] One patient in the PERK study received blunt trauma to the eyes on two occasions and did not experience a ruptured globe in either instance.[2]

There have been reports of ruptured globes following severe blunt trauma in patients after RK that resulted in globe perforation at the radial incision sites.[51,52] There have also been reported cases of globe perforation at alternate sites when the incision sites remained intact following severe blunt trauma.[53–55]

Animal studies are difficult to interpret, as many animal models, unlike the adult human, do not have the elaborate Descemet's membrane that provides much of the tensile strength to the human cornea. Additionally, many of these animal studies do not account for changes in corneal strength following wound healing.

All in all, it is prudent to advise patients to wear appropriate safety eye wear when engaging in contact sports and to discourage prospective patients whose occupational hazards include high-contact settings.

Endothelial Cell Loss

The original Sato procedure, incising across the endothelium from within the anterior chamber, resulted in a high incidence of bullous keratopathy.[56] There have been several studies evaluating endothelial cell loss following RK. Most studies report, on average, a cell loss of approximately 5%, without progression over time.[10,26,57,58] This degree of reported loss is well within the detection error of specular microscopy instrumentation and is not of direct clinical concern. To date, there have been no well-controlled prospective studies demonstrating significant endothelial cell loss in association with RK.

SIGHT-THREATENING COMPLICATIONS

Two types of sight-threatening postop complications are corneal stromal melting and infectious keratitis.

Stromal Melting

Stromal melting often develops in patients with crossed incisions (Fig 25–6) and may thus be prevented by exercising caution during the surgical procedure.[21] Corneal stromal melt is also an associated complication in patients with rheumatoid arthritis or other collagen vascular diseases that have concomitant severe keratoconjunctivitis sicca with diffuse punctate epitheliopathy. Patients with such advanced disorders are not viable candidates for incisional keratotomy. In patients with significantly diminished tear production, it may be necessary to perform punctal occlusion before considering incisional keratotomy.[32]

Keratitis

Although it is lower than the observed incidence in contact lens wearers, the most common sight-threatening complication associated with RK is infectious keratitis. (Fig 25–11) This generally occurs in the perioperative period,[59,60] although delayed cases,[61,62] several in association with contact lens wear,[63] have also been reported. Indeed, the only two cases of keratitis reported within the PERK study occurred in association with postop contact lens wear.[15]

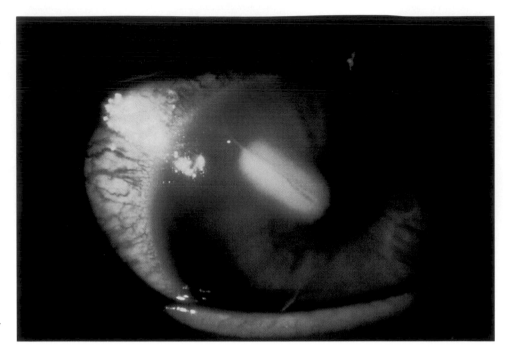

Figure 25–11. Acute infectious keratitis following RK.

It is possible to reduce the risk of infection by administering periop broad-spectrum prophylactic antibiotic drops. Prophylactic use of preop antibiotic drops beginning before the day of surgery may simply select for resistant organisms. Preexisting blepharitis should also be ruled out at the time of the preop ocular examination and, if present, treated preoperatively as needed.

Sterile technique should be observed during RK: the surgical field should be prepped with betadine and ophthalmic personnel within the operating room should wear sterile gloves and masks. Furthermore, patients must be instructed to avoid wearing eye makeup or exposing themselves to contaminated water, including swimming pools or hot tubs, for 1 week following the surgical procedure.

Patients should have a follow-up examination by the second or third postop day to rule out early keratitis. When infiltrates appear, they may be within the

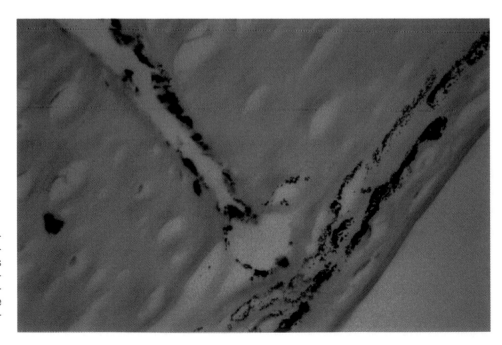

Figure 25–12. Light micrograph depicting infectious crystalline keratopathy with presence of numerous gram-positive cocci and absence of inflammatory cells. Patient had undergone corneal relaxing incisions while on chronic topical steroid therapy following penetrating keratoplasty.

deep stroma beneath intact overlying epithelium. Acute infiltrates are probably of bacterial origin. In such patients, the epithelium over the incision site should be opened and samples for culture and staining obtained from the side walls of the groove. Inoculate samples onto culture media of blood and chocolate agar for aerobic organisms, thioglycolate broth for anaerobic organisms, and Sabouraud's dextrose agar for fungi. Smears should include both a Gram and Giemsa stain.

Next, intensive broad-spectrum antibiotic therapy may include fortified ancef (50 mg/ml), fortified tobramycin (14 ng/ml), and ciprofloxacin or norfloxacin on an hourly basis, rotating every 20 minutes, while awaiting culture results. Administer a combination of 0.4 cc ancef (250 mg/ml) and 0.4 cc tobramycin (40 mg/ml) mixed with 0.1 cc of 2% lidocaine as a subconjunctival injection to the affected quadrant on a daily basis, until culture results are available. If the overlying epithelium covers the incisional groove, it is gently debrided for the first several days to enable high concentrations of antibiotic penetration into the deep stroma. In cases not responsive to antibacterial therapy, the presence of a fungal or other atypical microorganism should be considered. Steroids should not be used in the treatment of deep stromal keratitis (Fig 25–12)! The scar will eventually fade in most cases.

COMPLICATIONS ASSOCIATED WITH ADJUNCTIVE THERAPY

RK complications associated with adjunctive therapy include associated drug toxicity (Fig 25–13). Infectious keratitis may develop with subsequent contact lens wear or chronic steroid therapy. Steroids may also be associated with cataracts, elevated intraocular pressure, or even infectious crystalline keratopathy. RK management does not require prolonged topical steroid therapy.

A certain number of patients who undergo RK will subsequently develop cataracts. The standard SRK formulas coupled with keratometric corneal curvature analysis do not seem to provide predictable intraocular lens calculations for these patients. The change in refraction subtracted from the preradial keratotomy average K value may prove a more reliable estimated keratometry value for insertion into the SRK lens calculation.[64] It may, alternatively, be helpful to insert the computerized videokeratography value for the average 3-mm central corneal curvature.

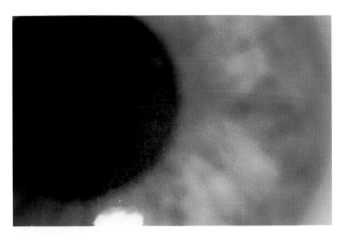

Figure 25–13. Diffuse epithelial toxicity associated with topical medical therapy following incisional keratotomy.

Adhering to Surgical Protocol Will Prevent Most Complications

In summary, one should remember not to ignore potential surgical pitfalls. These include crossing of incisions, incising to the limbus, redeepening the periphery of prior incisions (setting blades at the peripheral corneal thickness), and operating on a wet field.

REFERENCES

1. Salz JJ. How safe is radial keratotomy? *J Refract Surg.* 1987; 3:188–189.
2. Waring GO, Lynn MJ, Gelender H, et al: Results of the Prospective Evaluation of Radial Keratotomy (PERK) study five years after surgery. *Ophthalmology.* 1991;98:1164–1176.
3. Bourque LB, Cosand BB, Drews C, et al. Reported satisfaction, fluctuation of vision and glare among patients one year after surgery in the Prospective Evaluation of Radial Keratotomy (PERK) study. *Arch Ophthalmol.* 1986;104: 356–363.
4. Cross WD, Head WJ. Complications of radial keratotomy: an overview. In: Sanders D, Hofmann RF, Salz J, eds. *Refractive Corneal Surgery.* Thorofare, NJ: Slack, Inc; 1986: 347–399.
5. Waring GO. The changing status of radial keratotomy for myopia. Part II. *J Refract Surg.* 1985;1:119–137.
6. Waring GO, Lynn MJ, Gelender H, et al. Results of the Prospective Evaluation of Radial Keratotomy (PERK) study 4 years after surgery for myopia. *JAMA.* 1990;263:1083–1091.
7. Arrowsmith PN, Marks RG. Visual, refractive, and keratometric results of radial keratotomy: 1-year follow-up. *Arch Ophthalmol.* 1984;102:1612–1617.

8. Arrowsmith PN, Marks RG. Visual, refractive and keratometric results of radial keratotomy: five year follow up. *Arch Ophthalmol.* 1989;107:506–511.

9. Arrowsmith PN, Deitz MR, Marks RG, et al. *Radial Keratotomy: ARK Study Group.* Thorofare, NJ: Slack, Inc; 1984.

10. Deitz MR, Sanders DR, Marks RG. Radial keratotomy: an overview of the Kansas City study. *Ophthalmology.* 1984; 91:467–478.

11. Schanzlin DJ, Santos VR, Waring GO, et al. Diurnal change in refraction, corneal curvature, visual acuity and intraocular pressure after radial keratotomy in the PERK study. *Ophthalmology.* 1986;93:167–175.

12. Waring GO, Lynn MJ, Gelender H, et al. Results of the Prospective Evaluation of Radial Keratotomy (PERK) study one year after surgery. *Ophthalmology.* 1985;92:177–198.

13. Busin M, Yau CW, Avinil R., et al. The effect of changes in intraocular pressure on corneal curvature after radial keratotomy in the rabbit eye. *Ophthalmology.* 1986;93:331–334.

14. Ellis W. *Radial Keratotomy and Astigmatism Surgery.* Irvine, CA: Keith C. Terry and Associates; 1986:117–130.

15. Waring GO, Lynn MJ, Culbertson W, et al. Three-year results of the Prospective Evaluation of Radial Keratotomy (PERK) study. *Ophthalmology.* 1987;94:1339–1354.

16. Rowsey JJ, Bayeat HD. Radial keratotomy: preliminary report of complications. *Ophthalmic Surg.* 1982;13:27–35.

17. Sanders DR, Hofmann RF, Salz JJ, eds. *Refractive Corneal Surgery.* Thorofare, NJ: Slack, Inc; 1986.

18. Barker B, Swinger C. Complications of corneal refractive surgery. In: Schwab IR, ed. *Refractive Keratoplasty.* New York: Churchill-Livngstone; 1987:227–272.

19. Lewicky A, Salz J. Special report: radial keratotomy survey. *J Refract Surg.* 1986;2:32–33.

20. Assil, KK, Kassoff J, Schanzlin DJ, Quantock AJ. A novel combined incision technique of radial keratotomy: a comparison to centripetal and centrifugal incision techniques in human donor eyes. *Ophthalmology.* 1994.

21. Karr DJ, Grutzmacher RD, Reeh MJ. Radial keratotomy complicated by sterile keratitis and corneal perforation. *Ophthalmology.* 1985;92:1244–1248.

22. Schachar RA. Understanding radial keratotomy. *Ophthalmic Forum.* 1982;1:22–23.

23. Schachar RA. Indications, techniques and complications of radial keratotomy. *Int Ophthalmol Clin.* 1983;23:119–128.

24. Schachar RA, Levy NS, Schachar L. *Refractive Keratoplasty.* Denison, TX: LAL Publishing. 1983;328–396.

25. Sawelson H, Marks RG. Two-year results of radial keratotomy. *Arch Ophthalmol.* 1985;103:505–510.

26. Rowsey JJ, Balyeat HD. Preliminary results and complications of radial keratotomy. *Am J Ophthalmol.* 1982;93: 437–455.

27. Binder PS. Presumed epithelial ingrowth following radial keratotomy. *CLAO J.* 1986;12:247–250.

28. O'Day DM, Feman SS, Elliott JH. Visual impairment following radial keratotomy: a cluster of cases. *Ophthalmology.* 1986;93:319–326.

29. Ramsay RC, Knobloch WH. Ocular perforation following retrobulbar anesthesia for retinal detachment surgery. *Am J Ophthalmol.* 1978;86:61–64.

30. Davis DB. Retrobulbar and facial nerve block? No; peribulbar? Yes? *Ophthalmic Surg.* 1985;16:604.

31. Deitz MR, Sanders DR, Raanan MG. A consecutive series (1982–1985) of radial keratotomies performed with the diamond blade. II. *Am J Ophthalmol.* 1987;103:417–422.

32. Sawelson H, Marks RG. Three-year results of radial keratotomy. *Arch Ophthalmol.* 1987;105:81–85.

33. Arciniegas A, Amaya L, Velasquez G, et al. Corneal astigmatism induced by the combination of arc and radial keratotomies: experimental research in rabbits. *J Refract Corn Surg.* 1986;2:67–77.

34. Girard LJ, Wesson ME, Vesequlinovic A, Maghraby A. Case report: overcorrection of radial and arc keratotomies—two years postoperatively. *J Refract Surg.* 1985; 2:232.

35. Schivitz IA, Russell BM, Arrowsmith PH, Marks RG. Optical correction of postoperative radial keratotomy patients with contact lenses. *CLAO J.* 1986;12:59–62.

36. Nelson JD, Williams P, Lindstrom RL, Doughman DJ. Map–fingerprint–dot changes in the corneal epithelial basement membrane following radial keratotomy. *Ophthalmology.* 1985;92:199–205.

37. Binder PS, Nayak SK, Deg JK, et al. An ultrastructural and histochemical study of long-term wound healing after radial keratotomy. *Am J Ophthalmol.* 1987;103:432–440.

38. Jester JV, Villasenor RA, Miyashir J. Epithelial inclusion cysts following radial keratotomy. *Arch Ophthalmol.* 1983; 101:611–615.

39. Davis RM, Miller RA, Lindstrom RL, et al. Corneal iron lines after radial keratotomy. *J Refract Surg.* 1988;2: 174–178.

40. Steinert EB, Wilson LA, Waring GO, et al. Stellate iron lines in the corneal epithelium after radial keratotomy. *Am J Ophthalmol.* 1984;98:416–421.

41. Waring GO. Short-term results of the Prospective Evaluation of Radial Keratotomy (PERK) study. In: Sanders D, Hofmann RF, Salz J, eds. *Refractive Corneal Surgery.* Thorofare, NJ: Slack, Inc; 1986:313–346.

42. Assil KK, Quantock AJ, Schanzlin DJ. Corneal iron line associated with the intrastromal corneal ring. *Am J Ophthalmol.* 1993;116:350–356.

43. Condon PI, Hill DW. The testing of experimental corneal wounds stitched with modern corneal scleral sutures: experimental corneal wound healing. *Ophthalmol Res.* 1973; 5:137–150.

44. Gasset AR, Dohlman CH. The tensile strength of corneal wounds. *Arch Ophthalmol.* 1968;79:595–602.

45. Maurice DM. The biology of wound healing in the corneal stroma: Castroviejo lecture. *Cornea.* 1987;6:162–168.

46. Darakjian NE, Marchese A. Assessment of corneal strength post radial keratotomy in rabbit eyes. *Invest Ophthalmol Vis Sci.* 1982;22(suppl):26.

47. Larson BC, Kremer FB, Eller AW, Bernardino VB. Quantitated trauma following radial keratotomy in rabbits. *Ophthalmology.* 1983;90:660–667.

48. Luttrull JK, Jester JV, Smith RE. The effect of radial keratotomy on ocular integrity in an animal model. *Arch Ophthalmol.* 1982;100:319–320.

49. McKnight SJ, Fitz J, Giangiacoma J. Corneal rupture following radial keratotomy in cats subjected to BB gun injury. *Ophthalmic Surg.* 1988;19:165–167.

50. Rylander HG, Welch AJ, Fleming B. The effect of radial keratotomy in rupture strength of pig eyes. *Ophthalmic Surg.* 1983;14:744–749.

51. Binder PS, Waring GO, Arrowsmith PN, Wang CL. Traumatic rupture of the cornea after radial keratotomy. *Arch Ophthalmol.* 1988;106:1584–1590.

52. Simmons KB, Linsalata RP. Ruptured globe following blunt trauma after radial keratotomy. *Ophthalmology.* 1987; 94:148.

53. Forstot SL, Damiano RE. Trauma after radial keratotomy. *Ophthalmology.* 1988;95:833–835.

54. John ME, Schmitt TE. Traumatic hyphema after radial keratotomy. *Ann Ophthalmol.* 1983;15:930–932.

55. Spivak L. Case report: radial keratotomy incisions remain intact despite facial trauma from plane crash. *J Refract Surg.* 1987;3:59–60.

56. Waring GO. *Refractive Keratotomy for Myopia and Astigmatism.* St. Louis, MO: Mosby-Year Book; 1991.

57. Hoffer KJ, Darin JJ, Pettit TH, et al. Three years experience with radial keratotomy: the UCLA study. *Ophthalmology.* 1983;90:627–636.

58. Jester JV, Miyashiro JE, Fife L, Smith RE. Radial keratotomy in primate eyes: pathologic studies. *Invest Ophthalmol Vis Sci.* 1982;29(suppl):69.

59. Marmer RH. Radial keratotomy complications. *Ann Ophthalmol.* 1987;19:409–411.

60. Wilhelmus KR, Hamburg S. Bacterial keratitis following radial keratotomy. *Cornea.* 1983;2:143–146.

61. Cottingham AJ, Berkeley RG, Nordan LT, et al. Bacterial corneal ulcers following keratorefractive surgery: a retrospective study of 14,163 procedures, read before the Ocular Microbiology and Immunology Group Meeting; September 28, 1986; San Francisco.

62. Shivitz IA, Arrowsmith PN. Delayed keratitis after radial keratotomy. *Arch Ophthalmol.* 1986;104:1153–1155.

63. Mandelbaum S, Waring GO, Forster RK, et al. Late development of ulcerative keratitis in radial keratotomy scars. *Arch Ophthalmol.* 1986;104:1156–1160.

64. Consultations in Refractive Surgery. *Refract Corn Surg.* 1989;5:202–203.

SECTION V

Lamellar Refractive Surgery

CHAPTER 26

Lamellar Refractive Surgery

Stephen G. Slade ▪ Stephen A. Updegraff

HISTORY

In this chapter we review the history of lamellar corneal procedures for the correction of high myopia and hyperopia. We discuss patient selection, surgical techniques, and postoperative management of automated lamellar keratoplasty (ALK) and excimer laser in situ keratomileusis (LASIK).

The concept of altering the anterior corneal curvature by removing stromal tissue was originated and developed by José Ignacio Barraquer, MD, at his clinic in Bogotá, Colombia.[1] Although the concept of a stromectomy was first published in 1963,[2] no one pursued and perfected the technique as thoroughly as Barraquer. His work began in 1949 when he recognized the power of surgically manipulating the contour of the tear air interface (where two thirds of the dioptric power of the eye is located) and the importance of preserving each layer of the cornea by incorporating lamellar techniques.[3] The history of the evolution of design and technique leading to the present-day lamellar procedures is valuable, not only for our understanding of corneal wound healing,[4] but also for continued research and improvement in this expanding field of refractive surgery.

The term *keratomileusis* is derived from Greek roots meaning "cornea" and "carving." Barraquer initially performed the lamellar dissection freehand with a Paufique knife, creating a lamellar disc approximately 300 μm in depth. He attempted the refractive cut by removing stroma from both the lamellar bed and the disc. However, because of the imprecision of removing stroma from the bed (manually or with a keratome), he abandoned the "in situ" approach and focused his attention on refining the lamellar dissection and perfecting a more precise carving of the corneal lamellar disc.[5]

Barraquer discovered that by increasing intraocular pressure (IOP) with a pneumatic fixation ring, an oscillating razor blade mounted like a carpenter's plane could shave a round, parallel-faced corneal disc from the anterior corneal stroma (Fig 26–1). In order to achieve a true lamellar dissection, the IOP had to be greater than 65 mm Hg. He also recognized an important relation between IOP and resection diameter that directly affected the compression of the cornea by the microkeratome. The greater the IOP and/or the greater the diameter of the resected disc, the more the cornea is compressed beneath the plane of the microkeratome, resulting in a deeper resection. This relation determined his surgical approach. By using intraoperative applanation lenses, different-diameter suction rings, and various heights on the microkeratome track (which was part of the pneumatic ring), he could achieve a predetermined thickness and diameter of the lamellar disc.[5]

Even with these adjustments, he discovered that the speed with which the surgeon manually passed the

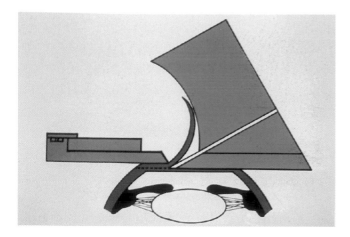

Figure 26–1. The keratome works on the principle of a carpenter's plane. An oscillating blade splits the cornea following a plane that applanates or flattens the cornea.

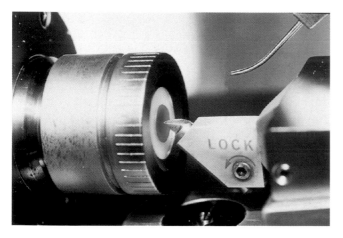

Figure 26–2. In keratomileusis the dyed corneal disc is placed on a lathe and frozen by liquid nitrogen in preparation for being cut by a cold tool.

microkeratome could dramatically affect the depth, quality, and shape of the lamellar disc. The greater the speed of the pass, the thinner the lamellar disc becomes. He stressed the importance of keeping constant contact between the microkeratome and the suction ring during a slow, uniform pass of the initial lamellar keratectomy. Any deviation greater than one hundredth of a millimeter could result in a nonparallel lamellar dissection. This could lead to interface scarring, an irregularly thin disc, and, ultimately, irregular astigmatism.[6] This critical step was overlooked by many surgeons learning the technique, primarily because of the somewhat overwhelming task of learning how to process the disc on the cryolathe. Overcoming this variable in the future was to permit the evolution to the present-day in situ techniques.

Barraquer refined the shaping of the resected corneal disc by incorporating freezing of the corneal lamellar disc and carving of the stromal side with a modified contact-lens lathe (Fig 26–2). He is a pioneer of cryosurgery, as this was the first time techniques originally designed for the frozen-section microtome were applied to performance of a surgical maneuver in humans. It was also the first time that part of a human organ was removed from the body to alter its function and then returned.

Without the advance of modern corneal pachymetry, Barraquer cleverly utilized an American Optical radiuscope to measure the central thickness of the lamellar disc with an error of $\pm$ 10 μm.[5] If there was significant error and the disc was thinner than measured, it could be perforated during lathing. If the disc was thicker than measured, a gross undercorrection could result.

After measuring thickness, the corneal disc tissue was placed in preservation media containing Kiton green 0.5%, which improved visualization during lathing.[5] The required corneal curvature to correct the ametropia was determined by the Littman formula:[7]

$$RF = \frac{1}{\dfrac{1}{RI} + \dfrac{DC}{332}} + (0.004095 \times DC)$$

where RF = the radius of curvature desired to correct the ametropia; RI = the original radius of curvature; and DC = the diopters of spectacle correction.

The lathe lap was then preground for the necessary radius of curvature the day before the surgery. The corneal lamellar disc was placed, epithelial side down, in the lathe lap, thus conforming to the contour (radius of curvature) of the lap by capillary attraction. Once mounted, the tissue and lap were frozen to $-30°$C. The stromal surface was then lathed from the periphery toward the center in the myopic cases so that more stroma was removed centrally (Fig 26–3). After thawing, the disc (no longer parallel) was placed on the host bed, and the anterior corneal curvature assumed a central flattening. Two interrupted sutures were placed to hold the disc to the bed, a conjunctival flap was placed over the disc, and a tarsorraphy was kept in place for 7 days.[5]

This would allow for a maximal myopic correction of 15 D at the spectacle plane if the preop radius of curvature was less than 7.5 mm. If it was 8 mm, the maximal correction would be only 12 D.[8] Barraquer identified the limit of the lenticle's deformity as a final radius of curvature of 10.6 mm (33 D). His in-

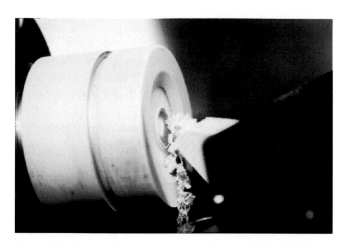

Figure 26–3. The lamellar corneal disc, with no power, is lathed with more tissue removed centrally than peripherally to produce a lens for correcting myopia.

strument had limits: it did not permit resection of corneas steeper than 7.3 mm or flatter than 8.5 mm. For hyperopic correction, he determined that the minimum radius of curvature to obtain good visual acuity was 5.82 mm. Hence, steeper radii of curvature distorted the image and also required a smaller optical zone.[9]

In 1961, Barraquer introduced his work to the ophthalmic community with a report of eight cases of keratophakia in human eyes.[10] The technique involved placing homoplastic stroma or alloplastic material on the stromal bed to ultimately steepen the central corneal curvature. This procedure would be the first of Barraquer's techniques to receive attention by surgeons in the United States, who took notice of his work only after the revolution of contact lenses and anterior chamber lenses made aphakia less acceptable.

By 1967, he published his technique for myopic keratomileusis in 100 patients with high myopia.[5] Although guidelines for reporting refractive surgery outcomes were not yet established in the literature,[11] his results indicated visual improvement in 80% of the patients.[5] There were reported problems of epithelium in the peripheral interface, foreign body debris of the interface, irregular astigmatism, and two infections.[5] However, the results were promising for patients with high myopia, and there was every indication that refinement of this procedure would proceed. He later demonstrated that the incidence of these complications was dramatically reduced in a group of 100 patients following his first 400 cases.[9] Admittedly, this was a telltale sign of extreme dependence on the individual surgeon's technique.

Over the next decade Barraquer extensively modified the contact lens lathe to include micrometer gauges and freezing circuits to shape the tissue more accurately. Improvements were also made in the microkeratome, most notably an increase of the blade oscillation to 10,000 excursions/min. He developed hyperopic and aphakic corrections of the lamellar corneal disc with the cryolathe.[9] By removing more stromal tissue from the periphery of the disc, he achieved a relative steepening of the central cornea. Thus, prior to its introduction to the United States, José I. Barraquer had designed and applied "classical" cryolathing for myopic keratomileusis (MKM), hyperopic keratomileusis (HKM), and keratophakia (KF).

In 1978, Troutman and Swinger brought these concepts to the United States and concentrated most of their early effort (1978–1980) on KF as a possible alternative to anterior chamber intraocular lens (IOL) implantation during intracapsular cataract extraction or to secondary IOL implantation.[12] Others also considered cryolathing to correct aphakia.[13–15]

With the groundswell of enthusiasm for Barraquer's novel technique, many ophthalmic surgeons ventured to Bogotá to learn the process.[16] Most were amazed by the complex nature of the procedure and the low margin for error, which were only overshadowed by stories of Barraquer having to transport the corneal disc to a facility for cryolathing. Once accomplished, the disc was brought back and placed on the lamellar stromal bed of the anxiously awaiting patient. The technical difficulty, steep learning curve, and expensive nature of the cryolathe discouraged many surgeons. This initially prevented the widespread use and acceptance of keratomileusis. There were even early reports of beginning surgeons making the mental error of leaving the plate (which determines the depth of the keratectomy) off the microkeratome, causing perforation into the anterior chamber and rupture of the lens. Because the keratectomies were done by hand, the success relied on a steady rate of passage, adequate suction, and good centration—all difficult for most surgeons new to the technique.

In 1979, Kaufman and Werblin, working together at the Louisiana State University Eye Center in New Orleans, developed the idea of using a corneal overlay made from human tissue, a "living contact lens."[17] This operation was called *epikeratophakia*, later renamed *epikeratoplasty*. In epikeratoplasty a disc of tissue was removed with a microkeratome from a donor eye, frozen, and lathed into a concave[18] or convex lens. This lens could then be lyophilized and stored for later use.[19]

Once the host cornea was de-epithelialized, a small peripheral keratotomy or keratectomy was made to fixate and suture the epikeratoplasty lenticle into place. With the lenticle held "tongue in groove" into the circumferential keratectomy, the host epithelium would gradually cover the surface and keratocytes would slowly repopulate the donor tissue.[20–26] Potential advantages of the surgery were minimal invasiveness and reversibility. In addition, surgeons would not have to deal with the microkeratome or cryolathe, as they only had to suture into place a lens that could be ordered from a facility that did the cryolathing and preparation.[27] The surgeon could specify the power to correct myopia, hyperopia, aphakia, and potentially even astigmatism.[28] Plano epikeratoplasty buttons were also employed to flatten the cornea in keratoconus to provide a more regular surface for contact lens wear.[29]

Meanwhile, with the acceptance of incisional keratotomy among corneal refractive surgeons to correct low to moderate myopia[30–32] and with the ensuing superiority of posterior chamber lens implantation during cataract surgery,[33] the focus of lamellar surgery shifted from correcting aphakia back to Barraquer's original work on high myopia. Several refractive surgery pioneers investigated the potential of lamellar techniques following Barraquer's guidelines. In 1984, Swinger and Barker conducted the first prospective evaluation of freeze MKM.[34] In 42 eyes, with an average follow-up of 10 months, no patient had an increase in astigmatism and no patient followed for more than 1 year had a decrease in best corrected visual acuity (BCVA). However, the majority of patients had some irregular astigmatism present immediately postop. Swinger and Barker reported the phenomenon of 63% of the patients having improved BCVA following surgery, averaging 1.5 Snellen lines more. This may be the result of increased asphericity of the paracentral cornea altering the light rays incident on the macula (exploiting the Stiles–Crawford effect in photopic conditions) or simply of a reduction of spectacle minification.[35]

In 1986, Lee Nordan initially operated on 74 consecutive nonamblyopic eyes; 80% of the cases had 20/40 or better uncorrected vision 6 weeks postop.[35] The operation did not greatly affect the amount of cylinder observed preoperatively, and for spherical corneas the procedure was fairly astigmatism neutral. However, he reported an irregular astigmatism rate of 9%, which was troublesome and constituted the primary cause for decreased BCVA. However, all of these patients achieved their preop BCVA once a hard contact lens over refraction was obtained. The irregularities induced by freeze MKM and suturing became more evident with the advent of corneal topography.[36] While irregular astigmatism was a problem, most of these patients improved if given sufficient time: between 1 and 2 years. This suggests a late remodeling and smoothing of the epithelial surface with freeze MKM. However, some patients did require either a homoplastic lenticle or a deep lamellar keratoplasty to solve the surface irregularity.[37] Similar results were achieved in one surgeon's series of his first 100 cases; however, the cornea of one patient was perforated owing to the lack of the plate in the microkeratome.[38]

Nordan also pointed out the usefulness of combining MKM with incisional keratotomy. Radial keratotomy (RK) flattens the central corneal curvature by a tectonic weakening without affecting thickness. He reported the first successful RK over an undercorrected MKM as well as the first homoplastic MKM over an undercorrected RK.[39] This is one of the earliest examples in the literature of using the different mechanical actions of refractive surgery techniques to complement each other to achieve the desired effect. For high myopes, it is not uncommon to plan for a slight undercorrection with lamellar refractive surgery. Six months later the eye can be titrated to the desired correction with incisional keratotomy.

Although the early MKM results were encouraging, only a handful of the hundreds of surgeons trained in freeze MKM were performing the procedure on a regular basis. In the mid 1980s there was a concomitant surge in the field of epikeratoplasty. Epikeratoplasty was much easier technically than MKM. Further, the surgeon did not have to own, operate, and maintain the microkeratome and the cryolathe.[19] Although many patients did very well, the accuracy varied, and some patients lost best corrected vision. In the Nationwide Study of Epikeratophakia for Aphakia, 48% of eyes lost at least one line of BCVA.[40] The Nationwide Study for Myopia revealed 28% of eyes losing at least one line of BCVA and a disturbing increase in astigmatism, from 1.4 ± 0.8 to 2.6 ± 2.1 D.[41] Even with the application of corneal topography[42] to aid in suture adjustment, irregular astigmatism was difficult to prevent—especially in the centrally thin myopic lenticules.[43] Significant regression was also reported between 6 and 12 months postop, although this tended to stabilize after 1 year.[44] While the epikeratoplasty buttons could be removed, on occasion there were changes in the patient's original refractive error so that complete reversibility was not obtained.[45,46]

Several modifications were explored in an attempt to improve epikeratoplasty. Lee Nordan developed a nonkeratectomy version of the procedure in

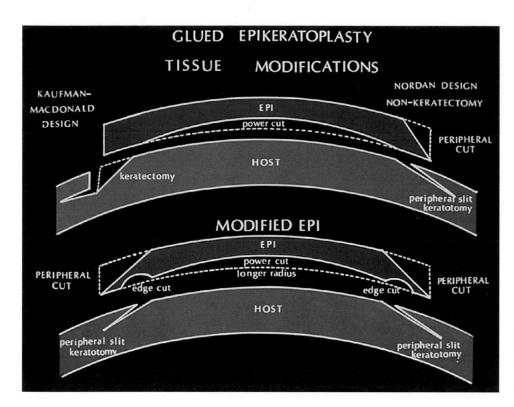

Figure 26–4. The design of the epikeratoplasty lens was modified extensively away from a keratectomy to allow a tapered edge to be inserted into a keratotomy.

which a knife-edged lenticle was slipped into an angled slit made in the peripheral cornea and then sutured (Fig 26–4). Slade et al worked with corneal tissue glues in an attempt to eliminate sutures from the procedure.[47] Goosey reported 20 cases of myopic epi keratoplasty without a keratectomy in an attempt to avoid the astigmatism and scarring associated with the standard technique.[48]

Another part of the inaccuracy of epikeratoplasty was believed to be caused by the changes and variables induced with the freezing of the tissue necessary for cryolathing. The tissue was also lyophilized for storage.[49] This processing may have been responsible for the characteristically long re-epithelialization, up to 25 days, seen following epikeratoplasty.[50] Persistent epithelial defects and decreased BCVA were the most common causes for a graft to be removed.[43]

To avert the healing problems inherent with heavily processed tissue, many investigators explored nonfreeze techniques.[51] Altmann et al reported on using the excimer laser with a small spot size and the cornea mounted on a movable platform to lathe the tissue.[52] In another approach to avoid freezing the tissue in order to shape it, Buratto and Ferrari used the Barraquer–Krumreich–Swinger system (BKS) (described below) technique to shape the epi lenticules without freezing.[53] The refractive outcome with this group was less predictable than desired, but the rate of visual recovery

was much faster than regular freeze epikeratoplasty. In the end, however, the difficulties could not be completely overcome. Epikeratoplasty was withdrawn from the market and its approval process with the FDA ended. However, the ease of epikeratoplasty, contrasted with the difficulty of MKM, inspired the investigation of ways to correct the highly myopic patient more readily.

In the quest to reduce the complexity of lamellar surgery, Drs Barraquer, Krumreich, and Swinger developed a system to perform nonfreeze keratomileusis, which bears their name. In 1985, Swinger and colleagues introduced the BKS system.[54] The BKS system included an improved microkeratome, a suction stand, and a set of dyes (Fig 26–5). A layer of tissue was removed from the eye and then draped over a preselected dye, which set the cornea up for a myopic or a hyperopic second resection to the undersurface of the disc. The BKS system produced some good results and had the advantage of not freezing the tissue. Mean UCVAs in some groups were reported at 20/50 at 6-month follow-up. However, visual rehabilitation was slow, and at least 12 months were required to recover best preop spectacle visual acuity. In some series, 30% of eyes lost two or more lines of BCVA.[55] As previously seen with the epi nonfreeze technique, there was a fair amount of variability in the results, but patients did recover faster. Thus, wound healing was reduced as a variable post-

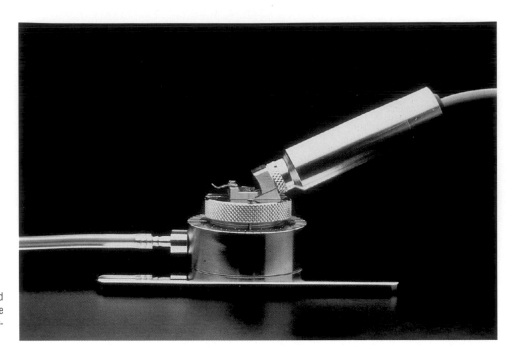

Figure 26–5. The BKS device featured an improved turbine microkeratome and a vacuum stand that held the corneal disc for a second shaping cut.

operatively, largely because of the nonfreeze nature of the surgery.

The elimination of the cryolathe increased the potential availability of the operation, but now two microkeratome cuts had to be performed. The manual microkeratome gave varied results mainly because two perfect keratectomies had to be performed. The initial resected piece of tissue had to be quite large—9 mm and 300 to 350 μm thick—making it a particularly difficult resection. Placing this large piece of tissue onto the suction stand and securing it was also technically difficult. More important, the accuracy of the technique refractively depended completely upon the thickness of the cornea cut by the microkeratome. Thus, the upper limit of myopic correction was approximately 16 D. Irregular astigmatism was present in several cases postoperatively, and predictability was not as good as that found in previous freeze MKM series. However, patients' comfortability with the nonfreeze technique and their rapid recovery were impressive, so that it presented a major advance in lamellar refractive surgery.

The desire to reduce high myopia predictably (without the dioptric limitation of carving a disc), as well as obtaining the quick recovery witnessed in nonfreeze techniques, prompted more research in keratomileusis in situ. This technique, as previously mentioned, relies on shaping the second resection upon the bed after the primary cap is resected. It was also developed by Barraquer and Luis Ruiz in Bogotá. Leo Bores performed the first cases in the United States of keratomi-

leusis in situ in November 1987, and he began further investigation of the technique. His patients had a more rapid recovery of vision and a more comfortable postop course.

The primary difference between keratomileusis in situ and classic keratomileusis is that the refractive excision of stroma to flatten the anterior corneal curvature is done upon the resected piece of tissue by the cryolathe in MKM and upon the bed using a microkeratome in keratomileusis in situ. Keratomileusis in situ, as originally envisioned, involved cutting a single lamellar disc of tissue as a cap and a second disc on the bed to thin out the central cornea (Fig 26–6). The first disc was replaced and would then "drape" into the resected bed, altering the anterior curvature of the cornea. The second disc removed is a lamellar section, as evidenced by electron microscope (EM) work (Fig 26–7). The advantage of the draping effect was a larger optical zone and a greater range of potential correction (up to −30 D) than that obtained in freeze MKM. However, the accuracy of the keratome is crucial for in situ MKM, where the thickness of the second resection is directly responsible for the power correction. The keratome is extremely dependent upon the speed of the pass to give the proper thickness for the second resection. In standard MKM, where the thickness of the resection does not determine the power, this was not as critical.

Early series of in situ MKM, where a manual keratome was used, resulted in a wide range of correction. Bas and Nano, reporting on 30 eyes, showed that only

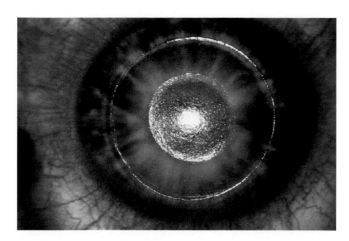

Figure 26–6. The cornea after the two cuts of keratomileusis in situ with the automated microkeratome displaying the smooth surface, circularity, and good centration.

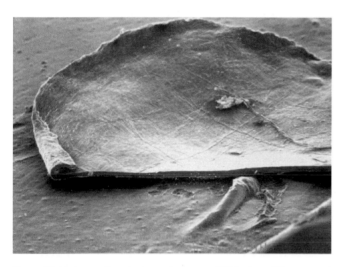

Figure 26–7. A scanning electron microscope (SEM) view of the removed second or refractive cut. This disc, which is 4.2 mm in diameter and 40 μm thick, has been transected to demonstrate the lamellar nature of the resection.

7% were able to obtain 20/40 or better without correction.[56] Arenas-Archila et al, reporting on 32 eyes with a mean follow-up of 128.7 days, reported an average reduction of myopia of 8.4 D. UCVA improved in all of the eyes, but in 14 eyes, it diminished. Four eyes lost two or more Snellen lines of BCVA, although many eyes had an improved corrected visual acuity. Several complications, including epithelium in the interface, undercorrection, and irregular astigmatism, were also reported. The authors felt that MKM as done with a manual keratome was not technically safe, precise, or predictable.[57] A refractive cut done with a hand-driven keratome produced considerable variability. Such a crucial role of the

keratome by MKM in situ led researchers to develop new and improved keratomes.[58] The Ruiz/Steinway, Drager, and Microprecision microkeratomes all embody attempts to improve the accuracy and reproducibility of the cuts. Smoothness of the keratectomy, ease of use, and reliability are also crucial requirements. While most systems were able to provide adequate resections, there was a need to improve the accuracy and reproducibility of the in situ technique.

In the late 1980s, Luis Ruiz developed a foot-operated automated geared keratome that controlled the speed of the pass across the eye so that more consistent cuts were possible (Fig 26–8). It also permitted a controlled reversal of the microkeratome without disturbing the lamellar cap. This advance in equipment has greatly popularized the technique. In addition, improvements to the suction ring increased the ease of the procedure. Keratectomies with this new device display a very fine smoothness (Fig 26–9).

Early on in the use of this technique, the first disc or corneal cap was sutured back into position. Later it became evident that sutures were not necessary. Cases can be done safely with topical anesthesia using this quick, simplified technique. The recovery time is improved, the patients have a more comfortable postop course, and there is less induced astigmatism. One-year data of 100 eyes enrolled in a multicenter prospective study of automated lamellar keratoplasty (ALK) reveal stable refractions, and 75% of patients have uncorrected vision within two lines of their preoperative BCVA. This has been a dramatic improvement for lamellar surgery. However, even though this procedure was beneficial for these patients with high myopia, predictability

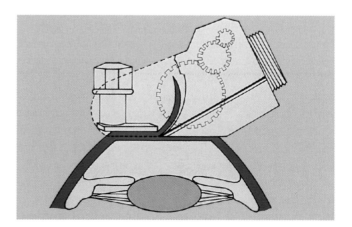

Figure 26–8. The Ruiz automated microkeratome, based on the Barraquer design, is geared so that the one motor that moves the blade also drives the keratome across the eye.

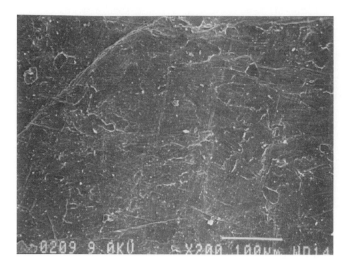

Figure 26–9. An SEM view of the corneal bed after a resection by the Ruiz keratome shows the smoothness obtained with the instrument.

needs improvement. The main concern with the technique is the refractive accuracy or depth obtained with the second resected disc. Improving the precision of the second disc resection is of primary importance. Improved keratome designs, which control the speed of the pass, calibration, and standardized blades, appear to be moving in this direction.

Disadvantages of this technique include potential irregular astigmatism. The reported irregular astigmatism rate is significantly lower than that reported for classic MKM, especially in the hands of surgeons new to lamellar surgery. Any irregular astigmatism is of concern, and removing the surgeon variable in creating a keratectomy appears to be a critical step toward eliminating it altogether. The reported loss of a cap has been reduced by returning to Barraquer's original keratomileusis in situ procedure using a flap technique.

The new keratome designed by Ruiz and the procedure built around it, automated lamellar keratoplasty, have provided ease of technique, rapid recovery, and a wide range of potential correction. The main goal remains to improve accuracy. While the microkeratome is superb at removing a disc of tissue, the second cut is not lenticular and is only accurate to within ± 5 μm. This has led researchers to explore other ways to make the second critical refractive cut.

Surgeons have begun to use the excimer laser to make the second cut for in situ MKM (Fig 26–10). In 1989 Peyman et al reported the first animal study in which a laser was used to remove stroma from a lamellar bed.[59] This work examined the potentially deleterious effect of permanently removing Bowman's layer:

the possibility, for example, of weak epithelial adhesion leading to possible recurrent epithelial erosions. Ioannis Pallikaris was the first investigator to perform excimer laser ablation under a corneal flap (LASIK) and to evaluate extensively the healing both histopathologically and in comparison to photorefractive keratectomy.[60] He proposed that stromal ablation could potentially avoid the regression of effect and stromal haze attributed to the well-documented activation of stromal keratocytes in PRK.[61–63] Lucio Buratto later reported the improvement of treating high myopia with excimer laser intrastromal keratomileusis in a large series of human eyes; however, the significant complications (23.2%) seen in this series appear to be related to manual keratectomy.[64] Prospective collaborative studies with an automated keratome are underway to explore this technique further. Brint and Slade first reported on this technique in the United States in 1992. In 1993 Slade combined the use of the automated keratome with the excimer to perform excimer ALK. Ruiz and Slade have reported on the early results of a prospective study of 120 patients randomized to ALK combined with PRK versus PRK alone for moderate to high myopia.[65] The reduced pain and earlier visual recovery in the combined groups is an advantage, however; longer-term follow-up will be needed to determine the efficacy and stability of these procedures. Hagen et al have demonstrated the difficulty of obtaining useful information in human cadaver eyes,[66] which underlines the need for prospective clinical trials in lamellar refractive procedures.[67]

The excimer laser potentially offers the accuracy to remove corneal tissue precisely as well as the ability to provide a lenticular, rather than a lamellar, cut and to correct astigmatism at the same time. Recent clinical trials suggest that frontal surface ablation with the excimer laser is best for patients with less than 6 D of myopia.[68] It appears that patients who received PRK for

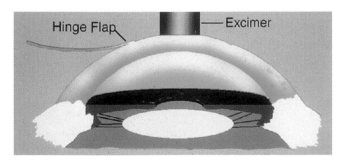

Figure 26–10. ALK/excimer flap technique using the excimer to make the second refractive keratectomy beneath a corneal flap (laser in situ keratomileusis, or LASIK).

high myopia, even with multizone ablation, have shown unpredictable responses, more haze, and late regression of effect. The automated microkeratome allows the ablation to be done in situ; therefore the ablated area is largely hidden from the normal healing processes of the eye that have played a key role in the problems associated with frontal excimer laser ablation or PRK in high myopia.

Lamellar refractive surgery has undergone a long evolutionary process. Fortunately, the early pioneers in this arena had the vision and persistence to strive for large, predictable corrections of ametropia without performing intraocular surgery. The potential risks of intraocular surgery are beginning to far outweigh those of lamellar surgery. However, in order for lamellar techniques to be the first choice for large refractive errors, the accuracy must approach that of an intraocular lens.[69] In manipulating the corneal surface, we are also obligated to achieve the degree of optical performance obtained by IOL implantation.[70] New ways of assessing optical quality of the corneal surface are on the horizon and will greatly benefit our patients.[71] Developing the current techniques, while keeping a watchful eye on the history of lamellar surgery, may lead to such refinements. The current forms of lamellar refractive surgery include automated lamellar keratoplasty (ALK) and excimer laser in situ keratomileusis (LASIK).

PATIENT SELECTION

In general, the patient should be over 18 years of age. Patients selected for ALK or LASIK should be in the range of −1 through −15 D. The upper limit of excimer MKM to the cap is −15 D. Limitations and predictability for hyperopic correction with these procedures is currently under evaluation and will be discussed in the sections on technique.

All patients should be screened for corneal disease. Detection of form fruste keratoconus and or corneal warpage is expedited with routine corneal topography.[72,73] If the patient has a history of contact lens wear, the lenses are to be discontinued for at least 1 week for soft lenses and 6 weeks for hard lenses. Serial examination of the patient should reveal a stable refraction and topography prior to surgery. Epithelial basement membrane disease or a history of recurrent erosions is considered a relative contraindication. Contraindications include a history of keratitis.

The patient is screened for retinal disease and should be treated if necessary before surgery. Prophylactic scatter photocoagulation is not currently recommended, as it has its own set of complications.[74]

The patient should have adequate exposure of the globe and be cooperative enough for local anesthesia. The suction ring (without suction) can be placed on the patient's eye after a drop of proparacaine is placed. This is a good way to assess the fit in the examination room, avoiding intraoperative surprises.

All patients should be thoroughly informed about the nature of the procedure and know what to expect intraoperatively and postoperatively.

AUTOMATED LAMELLAR KERATOPLASTY (ALK)

The keratome most commonly used today was developed by Luis Ruiz (Fig 26–11). This is the automated geared microkeratome, which controls the speed of the pass across the cornea so that a more consistent cut is possible. In addition, improvements to the suction ring increased the ease of the procedure. One suction ring is now adjustable to create any specific diameter so that different rings are no longer needed. When this instrument was initially used, the first disc or corneal cap was sutured back into position, but sutures were later found to be unnecessary. Various theories as to why the cap sticks into position have been proposed, including surface tension, the inherent stickiness of the glycoproteins, and the partial relative vacuum of the endothelial cell pump. Without sutures, there was less induced astigmatism, and the recovery time improved. Cases are now done safely with topical anesthesia. The patients have a more rapid recovery in vision and a more comfortable postop course, mainly because the tissue has not been overly manipulated, devitalized, or frozen. Another further advance is the flap technique. By not completely removing the covering cap and simply leaving a hinge, the risk of losing a cap has been markedly reduced (Fig 26–12).

Preoperative Preparation

The patient is brought to the operating room after signing the informed consent and having any questions answered. A mild sedative is administered. The patient is prepped and draped in the usual sterile fashion.

The automatic corneal shaper is removed from Cidex (where it has soaked at least 10 minutes for sterilization) and rinsed thoroughly in sterile water. The unit is inspected and the gears are turned to check for cleanliness. A new blade is inserted into

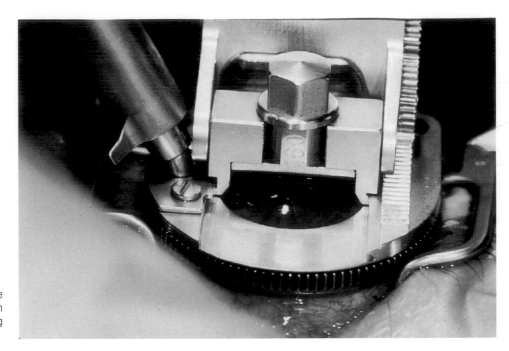

Figure 26–11. Frontal view of the Ruiz automated microkeratome in place on the adjustable suction ring before the keratectomy.

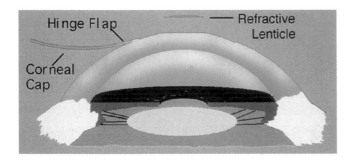

Figure 26–12. ALK for myopia with the flap technique leaves the first keratectomy hinged on to prevent total loss of the tissue and simplify the operation.

the blade holder of the shaper head. The shaper head is closed and the fit of the blade is checked by turning the blade holder with the probing shank. The blade is then inspected under the operating microscope. The motor is installed onto the shaper head and run through the suction ring for smoothness. The suction ring is checked for adequate suction of over 20 mm Hg.

The desired plates are removed from the kit and set aside. The first plate, 160 μm, is inserted into the shaper. The second plate is selected on the basis of the patient's target myopia, age, dominant or nondominant eye, and results of the first eye along the nomogram.

Procedure in Detail

After the patient has been prepped and draped, a lid speculum is placed to obtain maximum exposure of the globe. A locking speculum is preferred. All lashes and the eyelids must be out of the field of passage of the microkeratome. The patient is instructed to look at the microscope light, two drops of proparcaine are instilled, and the cornea is marked with the reference marker that has been inked with a sterile skin marker (Fig 26–13). The rings of the marker are centered over the patient's pupil, which is constricted by the microscope light. No pilocarpine is used.

The suction ring is then placed over the cornea and great care is taken to ensure perfect centration. The suction ring is pressed down on the globe and the suction engaged. The pressure of the eye is then checked with the tonometer to be over 65 mm Hg. The 7.2-mm applanation lens is then placed on the ring to ensure that an adequate diameter of cornea is exposed for the first keratectomy.

The keratome is then placed into the ring. The corneal stopper device is set for a myopic flap (Fig 26–14). The keratome is started and allowed to course across the ring to the stop and then reversed off the ring. The corneal flap is then inspected and laid over the suction ring (Fig 26–15). If a free cap is obtained, this cap is placed epithelial side down in the plastic chamber provided for this use and covered.

The keratome is then removed, and the plate is changed to the second or refractive plate. The ring is now adjusted with the adjustment wrench to the smaller or 4.2-mm-diameter resection, which is verified by an applanation lens.

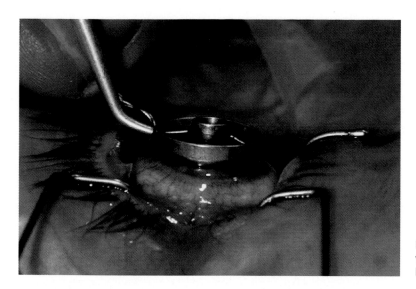

Figure 26–13. Before the keratectomy the cornea is marked with dye both to aid in centration of the suction ring and to help orient the cap or flap.

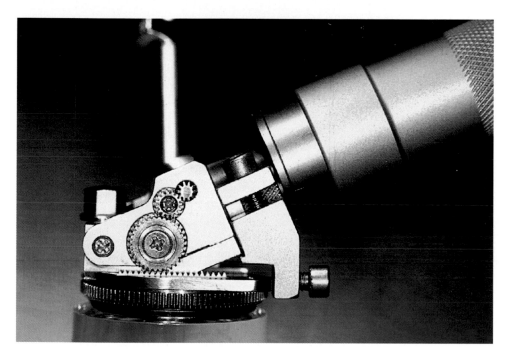

Figure 26–14. The keratome may be fitted with a travel limiter or corneal stop to automatically produce a corneal flap with the first resection.

Once the plate has been changed and the ring set for the smaller diameter, the keratome is passed again across the cornea for the second, or refractive, cut. After this cut, the suction ring is disengaged and removed from the eye. The second resection is then measured with the thickness gauge or the estimated thickness is entered onto the chart from subtraction pachymetry (Fig 26–16). The bed is then inspected and the centration, smoothness, and regularity of the resection is noted.

After the bed is rinsed and antibiotic drops instilled, the bed is lightly dried with oxygen while the flap is irrigated. The flap is then laid back into posi-

tion and allowed to seal into place. The flap or cap is considered adhered if striae from indenting the peripheral host radiate into the flap. Once this adherence is adequate, a clear shield is taped over the patient's open eye.

Postop Care

The patient is given mild pain medication and asked to return to the clinic the next day. On this first visit, the vision is tested and a slit lamp exam is performed. The patient is then started on a combination steroid antibiotic QID for 5 days. The patient is allowed to resume

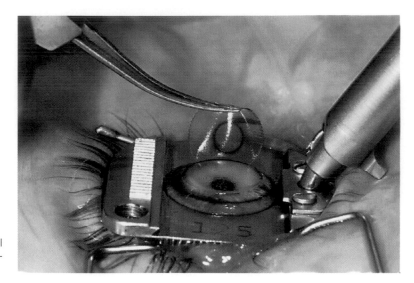

Figure 26–15. After the first resection, the 160-μm corneal flap, with the suction ring still in place, is laid over the platform prior to the second or refractive cut.

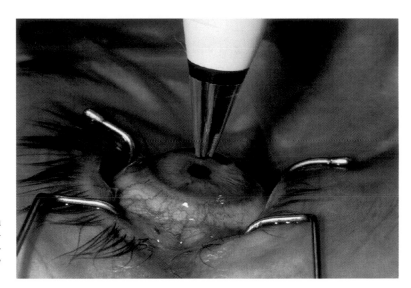

Figure 26–16. The corneal thickness is measured with a modified pachymeter prior to the first cut. A second measurement after the resection is then subtracted from the original reading to give the thickness of the first cut by subtraction.

normal activities but instructed to avoid hitting or trauma to the operated eye.

Early results have been reported by the ALK Study Group at the American Academy of Ophthalmology in 1993.[75] The Study Group prospectively evaluated 100 consecutive cases from 10 surgeons, typically their first cases with the procedure. Eight of these surgeons were not actively performing MKM. At 1-year follow-up, 75% of these eyes were within two Snellen lines of their preop BCVA. At 1 year, two eyes were reported as losing more than two lines relative to their preop BCVA because of irregular astigmatism. Seven eyes were reported as gaining more than two lines relative to their preop BCVA. These eyes gained visual acuity, most likely because of increased asphericity and decreased minification. The predictability was good, generally

within 1D of the planned correction. The refractive outcome was stable with little change throughout the 1-year follow-up. ALK appears to be "astigmatism neutral," affecting only the spherical component. The visual outcome was good, with 75% of the eyes achieving 20/40 or better uncorrected vision. Automated lamellar keratoplasty has reduced the complexity of lamellar refractive surgery, improved recovery times, and offers a wide range of potential correction. As currently done, ALK seems to be a reasonably safe, effective, and accurate technique for myopia ranging from 10 to 25 D.

The role of ALK for hyperopic correction is less well defined, primarily because the mechanical effect on the cornea is unique to this procedure (Fig 26–17). The technique requires a single, deep resection: approximately 300 to 400 μm, depending on the desired cor-

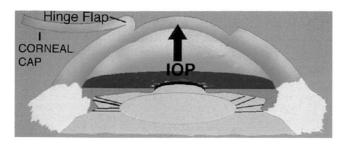

Figure 26–17. A thick (325 to 425 μm) corneal flap is created in ALK for hyperopia to allow the remaining cornea to bow forward to steepen the eye once the corneal flap is replaced.

rection. The depth and diameter of this resection determine the refractive effect by presumably creating a "controlled ectasia" of Descemet's membrane, thus reducing the hyperopia. Prospective controlled studies are underway to determine the efficacy and long-term stability of this procedure.

EXCIMER LASER IN SITU KERATOMILEUSIS (LASIK)

The precision of the excimer laser in shaping corneal stroma has been envisioned as a way to improve the results of lamellar refractive surgery. LASIK would ideally combine the accuracy of the excimer laser to remove corneal tissue and the keratome to access the inner stroma. This would preserve Bowman's layer and reduce the effect of wound healing.[59,60] LASIK is discussed in greater detail in Chapter 34. From the very first lamellar refractive procedures done by Barraquer, accuracy and predictability have been major concerns. Many different methods have been employed in the past to shape or remove stromal tissue. At this point, there are four main ways of shaping the corneal tissue with MKM: the cryolathe; the BKS system, which uses a mold or dye on a planar disc of tissue; the in situ method of Ruiz; and the excimer laser. Barraquer's initial methods of cryolathing were reasonably accurate but technically difficult. While using the manual microkeratomes to make a second refractive cut has proven to be inaccurate, using an automated microkeratome like that of Ruiz has been a vast improvement. However, even this technique, ALK, has not been completely accurate or predictable.

The original concept for using the excimer laser MKM was driven by the variable, and initially poor, results of using the excimer for frontal ablation in patients with high myopia (Fig 26–18). Because of the depth of the ablation required, wound healing played a very im-

portant role with these patients.[61–63] Scarring was more prominent, and regression caused by thick epithelium was also more of a problem. Retreatments were often necessary. There have been attempts to improve these results, such as multiple ablation zones. In general, however, results with the excimer laser in direct frontal ablation with high myopia have been poorer than those in low to moderate myopia.[68]

Perhaps the excimer laser, as other refractive operations, has a range of patients that it treats best. Wound healing has been theorized, from the work of Dan Durrie, to be a large variable in excimer laser results, perhaps 20% of the final effect. Although the stroma can be shaped with great precision, the epithelial healing response plays a large role in the final outcome. If the epithelium heals into the ablated area with a robust or vigorous healing response and fills in the stromal ablation too thickly, there will be an undercorrection. This is best demonstrated by early hyperopic ablations that created steep and deep peripheral corneal troughs that filled in over time with epithelium, thus negating the desired refractive effect. Conversely, if the patient heals rapidly with a thin, almost atrophic layer of epithelium over the stromal ablation, then he or she will remain overcorrected, as the assumed original normal thickness of the epithelium did not return. While these patients can be modified by removing the epithelium, this means an additional operation in which wound healing will also play a large role. The eye simply recognizes any epithelial abrasion and the stromal damage and attempts to heal the wound. Lamellar keratoplasty using the excimer laser presumes that the removed stroma would be "hidden" from the healing processes of the

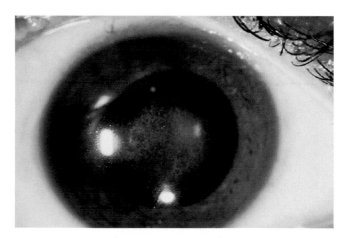

Figure 26–18. Corneas treated for high myopia with the excimer laser can result in increased scarring and regression, as in this case that was performed on a −16 D myope with a 5.5-mm OZ.

eye. There would be no large epithelial abrasion or defect, and the healing processes of the eye would not be as prominent a factor in the final result.

Once again, just as with ALK, the automated geared microkeratome developed by Ruiz is an integral part in refining the predictability of in situ keratomileusis and is of prime importance when assessing the potential advantage of utilizing the excimer laser for the second resection for myopia.

Preoperative Steps

The excimer is turned on and tested before the patient is brought into the operating room. A 300-µm plate is placed into the microkeratome after the entire system has been pretested. After the patient is prepped and draped, a lid speculum is chosen from a variety available to obtain maximum exposure. A corneal marker is centered over the visual axis to mark a 10-mm circle for centering the suction ring, a 3.5-mm mark to center over the visual axis, and a pararadial line to ensure proper alignment of the cap if it is removed completely (Figs 26–19 and 26–20).

Once good exposure has been obtained with a suitable lid speculum, an adjustable suction ring set to a diameter of 8.0 mm is placed on the eye. This suction ring both fixates the eye and raises the IOP to approximately 65 mm. This increased pressure aids a smooth, even keratectomy. The pressure is verified with a Barraquer tonometer. The eye is then wiped with a soaked Weck-cell sponge to irrigate and lubricate the cornea. The automated keratome is placed into the dovetail/groove system on the suction ring to lock it into position. The keratome is turned on with a foot switch and begins to pass across the cornea. The keratome pass of approximately 160 µm in depth is interrupted by watching the resection until the proper length of cut has been made. The keratome is then reversed off the ring. In this technique the patient is operated on beneath the excimer, or the patient is positioned close to the laser. The flap is then laid back and, after a standardized time to control hydration, the ablation is placed on the bed. An SEM view shows the ablation centered on a keratome bed in a bank eye (Fig 26–21). The patient is asked to fixate upon the He–Ne beam to provide centration, much as in PRK. If the patient has difficulty, the eye can be stabilized with two Weck cells or, in more difficult cases, the suction ring.

The ablated area is measured and checked for centration, then irrigated with filtered saline. The flap is then replaced, lightly dried, and adhesion is checked. With this technique no patch is used; just a clear shield is taped into position.[12]

LASIK patients, because of the intact epithelium and Bowman's membrane, have less postop discomfort than standard PRK patients. First-day uncorrected visions are often 20/40 or better. Large zones of central flattening are evident on corneal topography (Fig 26–22). The vision is usually more stable than with either PRK or RK as wound healing does not play as large a role. The haze seen in PRK is also avoided. LASIK offers the advantage of being able to treat astigmatism at the same time as the myopic ablation. We consider this operation, although still in development, a good choice for higher degrees of myopia.

Excimer laser MKM in a large series was first reported by Lucio Buratto of Milano. Buratto reported a prospective series of 30 consecutive eyes from −11.2 to −24.50 D that underwent excimer laser MKM.[64] A planocorneal disc was removed with a BKS microkeratome, followed by excimer ablation either of the resected disc (28 eyes) or on the stromal bed (2 eyes). The excimer laser nomogram was used as a standard PRK nomogram (see Figs 26–1 and 26–2). The disc was then sutured into position. Recovery was rapid, with 83% of the corneas clear by 3 weeks. Fifty-seven percent of the eyes were within 1 D of the intended refraction. Ten percent of the eyes were 20/40 or better uncorrected after surgery at 12 months, whereas 90% were 20/100 to 20/50. Significant irregular astigmatism and wrinkling of Bowman's layer were reported on two eyes while four other eyes had moderate irregular astigmatism. Interestingly, both of the patients treated with the in situ technique in which the ablation was done on the bed developed irregular astigmatism. This could have been a result of the greater difficulty in centering the optical zone with the in situ technique.

The next large series of excimer MKM to be done was the Summit FDA Protocol. This was started in New Orleans by Stephen Brint and Stephen Slade in the summer of 1991.[75] Sixty patients participated in this protocol.

Data on the Summit excimer laser series includes the original 60 patients treated with the laser. These patients ranged in myopia from 6 to 21 D. UCVAs at day 1 were excellent, with more than half of these patients seeing 20/40 or better. Visual acuities at 1 month continued to improve, with 13 out of the original 17 seeing 20/40 or better; those seeing 20/200 or worse were the patients with poor best corrected vision at the start of

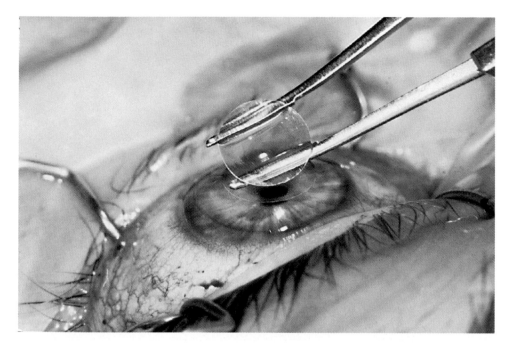

Figure 26–19. A thick disc of corneal tissue 300 to 350 μm is removed and the under or stromal surface is ablated using the excimer in the Burrato technique of excimer keratomileusis, which closely mimics classical freeze myopia keratomileusis.

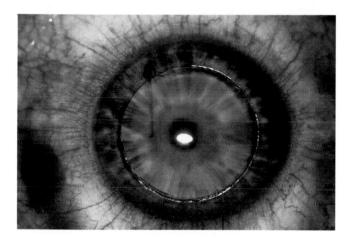

Figure 26–20. After the shaping resection is performed, the corneal cap is repositioned and oriented on the corneal bed.

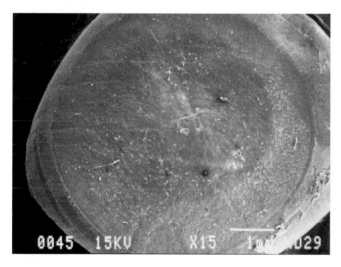

Figure 26–21. An SEM view of a cadaver eye that has been ablated centrally with the excimer after a keratectomy in the excimer keratomileusis technique.

the case. The excimer LK scattergram on 45 patients (Fig 26–23) shows a plot of the attempted diopteric change against achieved diopteric change, revealing a tight clustering along the ligher band within 1 D on the other side of plano. All lamellar patients tend to do better with time. Preop refraction ranges based on Stephen Brint's data with an initial range of −6.50 to −21.75 D have decreased to −0.81 to +1.87 D at 24 months. Postoperatively, the patients are in very little pain, usually far less than experienced by an RK patient. There does seem to be an original correction to the plus side, which

then levels out close to the intended correction and stabilizes. In contrast to some excimer data that show a continuing decreasing effect, our data suggest that at 12 and 24 months the effect is stable and does not continue to change (Fig 26–24).[68]

The operation does tend to be astigmatism neutral. The large flattening of the blue area is clearly demonstrated where the excimer ablation was made on the cap in this particular patient. Of course the ablation zone can be altered very readily by the excimer itself. As in PRK, corneal topography will be a valuable tool in as-

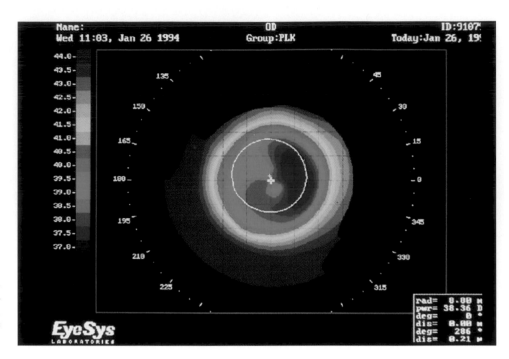

Figure 26–22. A corneal topography view at 1 day postop after excimer keratomileusis in situ with the flap technique shows the central zone of flattening.

sessing the accuracy of centration, ultimately leading to modifications to ensure reproducible ablations to the bed.[76]

The third large-group series used the Chiron/ Technolas excimer laser to treat astigmatic patients. One hundred and forty eyes on bilateral cases were enrolled, and the early results were very promising. Long-term follow-up is needed to judge the stability and efficacy of these procedures, but early results indicate minimal effect on the preexisting keratometric cylinder as well as a refractive effect similar to PRK alone. Another large series with George Waring in Jeddah is currently underway. There is considerable conjecture over which

technique would be better; performing the ablation on the cap or the bed. Ablating the cap has the advantage of perfect centration and a nonmoving target. Care must be taken to situate the cap perpendicularly, but otherwise there is no difficulty in centering this piece of tissue. A further advantage is that, in the event of a severe problem, the cap can be removed. Excimer ablation on the cap has another safety factor: if for some reason the cap is lost, a homoplastic piece of tissue may be carved with the excimer and placed on the eye, which has the same base curve as it had to begin with. This is not possible using the in situ technique, where the bed has been ablated with the excimer. Another inherent advantage of excimer ablation on the cap involves centration. If the optical center of the cornea is marked with dye before the keratectomy, then the ablation can be centered on the precise center, even though the keratome section may be slightly decentered. This is a further safety check with excimer ablation on the cap.

Obvious advantages to ablating the bed include the following:

1. A hinge technique is used, which is impossible with disc ablations.
2. The procedure can be performed under the laser, thus increasing speed and efficiency and in turn reducing hydration effects.
3. Toric and hyperopic ablations can be performed; once advancements are made in the centration during bed ablation, these are apt to be optically superior because there is minimal

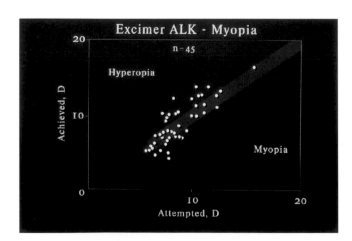

Figure 26–23. A scattergram of 45 patients with at least 6 months' follow-up after excimer MKM, showing achieved versus attempted correction. The lighter band is 1 D on either side of target.

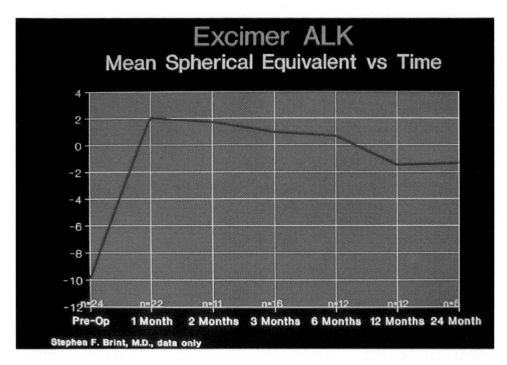

Figure 26-24. Excimer MKM mean spherical equivalent over time with the original Summit (NJ) patients shows an initial hyperopic shift, which decreases toward target over time. *(Data supplied by Stephen Brint, MD.)*

manipulation of the flap or disorientation of the disc.

4. Overall corneal stability may prove to be better maintained with the thinner 160-μm resection as opposed to the 300 μm required to make an ablatable cap.

Excimer ablation on the cap has safety factor: if, for some reason, the cap is lost, or the ablation is unsatisfactory, a homoplastic piece of tissue may be shaped with the excimer and placed on the eye, which has the same base curve as it had originally, as opposed to the in situ technique where the bed has been ablated with the excimer. The flap technique raises a 160-μm corneal flap and puts the excimer ablation on the bed itself. This mimics MKM in situ, while the excimer ablation on the cap mimics original freeze MKM. Centration with the flap technique must be done either by the patient voluntarily or by the surgeon fixating the eye. A poorly centered ablation is difficult to repair. There is a question of these ablations damaging endothelial cells closer to Descemet's membrane in the flap technique.

As excimers are investigated for the treatment of astigmatism, different methods can be used in a lamellar fashion. There are three main approaches for treating astigmatism currently with the major excimer laser protocols that can be used in LASIK: The Summit excimer laser study uses an ablatable mask, which could be positioned after the first cut is made. The VISX uses a pair of movable blades to lay down an ablation prefer-

entially over the astigmatic axis. The Nidek and Chiron/Technolas excimer laser uses a scannable beam, which tracks across the flat axis with a slowly expanding spot size and effects an astigmatic change.

LASIK patients, because of the virtually intact epithelium and Bowman's membrane, have less postop discomfort than standard PRK patients (Fig 26–14). First-day uncorrected visions are often 20/40 or better. Large zones of central flattening are evident on corneal topography. The vision generally stabilizes earlier than with either PRK or RK, as wound healing does not play as large a role. The standard PRK haze is rarely noted in this technique. The LASIK techniques also offer the advantage of being able to treat astigmatism on the bed or cap at the same time as the myopic ablation.

Excimer lamellar keratoplasty may offer advantages over even PRK. Lamellar refractive techniques are very much in evolution, as are keratomes, blades, and our knowledge of how best to use the excimer. Different spot sizes, optical zones, multizone treatments, and amounts of ablation parameters will all continue to change. Even at this early stage, however, excimer MKM and ALK are strong choices for myopia over 4 D.

COMPLICATIONS AND MANAGEMENT

Complications with MKM and lamellar keratoplasty include all the normal complications and risks inherent in eye surgery, along with specific problems like epithelial implantation of the stromal interface and irregular astigmatism. Epithelialization of the interface occurs because of turned-under edges of the corneal cap or inadequate irrigation of the stromal bed following resection, which allows inoculated epithelial cells to grow into the interface. It is not necessary in most cases to remove the cap in order to clear the interface of epithelial ingrowth. This can be done using the specially designed irrigating needles. Infiltrates and epithelial ingrowth can be minimized by avoiding excess manipulation of the cap and through adequate irrigation of the stromal/cap interface.

Infection rates were very low: approximately 2 in 7000 with Barraquer's original series. These two patients were part of a small series wearing a bandage contact lens without antibiotic coverage. Once the cap is epithelialized, which should be in only 4 to 8 hours, infection should not be a major problem. There have been no known cases reported in the United States of corneal infection following lamellar surgery. In the event of infection, the appropriate methods should be instituted, using culture and sensitivity and the appropriate topical antibiotics. If there is edema and/or inflammation of the cap, treatment with a topical steroid should be considered.

The dislocation of the cap tends to occur most frequently in hyperopes. Many surgeons simply elect to suture all totally resected apical caps. It is essential that the eye be taped shut. Pressure patches should be avoided. The eye should be allowed to move freely with no pressure that may force the cap off the eye. It is essential that the tape be removed very carefully on the first postop day. The dressing should be saved until it has been verified that the cap is in place. If the cap has dislocated into the tape, it may be very dehydrated, in which case it should be put into OptiSol. OptiSol should hydrate it without causing any swelling, but must be all removed before the cap is replaced. If the cap is dislocated on the globe, is normal in thickness, and is properly hydrated, it can be put directly onto the stromal bed. The cap should be sutured into place using an antitorque suture. If the cap is lost or is unsuitable for reuse, the surgeon can either do nothing and allow the epithelium to regenerate and evaluate postop visual recovery or attach a homoplastic piece of tissue. The cap should be secured using an antitorque suture.

The procedure can also result in over- or undercorrections. Significant over- and undercorrection has been reported. Most surgeons tend to achieve undercorrection for both myopia and hyperopia in the beginning.

Significant overcorrections are most commonly caused by inappropriate resection thickness and/or diameter. Enhancement procedures can be performed to correct most residual refractive errors.

The most significant problem with any lamellar surgery is irregular astigmatism. This is inherent in all lamellar keratoplasty and stems from a microscopic roughness or irregularity in the corneal surface. Computer analysis of these corneas is often able to diagnose irregular astigmatism; however, the most reliable method for diagnosis is by inspection of the mires of a manual keratometer.[1] The presence of irregular astigmatism may be confirmed by the use of a hard contact lens in a patient with overrefraction. For most of these patients, the only treatment available is time. If the vision is improving every month, it will probably reach a maximum improvement in about 90 days. However, if the patient has had stitches, or if there is an irregularity in the healing pattern of the edge of the cap, or if there have been problems with epithelium in the interface, a cap dissection generally cures the problem. With the pupil dilated, dissect the cap free with the blunt spatula angled at 45°, leaving a small hinge on one edge. It is helpful to leave that hinge at the 12 o'clock position. Reposition the cap and use balanced salt to irrigate any introduced particles. Dry the gutter. The cap is dried in position and the eye is taped overnight.

In some cases of irregular astigmatism, one might see a steep area on topography over one edge of the cap. The patient may have a more intensive fibrotic reaction in that one spot. This could be managed with a cap dissection as previously described, or the cornea can simply be freed in the affected quadrant. Dissect the edge of the cap only in the one quadrant that corresponds to the steep spot on the topography. Most of these patients will improve over the first year, and many become even better at year 2 compared to year 1. When irregular astigmatism does not improve and a patient is unable to wear a contact lens, a deep homoplastic graft is the only option available. The newer techniques have reduced the incidence of irregular astigmatism. The keratomileusis in situ prospective evaluation of 100 patients showed an irregular astigmatism rate of only 2%.[75]

Regular astigmatism can be induced, although in general ALK is astigmatism neutral. One should dissect the steep meridian 90° on each side, connecting in the center in a figure-8 pattern. Correction of 5 D of astigmatism can be obtained with this technique if the problem was caused by cap placement or if irregular fibrosis exists on the margin of the cap. This obviously does not work if the patient had the astigmatism before ALK.

Rare but potential complications include perforation of the globe and decentered cuts. The surgeon should be sure that the depth-plate nut, which attaches the depth plate to the shaper head, can be seen through the microscope and that the plate is fully seated before proceeding with the resection to prevent it from entering the anterior chamber. If decentration is noted after the myopic resection, nothing can be done. The surgeon should not try to fix the problem by recutting. The only solution for a significantly decentered cap is to allow the cornea to heal and return at a later date to repeat the procedure using a new set of refractive indices. Since decentration is a major problem, the best solution is to avoid it.

ALK cuts in hyperopic cases that are too deep (greater than 80%) can yield severe ectasia of the central cornea. This prolapse of the cornea appears similar to keratoconus, but without corneal thinning. Patients with corneal ectasia after hyperopic correction typically fall into one of the two categories. In the first, one can visibly tell at the slit lamp that the cut is deeper than 90%. In the second, the cut is of normal depth. Not uncommonly, these patients have had previous RK surgery to which they overresponded, and they now are overresponding to the hyperopic lamellar keratectomy. The treatment for this is to use eight radial interrupted 10-0 mersilene stitches to tighten the cap and to squash the cone. The sutures can be removed slowly over the next 2 to 6 months in order to titrate the amount of prolapse or flattening that is required. If low degrees of minus remain, then a myopic ALK or an RK can be done after 6 months.

Other common side effects can include haloes, glare, and fluctuating vision. Typically these side effects are moderate compared with those of other refractive surgery techniques or even of contact lenses, and they tend to get better with time. Given the potential side effects of ALK, the Committee on Ophthalmic Procedures Assessment/American Academy of Ophthalmology has recommended performing additional studies to evaluate the instrumentation and techniques of ALK and LASIK in order to improve the efficiency of these procedures and provide objective assessment of the technology.[77]

SUMMARY

Optimism about the future of lamellar refractive surgery is increasing rapidly. These procedures allow patients to be treated with a nonfreeze, nonsutured, minimally invasive operation under topical anesthesia. Lamellar refractive surgery lessens the role of wound healing. Although its accuracy must be improved, there is a rapid return to vision and excellent patient comfort. Irregular astigmatism rates are encouragingly low. The combination of the excimer laser for the refractive cuts and improved automated microkeratomes for the keratectomies may be fortunate. Further potential advances include intrastromal corneal lenses and improved solid state lasers. Investigators have also worked with laser microkeratomes. Perhaps the main advantage of lamellar refractive surgery is the ability to avoid wound-healing responses and to provide an "intrastromal ablation" effect at a time when the dream of true intrastromal ablation remains distant.

REFERENCES

1. Barraquer JI: Queratoplastia refractiva. *Estud Inform Oftal Inst Barraquer.* 1949;10:2–21.
2. Krawawicz T. Experimental operations of partial lamellar excision of corneal stroma for the correction of myopia. *Klin Oczna.* 1963;33:1.
3. Barraquer JI. Results of hypermetropic keratomileusis. In: Binder PS, ed. Refractive Corneal Surgery: The Correction of Aphakia, Hyperopia and Myopia. *Int Ophthalmol Clin.* 1983;23:25–44.
4. Binder PS. What we have learned about corneal wound healing from refractive surgery. Barraquer Lecture. *Refract Corneal Surg.* 1989;5:98–120.
5. Barraquer JI. Keratomileusis. *Int Surg.* 1967;48:103–117.
6. Barraquer JI. Results of myopic keratomileusis. *J Refract Surg.* 1987;3:98–101.
7. Littman H. Optic of Barraquer's keratomileusis. *Arch Oftal Optom.* 1966;6:1.
8. Krumeich JH. Indications, techniques, and complications of myopic keratomileusis. In: Binder PS, ed. Refractive Corneal Surgery: The Correction of Aphakia, Hyperopia and Myopia. *Int Ophthalmol Clin.* 1983;23:75–92.
9. Barraquer JI. Keratomileusis for myopia and aphakia. *Ophthalmology.* 1981;88:701–708.
10. Barraquer JI. Method for cutting lamellar grafts in frozen corneas: new orientations for refractive surgery. *Arch Soc Am Ophthalmol.* 1958;1:237.
11. Waring GO. Conventional standards for reporting results of refractive surgery. *Refract Corn Surg.* 1989;5:285–287.
12. Troutman RC, Swinger CA. Refractive keratoplasty: keratophakia and keratomileusis. *Trans Am Ophthalmol Soc.* 1978;76:329–339.
13. Taylor D, Stern A, Romanchuk K. Keratophakia: clinical evaluation. *Ophthalmology.* 1981;88:1141–1150.

14. Friedlander MH, Werblin TP, Kaufman HE. Clinical results of keratophakia and keratomileusis. *Ophthalmology.* 1981;88:716–720.

15. Jester JV, Rodrigues MM, Villasenor RA, et al. Keratophakia and keratomileusis: histopathologic, ultrastructural and experimental studies. *Ophthalmology.* 1984;91: 793–805.

16. Binder PS. Dedication. Refractive Corneal Surgery: The Correction of Aphakia, Hyperopia, and Myopia. *Int Ophthalmol Clin.* 1983;23:v–vi.

17. Kaufman HE. The correction of aphakia. XXXVI Edward Jackson Memorial Lecture. *Am J Ophthalmol.* 1980;89(1): 1–10.

18. Werblin TP, Klyce SD. Epikeratophakia: the correction of myopia: I. Lathing of corneal tissue. *Curr Eye Res.* 1982; 1:591.

19. Werblin TP. Epikeratophakia: techniques, complications and clinical results. *Int Ophthalmol Clin.* 1983;23: 45–58.

20. Barraquer JI. Modification of refraction by means of intracorneal inclusions. *Int Ophthalmol Clin.* 1966;6:53–78.

21. Rich LF, Friedlander MH, Kaufman HE, et al. Keratocyte survival in keratophakia lenticules. *Arch Ophthalmol.* 1981;99:677–680.

22. Googe JM, Palkama KA, Werblin TP. The histology of epikeratophakia grafts. *Invest Ophthalmol Vis Sci.* 1981;20:8.

23. Baumgartner SD, Bider PS, Deg JK, et al. Epikeratophakia: clinical and histopathologic evaluation in non-human primates. *Invest Ophthalmol Vis Sci.* 1983;24:148.

24. Samples JR, Binder PS, Zavala EY, et al. Epikeratophakia: clinical evaluation and histopathology of a non-human primate model. *Cornea.* 1984;3:51–60.

25. Binder PS, Zavala EY, Baumgartner SD, et al. Combined morphological effects of cryolathing and lyophilization on epikeratoplasty lenticles. *Arch Ophthalmol.* 1986;104:671–679.

26. Jaeger MJ, Berson P, Kaufman HE, Green WR. Epikeratoplasty for keratoconus: a clinicopathologic case report. *Cornea.* 1987;6:131–139.

27. Werblin TP, Kaufman HE, Friedlander MH, Sehon KL, et al. A prospective study of the use of hyperopic epikeratophakia grafts for the correction of aphakia in adults. *Ophthalmology.* 1981;88:1137.

28. Werblin TP, Blaydes JE, Kaufman HE. Epikeratophakia: the correction of astigmatism. *CLAO J.* 1983;9:61.

29. Kaufman HE, Werblin TP. Epikeratophakia: a form of lamellar keratoplasty for the treatment of keratoconus. *Am J Ophthalmol.* 1982;93:342.

30. Bores LD, Myers W, Cowden J: Radial keratotomy: an analysis of the American experience. *Ann Ophthalmol.* 1981;13:941–948.

31. Arrowsmith PN, Sanders DR, Marks RG. Visual, refractive and keratometric results of radial keratotomy. *Arch Ophthalmol.* 1983;101:873–881.

32. Deitz MR, Sanders DR, Marks RG. Radial keratotomy: An overview of the Kansas City study. *Ophthalmology.* 1984; 91:467–478.

33. Shearing SP. Posterior chamber lens implantation. *Int Ophthalmol Clin.* 1982;22:135–153.

34. Swinger CA, Barker BA. Prospective evaluation of myopic keratomileusis. *Ophthalmology.* 1984;91:785–792.

35. Nordan LT, Fallor MK. Myopic keratomileusis: 74 consecutive non-amblyopic cases with one year of follow-up. *J Refract Surg.* 1986;2:124–128.

36. Maguire LJ, Klyce SD, Sawelson H, McDonald MB, et al. Visual distortion after myopic keratomileusis: computer analysis of keratoscope photographs. *Ophthalmic Surg.* 1987;18:352–356.

37. Nordan LT. Keratomileusis. *Int Ophthalmol Clin.* 1991;31: 7–12.

38. Barraquer C, Guitierrez A, Espinosa A. Myopic keratomileusis: short term results. *Refract Corn Surg.* 1989;5:307–313.

39. Nordan LT, Havins WH. Undercorrected RK treated with MKM. *J Refract Surg.* 1985;1:56.

40. McDonald MB, Kaufman HE, Aquavella JV, et. al. The nationwide study of epikeratophakia for aphakia in adults. *Am J Ophthalmol.* 1987;103:350–365.

41. McDonald MB, Kaufman HE, Aquavella JV, et al. The nationwide study of epikeratophakia for myopia in adults. *Am J Ophthalmol.* 1987;103:375–383.

42. Reidy JJ, McDonald MB, Klyce SD. The corneal topography of epikeratophakia. *Refract Corn Surg.* 1990;6:26–31.

43. Wilson DR, Keeney AH. Corrective measures for myopia. *Surv Ophthalmol.* 1990;34:294–304.

44. Goosey JD, Prager TC, Goosey CB, et al. Stability of refraction during two years after myopic epikeratoplasty. *Refract Corneal Surg.* 1990;6:4–8.

45. Gilbert ML, Roth AS, Friedlander MH. Corneal flattening by shallow circular trephination in human eye bank eyes. *Refract Corneal Surg.* 1990;6:113–116.

46. Rozakis GW, Slade SG, et al. *Refractive Lamellar Keratoplasty.* 1994; Thorofare, NJ: Slack, Inc.

47. Slade SG, Strauss GH. Use of tissue adhesive (Tisseel) in epikeratophakia. *Invest Ophthalmol Vis Sci.* 1990;31:30.

48. Goosey JD, Prager TC, Marvelli TL, et al. Epikeratophakia without annular keratectomy. *Ann Ophthalmol.* 1987;19: 388–391.

49. Friedlander MH, Rich LF, Werblin TP, et al. Keratophakia using preserved lenticles. *Ophthalmology.* 1980;87:687–692.

50. Martel J. Intraepikeratophakia. *Ann Ophthalmol.* 1987;19: 287–292.

51. Zavala EY, Krumeich J, Binder PS. Laboratory evaluation of freeze vs nonfreeze lamellar refractive keratoplasty. *Arch Ophthalmol.* 1987;105:1125–1128.

52. Altmann J, Grabner G, et al. Corneal lathing using the excimer laser and a computer-controlled positioning system: Part I—lathing of epikeratoplasty lenticules. *Refract Corneal Surg.* 1991;7:377–384.

53. Buratto L, Ferrari M. Retrospective comparison of freeze and non-freeze myopic epikeratophakia. *Refract Corneal Surg.* 1989;5:94–97.

54. Swinger CA, Krumeich J, Cassiday D. Planar lamellar refractive keratoplasty. *J Refract Surg.* 1986;2:17–24.

55. Colin J, Mimouni F, Robinet A. The surgical treatment of high myopia: comparison of epikeratoplasty, keratomileusis and minus power anterior chamber lenses. *Refract Corneal Surg.* 1990;6:245–251.

56. Bas AM, Nano HD. In-situ myopic keratomileusis results in 30 eyes at 15 months. *Refract Corneal Surg.* 1991;7: 223–231.

57. Arenas-Archila E, Sanchez-Thorin JC, et al. Myopic keratomileusis in situ: a preliminary report. *J Cataract Refract Surg.* 1991;17:424–435.

58. Hofmann RF, Bechara SJ. An independent evaluation of second generation suction microkeratomes. *Refract Corneal Surg.* 1992;8:348–354.

59. Peyman GA, Badaro RM, Khoobehi B. Corneal ablation in rabbits using an infrared (2.9-mm) erbium:YAG laser. *Ophthalmology.* 1989;96:1160–1169.

60. Pallikaris IG, Papatzanaki ME, Stathi EZ, et al. Laser in situ keratomileusis. *Lasers Surg Med.* 1990;10:463–468.

61. Marshall J, Trokel SL, Rothery S, et al. Long term healing of the central cornea after photorefractive keratectomy using an excimer laser. *Ophthalmology.* 1998;95:1411–1421.

62. Tuft SJ, Zabel RW, Marshall J. Corneal repair following keratectomy. *Invest Ophthalmol Vis Sci.* 1989;30:1769–1777.

63. DelPero RA, Gigstad JE, Roberts AD, et al. A refractive and histopathological study of excimer laser keratectomy in primates. *Am J Ophthalmol.* 1990;109:419–429.

64. Buratto L, Ferrari M, Rama P. Excimer laser intrastromal keratomileusis. *Am J Ophthalmol.* 1992;113:291–295.

65. Slade SG, Ruiz L. A prospective single-center clinical trial to evaluate ALK and ALK combined with PRK using the excimer laser versus PRK alone for the surgical correction of moderate to high myopia. Bogota, Colombia. Unpublished data.

66. Hagen KB, Kim EK, Waring GO. Comparison of excimer laseer and microkeratome myopic keratomileusis in human cadaver eyes. *Refract Corneal Surg.* 1993;9:36–41.

67. American Academy of Ophthalmology. Ophthalmic procedures assessment. Keratophakia and keratomileusis: safety and effectiveness. *Ophthalmology.* 1992;99:1332–1341.

68. Waring GO: FDA Panel recommends conditional approval of excimer laser phototherapeutic keratectomy (PTK). *J Refract Corneal Surg.* 1994;10:77–78.

69. Holladay JT, Prager TC, Ruiz RS, et al. Improving the predictability of intraocular lens power calculations. *Arch Ophthalmol.* 1986;104:539–541.

70. Maguire LJ. Topographical principles in keratorefractive surgery. *Int Ophthalmol Clin.* 1991;31:1–6.

71. Camp JJ, Maguire LJ, Cameron BM, et al. A computer model for the evaluation of the effect of corneal topography on optical performance. *Am J Ophthalmol.* 1990;109: 379–386.

72. Maguire LJ, Bourne WM. Corneal topography of early keratoconus. *Am J Ophthalmol.* 1989;108:107–112.

73. Wilson SE, Lin DTC, Klyce SD, et al. Topographic changes in contact lens induced corneal warpage. *Ophthalmology.* 1990;97:734–744.

74. L'Esperance FA. Photocoagulation of ocular disease: application and technique. In: L'Esperance FA, ed. *Ophthalmic Lasers.* St. Louis, MO: CV Mosby Co; 1989.

75. Slade SG, et al. Keratomileusis in-situ: a prospective evaluation. *Ophthalmology.* 1993; 100(suppl).

76. Klyce SD, Smolek MK. Corneal topography of excimer laser photorefractive keratectomy. *J Cataract Refract Surg.* 1993;19:122–130.

77. American Academy of Ophthalmology. Automated lamellar keratoplasty. *Ophthalmology.* 1996;103:852–861.

CHAPTER 27

The Intrastromal Corneal Ring for the Correction of Myopia

Steven M. Verity ▪ David J. Schanzlin

INTRODUCTION

Several methods of altering the anterior corneal curvature to modify the refractive status of the eye have been advanced during the latter half of the twentieth century. Many of these techniques have incorporated the use of lenses or tissue implanted within the recipient corneal stroma to achieve the desired refractive effect.

Based upon the observations of Ridley and others that shattered pieces of plastic embedded in the corneas of dive bomber pilots were well tolerated, Stone and Herbert implanted annealed methyl methacrylate lenses in the corneal stroma of a series of rabbits.[1] The intralamellar implants were well tolerated with very little host reaction and a clear cornea for up to 2 years postoperatively. However, the problem of late extrusion of the implant prevented further development of this technique.

Krawicz introduced a technique to increase the refractive power of the cornea by implanting a small plastic lens within the corneal stroma for a period of 8 to 10 days.[2] The refractive effect of the implanted lens persisted after removal of the implant. Patients who underwent this procedure prior to cataract extraction tolerated the implant with no signs of undue irritation and maintained a clear cornea.

Belau and colleagues evaluated the clinical and histologic performance of several different materials implanted within the stroma of dogs for 7 to 155 days.[3] While silicone appeared to be the most suitable material, the polymethyl methacrylate (PMMA) lenses were also well tolerated. A slight peripheral haze was noted along the edges of the lenses in some animals. The authors concluded that this was due to a separation of the stromal surfaces, creating a space that was filled with new tissue. Histologically, there appeared to be minimal reaction to the implanted lenses.

Barraquer introduced the concept of intrastromal lenses composed of lathed corneal tissue.[4] The corneal lenticule was placed in the recipient stroma by means of a microkeratome resection. Although clinical studies utilizing this technique demonstrated adequate accuracy of refractive corrections, the period of visual rehabilitation after surgery was prolonged. Most patients required a year or longer to achieve a final, optimal visual acuity.[5] In addition, the complexity of the equipment and its high cost prevented widespread acceptance of this technique.

The contributions of Barraquer and an increased understanding of the principles of corneal topography led to the development of modern keratorefractive surgery. Previous studies, which demonstrated the feasibility of implanting plastic and tissue lenses within the corneal stroma, also verified the justification of intrastromal techniques to effect a change in the refractive status of the eye. However, all of these techniques require surgical intervention within the patient's visual axis. Long-term changes in the extracellular matrix caused by the disruption of collagen associated with keratectomy contribute to an extended period of visual rehabilitation after surgery.[6]

In 1987, Krasnov introduced a surgical technique that he called "circling keratorrhaphy."[7] In this procedure, a buried intracorneal suture was placed circumferentially that measured from 6 to 8 mm in diameter. The curvature at the corneal center was steepened by a peripheral ring of traction forces from the midperiphery toward the corneal center. When applied at the time of cataract extraction surgery in six patients, a central corneal steepening from 5.2 to 5.6 diopters was obtained. The initial effect decayed with time as the 9-0 nylon suture gradually eroded through the tissue.

The ideal intrastromal keratorefractive procedure should produce a change in the anterior corneal curvature without violating the central visual axis. Furthermore, the procedure should be reversible so that the corneal curvature returns to baseline levels upon removal of the implant.

Fleming and Reynolds et al introduced the intrastromal corneal ring (ICR) as a refractive device with the potential to correct myopic and hyperopic refractive errors.[8] The ICR device (Kera Vision, Inc, Fremont, CA) used in this study consisted of a PMMA ring with an outside diameter of 10.9 mm and an inside diameter of 9.4 mm. The ring was inserted in rabbit corneas at two thirds total stromal depth, utilizing a channeling device to create an intrastromal channel.[9] Significant central corneal flattening occurs as a result of the ICR thickness.[10] An average of 3.5 D of corneal flattening is obtained with ICRs of 0.31-mm thickness in eye bank eyes.

A phase I clinical trial/feasibility study in nonfunctional eyes, conducted under an investigational device exemption granted by the Food and Drug Administration, was initiated in July 1991 at Saint Louis University Health Sciences Center (St. Louis, MO). Ten patients each received the ICR implant in one eye and were followed for at least 1 year.[11] Based on the results of the phase I trial, patients were selected for a multicenter, phase II, sighted-eye trial of the ICR for mild to moderate myopia.

SURGICAL TECHNIQUE

The basic technique for implantation of the ICR has been published elsewhere.[10] In general, the procedure may be performed under general or topical anesthesia in cooperative patients. The visual axis is marked by in-

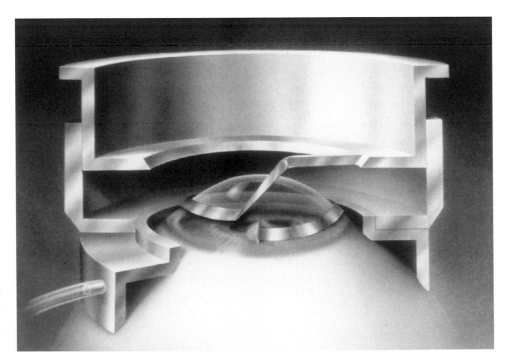

Figure 27–1. Artist's rendering of vacuum fixation device applied to the surface of the globe with stromal separator tool dissecting the intrastromal channel.

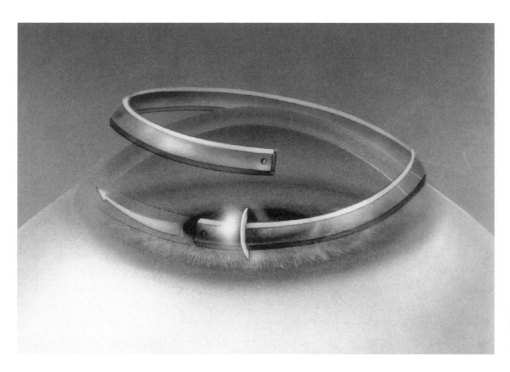

Figure 27–2. Artist's rendering of intrastromal corneal ring being dialed into the prepared intrastromal channel.

dentation of the epithelium with a Sinskey hook (Storz Instruments, St. Louis, MO). The peripheral corneal thickness is measured over the incision site at the 12 o'clock limbus by ultrasonic pachymetry. A diamond knife set to 66% of the peripheral corneal thickness is used to create an incision that will allow introduction of the channeling tool. A Suarez spreader (Storz Instruments) is used to create a small lamellar dissection. The intrastromal channel is created with a proprietary set of instruments (Kera Vision, Inc, Fremont, CA). A vacuum-centering device is applied to the globe. A stromal separator tool is then introduced through the incision in the clockwise direction to produce a 360° intrastromal channel in the midperipheral cornea (Fig 27–1) The suction fixation device is then removed, and the ICR is dialed into the intrastromal channel (Fig 27–2). The leading and trailing edges of the ICR are then sutured together with 10-0 Prolene™ suture. The corneal incision is closed with 10-0 nylon sutures. A bandage soft contact lens is placed on the eye for comfort and to aid in postop healing of the incision site.

RESULTS OF CLINICAL TRIAL WITH THE ICR

Nonfunctional Eye Study

In order to evaluate the safety and efficacy of the intrastromal corneal ring, a phase I clinical trial was initi-

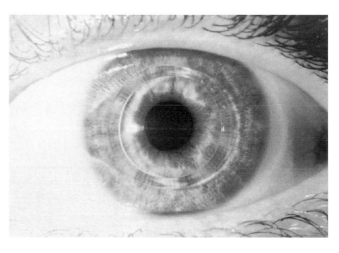

Figure 27–3. Nonfunctional eye patient 1 year after implantation of the ICR.

ated in July 1991. In this study, 10 patients each underwent surgical implantation of the ICR in one nonfunctional eye and were followed for at least 1 year.[11]

The ICR was well tolerated in all patients with no complications that necessitated its removal (Fig 27–3). There were no problems with wound healing after implantation of the device. There were no instances of implant extrusion, undue inflammation, or stromal thinning throughout the 12-month follow-up period.

Five patients developed a corneal epithelial iron line concentric with the ring's inner margin, inferiorly.[12] Three of the five patients had planned explants, and the pattern of iron deposition was noted to disappear or revert to a typical Hudson–Stähli type pattern within 3 months of the ICR's removal.

At the 12-month follow-up period, the ICR was noted to induce a mean keratometric flattening of 2.5 ± 1.1 D, compared with the preimplant average keratometry. Similarly, the retinoscopic spherical equivalence was reduced by an average of −2.4 ± 1.0 D. The keratometrically determined refractive effect of the ICR appeared stable throughout the follow-up period, with no evidence of progression or regression.

In order to evaluate the reversibility of the keratorefractive effect of ICR implantation, five of the ICRs in this nonfunctional eye study were explanted.[13] All five ICRs were easily removed without intraop complications, postop complications, or sequelae. Three months after removal of the ICR, the average change from preop keratometric spherical equivalent was −0.7 ± 0.3 D. The average change from the preop retinoscopic spherical equivalent was +0.1 ± 0.2 D. Longer-term follow-up after explantation of the ICR device has demonstrated that the reversal of ICR-induced keratorefractive effects is stable. One year after removal, the average change from the preop keratometric spherical equiva-

lent was −0.6 ± 0.5 D, and the average change in retinoscopic spherical equivalent was +0.09 ± 0.3 D[14] (Figs 27–4, 27–5).

Sighted Eye Study

Because the ICR was so well tolerated in the phase I study, and explantation of the device produced essentially complete reversal of the ICR-induced keratorefractive effects, a multicenter phase II sighted eye study in 90 patients was begun.

The first five myopic patients had preop refractive errors ranging from −2.75 to −3.75 D, and they underwent implantation of the ICR in one eye. All procedures were performed by one surgeon (DJS). All patients had a preop best-corrected spectacle visual acuity of 20/20 or better. Implanted ICRs measured 7.7 mm in outer diameter and 0.3 mm in sagittal thickness. Each patient participated in a routine follow-up schedule that included computer-assisted topographic analysis, manifest refraction, keratometry, and slit lamp biomicroscopy.

After 2 months of follow-up, four patients had an uncorrected visual acuity (UCVA) of 20/20 or better.

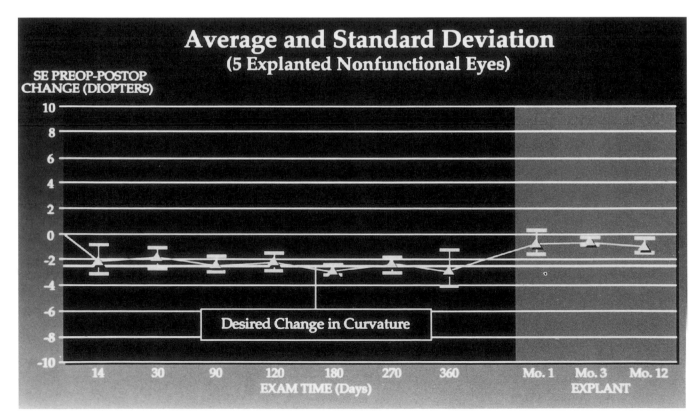

Figure 27–4. Average keratometric change after implantation and after explantation in five nonfunctional eyes.

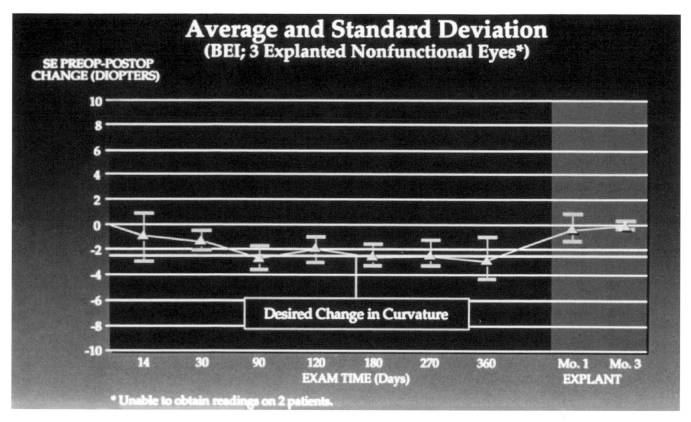

Figure 27–5. Average retinoscopic change after implantation and after explantation in five nonfunctional eyes. Note return to baseline levels after explantation.

The fifth patient had a UCVA of 20/50. This patient was noted to have a mild dehiscence of the wound at the ring insertion site, accounting for the poor UCVA. All patients retained a best-corrected spectacle visual acuity of 20/20 or better. The ICR produced a flattening of the keratometric spherical equivalence by an average of 1.62 ± 0.36 D. Myopic spherical equivalence, as determined by refraction, was reduced by an average of 1.97 ± 0.57 D in this group of patients. Significant findings in slit lamp biomicroscopy included faint peripheral corneal haze within the intrastromal channel and occasional gelatinous-appearing opacities, usually within the ICR suture holes. The peripheral haze is a consequence of stromal separation by the channeling tool; it fades with postop healing and does not appear to be clinically significant.

Brazil Sighted Eye Study

Longer-term follow-up data in sighted eyes is available from investigators at the São Paulo, Brazil, study site.[15] Ten patients with preop refractive errors ranging from −2.63 to −4.25 D underwent implantation of the intra-stromal corneal ring. In one early patient, a posterior corneal perforation was noted upon dissection of the stromal channel. Although the ICR was successfully inserted in this patient, the postop period was complicated by persistent focal corneal edema leading to excessive astigmatism and poor visual acuity. The ICR was explanted after 6 months of follow-up, with return of BCVA of 20/20.

For the remaining nine patients, the average reduction in myopic spherical equivalence as determined by manifest refraction was −2.25 ± 0.54 D at the 12-month follow-up period. All nine patients had a UCVA of 20/40 or better. All patients maintained a BCVA of 20/20 or better throughout the study period.

Two patients developed an infiltrate at the corneal incision site during the early postop follow-up period. These were successfully managed with topical antibiotic therapy without any untoward sequelae. Notable slit lamp findings included peripheral corneal haze along the stromal channel. This haze decreased with time and was not visually significant. Deposits were also noted within the lamellar channel, but they were nonprogressive and noninflammatory in nature. The

ICR implant was well tolerated without migration or extrusion throughout the 1-year follow-up period.

DISCUSSION

The results of ongoing studies of the safety and efficacy of the intrastromal corneal ring have verified the potential of this device as a method to alter the anterior corneal curvature and refractive status of the eye. The polymethyl methacrylate material of which the ring is composed appears to be very well tolerated, as demonstrated in both early and recent studies.[1,3,16] Long-term data with over 1 year of follow-up in nonfunctional eyes have demonstrated that the ICR is well tolerated without signs of corneal decompensation or extrusion of the device.[11,17] The surgical procedure does not cause substantial disruption of stromal collagen, nor does the ring produce deleterious alterations in the nutritional or metabolic activity in the cornea.[18] Analysis of deposits on the surface of explanted rings demonstrates that active stromal remodeling occurs as a re-

sult of normal corneal wound-healing mechanisms following ICR insertion. Scanning electron microscopy demonstrates that the deposits appear to be composed of somewhat disorganized fibrillar collagen. Wound-healing proteoglycans have also been identified within the stromal channels.[19]

There have been no significant alterations of intraocular pressure (IOP) associated with the ICR. Experimental studies have shown that placement of the ICR device does not interfere with accurate measurement of IOP. Additionally, there is no alteration in the facility of outflow associated with the ICR.[20]

The refractive effect of the ICR, as determined by keratometry and retinoscopy in nonfunctional eyes and by keratometry and manifest refraction in sighted eyes, appears to be remarkably stable without trends toward regression or progression of effect.[11,15,17] In this regard, the ICR appears to yield more favorable results than other keratorefractive procedures designed to flatten the anterior corneal curvature.[21]

Results of ICR implantation in sighted eyes have demonstrated improvement in UCVA in all patients. A

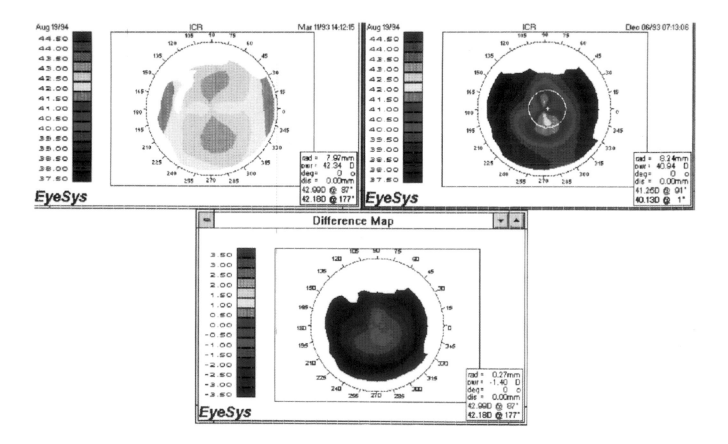

Figure 27–6. Computer-assisted corneal topographic data 9 months after implantation of ICR (sighted eye study). Note reduction of central corneal power and maintenance of normal anatomic positive asphericity.

unique feature of the ICR, compared with other keratorefractive surgical procedures, is the alteration of the corneal refractive power, reducing myopia, while maintaining physiologic corneal asphericity (Fig 27–6). This feature has been associated with better optical performance of the eye.[22] While refractive and visual acuity data may be good in many keratorefractive procedures, studies of topography and raytracing analysis have shown that topographic irregularities may be consistent with good visual acuity at the expense of other measures of optical performance.[23,24] The normal anatomic positive asphericity of the cornea is maintained with the ICR.[10] Studies with computer-assisted corneal topographic analysis have demonstrated that implantation of the ICR resulted in significant corneal flattening and no significant change in asphericity.[25] With the capacity to preserve physiologic corneal asphericity, the ICR may yield superior optical performance without the degradation of visual images and reduction of contrast sensitivity associated with other keratorefractive surgical procedures.[26]

The potential advantages of the ICR over other keratorefractive procedures include maintenance of positive asphericity, avoidance of surgical intervention in the central optical axis, maintenance of corneal integrity, stability of the refractive effect, and a reversible refractive effect. Additionally, it may be possible to titrate the keratorefractive effect of the ICR by performing exchange procedures with ICRs of different design parameters.

Although further studies are necessary, the intrastromal corneal ring appears to be a viable alternative in the surgical correction of refractive errors.

REFERENCES

1. Stone W, Herbert E. Experimental study of plastic material as a replacement for the cornea. A preliminary report. Part 2. *Am J Ophthalmol.* 1953;36:168–173.

2. Krawicz T. New plastic operation for correcting the refractive error of aphakic eyes by changing the corneal curvature. *Br J Ophthalmol.* 1961;45:59–63.

3. Belau PO, Dyer JA, Ogle KN, Hendersson JW. Correction of ametropia with intracorneal lenses. *Arch Ophthalmol.* 1964;72:541–549.

4. Barraquer JI. *Refractive Keratoplasty.* Bogota, Columbia: Instituto Barraquer de America; 1970: vol 1.

5. Troutman RC. Indication, techniques, and complications of keratophakia. In: Binder PS, ed. Refractive Corneal Surgery: The Correction of Aphakia, Hyperopia, and Myopia. *Int Ophthalmol Clin.* 1983;3:11–23.

6. Rawe IM, Tuft SJ, Meek KM. Proteoglycan and collagen morphology in superficially scarred rabbit cornea. *Histochem J.* 1992;24:311.

7. Krasnov MM. Circling keratorrhaphy: a new approach to surgical correction of aphakia. Preliminary communication. *Ann Ophthalmol.* 1987;19:423–427.

8. Fleming JF, Reynolds AE, Kilmer L, Burris TE, Abbott RL, Schanzlin DJ. The intrastromal corneal ring: two cases in rabbits. *J Refract Surg.* 1987;3:227–232.

9. Fleming JF, Wan LW, Schanzlin DJ. The theory of corneal curvature change with the intrastromal corneal ring. *CLAO J.* 1989;15:146–150.

10. Burris TE, Ayer CT, Evensen DA, Davenport JM. Effects of intrastromal corneal ring size and thickness on corneal flattening in human eyes. *Refract Corneal Surg.* 1991; 7:46–50.

11. Assil KK, Barrett AM, Fouraker BD, Schanzlin DJ, et al. One-year results of the intrastromal corneal ring in nonfunctional human eyes. *Arch Ophthalmol.* 1995;113:159–167.

12. Assil KK, Quantock AJ, Barrett AM, Schanzlin DJ. Corneal iron lines associated with the intrastromal corneal ring. *Am J Ophthalmol.* 1993;116:350–356.

13. Schanzlin DJ, Assil KK, et al. Corneal curvature analysis following explantation of the intrastromal corneal ring. *Invest Ophthalmol Vis Sci.* 1993;34(suppl):1240.

14. Schanzlin DJ, Assil KK, Barrett AM, Verity SM, et al. Corneal curvature analysis following explantation of the intrastromal corneal ring. *Ophthalmology.* 1993;100(suppl):126.

15. Nose W, Neves RA, Burris TE, Schanzlin DJ, Belfort R. The intrastromal corneal ring: twelve month sighted eye study. *Refract Corneal Surg.* Submitted.

16. D'Hermies F, Hartmann C, von Ey F, Holzkamper C, Renard G, Pouliguen V. Biocompatibility of a refractive intracorneal PMMA ring. *Fortschr Ophthalmol.* 1991;88: 790–793.

17. Nose W, Neves RA, Schanzlin DJ, Belfort R: Intrastromal corneal ring—one year results of first implants in humans: a preliminary nonfunctional eye study. *Refract Corneal Surg.* 1993;9:452–458.

18. Quantock AJ, Kincaid MC, Schanzlin DJ. Stromal healing following explantation of the intrastromal corneal ring. *Arch Ophthalmol.* 1995;113:208–209.

19. Quantock AJ, Assil KK, Schanzlin DJ. An electron microscopic evaluation of intrastromal corneal rings explanted from nonfunctional human eyes. *Refract Corneal Surg.* 1994;10:142–148.

20. Kreisberg AL, Barcolions N, Asbell PA. Intraocular pressure and the intrastromal corneal ring. *Refract Corneal Surg.* 1991;7:303–307.

21. Goosey JD, Prager TC, Goosey C, et al. Stability of refraction during two years after myopic epikeratoplasty. *Refract Corneal Surg.* 1990;6:4–8.

22. Patel S, Marshall J, Fitgke FW. Model for predicting the optical performance of the eye in refractive surgery. *Refract Corneal Surg.* 1993;9:366–375.

23. Maguire U, Klyce SD, Singer DE, et al. Corneal topography in myopic patients undergoing epikeratophakia. *Am J Ophthalmol.* 1987;103:404–416.

24. Maguire U, Zabel RW, Parker P, et al. Topography and ray-tracing analysis of patients with excellent visual acuity 3 months after excimer laser photorefractive keratectomy for myopia. *Refract Corneal Surg.* 1991;7:122–128.

25. Assil KK, Verity SM, Barrett AM, Schanzlin DJ, et al. The effects of intrastromal corneal ring implantation on corneal asphericity. In preparation.

26. Baron WS, Munnerlyn C. Predicting visual performance following excimer photorefractive keratectomy. *Refract Corneal Surg.* 1992;8:355–362.

CHAPTER 28

Intracorneal Alloplastic Inclusions

Johnny M. Khoury ▪ Dimitri T. Azar ▪ Tat Keong Chan

INTRODUCTION

Lamellar refractive surgical procedures that add tissue to the cornea include keratophakia, keratomileusis, epikeratophakia, and alloplastic lenticular implants. These procedures require lamellar keratectomy and have one common disadvantage: the difficulty of microkeratome resection. Furthermore, keratophakia, keratomileusis, and epikeratophakia have additional drawbacks.[1-4] Keratophakia uses a human donor cornea (lenticule) to produce an increase in the anterior curvature of the recipient cornea. The lenticule must be stained, frozen, lathed, and thawed before being replaced in an interlamellar pocket. The procedure has two optical interfaces and can correct up to 17 diopters. Both the donor and the recipient cornea undergo microkeratome sectioning. Keratomileusis requires cryolathing of the host cornea and can correct a maximum of 10 to 12 D. Moreover, the lenticule needs to be prepared intraoperatively, which increases the technical difficulty of the procedure. Epikeratophakia, designed to eliminate microkeratome resection of the recipient cornea, requires a donor cornea (as does keratophakia) and can correct 20 D. The replaced cornea's position anterior to the recipient cornea may lead to corneal epithelial healing problems.

The use of alloplastic lenticules has certain theoretical advantages over previous procedures: the unlimited supply, availability of prelathed lenticules, reducing of the potential risk of opacification, relative incompressibility compared with corneal tissue, standardized optical quality, and the capability of correcting large refractive errors.

Despite these advantages, at least two conditions remain to be fulfilled before "alloplastic keratophakia" gains approval: refining the lamellar keratectomy technique and finding the "ideal lens."

BACKGROUND

In 1949, José Barraquer described the inclusion of a lenticule within the corneal stroma to modify ametropia.[5] He speculated that the lenticule would modify both the anterior curvature of the cornea and the cornea's index of refraction. He first experimented with Flint glass lenses and later used transparent plastic (Plexiglas™). Because all the lenses were badly tolerated by the cornea and extruded, he abandoned the use of alloplastic materials, believing the best material for inclusion in the cornea to be the corneal parenchyma itself; he named the procedure *keratophakia*, from the Greek κερατοειλης, cornea, and φακος, lens.

Based on Barraquer's earlier work, Werblin (1980) and Kaufman (1981) developed the concept of epikeratophakia.[4,6] Although this form of lamellar refractive surgery is potentially reversible, as well as technically simpler than keratophakia and keratomileusis (pioneered by Barraquer), it is relatively unpredictable, requires months for full visual rehabilitation, and demands a normal anterior surface for its maintenance. With epikeratophakia, as with keratophakia and keratomileusis, a major difficulty exists in the preop analysis of the power and configuration of the lathed corneal lenses.

In an attempt to overcome some of these problems, researchers have turned to the potential use of alloplastic materials as intrastromal inclusions.

PRINCIPLES OF INTRACORNEAL LENSES

There are three major refracting surfaces in the eye: the anterior corneal surface and the two surfaces of the crystalline lens. The effect of the posterior corneal surface is negligible because the difference in refractive index between corneal stroma and aqueous humor is insignificant. The cornea, which has a refractive power three times that of the crystalline lens (approximately + 43 D compared with + 19 D for the crystalline lens), is an extremely important refracting element in the eye. The greater refractive power of the cornea is due to the difference in refractive index between air (1.000) and cornea (1.376), compared with the refractive index between aqueous and vitreous humour (1.336) and lens (1.406).

Intracorneal lenses (ICLs) affect the refractive power of the cornea in two ways: (1) by altering the radius of curvature of the anterior corneal surface and (2) by altering the refractive index of the cornea.[7,8] Alloplastic materials whose refractive indexes approximate corneal stroma affect refraction only when used in combination with a 360° lamellar keratectomy using a microkeratome dissection. This causes a significant change in the anterior corneal curvature, thus altering refraction. The reason for this effect becomes evident with the following example.

Figure 28–1 represents the surface powers of the cornea and a hydrogel implant. The hydrogel intracorneal lens (70% water content and 1.3853 refractive index) has a diopteric power of 15 at the surface interface in air (refractive index, 1.000). Located at mid-depth within the stroma, the ICL (with a 6-mm diameter) will have a total surface power of just 0.3 D because of the minor refractive index difference between the hydrogel (1.3853) and the stroma (1.376). Yet, when the lens is implanted on the bed of a microkeratome dissection, it can create a 12.2 D change in the corneal power by steep-

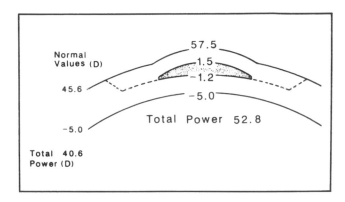

Figure 28–1. Surface powers of the cornea with a hydrogel implant. The power change induced by the implant is secondary to the anterior corneal curvature change. *(From McCarey BE. Current status of refractive surgery with synthetic intracorneal lenses: Barraquer lecture. Refract Corneal Surg. 1990;6[1]:40–46.)*

ening the anterior corneal curvature from 45.6 to 57.5 D. The anterior corneal curvature must undergo appreciable large alterations over a small optical zone to provide the necessary wide range of refractive corrections.

In this example, the cornea was steepened from a 7.4-mm radius to a 5.9-mm radius in order to create a 12.2 D change. A range of corneal refraction corrections from +20 to −20 D would require modification of the anterior curvature radius from 5.23 mm (64.5 D) to 12.35 mm (27.3 D), respectively, as determined with Watsky's algorithm.[8,9]

Based on elementary optical principles, Watsky and colleagues devised an algorithm to calculate the total corneal diopteric power change produced by a change in corneal thickness as a result of the implantation of a hydrogel ICL.[10] For example, a hyperopic implant designed to have a 5-mm–diameter, 0.001-mm edge thickness, 7.25-mm base radius, and 1.376 refractive index (equal to the cornea), and located at mid-depth in the cornea, will be effective in altering the corneal surface power by 1 D for each 11.3 μm of central implant thickness (Fig 28–2A). The preop corneal curvature was assumed to be 7.5 mm. A myopic implant will have minimal central thickness. In the example, we can set the central thickness to be 0.0001 mm and let the edge thickness increase according to the desired diopteric alteration of the cornea. Figure 28–2B demonstrates a 10-μm implant edge thickness per diopter of corneal refractive change.[9,18]

Materials with a refractive index greater than that of corneal stroma are effective in a freehand intralamellar pocket dissection. Using an ICL of the appropriate power, the original refractive error of the eye is cor-

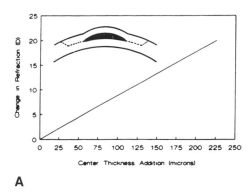

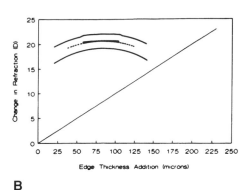

A   **B**

Figure 28–2. A. Relation between the change in stromal thickness over a 5-mm optical zone (OZ) of the cornea and the resulting refractive alteration of 11.3 μm/D. This value will be different for each OZ selected. **B.** A 10-μm implant edge thickness per diopter of corneal refractive change. *(From McCarey BE. Refractive keratoplasty with synthetic lens implants. Int Ophthalmol Clin. 1991;31[1]:87–99.)*

rected by a change in the inherent power of the lens itself, rather than by a change in the corneal curvature.[7,8]

PHYSIOLOGIC CONCERNS

Corneal clarity and thickness are determined by a corneal hydration control mechanism, which is a sodium-activated adenosine triphosphatase (ATPase) pump located in the endothelium (Fig 28–3). An impermeable ICL (such as one made of polysulfone) has the potential of causing corneal edema anterior to its location in the cornea. Fluid movement in and across the corneal stroma is significant not only for hydration control but also for corneal nutrition. The normal cornea is free of blood vessels and thus must receive and remove nutri-

ents via diffusion across the stroma. The three surfaces across which diffusion can take place are the anterior and posterior surfaces of the cornea and the limbus. The main source of nutrition is the aqueous humour, which supplies nutrients like glucose by diffusion through the posterior surface of the cornea. The limbus blood supply, as a route of corneal substance turnover, is significant to the cornea and extends in a peripheral ring 0.5 to 1.0 mm into the cornea. Central to this zone, diffusion through the posterior corneal surface is dominant.[8]

Based on these physiologic considerations, the ideal ICL would contain an inlay material that is (1) adequately permeable to metabolites like oxygen and glucose in solution, (2) of proven biocompatibility, (3) of high refractive index (so that inlays are as thin as possible because the thickness of the implant is inversely

The Corneal Environment Surrounding an ICL

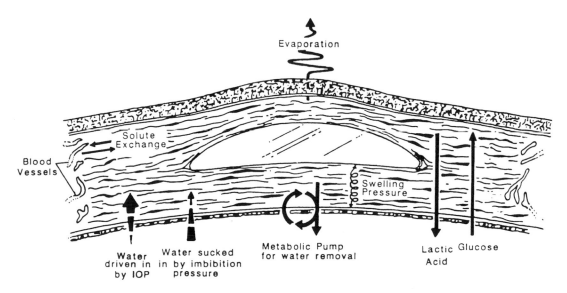

Figure 28–3. Stromal hydration is controlled passively via water evaporation from tear film and a metabolic pump located in the endothelium. The implant should not affect the movement of water or nutrients, stromal pH, osmolarity, or stromal swelling pressures. IOP = intraocular pressure. *(From McCarey BE. Refractive keratoplasty with synthetic lens implants. Int Ophthalmol Clin. 1991;31[1]:87–99.)*

proportional to the glucose diffusion through the implants), and (4) of good optical quality.[11]

Knowles and other investigators have demonstrated the importance of water and nutrient movement across the cornea from the aqueous humor using impermeable ICLs.[12] Brown and Mishima further observed that, within the cornea, an aqueous-to-tear movement of water was created by an increase in tear tonicity caused by evaporation during the intervals between blinks.[13] A water-impermeable intrastromal implant will therefore prevent the aqueous-to-stroma movement of water and will result in excessive concentration of the tear film, stromal thinning anterior to the implant, and epithelial and stromal breakdown (Fig 28–4). Maurice, in 1967, analyzed the epithelial glucose availability with an impermeable ICL material using a mathematical model.[14] He showed that implants larger than 4 mm in diameter, when placed in corneas of rabbit eyes, would lead to glucose starvation of the central epithelium anterior to the implant, eventually causing anterior stromal ulceration (Fig 28–5). Based on the experience of Knowles[12] and of Dohlman and Brown,[15] Maurice concluded that 5 mm was the maximum diameter for safe implantation of impermeable discs in

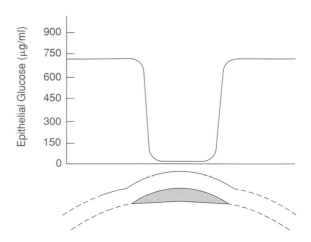

Figure 28–5. An impermeable ICL of 4 mm in diameter results in significant depletion of epithelial glucose. *(From Maurice DM. Nutritional aspects of corneal grafts and prosthesis. In: Raycroft PV, ed.* Corneo-plastic Surgery: Proceedings of the Second International Corneo-Plastic Conference, London, 1967. *New York: Pergamon Press; 1969:197–207.)*

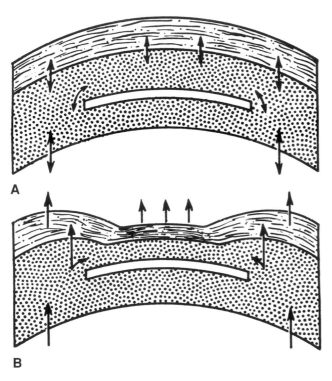

A

B

Figure 28–4. Illustration of water movement across intracorneal implants. **A.** Lids closed. **B.** Lids open. *Arrows* indicate direction of water movement. *(From Brown et al. Effect of intralamellar water impermeable membranes on corneal hydration.* Arch Ophthalmol. *1966;76:702–708.)*

humans. Therefore, with impermeable intrastromal implants, the diameter of the lens is crucial.

Fenestrations that allow nutrients to pass from the aqueous humor through the ICL to the anterior cornea greatly improve the safety margin of impermeable substances like polysulfone as an ICL material. However, microfenestrated lenses are required to maintain optical clarity, which makes the manufacturing process difficult and complex.[7,16]

In summary, the ICL material should not alter the posterior-to-anterior movement of water and nutrients. Furthermore, the implant should not interfere with the anterior-to-posterior movement of lactic acid from the epithelium. In addition, the stromal fluid pH, osmolarity, and stromal swelling pressures should not affect the stability of the lens material within the cornea.

LENSES

Early Nonpermeable Lenses

After experimenting on rabbits and cats using flint glass and Plexiglas implants in 1949, Barraquer found a poor tolerance to these lenses.[5] The implants resulted in anterior stromal necrosis, followed by extrusion of the implant. However, the posterior layer of the cornea, situated behind the lenticule, remained transparent.

In their search for an ideal intracorneal lens, Choyce, Belau, Krwawicz, Knowles, and others experimented with different lens materials (Table 28–1).

demonstrated the long-term (8.5 and 8 years, respectively) biocompatibility of hydrogel ICLs in nonhuman primates (Fig 28–8). The major histopathologic finding was some epithelial thinning over the implants.

In 1992, Werblin et al reported the first human experience with myopic Permalens hydrogel ICL implants (18 months' follow-up).[27] All surgeries were performed by José Barraquer in Bogotá, Colombia. Excellent corneal clarity was reported throughout the follow-up period (Fig 28–9). No decentration of the lenticule following implantation was observed. Corrections of up to −13 D were achieved. Corrections deviated from the predicted correction by a mean of −5.00 ± 2.10 D (range, −2.80 to −8.00 D). Visual recovery was rapid, usually achieving maximum acuity within 1 month. The major problem encountered in the study was the significant undercorrection of the preop refraction.

Polysulfone Lenses (Impermeable)

Polysulfone, a thermoplastic first synthesized in 1965 from Bisphenol A and 4,4′-dichlorophenylsulfone, is

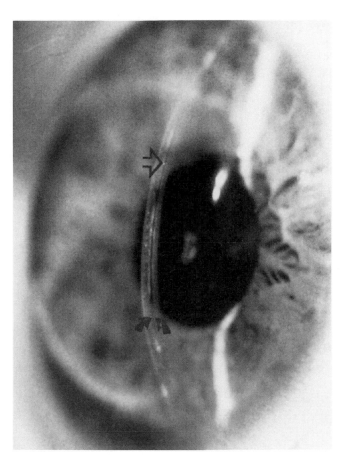

Figure 28–9. Hydrogel ICL in a human subject 4 months postop. The hydrogel appears as an optically void area at midstromal depth *(dark arrows).* One or two interface opacities can be seen *(open arrow)*, but the overall appearance of the cornea is very clear. *(From Werblin et al. Initial human experience with Permelens myopic hydrogel intracorneal lens implants.* Refract Corneal Surg. *1992;8[1]:23–26.)*

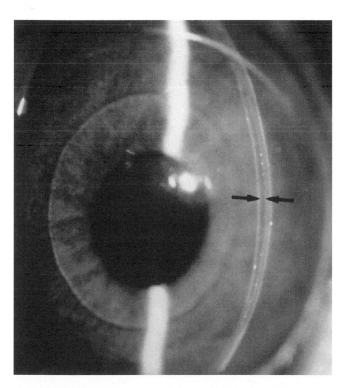

Figure 28–8. Nonhuman primate with hyperopic Permalens ICL in place, 7 years postop. The deep stromal position of the optically void hydrogel is demonstrated *(between arrows).* The surrounding cornea is clear with minimal interface debris. *(From Werblin et al. Eight years experience with Permalens intracorneal lenses in nonhuman primates.* Refract Corneal Surg. *1992;8[1]:12–22.)*

used as a microporous membrane in plasma separation. It is also used as an attachment vehicle for orthopedic and dental implants and has proven biocompatibility. In addition, polysulfone has excellent optical qualities and is sterilizable with wet and dry heat. A unique characteristic of polysulfone is its high refractive index (1.633), which allows the manufacture of very thin optical lenses. The lens is inserted into a pocket in the stroma following a deep lamellar dissection and centered over the visual axis.[8]

Attracted by these qualities, Choyce pioneered the use of this material in 1981 as an ICL for the correction of high refractive errors.[11] An independent retrospective review of Choyce's patients was reported, indicating that the procedure was effective. Complications included incisional scarring, refractile particles at the lens–cornea interface, Descemet's tears, wound dehiscence, blood vessels to the edge of the lens, inter-

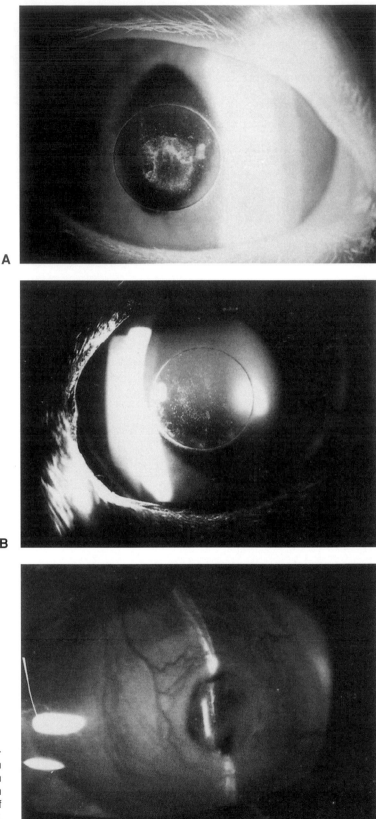

Figure 28–10. A. Clinical photograph of a visually significant nebular opacity. Posterior pole landmarks were not visualized through this opacity with a direct ophthalmoscope. **B.** Clinical photograph of nonvisually significant refractile particles. **C.** Clinical photograph of anterior corneal necrosis and vascularization in the presence of a polysulfone lens. *(From Lane et al. Polysulfone corneal lenses. J Cataract Refract Surg. 1986;12:50–60.)*

face nebular opacities, and irregular astigmatism. Based on Choyce's work, a protocol was established to study prospectively the safety and efficacy of polysulfone ICLs in a laboratory model. Monkeys, baboons, and cats were used to surgically implant 5- to 6-mm-diameter hyperopic and myopic lenses within the corneal stroma. Results of this study showed 70% of the cat corneas (n = 24) maintained clear media by ophthalmoscopic examination at follow-ups ranging from 3 to 6 months. However, complications including interface opacification, interface refractile particles, epithelial dimple formation, irregular astigmatism, anterior corneal necrosis, vascularization, and lens extrusion were encountered (Fig 28–10). The reversibility of polysulfone corneal lenses was also investigated because of these complications. The opacification noted preoperatively was reversed, with only mild, nonvisually significant, midstromal scarring 3 months after removal of the lens. In the baboon model (n = 8), the majority of the procedures were considered failures owing to complications that included lens extrusions, anterior stromal necrosis, interface opacification, and anterior corneal edema with neovascularization. All the monkeys tested (n = 4) tolerated the polysulfone ICL well without any significant complication. When the specimens with nebular opacities and refractile particles were examined histologically, multiple, discrete, oil-red

O-positive deposits were noted at the same corneal depth as the opacities seen clinically. The authors believe that these lipid deposits originated from keratocytes that were compromised as a result of inadequate nutrition anterior to the impermeable ICL.[7,8,28]

The concept of making the lens fenestrated was introduced in an attempt to overcome this barrier of nonpermeability. Five-millimeter fenestrated polysulfone lenses (35-μm fenestrations) were surgically implanted within the corneal stroma of six cats to investigate this hypothesis. An otherwise identical, nonfenestrated 5-mm polysulfone lens was placed at the same corneal depth in the fellow eye. While all the corneas that received a fenestrated lens remained clear, 33% showed peripheral nebular opacification in some areas over the nonfenestrated portion of the lens. One eye had multiple clear areas directly overlying open fenestrations of the peripheral lens within the area of peripheral nebular opacification (Fig 28–11). This supports the hypothesis of nutritional stress as the etiology for the nebular opacification. The clear stromal areas overlying the fenestrations represent adequately nourished cornea surrounded by opaque, inadequately nourished cornea. None of the nonfenestrated lens eyes achieved ophthalmoscopically clear media at 1 year, whereas 100% of the fenestrated eyes showed some degree of interface change. Complications seen in the nonfenestrated lens

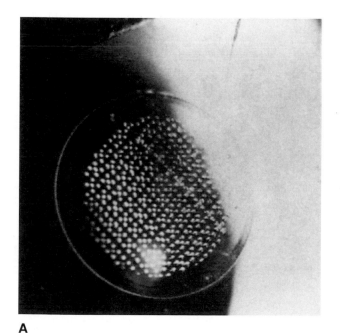

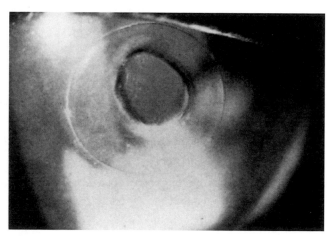

A   **B**

Figure 28–11. A. Fenestrated polysulfone lens in right cornea of a cat with no evidence of interface opacification at 1 year. **B.** Nonfenestrated polysulfone lens in left cornea of a cat with significant central opacities at lens–cornea interface and a large central opacity melt at 1 year. *(From Lane et al. Polysulfone intracorneal lenses.* Refract Corneal Surg. *1990;6[1]:32–37.)*

eyes included nebular interface opacities (100%), refractile particles (100%), anterior thinning (50%), extrusion of lens (33%), vascularization (33%), and anterior corneal necrosis (17%). These complications were not noted in the fenestrated lens group. Histopathologic evaluation of these fenestrated specimens revealed the presence of normal keratocytes and stroma within the fenestrations. The endothelium and epithelium were examined and found to be normal, with no central epithelial thinning or peripheral epithelial thickening.[7]

Although this study indicated that the fenestrations were safe, the lenses proved to be optically unsatisfactory. Both direct ophthalmoscopy and ophthalmoscopic photographs of the cats' posterior poles with the fenestrated lenses in situ revealed a poor view of retinal structures. Theoretically, smaller fenestrations (microfenestration) would prove successful from both an optical and safety standpoint. Results from a pilot series using fenestration diameters of less than 10 μm have been encouraging.[7]

Polymethyl Methacrylate Lenses (Impermeable)

Polymethyl methacrylate (PMMA) is the most widely used material for optical lens construction. PMMA is produced by addition or free radical polymerization of methacrylic acid methylester, which is derived from acrylic acid. Polymethyl methacrylate is light (specific gravity 1.19) and durable, with a high resistance to aging and climatic change. It is as clear as glass and has a refractive index of 1.49. There is no evidence that PMMA degrades within the eye, and it is a time-tested, well-tolerated intraocular lens (IOL) material that has been used extensively for almost four decades.[29]

Recently, polymethyl methacrylate has been used for ICLs. Rodrigues et al, in 1990, evaluated PMMA ICLs (5-mm diameter) in rhesus monkey eyes that were followed for 3 years.[30] Myriad crystalline aggregates in the deep corneal stroma behind the implant were noticed (Fig 28–12). These crystalline deposits stained positively with oil-red O and with filipin, indicating the presence of neutral fat as well as unesterified cholesterol. Electron microscopy revealed dissolved lipid aggregates and laminated electron-dense material that were most abundant posterior to the implant where the keratocytes appeared disintegrated. The authors reported that PMMA lenses appeared to induce lipid keratopathy.

In the same year, Kirkham and Dangel compared a newly designed PMMA intracorneal keratoprosthesis, covalently coated with type 1 collagen, with an identical, uncoated keratoprosthesis in 12 rabbits.[31] Although both keratoprostheses were retained for 15 months, the uncoated implants had more extensive adjacent corneal melting, a greater inflammatory response, and more epithelial downgrowth than their collagen-coated

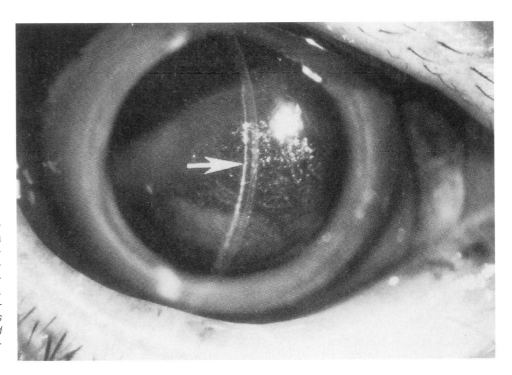

Figure 28–12. Slit lamp biomicroscopic photograph of monkey cornea with PMMA ICL 18 months after surgery shows deposits of whitish crystalline material posterior to the lenticule *(arrow)*. *(From Rodrigues et al. Lipid deposits posterior to impermeable intracorneal lenses in rhesus monkey: clinical, histochemical, and ultrastructural studies.* Refract Corneal Surg. *1990;6[1]:32–37.)*

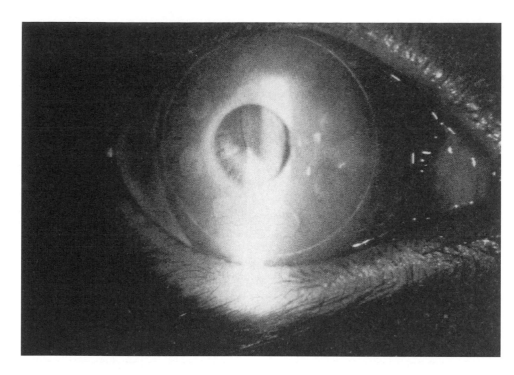

Figure 28–13. Opacification occurring in an uncoated keratoprosthesis 4 months after surgery. *(From Kirkham et al. The keratoprosthesis: improved biocompatability through design and surface modification.* Ophthalmic Surg. *1991;22[8]: 455–461.)*

counterparts (Fig 28–13). Electron microscopy showed that stromal collagen fibers had attached to the surface of the coated implants, but not to the surface of the uncoated ones. The authors reported that intracorneal keratoprostheses covalently coated with type 1 collagen may offer superior biocompatibility and become incorporated into corneal tissues.

CONCLUSION

The use of intracorneal lenses for the correction of refractive errors is a relatively new concept that is still under investigation. Many variables play a crucial role in this surgical procedure, some of which are biocompatibility of the material used, diameter and thickness of the lens, the corneal depth at which the lens is implanted, permeability of the lens with pore diameter when applicable, refractive index of the material used, power (diopters) and shape of the lens, and the specific surgical technique used for lens implantation. Determination of the predictability and long-term outcome of alloplastic intracorneal inclusions is of utmost importance. Ideally, the refractive power correction should be derived from the optics of the implant, comparable to IOL diopteric power correction within the aqueous, and the surgical procedure should be simplified, for example, by using a lamellar pocket dissection or a corneal flap.

REFERENCES

1. Binder PS, Deg JK, Zavala EY, Grossman KR. Hydrogel keratophakia in non-human primates. *Curr Eye Res.* 1981–1982;1(9):S35–S42.
2. Wilson DR, Keeney AH. Corrective measures for myopia. *Surv Ophthalmol.* 1990;34(4):294–304.
3. Binder PS. What's new in the subspecialities? II. Current concepts of lamellar refractive surgery. *Ophthalmic Forum.* 1982;(1):66–67.
4. Werblin TP, Kaufman HE. Epikeratophakia: the surgical correction of aphakia. II. Preliminary results in a non-human primate model. *Curr Eye Res.* 1981;1:131.
5. Barraquer JI. Modification of refraction by means of intracorneal inclusions. *Int Ophthalmol Clin.* 1966;6:53–78.
6. Werblin TP, Kaufman HE. Epikeratophakia: the surgical correction of aphakia. I. Lathing of corneal tissue. *Curr Eye Res.* 1981;1:123.
7. Lane SS, Lindstrom RL. Polysulfone intracorneal lenses. *Refract Corneal Surg.* 1990;6(1):32–37.
8. McCarey BE, Lane SS, Lindstrom RL. Alloplastic corneal lenses. *Int Ophthalmol Clin.* 1988;28:155.
9. McCarey BE. Refractive keratoplasty with synthetic lens implants. *Int Ophthalmol Clin.* 1991;31(1):87–99.
10. Watsky MA, McCarey BE, Beekhuis WH. Predicting refractive alterations with hydrogel keratophakia. *Invest Ophthalmol Vis Sci.* 1985;26:240.
11. Choyce DP. The correction of refractive errors with polysulfone corneal inlays. *Trans Ophthalmol Soc UK.* 1985; 104:332.

12. Knowles WF. Effect of intralamellar plastic membranes on corneal physiology. *Am J Ophthalmol.* 1961;51:1146–1156.

13. Brown SI, Mishima S. Effect of intralamellar water impermeable membranes on corneal hydration. *Arch Ophthalmol.* 1966;76:702–708.

14. Maurice DM. Nutritional aspects of corneal grafts and prosthesis. In: Raycroft PV, ed. *Coreno-Plastic Surgery: Proceedings of the Second International Corneo-Plastic Conference, London, 1967.* New York: Pergamon Press; 1969:197–207.

15. Dohlman CH, Brown S. Treatment of corneal edema with a buried implant. *Trans Am Acad Ophthalmol Otolaryngol.* 1966;70:267–279.

16. Lane SS, Lindstrom RL, Midrup EA, Cameron JD. One year follow-up of fenestrated intracorneal lenses. Complications, reversibility, and histopathology. *Invest Ophthalmol Vis Sci.* 1988;29(suppl):311.

17. Choyce DP. The present status of intracameral and intracorneal implants. *Can J Ophthalmol.* 1968;3:295–311.

18. Choyce DP. Management of endothelial corneal dystrophy with acrylic corneal inlays. *Br J Ophthalmol.* 1965; 49:432.

19. Belau PG, Dyer JA, Ogli KN, et al. Correction of ametropia with intracorneal lenses. *Arch Ophthalmol.* 1964;72: 541–547.

20. McCarey BE. Current status of refractive surgery with synthetic intracorneal lenses: Barraquer lecture. *Refract Corneal Surg.* 1990;6(1):40–46.

21. Dohlman CH, Refojo MF, Rose J. Synthetic polymers in corneal surgery: I. Glyceryl methacrylate. *Arch Ophthalmol.* 1967;77:252–257.

22. Mester U, Heimig D, Dardenne MU. Measurement and calculation of refraction in experimental keratophakia with hydrophilic lenses. *Ophthalmic Res.* 1976;8:111–116.

23. McCarey BE, Andrews DM. Refractive keratoplasty with intrastromal hydrogel lenticular implants. *Invest Ophthalmol Vis Sci.* 1981;21:107–115.

24. Samples JR, Binder PS, Zavala EY, Baumgartner S, Deg JK. Morphology of hydrogel implants used for refractive keratoplasty. *Invest Ophthalmol Vis Sci.* 1984;25:843–850.

25. Parks RA, McCarey BE. Hydrogel keratophakia: long-term morphology in the monkey model. *CLAO J.* 1991; 17(3):216–222.

26. Werblin TP, Priffer RL, Binder PS, McCarey BE, Patel AS. Eight years' experience with Permalens intracorneal lenses in nonhuman primates. *Refract Corneal Surg.* 1992; 8;(1):12–22.

27. Werblin TP, Patel AS, Barraquer JI. Initial human experience with Permalens myopic hydrogel intracorneal lens implants. *Refract Corneal Surg.* 1992;8(1):23–26.

28. Lane SS, Lindstrom RL, Cameron JD, et al. Polysulfone corneal lenses. *J Cataract Refract Surg.* 1986;12:50–60.

29. Apple DJ, Kinkaid MC, Mamalis N, Olson RJ. *Intraocular Lenses: Evolution, Designs, Complications, and Pathology.* Baltimore: Williams & Wilkins; 1989:422–426.

30. Rodrigues MM, McCarey BE, Waring GO, Hidayat AA, Kruth HS. Lipid deposits posterior to impermeable intracorneal lenses in rhesus monkey: clinical, histochemical, and ultrastructural studies. *Refract Corneal Surg.* 1990;6(1): 32–37.

31. Kirkham SM, Dangel ME. The keratoprosthesis: improved biocompatability through design and surface modification. *Ophthalmic Surg.* 1991;22(8):455–461.

CHAPTER 29

Epikeratoplasty

Michael D. Wagoner

Epikeratophakia is a form of onlay lamellar kerato-plasty in which a lens made of human corneal tissue is sutured onto the anterior surface of the cornea to change the anterior curvature and refractive properties of the cornea (Fig 29–1).[1,2] More appropriately referred to as epikeratoplasty (EKP), it was originally introduced by Dr Herbert Kaufman at the Jackson Memorial Lecture at the American Academy of Ophthalmology in 1979[3] as a new form of refractive surgery based on the pioneering work of Joaquin Barraquer[4] in the development of keratophakia and keratomileusis.

Keratophakia, which is used to correct aphakia, and keratomileusis, which is used primarily for the correction of myopia, require dissection and removal of a portion of the central cornea, as well as a technically complex lathing procedure that depends on expensive equipment. The objective of EKP is to provide the refractive benefits of these procedures, but with less cost, technical complexity, and complications. Kaufman accomplished this by recommending the use of a commercially prepared corneal donor lens, or "lenticule," of prespecified dioptric power onto a recipient eye from which the central epithelium has been removed but Bowman's layer has been left undisturbed. By providing commercially prepared lenses, the expense and difficulty of lathing the lenticules is eliminated. By not requiring dissection of the central portion of the recipient cornea, the technical

complexity of the procedure is reduced, as is the risk of interface scarring and opacification. Finally, EKP is potentially reversible because the central cornea is not disturbed by the procedure.

After the introduction of EKP, lenticules were commercially prepared by Allergan Medical Optics and tested at the Department of Ophthalmology at Louisiana State University.[3,5–12] In 1985, a nationwide study was initiated that recruited 234 "general ophthalmologists," who had received an intensive two-day training course, to evaluate the use of EKP for four indications (adult aphakia, pediatric aphakia, myopia, and keratoconus) in preparation for market approval by the US Food and Drug Administration (FDA) for general commercial use.[13–17] Following a discussion of the surgical technique and prognostic factors common to all four indications, the experience of EKP for each of these indications will be discussed separately.

In theory, the use of a commercially prepared lenticule of precise power (or "living contact lens") and the utilization of a surgical technique that provides for complete reversibility in the "worst-case scenario" of lenticule failure for refractive or mechanical reasons should have made EKP the ideal refractive surgical procedure for the correction of both hyperopia and myopia. As will be seen, EKP does have a role in refractive surgery, but the original optimism after its introduction was not fully realized in clinical trials.

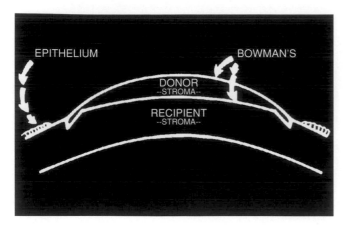

Figure 29–1. Schematic representation of epikeratoplasty. *(Courtesy of Allergan Medical Optics.)*

SURGICAL TECHNIQUE

Patient Selection

The original indication for which EKP was recommended was for contact lens–intolerant, monocularly aphakic adults,[3] in whom secondary intraocular lens implantation was contraindicated.[7,11–12] The indications were later expanded to include the correction of bilateral aphakia in spectacle and contact lens–intolerant adults,[2,14,18–22] pediatric aphakia,[16–17,20,21,23–32] phakic hypermetropia,[33] and myopia.[2,15,20,21,34–39] Finally, it was introduced for the treatment of keratoconus[1,5,6,13,20,21,40–47] and other ectatic corneal disorders.[48–51]

Donor Lenticule

All EKP lenticules used in the original studies were commercially prepared (Allergan Medical Optics, Irvine, CA). The corneal tissue was supplied by eye banks and had been stored in McCarey–Kaufman medium for 4 to 14 days prior to processing. The tissue was screened by eye banks based on the same criteria used for the selection of routine penetrating keratoplasty; however, the EKP lenticules were made from tissue deemed unsuitable for penetrating keratoplasty (PKP) because of inadequate endothelial cell counts, length of storage, or other reasons. To prepare the lenticule, the donor tissue (Bowman's layer and anterior stroma) is stained with a temporary dye to enhance visibility, lyophilized, lathed to a specified power based upon the patient's spherical equivalent corrected to the corneal plane (with the exception of keratoconus, which was lathed to plano power), placed in a vacuum-sealed container (Fig 29–2), and shipped to the surgeon within 2

months of the date of manufacture.[13–17] The most recent designs use a 8.5-mm donor lenticule for aphakia and myopia, and a 9-mm donor lenticule for keratoconus.

Recipient Preparation

Most surgeons prefer to perform EKP with retrobulbar or peribulbar anesthesia, although topical anesthesia may be used in a very cooperative patient. The surgeon may either mark the visual axis according to his or her method of choice or merely center the lenticule on a constricted pupil. Total epithelial debridement in the area of the proposed graft is essential for the success of the procedure. The epithelium is debrided at least 1 to 1.5 mm beyond the edge of the anticipated trephination with a dull spatula (never a sharp instrument), facilitated by topically applied 4% cocaine, if necessary. Many surgeons leave a small area of central epithelium corresponding to the visual axis until after trephination.

After epithelial removal, a Hessburg–Barron trephine[52] is centered on the visual axis, and trephination is performed approximately 200 to 225 μm into the corneal stroma. For adult and pediatric aphakia, a 7-mm trephine is used; for keratoconus, an 8.5-mm trephine is required. An annular keratectomy of approximately 0.5 mm in diameter may be performed on the inner aspect of the trephine incision with Vannas scissors. This annular keratectomy provides additional donor-stromal to recipient-stromal contact and facilitates keratocyte migration into the donor lenticule. It also provides additional surface area of adhesion between the graft and recipient and may create a smoother transition of the lenticule into the lamellar pocket. Many investigators have dropped this step from the procedure without significantly altering the results. Next, a 360°, 1-mm lamellar pocket is dissected at the base of the trephination groove and extended into the recipient cornea peripheral to the trephination mark.

Suture Techniques

The donor lenticule is rehydrated for 20 minutes in a balanced salt solution, with an antibiotic like gentamycin 100 μg/ml prior to suturing. Prior to securing the lenticule on the eye, it is imperative to ensure that no epithelium or foreign material (eg, remnants of the Weck-cell sponge) remain on the recipient cornea where the lenticule is to be placed.

For the treatment of aphakia or myopia, the lenticule is sutured into the lamellar pocket. The placement of a 1.5-mm oversized graft into a lamellar pocket

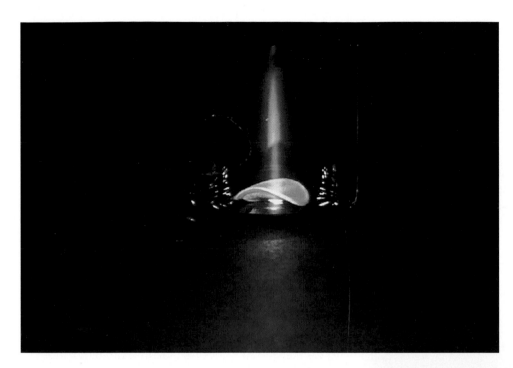

Figure 29–2. Commercially prepared, lyophilized, and vacuum-packed EKP lenticule. *(Courtesy of Allergan Medical Optics.)*

seems to be the optimal technique to eliminate flattening of the host cornea and induction of undesirable refractive changes, which are more likely to occur when 0.5- or 1.0-mm oversized lenticules are used.[2] Conversely, a 0.5-mm oversized lenticule is used in the management of keratoconus to flatten the host cornea.[13]

Proper suturing techniques are critical to preventing the induction of unwanted myopia, hyperopia, and astigmatism. Initially, four to eight cardinal 10-0 nylon sutures, followed by a 16-bite 10-0 running nylon suture, were used to secure the lenticule in the lamellar pocket. Later, this was modified to the current preferred technique of 16 interrupted 10-0 nylon sutures. The needles must be placed through the 0.13-mm-thick wing of the lenticule to ensure proper placement of the lenticule into the lamellar pocket. The sutures are tied loosely to avoid excessive tension on the graft, which would result in overcorrection in hyperopia and undercorrection in myopia. If these abnormalities are detected in the postop period, it is imperative to remove the sutures as soon as possible. If the sutures are removed before a tight, secure scar forms in the lamellar pocket and along the stromal–stromal interface in the annular keratectomy, it is possible to reverse the induced refractive errors by excessively tight sutures. If the sutures are retained too long, the induced refractive changes may persist.

The placement of the lenticule and the suture technique are somewhat different for the treatment of kera-

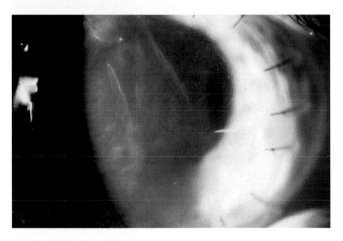

Figure 29–3. Folds in Descemet's membrane immediately following EKP for keratoconus. *(From Mandel E, Wagoner MD. Atlas of Corneal Disease. Philadelphia: WB Saunders; 1989: 91. Reproduced by permission.)*

toconus. Unlike the technique for aphakia and myopia, the cornea peripheral to the trephination is not undermined. The donor lenticule is sutured tightly right to the edge of recipient cornea with 16 or 24 interrupted 10-0 nylon sutures, using sufficient tension to flatten the cone. Folds should be seen in Descemet's membrane at the conclusion of the procedure (Fig 29–3). These usually vanish after suture removal (Fig 29–4).

Some surgeons[53,54] have advocated "no-stitch" techniques to reduce some of the problems induced by lenticule suturing. Cotter[53] successfully performed 24 aphakic EKPs on 26 eyes (92.3%) by merely tucking the lenticule into the peripheral pocket and allowing the sutureless lenticule to re-epithelialize postoperatively. Five of these eyes did develop partial wound dehiscences postoperatively. Three were successfully reposited at the slit lamp; two required suturing.

More recently, Robin et al[54] have employed a mussel adhesive protein from the common blue mussel (*Mytilus edulis*) as an alternative to sutures in experimental animal models. The clinical application of this technique has not been investigated.

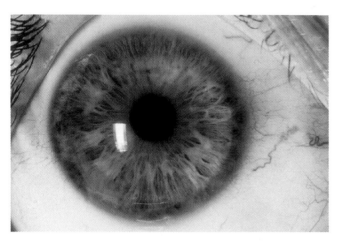

Figure 29–4. Same patient as in Figure 29–3. Appearance of clear lenticule with no folds in Descemet's membrane 5 years following EKP for keratoconus. *(From Mandel E, Wagoner MD. Atlas of Corneal Disease. Philadelphia: WB Saunders; 1989:91 Reproduced by permission.)*

Postoperative Care

Postoperatively, meticulous attention is given to facilitating prompt re-epithelialization and to preventing the loss of graft clarity that invariably accompanies persistent epithelial defects. To facilitate re-epithelialization, most surgeons use bandage soft contact lenses or pressure patching. A temporary tarsorrhaphy is performed if epithelial migration is delayed or arrests before completion.[13-17] Unfortunately, late tarsorrhaphy usually fails to reverse the inexorable downhill course of lenticules with persistent epithelial defects still present after 7 to 10 days.

Recent evidence[55] suggests that the optimal postop management following EKP is achieved with placement of a temporary tarsorrhaphy at the conclusion of every procedure. In this study, the mean re-epithelialization time of all eyes treated with a temporary tarsorrhaphy at the time of surgery was 4.61 days, compared to 8.03 days with pressure patching ($P<0.01$) and 13.2 days ($P<0.005$) with bandage soft contact lenses. Caporossi and Manetti[56] have reported similar favorable results when topical epidermal growth factor is used, but this remains investigational. Examinations should be conducted every 24 to 48 hours until re-epithelialization is complete. Topical antibiotics (eg, polysporin ophthalmic ointment TID) are used until re-epithelialization is complete.

Topical steroids (eg, prednisolone acetate 1% TID) are used to prevent premature suture vascularization

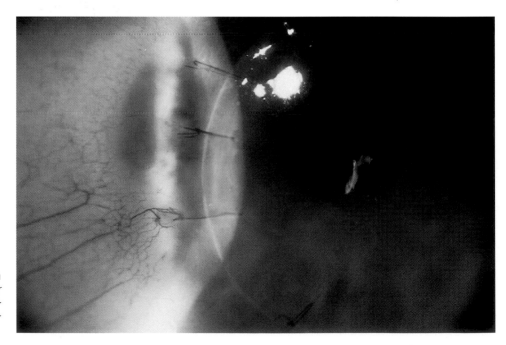

Figure 29–5. Early suture vascularization and loosening. *(From Mandel E, Wagoner MD. Atlas of Corneal Disease. Philadelphia: WB Saunders; 1989:91. Reproduced by permission.)*

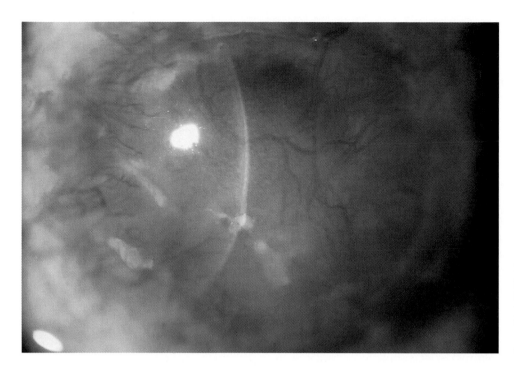

Figure 29–6. Severe superficial and deep stromal vascularization associated with severe postop inflammation and inappropriate retention of lenticule following EKP for keratoconus. *(Courtesy of Dr George Waring, Department of Ophthalmology, Emory University School of Medicine.)*

and loosening. This is particularly important following EKP for keratoconus, where early loosening and removal of sutures (Fig 29–5) can result in the development of irregular astigmatism. In uncomplicated cases, all sutures are removed at 2 to 3 weeks for pediatric aphakia and at 8 weeks for adult aphakia and myopia.[13–17] For keratoconus, suture removal was originally recommended at 3 months.[13] Current opinion is that better results can be obtained by retaining the sutures for 4 to 6 months.[21,47] Nevertheless, vascularized sutures must be removed promptly to prevent severe corneal vascularization (Fig 29–6), which can greatly reduce the prognosis of potential future PKP.

Suture removal should always be performed so that the knot exits from the corneal side to avoid dehiscing the lenticule. If lenticule dehiscence does occur during suture removal, it is important to tuck the lens back into place either at the slit lamp or in the minor treatment room. If the lens will not remain in place spontaneously, the area of dehiscence must be re-sutured.

PROGNOSTIC FACTORS AND COMPLICATIONS

A number of factors play a role in the ultimate success of EKP.[57–89] Of paramount importance are the preparation and proper function of the donor lenticule, prompt re-epithelialization of the donor lenticule, and elimination or reduction of adverse alterations of the host cornea resulting from the operative procedure or postop complications.

Donor Lenticule

The donor lenticule must have the following characteristics:

1. Be of predictable size and power
2. Have optical clarity
3. Support epithelial migration and adhesion
4. Be permeable to solutes
5. Resist enzymatic digestion

Precise lathing of EKP lenticules was initially difficult because the lathing tools expanded unpredictably during freezing and corneal tissue became swollen before it was lathed,[90] resulting in considerable dioptric unpredictability. Modifications were introduced to compensate for the changes in the dimensions of the cryolathe during freezing,[83] and a corneal press was developed to return the swollen postmortem cornea to its normal state of hydration before it is frozen and lathed[84]; both of these precautions vastly improved the dioptric precision of lenticule preparation.[2]

Preservation and maintenance of the optical clarity properties of the original corneal donor tissue is as critical to final visual function as the provision for proper power. Lyophilization destroys viable keratocytes and produces changes in the interfibrillar collagen distance as well as increasing the fibril diameter.[62] The impact of the early absence of viable keratocytes cannot be overemphasized, as this factor leaves the donor lenticule without the repair mechanisms necessary to avoid any enzymatic degradation that may be initiated in the presence of a persistent epithelial defect.[85]

If the graft remains clear until re-epithelialization, gradual ingrowth of keratocytes into the donor lenticule results in improved optical clarity (Fig 29–4) and restoration of more normal corneal histology and function.[59,60,67,70] Despite this, some histopathologic abnormalities remain[70,72] in lenticules that are clinically normal in appearance. Often there are breaks in the recipient's Bowman's membrane that are associated with the ingrowth of keratocytes and irregular collagen, often accompanied by accumulation of an electron-dense fibrocellular material.[70] Keratocyte numbers are usually reduced, even in long-standing grafts, and the distribution remains irregular. A periodic-acid–Schiff positive, electron-dense fibrogranular material is sometimes seen at the interface between the lenticule and the recipient's Bowman's membrane.[72]

A number of modifications have been tried to overcome some of the problems associated with lyophilization of the donor tissue. Altman et al[90] tried excimer laser ablation of the posterior surface of the donor lenticules to eliminate the need for cryolathing and to preserve as many viable keratocytes near the epithelial surface as possible. Krumeich and Swinger[37] and Armesto[26] tried noncryolathing techniques to prepare donor lenticules for the treatment of myopia and aphakia, respectively. Their results, however, do not differ significantly from other published series using lyophilized tissue.[13–17]

Some investigators have attempted to eliminate the problems associated with acquisition and preparation of human corneal tissue by investigating the use of synthetically prepared collagen lenticules.[91–94] To date, experimental work with lenticules prepared from types I, III, and IV collagen have been reported,[92–94] as well as early work with solid-state UV ablation (213 nm) of lenticules prepared from type I collagen.[91] This work is still investigational, and it remains to be seen if excimer-ablated, synthetic collagen lenticules have a future in refractive surgery.

Corneal Epithelium

The corneal epithelium is important for proper ocular function, as is the restoration of an intact epithelium in those situations where it is absent.[85,86] An intact epithelium is essential as a barrier to microbial penetration into the corneal stroma.

The epithelium must be regular in order to provide proper refractive function at the air–tear interface.[82] A phenotypically normal epithelium is essential for proper regulation of corneal keratocytes in the maintenance of appropriate corneal repair and responses to injury.[87–89] It is recognized that alteration of normal epithelial–stromal interactions in the setting of a per-

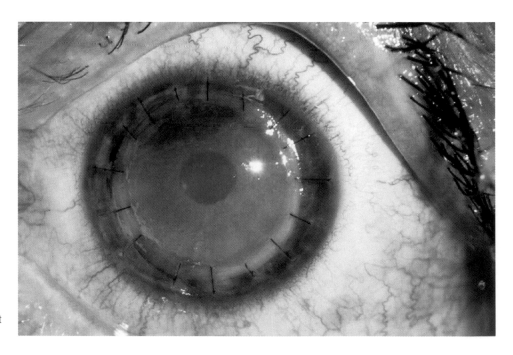

Figure 29–7. Persistent epithelial defect 2 weeks after EKP.

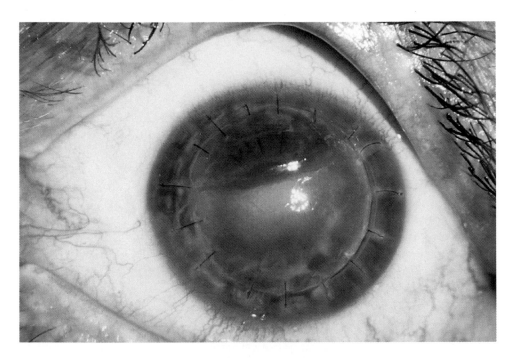

Figure 29–8. Same patient as in Figure 29–7. Sterile ulceration and loss of clarity 3 weeks after EKP.

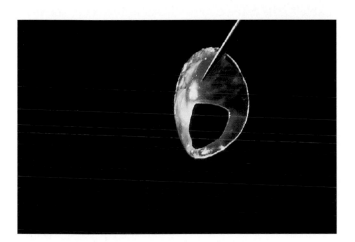

Figure 29–9. Complete loss of lenticule stroma in area corresponding to total epithelial defect 3 weeks following EKP for myopia. *(From Mandel E, Wagoner MD.* Atlas of Corneal Disease. *Philadelphia: WB Saunders; 1989: 92. Reproduced by permission.)*

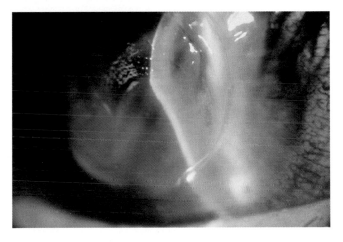

Figure 29–10. Same patient as in Figure 29–9. Extensive sterile ulceration of recipient cornea in same distribution as persistent epithelial defect and sterile ulceration of the overlying epikeratoplasty lenticule. *(From Mandel E, Wagoner MD.* Atlas of Corneal Disease. *Philadelphia: WB Saunders; 1989: 92. Reproduced by permission.)*

sistent epithelial defect is often associated with sterile stromal ulceration,[85–89] particularly after EKP when there are no viable keratocytes in the lenticule. Enzymatic degradation and loss of graft clarity may be seen as soon as 2 to 3 weeks postoperatively if epithelial closure is not complete (Figs 29–7, 29–8). This is the most common complication, resulting in graft failure,[59,60,67] with an incidence of 5% to 10%.[13–17] When sterile ulceration of the graft occurs it should be considered irreversible. Prompt removal of the lenticule (Fig 29–9) is

essential to allow re-epithelialization of the host cornea and to prevent extension of potentially sight-threatening ulceration into the recipient cornea (Fig 29–10).

Persistent epithelial defects occur most frequently in patients with preexisting ocular surface disease such as severe keratoconjunctivitis sicca, blepharitis, or atopy, or with uncorrected lid–globe abnormalities such as entropion or lagophthalmos. Patients with these disorders should not undergo EKP unless there are no other surgical alternatives, the underlying disease is well controlled, and all lid–globe abnormalities have been corrected.

In Azar's classic study of failed EKP lenticules,[58] distinct differences were observed between lenticules that were removed for inaccurate refractive correction ("anatomic success") and those that were removed because graft clarity was lost owing to problems with re-epithelialization ("anatomic failure"). In anatomically successful cases, the epithelium is fairly regular and near normal hemidesmosome formation is present, although there is some reduction in basement membrane. In anatomically failed cases, the epithelium is often absent in large areas of the graft and thickened in areas where it is present. There are few epithelium–basement membrane complexes, basement membrane is absent or reduced, and the donor Bowman's membrane is often disrupted. Frangieh et al[67] correlated findings of epithelial abnormalities with changes in the basal lamina, Bowman's layer, and underlying stroma. Epithelial defects correlated directly with various degrees of sterile stromal ulceration of the underlying lenticule, confirming clinical observations.

Recipient Cornea

In theory, EKP should not induce any significant changes in the recipient cornea. Unfortunately, alterations in the recipient cornea occurring at the time of surgery or postoperatively can play a role in final corneal function and refractive function following EKP.[60,71,74,76,78,80,95]

Interface opacification may be seen that is caused by retention of epithelium or foreign material beneath the lenticule during the surgical procedure. Late interface scarring and opacification may occur (Fig 29–11), even though Bowman's membrane is theoretically not damaged by the surgical technique.[74,78] Finally, infectious keratitis involving the interface or deeper layers of the cornea may result in irreversible scarring of the recipient cornea.[71] Sterile ulceration of the lenticule and recipient stroma has been reported, even in the presence of an intact epithelium,[60] although this is very rare.

Trephination, which is essential for performing EKP, may induce steepening of the recipient cornea[75,76] in a manner similar to that seen with hexagonal keratotomy. This may not be distressing to the hyperopic patient, who may be less hyperopic after lenticule removal. In the case of myopia, it is particularly distressing when removal of the lenticule may be accompanied by a 2- to 5-diopter worsening of the preexisting myopic error.[21,75,76]

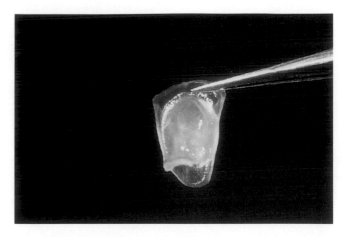

Figure 29–11. Dense interface opacification occurring in EKP performed for pediatric aphakia. *(From Mandel E, Wagoner MD. Atlas of Corneal Disease. Philadelphia: WB Saunders; 1989:91. Reproduced by permission.)*

Rao et al[80] have shown endothelial changes (attenuation of cells, irregular shape, and decreased density with poor interdigitation) after EKP. This may be attributable to the corneal hypesthesia induced by trephination of the anterior corneal nerves. The clinical significance of these findings has yet to be determined.

EPIKERATOPLASTY FOR ADULT APHAKIA

Indications

Epikeratoplasty was initially conceived as an alternative to secondary intraocular lens (IOL) implantation in contact lens–intolerant, monocularly aphakic adults.[3] At the time of its introduction in 1979, the occurrence of monocular (or binocular) aphakia was not uncommon. There were many aphakic patients in the pre-IOL era. Many patients did not receive IOL implantation because surgeons were often reluctant to use the iris-plane and anterior-chamber IOLs that were available at that time. Relative contraindications for the implantation IOLs in patients with significant anterior segment pathology (Fig 29–12)—chronic glaucoma, uveitis, or retinal pathology—were enforced by human investigation committees that regulated IOL use in many centers.

As a result, EKP offered many patients with monocular aphakia who were contact lens intolerant an opportunity to obtain useful, binocular vision. In addition, it was available for bilateral use in patients with the newly recognized disease of "spectacle intolerance," whose emergence corresponded closely with the rapidly developing field of keratorefractive surgery.

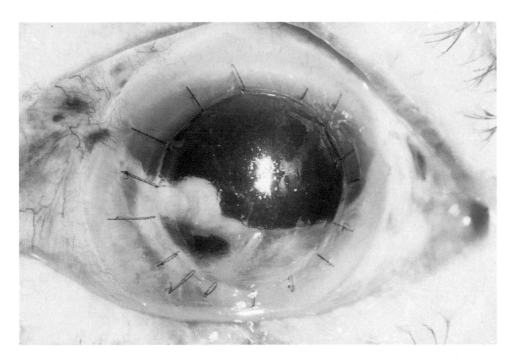

Figure 29–12. EKP for monocular aphakia in an adult with extensive superior iridodialysis that occurred following an intracapsular cataract extraction 10 years previously.

Clinical Results

The criteria by which EKP for adult aphakia is judged are dependent upon the preop diagnosis and patient expectations. In the case of the monocularly aphakic patient who is truly contact lens intolerant, sufficient reduction of the anisometropic error to permit the comfortable wearing of spectacles will restore satisfactory binocular vision and a profound improvement in overall function. This is the case even if the uncorrected acuity in the operative eye is less than satisfactory or there is a mild loss of best corrected visual acuity (BCVA). On the other hand, the same result may not be as satisfactory to the monocular aphake who is "contact lens weary" and is looking to eliminate dependence on contact lenses or spectacles altogether. In this case, even a mild residual refractive error or a loss of one or two lines of BCVA will result in a decrease in the level of preop function.

For the bilateral aphake who is truly spectacle intolerant, the reduction but not complete elimination of the refractive error may be satisfactory even when there is loss of one or two lines of BCVA because aberrations associated with aphakic spectacle wear have been eliminated. Conversely for the bilateral aphake who is a successful contact lens wearer, the predictability and retention of BCVA must be highly reliable to avoid a setback relative to preop function.

In all four situations, the results of EKP must be judged against the predictability, improvement in UCVA, maintenance of BCVA, contrast sensitivity, and surgical complication rate of the other major surgical alternative: secondary IOL implantation.[19]

Most large series[2,14,18–21,96] have reported similar results for this indication for EKP. Anatomic success is achieved in 95%, with persistent epithelial defects and loss of graft clarity being the major reason for graft failure. Over 90% of grafted eyes have an improvement in UCVA. Approximately 75% of eyes have final refractive errors within 3 D of emmetropia and are considered "refractively successful."

The two major functional limitations are the rate of recovery of BCVA and relatively poor contrast sensitivity. There is usually some delay in restoration of normal corneal hydration and clarity (especially in the very elderly). Although all studies[2,14,18–21] indicate that most eyes achieve an acuity within two lines of their BCVA within 2 months postoperatively, a few patients may require 6 to 12 months to achieve their BCVA.[14,21] While approximately 25% of eyes lose one line of BCVA, losses of two or more lines occur in less than 1% of cases.[14]

Although anatomic and refractive success is quite good, there seems to be a significant subjective disparity between recorded Snellen acuity and visual function in many patients. Carney and Kelley[63] demonstrated a statistically significant decrease in contrast sensitivity in patients who were treated with EKP compared to those treated with either IOL or contact lens therapy.

Summary

When judged by the criteria of providing significant improvement in UCVA, significant reduction in anisometropia, preservation of most or all of best corrected preop visual acuity, and having an acceptably low rate of significant, irreversible complications, EKP may be an effective and safe therapeutic modality in the management of aphakia. There various reasons, however, why it is seldom employed for this indication today.

The near universal use of primary IOL implantation has made monocular aphakia a rare disorder. In such occasions, a number of factors favor the use of secondary IOL implantation. First, the technical contraindications to IOL implantation in anterior segment abnormalities (eg, absent posterior capsule, chronic open-angle glaucoma) have been eliminated to a large degree by the technique of sutured posterior chamber IOLs. Second, the superior contrast sensitivity following secondary IOL implantation (despite similar Snellen acuity) makes this technique subjectively much more satisfactory to patients. Third, visual rehabilitation is much more rapid with secondary IOL implantation. For these reasons, the current application for EKP for aphakia is restricted to the contact lens–intolerant, monocular aphake in whom secondary IOL implantation is truly contraindicated or undesirable and improved visual function is required.

EPIKERATOPLASTY FOR PEDIATRIC APHAKIA

Indications and Contraindications

Compliance with optical and occlusive therapy is the major problem facing the ophthalmologist and family of a unilaterally aphakic child. For such children, who are unable to wear contact lenses, EKP and secondary IOL implantation are the only alternatives to abandoning therapy. The potential usefulness of EKP lies in eliminating the problems with optical noncompliance related to hyperopic anisometropia without exposing the eye to the risks and poorly defined long-term effects of secondary IOL implantation.[2,8,9,16,17,21–33]

Epikeratoplasty is generally recommended for children over the age of 1. It is especially useful in cases of unilateral aphakia for which contact lenses are not possible owing to intolerance or socioeconomic conditions that discourage successful contact lens use. It is particularly useful for unilateral traumatic aphakia and can even be used if corneal scars are present, as long as the visual axis is not involved (Fig 29–13). In cases of bilateral aphakia where spectacle therapy is unsuccessful, it can be used bilaterally to minimize the risk of amblyopia from optical noncompliance.

Clinical Results

Because operative intervention should only be contemplated when more conservative measures like specta-

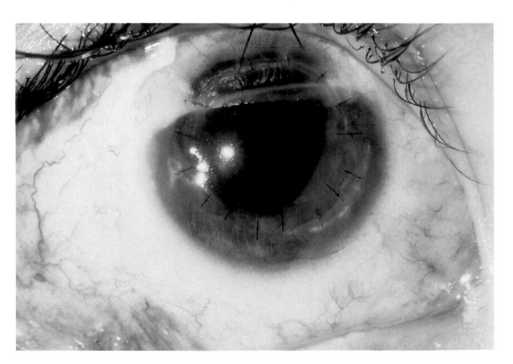

Figure 29–13. EKP for monocular pediatric traumatic aphakia with a full-thickness corneal stromal scar.

cles or contact lens therapy have failed, the results of EKP must be compared against abandonment of therapy altogether. As such, the criterion by which the success of EKP for pediatric aphakia should be judged is its ability to achieve a refractive result that permits the successful initiation of amblyopia therapy. Comparison with secondary IOL implantation is difficult because of the length of time required to fully assess the long-term complications of IOL insertion in this age group.

The anatomic and refractive results for pediatric aphakia are similar to those for adult aphakia.[2,8,9,16,17,21–33,66] Anatomic success may be as high as 95%, while refractive success (within 3 D of emmetropia) is achieved in approximately 75% of eyes. EKP lenticules clear much faster in children than in adults, presumably because of their superior endothelial function. Occlusive therapy may be initiated as soon as 1 to 2 weeks following suture removal (4 to 5 weeks postoperatively).

The visual results of EKP in the pediatric patient are hard to assess. The young age of many of the patients makes vision testing impossible. In addition, many of the early patients were enrolled in investigational trials after amblyopia had already been established because previous therapy had failed. With early and more aggressive use of EKP (or secondary IOL implantation), this problem should be reduced in the future.

As with other indications for EKP, persistent epithelial defect is the most common cause of graft failure in pediatric patients, resulting in a failure rate of 5% to 10%.[16,66] In most cases, repeat EKP is successful.[16] Inasmuch as it is extremely unusual for concomitant ocular surface disease to be present in these patients, poor compliance with pressure patching, bandage soft contact lenses, and postop antibiotic use is probably the most likely explanation for these failures. The incidence of this complication has been significantly reduced when a temporary tarsorrhaphy is performed at the time of surgery.[55]

Summary

The combination of significant reduction of refractive error and the rapidity of optical clarity greatly simplify the optical maneuvers necessary to initiate amblyopia therapy in this patient population. Many of the factors that give secondary IOL implantation an edge over EKP in adults (more rapid visual recovery, better contrast sensitivity) do not apply to the pediatric age group whose grafts clear much more rapidly. Concerns about

the long-term complications of implanting IOLs into immature eyes still remain.

Epikeratoplasty offers a safe and effective means of reducing the refractive error in the pediatric aphake and has been approved by the US Food and Drug Administration. At the present time, pediatric aphakia is the leading indication for the use of EKP. It should remain an integral part of the management of monocular pediatric aphakia. Its use should be reserved not only for cases where other optical maneuvers have failed, but also early on in situations of anticipated contact lens failure and when there is the opportunity to avoid the development of dense amblyopia.

EPIKERATOPLASTY FOR KERATOCONUS

Indications and Contraindications

Lamellar keratoplasty has long been used to reinforce thin, ectatic corneas in patients with keratoconus, keratoglobus, and pellucid marginal degeneration.[1] Compared with penetrating keratoplasty (PKP), lamellar keratoplasty is extraocular, reducing or eliminating the potential for many of the serious complications of intraocular surgery like expulsive hemorrhage or endophthalmitis. By preserving the recipient endothelium, which is often normal in these young and otherwise healthy corneas, the probability of maintaining corneal clarity is improved, and the risk of endothelial rejection, which is seen in 8% to 39% of penetrating keratoplasties,[97-99] is eliminated. While the risk of stromal rejection remains,[77] this complication is far less serious than endothelial rejection. Unfortunately, the visual results with PKP proved to be superior to those of lamellar keratoplasty. As a result, PKP became the treatment of choice for ectatic disorders of the cornea.

In 1982, Kaufman described EKP as an improvement in standard lamellar keratoplasty for treatment of keratoconus and a potential alternative to PKP.[5] Because dissection of the central cornea is not required with EKP, the visual results were expected to be better than with lamellar keratoplasty. In addition, there is the additional safety of an extraocular procedure and the reduced risk of serious rejection episodes compared with PKP.

EKP is best suited for keratoconus patients who have poor spectacle acuity, a BCVA with a hard contact lens of 20/40 or better, and an inability to tolerate contact lens wear because of severe corneal distortion. Because the procedure may flatten and shift the position of the cone, it is best to avoid eyes whose central as well as paracentral opacities are within 1 mm of the visual axis, as these may be shifted into the optical center postoperatively. Exceptions can be made in cases like Down's syndrome, where the advantages of an extra-ocular procedure may outweight the disadvantages of a "less than perfect" visual result if the procedure is performed in eyes with mild to moderate central scarring. Although there were no limitations on corneal steepness for which correction can be attempted, some observers have found that patients with cones <60 D seem to benefit more from EKP than those with steeper cones.[21,47]

After its successful introduction for the treatment of keratoconus, the procedure was successfully expanded for other ectatic corneal disorders like keratoglobus[48,49] and pellucid marginal degeneration.[50] In cases of keratoglobus or other ectatic disorders, custom-made lenses up to 12.5 mm in diameter may be ordered, but the graft should never be oversized by more than 0.5 mm to achieve maximum tightness and flattening of the cone at the conclusion of the procedure. If adequate visual results are not obtained, it is possible to perform a smaller (<8 mm) central penetrating keratoplasty because of the increased ease of suturing the edge of the donor button into the peripheral cornea after its thickness has been augmented by the 300-μm–thick EKP lenticule.

Results

Because EKP is offered in some cases rather than PKP, it is important not only to examine the improved safety of EKP but also to weight this reduction in surgical risk against any difference in visual results between the two techniques. Despite its potential complications, PKP for keratoconus is one of the most successful corneal procedures.[97–99]

The largest series to date to study this—and other—indications for epikeratoplasty was the nationwide study for keratoconus.[13] Of the 82 eyes for which follow-up of 1 month or more was available after suture removal, UCVA improved in 80 of 82 (97.5%). Only 9% had a UCVA of 20/100 or better preoperatively, whereas 64.2% had a UCVA of 20/100 or better postoperatively. The mean flattening of keratometric astigmatism was 9.36 D (SD = 0.68 D), and the mean reduction in spherical equivalent was −8.62 D (SD = 0.84). Eighty of 82 were within one line of preop BCVA. Other studies have found results similar to the original study.[20,21,41–47]

In one study,[47] a striking feature was not only substantial improvement in UCVA from a preop mean of 20/260 to 20/134, but also improvement in spectacle acuity from a preop mean of 20/260 to 20/30. In seven of nine patients, the spectacle acuity was equivalent to that of a hard contact lens refraction. For many patients who have been absolutely dependent upon contact lens wear for acceptable functioning, the opportunity to achieve adequate vision with spectacles alone is a major improvement in the quality of their lives. For those patients who wish to continue wearing contact lenses for cosmetic or athletic purposes, or for convenience, contact lens wear seems to be well tolerated in the setting of an EKP lenticule.[58]

A number of studies have compared the visual results of EKP and PKP.[40,43,44,46,47,65] In looking at 30 PKPs versus 30 EKPs followed for 3 to 6 years, Fronterre and Portesani[41,43] found similar mean UCVA (20/63 vs 20/52), spectacle-corrected visual acuity (20/22 vs 20/23), and contact-lens–corrected visual acuity (20/20 vs 20/21). Steinert and Wagoner[47] found similar results in a comparison of 10 PKPs versus 10 EKPs, with a mean spectacle-corrected visual acuity of 20/32 versus 20/27. One interesting finding in this study was that not a single patient who received an EKP had a BCVA of 20/20. Goosey et al[44] made a similar observation: 93% of their patients who had received either a PKP or an EKP had a BCVA of 20/40 or better, 73% of patients with a PKP achieved a BCVA of 20/20, while only 23% of patients with an EKP had a similar result.

The contrast between the results of PKP and EKP for keratoconus intensifies when contrast sensitivity is analyzed. Carney and Lembach[65] compared EKP with PKP and rigid gas-permeable contact lens therapy in patients with keratoconus in the presence and absence of glare. In both situations, patients with EKP had statistically significantly poorer results than those treated with the other two modalities.

The major complications of EKP for keratoconus include primary graft failure from failure to re-epithelialize and persistent irregular astigmatism caused by premature suture loosening or removal, and residual myopia.[13,47] Although secondary refractive procedures like radial keratotomy[101] or relaxing incisions[42] have produced improvement in some cases, it is often best to proceed to PKP in situations where the visual results are suboptimal.[13,47,102] Although there are not enough patients to make absolute statements, the presence of a previous EKP does not seem to adversely affect the prognosis for subsequent PKP.[13,47,68,72,100] To maximize the chances of future PKP, it is the responsibility of the surgeon who performs EKP to avoid complications that will worsen the prognosis in future PKP. Such mistakes include failure to remove a lenticule that does not re-epithelialize before ulceration of the recipient cornea, failure to utilize topical steroids, removal of loose sutures to prevent corneal vascularization (Fig 29–5), and failure to remove lenticules in cases where suture removal and steroids do not halt the progression of vascularization into the graft–host interface (Fig 29–6).

Summary

For keratoconus, EKP offers a potential alternative for the patient who falls "between the cracks" of having enough corneal warpage to preclude comfortable or adequate hard contact lens wear, but does not have enough central corneal scarring or sufficient motivation to assume the potential morbidity associated with a PKP. Because the visual results with EKP are slightly poorer than with successful PKP (see below), many ophthalmologists limit the selection of this procedure to patients who have specific reasons for not undergoing PKP (ie, bad experience with a PKP in the other eye, inability to restrict activity postoperatively owing to occupational requirements). The prognosis of subsequent PKP does not seem to be compromised in patients who have had unsuccessful EKP for keratoconus.[100] Thus, like other indications, EKP used for keratonus appears to be potentially reversible.

As such, it is infrequently used in the management of keratoconus. In a large series of 746 eyes of 417 patients with keratoconus referred to major university centers for therapy, Lass and colleagues[45] reported that 74% of patients with keratoconus were managed successfully with contact lenses or spectacles, whereas 21% either received or were recommended for PKP, and only 4% were managed with EKP. While this indication for EKP remains rare in countries where donor tissue is readily available for transplantation and compliance with postop follow-up is relatively easy, it remains useful in developing countries where there is limited access to donor tissue or where patient follow-up and compliance are problems.

EPIKERATOPLASTY FOR MYOPIA

Indications and Contraindications

Epikeratoplasty was introduced for myopia in the hope that the procedure would provide predictability similar to that of a contact lens and complete reversibility in cases of anatomic or refractive complications. Because of the large population of moderate and high myopes, compared to that with monocular aphakia and keratoconus, it was originally believed that the treatment of myopia would become the major indication for EKP. Following its introduction, lenticules were provided for −5 D to −30 D of correction.

Clinical Results

The early optimism[15] of the potential for EKP in managing myopia was tempered by the results seen by most investigators.[20,21,34–39,64,95,103–105] The major postop problem is one of regression of refractive effect, defined as greater than 2 D of myopic shift more than 4 months postoperatively. This seems to increase in direct proportion to the amount of attempted correction. In the nationwide study,[15] 12% of eyes with initial refractive errors between −3.75 D and −11.75 D had refractive regression, compared with 18% of eyes between −12.00 D and −17.75 D and 32% of eyes between −18.00 D and −32.50 D. Inasmuch as only 134 of 352 treated eyes had undergone 6 months' follow-up at the time of this report, and given that subsequent studies[21,69] showed that most of the refractive regression occurs between 6 and 12 months postoperatively, these initial disappointing results proved to underestimate the severity of the problem. Regression was often to the original refractive error and was highly inconsistent between the two eyes of bilaterally treated patients, introducing new problems with iatrogenic anisometropia.

Among patients with anatomically successful lenticules in whom significant regression did not occur, the percentage of eyes with uncorrected Snellen acuity of 20/40 or better is unacceptably low. In the nationwide study,[15] only 33% of treated eyes were better than 20/40 without correction, and 31% were 20/200 or worse. Among patients with acceptable refractive and Snellen acuity, contrast sensitivity, in both the presence and absence of a glare source, is significantly worse than those treated with spectacles or contact lenses or with other refractive procedures like radial keratotomy.[64]

Various theories were proposed to explain the phenomenon of refractive regression in an attempt to provide appropriate therapeutic intervention. These include epithelial hyperplasia,[106] excessive tension at the keratectomy site, or steepening of the recipient cornea due to the annular keratectomy. Attempted surgical corrections of refractive regression have included epithelial debridement, retrephination of the original groove to release tension between the lenticule and recipient stroma,[39,103] and excimer photorefractive keratectomy.[104,105] All of these techniques have proven unsuccessful in permanently reversing the problem of refractive regression. For instance, Choi and Choi[103] had uniformly good initial results in reducing large myopic refractive errors with retrephination of the graft–host junction, but they experienced complete regression to preop levels by 6 months in all eyes treated. Similarly, excimer photorefractive keratectomy improved refractive results, but produced such significant haze and reduction in BCVA that, in one series,[104] 100% of treated lenticules had to be removed.

Finally, the procedure is not truly reversible in this patient population. Following annular keratectomy, there may be steepening of the recipient cornea,[21,75,76] which has resulted in increased myopia ranging from -2.40 D[75] to -5.00 D[21] following lenticule removal. In addition, progressive stromal scarring in the recipient cornea has been reported following lenticule removal.[78]

Summary

For any refractive procedure to be considered safe and effective, it must meet rigid standards of predictability, improve UCVA to acceptable levels in a majority of patients, and subject patients to minimal risk of loss of BCVA. On all counts, EKP for myopia is a failure. The high incidence of regression in anatomically successful EKP implies that bilateral symmetry cannot be ensured. The low percentage of patients achieving acceptable levels of UCVA, as well as the poor contrast sensitivity that results compared with other keratorefractive techniques like radial keratotomy and photorefractive keratectomy, makes EKP an unworthy addition to the refractive arena for the correction of myopia. At the present time, EKP is not approved for this clinical use by the FDA in the United States.

REFERENCES

1. McDonald MB. Onlay lamellar keratoplasty. In: Kaufman HE, Barron BA, McDonald MB, Waltman SR, eds. *The Cornea.* New York: Churchill-Livingstone; 1988:697–711.
2. McDonald MB, Morgan KS. Epikeratophakia for aphakia and myopia. In: Kaufman HE, Barron BA, McDonald MB, Waltman SR, eds. *The Cornea.* New York: Churchill-Livingston; 1988:823–847.
3. Kaufman HE. The correction of aphakia. *Am J Ophthalmol.* 1980;89:1–10.
4. Barraquer JI. Keratomileusis and keratophakia. In: Rycroft PV, ed. *Corneoplastic Surgery: Proceedings of the 2nd International Cornea–Plastic Conference.* New York: Pergamon; 1969.
5. Kaufman HE, Werblin TP. Epikeratophakia for the treatment of keratoconus. *Am J Ophthalmol.* 1982;93:342–347.
6. McDonald MB, Koenig SB, Safir A, Kaufman HE. Onlay lamellar keratoplasty for the treatment of keratoconus. *Br J Ophthalmol.* 1983;67:615–618.
7. McDonald MB, Koenig SB, Safir A, et al. Epikeratophakia: the surgical correction of aphakia. Update, 1982. *Ophthalmology.* 1983;90:668–672.
8. Morgan KS, Werblin TP, Asbell PA, et al. The use of epikeratophakia grafts in pediatric monocular aphakia. *J Pediatr Ophthalmol Strabismus.* 1981;18(6):23–29.
9. Morgan KS, Asbell PA, McDonald MB, et al. Preliminary visual results of pediatric epikeratophakia. *Arch Ophthalmol.* 1983;101:1540–1544.
10. Werblin TP, Kaufman HE, Friedlander MH, et al. A prospective study of the use of hyperopic epikeratophakia grafts for the correction of aphakia in adults. *Ophthalmology.* 1981;88:1137–1140.
11. Werblin TP, Kaufman HE, Friedlander MH, Granet N. Epikeratophakia: the surgical correction of aphakia. III. Preliminary results of a prospective clinical trial. *Arch Ophthalmol.* 1981;99:1957–1960.
12. Werblin TP, Kaufman HE, Friedlander MH, et al. Epikeratophakia: the surgical correction of aphakia. Update, 1981. *Ophthalmology.* 1982;89:916–920.
13. McDonald MB, Kaufman HE, Durrie DS, et al. Epikeratophakia for keratoconus: the nationwide study. *Arch Ophthalmol.* 1986;104:1294–1300.
14. McDonald MB, Kaufman HE, Aquavella JV, et al. The nationwide study of epikeratophakia for aphakia in adults. *Am J Ophthalmol.* 1987;103:358–365.
15. McDonald MB, Kaufman HE, Aquavella JV. The nationwide study of epikeratophakia for myopia. *Am J Ophthalmol.* 1987;103:375–383.
16. Morgan KS, McDonald MB, Hiles DA, et al. The nationwide study of epikeratophakia for aphakia in children. *Am J Ophthalmol.* 1987;103:366–374.
17. Morgan KS, McDonald MB, Hiles DA, et al. The nationwide study of epikeratophakia for aphakia in older children. *Ophthalmology.* 1988;95:526–531.
18. Arffa RC, Busin M, Barron BA, et al. Epikeratophakia with commercially prepared tissue for the correction of aphakia in adults. *Arch Ophthalmol.* 1986; 104:1467–1472.
19. Durrie DS, Habrich DL, Dietze TR. Secondary lens implantation vs. epikeratophakia for the treatment of aphakia. *Am J Ophthalmol.* 1987;103:384–391.
20. Lass JH, Stocker EG, Fritz ME, et al. Epikeratoplasty: the surgical correction of aphakia, myopia, and keratoconus. *Ophthalmology.* 1987;94:912–925.
21. Wagoner MD, Steinert RF. Epikeratoplasty for adult and pediatric aphakia, myopia, and keratoconus: the Massa-

chusetts Eye and Ear Infirmary experience. *Acta Ophthalmol.* 1989;67(suppl 192):38–45.

22. Werblin TP, Pieffer RL, Patel AS. Synthetic keratophakia for the correction of aphakia. *Ophthalmology.* 1987;94: 926–934.

23. Arffa RC, Marvelli TL, Morgan KS. Keratometric and refractive results of pediatric epikeratophakia. *Arch Ophthalmol.* 1985;103:1656–1659.

24. Arffa RC, Mavelli TL, Morgan KS. Long term follow-up of refractive and keratometric results of pediatric epikeratophakia. *Arch Ophthalmol.* 1986;104:668–670.

25. Arffa RC, Donzis PB, Morgan KS, Zhou YJ. Prediction of aphakic refractive error in children. *Ophthalmic Surg.* 1987;18:581–584.

26. Armesto DM, Lee AM, Prager TC. Epikeratoplasty with nonlyophilized tissue in children with aphakia. *Am J Ophthalmol.* 1991;111:407–412.

27. Collie DM. Pediatric aphakic epikeratoplasty: early Australian experience. *Aust NZ J Ophthalmol.* 1989;17: 233–237.

28. Kelley CG, Keates RH, Lembach RG. Epikeratophakia for pediatric aphakia. *Arch Ophthalmol.* 1986;104:680–682.

29. Morgan KS, Stephenson GS, McDonald MB, Kaufman HE. Epikeratophakia in children. *Ophthalmology.* 1984;91: 780–784.

30. Morgan KS, Stephenson GS. Epikeratophakia in children with corneal lacerations. *J Pediatr Ophthalmol Strabismus.* 1985;22:105–108.

31. Morgan KS, Marvelli TL, Ellis GS, Arffa RC. Epikeratophakia in children with traumatic cataracts. *J Pediatr Ophthalmol Strabismus.* 1986;23:108–113.

32. Morgan KS, Arffa RC, Marvelli TL, Verity SM. Five year follow up of epikeratophakia in children. *Ophthalmology.* 1986;93:423–431.

33. Hiles DA, Cheng KP. Bilateral phakic hypermetropic epikeratoplasty for accommodative esotropia. *J Cataract Refract Surg.* 1990;16:361–366.

34. Keates RH, Kelley CG. Epikeratophakia for myopia: preliminary considerations. *J Refract Surg.* 1985;1:25.

35. Keates RH, Watson SA, Levy SN. Epikeratophakia following previous refractive keratoplasty surgery: two case reports. *J Cataract Refract Surg.* 1986;12:536–540.

36. Kim WJ, Lee JH. Long term results of myopic epikeratoplasty. *J Cataract Refract Surg.* 1993;19:352–355.

37. Krumeich JH, Swinger CA. Nonfreeze epikeratophakia for the correction of myopia. *Am J Ophthalmol.* 1987;103: 397–403.

38. McDonald MB, Klyce SD, Suarez H, et al. Epikeratophakia for myopic correction. *Ophthalmology.* 1985;92: 1417–1421.

39. Suarez E, Arffa RC, Salmeron B, et al. Efficacy of surgical modifications in myopic epikeratophakia. *J Refract Surg.* 1985;1:156.

40. Dietz TR, Durrie DS. Indications and treatment of keratoconus using epikeratophakia. *Ophthalmology.* 1988;95: 236–244.

41. Fronterre A, Portesani GP. Epikeratoplasty for keratoconus. Report of 40 cases. *Cornea.* 1989;8:236–239.

42. Fronterre A, Portesani GP. Relaxing incisions with compression sutures to reduce astigmatism after epikeratoplasty. *Refract Corneal Surg.* 1990;6:413–417.

43. Fronterre A, Portesani GP. Comparison of epikeratoplasty and penetrating keratoplasty for keratoconus. *Refract Corneal Surg.* 1991;7:167–173.

44. Goosey JD, Prager TC, Goosey CB, et al. A comparison of penetrating keratoplasty to epikeratoplasty in the management of keratoconus. *Am J Ophthalmol.* 1991;111: 145–151.

45. Lass JH, Lembach RAG, Park SB, et al. Clinical management of keratoconus. A multicenter analysis. *Ophthalmology.* 1990;97:433–435.

46. McDonald MB, Safir A, Waring GO, et al. A preliminary comparative study of epikeratophakia or penetrating keratoplasty for keratoconus. *Am J Ophthalmol.* 1987; 103:467.

47. Steinert RF, Wagoner MD. Long term comparison of epikeratoplasty and penetrating keratoplasty for keratoconus. *Arch Ophthalmol.* 1988;106:493–496.

48. Cameron JA. Epikeratoplasty for keratoglobus associated with blue sclera. *Ophthalmology.* 1991;98:446–452.

49. Cameron JA. Keratoglobus. *Cornea.* 1993;12:124–130.

50. Fronterre A, Portesani GP. Epikeratoplasty for pellucid marginal degeneration. *Cornea.* 1991;10:450–453.

51. Maguen E, Nesburn AB. Bilateral epikeratoplasty for variable diurnal vision and keratoglobus. *J Refract Surg.* 1987;3:12.

52. Hessburg PC, Barron M. A disposable corneal trephine. *Ophthalmic Surg.* 1980;11:730–733.

53. Cotter JB. No-suture aphakic epikeratoplasty. *Refract Corneal Surg.* 1992;8:27–32.

54. Robin JB, Picciano P, Kusleika RS, et al. Preliminary evaluation of the use of mussel adhesive protein in experimental epikeratoplasty. *Arch Ophthalmol.* 1988;106: 973–977.

55. Wagoner MD, Steinert RF. Temporary tarsorrhaphy enhances reepithelialization following epikeratoplasty. *Arch Ophthalmol.* 1988;106:13–14.

56. Caporossi A, Manetti C. Epidermal growth factor in topical treatment following epikeratoplasty. *Ophthalmologica.* 1992;205:121–124.

57. Binder PS, Zavala EY. Why do some epikeratoplasties fail? *Arch Ophthalmol.* 1987;105:63–69.

58. Azar DT, Spurr-Michaud SJ, Tisdale AS, et al. Reassembly of the corneal epithelial adhesion structure following human epikeratoplasty. *Arch Ophthalmol.* 1991;109: 1279–1284.

59. Bechara SJ, Grossniklaus HE, Waring GO. Subepithelial fibrosis after myopic epikeratoplasty. Report of a case. *Arch Ophthalmol.* 1992;110:228–232.

60. Bechara SJ, Grossniklaus HE, Waring GO. Sterile stromal melt of epikeratoplasty lenticule. *Arch Ophthalmol.* 1992; 110:1528–1529.

61. Binder PS, Baumgartner SD, Fogle JA. Histopathology of a case of epikeratophakia (aphakic epikeratoplasty). *Arch Ophthalmol.* 1985;103:1357–1363.

62. Binder PS, Zavala EY, Baumgartner SD, Nayak SK. Combined morphologic effects of cryolathing and lyophilization on epikeratoplasty lenticules. *Arch Ophthalmol.* 1986;104:671–679.

63. Carney LG, Kelley CG. Visual performance after aphakic epikeratoplasty. *Curr Eye Res.* 1991;10:939–945.

64. Carney LG, Kelley CG. Visual losses after myopic epikeratoplasty. *Arch Ophthalmol.* 1991;109:499–502.

65. Carney LG, Lembach RG. Management of keratoconus: comparative visual assessment. *CLAO J.* 1991;17:52–58.

66. Cheng KP, Hiles DA, Biglan AW, et al. Risk factors for complications following epikeratoplasty. *J Cataract Refract Surg.* 1992;18:270–279.

67. Frangieh GT, Kenyon KR, Wagoner MD, John TJ, Hanninen LA, Steinert RF. Epithelial abnormalities and sterile stromal ulceration in epikeratoplasty grafts. *Ophthalmology.* 1988;95:213–227.

68. Goodman GL, Pfeiffer RL, Werblin TP. Failed epikeratoplasty and penetrating keratoplasty for keratoconus. *Cornea.* 1986;5:29–34.

69. Goosey JD, Prager TC, Goosey CB. Stability of refraction during two years after myopic epikeratoplasty. *Refract Corneal Surg.* 1990;6:4–8.

70. Grossniklaus HE, Lass JH, Jacobs G. Light microscopic and ultrastructural findings in failed epikeratoplasty. *Refract Corneal Surg.* 1989;5:296–301.

71. Hemady RK, Bajart AM, Wagoner MD. Interface abscess after epikeratoplasty. *Am J Ophthalmol.* 1990;109:735–736.

72. Jaeger MJ, Berson P, Kaufman HE, Green WR. Epikeratoplasty for keratoconus. A clinicopathologic case report. *Cornea.* 1987;6:131–139.

73. Kaufman HE, McDonald MB. Clinical and histopathologic changes in the host cornea after epikeratoplasty for keratoconus. *Am J Ophthalmol.* 1993;115:121–123.

74. Morgan KS, Beuerman RW. Interface opacities in epikeratophakia. *Arch Ophthalmol.* 1986;104:1505–1508.

75. Nirankari VS. Corneal steepening after epikeratoplasty. *Cornea.* 1989;8:240–246.

76. Nirankari VS, Rodrigues MM, Bauer SA, et al. Effects of epikeratoplasty on the host cornea. An experimental study. *Cornea.* 1990;9:211–216.

77. Pepose JS, Benevento WJ. Detection of HLA antigens in human epikeratophakia lenticules. *Cornea.* 1991;10:105–109.

78. Price FW, Binder PS. Scarring of a recipient cornea following epikeratoplasty. *Arch Ophthalmol.* 1987;105:1556–1560.

79. Rodrigues M, Nirankari V, Rajagopalan S, et al. Clinical and histopathologic changes in the host cornea after epikeratoplasty for keratoconus. *Am J Ophthalmol.* 1992;114:161–170.

80. Rao GN, Ganti S, Aquavella JV. Specular microscopy of corneal epithelium after epikeratophakia. *Am J Ophthalmol.* 1987;103:392–396.

81. Shands PR, Lass JH. Severe anterior segment inflammation following corneal surgery for keratoconus. *Ophthalmic Surg.* 1990;21:645–646.

82. Simon G, Ren Q, Kervick GN, Parel JM. Optic of corneal epithelium. *Refract Corneal Surg.* 1993;9:42–50.

83. Safir A, McDonald MB, Friedlander MH, et al. Compensating for thermally caused dimensional changes in the cryolathe. *Ophthalmic Surg.* 1984;15:306.

84. Safir A, McDonald MB, Klyce SD, et al. The cornea press: restoring donor corneas to normal dimensions and hydration before cryolathing. *Ophthalmic Surg.* 1983;14:327–331.

85. Wagoner MD, Kenyon KR. Noninfected corneal ulceration. In: *Focal Points: Modules for Ophthalmologists.* San Francisco: American Academy of Ophthalmology; 1985;3(7).

86. Kenyon KR, Starck T, Wagoner MD. Corneal epithelial defects and noninfectious ulceration. In: Albert DM, Jakobiec FA, eds. *Principles and Practice of Ophthalmology.* Philadelphia: WB Saunders; 1994;1:218–234.

87. Wagoner MD, Kenyon KR. Chemical injuries of the eye. In: Albert DM, Jakobiec FA, eds. *Principles and Practice of Ophthalmology.* Philadelphia: WB Saunders; 1994;1:234–245.

88. Johnson-Muller B, Gross J. Regulation of corneal collagenase production: epithelial-stromal cell interactions. *Proc Natl Acad Sci USA.* 1978;75:4417.

89. Johnson-Wint B. Regulation of stromal cell collagenase production in adult rabbit corneas: in vitro stimulation and inhibition by epithelial cell products. *Proc Natl Acad Sci USA.* 1980;77:5531.

90. Altmann J, Grabner G, Husinsky W, et al. Corneal lathing using the excimer laser and a computer-controlled positioning system. Part I: Lathing of epikeratoplasty lenticules. *Refract Corneal Surg.* 1991;7:377–384.

91. Gailitis RP, Ren QS, Thompson KP, et al. Solid state ultraviolet (213 nm) ablation of the cornea and synthetic collagen lenticules. *Lasers Surg Med.* 1991;11:556–562.

92. Thompson KP, Hanna K, Waring WO. Emerging technologies for refractive surgery: laser adjustable synthetic epikeratoplasty. *Refract Corneal Surg.* 1989;5:33–38.

93. Thompson KP, Hanna K, Waring GO, et al. Current status of synthetic epikeratoplasty. *Refract Corneal Surg.* 1991;7:240–248.

94. Thompson KP, Hanna KD, Gipson IK, et al. Synthetic epikeratoplasty in rhesus monkeys with human type IV collagen. *Cornea.* 1993;12:35–45.

95. Goodman DF, Gottsch JD, Smith PW, et al. Lamellar keratectomy and repeat epikeratoplasty. A clinicopathologic report. *Cornea.* 1989;8:295–298.

96. Burillon C, Durand L, Gourrand A. Combined epikeratoplasty and homoplastic keratophakia for correction of

aphakia: double curve effect. *Refract Corneal Surg.* 1993;9: 214–218.

97. Chandler JW, Kaufman HE. Graft rejections after keratoplasty for keratoconus. *Am J Ophthalmol.* 1974;77: 543–547.

98. Donshik PC, Cavanaugh HD, Boruchoff SA, Dohlman CH. Effect of bilateral and unilateral grafts on the incidence of rejection in keratoconus. *Am J Ophthalmol.* 1979; 87:823–826.

99. Young SR, Olson JR. Results of double running suture in penetrating keratoplasty performed on keratoconus patients. *Ophthalmic Surg.* 1985;16:779–786.

100. Frantz JM, Limberg MB, Kaufman HE, McDonald MB. Penetrating keratoplasty after epikeratophakia for keratoconus. *Arch Ophthalmol.* 1988;106:1224–1227.

101. Casebeer JC, Shapiro DR. Radial keratotomy in intact epikeratoplasty graft. *Refract Corneal Surg.* 1993;9: 133–134.

102. Asbell PA, Werblin TP, Loupe DN, et al. Secondary surgical procedures after epikeratophakia. *Ophthalmic Surg.* 982;13:555–557.

103. Choi YS, Choi SK. Trephination with a vacuum trephine in undercorrection of myopic epikeratoplasty. *Korean J Ophthalmol.* 1993;7:16–19.

104. Colin J, Sangiuolo B, Malet F, Volant A. Photorefractive keratectomy following undercorrected myopic epikeratoplasties. *J Fr Ophthalmol.* 1992;15:384–388.

105. Teichman KD. Combining epikeratoplasty and photorefractive keratectomy. *J Cataract Refract Surg.* 1991;17:867.

106. Trocme SA, Wagoner MD, Steinert RF, Frangier GF, Kenyon KR. Epithelial hyperplasia and myopic regression following epikeratoplasty. *Saudi J Ophthalmol.* 1995;8:25–28.

CHAPTER 30

Synthetic Epikeratoplasty

Keith P. Thompson ▪ Jan Daniel

DEFINITION

Synthetic epikeratoplasty (EKP) is an investigational procedure whereby a biocompatible synthetic lenticule is attached to the anterior surface of a de-epithelialized host cornea. Epithelialization of the lenticule restores the ocular surface. Thus, the radius of the anterior corneal surface can be changed and the optical power of the host cornea modified, allowing treatment of myopia, hyperopia, and astigmatism.

BACKGROUND

Epikeratoplasty using human donor tissue was first described by Werblin and Kaufman in the early 1980s,[1,2] and extensive efforts to refine this technique were made by McDonald and colleagues.[3,4] This technique employs lenticules harvested from lyophilized corneal tissue or fresh cadaver eyes with a microkeratome. The lenticule is shaped using the cryolathe invented by Barraquer, the Barraquer–Krumeich–Swinger nonfreezing lathe, or more recently, the excimer laser. After shaping, the graft lenticule containing an intact Bowman's layer and anterior corneal stroma is sutured to the de-epithelialized recipient cornea within a circular keratotomy. Attempts to attach the lenticule without sutures have not been successful.[5–7]

The patient's epithelium recovers the lenticule, usually within 1 week.

Compared with classical keratomileusis or keratophakia, EKP offers some distinct advantages: it is less invasive, and the avoidance of the intrastromal cut with the microkeratome decreases the risk of severe complications. The procedure is less technically demanding and easier to learn. The use of suitable methods of tissue preservation allowed for manufacture by an off-site commercial firm of the graft lenticule based on reproducible quality standards, which improved the uniformity and quality of the lenticules. In addition, it eliminated the need for lathing procedures at the time of surgery. EKP does not violate the optical zone, and therefore it is partially reversible. Because the lenticule is attached to the host cornea peripherally and superficially, it can be removed easily.

Nevertheless, this procedure suffers from several unsolved problems. EKP depends on a limited supply of human donor lenticules. Widespread commercial use of human donor tissue may cause ethical problems. There is some risk of transmission of infectious agents. Like keratomileusis, the time for visual recovery is prolonged; many patients require up to 1 year to achieve their best corrected visual acuity. Because of possible distortions occurring with shaping and placing the lenticule intraoperatively[8] and cellular remodeling postoperatively,[9] the refractive outcome of EKP has been poorly predictable. Consequently, many patients have lost best corrected visual acuity (BCVA) after EKP, most commonly because of irregular astigmatism. Unpredictable refractive results occur commonly, which makes careful patient selection mandatory. After extensive clinical trials during the 1980s that revealed the deficiencies of the EKP procedure, and because the procedure never gained approval by the FDA in the United States, it is no longer used routinely to treat ametropia and is used rarely in the management of aphakic patients in whom an intraocular lens (IOL) is contraindicated. Therefore, Allergan Medical Optics no longer manufactures lenticules for EKP. In the United States, EKP is still monitored by the Food and Drug Administration (FDA), and it is performed on an investigational device exemption at only two clinical centers.

Many of the deficiencies of EKP are associated with the use of tissue lenticules, and may be avoided by the employment of a suitable synthetic material.[10,11] The use of synthetic material could allow performance of this procedure virtually without any limitations, eliminating the risk of transmission of infectious diseases by donor tissue. Because the synthetic lenticule would not contain keratocytes, postop synthesis of collagen fibers, which results in scarring, and changes in the shape of the lenticule, caused by tissue remodeling, may be avoided. Synthetic material may even provide better optical properties than tissue lenticules. In addition, synthetic lenticules could be shaped much more precisely than human tissue lenticules.

A synthetic lenticule attached to the cornea could be ablated with an excimer laser system for adjustment of its optical power and refinement of the refractive error.[12] Because this ablation would affect the acellular lenticule rather than the native recipient cornea, the patient's Bowman's layer would not be violated. Therefore, postop haze in the ablation area and regression of the refractive effect that occurs frequently after excimer laser photorefractive keratectomy (PRK) may be avoided. This adjustment could be performed either immediately after the attachment to correct for inaccuracies in the optical power of the lenticule, or later to correct for changes in the refraction of the eye.

If a method could be devised whereby the synthetic lenticule could be attached directly to Bowman's layer, several additional benefits would accrue. Maintenance of an intact Bowman's layer may allow the whole procedure to be completely reversible. Confining the procedure to the area anterior to Bowman's layer would preserve the structural integrity of the cornea. This may allow the refractive outcome of synthetic EKP to be in-

dependent of corneal stromal wound healing, thereby avoiding what is considered to be a major limiting factor in the predictability of corneal refractive procedures currently in use.[13]

POTENTIAL BIOMATERIALS FOR SYNTHETIC EPIKERATOPLASTY

The requirements that a synthetic material suitable for EKP should meet are summarized in Table 30–1. Based on these criteria, several potential biomaterials for investigation were selected and listed in Table 30–2.

Since types I and III collagen are the primary components of Bowman's layer,[14] collagen-containing or collagen-derived materials should be evaluated regarding their properties for EKP. Collagen supports epithelial migration and attachment. Successful synthesis of copolymers consisting of 2-hydroxyethyl methacrylate (HEMA) and collagen have been reported.[15] Those copolymers may combine the advantages of both components: the biologic activity of collagen and the superior optical performance of HEMA. Collagen synthetic copolymers may be a suitable material for synthetic EKP. However, the use of collagen-containing biomaterials will increase the vulnerability of the lenticule to breakdown by proteolytic enzymes released by corneal and immunologic cells.

Extensive use of HEMA for lens implants in cataract surgery has shown this biomaterial to be stable and well tolerated,[16] making hydrogel biomaterials potentially suitable for synthetic EKP. Hydrogels are not susceptible to enzymatic degradation. However, to ensure sufficient spreading and stable attachment of the corneal epithelium, the HEMA lenticule must be coated with a suitable biomaterial substrate to support cell attachment. Successful epithelialization of a polyvinyl alcohol copolymer lens coated in this manner has been achieved both in vitro and in an animal model.[17] However, whether or not coated hydrogel polymers allow long-term epithelial adhesion in vivo remains unknown.

TABLE 30–1. REQUIREMENTS FOR BIOMATERIALS USED FOR SYNTHETIC EPIKERATOPHAKIA

Optically clear
Support epithelial spreading and attachment
Permeable to nutrients and metabolites
Biocompatible
Stable

TABLE 30–2. POTENTIAL BIOMATERIALS FOR SYNTHETIC EPIKERATOPHAKIA

Materials	Examples	Advantages	Disadvantages
Pure collagen	Cross-linked human type IV collagen (nonfibrillar)	Clear	Susceptible to proteolysis
	Cross-linked bovine type I or III collagen (fibrillar)	Strong epithelium affinity	Fibrillar collagen is less transparent
Collagen synthetic copolymers	HEMA-collagen composites	Good optical properties, potentially more stable	Susceptible to proteolysis, brittle
Coated synthetics	Laminin-, fibrin-, or fibronectin-coated HEMA	Proven biocompatibility of hydrogels, not susceptible to proteolysis	Dependent on attached coating; difficult to achieve stable epithelial attachment
Bioactive synthetics	Blown synthetic microfibers	Resistant to proteolysis	Difficult to achieve stable epithelial attachment

Abbreviation: HEMA, 2-hydroxyethyl methacrylate.

Recently, a blown mixture of polypropylene and polybutylene microfibers has been employed to imitate the structure of the extracellular matrix (ECM).[18] Although this material does not contain collagen, it may support epithelial migration and attachment to its surface. However, this approach serves as an experimental device, and a suitable bioactive synthetic material has yet to be developed.

IN VITRO TRIALS FOR EVALUATION OF POTENTIAL BIOMATERIALS

Optical Characteristics

Excellent optical performance is an apparent prerequisite for an appropriate biomaterial that covers the central corneal surface. Therefore, the transmission of light in the visible spectrum must be measured by spectroscopy in potential biomaterials. In contrast to donor-tissue lenticules, synthetic materials do not require keratocytes to maintain optical clarity.

Support of Epithelial Migration

The capability to support epithelial migration and cell attachment is one of the most important characteristics of a potential biomaterial for synthetic EKP. Presumably, to ensure stable, long-term adhesion, the epithelium must form normal attachment complexes to the synthetic lenticule. These subcellular components have been described elsewhere and include hemidesmosomes, basement membrane, and anchoring fibrils.[19] In order to screen a potential biomaterial for its ability to support cell migration and attachment, rabbit corneal epithelium is removed from the cornea by the dispase method. The cells are cultured at the surface of potential biomaterial in cell culture medium for an appropri-

ate period. Afterward, the cell sheet is examined by shaking. If the epithelium remains attached to the synthetic surface, the cell-lenticule sheet may be processed for transmission electron microscopy (TEM) and immunohistochemistry. The typical epithelial attachment structures should be evident in both exams.

Permeability

Because the corneal epithelium derives its nutrition from the aqueous humor, a suitable lenticule for EKP must be permeable to nutrients and metabolites. Preliminary in vivo studies with intracorneal lenses have shown that impairment of intracorneal diffusion caused by impermeable implants may lead to epithelial thinning or even aseptic necrosis. Glucose has been used to determine its diffusion rate in potential synthetic materials. However, glucose is a small molecule and does not necessarily represent the diffusion rate of more complex proteins like neurotrophic factors released from intracorneal nerves or cytokines produced by keratocytes, which may be necessary for long-term epithelial viability.

Kim and colleagues have investigated the permeability of the cornea to radiolabeled inulin (molecular weight [MW] about 7000 D) and dextran (MW about 50,000 D).[20] This method was deemed a suitable approach for testing the permeability of potential synthetic materials. Data obtained from the native rat corneas served as a control. The results of a preliminary study are shown in Table 30–3.

Stability

To ensure long-term refractive stability, the synthetic lenticule must be capable of withstanding erosion and breakdown caused by naturally occurring corneal enzymes. Two major types of proteolytic enzymes are

TABLE 30–3. COEFFICIENTS OF PERMEABILITY IN POTENTIAL BIOMATERIALS[a]

Materials	Inulin	Dextran
Corneal stroma (rat model)	7.0 ± 0.2	5.0 ± 0.1
Collagen type IV	8.3 ± 0.5	4.0 ± 0.4
Collagen type I	8.7 ± 0.3	15.0 ± 0.2
HEMA-type IV collagen	33.1 ± 15.1	19.8 ± 14.7

[a]mm/sec × 10⁻⁵.
Abbreviation: HEMA, 2-hydroxyethyl methacrylate.

present in the cornea: (1) collagenases released by keratocytes, which are capable of breaking down native interstitial collagen molecules; and (2) neutral proteases secreted by both keratocytes and epithelial cells, which break down denatured collagen so that it loses its typical helical structure. Consequently, epithelial cells exposed to denatured collagen have the capability to remodel it. For this reason, collagen synthetic copolymers like HEMA–collagen composites may be susceptible to epithelial proteolytic enzymes.

Like avascular hyaline cartilage, the cornea has a low turnover rate of collagen, and there is no collagenase detectable in the normal cornea.[21] Bowman's layer, which separates the corneal epithelium from the stroma, is probably synthesized by the epithelium during embryogenesis. This layer remains the same thickness throughout life unless it is destroyed or damaged by diseases or injuries. A potential biomaterial for synthetic EKP will be required to provide a stable refrac-

tive effect similar to that of Bowman's layer. A synthetic lenticule composed of a material that is susceptible to breakdown may induce intracorneal pathologic processes, such as proteolysis, resulting in breakdown of Bowman's layer and remodeling of stromal collagen.

In order to test the stability of potential materials, an in vitro approach was used in which these materials were exposed to corneal enzymes (collagenases and proteases) for a defined period. Figure 30–1 shows the stability of human type IV collagen copolymer compared with native rabbit stroma after 20 hours of exposure to different enzymes.

Excimer Laser Ablation Characteristics

Appreciating past experience with refractive surgery, it seems unlikely that these procedures will be capable of correcting refractive errors as accurately and predictably as glasses or contact lenses. These virtually allow a BCVA of 20/20 in the otherwise healthy eye. Furthermore, the refractive status of the eye may be subject to change in the postop period. For these reasons, it could be desirable to reshape the lenticule surface either immediately following the synthetic EKP procedure in order to adjust the optical power of the synthetic lenticule, or later to correct for refractive changes.

Results of excimer laser PRK suggest that the excimer laser may be capable of precise ablation of the synthetic lenticules. Because the photoablation would be performed in an acellular synthetic lenticule, the haze

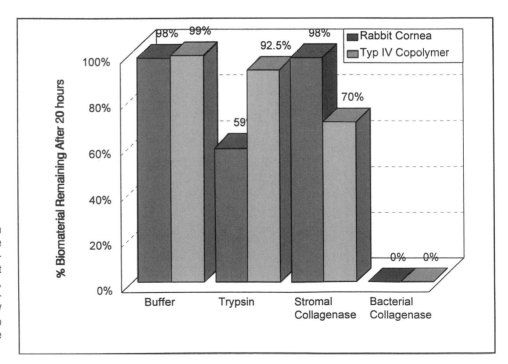

Figure 30–1. Biostability of human type IV collagen compared with native rabbit stroma. Both materials were incubated in buffer, trypsin, rabbit stromal collagenase (V collagenase), and bacterial collagenase (B collagenase). The data suggest that type IV collagen is much more susceptible to trypsine, a neutral protease, than the native rabbit stroma.

and collagen remodeling occurring after PRK could be avoided. Therefore, modification of the lenticule surface could be repeated without danger of corneal scarring or regression of the refractive effect.

Preliminary experiments engendered confidence that collagen-containing synthetic biomaterials for EKP could be successfully shaped using the excimer laser, resulting in a smooth surface, reproducible ablation depth, and minimal structural damage of the molecules adjacent to the ablation area.[22]

ATTACHMENT OF THE SYNTHETIC LENTICULE TO THE CORNEA

The attachment of the synthetic lenticule to the corneal surface presents a major challenge. An appropriate procedure must attach the lenticule in an exactly centered position in a reproducible fashion. To ensure the reversibility of synthetic EKP, the lenticule should be attached directly to the cornea without damaging Bowman's layer or the underlying corneal stroma. Finally, the lenticule must be attached securely for an indefinite period.

Intrastromal Pocket

For experimental purposes, Albinet and coworkers have used a sutureless approach to attach synthetic type IV lenticules to the host cornea.[23] They performed a 4-mm circular keratotomy and inserted an oversized synthetic lenticule measuring about 7.5 mm in diameter into the corneal pocket created with a trephine and scalpel. Using this technique, the integrity of Bowman's layer and of the corneal stroma are violated. This results in wound-healing processes within and around this pocket that may modulate the refractive outcome. Furthermore, the surgical dissection of the stroma, which is necessary to create the 2-mm–wide stromal pocket, appears difficult to standardize. Thus, it may induce unpredictable changes to the shape of the lenticule and the cornea. For this reason, Hanna introduced a rotating device that he derived from his trephine used for penetrating keratoplasty (PKP).[24] This instrument is capable of creating an angled keratotomy (42° to the surface) in the cornea to seat a suitably designed synthetic EKP lenticule.

Laser Welding

The successful use of CO_2 laser welding for fusion of blood vessels, nerves, and other collagenous struc-

tures[25,26] suggested this approach for lenticule attachment. However, laser welding of tissue[6] or synthetic biomaterials[27] to the cornea proved unsuccessful. Even with the application of adjunct biologic solder, a reliable attachment was not achieved. Probably the dense collagenous matrix of Bowman's layer and the relative paucity of connective tissue prevent a suitable attachment.

Biologic Adhesives

First attempts to employ biologic adhesives for attachment of synthetic lenticules were reported by Robin and coworkers in 1988.[28] Further experiments were conducted by Rostron and coworkers, who performed experimental EKP with a fibrin-based bioadhesive.[29] However, in both approaches, the lenticule failed to epithelialize, presumably either because of the toxicity of the adhesive or the poor edge design of the lenticule. Recently, collagen-based adhesives have been employed successfully in corneal surgery, which makes the properties of collagen-derived bioglues for lenticule attachment an interesting subject for further investigation.[30]

Suturing

Past experience with EKP using human tissue-donor lenticules provided evidence that suturing the lenticule with a nonabsorbable material onto the de-epithelialized host cornea is a feasible approach. However, in synthetic EKP, most of the tested potential biomaterials were found to be unsuitable for suturing because the sutures (cheesewire) cut through the lenticules. Improvement of its mechanical properties or incorporation of fibrillar collagen might allow successful suture placement.

Molecular Linking

Most desirable is an attachment technique that avoids any damage to Bowman's layer and the corneal stroma. A possible approach for this may be molecular linking of the synthetic biomaterial to Bowman's layer. The biomaterial might be applied in a liquid or gel form to the cornea, where it polymerizes and links to the collagen fibers of Bowman's layer. Polymerization and linking may be supported by adjuvants like lysyl oxidase or ultraviolet light. Shaping of the synthetic lenticule to the desired surface specifications could be achieved by an appropriate mold (eg, back-side surface of a rigid contact lens), which is attached to the patient's eye by a suction ring. However, the feasibility of this approach has yet to be demonstrated.

PRELIMINARY STUDY IN THE MONKEY EYE

To test the feasibility of the synthetic epikeratoplasty in vivo, we conducted an experimental study with lenticules made from synthetic human type IV collagen involving seven rhesus monkeys. First results were reported in 1993. Monkeys were selected as an experimental model because of the anatomic and physiologic similarity of rhesus monkey eyes to humans and the failures encountered by other investigators with rabbits. (Rabbits blink infrequently, making them a poor model for encouraging re-epithelialization of a synthetic lenticule.) All experiments followed the guidelines of the resolution by the Association for Research in Vision and Ophthalmology on the use of animals in research.

The Biomaterial

Type IV collagen extracted from the supernatant of human placental preparations was filtered and dried to a powdered form. Prior to use, the collagen was rehydrated and injected into flat discs or curved lenticules with a diameter of 7.5 mm. Cross-linking of the collagen fibers was achieved by adding glutaraldehyde. The lenticules created were 250 μm thick and had an optical power of +10 and −10 D.

Before starting the experiments on the rhesus monkeys, we performed in vitro tests to ensure that our synthetic lenticules were capable of supporting epithelial spreading and attachment. Corneal buttons with a diameter of 6 mm were harvested from adult New Zealand rabbits. After peeling off the epithelium, the corneal epithelial sheet was applied to the synthetic lenticule and incubated in modified Eagle's minimum essential medium (MEM). If the cell sheet appeared adherent after 24 hours, the culture was continued for a total of 4 days. Afterward, the specimens were processed for immunohistochemistry and electron microscopy. For immunohistochemical detection of the epithelial adhesion components, bullous pemphigoid antisere, laminin antibodies, and type VII collagen antibodies were employed.

Surgical Technique

Seven eyes of seven rhesus monkeys underwent uncomplicated synthetic EKP with the collagen type IV lenticules. The surgical procedure has been described by Albinet and coworkers[23] and is demonstrated in Fig 30–2. To prevent the lenticules from mechanical damage and infection secondary to eye rubbing, the hands of monkeys 5, 6, and 7 were immobilized temporarily by means of plaster casts. The restraints and tarsorrhaphy were removed after 1 week. All animals underwent slit lamp biomicroscopic examination each day for the first week, once a week for 3 months, and monthly thereafter.

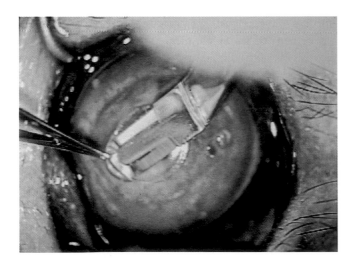

A

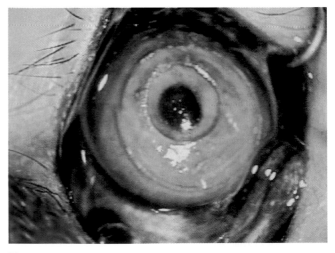

B

Figure 30–2. Surgical technique for synthetic epikeratoplasty. **A.** After removal of the epithelium centrally, a 4-mm guarded trephine set to 0.1-mm depth is used to make a circular keratotomy. **B.** A 2-mm peripheral stromal pocket is created with a number 66 beaver blade. The lenticule is placed onto the cornea and, subsequently, it is guided into the stromal pocket with a Weck sponge. The lenticule is centered within its stromal pocket leaving an optical zone of 4 mm.

All animals were killed by an intravenous application of a lethal overdose of pentobarbital. The cornea–synthetic lenticule button was harvested, and half of the specimen from each animal was processed for TEM. The remaining tissue of animals 3, 4, 5, and 7 was prepared for immunohistochemistry.[31] Half of the specimen of animal 6, which revealed an erosion, was tested for endogenous collagenases and neutral proteases.

Results

In Vitro Tests

In the epithelial cell cultures, all three antigens were detected along the basal cells of the epithelium cultured on the surface of the synthetic type IV collagen lenticule in MEM for 4 days. With EM, a normal basement membrane or cross-banded anchoring fibrils were not found. However, electron densities were seen along the basal cell membrane. Presumably, culturing in an artificial medium for a period of 4 days may not allow prediction of whether the corneal epithelium, which is exposed to the surface of a synthetic lenticule, will be capable of producing normal adhesion structures like basement membrane, hemidesmosomes, and anchoring fibrils. Nevertheless, the results indicate that type IV collagen lenticules may have suitable properties to support epithelial attachment in vitro.

In Vivo Tests

Incomplete Epithelialization

The clinical results of synthetic EKP in seven rhesus monkeys are summarized in Table 30–4. Because of extensive eye rubbing in animals 1 and 2, resulting in expulsion of the lenticule on the first and third postoperative day, respectively, we excluded them from the study and stopped further follow-up exams.

According to reports of the animal care personnel, animals 3 and 4 were observed to rub their eyes frequently. Consequently, these animals did not achieve complete epithelialization of their lenticules. In the follow-up exams, their periorbital skin appeared scaly and erythematous. Additionally, the synthetic lenticules were epithelialized in different areas, as observed in consecutive slit lamp examinations. Postop thinning of the synthetic lenticules was seen in both animals 4 and 6 weeks postoperatively, respectively. Because the areas of lenticule thinning were free of infiltration and no conjunctival injection was seen in either eye, the thinning areas were supposed to be sterile. Both animals were sacrificed 4 weeks and 6 weeks postoperatively, respectively, when the progressive thinning of the lenticules had reached 90% of the original thickness.

Light microscopic examination confirmed the clinical findings of incomplete epithelialization of the lenticule. In epithelialized areas, the epithelium was found to be three cell layers thick. Furthermore, several areas of lenticule thinning were found. However, thinning occurred particularly close to the intrastromal pocket. In one specimen, the lenticule was thinned completely to Bowman's layer. Basal epithelial cells above the thinning areas revealed considerable vacuolization. Bowman's layer beneath the synthetic lenticule appeared normal. Although the corneal stroma contained activated keratocytes near the edge of the stromal pocket, there was no evidence of infiltration of inflammatory cells. In the middle and posterior portion of the stroma, activated keratocytes were not observed.

TEM confirmed vacuolization of the basal epithelium cells and an electron-dense structure, which ap-

TABLE 30–4. SUMMARY OF THE POSTOP OUTCOME

Animal	Complete epithelialization of the lenticule	Use of hand restraints	Postop outcome	Animal status
1	—[a]	No	Lenticule expulsed day 1	Removed from study
2[b]	—[a]	No	Lenticule expulsed day 3	Removed from study
3	No	No	Erosion of lenticule, 4 weeks	Sacrificed 4 weeks po
4[b]	Partial	No	Erosion of lenticule, 6 weeks	Sacrificed 6 weeks po
5	Yes	Yes	Peripheral focal erosion of lenticule, 4 months	Sacrificed 4 months po
6	Yes	Yes	Peripheral focal erosion of lenticule, 4 months	Sacrificed 4 months po
7[b]	Yes	Yes	Lenticule stable over 42 months	Sacrificed 42 months po

[a]Extensive eye rubbing.
[b]Anterior surface of the lenticule was ablated with an excimer laser prior to the attachment.
Abbreviation: po, postoperative.

peared to be lenticule material incorporated within intracytoplasmic vesicles. At the epithelium–lenticule interface, electron-dense structures were seen. Keratocytes located close to the intrastromal pocket revealed plump nuclei, prominent nucleoli, and abundant rough endoplasmic reticulum.

As seen in vitro, immunohistochemistry detected epithelium attachment components, including bullous pemphigoid antigen and type VII collagen, in areas where the lenticule was epithclialized successfully. By contrast, these complexes were not seen over thinned portions.

Complete Epithelialization

The unsatisfactory results in the first four animals forced us to immobilize both hands of the remaining monkeys for 7 days postoperatively. Consequently, all EKP lenticules in these eyes epithelialized completely within 7 days. After removing the hand casts, the animals did not resume frequent eye rubbing. In the slit lamp examination, the conjunctiva showed no injection or other signs of inflammation, and the epithelial layer remained stable during the follow-up period. The synthetic lenticule remained clear throughout the follow-up period.

At the 3-month follow-up examination of animal 5, anterior thinning of the lenticule appeared in three focal areas of oval shape that were located close to the stromal pocket. Although the epithelium remained intact, the thinning progressed during the following 4 weeks, reaching a maximum estimated depth of 20%

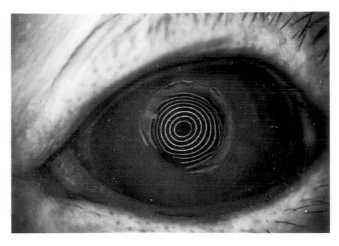

Figure 30–4. Keratoscope photograph following synthetic epikeratoplasty in animal 7 at 21 months postoperatively. Although there is a slight astigmatism evident, the regular mires indicate an acceptable corneal surface centrally.

lenticule thickness and a diameter of 1.25 × 1.5 mm. Thinning of the lenticule portion inserted into the intrastromal pocket was not observed. There was no infiltrate or thinning of the host cornea. The animal was sacrificed 4 months postoperatively.

Except for the number of thinning areas, the postop course was similar in animal 6. At 3 months, an oval thinning area 1.0 × 1.5 mm in diameter covered by an intact epithelial layer was evident. Like animal 5, the thinning occurred close to the intrastromal pocket. Animal 6 was sacrificed 4 months postoperatively.

Following complete epithelialization of the synthetic lenticule in animal 7, the postop course remained free of complications, such as recurrent epithelial erosions, lenticule thinning, detachment of the synthetic lenticule, infiltration, or neovascularization, for 42 months postoperatively (Figs 30–3, 30–4).

In the light microscopic examination, we found the epithelium to be about three cell layers thick. In animals 5 and 6, where lenticule thinning occurred, basal epithelial cells beneath thinning areas were vacuolized. In animal 7, basal epithelium was generally nonvacuolized. The thinning of the lenticule in animals 5 and 6 was located close to the intrastromal pocket, and the epithelium in these areas appeared thickened. Bowman's layer underlying the synthetic lenticule was normal. There was no evidence of activated keratocytes except close to the intrastromal pocket where keratocytes were found in increased size and number (Fig 30–5). Few specimens revealed invasion of keratocytes into the lenticule. The middle and posterior stromal portion, as well as Descemet's membrane and the endothelium, were found to be normal.

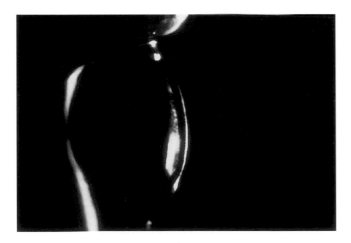

Figure 30–3. Slip-lamp photomicrograph of a human derived type IV collagen lenticule in animal 7 at 42 months after epikeratoplasty. The epithelium covers the synthetic lenticule completely and there is no evidence of epithelial erosions. The lenticule remains stable with respect to its thickness. Note the superior optical performance of the synthetic material compared to the native host cornea.

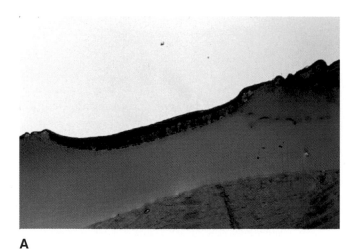
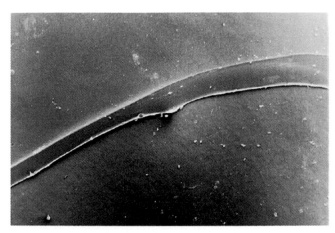

A   B

Figure 30–5. A. Light micrograph of a specimen of animal 7 sacrificed 42 months after synthetic epikeratoplasty ($\times$ 187.5). The specimen was harvested from the region where the lenticule is inserted into the intrastromal pocket. The overlaying epithelium layer appears thickened. **B.** Electron micrograph of the intrastromal pocket of animal 7 ($\times$ 13.200). The keratocytes adjacent to the synthetic lenticule appear not activated. They reveal the typical long and flat form and are embedded in collagen fibers. The basal epithelial cells reveal normal attachment complexes.

In the EM examination, we found one specimen (animal 5) with cells that presumably contained intracytoplasmic inclusions of lenticule fragments. Basal epithelial cells were found with hemidesmosomes, and focal segments of basement membrane were apparent. All physiologic components of the epithelial adhesion complex were localized immunohistochemically at the epithelial lenticule interface. In the specimens of animal 6 tested for collagenolytic enzymes we did not find interstitial collagenase (MMP-1), polymorphonuclear (PMN) collagenase (MMP-8), or stromalysin (MMP-3). However, the zymogram of the fragments contained four major bands, indicating the presence of at least four different gelatin-degrading enzymes. In addition, one specimen contained a caseinolytic neutral protease.

COMMENTS

The results of preliminary studies of synthetic EKP in nonhuman primates suggest that this new approach may be feasible. However, research is still in an early experimental stage, and further efforts will be needed to find a synthetic material with suitable properties and to refine the attachment procedure. Synthetic type IV collagen was found to support attachment and migration of the corneal epithelium both in vitro and in vivo. The appearance of hemidesmosomes, anchoring fibril components, and basement membrane is promising because the production of normal attachment complexes is considered a prerequisite for stable, long-term attachment of the corneal epithelium to the lenticule surface. There was no evidence of epithelial toxicity, recurrent epithelial erosions, infiltration, neovascularization, or other adverse complications. Additionally, the optical properties of type IV collagen were even superior to the human native corneal stroma. This may be attributed to cross-linked matrix, which does not contain continuous helical collagen fibers. We found no difference in results between ablated and nonablated lenticules. Therefore, it may be possible to adjust the anterior curvature or surface characteristics of the synthetic lenticule by means of an excimer laser.

However, the type IV collagen lenticules were found to thin gradually in most of our animals. Frequently, these thinning areas were located close to the intrastromal pocket, which may give rise to the assumption that activated keratocytes released proteolytic enzymes degrading the type IV collagen molecules of the synthetic lenticule.[32,33] Other possible sources of the proteolytic enzymes are epithelial cells and leukocytes. The biochemical examination of the specimen harvested from animal 6 with respect to collagenases revealed that at least four neutral proteases with activity for gelatin, and therefore for type IV collagen,[34] were present in the lenticule, two of which were found in the active form.[35] The exact nature of these enzymes is unknown, although the measured molecular weights referred to different type IV collagenases. These proteases degrade type IV collagen but do not break down type I collagen, which is a major component of the native human cornea. Type I collagen is uniquely degraded enzymatically by interstitial and PMN collagenases.[34] Because we did not find these enzymes either in the thinned lenticule or the host cornea, we conclude that synthetic lenticules consisting of type I collagen may achieve acceptable stability.

Past experience with use of synthetic intracorneal implants to change the refractive status of the eye has shown that the surgeon must be very careful to avoid impairment in intracorneal diffusion of nutrients and metabolites, as this may result in epithelial thinning or even aseptic necrosis. We found the epithelium overlying the synthetic lenticule to be thinned generally to three cell layers. Whether this change was caused by diminished diffusion or insufficient reinnervation of the epithelium covering the lenticule remains to be determined. Corneal nerves or neurotrophic agents have been shown to support normal epithelial morphology and physiology.[36] Nevertheless, stable epithelialization has been observed over completely or partially denervated corneal grafts and human EKP lenticules. Furthermore, the synthetic collagen matrices have demonstrated their potential capability of allowing epithelial reinnervation.[37]

Synthetic EKP is not expected to offer safe and predictable correction of ametropia in humans in the near future. However, the shortcomings of all refractive procedures in current use and the potential advantages of this new approach support further research. Increasing the biostability of synthetic biomaterials, while maintaining the support for epithelial spreading and attachment, and refining the lenticule attachment method will be the focus of further experimental studies.

ACKNOWLEDGMENTS

This study was supported in part by NIH grant no EY007388-02; Yerkes Primate Research Center core grant no RR-00165; Research to Prevent Blindness, Inc; NIH departmental core grant no P30 EY06360; a research grant from General Electric Medical Systems, Milwaukee, Wisconsin, USA; and Domilens, Inc, Lyon, France. The data have been presented partially in a paper published in *Cornea*.

REFERENCES

1. Werblin TP, Klyce SD. Epikeratophakia: the surgical correction of aphakia. I. Lathing of corneal tissue. *Curr Eye Res.* 1981;1:123–129.
2. Werblin TP, Kaufman HE. Epikeratophakia: the surgical correction of aphakia. II. Preliminary studies in a nonhuman primate model. *Curr Eye Res.* 1981;1:131–137.
3. McDonald MB, Klyce SD, Schwarz H, Kandarakis N, Friedlander MH, Kaufman HE. Epikeratophakia for myopia correction. *Ophthalmology.* 1985;92:1417–1422.
4. McDonald MB, Kaufman HE, Aquavella JV, et al. The nationwide study of epikeratophakia for aphakia for adults. *Am J Ophthalmol.* 1987;103:358–365.
5. Grabner G. Myopic epikeratophakia. Results, complications, and new techniques. In: Schachar RA, Levy NS, Schachar U, eds. *Keratorefractive Surgery.* Denison, TX: LAL; 1990:157.
6. Keates RH, Fried S, Levy SN, Morris JR. Carbon dioxide laser use in wound healing and epikeratophakia. *J Cataract Refract Surg.* 1987;13:290–295.
7. Rostron CK. Epikeratophakia grafts glued with autologous cryoprecipitate. *Eur J Implant Refract Surg.* 1989; 1:105.
8. Barrett G, Moore MB. A new method of lathing corneal lenticules for keratorefractive procedures. *J Refract Surg.* 1988;4:142–147.
9. Grabner G. Complications of epikeratophakia for the correction of aphakia, myopia, hyperopia, and keratoconus. *Fortschr Ophthalmol.* 1991;8:4–11.
10. McDonald MB. The future direction of refractive surgery. *Refract Corneal Surg.* 1988;4:158–167.
11. Thompson KP, Hanna K, Waring GO. Emerging technologies for refractive surgery: laser adjustable synthetic epikeratoplasty. *Refract Corneal Surg.* 1989;5:46–48.
12. Thompson KP, Hanna K, Waring GO, et al. Current status of synthetic epikeratoplasty. *Refract Corneal Surg.* 1991;7: 240–248.
13. Thompson KP. Will the excimer laser resolve the unsolved problems with refractive surgery? *Refract Corneal Surg.* 1990;6:315–317.
14. Nimni ME, Harkness RD. Molecular structures and functions of collagen. In: Nimni ME, ed. *Collagen.* Boca Raton, FL: CRC Press, Inc; 1988;1:51.
15. Rao KP, Joseph KT. Collagen graft copolymers and their biomedical applications. In: Nimni ME, ed. *Collagen: Biotechnology.* Boca Raton, FL: CRC Press Inc; 1988;3:63–86.
16. McCarey BE, Storie BR, VanRij G, Knight PM. Refractive predictability of myopic hydrogel intracorneal lenses in nonhuman primate eyes. *Arch Ophthalmol.* 1990, 108: 1310–1315.
17. Trinkaus-Randall V, Capecchi J, Newton A, Vadasz A, Leibowitz H, Franzblanc C. Development of a biopolymeric keratoprosthetic material: evaluation in vitro and in vivo. *Invest Ophthalmol Vis Sci.* 1988;29:393–400.

18. Trinkaus-Randall V, Capecchi J, Sanmon L, Gibbons D, Leibowitz HM, Franzblau C. In vitro evaluation of fibroplasia in a porous polymer. *Invest Ophthalmol Vis Sci.* 1990;31:1321–1326.

19. Gipson IK, Spurr-Michaud S, Tisdale A, Keough M. Reassembly of the anchoring structures of the corneal epithelium during wound repair in the rabbit. *Invest Ophthalmol Vis Sci.* 1989;30:425–434.

20. Kim JH, Green K, Martinez M, Paton D. Solute permeability of the corneal endothelium and Descemet's membrane. *Exp Eye Res.* 1971;12:231–238.

21. Brown SI, Weller CA. Cell origin of collagenases in normal and wounded corneas. *Arch Ophthalmol.* 1970;83:74–87.

22. Hanna KD, Thompson KP, Fantes FE, et al. Interaction of type IV collagen with a 193 nm excimer laser. *Invest Ophthalmol Vis Sci.* 1989;30:189(suppl).

23. Albinet P, Romanet JP, Mouillon M, et al. Epikeratoplastie sans suture ava lentille de Collagene IV chez le singe: description de la technique chirurgicale. *J Fr Ophtalmol.* 1990; 109–114.

24. Waring GO, Hanna KD. The Hanna suction punch block and trephine system for penetrating keratoplasty. *Arch Ophthalmol.* 1989;107:1536–1539.

25. Bailes JE, Quigley MR, Cerullo LJ, Kwaan HC. Review of tissue welding applications in neurosurgery. *Microsurgery.* 1987,8:242–244.

26. Flemming AFS, Colles MJ, Guillianotti R, Brough MD, Brown SG. Laser assisted microvascular anastomosis of arteries and veins: laser tissue welding. *Br J Plast Surg.* 1988;41:378–388.

27. Gailitis RP, Thompson KP, Ren QR, Morris J, Waring GO. Laser welding of synthetic epikeratoplasty lenticules to the cornea. *Refract Corneal Surg.* 1990;6:430–436.

28. Robin JB, Picciano P, Kusleika RS, Salazar J, Benedict C. Preliminary evaluation of the use of mussel adhesive protein in experimental epikeratoplasty. *Arch Ophthalmol.* 1988;106:973–977.

29. Rostron CK, Brittain PH, Morton DB, Rees JE. Experimental epikeratophakia with biological adhesive. *Arch Ophthalmol.* 1988;106:1103–1106.

30. De Toledo AR, Witlock DR, Kaminski LA, Robin JB. Preliminary evaluation of a new collagen-derived bioadhesive. *Invest Ophthalmol Vis Sci.* 1990;31:317(suppl).

31. Gipson IK, Spurr-Michaud SJ, Tisdale AS. Hemidesmosomes and anchoring fibril collagen appear synchronously during development and wound healing. *Dev Biol.* 1988;126:253–262.

32. Johnson-Muller B, Gross J. Regulation of corneal collagenase production: epithelial-stromal cell interactions. *Proc Natl Acad Sci USA.* 1978;75:4417–4421.

33. Johnson-Wint B, Gross J: Regulation of connective tissue collagenase production: stimulators from adult and fetal epidermal cells. *J Cell Biochem.* 1984;98:90–96.

34. Matrisian LM. Metalloproteinases and their inhibitors in matrix remodeling. *Trends Genet.* 1990;6:121–125.

35. Emonard H, Grimaud J-A. Matrix metalloproteinases: a review. *Cell Mol Biol.* 1990;36:131–153.

36. Beuerman RW, Tanelian DL, Schimmelpfennig B. Nerve tissue interactions in the cornea. In: Cavanagh HD, ed. *The Cornea: Transactions of the World Congress on the Cornea.* New York: Raven Press; 1988;3:59–62.

37. Akelman E, Cannistra LM, Tang M, Williams S, Mares F. Regeneration of a peripheral nerve through a bioresorbable nerve guide in primate: a preliminary study. In: *Proceedings of 34th Annual Meeting of the Orthopedic Research Society;* 1988:468.

SECTION VI

Corneal Laser Surgery

CHAPTER 31

Excimer Laser Photorefractive Keratectomy for Myopia

Vance Thompson ■ Theo Seiler

HISTORY OF EXCIMER LASER DEVELOPMENT

The early history of excimer laser development at the beginning of the 1970s was characterized by experiments utilizing pure rare-gas excimer lasers that relied on xenon, krypton, and argon as the laser medium. Subsequent efforts concentrated on developing excimer lasers that used rare-gas–halogen combination molecules, called *dimers*, as the laser medium. These early experiments were among the first attempts to produce lasers in the visible portion of the electromagnetic spectrum, more specifically the ultraviolet (UV) range. Research ensued in the mid-1970s to develop more efficient excimer lasers by studying various rare-gas–halogen mediums, which, upon electric stimulation, led to an unstable bond between the rare-gas and halogen molecule. There was great excitement in the laser community when there was immediate dissociation of this dimer with subsequent fluorescence of UV energy, which, when properly harnessed through sophisticated optical focusing mechanisms, produced a laser beam of considerable energy.[1] Different rare-gas–halogen excimer laser combinations produced different wavelengths of UV laser light (Table 31–1).

Trokel, working with Srinivasan at the IBM Watson Research Center, was the first to suggest that the excimer laser had unique qualities for performing corneal surgery.[2,3] They found that the argon fluoride (ArF) excimer laser at 193 nm produced optimal biologic effects by minimizing thermal damage to adjacent tissues and maximizing accuracy and preciseness of tissue removal. They termed this process *ablative photodecompensation* because of the ability of the laser UV light to cleave chemical bonds and thus to vaporize tissue accurately. In their 1983 publication, they suggested that this laser could be used to remove a lamellar portion of tissue to reshape the corneal curvature and also to perform precisely placed incisions in the cornea. This early work stimulated considerable interest and research activity in laser corneal surgery with the excimer laser.[4]

Theo Seiler was the first to use the excimer laser on a human eye, utilizing it to perform astigmatic keratotomy in 1985.[5] In 1986 Seiler was also the first to use the excimer laser to perform phototherapeutic keratectomy (PTK).[6] Subsequently, Marshall and colleagues suggested the technique of anterior surface ablation to reprofile the anterior corneal curvature.[7] A computer-generated algorithm relating the treatment zone diameter with the depth of ablation to affect a specific

TABLE 31–1. EXCIMER LASER WAVELENGTHS

Laser Medium	Wavelength (nm)
Argon fluoride	193
Krypton chloride	222
Krypton fluoride	248
Xenon chloride	308
Xenon fluoride	351

dioptric change was developed and published by Munnerlyn and colleagues.[8] McDonald was the first to perform photorefractive keratectomy (PRK) on a sighted, myopic eye.[9] Since then immense effort has been focused on excimer laser PRK.[10,11]

EXCIMER LASER PHYSICS

The word *excimer laser* is derived from two words, *excited dimer*. Literally the word *dimer* means "two of the same thing." Obviously the ArF dimer is not made up of two of the same thing, but rather of two different things. In organic molecular physics this type of molecular structure, which is composed of two different molecules, is called an *exciplex*. Some feel that the misnomer *excimer laser* persisted because it is much easier to say than exciplex laser.

A simplified description of an excimer laser system includes a laser cavity with rare-gas and halogen-gas molecules filling it (Fig 31–1). A high-voltage electric discharge is sent into the laser cavity, which causes an unstable bond to be formed between these different types of molecules, resulting in dimers that spontaneously dissociate. Upon separation, a photon of energy is released. These photons of energy are harnessed through a series of focusing lenses and mirrors that make up the excimer laser beam utilized to treat the corneal surface.[12]

Before exiting the laser, the excimer laser beam can be shaped by various methods. Small excimer laser beams can be scanned over the corneal surface in a multitude of patterns. PRK procedures utilizing a scanning technique typically take longer than those utilizing the large-area photoablation technique. Many techniques of large-area photoablation can be utilized to flatten the corneal curvature, the most common being an expanding or contracting iris diaphragm that flattens the cen-

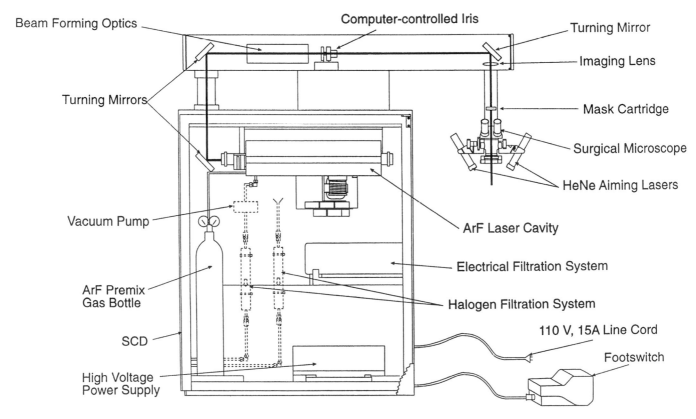

Figure 31–1. Schematic of the Summit Technology UV200 Excimer Laser System.

ter of the cornea more than the periphery. The typical iris diaphragm opens or closes with each pulse of the laser, resulting in small steps seen on electron microscopy (EM) and etched into the corneal surface (Fig 31–2).

Typical lasers utilized in eye surgery require a high number of photons converging to a focal point to provide enough energy to achieve the desired reaction.[13] This is because most lasers have a low amount of energy per photon. Excimer lasers have several desirable characteristics for corneal surgery. The energy per photon is very high, 6.4 electron volts (ev), which easily overcomes intermolecular bond energies (carbon–carbon bonds equal 3.4 ev and peptide bonds equal 3.0 ev) at the corneal surface, thus allowing accurate layer-by-layer tissue removal on a molecular level. The penetration depth of each laser pulse is also minimal so that adjacent tissue damage is minimized.[14] These unique features give accuracy on the micron level and control to lamellar corneal surgery never seen previously because a single pulse of the laser removes approximately 0.22 to 0.25 μm of tissue, depending on the laser parameters utilized. Various excimer laser wavelengths have been studied in the past, but it is the ArF excimer laser at 193 nm that has been shown to be the best for performing PRK.[15]

PREOP EVALUATION

The importance of a thorough examination and counseling session with any refractive surgery patient preoperatively cannot be overemphasized. All patients considered for PRK need to have a complete examination of their anterior and posterior segment. Excimer laser PRK, alternatives to the procedure, and the topic of informed consent should be discussed. An educational video can also be shown, but we feel that this should only be used to reinforce a personal discussion so that each patient understands and clarifies his or her goals and expectations.

Initially the evaluation should include history taking and a statement on why the patient has come in for a refractive surgical evaluation. Particular attention should be paid to statements such as "I want to have this procedure done so I never need to use glasses or contacts again." With counseling on the proper goals and expectations of refractive surgery, which emphasizes "reduced dependence on optical devices but not their elimination from life," most patients with unrealistic expectations can be guided toward more realistic goals, which ultimately results in happier patients.

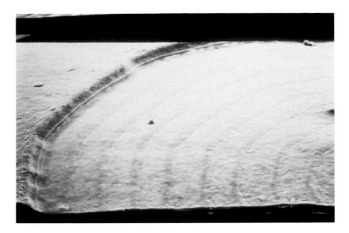

Figure 31–2. Scanning electron micrograph shows small steps seen from the opening iris-diaphragm technique of PRK on this PMMA disc.

Contact lens status, general health history, eye health history, medications review, and allergy history are also documented. Patients with collagen-vascular diseases like systemic lupus erythematosis (SLE) are contraindicated from undergoing PRK because of potential problems with delayed epithelial healing and potential corneal melting. Ocular dominance is checked using a small piece of white cardboard with a 2.5- to 3.0-cm hole or just by having the patient make a small circle with his or her index finger and thumb to look through. The patient fixates with both eyes upon a distant object (we use a distant, red fixation light), then brings the cardboard up into their visual axis and centers the red light in the hole while keeping both eyes open. Keeping both eyes wide open, the patient follows the instruction to bring the piece of cardboard closer to his or her face until it rests in front of one eye, thereby indicating that this is the dominant eye. Manifest refraction is then performed to obtain the best corrected spectacle vision. Cycloplegic refractions are also performed on every patient to make sure he or she is not accommodating or inducing myopia. Patients who cannot be refracted to 20/20 or better need close evaluation. If the cornea, lenses, maculae, and optic nerves appear fine, a rigid contact lens overrefraction can be performed to rule out irregular astigmatism. If this yields better results, a search for keratoconus or contact lens–induced corneal warpage is undertaken. This evaluation is best made with computed topographic analysis. Because patients with permanent irregular astigmatism often yield poor results after refractive surgery, it is considered a contraindication for refractive surgery.

A thorough slit lamp examination is then performed. Blepharitis should be ruled out and, if present, treated aggressively before scheduling PRK. An evaluation for dry eyes is performed, looking for a healthy tear strip and no evidence of any punctate staining of the epithelium with fluorescein. The cornea is evaluated for evidence of keratoconus such as a Fleischer's ring or Vogt's lines. Stromal scars are evaluated closely and old herpetic disease is considered. If herpetic disease is felt to be a possibility, refractive surgery is not recommended. A quiet anterior chamber is expected, and the lens is thoroughly evaluated for any cataractous change. The main factor that limits the upper age of our patients with healthy eyes requesting PRK is their lenticular status. If they have a cataract, refractive surgery is not recommended. If myopia is present after cataract surgery, the patient can still be a good candidate for PRK. The vitreous and retina are evaluated thoroughly for any evidence of retinal pathology, such as macular disease or peripheral retinal pathology. Intraocular pressure (IOP) is evaluated because myopes are at increased risk for developing glaucoma and also because steroids may be used postoperatively. In the event of a steroid-induced pressure rise, documentation of a normal IOP preoperatively is important.

Central keratometry is performed on all patients. Although this information is limited to the central cornea, it can still be useful. Computed corneal topography is utilized to evaluate the curvature of the majority of the cornea and is very useful in ruling out keratoconus. Those patients with keratoconus are contraindicated for PRK.

PATIENT COUNSELING

After the examination and review of corneal topography, the patients are counseled thoroughly. Alternative refractive procedures like radial keratotomy (RK) are reviewed. A brief review of the history and current regulatory status of the excimer laser is given. In the United States the patient should understand the phases of clinical study that PRK is undergoing in its current Food and Drug Administration (FDA) status as an investigational device. The surgeon reviews a typical PRK procedure, emphasizing that topical anesthesia is used and that there is no pain during the treatment. Pain after the anesthesia wears off is discussed, as are the techniques for treating it. Visual return is discussed, including the poor vision that occurs early on, followed by gradual improvement after re-epithelialization (typically within 48 to 72 hours), the appearance of functional vision typically 2 to 3 weeks postoperatively, and

the establishment of best vision 1 to 3 months postoperatively. The early hyperopic period during the first few weeks to a month is discussed; presbyopes are counseled to expect more blur at all distances than they experienced before the procedure. Monovision is discussed and offered as an option. Typically the nondominant eye is treated first and undercorrected by 0.75 diopters (D) to 1.25 D if this approach is requested. In the 6 D and under range, patients are told that they have a 90% to 94% chance of 20/40 or better uncorrected vision after PRK with one treatment. Increasingly higher dioptric corrections are recommended to counteract less successful results with lower dioptric corrections.

Risks of infection with the potential for ulceration, scarring, and loss of best corrected vision are reviewed. The rare chance of needing a corneal transplant with a visually significant scar formation is discussed. The normal stromal and subepithelial healing response is reviewed and haze is described. The risk of overhealing and scar formation is explored. The incidence of enough haze formation to develop a sight-impairing scar is presented as occurring at a rate of approximately 1 out of 100 patients. The techniques for treating overhealers with topical steroids, mechanical scraping at the slit lamp, and phototherapeutic–refractive type excimer procedures are reviewed. The risks of under- and overcorrection are discussed, as is the potential for glare and haloes, especially at night. The risks of topical steroids, including cataracts and IOP elevation, which is rarely permanent, are discussed.

The need for reading glasses after PRK is reviewed with presbyopes and patients near presbyopic age. Patients are offered the chance to talk with other patients who have undergone the procedures. Their questions are then answered, and if the patients' goals and expectations, and their understanding of the process, seem in order, then the PRK procedure is scheduled.

PATIENT SELECTION

The most predictable level of refractive error treatable with the excimer laser continues to be in the low to moderate levels of myopia (1.5 to 6.0 D).[16] Success rates of greater than 90% of patients achieving 20/40 or better uncorrected vision are common at this level of myopia with a single treatment.[11,17]

Patients with greater than 6 D of myopia should be counseled on the increased rate of regression with higher attempted corrections. Gartry et al reported PRK results on 120 eyes with 7 D and under of myopia:

the percentage achieving 20/40 or better uncorrected vision was 90% in the 2-D group, 78% in the 3-D group, 59% in the 4-D group, 50% in the 5-D group, 63% in the 6-D group, and 25% in the 7-D group. Treatment zones in this study were 4 mm in diameter, and the overall rate of 20/40 or better in this group was 70%.[18] Tally et al reported on 91 eyes with a similar range of myopia (−1.00 D to −7.50 D) with achieved results of 20/40 or better uncorrected vision occurring in 93% of patients and 72% achieving 20/25 or better.[19] Treatment zones ranged from 6 to 7 mm. Improved results are thought to be obtained in the higher dioptric range with larger ablation zones and/or peripheral blend zones.[20]

It is notable that patients with greater than 6 D attempted PRK treatments should have a vertex distance correction calculated for entry into the laser computer. After preop spectacle best corrected vision is obtained, the vertex distance should be measured and the appropriate, converted number obtained using vertex conversion charts to make the correct surgical decision in any patient with a greater than 6 D attempted correction.

SURGICAL TECHNIQUE OF PRK

We utilize the Summit Technology OmniMed™ excimer laser system. Thus the technique will reflect the use of this system, although many of the steps presented here are similar in all excimer laser systems.

At the start of each operating day, testing should be performed to assure adequate beam profile and alignment. Various manufacturers utilize different testing methods to evaluate three major factors. Beam homogeneity is first evaluated to ensure that there are no "hot" or "cold" spots in the laser but, rather, a homogenous beam. The second important parameter is the power output, which should be specific in an excimer system so that the algorithm relating number of pulses to depth of ablation is consistent from patient to patient. It is also important to assure appropriate beam alignment by assessing that the helium–neon (HeNe) beam target centration is exactly aligned with the excimer laser beam for centration. Typically the testing of the laser is only done at the beginning of an operative day, not between each case.

After ensuring accurate laser parameters, the patient is brought into the room and positioned under the microscope by reclining on a chair. The nonoperative eye is patched to maximize patient fixation with the operative eye. A patch can also be placed alongside the operative eye to catch excess fluids like tears or topical anesthetic (Fig 31–3).

Topical anesthetic and topical antibiotic placement are performed preoperatively. The surgeon can choose whether or not to constrict the pupil with pilocarpine. Topical anesthesia may be helpful in the nonoperative eye to relax any reflex tearing or discomfort to the patient. A lid speculum is then placed in the operative eye,

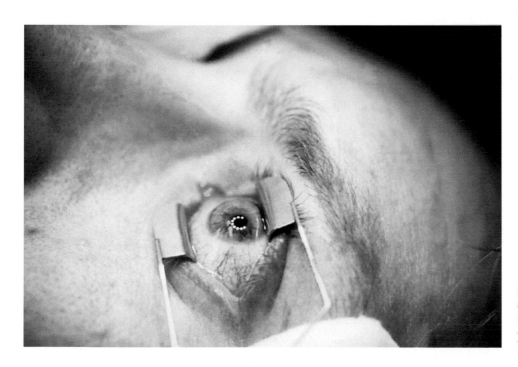

Figure 31–3. The patient's nonoperative eye is patched to maximize proper fixation with the operative eye. A patch along the side of the operative eye can improve patient comfort.

and topical anesthesia is reapplied. The HeNe aiming beams are then positioned. Studies have shown improved PRK centration when the procedure is focused on the center of the pupil rather than on the corneal light reflex.[21,22] Upon precise focusing, one HeNe beam spot is seen in the center of the pupil; these beams diverge and are seen as two red dots equally spaced at the 3 o'clock and 9 o'clock position of the pupillary border. During this whole beginning process, the physician should explain to the patient in detail what is occurring and also what will be occurring during laser energy delivery. It is important to emphasize to the patient that the eye must be fixated on the fixation light in the laser at all times. The patient should be told that the light may blur during the ablation, but he or she should be able to see it at all times. Patients should also be told that the laser will produce a certain noise and smell, which they will be introduced to during the preliminary testing before treatment.

At this time a training session is performed to familiarize the patient with the PRK procedure. First a drop of 1% methylcellulose is applied on the entire corneal surface, and test shots are fired to make sure that the patient fixates well during the laser delivery. This test also familiarizes them with the sounds of the laser (Fig 31–4). It is then repeated on the bare epithelium to acquaint the patient with the louder and more snapping sound of tissue ablation and also with the smell of tissue ablation. Before the epithelial test, the patient is warned that the sounds of the laser will be louder than

during the methylcellulose test but not to worry and to continue fixation. From the surgeon's point of view the imprint left by the laser on the bare epithelium during the epithelial test is easily visualized and serves as a nice secondary check that the laser ablation is appropriately centered over the patient's entrance pupil.

At this point, the testing phase is complete if the patient has maintained appropriate fixation during the test. The methylcellulose test can be repeated until appropriate fixational abilities are documented by the patient. After the surgeon is convinced that the patient can fixate well, the desired refractive correction and the treatment-zone diameter are entered into the laser computer, which determines the number of pulses to be delivered. After documenting that the laser has accepted the parameters of refractive correction and treatment-zone diameter, the epithelium can be removed. It is always prudent to document that the laser is armed, tested, and ready to go with the patient's correction before removing any epithelium.

At this point, an optical-zone marker 1 mm larger than the desired PRK optical-zone treatment is centered, and an imprint is made on the epithelial surface (Fig 31–5). The epithelium is then removed out to the optical-zone mark, utilizing either a number 64 Beaver blade or a Paton spatula (Fig 31–6).

In the past it was felt that removal of epithelium improves the accuracy of the procedure because of variable ablation rates between epithelium, Bowman's membrane, and stroma.[23] The epithelium also varies in

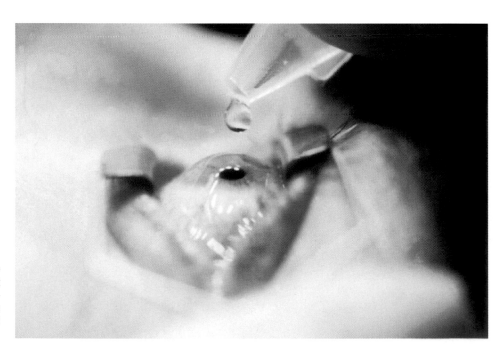

Figure 31–4. One percent methylcellulose is placed on the cornea so that test pulses can be performed to familiarize the patient with the sounds of the laser. This test is then repeated on the bare epithelium.

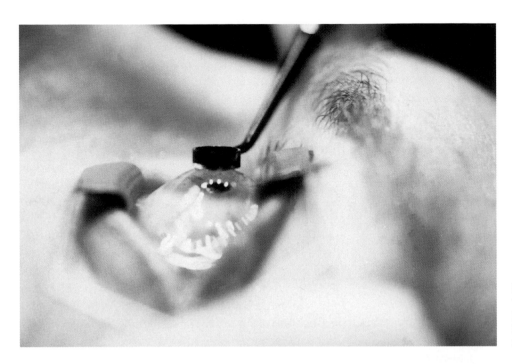

Figure 31–5. An optical-zone mark 1 mm larger than the desired treatment zone is centered and an epithelial imprint is made to guide epithelial removal.

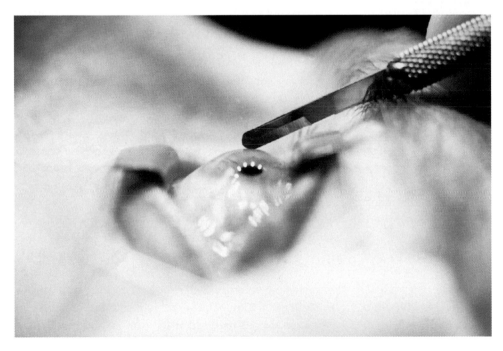

Figure 31–6. Mechanical epithelial removal is facilitated with a Paton spatula or, as in this figure, a number 64 Beaver blade. When utilizing a sharp-edged instrument, a "dragging" rather than a "pushing" motion will help lessen the chance of damaging Bowman's layer.

thickness from one patient to the next, again supporting the notion that removing the epithelium may improve the accuracy of the procedure. Studies are currently underway to assess the need for epithelial removal. Since the epithelium fluoresces to UV light, one can use the excimer laser beam to remove the epithelium with the laser until all remaining fluorescence disappears. Then the PRK procedure can be performed after laser epithelial removal. Well-controlled clinical trials are needed to prove the existence of a clinical difference between mechanical versus laser epithelial removal. At the time of this writing, we both still prefer mechanical epithelial removal.

The epithelial removal time should be less than 5 minutes, and preferably less than 2 minutes, because hydration changes in the cornea can occur that can affect the algorithms and increase the chance of a less accurate refractive correction. A microsurgical sponge is utilized to ensure removal of all the epithelium; a drop of methylcellulose is applied and wiped off with a dry sponge to ensure that all epithelial debris has been removed. The HeNe beams are then recentered, the patient is again instructed on the importance of continual fixation, the laser footpedal is depressed, and the laser procedure is begun. During the procedure the patient's fixation is monitored very closely. If the patient moves, the laser procedure is stopped by lifting the foot off the laser activation pedal, the patient is instructed to refixate, and the laser procedure is then continued because the computer restarts the procedure where it left off. The typical wide-area photoablation procedure involves 15 to 30 seconds of lasing time.

PRK POSTOP CARE

After completion of the procedure, antibiotic/steroid ointment or antibiotic-only ointment is instilled and the eye is patched. Topical antibiotic coverage in the form of ointment or drops is utilized until re-epithelialization occurs, which typically takes less than 72 hours. Postop pain usually occurs. This pain typically is most prominent the first evening of the PRK treatment, gradually improving over the ensuing 24 hours. Oral pain medications like Mepergan Fortis can be helpful in controlling the pain. Topical nonsteroidal anti-inflammatory drugs (NSAIDs) with or without the use of a bandage lens have been reported by some as an effective treatment for pain control.[24,25] Studies are under way to document both this and the effect, if any, of these treatment modalities on refractive outcome in well-controlled clinical trials.

Following re-epithelialization, which typically occurs within 72 hours, the decision of whether or not to use topical steroids is made. We currently use topical FML 0.1%, 1 drop to the operative eye TID for the first month postoperatively, tapering gradually over a 3-month period. In Summit Technology's US clinical trial, a semirigid steroid regimen has been established to enhance the statistical reliability of the results in the FDA-monitored PRK clinical trials. The efficacy of steroid use remains to be proven in randomized clinical trials. Some investigators have concluded that steroids are not needed and that they delay the normal healing response and visual recovery.[26] Others feel that steroids not only help improve the refractive outcome and lessen haze but also are beneficial in patients with late postop regressions that can respond to steroids positively.[27,28] Research is under way to establish a dioptric

cutoff below which steroids may not be needed. Our current impression is that the majority of patients with low to moderate myopia (4 D and under) treated with PRK most likely do not need topical steroids postoperatively.

PRK COMPLICATIONS

Complications can occur intraoperatively or postoperatively. Incomplete epithelial removal could be a cause of an irregular refractive result. Because epithelium fluoresces upon exposure to UV radiation, one can immediately tell if there is any residual epithelium. If the epithelium is not completely removed, an incomplete photokeratectomy will occur. Delayed removal of the epithelium can lead to hydration changes in the corneal stroma and unpredictable refractive results. We recommend performing excimer ablation within 2 minutes after the epithelium is removed.

Loss of patient fixation can lead to eccentric ablation and can occur in one of two forms. The first is a rapid and obvious loss of patient fixation. If the patient briefly loses fixation and refixates immediately, the ablation can continue uninterrupted. But if rapid loss of fixation occurs without an immediate refixation, the laser ablation should be immediately stopped. The laser computer remembers where it left off, so that by simply instructing the patient to be calm and refixate one can reinstitute the ablation without causing any problems. Problems occur when the ablation is not stopped and is allowed to continue.

The second type of loss of fixation is a slow drift, which can be more difficult for the surgeon to recognize. It is helpful for the surgeon to concentrate on the patient's entrance pupil and to make sure that the fixation HeNe beams are well centered on the pupil during the whole ablation. An inexperienced excimer laser surgeon sometimes tends to watch the ablation of the expanding iris diaphragm so that a slow drift of the HeNe beams from the center of the pupil may not be recognized. However, by concentrating on the HeNe beam and proper centration, a slow drift can be easily recognized and corrected. Studies have shown that PRK centration is optimized by localization of the aiming beam on the center of the entrance pupil.[22] Uncorrected and best corrected vision can be degraded with eccentric ablations that are more than 1 mm decentered.[29] Symptoms of blurred vision, glare, ghost images, and poor contrast sensitivity can occur with a decentered ablation.

Tracking systems are being evaluated to potentially maximize PRK centration. They are being studied in various excimer laser systems and generally come in two forms. One form involves highly sensitive tracking equipment that fixates the desired point of centration on the cornea, locks in on it in the three-dimensional sense, and moves the excimer beam system to stay in the correct position on the cornea during the ablation. In the other type of tracking system, parameters are set that allow micromovements of the eye during ablation. However, should there be a movement beyond the parameters set, such as loss of fixation, the laser temporarily stops ablation and does not restart until the patient's fixation is back. The importance of tracking systems will become more obvious through well-controlled clinical trials. We feel that a tracking system is probably more important in a scanning excimer laser system than in wide-area photoablation with an expanding iris diaphragm because the scanning technique takes longer, increasing the likelihood of loss of fixation.

During an iris-diaphragm–wide area photoablation procedure, centration is most critical at the point when the iris diaphragm is at its smallest point. The pulses that come out of the laser at this point are very small in diameter so that any decentration would take them away from the center of the pupil. Our clinical observations reflect more solid patient fixation at the beginning of the excimer procedure when the fixation light appears the most crisp to the patient and the patient is not fatigued. This issue becomes critical when assessing whether or not an opening or closing iris diaphragm is better for wide-area photoablation. It is our opinion that, because the patient's fixational abilities appear to be best at the beginning of the ablation, the opening iris diaphragm makes the most sense because those first, smaller pulses that need to be centered crucially will occur during the period of best patient fixation, that is, at the beginning of the procedure. When the iris diaphragm is wide open, the diameter of the pulses is very large; the possibility of any slight patient movement is less significant during this portion of the procedure. This is why we feel an opening iris diaphragm is advantagous in wide-area photoablation.

Another issue is globe fixation. Better centration is obtained with patient self-fixation during wide-area photoablation. It is possible for the operating surgeon to center the HeNe beams on what looks like the center of the pupil, but not to be treating the cornea over the center of the pupil if the patient is not fixating. This is because the cornea is a clear structure and parallax can lead to this type of problem. Thus patient fixation while the surgeon concentrates on focusing the guiding HeNe beams on the pupillary center optimizes centration of the PRK procedure.

Early postop complications include delayed re-epithelialization. The majority of PRK patients are re-epithelialized within 72 hours. During this period the patient is monitored for any development of infectious infiltrates. Infectious infiltrates after PRK are rare but have been reported.[30] Because of the large area of epithelial removal, patients with known epithelial healing disorders should not undergo PRK. Seiler reported on a 62-year-old patient with undiagnosed SLE who underwent PRK and required 10 days for the epithelium to close.[6] One month after the procedure the patient presented with a painless, perforated, sterile corneal melt, which necessitated emergency penetrating keratoplasty. PRK is absolutely contraindicated in patients with autoimmune and connective tissue diseases known to be associated with delayed corneal epithelial healing.

Early on there was concern that ablation of the anterior corneal stroma and Bowman's membrane might lead to epithelial disorders. Normal epithelial patterns emerge after PRK, however, and the excimer laser does not affect the morphologic characteristics of the superficial epithelium.[31] Hemidesmosomal attachments also occur between the epithelium and the new anterior stromal bed (Fig 31–7). In fact, the excimer laser has been effective in treating recurrent corneal erosion that has been unresponsive to other treatment modalities.[32]

Surface elevations, seen topographically and described as "central islands," have been reported recently in some patients.[33] These abnormalities can be associated with monocular diplopia, ghost images, and

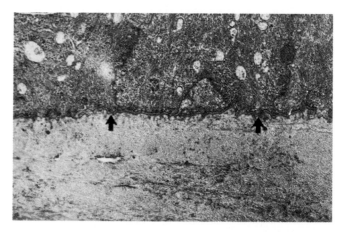

Figure 31–7. Histologic photo demonstrating reestablishment of hemidesmosomal attachments between regenerated corneal epithelium and ablated anterior stroma.

decreased contrast sensitivity. Current efforts are being directed to unravel the cause of these central elevations. Some have suggested corneal moisture buildup during ablation, possible laser-beam–quality problems, or maybe a gradual degradation of the optics of the excimer laser system over time. We believe that central islands are related to larger optical-zone and/or high dioptric treatments, in which greater depth of ablation must be obtained to satisfy the algorithms for these treatments, resulting in increased central buildup of tissue-ablation corneal moisture and thereby lessening the amount of central tissue that is ablated. This theory should be documented in well-controlled clinical trials. The current definition of a topographic central island is an elevation of at least 1 mm in size and 1 D in topographic height.

Other possible side effects after excimer laser can include ptosis, possibly lid-speculum or steroid related, and anisocoria, most likely due to topical steroids. Patients should be instructed on these potential complications as well as the other risks of topical steroids like cataracts, glaucoma (potentially permanent), and increased risks of infection or reactivation of herpes simplex keratitis.

Haloes around bright sources of light can occur at night. Glare also may occur at night. Haloes may be associated with a treatment zone that is smaller than the pupil diameter in low light conditions. One study comparing 4- and 5-mm ablation zones showed significantly fewer haloes in the 5-mm ablation zone treatments.[34] It has been suggested that the optical zone diameter should match the entrance pupillary diameter in low light conditions.[35] Greater ablation zones would probably solve the halo symptoms. There is a tradeoff, however, as the larger the optical zone, the deeper the amount of ablation.[8] And there is some clinical evidence that deeper ablations result in a higher incidence of regression and scar formation. Also, aspheric corrections, including a peripheral blend zone, can be performed to create greater effective optical zones and minimize halo effects.[20]

Subepithelial haze formation, which peaks at 3 months, may also contribute to glare symptoms and to reduction in low light-contrast sensitivity, peaking around 3 months postoperatively and returning toward preop levels by the 6-month postop visit.[36] Lohman et al have developed a device utilizing a CCD camera fixed to a slit lamp microscope and a computer, which provided objective measurements of haze formation and transparency reduction by measuring corneal light scattering.[37] Back-scattered light (what the surgeon sees) and forward-scattering light (what the patient views and experiences) can also be measured. When these two variables are utilized for quantitating measurements of glare and haloes, spectacles, hard contact lenses, and excimer laser surgery have all been shown to be superior to soft contact lenses in terms of light scatter and low-contrast visual acuity.[36]

A number of studies have evaluated the corneal endothelium after PRK. Amano and Shimuzu performed specular microscopy on 26 eyes after myopia PRK and found no statistical differences in mean cell density or coefficient of variation of mean cell area between preop, 1 month, and 1 year.[38] They felt that PRK does not markedly affect the corneal endothelial cell density. Dehm et al looked at the corneal endothelium in rabbits and found that 193-nm excisions to 90% of corneal depth produced endothelial alterations similar to those seen underlying diamond-knife incisions of a similar depth in which the sheet of endothelial cells remains continuous.[39] Perez-Santonja et al studied endothelial-cell density, coefficient of variation in cell size, and hexagonality in 14 eyes after excimer laser preoperatively and 6 months postoperatively and concluded that no endothelial abnormalities were found after PRK.[40]

CORNEAL HEALING AFTER PRK

Even though the typical wide-area photoablation PRK procedure takes in the range of 20 to 30 seconds of laser time and the epithelium grows in rather quickly, that is, typically within 72 hours, it is the ensuing months of slow and continuous healing in the anterior stromal and subepithelial layers that balances out the initial surgical effect to provide the patient with a final refractive error that often depends on individual wound-healing characteristics. The excimer laser provides a consistent dioptric flattening from patient to patient in a fashion more predictable than any other refractive surgery technique developed thus far, but the subsequent wound healing can vary from patient to patient, sometimes impressively.

The majority of the patients after PRK developed a trace to mild subepithelial corneal haze. This haze begins to show up at around 1 month postoperatively and typically peaks at the 3- to 6-month visit.[40–42] It then decreases gradually, and at about 18 months postoperatively most corneas are clear except for some that may show a trace residual haze and often a central epithelial iron line in the treatment area. The haze should be followed and documented at each postop visit (Fig 31–8).

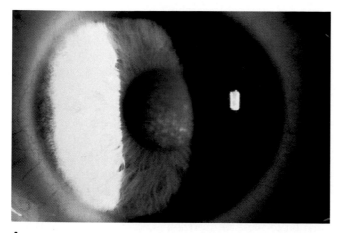

A

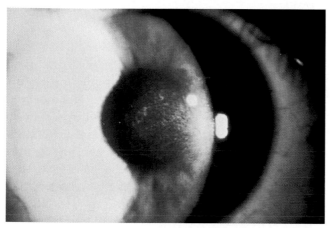

B

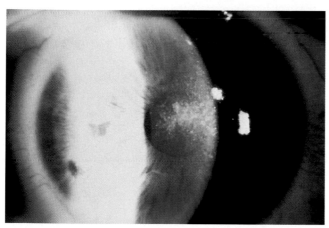

C

Figure 31–8. Grading of postop haze formation: **A.** Trace haze. **B.** Mild haze. **C.** Moderate haze.

Intense haze formation, to the level that would be considered an anterior stromal scar, with significant regression of effect, occurs in approximately 1 out of 100 patients. Best corrected vision is reduced in these patients. The treatment of these intense haze-forming patients can be challenging. It is best to approach these patients in a stepwise fashion. We first treat patients with intense haze by placing them back on topical steroids. Early on, this haze formation and mild regression can be quite steroid responsive.[28] If no, or minimal, response is noted with topical steroid therapy after approximately 1 month, a corneal scraping with a number 64 Beaver blade can be effective in removing this subepithelial fibrous material. After too long a wait, this material adheres more tightly to the anterior stroma and can be more difficult to remove. After scraping the surface and removing the superficial tissue, the steps of the original ablated bed are often still present. Early reports of this scraped material demonstrate a heavy concentration of glycosaminoglycans (John Marshall, PhD, personal communication, September 1993). In cases where the haze proves unresponsive to both steroids and a scraping procedure (too much time may have elapsed since initial therapy), the adherent remaining scar tissue may be removed with repeat excimer laser therapy. In one study of 11 patients with significant scar formation who were retreated, only one showed a repeated mild scar formation 6 months after the operation.[44] Thus repeat excimer laser can be beneficial in cases of aggressive healing that have not been responsive to topical steroids or mechanical scraping.

Durrie et al[44] have nicely described three wound-healing types, which can be helpful in following the PRK patients postoperatively. Type 1 healers comprise the majority of patients, following the trace to mild haze formation that begins at 1 month, peaks at 3 to 6 months, and gradually dissipates. Type 2 healers are known as underhealers, and clear corneas to trace haze is often seen during the 3- to 6-month period. These patients are at risk for overcorrection. Type 3 healers are the more aggressive healers, who are at risk for moderate to severe haze formation. How each one of these wound-healing types is handled can optimize the result after PRK.

The question of whether or not type 1, or average, responders, who constitute the majority of patients, need topical steroids or not is still unanswered. These patients may do fine without topical steroid therapy. The overhealers, however, can receive great benefit from topical steroid therapy to blunt their aggressive healing response. The underhealers can also be helped by stopping their steroids in order to stimulate a wound-healing response. If the cornea remains clear and the patient remains overcorrected, a corneal scraping combined with bandage lens placement can be beneficial in stimulating a wound-healing response, subsequent lessening of hyperopia, and improvement of their refractive state.[44]

The same haze that once worried investigators about excimer laser PRK now elicits relief when it occurs in its trace to mild form because it tells the examiner that the patient is following a normal healing response and should end up with a nice result.

ERODIBLE-MASK PRK

Most excimer laser systems employ combinations of mechanical irises, slits, and/or apertures to deliver the appropriate amount and distribution of the excimer beam to the eye. The ability to treat simple refractive errors like myopia has not been too difficult, but the ability to perform toric ablations for astigmatism and compound refractive errors has not been as easy to attain. The excimer laser in combination with the erodible mask enables toric ablations to be performed. The use of an erodible mask to perform PRK also offers potential advantages in the procedure, including a smoother surface, without the steps associated with iris diaphragm delivery. Furthermore, any refractive state that can be numerically described could theoretically be sculpted onto the eye.

The concept of using an erodible mask to perform PRK was first suggested by Muller,[45] with preclinical trials[46]; sighted-eye studies have since been conducted.[47,48] The erodible mask consists of a precisely shaped, plastic button made out of polymethyl meth-

acrylate (PMMA), which exhibits an ablation rate similar to that of corneal tissue. The mask is mounted on a quartz substrate that is transparent to photons at 193 nm (Fig 31–9). The excimer laser beam is designed in an erodible-mask technique to illuminate the entire erodible mask. The first few pulses of the laser energy are totally absorbed by the mask material. Erosion through the mask material occurs in its thinner areas first (in the center for a myopic correction, and just the opposite for a hyperopic correction), thus distributing the laser energy on the anterior corneal surface in the desired pattern (Fig 31–10). The mask template can theoretically be shaped to treat any refractive error, including myopia, astigmatism, hyperopia, or complex compound refractive errors. Current visual and refractive results with myopic masks closely approximate those of standard iris-diaphragm PRK.[49]

Clinical studies have thus far utilized a hand-held technique that requires surgeon expertise and an accompanying learning curve to achieve optimal results. This system has been difficult to use for alignment reasons. The development of the coaxial microsoft in the OmniMed excimer laser system has eased the alignment difficulties that arose with the hand-held erodible-mask system. Variations on the hand-held technique of erodible-mask PRK have also been developed.[50]

Phase IIB erodible-mask myopia results have closely approximated those of phase III iris-diaphragm PRK in a group of 14 patients at 3 months, which showed 79% having uncorrected vision of 20/20 or better and 100% with uncorrected vision of 20/30 or better; the entire group was within ± 1 D manifest refraction. Six-month phase IIB astigmatism studies demonstrate 90% within ± 1 D of intended sphere and residual astigmatism, or less than 1 D in 75% of the patients.[16] Hyperopia erodible-mask trials in the United States are ap-

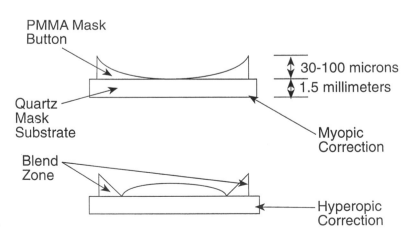

Figure 31–9. The erodible-mask assembly.

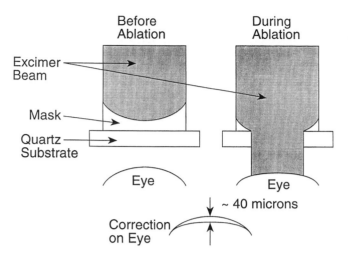

Figure 31–10. Shape transfer with an erodible mask.

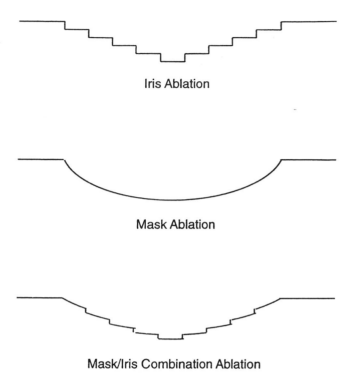

Figure 31–11. Comparison of iris ablation, mask ablation, and combined mask–iris ablation.

proximately 6 months into the phase IIA clinical trials. Three-month results on this first group of patients treated in the United States show an achieved versus attempted correction of 60% to 65% in the +1.5-D to +4.0-D range. Vision without correction is 20/50 or better in 100% of the patients, and 90% have less than 1.5 D of residual hyperopia.[16]

A procedure that is showing early promise is combination iris–diaphragm ablations for myopia in tandem with use of the erodible mask for the toric portion of the ablation. An advantage to this type of approach is that only a small inventory of mask types is needed to treat the majority of astigmatic corrections in combination with myopic refractive error. In the combination mask–iris technique, the first step is to perform the myopic iris–diaphragm correction into the polymethyl methacrylate astigmatic button and then complete the mask ablation at the full diameter of the mask's ablation zone.[51] A specially designed endpoint detection system ensures that the mask is completely ablated. Microscopic steps are seen on the polymethyl methacrylate button, but the differential ablation rate of the PMMA material at the edge of the ablation zone smooths out the stepped profile of the iris–diaphragm steps (Fig 31–11).

The erodible mask appears to be a safe and effective technique for the combination of myopia, hyperopia, and astigmatism. Future possibilities include the ability to produce a customized mask based on computerized corneal topography to treat both refractive error and corneal irregularities such as irregular astigmatism. The elimination of the surgeon variable with the newly developed erodible mask in the optical rail design, the inherent advantages of producing a

smoother ablated surface, and the ability to transfer complex shapes to the corneal surface, thereby correcting an infinite number of complicated refractive errors, will make this technique a very important part of future PRK surgery.

CONCLUSION

Photorefractive keratectomy has been shown to be a safe and effective technique for the treatment of 6 D and under of myopia. Its predictability from surgeon to surgeon is unrivaled. Current research is making great strides toward more predictable treatments in higher amounts of myopia and astigmatism as well as hyperopia. Treating postop pain and manipulation of wound healing are two critical areas of research that have achieved a good deal. Tear-film analysis to identify key immune mediators may play a role in the future in not only deciding who may be the best candidates for PRK, but also in helping manipulate postop pharmacologic control. Combination techniques like the iris–diaphragm–erodible-mask technique will continue to be developed, and the optimal treatment of complex refractive errors will be defined. Despite the excimer laser's being a relatively new technique for treating refractive error, it has etched its place in history. The goal now will be to take a beautiful instrument for changing corneal curvature to the next level of maximal predictability to treat large ranges of refractive error in a comfortable fashion.

REFERENCES

1. Ewing JJ. In: *Laser Pioneer Interviews,* 1st ed. Torrance, CA: High Tech Publications; 1985:243–256.
2. Trokel SL. Evolution of excimer laser corneal surgery. *J Cataract Refract Surg.* 1989;15:373–383.
3. Trokel SL, Srinivasan R, Braren B. Excimer laser surgery of the cornea. *Am J Ophthal.* 1983;96:710–715.
4. Marshall J, Trokel SL, Rothery S, et al. A comparative study of corneal incisions induced by diamond and steel knives and two ultraviolet radiations from an excimer laser. *Br J Ophthalmol.* 1986;70:482–501.
5. Seiler T, Wollensak J. In vivo experiments with the excimer laser—technical parameters and healing processes. *Ophthalmologica.* 1986;192:65–70.
6. Seiler T. Photorefractive keratectomy: European experience. In: Thompson FB, McDonnell PJ, eds. *Excimer Laser Surgery: The Cornea.* New York: Igaku-Shoin; 1993:53–62.
7. Marshall J, Trokel SL, Rothery S, et al. Photoablative reprofiling of the cornea using an excimer laser: photorefractive keratectomy. *Lasers Ophthalmol.* 1986;1:21–48.
8. Munnerlyn CR, Koons SJ, Marshall J. Photorefractive keratectomy: a technique for laser refractive surgery. *J Cataract Refract Surg.* 1988;14:46–52.
9. McDonald MB, Kaufman HE, Frantz JM, et al. Excimer laser ablation in a human eye. *Arch Ophthalmol.* 1989;107:641–642.
10. Seiler TS, Kahle G, Kriegerowski M. Excimer laser (193 nm) myopic keratomileusis in sighted and blind human eyes. *Refract Corneal Surg.* 1990;6:165–173.
11. Seiler TS, Wollensak J. Myopic photorefractive keratectomy (PRK) with the excimer laser—one year followup. *Ophthalmology.* 1991;98:1156–1163.
12. Waring GO. Development of a system for excimer laser corneal surgery. *Trans Am Ophthalmol Soc.* 1989;87:854–983.
13. Durrie DS, Thompson VM. Excimer laser and its uses in refractive surgery. *Ophthalmic Practice.* 1991;9:117–122.
14. Marshall J, Trokel SL, Rothery S, et al. A comparative study of corneal incisions induced by diamond and steel knives and two ultraviolet radiations from an excimer laser. *Br J Ophthalmol.* 1988;70:482–501.
15. Puliafito CA, Wong K, Steinert RF. Quantative and ultrastructural studies of excimer laser ablation of the cornea at 193 and 248 nanometers. *Lasers Surg Med.* 1987;7:155–159.
16. Thompson V, Gordon M. Use of the excimer laser in refractive surgery. *Semin Ophthalmol.* 1994;9(2):91–96.

17. Tengroth B, Epstein D, Fagerholm P, et al. Excimer laser photorefractive keratectomy for myopia: clinical results in sighted eyes. *Ophthalmology.* 1993;100:739–745.
18. Gartry DS, Kerr Muir MG, Marshall J. Photorefractive keratectomy with an argon fluoride excimer laser: a clinical study. *Refract Corneal Surg.* 1991;7:1–16.
19. Tally AR, Sher NA, Kim MS, et al. Use of the 193 nm excimer laser for photorefractive keratectomy in low to moderate myopia. *J Cataract Refract Surg.* 1994;20:5239–5241.
20. Thompson KP. Photorefractive keratectomy. *Ophthalmol Clin N America.* 1992;5(4):745–751.
21. Jozato H, Guyton DL. Centering corneal surgical procedures. *Am J Ophthalmol.* 1987;103:264–275.
22. Cavanaugh TB, Durrie DS, Riedel SM, et al. Topographical analysis of the centration of excimer laser photorefractive keratectomy. *J Cataract Refract Surg.* 1993;19:136–143.
23. Seiler T, Kriegerowski M, Schnoy N, et al. Ablation rate of human corneal epithelium and Bowman's layer with the excimer laser (193 nm). *Refract Corneal Surg.* 1990;6:99–102.
24. Sher NA, Frantz JM, Talley A, et al. Controlling ocular pain after excimer laser PRK. Third American–International Congress on Cataract, IOL, and Refractive Surgery; May 1993:25. Abstract.
25. Arshinoff SA, Sadler C, D'Addario D. The effect of topical non-steroidal anti-inflammatory drugs (NSAIDs) on pain and myopic regression in excimer laser photorefractive keratectomy. Third American–International Congress on Cataract, IOL, and Refractive Surgery; May 1993:19. Abstract.
26. Gartry DS, Kerr-Muir MG, Lohman CP, et al. The effect of topical corticosteroids on refractive outcome and corneal haze after photorefractive keratectomy. *Arch Ophthalmol.* 1982;110:944–952.
27. Fitzsimmons TD, Fagerholm P, Tengroth B. Steroid treatment of myopic regression: acute refractive and topographic changes in excimer photorefractive keratectomy patients. *Cornea.* 1993;12:358–361.
28. Carones F, Brancato R, Venturi E, et al. Efficacy of corticosteroids in reversing regression after photorefractive keratectomy for myopia. *Refract Corneal Surg.* 1993;10:552–560.
29. Maloney RK. Corneal topography and optical zone location in photorefractive keratectomy. *Refract Corneal Surg.* 1990;6:363–371.
30. McDonald MB, Frantz JM, Klyce SD, et al. Central photorefractive keratectomy for myopia. The blind eye study. *Arch Ophthalmol.* 1990;108:799–808.
31. Amano S, Shimizu K, Tsubota K. Corneal epithelial changes after excimer laser photorefractive keratectomy. *Am J Ophthalmol.* 1993;115:441–443.
32. Forster W, Grewe S, Atzler V, et al. Phototherapeutic keratectomy in 13 eyes with superficial corneal diseases. *Refract Corneal Surg.* 1993;9:465–467.

33. Lin D, Sutton HF, Berman M. Corneal topography following excimer laser photorefractive keratectomy for myopia. *J Cataract Refract Surg.* 1993;19:149–154.

34. O'Brart DPS, Gartry DS, Lohman CP, et al. Photorefractive keratectomy for myopia: comparison of 4.0 mm and 5.0 mm ablation zones. *Refract Corneal Surg.* 1994;10:530.

35. Roberts CW, Koester CJ. Optical zone diameters for photorefractive corneal surgery. *Invest Ophthalmol Vis Sci.* 1993;34:2275–2281.

36. Lohman CP, Fitzke F, O'Brart D. Corneal light scattering and visual performance in myopic individuals with spectacles, contact lenses, or excimer laser photorefractive keratectomy. *Am J Ophthalmol.* 1993;115:444–453.

37. Lohman CP, Timberlake GT, Fitzke FW. Corneal light scattering after excimer laser photorefractive keratectomy: the objective measurement of haze. *Refract Corneal Surg.* 1992;8:114–121.

38. Amano S, Shimuzu K. Corneal endothelial changes after excimer laser photorefractive keratectomy. *Am J Ophthalmol.* 1993;116:692–694.

39. Dehm EJ, Puliafito CA, Adler CM, et al. Corneal endothelial injury in rabbits following excimer laser ablation at 193 nm and 248 nm. *Arch Ophthalmol.* 1986;104:1364–1368.

40. Perez-Santonja JJ, Meza J, Moreno E, et al. Short term corneal endothelial changes after photorefractive keratectomy. *J Refract Corneal Surg.* 1994;10:194–198.

41. Hanna KD, Pouliquen Y, Waring GO, et al. Corneal stromal wound healing in rabbits after 193 nm excimer laser surface ablation. *Arch Ophthalmol.* 1989;107:895–901.

42. Fantes FE, Hanna KD, Waring GO, et al. Wound healing after excimer laser keratomileusis (photorefractive keratectomy) in monkeys. *Arch Ophthalmol.* 1990;108:665–675.

43. Seiler T, Derse M, Pham T. Repeated excimer laser treatment after photorefractive keratectomy. *Arch Ophthalmol.* 1992;110:1230–1233.

44. Durrie DS, Lesher MP, Hunkeler JD. Treatment of overcorrection after myopic photorefractive keratectomy. *J Refract Corneal Surg.* 1994;10:295.

45. Muller DF. Laser reprofiling system and methods. US patent number: 4,856,513.

46. Maloney RK, Friedman M, Harmon T, et al. A prototype ablatable mask delivery system for the excimer laser. *Ophthalmology.* 1993;100:542–549.

47. Seiler T. Der Excimerlaser—ein Instrument für die Kornhaut–chirurgie. *Ophthalmologe.* 1992.

48. Gordon M, Seiler T, Carey JP, et al. Photorefractive keratectomy (PRK) at 193 nm using an erodible mask. *SPIE Proc Ophthalmic Technol.* 1992;2:1664–1652.

49. Gordon M, Seiler T, Carey JP, et al. Photorefractive keratectomy (PRK) at 193 nm using an erodible mask; new developments and clinical progress. *SPIE Proc Ophthalmic Technol.* 1993:3:1877.

50. Brancato R, Carones F, Trabuech G, et al. The erodible mask in the correction of myopia and astigmatism. *Refract Corneal Surg.* 1993;9:1–6.

51. Friedman MD, Bettenson S, Brodsky L. OmniMed II: A new system for use with the emphasis erodible mask. *J Refract Corneal Surg.* 1994;10:5267–5273.

CHAPTER 32

Photoastigmatic Refractive Keratectomy (PARK)

Johnny M. Khoury ▪ Walter J. Stark ▪ Dimitri T. Azar

INTRODUCTION

Disabling astigmatism can result from different surgical procedures (eg, penetrating keratoplasty, cataract extraction, and refractive surgical procedures like radial keratotomy), or it can be naturally occurring. Conventional treatments include spectacle or contact lens wear. Some patients however, may be contact lens intolerant or unable to tolerate the high cylindrical prescription in their spectacles. The concept of surgically treating corneal astigmatism was first introduced by Schiotz in 1885.[1] Before excimer laser technology was developed, incisional procedures (relaxing incisions), suture removal, and wedge resection were the mainstays of surgical correction of astigmatism.

In 1983, Trokel and associates introduced excimer laser surgery to the field of ophthalmology.[2] The excimer laser emits short-wavelength (193-nm), high-energy UV radiation capable of ablating the surface layer of exposed tissue with minimal damage to neighboring tissues.[3,4] Photorefractive keratectomy (PRK) with the excimer laser is currently under investigation as a means of correcting refractive errors. Good results have been reported for PRK in low myopia of up to −6 diopters.[5–7] The results of PRK for higher degrees of myopia, however, are more variable.[8,9] PRK is radially symmetric surgery that is performed with greater ablation depth in the center, rather than the periphery, of the cornea.

Recently, the excimer laser has been used for the correction of astigmatism. This procedure requires a nonradially symmetric approach to tissue ablation, with selective flattening of the steep meridian or, alternatively, steepening of the flat meridian (Fig 32–1). While the results seem promising, they are based on reports of a relatively small number of cases.

SURGICAL TECHNIQUES

Correction of astigmatism utilizing the energy of the excimer laser is possible, and several surgical techniques have been described. These include the whole-field, the scanning, and the erodible-mask techniques.

The whole-field technique is the most commonly used, and was first described by McDonnell et al in 1991.[10] The 193-nm excimer laser (TwentyTwenty, VISX, Inc, Santa Clara, CA) software and hardware were modified to perform toric ablations designed to

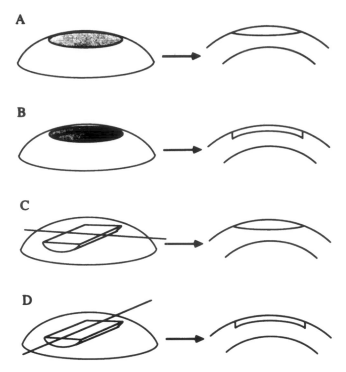

Figure 32–1. A. Schematic illustration of PRK for myopia. **B.** PTK with uniform ablation depth. **C.** Astigmatic keratectomy sectioned in meridian of desired flattening. **D.** Meridian of no intended refractive change. *(From Shieh et al. Quantitative analysis of wound healing after cylindrical and spherical excimer laser ablations.* Ophthalmology. *1992;99:1050–1055.)*

In addition to cylindrical correction, the diaphragm movements can be controlled by computer software to perform elliptical or sequential spherocylindrical treatments. In an elliptical treatment, the computer-controlled mechanism built into the laser expands both the slit and the iris diaphragm simultaneously, ablating an elliptical area of the cornea and flattening the corneal curvature along the meridian of the slit expansion. In a sequential treatment, the cylinder is usually treated first, followed by the sphere.

The scanning and erodible-mask techniques are in the early investigational stages. The scanning technique involves a preprogrammed scan that is used to remove a spherocylindrical tissue lenticule from the corneal stromal surface. In such a procedure, the beam is transmitted to the anterior stroma when the thinnest part of the mask is ablated. At the end of the procedure, the shape of the mask is transformed to the cornea, producing the desired astigmatic correction (Fig 32–3). Thus,

correct cylindrical errors. Therefore, a cylindrical-lens shape rather than a spherical-lens shape is carved onto the cornea. To correct astigmatism, a large-diameter (5.3-mm) laser beam is passed between a set of parallel blades. The separation between the blades is controlled by computer (with the slit opening during the procedure), and the resultant variable slit is used to control the laser delivery, much as the iris diaphragm is used for correction of myopia. As in laser treatment to correct myopia, 240 steps are used. By using the slit, the resultant corneal flattening is only in the meridian perpendicular to the long axis of the slit (termed the mechanical axis); no refractive change is intended along the mechanical axis (long axis of the slit). Alignment of the mechanical axis with the astigmatic axis of the patient (with the refractive error expressed in the minus cylinder form) is achieved by rotating the slit mechanism with computer control. A "transition zone" of 0.3 mm is generated at the ends of the slit to form a sigmoidal transition between unoperated and ablated cornea (Fig 32–2). To calibrate the laser, toric ablations in polymethyl methacrylate blocks are performed, and the induced cylindrical change is measured with a lensometer.

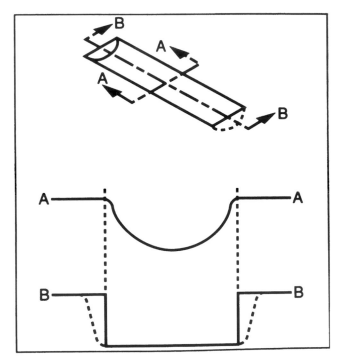

Figure 32–2. Schematic illustration of toric superficial ablation using a beam that begins as a narrow slit (mechanical axis perpendicular to the corneal meridian to be flattened) and widens gradually to the ablation zone of 4.5 mm in diameter. **A.** A cross-section of the ablation zone perpendicular to the mechanical axis shows a curved ablation profile with greater tissue ablation centrally than peripherally, flattening the cornea in this meridian. **B.** A cross-section of the ablation zone parallel to the mechanical axis of the slit shows straight-edged ablation with 0.3-mm transition at the ends; there is no intended refractive change in this meridian. *(From McDonnell PJ, Moreira H, Garbus J, et al. Photorefractive keratectomy to create toric ablations for corrections of astigmatism.* Arch Ophthalmol. *1991;109:710–713.)*

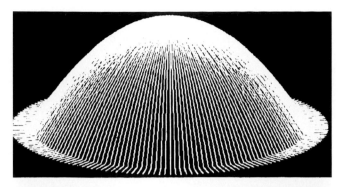

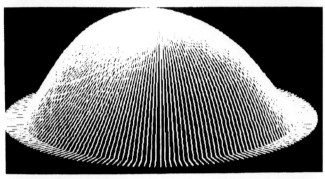

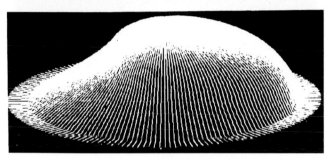

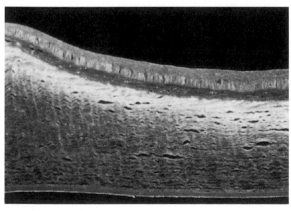

Figure 32–3. Computer-simulated profile of the ablated tissue for correcting myopia *(upper)*, astigmatism *(middle)*, and irregular astigmatism *(lower)*. *(From Dausch et al. Photorefractive keratectomy to correct astigmatism with myopia or hyperopia. J Cataract Refract Surg. 1994;20([suppl]).252–257.)*

these techniques are not limited to the correction of astigmatism with toric ablations only, but can potentially be utilized to carve a variety of desirable shapes onto the cornea, rendering feasible the correction of irregular astigmatism.

Preop evaluation and postop management are similar to those followed in PRK. Essentially, a complete ophthalmologic exam is performed prior to surgery as part of the evaluation. This usually includes visual acuity, visual potential, pupil size, slit lamp biomicroscopy, and dilated fundus examination. Postoperatively, the eye is patched and the patients are examined every 24 to 48 hours until re-epithelialization occurs. Postop topical medications include prophylactic antibiotics, anti-inflammatory agents (prednisolone acetate or fluorometholone), and a cycloplegic agent. Topical steroids are then slowly tapered over several months.

CORNEAL WOUND HEALING AFTER PARK

The corneal wound healing that follows cylindrical excimer laser ablations was studied by Shieh et al in 1991.[11] Rabbit corneas treated with spherical and cylindrical ablations at depths of 2, 4, 6, and 8 D were examined histologically, using a dichlorotriazinyl aminofluorescein stain for collagen 12 weeks postoperatively. The results were quantified using a digital videoimage analysis system. The epithelial thickness and the thickness of the newly laid collagen correlated with the depth of ablation, following spherical ablations. However, epithelial

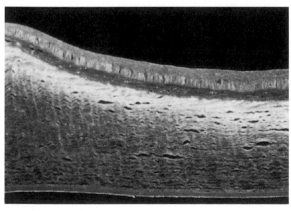

A

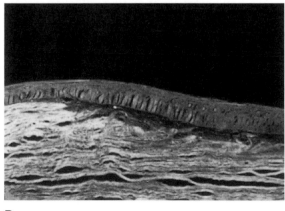

B

Figure 32–4. A. Fluorescence micrograph of edge of 6 D astigmatic ablation sectioned in the meridian of desired flattening demonstrates gently sloping edge and zone of new collagen between thickened epithelium and normal stroma (original magnification, ×55). **B.** Higher power of periphery of ablation zone demonstrates interweaving of new (unstained) and old (fluorescent) collagen (original magnification, ×110). *(From Shieh et al. Quantitative analysis of wound healing after cylindrical and spherical excimer laser ablations. Ophthalmology. 1992;99:1050–1055.)*

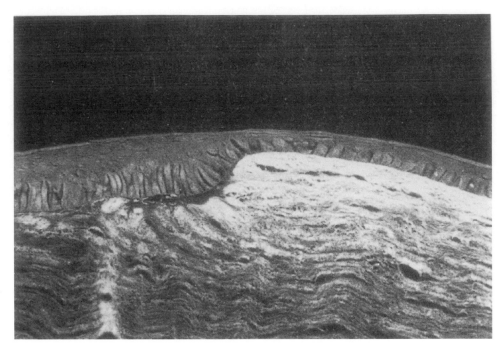

Figure 32–5. Fluorescence micrograph of edge of 8 D astigmatic ablation sectioned in the meridian of no intended refractive change demonstrates steep edge and lack of sharply defined new collagen at the edge (original magnification, ×110). *(From Shieh et al. Quantitative analysis of wound healing after cylindrical and spherical excimer laser ablations.* Ophthalmology. *1992;99:1050–1055.)*

thickness and new collagen formation correlated with ablation depth in one axis only, following cylindrical ablations. Comparison of the two meridians of the astigmatic ablation revealed contrasting morphology. A smooth, sloping edge, with new collagen present at the margin and the center of the ablation, was seen in the meridian of intended flattening (Fig 32–4). A more abrupt, flatter edge, with a less well-defined layer of new collagen, was observed in the meridian where no refractive correction was intended (Fig 32–5). These results suggest that radially asymmetric stromal ablations produce quantitatively asymmetric wound healing.

TABLE 32–1. CLINICAL OUTCOME FOLLOWING PHOTOASTIGMATIC REFRACTIVE KERATECTOMY

Study (year)	Laser	Eyes (no)	Follow-up (mo, range)	Treated refractive error (range, D)	Etiology	Treatment
McDonnell, 1991[12]	VISX	4	8–24	Astigmatism (5.5–12)	Postkeratoplasty Ulcer Naturally occurring	Cylindrical
Campos, 1992[13]	VISX	12	6–14	Astigmatism (2.25–12)	Postkeratoplasty	Cylindrical
Taylor, 1993[14]	VISX	54 PARK 66 PRK	1–6	Astigmatism <-6 Myopia <-6	Naturally occurring	Sequential
Pender, 1994[15]	VISX	8	12–18	Astigmatism (0.75–2.25)	Naturally occurring	Cylindrical
Kim, 1994[16]	VISX	168	3–6	Astigmatism (0.5–4.25) Myopia (2.5–17.25)	Naturally occurring	Elliptical
Taylor, 1994[17]	VISX	139 PARK 107 PRK	3–12	Astigmatism ≤-6 Myopia <-18	Naturally occurring	Sequential/elliptical
Spigelman, 1994[18]	VISX	70	6–12	Astigmatism (0.75–4.5) Myopia (1–6)	Naturally occurring	Sequential
Dausch, 1994[19]	MEL 60-Meditec	73	3–13	Astigmatism Myopia Hyperopia Irregular astigmatism	Naturally occurring Postkeratoplasty Postcataract Postpterygium Postkeratoconjunctivitis	Erodible mask

Clinically, several studies have indicated that the rate of re-epithelialization and the development of haze following PARK are similar to those following PRK.[12–15]

CLINICAL OUTCOME

To date, clinical outcomes of 528 eyes, treated for astigmatism with excimer laser PARK, have been published in eight reports (Table 32–1; search limited to the literature published in the English language).[12–19] Two excimer lasers have been used: TwentyTwenty and MEL 60 (Aesculap Meditec, Heroldsberg, Germany). Ninety-six percent (507) of the eyes were treated for naturally occurring astigmatism, 3% (17) for astigmatism resulting from penetrating keratoplasty (PKP), and one eye for astigmatism resulting from each of the following surgical procedures or eye pathology: cataract extraction, pterygium excision, corneal ulcer, and epidemic keratoconjunctivitis.

Wide variations in postop astigmatism ranging from a 100% reduction to an increase were noted by Kim et al.[16] At the 6-month follow-up, 67 eyes (75.3%) showed a reduction in astigmatism, 12 (13.5%) had no change, and 10 (11.2%) had increased astigmatism. The overall improvement in astigmatic cylinder was 55.6% (53.5% and 68.8% for eyes with preop astigmatism of 1.0 to 1.75 D and 3.0 to 4.25 D, respectively). This shows

that the greater the amount of preop astigmatism, the more effective the toric ablation. However, the greater the preop cylinder, the higher the amount of residual astigmatism (0.6 D $\pm$0.58 in patients with a preop astigmatism of 1.0 to 1.75 D, compared to 1.04 $\pm$ 0.62 D in those with a preop astigmatism of 3.0 to 4.25 D). Astigmatism 6 months after surgery was within 10° of the preop axis in 46.1% of the eyes, and 11 eyes (12.4%) had a postop axis 80° to 90° off the preop one.

To compensate for the hyperopic shift associated with the sequential astigmatic excimer laser treatment, Taylor et al calculated the amount of expected hyperopic shift by subtracting 1 D from the amount of cylinder and then halving the remaining amount of cylinder.[14,17] This amount was then subtracted from the spherical component to determine the amount of minus sphere to be treated. Utilizing the vector method to determine surgically induced astigmatism (SIAG), Taylor et al found that an analysis of the variance between the target induced astigmatism (TIAG) and the SIAG for PARK shows a consistent trend of undercorrection of magnitude of astigmatism.[17] The ratio of the TIAG to the SIAG, the coefficient of adjustment, was equal to 1.2.

Campos et al, studying the effect of PARK on post-PKP astigmatism (n = 12), noticed a significant reduction in refractive cylinder 1 month postoperatively, followed by a slight regression of the initial effect; the average correction was 38%.[13] Mean shift in

Preop astigmatism (mean ± SD)	Postop astigmatism (mean ± SD)	Preop spherical equivalent (mean ± SD)	Postop spherical equivalent (mean ± SD)	Percentage within 1 D intended correction	UCVA (% <20/40)
7.56 ± 3.00	2.25 ± 2.52	−3.97 ± 1.28	1.06 ± 1.57	—	—
7 ± 3.6	4.30 ± 2.90	−7.40 ± 4.20	−3.30 ± 4.4	—	17
−1.39 ± 1.33	−0.61 ± 0.53	—	—	85 (PARK) 88 (PRK)	95 (PARK) 88 (PRK)
1.28	0.46	−4.06	−0.03	—	62.5
1.51 ± 0.81	0.67 ± 0.60	—	—	79.8	91
—	—	—	—	68 (PARK) 87 (PRK)	72 (PARK) 90 (PRK)
−1.52	−0.54	−4.96	−0.14	—	71
−3.3 ± 2.4[a] −2.1 ± 0.93[b]	−0.3 ± 0.58[a] −0.08 ± 0.23[b]	— −6.1 ± 3.7[b]	— −0.12 ± 1.05[b]	86.7[a] 84[b]	80[a] 54[b]

[a]Astigmatism only (n = 30).
[b]Myopic astigmatism (n = 36).
Abbreviations: PARK, photoastigmatic refractive keratectomy; PRK, photorefractive keratectomy; UCVA, uncorrected visual acuity.

the axis of cylinder was 58° ± 62° with a range of 1 to 173. Four patients had overcorrection of their astigmatism, with a shift in the cylinder axis of more than 100°. Nine of the 12 patients had a reduction in refractive cylinder to a level that was tolerable with spectacles.

Pender et al, looking at the effect of PARK on naturally occurring astigmatism (n = 8), found a reduction in the refractive cylinder in seven of eight eyes.[15] The shift in cylinder axis in six patients varied between 5° and 10° from the preop cylinder axis; in one eye with an eccentric ablation, the axis changed by 40°. The procedure was found to be effective; however, some residual astigmatism remained in most patients. Patient satisfaction was assessed on a scale of 1 to 10 (1 = very disappointed; 10 = very satisfied with the procedure), and a mean score of 8.2 was registered. Similarly, patients' expectations from the surgery registered a mean score of 7.2 on a scale of 1 to 10 (1 = nowhere near the expectation; 10 = much more than expected).

Dausch et al were the first to use PARK to treat patients with mixed astigmatism (n = 5) and irregular astigmatism (n = 2).[19] To perform asymmetric ablations, a special asymmetric mask was designed, based on the videokeratographic images. The result of only one patient with mixed astigmatism was reported. The patient's manifest refraction changed from +3.75 −5.50 × 165 preoperatively, to +0.75 3 months postoperatively. The two patients with irregular astigmatism had a preop refraction of +2.0 −1.25 × 90 and +1.25 −7.0 × 130. Three months af-

ter surgery, their refraction was +0.75 −0.5 × 168 and +0.5 −1.5 × 180, respectively.

LIMITATIONS TO PARK

Correction of naturally occurring or surgically induced astigmatism with the excimer technology is plausible. Complications and side effects of PARK are similar to those observed with PRK, suggesting that toric ablations result in no special risk to the cornea.[13–19] In brief, these include immediate postop pain, undercorrection or overcorrection, and the development of subepithelial haze. However, exact axis alignment is a major additional concern in PARK. Preoperatively, the axis of astigmatism determined by manifest refraction may differ from that obtained through cycloplegic refraction or corneal topography. In such cases, it is unclear which axis should be used in performing the surgery. Moreover, it is difficult to ensure exact placement of the beam axis on the corneal astigmatic axis, especially since cyclotorsion or drift of the eye may occur during treatment. Calculations reveal that an alignment error of even 5° will result in a loss of 17% of the astigmatic treatment effect (Fig 32–6). When the treatment is exactly "on axis," the vector difference can be obtained either by simple subtraction or by performing difference maps (Fig 32–7). In addition, there are several sources of astigmatism besides the anterior corneal surface, none of which is altered by PARK. These include the posterior corneal surface, the anterior and posterior surfaces of

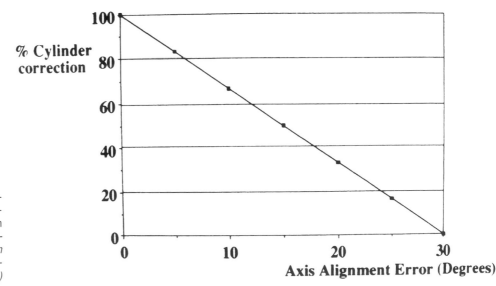

Figure 32–6. Effect of axis misalignment in optical neutralization of cylinder lenses (calculated by William Telfair, MD). *(From Kim et al. Photoastigmatic refractive keratectomy in 168 eyes: six-month results.* J Cataract Refract Surg. *1994;20:387–391.)*

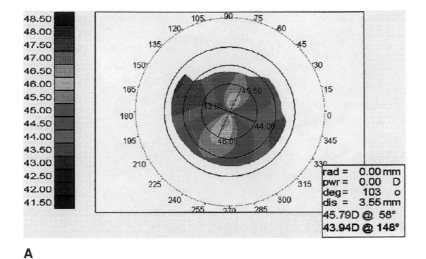

A

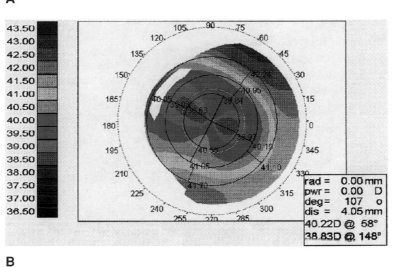

B

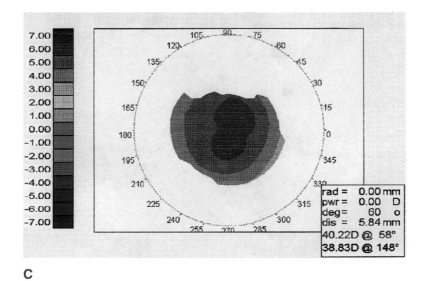

C

Figure 32–7. A. Preop topographic map of patient undergoing PARK and PRK. Preop axis of astigmatism corresponded to the treatment axis of 58°. **B.** Postop topographic map showing reduction of astigmatism at the 58° meridian. **C.** Subtraction map showing the overall effect of combined PARK and PRK.

the lens, lenticular lamellar zones, lenticular decentration, and foveal position.

A correcting cylinder of equal magnitude to the cylinder present, but axis misaligned produces a resultant cylinder and a small misalignment produces a large rotation in the axis of the resultant cylinder. At an axis misalignment of 30° there is no reduction at all in the magnitude of the original cylinder. When axis error is present the optimal correcting cylinder is not a cylinder of the same magnitude as the original cylinder, a cylinder of less magnitude can provide less resultant-cylinder and smaller amount of induced axis change. Overcorrection of a cylinder results in marked axis swing if there is axis misalignment, and may leave residual cylinder at an undesired oblique axis. Hence the slight undercorrecting tendency of current excimer laser astigmatic treatment has the benefit of compensating for small angles of axis error. Increasing cylinder treatment power may result in marked axis swing of resultant cylinder.[20] Stevens and coworkers found that off-axis tilt and a vector axis error between 6° and 20° and a magnitude of treatment greater than intended, had a near axis shift due to treatment of 43° and 15° in cases with magnitude less than intended.[21]

REFERENCES

1. Schiotz H. Ein Fall von hochgradigem Horn-hautastigmatismus nach Staarextraction. Besserung auf operativem Wege. *Arch. Augenheilkd.* 1885;15:178.

2. Trokel SL, Srinivasan R, Barron B. Excimer laser surgery of the cornea. *Am J Ophthalmol.* 1983;96:710–715.

3. Marshall J, Trokel S, Rothery S, Schubert H. An ultrastructural study of corneal incisions induced by an excimer laser at 193 nm. *Ophthalmology.* 1985;92:749–758.

4. Kruger RR, Trokel SL, Shubert HD. Interaction of ultraviolet light with the cornea. *Invest Ophthalmol Vis Sci.* 1985;26(suppl):1455–1464.

5. Seiler T, Kahle G, Kriegerowski M. Excimer laser (193 nm) myopic keratomileusis in sighted and blind human eyes. *Refract Corneal Surg.* 1990;6:165–173.

6. McDonald MB, Liu JC, Byrd TJ, et al. Central photorefractive keratectomy for myopia: partially sighted and normally sighted eyes. *Ophthalmology.* 1991;98:1327–1337.

7. Lawless MA, Cohen P, Rogers C. Excimer laser photorefractive keratectomy: first Australian series. *Med J Aust.* 1992;156:812.

8. Lindstrom RL, Sher NA, Chen V, et al. Use of the 193-nm excimer laser for myopic photorefractive keratectomy in sighted eyes: a multicenter study. *Trans Am Ophthalmol Soc.* 1991;89:155–182.

9. Sher NA, Barak M, Daya S, et al. Excimer laser photorefractive keratectomy in high myopia: a multicenter study. *Arch Ophthalmol.* 1992;110:935–943.

10. McDonnell PJ, Moreira H, Garbus J, et al. Photorefractive keratectomy to create toric ablations for corrections of astigmatism. *Arch Ophthalmol.* 1991;109:710–713.

11. Shich E, Moreira H, D'Arcy J, et al. Quantitative analysis of wound healing after cylindrical and spherical excimer laser ablations. *Ophthalmology.* 1992;99:1050–1055.

12. McDonnell PJ, Moreira H, Clapham TN, et al. Photorefractive keratectomy for astigmatism: initial clinical results. *Arch Ophthalmol.* 1991;109:1370–1373.

13. Campos M, Hertzog L, Garbus J, et al. Photorefractive keratectomy for severe postkeratoplasty astigmatism. *Am J Ophthalmol.* 1992;114:429–436.

14. Taylor HR, Guest CS, Kelly P, et al. Comparison of excimer laser treatment of astigmatism and myopia. *Arch Ophthalmol.* 1993;111:1621–1626.

15. Pender PM, Excimer Laser Study Group. Photorefractive keratectomy for myopic astigmatism: phase IIA of the Federal Drug Administration study (12 to 18 months follow-up). *J Cataract Refract Surg.* 1994;20(suppl):262–264.

16. Kim YJ, Sohn J, Tchah H, Lee CO. Photoastigmatic refractive keratectomy in 168 eyes: six-month results. *J Cataract Refract Surg.* 1994;20:387–391.

17. Taylor HR, Kelly P, Alpins N. Excimer laser correction of myopic astigmatism. *J Cataract Refract Surg.* 1994;20(suppl):243–251.

18. Spigelman AV, Albert WC, Cozean CH, et al. Treatment of myopic astigmatism with the 193 nm excimer laser utilizing aperture elements. *J Cataract Refract Surg.* 1994;20(suppl):258–261.

19. Dausch D, Klein R, Landesz M, Schroder E. Photorefractive keratectomy to correct astigmatism with myopia or hyperopia. *J Cataract Refract Surg.* 1994;20(suppl):252–257.

20. Stevens JD. Astigmatic excimer laser treatment: theoretical effects of axis misalignment. *Eur J Implant Ref Surg.* 1994;310–317.

21. Stevens JD, Steele ADMcG, Ficker LA, et al. Astigmatic axis changes after excimer laser photoastigmatic refractive keratectomy for compound myopia and astigmatism. Presented at the AAO meeting, Atlanta, Georgia, October 1995.

CHAPTER 33

Clinical Results of Excimer Laser Photorefractive Keratectomy for the Treatment of Myopia

Charles W. Flowers ■ Peter J. McDonnell

INTRODUCTION

Excimer laser photorefractive keratectomy (PRK) is one of the most promising refractive surgical procedures for the correction of myopia. Since its use was introduced into the ophthalmic community by Trokel and associates[1] in 1983, use of the excimer laser has rapidly evolved from experimental laboratory studies to clinical applications.

Because ophthalmic application of the excimer laser is relatively new, many of the results pertaining to its efficacy and safety are just beginning to appear in the literature. As with any new clinical breakthrough, many of the initial reports constitute preliminary observations on small series, series with short follow-up periods or high percentages of loss to follow-up, and series published without peer review. Despite these shortcomings, initial studies provide a basis on which to evaluate new clinical technologies. In recent years, reports of several prospective studies of PRK with large series of patients and reasonable follow-up periods have been published.[2–10] These studies, in conjunction with previous reports, provide valuable insights into the efficacy, safety, predictability, and stability of excimer laser PRK for treatment of myopia. Initial results are generally regarded as promising, but an additional 3 to 4 years will probably be necessary to determine the adequacy of this procedure. The most definitive insights will surely come from the Food and Drug Administration (FDA)-supervised phase III clinical trials, which are currently ongoing.

The goal of this chapter is to summarize the clinical results of excimer laser PRK for the treatment of myopia. In order to make the information on efficacy, safety, predictability, and stability easy to interpret, we have organized it in accordance with the guidelines for the reporting of refractive surgery results set forth by Waring.[11] In so organizing the material, we also strive to have it serve as a reference for comparing excimer laser PRK with other refractive procedures used to correct myopia.

Although three distinct techniques for performing excimer laser PRK for myopia have evolved, the results summarized here pertain only to the technique of wide-area surface ablation with a large-diameter beam. This technique has been most widely used, and the majority of published results are based on PRK performed in this manner. The scanning slit technique is used primarily in Europe and, to date, only one report of a prospective trial using this technique has been published in the international literature. The erodible-mask technique is still in the early experimental stages, and thus insufficient clinical data are available.

CLINICAL RESULTS

In reviewing the clinical results of any new device or procedure, one seeks to answer whether it is safe and effective. In the case of excimer laser PRK for myopia, making this determination is difficult because of the wide variability in patient selection, follow-up, and definition of "success" in the studies that have been reported. Many of the reports differ in terms of the outcome measures used to determine effectiveness; most studies use some combination of postop uncorrected visual acuity (UCVA), postop refractive error, postop keratometry, and postop pachymetry. In addition, the studies vary in duration of follow-up, ranges of myopia treated, and ablation-zone diameters utilized, making it difficult to compare various studies and to draw conclusions about the efficacy and safety of excimer laser PRK. To simplify this process, we have chosen several critical outcome measures, used frequently in the keratorefractive literature, as a basis for evaluating the outcome of excimer laser PRK in the treatment of myopia (Table 33–1). The measure of visual outcome used most extensively in the literature on PRK is postop UCVA, with visual success defined in terms of the percentage of eyes achieving a UCVA of 20/40 or better.

The refractive outcome measures used most commonly have been the predictability and long-term stability of the postop refractive effect. The measure of predictability used to define refractive success has been the percentage of eyes with manifest postop refractions within plus or minus 1 diopter of the attempted correction. The measure of stability used to define a successful refractive outcome is the percentage of eyes showing significant regression of myopia.

The safety of excimer laser PRK has been evaluated primarily in terms of two parameters: the percentage of eyes losing two or more lines or best spectacle-corrected visual acuity and the occurrence of vision-threatening complications. An equally important measure of safety is the occurrence of visually compromising complications, which has also received considerable attention in the photorefractive literature.

TABLE 33–1. OUTCOME MEASURES USED TO ASSESS EXCIMER LASER PHOTOREFRACTIVE KERATECTOMY

Efficacy
  Visual outcome
    · Uncorrected postop visual acuity
      Percentage of eyes 20/40 or better
  Refractive outcome
    · Predictability
      Percentage of eyes within ±1 D of emmetropia or attempted correction
    · Stability
      Percentage of eyes showing significant myopic regression
Safety
    · Loss of best spectacle-corrected visual acuity
      Percentage of eyes losing two or more Snellen lines of acuity
    · Visually compromising complications
      Haze and scarring
      Halo effect
      Decreasedd contrast sensitivity
      Decentration of ablation
      Elevated intraocular pressure
      Recurrent erosion and delayed epithelial healing
      Loss of corneal sensitivity
      Diurnal fluctuation
    · Vision-threatening complications
      Corneal perforations
      Infectious keratitis

Efficacy

Visual Outcome

One of the most consistent findings regarding visual outcome after excimer laser PRK is the degree to which visual success depends on the attempted refractive correction. Lui and coworkers[12] were among the first to point this out. In a retrospective study of excimer laser PRK in myopes, these investigators found that the larger the attempted correction, the less chance there was of attaining a UCVA of 20/20. Subsequent to this report, other investigators have identified specific levels of attempted correction or baseline myopia that yield the best visual results. From the prospective studies published to date, patients with low to moderate myopia (less than or equal to 6 D) appear to have the best visual results; of these, patients in the low myopia group (less than or equal to 3 D) have the best visual results overall. Studies have shown that from 78% to 100% of eyes with 3 D or less of myopia will attain UCVA of 20/40 or better following excimer laser PRK.[2,3,13–17] Similarly, in the moderate myopia group (−3.10 to −6.00 D), high visual success rates have been reported following excimer laser PRK, with 91% to 97% of eyes achieving a UCVA of 20/40 or better.[2,15–17] For myopia greater than 6 D, however, reported visual results have been highly variable, with success rates ranging from 25% to 83% in this group.[8,13,14,16,18–20] Table 33–2 summarizes the visual results from published prospective series of excimer laser PRK.

Although the level of Snellen acuity is an important measure of visual function, it provides only partial information regarding visual performance. An equally important component of visual function is contrast sensitivity, which is critical under conditions of reduced illumination. Conventional Snellen visual-acuity assessment is a high-contrast test that is insensitive to many subtleties of daily visual function. Snellen acuity provides no information on visual performance under reduced lighting conditions (ie, night driving, overcast day), and patients with good Snellen acuities can be significantly handicapped under suboptimal lighting. Therefore, uncorrected Snellen acuity cannot, and should not, be used as the sole measure of visual success for excimer laser PRK, or for any refractive procedure for that matter. Unfortunately, contrast sensitivity has not been systematically studied or reported in the photorefractive literature, so we have very limited data regarding the impact of excimer laser PRK on this aspect of visual function. Future studies will have to address this issue if we are to obtain a more complete understanding of excimer laser PRK's complete effect on visual function.

Refractive Outcome

Predictability

As with visual outcome, the refractive outcome has been shown to depend strongly on the attempted refractive correction. Studies have demonstrated that higher refractive success rates are achieved for patients with low to moderate myopia. A review of the literature reveals that from 71% to 97% of eyes with baseline refractions less than or equal to 6 D achieve manifest postop refractions within ± 1 D of the attempted correction 1 year after surgery[2–4,6,15,21–25] (Table 33–2). Seiler and Wollensak,[2] reporting the 1-year follow-up of 193 eyes that underwent excimer laser PRK, found that 97.6% of eyes in the low myopia group (less than or equal to 3 D) attained postop refractions within ± 1 D of the attempted correction, as did 91.2% of eyes in the moderate myopia group (3.10 to 6.00 D). Similarly, Salz et al[3] found that 84% of eyes with 1 to 6 D of myopia achieved refractions within ± 1 D of the intended correction at 1 year, and 11 of 12 (91.6%) eyes did so at 2 years.

In contrast, prospective series reporting the results of excimer laser PRK in higher myopia groups (greater than 6 D) have found significantly lower levels of predictability. Kim et al[8] found that only 52% of eyes with preop myopia ranging from −7.25 to −13.50 D achieved refractive correction within ± 1 D of the expected result at 1 year after surgery. Brancato et al,[9] in a multicenter study, similarly found significantly poorer predictability in eyes undergoing myopic correction of greater than 6 D. In this series, 35% of eyes with 6.10 to 9.90 D of attempted myopic correction and only 28% of eyes with 10 to 25 D of attempted myopic correction were within ± 1 D of the intended result at 1-year follow-up. In this same series, 71% of eyes with attempted corrections less than or equal to 6 D were within ± 1 D of the intended correction.

Stability

The postop refraction following excimer laser PRK evolves in a characteristic pattern over a period of several months (Fig 33–1). In the early postop period there is an overcorrection, followed by an asymptomatic reduction in refractive effect (regression) toward a plateau, where the refraction stabilizes. This process occurs in all patients and is a result of corneal wound healing. If regression of the refractive effect progresses beyond the 1-D limit used to define a successful refractive outcome, this phenomenon is referred to as *myopic regression*. Myopic regression has also been shown to depend on the attempted myopic correction, with most studies demonstrating myopic regression in patients whose myopia exceeds 6 D.[2,5,9,10,12,15,19,21,22,24] In a recent report, Seiler et al[10] presented the results of PRK in 193 eyes followed for 2 years after a single procedure, and noted that eyes with baseline refractions up to −3 D did not show continued regression of 1 D or more during the second year after surgery. However, 8.6% of eyes with baseline refractions between −3.1 and −6.0 D, 20% of eyes with baseline refractions between −6.0 and −9.0 D, and 100% of eyes with baseline refractions of greater than −9.0 D did continue to show myopic regression of 1 D or more during the second year after surgery.

Reports vary regarding the temporal endpoint of refractive stabilization. This variability arises because the time required for stabilization appears to vary according to patient age, attempted myopic correction, laser fluence, and ablation-zone diameter. Seiler and Wollensak[21] noted that the early postop regression that occurs in all eyes following excimer laser PRK devel-

TABLE 33–2. VISUAL RESULTS FROM PUBLISHED PROSPECTIVE STUDIES OF EXCIMER LASER PHOTOREFRACTIVE KERATECTOMY

Study	Eyes (no)	Follow-up correction months	Attempted emmetropia (D)	±1 D of emmetropia (%)	20/40+ uncorrected (%)	Eyes losing 2+ lines of BCVA[a] (%)	Increased IOP
McDonald (1991)[22]	7	12 mo	−2 to −5	57	86	0	NR
	10	12 mo	−5 to −8	18	18	11	
Gartry (1991)[23]	120	8–18 mo; med = 12	−1.5 to −7	50	61	2.5	12% > 25 mm Hg
Seiler (1991)[21]	26	12 mo	−1.4 to −9.25	92	96	0	8% rise of >5 mm Hg
Sher (1991)[13]	31	6 mo	−4 to −12	55	45	0	6% > mid-20s
Ehlers (1992)[20]	22	6 mo	−5 to −8	32	NR	0	NR
	18	6 mo	−9 to −12	33		17	
Tengroth (1993)[30]	420	12 mo	−1.5 to −7.5	86	91	NR	13% > 24 mm Hg
	(194)[b]	15 mo		87	87	NR	
Salz (1993)[3]	71	12 mo	−1.25 to −7.5	84	91	1.4	3% > 24 mm Hg
	(12)[b]	24 mo		92	100	0	
Machat (1993)[16]	119	3–11 mo; med = 8	−1.75 to −5.9	66	93	0	22% > 21 mm Hg
	28		−6 to −8.75	17	68		
Kim (1993)[8]	135	12 mo	−2.0 to −7.0	91	99	8.1	14%
	67		−7.25 to −13.5	52	63	17.9	24%
Brancato (1993)[9]	146	12 mo	−0.8 to −6	71	NR	1.4	25% > 25 mm Hg
	145	12 mo	−6.1 to −9.9	35	NR	2/1	1.6% > 32 mm Hg
Eiferman (1991)[43]	6	6 mo	−4 to −8	67	83	0	NR
Lavery (1993)[7]	99	12 mo	−1.25 to −9.6	93	84	0.6[c]	NR
Gimbal (1993)[39d]	52	med = 15.5 mo	−5.6 ± 1.6	43	96	NR	NR
	52	med = 9 mo	−5.9 ± 1.5	45	92	NR	NR
Tutton (1993)[26]	95	6 mo	−1 to −6	88	100	2	NR
Weinstock (1993)[17]	57	6 mo	−1 to −3	87	NR	NR	NR
	90	6 mo	−3.1 to −6	84			
	39	6 mo	−6.1 to −9	62			
	7	6 mo	−9 +	43			
Salorio (1993)[25]	88	3–18 mo; med = 13	<−6	NR	NR	NR	NR
	90		>−6				
Pallikaris (1993)[55]	96	NR	NR	NR	NR	NR	9% 5–6 mm
Weinstock (1993)[38]	46	3–6 mo	−1 to −8.38	74	96	0	46% > 21 mm Hg 11% > 30 mm Hg
Piebenga (1993)[4]	21	36 mo	−2 to −8 < 1.5 astig		60	70	0% 3/129 > 21 mm Hg
	25	24 mo	−1 to −5 < 1 astig		58	67	0%
	70	12 mo	−1 to −6 < 1 astig	71	75	0	
	17	6 mo	−1 to −6 < 1 astig − N2		88	100	0%
Gartry (1992)[32]	113	>1 y	−3 and −6	NR	NR	15 (22/96?)	
Duff	47	12 mo	−1.5 to −6.1	80	94	0	5/47 > 22 mm Hg
FDA–study SUMMIT	544	12 mo	−1.0 to −6.0	76	91	NR	NR
FDA–study VISX	691	12 mo	−1.0 to −6.0	79	86	1	3% > 5 mm Hg
	691	24 mo	−1.0 to −6.0	79	85	1	0.2% > 10 mm Hg

[a]The choice of two or more lines of vision required for significant visual loss was determined by others.[56]
[b]This group is a subset of 240 eyes.
[c]For all cases.
[d]Bilateral excimer for all 52 patients.
Abbreviations: Astig, astigmatism; BCVA, best corrected visual acuity; IOP, intraocular pressure; med, median; −N2, no nitrogen gas blowing used; NR, not reported.

oped more slowly in older patients. Gartry et al[24] found that patients with 5 D or less of myopia achieved stable refractions by 4 months postoperatively, whereas patients with 7 D or greater of myopia continued to show regression up to 1 year. Sher et al,[13] utilizing dif-

ferent laser parameters than other investigators, demonstrated insignificant regression within 6 months after surgery in a multicenter study of 16 highly myopic eyes (myopia ranging from −8.62 to −14.50 D). In this study, larger ablation diameters of 5.5 to 6.0 mm were

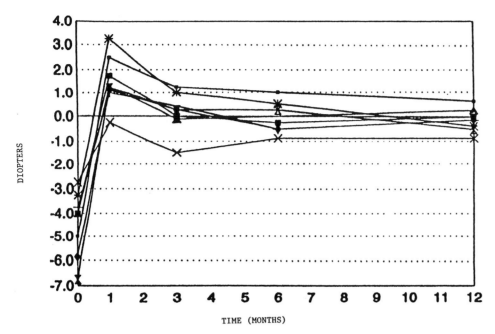

Figure 33–1. Evolution of the manifest refraction over time following excimer laser PRK. *(From Thompson KP. Photorefractive keratectomy. Ophthalmol Clin North America. 1992; 5:745–751.)*

used, and ablations were conducted at a relatively low fluence of 120 mJ/cm^2. Many of the published reports of prospective clinical series of PRK have utilized ablation-zone diameters of 3.5 to 5.0 mm, and laser fluences from 160 to 200 mJ/cm^2. Therefore, given these factors, the time to refractive stability has been variously reported as 3 months,[3,13] 6 months,[4,6,8,18,24] and 12 months.[2,15–18,22–24,26] Based on the majority of clinical data collected thus far, postop refraction appears to stabilize within 1 year after surgery for attempted corrections of 6 D or less.[2,5,15–17,21,26] Seiler et al[10] have shown small, statistically insignificant changes in the manifest refraction between the 1-year and 2-year visits in eyes with myopic corrections of less than 6 D. For attempted corrections greater than 6 D, there is clinical evidence that refractive stabilization is not achieved by 1 year. Brancato et al,[9] in a multicenter study, found that eyes with attempted corrections greater than 6 D continued to show regression at 12 months postoperatively. Similarly, Buratto and Ferrari,[19] in a retrospective study of 40 eyes with myopia ranging from −6 to −10 D and follow-up of 24 months, observed myopic regression that continued up to 24 months after surgery in 65% of the eyes.

The use of corticosteroids to limit myopic regression remains controversial. The initial impetus for using topical steroids after PRK came from the results of an early study in which postop steroid treatment was reported to reduce both stromal haze and new collagen production in a rabbit model.[27] Further support for the use of corticosteroids in the treatment of myopic regres-

sion came from an early blind-eye study by Seiler et al,[28] who observed myopic shifts of 0.50 to 1.0 D within days of discontinuing steroid use. Zabel et al,[29] in another early report, noted a significant regression in the refractive effect in two patients who discontinued topical corticosteroid use before completing the recommended course. In one of the patients, steroid therapy was reinstituted and regression stopped. Following these initial reports, several studies were published that demonstrated a benefit to using corticosteroids for reducing or reversing myopic regression.[5,27,30,31] In one study the use of corticosteroids was shown to reverse delayed myopic regression in six eyes that underwent PRK for the correction of myopia ranging from −6 to −8 D.[31] In this report, all eyes had completed a full course of postop steroid therapy of at least 2 months', but no more than 6 months', duration. Steroids were discontinued in each case when the refraction seemed stable and the cornea was clear. After cessation of steroids, an increase in myopia occurred, ranging from 1.00 to 3.50 D. Corticosteroid therapy was then reinstituted and five of the six eyes regained the attempted correction when the corticosteroids were stopped (±0.50 D). Tengroth et al[30] retrospectively compared results in eyes receiving topical dexamethasone 0.1% for 3 months with eyes receiving no steroids and found that there was statistically less regression in the steroid-treated group.

Despite the findings of Seiler and others, Gartry et al,[32] in a double-masked, placebo-controlled trial of 113 patients treated with ablations to correct either 3 or 6 D of myopia, found no statistically significant difference in refractive changes at 6 and 12 months between the corticosteroid- and the noncorticosteroid-treated group. Piebenga et al,[4] in a prospective study of 133 eyes undergoing PRK to correct from 1 to 6 D of myopia, also found no statistically significant difference in refractive or visual outcome at 6 months between patients receiving 0.1% fluorometholone and patients using no steroids. Thus, prolonged corticosteroid use following excimer laser PRK is of questionable benefit in the treatment of myopic regression, and more well-controlled prospective studies are needed to fully address this issue.

Safety

Loss of Best Spectacle-Corrected Acuity

A review of the literature reveals that from 0% to 18% of patients across all myopia groups experience a loss of two or more Snellen lines of best spectacle-corrected acuity following excimer laser PRK[2–4,6,15,21–24] (Table 33–2). This complication shows a strong dependence on the amount of attempted correction, with 0% to 8.1% of eyes with myopia less than or equal to 5 to 7 D manifesting this level of visual loss, and 2.1% to 18% of eyes with myopia greater than 5 to 7.5 D.

The loss of best spectacle-corrected acuity also appears to be a function of length of follow-up; with increasing length of time following surgery, fewer patients experience this level of visual loss. In a 2-year follow-up of 176 eyes, Seiler et al[10] reported that 2 eyes (1.1%) experienced a loss of two or more lines of Snellen acuity at the 1-year follow-up. By 2 years, one of these two eyes regained baseline BCVA, thus reducing the incidence of visual loss to 0.6%. Brancato et al[9] similarly showed this trend for patients to regain their level of baseline best corrected Snellen acuity with increasing length of time from surgery, irrespective of level of attempted correction. This is nicely illustrated in Table 33–3. In each of the myopia groups listed in the table, the percentage of patients losing one or more lines of best spectacle-corrected visual acuity decreased between the 6- and 12- month follow-up.

Visually Compromising Complications

HAZE AND SCARRING

Faint subepithelial opacification, commonly referred to as haze, occurs in the majority of patients following excimer laser PRK. This represents a transient phenomenon in most cases and follows a characteristic time course; this opacity is the clinically visible manifestation of corneal healing.[33–35] The subepithelial haze first

TABLE 33–3. CHANGE IN BEST SPECTACLE-CORRECTED VISUAL ACUITY AFTER EXCIMER LASER PHOTOREFRACTIVE KERATECTOMY

Attempted correction: −0.80 to −6.00 D

| | Time after Surgery (Total Eyes) | |
| | 6 m (294) | 12 m (146) |
Snellen Lines	Eyes (%)	Eyes (%)
Gained	35 (12.1)	37 (25.3)
Unchanged	202 (68.8)	92 (63)
Lost 1 line	54 (18.4)	15 (10.3)
Lost 2 lines	1 (0.3)	2 (1.4)
Lost 3 or more lines	0 (0)	0 (0)

Attempted correction: −6.10 to −9.90 D

| | 6 m (314) | 12 m (145) |
	Eyes (%)	Eyes (%)
Gained	57 (18.1)	32 (22.1)
Unchanged	158 (68.8)	76 (63)
Lost 1 line	78 (18.4)	34 (10.3)
Lost 2 lines	17 (0.3)	3 (1.4)
Lost 3 or more lines	4 (1.3)	0 (0)

Attempted correcttion: −10.00 to −25.00 D

| | 6 m (144) | 12 m (39) |
	Eyes (%)	Eyes (%)
Gained	36 (25.0)	10 (25.6)
Unchanged	67 (46.5)	18 (46.1)
Lost 1 line	30 (20.8)	8 (20.6)
Lost 2 lines	6 (4.2)	3 (7.7)
Lost 3 or more lines	5 (3.5)	0 (0)

From: Brancato R, Tavola A, Carones F, et al. Excimer laser photorefractive keratectomy for myopia: results in 1165 eyes. *Refract Corneal Surg.* 1993:95–104.

appears at about 1 month after surgery and increases in intensity over the next several months. The haze reaches a peak at approximately 3 to 6 months postoperatively and then gradually declines until it either completely resolves or reaches an imperceptible level, which usually occurs by about 18 months postoperatively[36] (Fig 33–2). Most studies that have evaluated postexcimer haze have used a subjective grading system based on slit lamp examination in an effort to quantify the severity and extent of subepithelial haze, equating changes in acuity with different amounts of haze. Given the subjective and arbitrary nature of these various grading systems, useful comparisons regarding the incidence and severity of haze between studies are difficult to make. More recently, a new device has been developed to analyze postop haze with objective and optical criteria, but clinical experience with this device is very limited.[37]

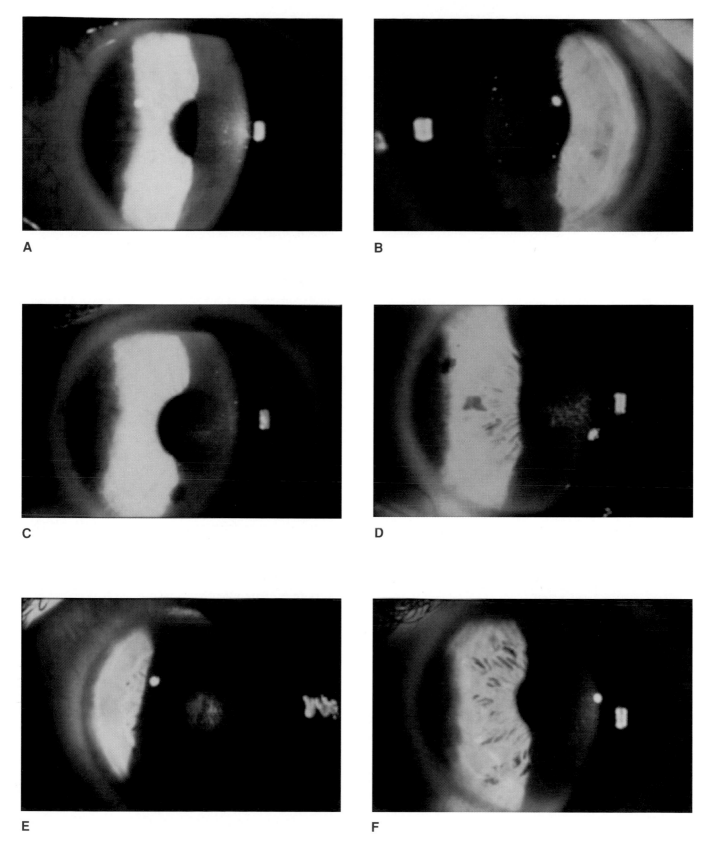

Figure 33–2. The evolution of corneal haze following PRK: postop haze at its maximal expression (after 3–6 months). **A.** Trace haze. **B.** Haze grade +1. **C.** Haze grade 1.5+. **D.** Haze grade 2+. **E.** Haze grade 4+. **F.** Clear cornea 12 months after PRK. *(From Seiler T. Photorefractive keratectomy: European experience. In: Thompson FB, McDonnell PJ, eds.* Color Atlas/Text of Excimer Laser Surgery. The Cornea. *New York: Igaku-Shoin Medical Publishers Inc; 1993:53–62.)*

Factors that increase the incidence and severity of corneal haze following excimer laser PRK are the amount of attempted correction and the ablation-zone diameter. In a retrospective analysis of 285 myopic eyes treated with excimer laser PRK, Caubet[33] examined the clinical significance of subepithelial corneal haze based on a subjective grading system. From his analysis, Caubet found the factors that significantly influenced the rate and severity of corneal haze after excimer laser PRK to be the amount of attempted correction, with deeper ablations for the correction of high myopia (> 6 D) eliciting more clinically significant haze, and an ablation-zone diameter less than 4.5 mm. Numerous prospective series have reported similar observations.[5,8,9,16,17,21,22,24,26,38] In one study, 17% of patients with myopia ranging from 9 to 12 D developed moderate-to-severe haze at 6 months' follow-up.[20]

The visual significance of subepithelial haze is minimal in the overwhelming majority of cases, with only a small percentage of patients experiencing decreases in their BCVA, which subsequently improves as the haze clears.[5,8,9,16,17,21,22,24,26,38] In most instances the corneal haze is more disturbing to the examiner than to the patient. However, in a small percentage of cases, the haze can progress to become a visually significant scar. One estimate is that visually significant corneal scarring occurs in 1% of cases following PRK.[35] The factor most commonly associated with the development of scarring following excimer PRK is high myopia.[10,35] These higher myopic corrections appear to increase the risk of scarring because they require deeper tissue ablations. In one report, the incidence of manifest scars after excimer laser PRK was significantly higher following corrections greater than 6 D[10] (Table 33–4).

In addition to visual consequences, corneal haze appears to have refractive consequences as well. A number of studies have documented that the appearance of haze is accompanied by at least partial regression of myopia.[5,23,34] Gartry et al,[23] in a prospective series of 120 eyes with myopia ranging from 2 to 7 D that underwent excimer laser PRK, found a good correlation between the magnitude of haze assessed subjectively and regression toward the preop refraction. Tengroth et al,[5] in their series of 420 eyes with myopia ranging from −1.25 to −7.50 D, similarly noted that haze in the +3 to +4 range always correlated with regression of myopia.

The role of corticosteroids in the treatment of corneal haze and scarring has not been firmly established. Although most investigators use corticosteroids to treat corneal haze and scarring after excimer laser PRK, there are no convincing data to show that corticosteroids are

TABLE 33–4. INCIDENCE OF MANIFEST SCARS AFTER PHOTOREFRACTIVE KERATECTOMY

Myopia Group	Baseline Refraction (D)	Eyes with Manifest Scars [no (%)]
Lower	≤−3.0	0 (0)
Middle	−3.1 to −6.0	1 (1.1)
High	−6.1 to −9.0	7 (17.5)
Highest	≥−9.1	2 (16.7)

From: Seiler T, Holschbach A, Derse M, Jean B, Genth U. Complications of myopic photorefractive keratectomy with the excimer laser. *Ophthalmology.* 1994;101:153–160.

effective in this situation. In fact, the one prospective, randomized, double-blind trial performed to date showed that steroids had no statistically significant effect on anterior stromal haze.[32] Contrary to this finding, several investigators have reported favorable results with the use of corticosteroids for the treatment of postexcimer corneal haze.[5,8,21,28] Additional well-controlled, randomized trials are required to convincingly define the role of steroids in the management of corneal haze.

HALOES

The presence of haloes around light sources is one of the most common side effects of excimer laser PRK. Many patients experience this phenomenon, particularly at night, and symptoms tend to be most marked during the early postop period.[8,13,16,18,21,23,24,38,39] Gartry et al[23] found that on direct questioning of patients following excimer laser PRK, 78% (94 of 120) reported haloes around sources of light at night in the early postop period. This effect diminished with time, and by 1 year had either disappeared completely or was regarded as only a minor problem by 82 of these patients. In 12 (10%) patients, however, the halo effect was persistent and sufficiently debilitating to prevent the patients from proceeding with PRK in the other eye.

The primary determinants of the halo effect appear to be the ablation-zone diameter, pupil size, and the amount of induced refractive change.[5,21,23,24,40] The halo effect after excimer laser PRK is generated by the differential refraction of light through the treated (flattened) central cornea and the untreated (still myopic) paracentral cornea. When the pupil is larger than the diameter of the ablation zone, light rays passing through the paracentral cornea, which are normally blocked by the iris, now fall on the perifoveal retina and create a defocused annulus of light around the focused image on the fovea. This optical aberration results in a myopic blur circle superimposed on the corrected image from the central cornea. Therefore, under scotopic conditions, when the pupil dilates, the halo effect tends to be more pronounced, particularly in patients with small ablation-zone diameters. Seiler and Wollensack,[21] for example, reported significant halo effects at night in patients with 3.5-mm–diameter ablation zones. In their study, 34% of patients reported haloes at 9 months. In contrast, Sher et al,[13] utilizing ablation-zone diameters of 5.2 to 6.0 mm, reported minimal complaints about night glare.

The magnitude of the halo effect has also been shown to be highly correlated with large, induced refractive changes. Patients with greater overcorrection in the early postop period have been shown to experience the most marked halo effects.[23] With the onset of regression during the first 3 months after surgery, the magnitude of the halo effect lessens.

DECREASED CONTRAST SENSITIVITY

At the present time, information regarding the effect of excimer laser PRK on contrast sensitivity is very limited. From the few studies conducted thus far, it is difficult to draw any general conclusions about the effect of excimer laser PRK on contrast sensitivity.[4,13,14,41–43] The studies have differed in the technique utilized to measure contrast sensitivity, and the results have been variable. In one study, contrast sensitivity was shown to decrease in the highest frequencies after the correction of myopia of greater than 6 D, but to return to baseline by 6 months after surgery.[41] In this study, eyes with corrections less than 6 D showed only a modest decrease in contrast sensitivity at the highest frequencies 2 months after PRK, but returned to baseline by 3 months after surgery. No correlation between the reduction of contrast sensitivity and corneal haze was demonstrated for this group of patients. A multicenter study of 31 eyes with myopia ranging from −4 to −12 D and 6-month follow-up found no difference in contrast sensitivity from baseline at 3 months after PRK.[13] In another multicenter study of highly myopic eyes, with myopia ranging from −8.62 to −14.50 D and 6-month follow-up, contrast sensitivity was shown to be unchanged from baseline at 6 months after surgery.[14] Contrary to the findings of these studies, one study found contrast sensitivity to be depressed at 6 months in eyes that underwent PRK compared with the unoperated eyes, but this depression was no longer measurable at 12 months after PRK.[42] In another study, a prolonged decrease in contrast sensitivity was noted in high frequencies at 1 year in patients treated with nitrogen gas blowing across the cornea intraoperatively, compared to those not treated with nitrogen.[4]

DECENTRATION OF ABLATION

The true incidence of eccentric ablation associated with excimer laser PRK is currently unknown; however, several investigators have reported this complication to occur in approximately 1% to 11% of patients.[9,23,24,36] In the technique commonly employed to center the ablation for excimer laser PRK, the ablation zone is centered over the midpoint of the entrance pupil while the patient is fixing coaxially with the surgeon.[44,45] Improper alignment of the ablation zone has been shown to lead to significant astigmatism, increased halo effect, and degradation in visual performance[3,15,22–24,36] (Fig 33–3). Surgical, patient, and instrument variables all interplay to cause decentration. Surgeon inexperience has been identified as a major cause of decentration,[15,46] and patient anxiety and failure to fixate on the appropriate target has also led to improper alignment of the ablation zone.[10,23,24] The amount of attempted correction has also been shown to be a contributory factor in decentration. In a study analyzing the corneal topography of 175 eyes that had undergone excimer laser PRK, the investigators found that higher attempted corrections resulted in greater amounts of decentration.[47] Although no apparent cause for this effect could be identified, the investigators postulated that these patients may have greater difficulty in maintaining fixation during treatment, either because of their larger degree of myopia or because of the longer time required for the laser treatment. Misalignment of the optics of the laser delivery system can also cause decentration.

One of the main unknowns regarding decentration is the point at which decentration of the ablation zone becomes clinically significant. Several studies have demonstrated that patients can maintain relatively good spectacle-corrected visual acuity despite relatively large amounts (≥ 1.5 mm) of decentration.[47–49] In each of these studies, no demonstrable correlation was found between the magnitude of decentration and the Snellen acuity. It is generally accepted that decentrations less than, or equal to, 0.5 mm have no impact on vision or refractive outcome, but that eccentricity of 0.5 to 1.0 mm results in an increased halo effect.[15] Seiler et al[10] reported, in a large series of 193 eyes, that eccentricity of the ablation zone between 0.5 and 1.0 mm occurred in 22.7% of eyes, but had no effect on best spectacle-corrected visual acuity or refractive astigmatism.

ELEVATED INTRAOCULAR PRESSURE

Increased intraocular pressure (IOP) following excimer laser PRK has been caused solely by the prolonged use of topical steroids postoperatively. The reported incidence of steroid-induced glaucoma ranges from

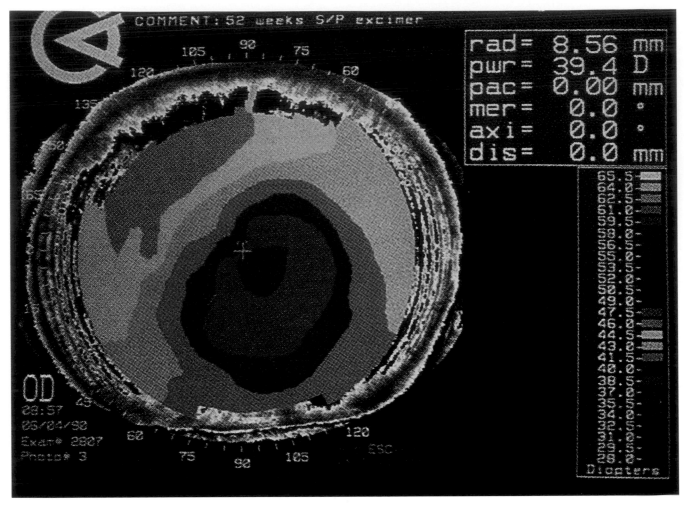

Figure 33–3. Decentration of the ablation zone inferiorly. *(From Klyce SD. Corneal topography in refractive keratectomy. In: Thompson FB, McDonnell PJ, eds.* Color Atlas/Text of Excimer Laser Surgery. The Cornea. *New York: Igaku-Shoin Medical Publishers Inc; 1993:19–36.)*

11%[23,32,38] to 30%.[9,10,36] Significant rises in IOP have been recorded, with one study reporting pressure rises to as high as 45 mm Hg in 1.6% of patients.[24] In several reports, a higher incidence of steroid-induced glaucoma was noted in patients with high myopic corrections[8,10,15]; however, this has not been a consistent finding in all studies. The onset of IOP elevation in most reports has occurred between 2 and 6 weeks after surgery.[10,23,24] In all reported cases, the IOP elevation has responded promptly to discontinuation of the steroid medication or to a short course of topical beta-blockers.

RECURRENT EROSION AND DELAYED EPITHELIAL HEALING

Despite removal of Bowman's layer, excimer laser PRK has caused an extremely low incidence of recurrent erosion and delayed epithelial healing. In the overwhelming majority of cases, epithelial healing occurs rapidly and is complete within 3 to 5 days after excimer laser PRK.[2,4,5,8,10,15,21,22] In a series of 255 eyes, Seiler and Wollensak[21] found that complete re-epithelialization occurred within 3 days in 88% of treated eyes. In this same study, only 4 of the 255 (0.8%) eyes had a delay in epithelial healing. Similarly, a multicenter study of excimer laser PRK in 1236 eyes found that only 106 (9.4%) eyes required more than 4 days for re-epithelialization.[9]

This low rate of persistent epithelial defects is paralleled by an equally low incidence of recurrent erosion. The majority of published prospective studies report no episodes of recurrent erosions.[4,5,8,9,16,19,38] In one series of 120 eyes, Gartry et al[24] reported that 18% of patients experienced symptoms of foreign body sensation upon awaking and tenderness on eye rubbing, but this subsequently resolved within a 6- to 9-month period.

Loss of Corneal Sensation

Campos et al[50] found a prolonged decrease in central corneal sensitivity in 14 patients following excimer laser PRK. Peripheral corneal sensitivity (outside the ablation zone) remained intact. The time required for recovery of corneal sensitivity to baseline appeared to be a function of the amount of attempted correction. Within the first 3 months, patients operated on for correction of compound astigmatism recovered 96% of baseline corneal sensitivity, while patients treated for severe myopia recovered 86% of baseline sensitivity. None of the patients experienced delayed epithelial healing or recurrent corneal erosion during the time of decreased corneal sensitivity. These findings imply that patients may be at risk for the complications associated with neurotrophic keratitis for several weeks after PRK, and patients undergoing deep stromal ablations may be at even higher risk.

Diurnal Fluctuation

In a recent report, Seiler et al[51] have, for the first time, documented a diurnal variation in refraction after excimer laser PRK. In this study, 10 patients who had undergone PRK were shown to have a significant fluctuation in their manifest refraction from morning to evening, compared with a control group. Prior to this report, diurnal changes following PRK had been inferred from subjective complaints of patients who reported fluctuation of their vision.[8,52]

Vision-Threatening Complications

Corneal Perforation

The incidence of vision-threatening complications associated with excimer laser PRK is extremely rare. To date, there are no reports of intraoperative corneal perforations. There has been only one reported case of sterile ulceration; this occurred 1 month after surgery and required corneal transplantation. It should be noted, however, that this patient was subsequently diagnosed as having systemic lupus erythematosus.[21]

Infectious Keratitis

Only two cases of infectious bacterial keratitis following excimer laser PRK have been reported. One case occurred in the immediate postop period,[53] and the other occurred 6 months after surgery.[7] Both cases were effectively managed medically, and no permanent sequelae resulted.

McDonnell et al[54] reported reactivation of herpetic keratitis as a complication of excimer laser PRK in a patient treated for high postkeratoplasty astigmatism. This patient had originally undergone penetrating keratoplasty for corneal scarring that developed secondary to a herpetic stromal keratitis. Four weeks after PRK, recurrent dendritic keratitis was noted.

SUMMARY

Based on the results reported to date, excimer laser PRK compares favorably with radial keratotomy for the correction of myopia. As with radial keratotomy, excimer laser PRK yields the best results in patients with 6 D or less of myopia. Refractive results that are reasonably predictable and that remain stable for at least 2 years can be obtained in this group of patients. Refractive results in patients with greater than 6 D of myopia tend to be highly variable and undergo much more regression.

Excimer laser PRK appears to offer a high level of safety, as does radial keratotomy, with vision-threatening complications being exceedingly rare. However, PRK does not weaken the cornea and predispose it to rupture from blunt trauma, as does radial keratotomy. PRK can, however, lead to complications (haze, haloes) that significantly compromise vision and, although infrequent following the treatment of low myopia, may reach intolerable levels following treatment of high myopia.

Overall, the results of excimer laser PRK are encouraging and should improve as we gain more experience with this technique and develop a better understanding of the laser–tissue interactions.

ACKNOWLEDGEMENT

This study was supported in part by an unrestricted grant from Research to Prevent Blindness Inc, New York, NY. Dr McDonnell is a Research to Prevent Blindness William and Mary Greve International Research Scholar.

REFERENCES

1. Trokel SL, Srinivasan R, Braren B. Excimer laser surgery of the cornea. *Am J Ophthalmol*. 1983;96:710–715.
2. Seiler T, Wollensak J. Results of a prospective evaluation of photorefractive keratectomy at 1 year after surgery. *Ger J Ophthalmol*. 1993;2:135–142.

3. Salz JJ, Maguen E, Nesburn AB, et al. A two-year experience with excimer laser photorefractive keratectomy for myopia. *Ophthalmology.* 1993;100:873–882.

4. Piebenga LW, Matta CS, Deitz MR, Tauber J, Irvine JW, Sabates FN. Excimer photorefractive keratectomy for myopia. *Ophthalmology.* 1993;100:1335–1345.

5. Tengroth B, Epstein D, Fagerholm P, Hamberg-Nystrom H, Fitzsimmons TD. Excimer laser photorefractive keratectomy for myopia. Clinical results in sighted eyes. *Ophthalmology.* 1993;100:739–745.

6. Salz JJ, Maguen E, Macy JI, Papaioannou T, Hofbauer J, Nesburn AB. One-year results of excimer laser photorefractive keratectomy for myopia. *Refract Corneal Surg.* 1992;8:269–273.

7. Lavery FL. Photorefractive keratectomy in 472 eyes. *Refract Corneal Surg.* 1993;9:S98–S100.

8. Kim JH, Hahn TW, Lee YC, Joo CK, Sah WJ. Photorefractive keratectomy in 202 myopic eyes: one year results. *Refract Corneal Surg.* 1993;9:S11–S16.

9. Brancato R, Tavola A, Carones F, et al, Italian Study Group. Excimer laser photorefractive keratectomy for myopia: results in 1165 eyes. *Refract Corneal Surg.* 1993;9:95–104.

10. Seiler T, Holschbach A, Derse M, Jean B, Genth U. Complications of myopic photorefractive keratectomy with the excimer laser. *Ophthalmology.* 1994;51:1929.

11. Waring GO III: Standardized data collection and reporting for refractive surgery. *Refract Corneal Surg.* 1992;8(suppl):1–45.

12. Liu JC, McDonald MB, Varnell R, Andrade HA. Myopic excimer laser photorefractive keratectomy: an analysis of clinical correlations. *Refract Corneal Surg.* 1990;6:321–328.

13. Sher NA, Chen V, Bowers RA, et al. The use of the 193-nm excimer laser for myopic photorefractive keratectomy in sighted eyes. A multicenter study. *Arch Ophthalmol.* 1991;109:1525–1530.

14. Sher NA, Barak M, Daya S, et al. Excimer laser photorefractive keratectomy in high myopia. A multicenter study. *Arch Ophthalmol.* 1992;110:935–943.

15. Seiler T. Photorefractive keratectomy: clinical experience. *Ophthalmol Clin North America.* 1993;6:393–398.

16. Machat JJ, Tayfour F. Photorefractive keratectomy for myopia: preliminary results in 147 eyes. *Refract Corneal Surg.* 1993;9:S16–S19.

17. Weinstock SJ. Excimer laser keratectomy: one year results with 100 myopic patients. *CLAO J.* 1993;19:178–181.

18. Lindstrom RL, Sher NA, Barak M, et al. Excimer laser photorefractive keratectomy in high myopia: a multicenter study. *Trans Am Ophthalmol Soc.* 1992;90:277–301.

19. Buratto L, Ferrari M. Photorefractive keratectomy for myopia from 6.00 D to 10.00 D. *Refract Corneal Surg.* 1993;9:S34–S36.

20. Ehlers N, Hjortdal JØ: Excimer laser refractive keratectomy for high myopia. 6-month follow-up of patients treated bilaterally. *Acta Ophthalmol (Copenh).* 1992;70:578–586.

21. Seiler T, Wollensak J. Myopic photorefractive keratectomy with the excimer laser. One-year follow-up. *Ophthalmology.* 1991;98:1156–1163.

22. McDonald MB, Liu JC, Byrd TJ, et al. Central photorefractive keratectomy for myopia. Partially sighted and normally sighted eyes. *Ophthalmology.* 1991;98:1327–1337.

23. Gartry DS, Muir MGK, Marshall J. Excimer laser photorefractive keratectomy. 18-month follow-up. *Ophthalmology.* 1992;99:1209–1219.

24. Gartry DS, Muir MGK, Marshall J. Photorefractive keratectomy with an argon fluoride excimer laser: a clinical study. *Refract Corneal Surg.* 1991;7:420–435.

25. Salorio DP, Costa J, Larena C, et al. Photorefractive keratectomy for myopia: 18-month results in 178 eyes. *Refract Corneal Surg.* 1993;9:108–110.

26. Tutton MK, Ramsell TG, Garston JB, et al. Photorefractive keratectomy for myopia: 6-month results in 95 eyes. *Refract Corneal Surg.* 1993;9:S103–S104.

27. Fitzsimmons TD, Fagerholm P, Tengroth B. Steroid treatment of myopic regression: acute refractive and topographic changes in excimer photorefractive keratectomy patients. *Cornea.* 1993;12:358–361.

28. Seiler T, Kahle G, Kriegerowski M. Excimer laser (193 nm) myopic keratomileusis in sighted and blind human eyes. *Refract Corneal Surg.* 1990;6:165–173.

29. Zabel RW, Sher NA, Ostrov CS, Parker P, Lindstrom RL. Myopic excimer laser keratectomy: a preliminary report. *Refract Corneal Surg.* 1990;6:329–334.

30. Tengroth B, Fagerholm P, Soderberg P, et al. Effect of corticosteroids in postoperative care following photorefractive keratectomies. *Refract Corneal Surg.* 1993;9:S61–S64.

31. Carones F, Brancato R, Venturi E, et al. Efficacy of corticosteroids in reversing regression after myopic photorefractive keratectomy. *Refract Corneal Surg.* 1993;9:S52–S58.

32. Gartry DS, Muir MGK, Lohmann CP, Marshall J. The effect of topical corticosteroids on refractive outcome and corneal haze after photorefractive keratectomy: a prospective, randomized, double-blind trial. *Arch Ophthalmol.* 1992;110:944–952.

33. Caubet E. Cause of subepithelial corneal haze over 18 months after photorefractive keratectomy for myopia. *Refract Corneal Surg.* 1993;9:S65–S70.

34. Fantes FE, Hanna KD, Waring GO III, Pouliquen Y, Thompson KP, Savoldelli M. Wound healing after excimer laser keratomileusis (photorefractive keratectomy) in monkeys. *Arch Ophthalmol.* 1990;108:665–675.

35. Seiler T, Derse M, Pham T. Repeated excimer laser treatment after photorefractive keratectomy. *Arch Ophthalmol.* 1992;110:1230–1233.

36. Seiler T. Photorefractive keratectomy: European experience. In: Thompson FB, McDonnell PJ, eds. *Color Atlas/Text*

of Excimer Laser Surgery. The Cornea. New York: Igaku-Shoin Medical Publishers Inc; 1993:53–62.

37. Lohmann CP, Timberlake GT, Fitzke FW, Gartry DS, Muir MK, Marshall J. Corneal light scattering after excimer laser photorefractive keratectomy: the objective measurements of haze. *Refract Corneal Surg.* 1992;8:114–121.

38. Weinstock SJ, Machat JJ. Excimer laser keratectomy for the correction of myopia. *CLAO J.* 1993;19:133–136.

39. Gimbel HV, Van Westenbrugge JA, Johnson WH, Willerscheidt AB, Sun R, Ferensowicz M. Visual, refractive, and patient satisfaction results following bilateral photorefractive keratectomy for myopia. *Refract Corneal Surg.* 1993;9:S5–S10.

40. Lohmann CP, Fitzke FW, O'Brart D, Muir MK, Marshall J. Halos—a problem for all myopes? A comparison between spectacles, contact lenses, and photorefractive keratectomy. *Refract Corneal Surg.* 1993;9:S72–S75.

41. Esente S, Passarelli N, Falco L, Passani F, Guidi D. Contrast sensitivity under photopic conditions in photorefractive keratectomy: a preliminary study. *Refract Corneal Surg.* 1993;9:S70–S72.

42. McDonald MB, Leach DH: Myopic photorefractive keratectomy: US experience. In: Thompson FB, McDonnell PJ, eds. *Color Atlas/Text of Excimer Laser Surgery. The Cornea.* New York: Igaku-Shoin Medical Publishers Inc; 1993: 37–51.

43. Eiferman RA, O'Neill KP, Forgey DR, Cook YD. Excimer laser photorefractive keratectomy for myopia: six-month results. *Refract Corneal Surg.* 1991;7:344–347.

44. Maloney RK. Corneal topography and optical zone location in photorefractive keratectomy. *Refract Corneal Surg.* 1990;6:363–371.

45. Uozato H, Guyton DL. Centering corneal surgical procedures. *Am J Ophthalmol.* 1987;103:264–275.

46. Wilson SE, Klyce SD, McDonald MB, Liu JC, Kaufman HE. Changes in corneal topography after excimer laser photorefractive keratectomy for myopia. *Ophthalmology.* 1991;98:1338–1347.

47. Cantera E, Cantera I, Olivieri L. Corneal topographic analysis of photorefractive keratectomy in 175 myopic eyes. *Refract Corneal Surg.* 1993;9:S19–S22.

48. Maguire LJ, Zabel RW, Parker P, Lindstrom RL. Topography and raytracing analysis of patients with excellent visual acuity 3 months after excimer laser photorefractive keratectomy for myopia. *Refract Corneal Surg.* 1991; 7:122–128.

49. Klyce SD. Corneal topography in refractive keratectomy. In: Thompson FB, McDonnell PJ, eds. *Color Atlas/Text of Excimer Laser Surgery. The Cornea.* New York: Igaku-Shoin Medical Publishers Inc; 1993:19–36.

50. Campos M, Hertzog L, Garbus JJ, McDonnell PJ. Corneal sensitivity after photorefractive keratectomy. *Am J Ophthalmol.* 1992;114:51–54.

51. Seiler T, Hell K, Wollensak J. Diurnal variation in refraction after excimer laser photorefractive keratectomy. *Ger J Ophthalmol.* 1992;1:19–21.

52. Kim JH, Hahn TW, Lee YC, Sah WJ. Clinical experience of two-step photorefractive keratectomy in 19 eyes with high myopia. *Refract Corneal Surg.* 1993;9:S44–S47.

53. McDonald MB, Frantz JM, Klyce SD, et al. Central photorefractive keratectomy for myopia. The blind eye study. *Arch Ophthalmol.* 1990;108:799–808.

54. McDonnell PJ, Moreira H, Clapham TN, D'Arcy J, Munnerlyn CR. Photorefractive keratectomy for astigmatism. Initial clinical results. *Arch Ophthalmol.* 1991;109:1370–1373.

55. Pallikaris IG, Lambropoulos IE, Kolydas PK, Nicolopoulos NS, Kotsiras IE. Excimer laser photorefractive keratectomy for myopia: clinical results in 96 eyes. *Refract Corneal Surg.* 1993; 9(suppl):S101–S102.

56. Nizam A, Waring GO III, Lynn MJ, et al. Stability of refraction and visual acuity during 5 years in eyes with simple myopia. *Refract Corneal Surg.* 1992;8:439–447

CHAPTER 34

Excimer Laser Intrastromal Keratomileusis (LASIK)

Paolo Rama ▪ Wallace Chamon ▪ C. Genisi ▪ Dimitri T. Azar

INTRODUCTION

Excimer laser intrastromal keratomileusis combines the techniques of lamellar corneal surgery using a microkeratome and the precision of the excimer laser for tissue removal. This keratome-laser combination was reported in 1990 independently by Burrato, who performed photokeratomileusis (PKM), and by Pallikaris, who performed excimer laser in situ keratomileusis (LASIK). Burrato's technique involves removal of a keratomileusis cap and performing PKM on the cap, while Pallikaris' LASIK technique involves raising a hinged flap and treating the stromal bed with the excimer laser.

HISTORY

In 1964 José Barraquer introduced the keratomileusis technique (*myopic keratomileusis,* or MKM) for correcting myopia.[1] This technique alters the refractive state of the eye by carving the corneal stroma. A certain amount of stroma is removed from the central part of the cornea, depending on the degree of myopia that is to be corrected. This results in a flattening of the anterior profile, which reduces the dioptric power of the cornea and corrects the myopia. In Barraquer's original

technique a cap of the cornea was removed by the microkeratome and the stroma was then processed with a lathe especially designed for this operation (*cryolathe technique*) (Fig 34–1).[1–3] This method had several drawbacks, mostly related to the tissue freezing and the complex preparation of the lenticule.[4–9] The refractive results were often imprecise, resulting in hypo- and hypercorrections, and the recovery was slow, sometimes taking 6 to 12 months for the cornea to regain transparency. Irregular astigmatism was one of the main problems.[10–18]

To avoid the problems associated with the cryolathe, Krumeich designed a technique known as *non-freeze keratomileusis,* which permitted work to be done on the corneal cap without freezing it.[5,19] The necessary surgical set is called BKS 1000, named for the initials of the creators: Barraquer, Krumeich, and Swinger. The cap of the cornea is removed with a microkeratome similar to Barraquer's and then placed on a special bench with the epithelium facing down. This bench has Teflon dies, concave or convex, that expose the stroma to a second keratectomy (*refractive keratectomy*) using the same microkeratome. When a concave die is used, the microkeratome removes a peripheral portion of the stroma, steepening the anterior surface of the cornea (*hyperopic keratomileusis);* with a convex die, a central part of the

455

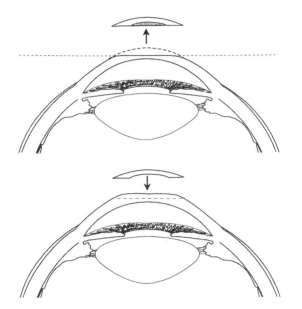

Figure 34–1. Myopic keratomileusis (MKM). The secondary keratectomy is performed using the cryolathe (Barraquer technique). The microkeratome is on the bench (Krumeich technique) and the remaining stroma is "in situ" (Ruiz technique).

stroma is removed, which leads to a flattening of the anterior profile *(myopic keratomileusis)* (Fig 34–1). This technique has overcome many of the problems inherent in Barraquer's classic method, permitting rapid recovery of visual acuity, better refractive results, and better predictability.[20–25] Its negative aspects include traumas related to the manipulation of the cap when the refractive keratectomy is done on the bench. Moreover, with this technique, it is impossible to perfectly control the centering of the refractive keratectomy.

To simplify this method, and to avoid the traumas and manipulation of the cap during the refractive keratectomy, Ruiz and Rowsey proposed the "in situ" technique a few years later.[26] The refractive keratectomy is done directly on the cornea, instead of on the cap. The primary keratectomy is performed with the microkera-

tome, as in nonfreeze keratomileusis. Then the microkeratome slices the central part of the remaining stroma while the cap remains untouched in a Petri dish. The thickness of the lenticule (refractive keratectomy disc) is proportional to the degree of myopia to be corrected, and it is determined by a nomogram that Ruiz proposed. After the stromal lenticule has been removed, the cap is replaced over the treated cornea (Fig 34–1). This technique has had good results, but it is not without risks.[8,27–29] Possible errors or malfunctioning of the instrument during the secondary keratectomy can cause surface irregularities, or even perforations. In addition, as in nonfreeze keratomileusis, it is not possible to perfectly control the centering of the refractive keratectomy. Thus, errors in the intended correction can occur because the microkeratome performs the secondary keratectomy imprecisely.

The use of the excimer laser in ophthalmology was first presented by Toboada and Archibald in 1981.[30] In 1993 Trokel and colleagues described the capacity of the excimer laser to remove tissue precisely.[31] The ultraviolet radiation of the excimer laser can remove tissue through photoablation; this peculiarity was utilized to correct myopia by removing tissue from the anterior surface of the cornea *(photorefractive keratectomy,* or PRK).[32–36] While PRK has good results, moderate predictability, and rare complications when correcting mild to moderate myopia (up to 6 D), the results above 6 D are unpredictable because of haze and regression.[37]

In 1990 Buratto presented the first results of keratomileusis using the excimer laser *(photokeratomileusis— Buratto technique)* for the refractive treatment (Lucio Buratto, personal communication: First International Meeting on Keratomileusis, Venice, Italy, June 1990). Buratto proposed removing the cap with the microkeratome and then treating the stromal face of the cap with the excimer laser (Fig 34–2). The rationale was to combine the techniques of keratomileusis and PRK in order

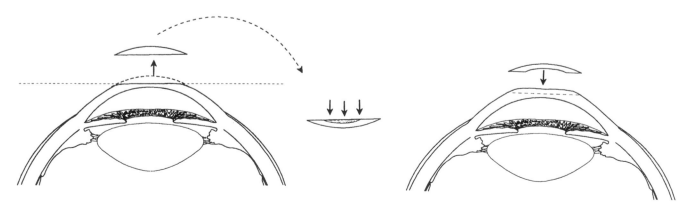

Figure 34–2. Buratto technique: the secondary keratectomy is done with the excimer laser on the stromal face of the cap.

to take advantages of the high corrective capacity of the first technique and the excimer laser's precision in tissue removal.[38,39]

Also in 1990, Pallikaris proposed to treat the stroma "in situ" with the excimer laser *(laser in situ keratomileusis—LASIK)*.[40,41] The microkeratome slices the cornea, but stops before completing the keratectomy. The corneal flap is raised and the remaining stroma is treated with the excimer laser (Fig 34–3).

According to Buratto, photokeratomileusis (PKM) follows the theoretical and mathematical principles of

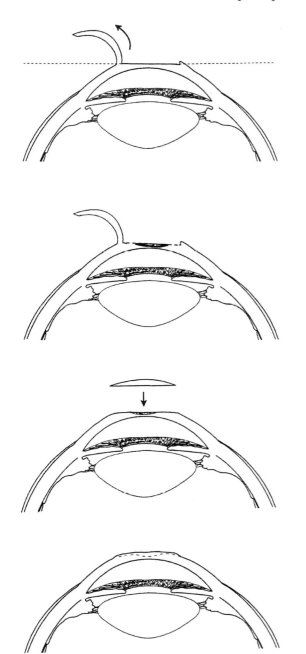

Figure 34–3. Pallikaris technique: the excimer laser treatment is performed on the remaining stroma in situ, raising the corneal flap.

traditional keratomileusis in terms of the primary keratectomy using a microkeratome. The secondary keratectomy is performed with the excimer laser on the cap or on the stroma in situ, and the refractive correction is achieved utilizing the same protocol as PRK.[25–42] Compared with PRK, PKM has not resulted in haze and regression, and it is effective for myopia ranging from 8 to 25 D.[43–45]

Advantages of Laser Intrastromal Keratomileusis

Trauma

Excimer laser treatment makes it possible to avoid the trauma of removing the refractive corneal cut. The laser beam removes tissue without manipulating the cap.

Precision

The excimer laser can apply submicron precision to the removal of tissue. Because the precision is notably greater than any mechanical instrument, the results are more predictable and the technique more reproducible.

Rapidity

Refractive treatment is rapid, ranging from 30 to 60 seconds. This is an important factor because variations in the hydration of the cap can influence the final result.

Risks

There is minimal risk of damaging the cap or perforating the cornea, which were possibilities in the early keratomileusis methods described above. Moreover, the quality of the excimer laser is much higher and it is more expensive than refractive keratectomy with the microkeratome (Krumeich and Ruiz techniques) or the cryolathe (Barraquer technique).

Choice of the Optical Zone

This technique enables the surgeon to choose the diameter of the optical zone according to the degree of myopia, age, pupil diameter, corneal thickness, and other factors, which was not possible with earlier methods.

Centration

When the refractive keratectomy is done with the microkeratome, perfect control over the centering is not possible. But with Buratto's technique, the cornea is first marked on the epithelium and the treatment is then undertaken while centering the laser on the mark, which is visible in transparency. In the Pallikaris technique, centration on the entrance pupil is achieved in the same way as in regular PRK. In both techniques of excimer-laser secondary keratectomy, the refractive correction can be centered even when the first cut is slightly off center (Fig 34–8H).

Nondependence on a Perfect First Keratectomy

Earlier techniques of keratomileusis depended on the thickness and diameter of the cap obtained during the primary keratectomy. Using the excimer laser, the refractive treatment can always be done, even when, for example, the cap is thinner than planned. In PKM the thickness of the corneal cap is measured with a micrometer after the keratectomy. If the calculated thickness after the ablation is more than 130 μm, the cap should be treated under the excimer laser. If the calculated thickness is less than 130 μm, the patient should be moved under the excimer laser and the treatment done on the remaining stroma of the cornea (in situ). The idea of leaving at least 130 μm of untreated stroma over the cornea is to avoid any complication related to a thin cap, such as wrinkles and irregular astigmatism.

Regularization of the Surface

If the first keratectomy leaves an irregular surface, it can be regularized using the excimer laser in a phototherapeutic approach with a masking fluid *(PTK technique)*.

Correction of Astigmatism

The latest generation of excimer lasers allows the surgeon to treat the astigmatism as well. It is important to remember, when treating the cap (Buratto's technique), that because the cap will be treated upside down, the axis of the astigmatism must be changed. The cornea must be marked on the epithelium at 90° and 180° to indicate which axis to treat.

SURGICAL TECHNIQUES

Anesthesia

Although the operation can be carried out with general, local, or topical anesthesia, most surgeons perform the procedure with topical anesthesia. Retrobulbar injection may be helpful in some patients to expose the globe and prevent the microkeratome movement from being limited by the orbital rim.

Centration

One drop of pilocarpine 2% may be instilled 30 minutes before the surgery. The center of the entrance pupil can

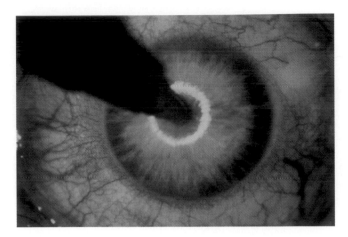

Figure 34–4. The cornea is marked on the entrance pupil with a pen.

be located with a marking pen on the cornea under the microscope (Fig 34–4). The patient should be looking at the fixation light in the recommended manner (see Chapter 19).[46–48] The same marking pen is used to trace a transverse line on the cornea at the edge of the cap in order to reposition it with the same orientation after the excimer laser treatment (Fig 34–5). Another method is to mark the center of the entrance pupil with the excimer laser as well. The excimer laser marks the epithelium while the patient looks at the fixation light; 20 or 30 shots of 2 mm in diameter are sufficient to create a methylene-blue–stained marking spot (Fig 34–6).

Primary Lamellar Keratectomy

The microkeratome is required to perform the primary keratectomy. A corneal lamella of predetermined diameter and thickness is elicited. This cap or flap does not have any dioptric power. Microkeratome precision is extremely important because the success of the procedure depends largely on the quality of the keratec-

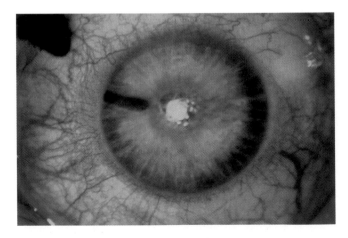

Figure 34–5. A transverse marking line is made to reposition the cap with the same orientation after the excimer laser treatment.

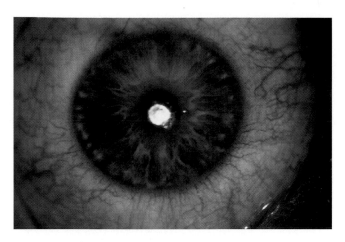

Figure 34–6. Twenty shots of excimer laser mark the epithelium while the patient looks at the fixation light.

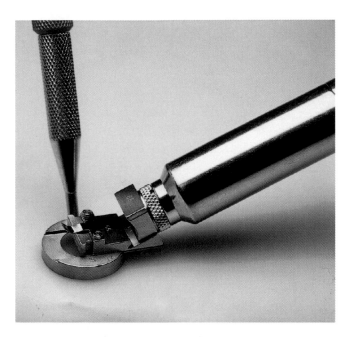

Figure 34–7. A Krumeich microkeratome.

tomy. The ideal instrument is easy to use and obtains the precise depth and diameter that were determined for the cap. The cost of the instrument has to be considered. One reason why keratomileusis is not frequently performed is that it requires a long learning curve. In fact, the accuracy of the keratectomy greatly depends upon the surgeon's skill. Greater velocity of the microkeratome movement means a thinner cap, whereas more or less pressure on the suction ring can influence the predetermined values of diameter and thickness. Therefore, technical research strove to make instruments that would better control the suction (see Chapter 18). Automatic movement of the microkeratome is an important tool to reduce the variables associated with the surgeon's experience. It is very important to take good care of the microkeratome: the instrument must be cleaned and dried properly after the procedure and carefully assembled and checked beforehand.

LASIK Using Krumeich or SCMD Microkeratome

The Krumeich and SCMD instruments are based on Barraquer's original microkeratome and comprise a motor that moves the blade, a plate that is inserted in the head of the microkeratome for applanating the cornea, and a pneumatic suction ring (Fig 34–7). This ring fixes the globe during the operation, predeterminates the diameter of the cap, and permits the microkeratome to slide (see Table 18–2). The electric motor of the Krumeich machine, which revolves at 12,000 to 15,000 rpm, is in the instrument's handle and is controlled by a foot switch. The SCMD microkeratome has an advantage of being turbo-driven (pneumatic instead of electric motor). The blade alternates when it moves. The blades, which are made of steel, should be replaced after any cut and checked under the microscope before they are

used. Sapphire and diamond blades also exist; while they produce an even better keratectomy, they have the disadvantage of being fragile and very expensive. The microkeratome contains three interchangeable plates beneath the head, which are marked by a number corresponding to the depth of the desired keratectomy (0.30, 0.36, and 0.42 mm). It is very important to insert them correctly because if the plate is missed or incorrectly inserted, the keratectomy will be done full thickness and the cornea will be perforated. There are four suction rings (nos 3, 4, 5, and 6), connected by a tube to the vacuum pump; these are chosen according to the keratometric values of the patient and they regulate the cap diameter: the more the cornea extrudes from the ring, the larger is the diameter of the cap. The advantage of the turbo-driven SCMD machine is that the vibrations allow for smooth lenticule resection. The microkeratome's movement across the cornea is manual and the results obtained with its use have been highly predictable. These instruments have two major drawbacks: the possible perforation of the cornea if the applanation plate is forgotten or incorrectly positioned and the manual drag of the microkeratome, which adds a variable to the procedure.

Technique

The suction ring is chosen on the desired diameter of the cap, according to the keratometric values of the patient. Numbers 5 and 6 are more often used. Then the

EAST GLAMORGAN GENERAL HOSPITAL
CHURCH VILLAGE, near PONTYPRIDD

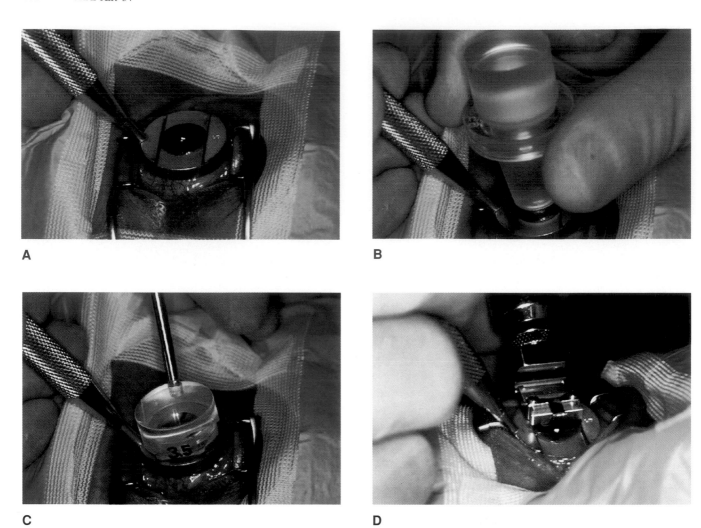

A

B

C

D

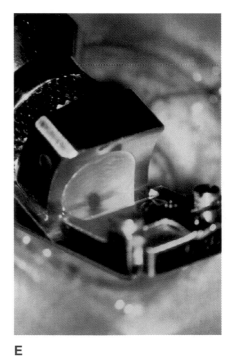

E

Figure 34–8. Surgical procedure with the Krumeich microkeratome. **A.** Fixation ring. **B.** Tonometry. **C.** Applanation. **D.** Primary keratectomy. **E.** The cap after the keratectomy.

applanation plate is chosen and inserted in the head of the microkeratome. This keratectomy is planned to give a 360-μm–thick lamella (plate no. 0.36). Before starting the operation, the instrument is checked: first the suction is controlled by occluding the pneumatic ring with a finger; the suction has to reach at least 700 millibars. Then the blade functioning is checked. The pneumatic ring is placed on the patient's eye and centered on the pupil (Fig 34–8A). The vacuum must raise the intraocular pressure (IOP) to 60 to 65 mm Hg in order to ensure a precise and regular keratectomy (Fig 34–8B). It has been accepted that this temporary suction has no secondary effects on the ocular globe.[49] The applanation is carried out to confirm that the diameter of the keratectomy corresponds to what is desired (Fig 34–8C). Once the suction ring has been placed and the microkeratome checked, the guides are moistened with distilled water to ensure smooth sliding. The surgeon must find the right position for his arm and hand so that he can perform the entire cutting procedure without moving. The movement of the microkeratome must be regular and at a constant speed of approximately 1 mm per second (Fig 34–8D). Once the keratectomy has been made, it is essential to stop the blade immediately to prevent damage to the cap (Fig 34–8E). The diameter is then measured and the thickness checked with a micrometer. If the flap extends to become a cap, it is viewed under the microscope in order to control the quality of the keratectomy. It is advisable to protect the stroma from being dehydrated by keeping the flap covered while the patient is transported to the excimer.

LASIK USING RUIZ (CHIRON) MICROKERATOME

In attempting to reduce the variable associated with the operator's hand, Ruiz introduced a new microkeratome with an automatic movement (Fig 34–9).[50] A gear placed on the microkeratome's head meets a track on the suction ring. The motor, placed in the handle of the instrument, drives either the oscillation of the blade or the rotation of the gear that moves the microkeratome forward on the cornea. In addition to the suction ring, a screw regulates the corneal exposure allowing for choice of the diameter of the keratectomy (see Chapters 18 and 26). This instrument represents an improvement on earlier ones because the microkeratome moves automatically across the cornea. Moreover, it is relatively easy to prepare a corneal flap with this microkeratome when performing the in situ technique: the instrument is set to stop before the keratectomy is completed.

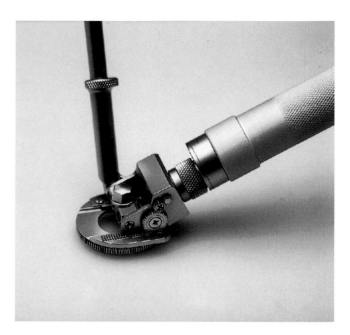

Figure 34–9. A Ruiz automatic microkeratome.

Technique

The first steps are similar to the Krumeich-instrument technique described above: the instrument must be checked, the applanation plate inserted, and the tonometry and applanation performed before starting the keratectomy. This procedure differs in that the diameter of the desired keratectomy is obtained without changing the suction ring. After the applanation, the surgeon can use the screw to raise or lower the suction ring: the suction ring should be lowered to obtain a smaller cap and raised for a larger diameter. The microkeratome is gently inserted on the suction ring and is pushed forward until the gear touches the track. When the surgeon presses the foot switch the microkeratome moves forward automatically, and it stops as soon as the stop reaches the end of the track.

LASIK USING DRAEGER OR PHOENIX MICROKERATOMES

These instruments present distinct innovations (Fig 34–10).[51–53] Two important features of the Draeger microkeratome are, first, that it has a rotating circular blade instead of an oscillating rectangular blade, and, second, that the automatic movement for slicing the cornea is applied only to the blade and to the applanation plate, not to the entire instrument (see Chapter 18). The use of a circular blade produces a smooth surface, and

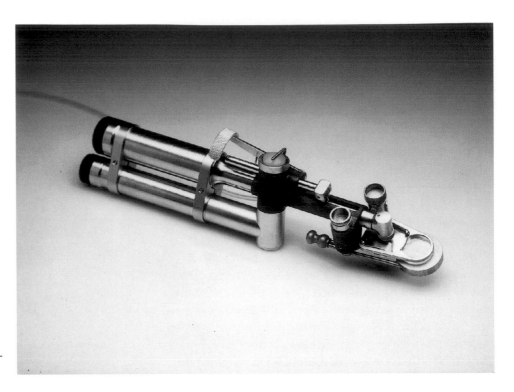

Figure 34–10. A Draeger microkeratome.

the movement of only a small part of the instrument produces a constant cutting speed. The Phoenix machine is very similar to the Draeger microkeratome except that an oscillating blade replaces the rotating circular blade.

The Draeger microkeratome utilizes two separate, armor-plated electric engines that fit in the handle of the instrument. One is responsible for the rotating movement of the blade and the other, for the forward movement of the applanation plate and blade. The rotating movement is controlled using the foot switch; the forward movement is controlled by a button localized in the handle. The Phoenix and Draeger microkeratomes' applanation plates are transparent, allowing the surgeon to see through the plate while cutting. The plate has millimetric landmarks that permit precise measurement of the applanated cornea (expected diameter of the cap) during the procedure. The diameter of the applanated cornea is regulated by a micrometric screw. The Draeger instrument has only one suction ring that theoretically fits all eyes. The thickness of the cut is changed using different spacers between the applanation plate and blade. The microkeratome allows the surgeon to choose three different thicknesses of the keratectomy (0.15, 0.25, and 0.35 mm). Two tubes are connected to the instrument: one for suction and the other for lubricating and irrigating the procedure. The whole instrument is autoclavable, and the engines are inserted in its handle at the time of the surgery without contaminating it.

The Draeger instrument offers several improvements: it is easy to use, the quality of the cut is extremely good, and the diameter of the cut is very precise.[54,55] On the negative side, we have experienced some difficulty in centering the instrument because of the size of its suction ring and the quality of the electric connections, which sometimes cause the movement of the instrument to stop. The main difficulty that we have encountered is variability of the cap thickness, resulting in errors of up to 50 to 60 μm.[56]

Technique

After choosing the correct spacer for the intended thickness, the instrument is placed on the eye and centered on the pupil. The diameter of the presumed keratectomy is checked, using the landmarks visible in the glass applanation plate and regulated through the micrometric screw. The rotational movement of the blade is started with the foot switch, and the assistant irrigates the instrument. When the surgeon presses the button the blade moves forward. This movement is stopped before the complete cut of the cap, leaving a small flap still connected to the cornea to treat the stroma in situ *(Pallikaris LASIK technique).*

REFRACTIVE KERATECTOMY

The refractive treatment is carried out with the excimer laser directly on the stroma instead of through the Bowman's layer as occurs in surface PRK. The photoablation is usually performed on the remaining stromal bed of the cornea (in situ).

Most excimer laser systems require a modification of the operating microscope to increase the working distance for the operation of the microkeratome. Some excimer laser systems, however, have a large enough working distance to allow for the lamellar keratome to be placed directly under the laser without modification and thus allowing the entire LASIK procedure to be performed without moving the patient. If the patient has to be transported, the corneal flap should be repositioned onto the stromal bed during the move to prevent trauma to the flap and to prevent stromal dehydration. The patient's head is aligned under the excimer laser so the chin and forehead are in the same frontal plane. Once positioned properly, the corneal flap can be folded over to expose the stromal bed. At this point, the surgeon can proceed to ablate the stromal bed with the excimer laser. Stromal hydration remains adequate during LASIK only if the laser treatment is performed in a timely manner. This is possible if adequate preparation for the laser treatment begins prior to lifting of the flap. The excimer laser treatment is centered on the pupil even if the initial lamellar keratectomy is slightly decentered. When the ablation is completed, the backside of the flap and the stromal bed are irrigated with balanced salt saline solution to remove any particulate debris. The flap is then replaced onto the stromal bed and the interface is allowed to dry for several minutes. To check for proper apposition of the flap, a blunt tip instrument, such as forceps, is used to depress the cornea approximately 1 mm outside the interface. Proper adhesion is achieved if depression striae are seen extending from the peripheral cornea to inner aspect of the flap. After removing the lid speculum and surgical draping, the eye should be reexamined one last time to make certain the flap is in proper position.

Many surgeons perform ultrasonic pachymetry of the corneal bed prior to excimer laser keratectomy to determine the thickness of the flap by subtracting the former from the total corneal thickness. The Burrato technique of laser treatment of the cap instead of the stromal bed may be necessary if the flap is detached, especially if the depth of the keratectomy exceeds 250 μm. Some surgeons prefer the Burrato technique and routinely treat the cap (Fig 34–11).

Marking the epithelium on the optical zone before the operation allows the cap to be treated by centering the laser on the mark, which is visible in transparency. Treating the cap avoids the risk of patient movement during the ablation and does not require an excimer laser at the operating room. The in situ technique (LASIK) may still be necessary if the calculated thickness of the cap (cap thickness minus total depth of the photoablation) is less than 130 μm.

The depth and diameter of the ablations influence the outcome of the procedure. Deeper ablations can distort the anterior corneal surface. Small diameters of ablation may lead to a small functional optical zone, resulting in night vision complaints of glare and haloes. When performing the cap treatment, we program a 360-μm–thick cap, and we program the excimer laser to treat patient's spherical equivalent (at corneal plane) in two steps. Fifty percent of the total intended treatment is done in a 3.5-mm optical zone ablation, and the other 50% is done in a 5-mm optical zone. When treating the stroma in situ (LASIK), it is advisable not to perform deep ablations in order to avoid damage to the endothelium.

Lenticule Detachment

The lenticule is repositioned on the cornea so that the original orientation follows the earlier mark on the epithelium (Fig 34–11D). After experimenting with the single running suture, we now use an "overlay" rectangular suture (nylon 10-0) similar to that proposed by Guimarães (Fig 34–11E).[57] The needle is passed through the cornea on its portion outside of the keratectomy to avoid trauma to the cap (Fig 34–11D). The suture is removed after 7 days and leaves no signs. We have also achieved the same results with the sutureless technique proposed by Guimarães. We dry the stroma with filtered oxygen before repositioning the cap on the cornea, and we then dry the border of the keratectomy as well. A pressure patch is kept in place for 48 hours.

Postop Treatment

Topical antibiotics are used until complete re-epithelialization. Eyedrops of 0.1% of dexamethazone are

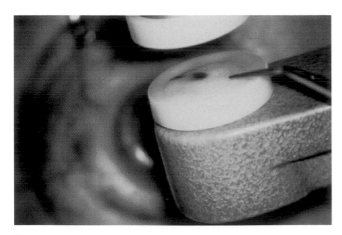

A

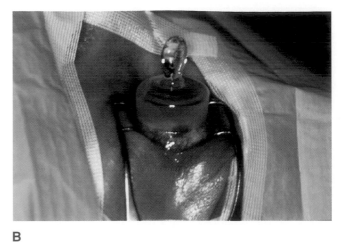

B

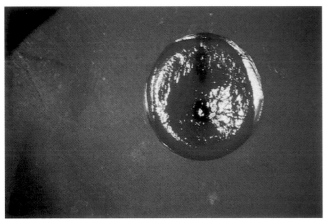

C

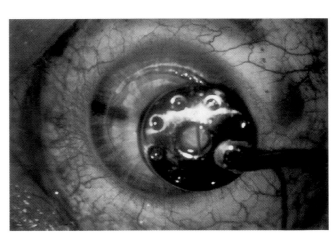

D

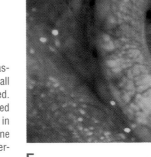

E

Figure 34–11. Surgical procedure with Krumeich microkeratome. **A.** Measurement of the cap with the micrometer: 340-μm–thick cap. **B.** A small glass cover placed on the eye prevents the stroma from being dehydrated. **C.** The cap after the excimer laser treatment. The treated area is decentered on the lenticule but well centered on the marking spot that is visible in transparency. **D.** The cap is repositioned on the cornea. The transverse line allows the surgeon to respect the same orientation of the cap. **E.** An "overlay" rectangular suture.

used QID for 2 weeks. Artificial tears are used according to patient need up to 6 times a day.

COMPLICATIONS

Intraoperative Complications

Complications during the operation are rare, and they can be avoided if the surgeon gains confidence by practicing with the microkeratome on banking or animal eyes. It is important to check the instrument carefully before the surgery.

Corneal Perforation

This is the most serious complication, and it is rare. It can occur if the applanation plate of the Krumeich microkeratome is missed or incorrectly inserted or if the cornea is very thin or irregular (keratoconus or irregular leukoma). Ultrasonic pachymetry and corneal topography should be performed in all patients before the procedure in order to minimize the risk of perforation. The danger of corneal perforation is aggravated when the high pressure is followed by hypotony upon opening of the anterior chamber. The damage caused by this sudden hypotony can range from the perforation to more serious consequences, such as lesions of the iris or the lens or even an expulsive hemorrhage. In case of perforation, the surgeon must immediately stop the suction. The corneal flap is resutured with mononylon 10-0, and the anterior chamber is reformed with a balanced salt solution or with viscoelastic substances. If the anterior segment is not damaged, the surgery can be undertaken after at least 4 or 5 months, using a donor cornea to prepare the cap.

Irregular Keratectomy

Irregularity of the primary keratectomy can generate irregular astigmatism and reduce best-corrected visual acuity (BCVA). An irregular keratectomy has several causes. The blade should always be checked under the microscope to detect irregularities of the cutting wire. Mechanical defects like motor malfunction or incorrect sliding of the microkeratome on the cornea can be avoided by carefully inspecting the instrument before the procedure. Irregular sliding of the microkeratome can also be secondary to friction on the guide as a result of deposits or insufficient lubrication. It is important to clean the instrument properly after the surgery. Another reason for an irregular keratectomy is a poor suction. IOP must be raised up to 65 mm Hg to ensure a regular cut with the microkeratome. When the surface after the keratectomy is very irregular, it is better to suture the cap back on the cornea. After 5 months the surgery can be repeated after planning a deeper keratectomy and using donor tissue for the new cap. If the irregularities are mild, it is possible to regularize both surfaces with the excimer laser (PTK treatment).

Errors in Thickness or Diameter

The use of an excimer laser for the refractive keratectomy minimizes the importance of an accurate control of thickness and diameter. The photoablation can be performed after primary keratectomies of diameters as small as 6 mm. If for any reason the thickness of the cap exceeds 360μm, the Burrato technique of treating the cap should be considered (Fig 34–12). The surgery can still be carried out without problems after completion of the keratectomy.

Decentered Keratectomy

When the first keratectomy is slightly decentered, the PKM technique, rather than the traditional keratomileusis, can surmount the problem by decentering the laser treatment. Marking the cornea on the optical zone before the operation allows the surgeon to treat the stroma on the epithelial mark that is visible in transparency. A more pronounced decentration, however, can cause an irregular secondary astigmatism.

Incomplete Keratectomy

An incomplete keratectomy can occur if the motor of the microkeratome stops during the procedure. The results differ depending on whether or not the optical

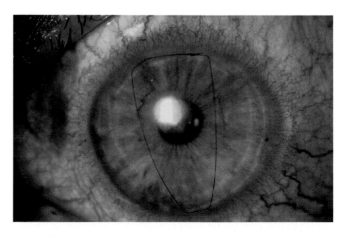

Figure 34–12. One day following LASIK requiring suturing.

zone is affected. If the keratectomy stops before the optical zone, the cap can be resutured and the surgery reperformed after the healing process (5 months). If the keratectomy stops within the optical zone, the cap should be resutured and the surgery reperformed after the cornea heals, using donor tissue for the cap. If the surgery stops after leaving the optical zone, the surgeon can complete the keratectomy manually and proceed with the photoablation. In this case the flap must be lifted and the bed of the keratectomy treated with the laser (*Pallikaris technique*).

Destruction of the Cap

The cap can be destroyed if the blade captures the cap once the keratectomy is finished. The surgeon must remember to stop moving the blade immediately after the cutting is finished.

Decentered Refractive Treatment

Improper centration of the photoablation with the excimer laser can cause monocular diplopia and haloes. It results either from an error in marking the optical zone before the operation or a malfunction of the alignment system of the excimer laser.

Postop Complications

Epithelial Growth on the Interface

Because the keratectomy is done without removing the epithelium, the blade might "seed" epithelial cells in the interface. Despite even the most careful washing of the surface, epithelial cells can remain within the bed. If the epithelial island is not within the optical zone and does not alter the corneal topography, clinical control is sufficient. However, when the optical zone is involved, the epithelial inclusion should be removed as soon as possible. For this purpose, the cap is carefully raised to the periphery, and the island is removed with a spatula; the surface must be generously irrigated to eliminate any remaining cells.

Irregular Astigmatism

This can be caused by an irregular primary keratectomy, by errors in marking the optical zone, and by decentered photoablation. Because suture of the cap was one of the most frequent causes of secondary astigmatism, it was replaced by an "overlay" suture, or a sutureless technique, to avoid traction and trauma to the tissue.

Epithelial Defects

Re-epithelialization of the edge of the cap occurs normally within 48 hours after the procedure. However, patients with dry eyes may have persistent epithelial defects that can be treated with a pressure patch, therapeutic contact lenses, or artificial tears. It is good practice to evaluate and treat patients with dry eyes before the surgery.

Deposits in the Interface

Not infrequently impurities are found on the interface of the keratomileusis that are caused by incorrect use of materials like gauze, glove powder, and cotton tips, or by metallic debris from the blade of the microkeratome. These deposits, even when visible at the slit lamp, usually have no effect on the quality of vision.

Infection

This is a rare complication as in any other lamellar keratoplasty. When infection is suspected, aggressive topical antibiotic treatment should be immediately initiated based on laboratory findings. Careful follow-up is necessary to evaluate the need to remove the cap to improve antibiotic penetration.

Hypo- and Hypercorrections

These can be caused by errors in the surgical procedure, poor functioning of the excimer laser, regression, or individual variations. Regression is not as critical a factor in excimer laser keratomileusis, as it is in PRK.

Glare

Glare depends on the diameter of the refractive treatment, size of the pupil, age, and surface regularity.

Haze

A mild haze is seen in a few cases, which disappears spontaneously in some weeks. Steroid treatment is not required.

CONCLUSIONS

The introduction of the excimer laser in refractive surgery raises new interest in keratomileusis. This technique was not widely used in the past, mainly because of the complexity of the procedure and the steep learning curve. The recently created opportunities to perform refractive keratectomy with the excimer laser

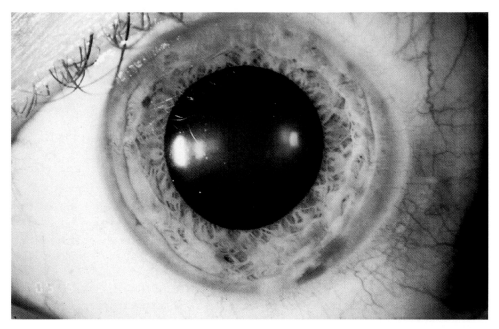

A

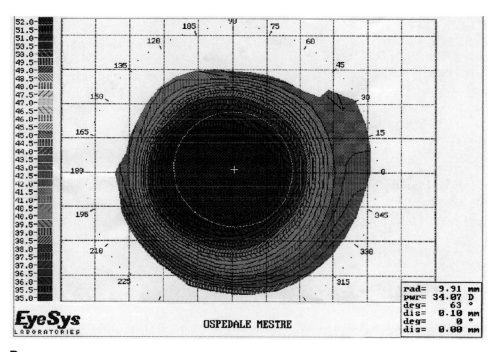

B

Figure 34–13. Left eye of a 30-year-old patient with −15 D of myopia. **A.** Preop visual acuity 0.6 with spectacles, intolerant of contact lenses. Intended correction −15 D. Treated 7.5 D with 3.5-mm optical zone and 7.5 D with 5.0-mm optical zone. Three weeks from the surgery, visual acuity 0.5 without correction and 0.6 with −1 D. **B.** The corneal map shows a well-centered and smooth treatment.

simplify the procedure. Its predictability and reproducibility improved because of the precision of the excimer laser in removing tissue. Photoablation of the stroma, instead of a secondary keratectomy with the microkeratome, makes LASIK safer and avoids trauma to the cap. In contrast to PRK, photokeratomileusis and LASIK produce neither regression nor haze, and steroid treatment is not required. The new generation of excimer lasers allows the astigmatism to be treated with even more precision than in the past. Indications for this procedure have therefore expanded, and we consider keratomileusis to be a safe and predictable procedure for myopia ranging from 6 to 23 D.

Some controversy remains about the first keratectomy, which is carried out with microkeratomes that are not very different from the first instrument produced in the 1960s (Chapter 18). The high cost of the procedure has to be considered as well because it includes both the excimer laser and the microkeratome. We hope that the renewed interest in keratomileusis will improve the microkeratomes even more.

REFERENCES

1. Barraquer JI. Queratomileusis para la correccion de la miopia [in Spanish]. *Arch Soc Am Oftalmol Optom.* 1964; 5:27–48.

2. Barraquer JI. Bases de la queratoplastia refractiva [in Spanish]. *Arch Soc Am Oftalmol Optom.* 1965;5:179.

3. Barraquer JI. *Queratomileusis y Queratofaquia* [in Spanish]. Bogotá: Litografia Arco; 1980.

4. Schanzlin DJ, Jester JV, Eunduck K. Cryolathe corneal injury. *Cornea.* 1983;2:57–68.

5. Swinger CA, Krumeich J, Cassidy D. Planar lamellar refractive keratoplasty. *J Refract Surg.* 1986;2:17–24.

6. Zavala EY, Krumeich J, Binder PS. Laboratory evaluation of freeze vs nonfreeze lamellar refractive keratoplasty. *Arch Ophthalmol.* 1987;105:1125–1128.

7. Maxwell WA, Nordan LT. Optical and wound complications of keratomileusis: incidence and treatment. In: Cavanagh HD, ed. *The Cornea: Transactions of the World Congress on the Cornea. III.* New York: Raven Press; 1988: 597–601.

8. Hagen KB, Kim EK, Waring III GO. Comparison of excimer laser and microkeratome myopic keratomileusis in human cadaver eyes. *Refract Corneal Surg.* 1993;9: 36–41.

9. American Academy of Ophthalmology. Ophthalmic procedures assessment. Keratophakia and keratomileusis: safety and effectiveness. *Ophthalmology.* 1992;99:1332–1341.

10. Barraquer JI: Cirugia Refractiva de la Cornea [In Spanish]. Tomo I. Bogotá, 1989:467–480.

11. Krumeich JH. Indications, techniques, and complications of myopic keratomileusis. *Int Ophthalmol Clin.* 1983; 23:75–92.

12. Swinger CA, Barraquer JI. Keratophakia and keratomileusis: clinical results. *Ophthalmology.* 1981;88:709–715.

13. Swinger CA, Barker BA. Prospective evaluation of myopic keratomileusis. *Ophthalmology.* 1984;91:785–792.

14. Dossi F, Bosio P. Myopic keratomileusis: results with a follow-up over one year. *J Cataract Refract Surg.* 1987;13:417–420.

15. Maxwell WA. Myopic keratomileusis: initial results and myopic keratomilusis combined with other procedures. *J Cataract Refract Surg.* 1987;13:518–524.

16. Nordan LT, Fallor MK. Myopic keratomileusis: 74 consecutive non-amblyopic cases with one year of follow-up. *J Refract Surg.* 1986;2:124–128.

17. Saragoussi J, Hanna K, Jobin D, et al. Resultats du keratomileusis myopique [In French]. *J Fr Ophtalmol.* 1988;11: 311–316.

18. Krumeich JH, Swinger CA, Boyd B. The planar non-freeze lamellar refractive keratoplasty techniques. Non-freeze keratomileusis, non-freeze epikeratophakia. In: Boyd B, ed. *Refractive Surgery with the Masters.* Coral Gables, FL: Highlights of Ophthalmology; 1987;122–136.

19. Swinger CA, Krumeich JH, Cassiday D. A new device for viable refractive keratoplasty. *Invest Ophthalmol Vis Sci.* 1985;26(suppl):151.

20. Laroche L, Martinsky M, Scarano M, et al. Non-freeze myopic keratomileusis: visual and corneal evolution. *Eur J Implant Ref Surg.* 1989;1:178–180.

21. Couderc JLR, Lozano Mouri F. Freeze or non-freeze myopic keratomileusis: which is the best? *Eur J Implant Ref Surg.* 1989;1:175–177.

22. Durand L, Burillon C, Mutti P. Correction de la myopie forte par la kératoplastie lamellaire réfractive sans congélation [In French]. *J Fr Ophtalmol.* 1991;14:167–175.

23. Bosc JM, Montard M, Delbosc B, et al. Kératomileusis myopique non gel. Etude rétrospective de 27 interventions consécutives [In French]. *J Fr Ophtalmol.* 1990;13:10–16.

24. Colin J, Minoumi F, Robinet A, et al. The surgical treatment of high myopia: comparison of epikeratoplasty, keratomileusis and minus power anterior chamber lenses. *Refract Corneal Surg.* 1990;6:245–251.

25. Buratto L, Genisi C, Ferrari M. Cheratomileusi miopica. In: Rama G, Buratto L, Dal Fiume E, Merlin U. *Chirurgia della Cornea* [In Italian]. Milano: Fogliazza; 1993:607–608.

26. Ruiz LA, Rowsey JJ. In situ keratomileusis. *Invest Ophthalmol Vis Sci.* 1988;29(suppl):392.

27. Bas MA, Nano HD, Jr. In situ myopic keratomileusis results in 30 eyes at 15 months. *Refract Corneal Surg.* 1991;7: 223–231.

28. Arenas-Archila E, Sanchez-Thorin JC, Naranjo-Uribe JP, Hernandez-Lozano A. Myopic keratomileusis in situ: a preliminary report. *J Cataract Refract Surg.* 1991;17:424–435.

29. Buratto L, Ferrari M. Cheratomileusi in situ. Tecnica di Ruiz. In: Buratto L, Ferrari M. *Chirurgia della Miopia Assile Mediante Cheratomileusi* [In Italian]. Milano: CAMO; 1993: 53–70.

30. Toboada J, Archibald CJ. An extreme sensitivity in the corneal epithelium to far UV ArF excimer laser pulses. In: Proceedings of the 52nd Annual Meeting of Aerospace Medical Association; Washington, DC, 1981:98–99.

31. Trokel SL, Srinivasan R, Braren B. Excimer laser surgery of the cornea. *Am J Ophthalmol.* 1983;96:710–715.

32. Seiler T, Marshall J, Rothery S, Wollensak J. The potential of an infrared hydrogen fluoride gas (HF) laser for corneal surgery. *Lasers Ophthalmol.* 1986;1:49–60.

33. Marshall J, Trokel SL, Rothery S, Krueger RR. Photoablative reprofiling of the cornea using an excimer laser:

photorefractive keratectomy. *Lasers Ophthalmol.* 1986; 7:21–48.

34. Trokel SL. Evolution of excimer laser surgery. *J Cataract Refract Surg.* 1989;15:373–382.

35. Munnerlyn CR, Koons SJ, Marshall T. Photorefractive keratectomy: a technique for laser refractive surgery. *J Cataract Refract Surg.* 1988;14:46–52.

36. L'Esperance FA, Taylor DM, Warner JW. Human excimer laser keratectomy: short term histopathology. *J Refract Surg.* 1988;4:118–124.

37. Seiler T, Holschbach A, Derse M, et al. Complications of myopic photorefractive keratectomy with the excimer laser. *Ophthalmology.* 1994;101:153–160.

38. Buratto L, Ferrari M. Excimer laser intrastromal keratomileusis: case reports. *J Cataract Refract Surg.* 1992;18:37–41.

39. Buratto L, Ferrari M, Rama P. Excimer laser intrastromal keratomileusis. *Am J Ophthalmol.* 1992;113:291–295.

40. Pallikaris IG, Papatzanaki ME, Stathi EZ, et al. Laser in situ keratomileusis. *Lasers Surg Med.* 1990;10:463–468.

41. Pallikaris IG, Papatzanaki ME, Siganos DS, et al. A corneal flap technique for laser in situ keratomileusis. Human study. *Arch Ophthalmol.* 1991;145:1699–1702.

42. Buratto L, Ferrari M. Cheratomileuisi con laser ad eccimeri. Tecnica di Buratto [In Italian]. In: *Chirurgia della Miopia Assile.* Milano: CAMO ed; 1993.

43. Chamon W, Rama P, Tyson FC, et al. Excimer laser intrastromal keratomileusis using a rotating blade microkeratome. *Invest Ophthalmol Vis Sci.* 1993;34(suppl):894.

44. Buratto L, Ferrari M, Genisi C. Keratomileusis for myopia with the excimer laser (Buratto technique): short-term results. *Refract Corneal Surg.* 1993;9(suppl):130–133.

45. Buratto L, Ferrari M, Genisi C. Myopic keratomileusis with the excimer laser: one-year follow up. *Refract Corneal Surg.* 1993;9:12–19.

46. Uozato H, Guyton DL. Centering corneal surgical procedure. *Am J Ophthalmol.* 1987;103:264–275.

47. Walsh PM, Guyton DL. Comparison of two methods of marking the visual axis on the cornea during radial keratotomy. *Am J Ophthalmol.* 1984;97:660–661.

48. Maloney RK. Corneal topography and optical zone location in photorefractive keratectomy. *Refract Corneal Surg.* 1990;6:363–371.

49. Mendez A, Valdez J, Trevino E, et al. Keratomileusis in situ, morphometric corneal endothelial cell changes. *Invest Ophthalmol Vis Sci.* 1992;33(suppl):1000.

50. Ruiz LA. Cheratomileusi automatizzata in situ. In: Buratto L, Ferrari M. *Chirurgia della Miopia Assile Mediante Cheratomileusi* [In Italian]. Milano: CAMO ed; 1993:137–142.

51. Draeger J. Cheratomo rotante secondo Draeger. In: Buratto L, Ferrari M. *Chirurgia della Miopia Assile Mediante Cheratomileusi* [In Italian]. Milano: CAMO ed; 1993:143–148.

52. Draeger J, Böhnke M, Klein L, Kohlhaas M. Experimentelle untersuchungen zur prazision lamellarer hornhautschnitte [In German]. *Fortschr Ophthalmol.* 1989;86:272–275.

53. Draeger J, Böhnke M, Grabner G, et al. Neue wege der refraktiven hornhautchirurgie. Experimentelle untersuchungen [In German]. *Klin Monatsbl Augenheilkd.* 1988;192:458–461.

54. Draeger J, Grabner G, Böhnke M, et al. Uberlegungen für eine optimierte lamellare schneidetechnik [In German]. *Fortschr Ophthalmol.* 1988;85:251–254.

55. Hofmann RF, Bechara SJ. An independent evaluation of second generation suction microkeratomes. *Refract Corneal Surg.* 1992;8:348–354.

56. Genisi C. Esame comparativo delle strumentazioni per cheratomileusis. In: Buratto L, Ferrari M. *Chirurgia della Miopia Assile Mediante Cheratomileusi* [In Italian]. Milano: CAMO ed; 1993:149–153.

57. Guimarães RQ, Rowsey JJ, Reis-Guimarães MF, et al. Suturing in lamellar surgery: the BRA-technique. *Refract Corneal Surg.* 1992;8:84–87.

CHAPTER 35

Intrastromal Lasers for Myopia and Hyperopia

Mark G. Speaker ▪ Maged S. Habib

Intrastromal lasers are a new technology in refractive surgery that are designed to remove corneal stromal tissue, effecting refractive changes without altering the integrity of the epithelium and Bowman's layer. Disruption of the epithelium and Bowman's layer by surface ablation procedures (eg, excimer laser) activates corneal wound-healing responses, which can lead to stromal scarring and regression of the refractive effect.[1,2] Intrastromal surgery is attractive because of its potential for minimizing wound-healing responses, thereby possibly reducing regression and increasing predictability. With an intact surface, or in combination with keratomileusis, intrastromal laser surgery should also reduce the risk of infection postoperatively. Another appealing feature of intrastromal keratectomy with an infrared laser is that it is a painless procedure that can be performed under topical anesthesia. The feasibility of effecting myopic corrections up to 25 diopters through removal of stromal tissue has been demonstrated with keratomileusis techniques, LASIK and automated lamellar keratoplasty (ALK). The use of an intrastromal laser in combination with keratomileusis is a particularly exciting approach to this method of correcting myopia because it avoids the hazards and unpredictability of the "second pass" of keratomileusis surgery.

Intrastromal photorefractive keratectomy (IPRK) with the neodymium:YLF picosecond laser (Intelligent Surgical Lasers, San Diego, CA) and laser thermal keratoplasty (LTK) with the holmium:YAG laser (Sunrise Technologies, Fermont, CA) are the principal intrastromal procedures with the most up-to-date available information. This chapter will review the current status of intrastromal surgery using the picosecond laser, and LTK will be discussed in Chapter 37.

THE PICOSECOND LASER

The picosecond laser is a pulsed, infrared laser. The infrared laser beam is invisible, penetrating tissues without being significantly absorbed. The laser effect is produced only at the focal point. In corneal applications, this permits the laser energy to pass through the epithelium and Bowman's layer without damaging them; photodisruption of the stromal tissue occurs at the focal point. Photodisruption converts stromal tissue to gas, which either diffuses through the surface, is reabsorbed, or both. Subsequently, the stromal cavities that have been created collapse and the cornea is thinned. The resulting tissue removal results in the desired refractive change.

Intrastromal photorefractive keratectomy was first described by Troutman in 1986, using the ALS (Automated Laser Systems, Inc) computer-aided laser microsurgery unit (CALM™), which operated at a wavelength of 595 nm.[3] During the early phase of work with intrastromal lasers, Dr Troutman and colleagues used postmortem cadaver eyes in which the cornea and the extraocular muscle tendon sheath were exposed to laser treatments. In all their specimens a pulse duration of 10 picoseconds was delivered at a cone angle of 30° to 40°. This was focused into a spot size of 2 μm, creating a power density of 10^{15} W/cm^2. They reported that the two eye-bank corneal specimens treated with the laser demonstrated that Bowman's layer, the superficial stroma, the stroma deep to the treated area, Descemet's membrane, and the corneal endothelium all appeared to be unaffected at the light microscopic level by treatment. On electron microscopic examination of these corneas, the collagen strands appeared to be broken at the site of the laser treatment, and moderate amounts of electron-dense fragments were present in the field. The extraocular muscle tendon treated with laser energy revealed an intratendinous cavity where a 6-0 silk suture had been present for marking purposes, and considerable thinning of the epitendinous connective tissue sheath was evident.

The work by Troutman and colleagues on eye-bank cadaver corneas demonstrated the feasibility of intrastromal laser surgery by showing that intrastromal lasers can produce well-localized lesions within the corneal stroma that spare surrounding stroma as well as Bowman's and Descemet's membranes.

Research with intrastromal lasers was continued by Hoh and colleagues, who described their work with a Q-switched Nd:YAG laser focused in the posterior third of rabbit corneas.[4] They reported that the procedure was painless and did not require local or general anesthesia. They described the development of air cavities in the cornea "frostwork," the size of which were proportional to the amount of energy per pulse. This approach close to the epithelium produced corneal edema after the laser treatment, which lasted for a few days and then resolved. This presumably was the result of injury to the endothelial cells from shock waves. Hoh's work with rabbit corneas produced refractive effects: initially, a hyperopic shift of up to 2.5 D, followed by myopic change after 4 months with a corresponding flattening of the cornea. He concluded that increasing the energy per pulse does not increase the refractive effect, but on the other hand increases endothelial cell

damage with subsequent corneal edema and decompensation.

The introduction of an ultrashort (40 picosecond), pulsed, solid-state Nd:YLF (neodymium:yttrium lithium fluoride) picosecond laser (Intelligent Surgical Lasers, San Diego, Fig 35–1) operating in the infrared range at 1053 nm has allowed the development of a system for intrastromal corneal laser refractive surgery. The picosecond laser is quite different from a 193-nm excimer laser whose photons are strongly absorbed by tissues and have enough energy (6.4 eV) to break molecular bonds on the surface of the tissue to be ablated. The energy of the photons generated by the Nd:YLF picosecond laser (1.2 eV) is insufficient to break molecular bonds, and at 1053 nm the absorption coefficient is low.[5–17] In contrast to surface ablation with UV excimer lasers, where ablation results from direct absorption of photons, leading to breakage of molecular bonds, tissue removal by the picosecond laser is accomplished by plasma-mediated photodisruption at the focal point of the laser, analogous to the commercially available nanosecond-pulsed Nd:YAG lasers used for capsulotomy.[7,8] We have adopted the term *intrastromal photorefractive keratectomy* (intrastromal PRK, or IPRK) to describe this procedure as a replacement for *intrastromal ablation* because ablation refers to a process in which direct absorption of photons leads to tissue removal.[18,19]

The low absorption coefficient of the picosecond laser at 1053 nm allows the laser to be focused, with photodisruption and tissue removal occurring at any depth within transparent media such as corneal tissue. This means that the laser radiation travels through transparent media without causing any tissue effects until it reaches its focal point, where tissue removal occurs. The picosecond Nd:YLF laser is preferred over a nanosecond-pulsed Nd:YAG laser for intrastromal PRK because the ultrashort pulse width allows optical breakdown and tissue removal to occur at low threshold energies of 6 to 21 μJ in corneal tissue, compared to 100 μJ or greater with nanosecond lasers. The diameter of the damage zone (d) and the cavitation bubble produced by a laser pulse are proportional to the cube root of the energy (E): $d = E^{1/3}$. The tissue effects at the low pulse energies required for optical breakdown with picosecond pulses are confined to approximately 10 μm, thereby minimizing thermal effects and collateral damage to sensitive structures like epithelium and endothelium. Nanosecond lasers produce effects over a zone of 1 mm in diameter. Histologic and ultrastructural studies in rabbit and cat eyes have not demon-

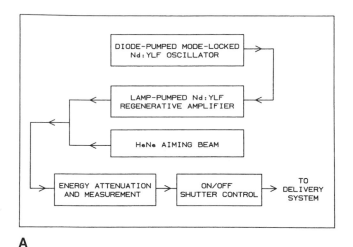

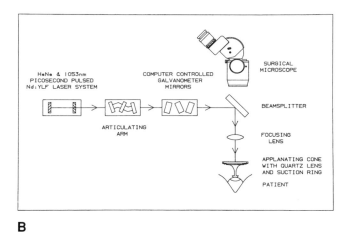

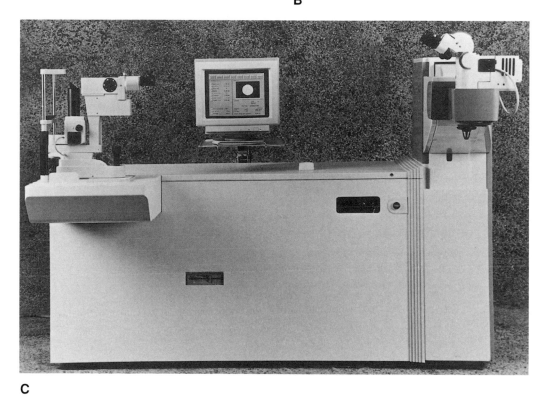

Figure 35–1. A. Schematic of Nd:YLF oscillator and regenerative amplifier laser generating 40-picosecond pulses of wavelength 1053 nm at 1000 Hz. **B.** Schematic of operating microscope with applanating lens delivery system. **C.** Appearance of Intelligent Surgical Lasers, Model 4000, Nd:YLF picosecond laser.

strated any thermal effects in corneal tissue, and our studies in rabbit and cat corneas have not uncovered any evidence of endothelial damage when the laser is focused within the anterior one third of the cornea at threshold energies. Our studies in rabbits have demonstrated damage at threshold energies when the laser is focused within the posterior one third, confirming the work of Hoh.[4]

In our investigational studies, a diode-pumped, mode-locked, regeneratively amplified Nd:YLF laser

(Intelligent Surgical Lasers, Model 4000, "The Eye Laser," San Diego, CA) was used to perform myopic IPRK in cat corneas (Fig 35–1). The laser generates pulses at 1053 nm with a duration of 40 picoseconds and a repetition rate of 1 to 2 kHz, permitting plasma generation in the range of 10 to 350 μJ with a 10-μm spot size. Because the size of the laser effect from each pulse is measured in micrometers, thousands of pulses are required to remove sufficient tissue to produce a refractive effect in the cornea. Therefore, in order to take advantage of the obvious benefits on intrastromal-laser PRK, the challenge of developing a delivery system that meets these requirements had to be met. The delivery system currently consists of a modified Möller operating microscope capable of scanning the laser beam in the X, Y, and Z axes. A computer calculates three-dimensional treatment patterns according to user-defined specifications and controls a series of galvanometers in the delivery system that scan the beam during treatment (Fig 35–2A). Because the laser produces an effect of only 10 μm in size, the effect is precise and well localized, but it also means that the laser must scan over a large area. This requires the cornea to be immobilized or an effective tracking system to be available. Attempts to develop an effective tracking system held up development of this laser system for some time, and an alternative approach was developed. In the current configuration the cornea is stabilized during treatment by a cone containing a quartz applanating lens and a limbal suction ring that couples the cornea to the delivery system. With the cornea immobilized in the X, Y, and Z directions, precise and reproducible scanning can be achieved. Prior to research on refractive effects in animals, considerable investigation using human corneas was required to determine the best treatment parameters for corneal tissue removal. The investigation focused on the distance between pulses, the distance between layers, and the energy per pulse (Fig 35–2B).

Tissue removal results from the effect of the laser plasma on tissue in the focus of the beam. Intrastromal PRK is achieved by placing a series of laser pulses into adjacent tissue volumes. It follows that the most efficient tissue removal can be achieved by packing the plasma balls adjacent to one other. However, secondary effects, namely cavitation bubbles, may decrease the surgical effect of the laser. For example, if the cavitation bubble generated by the first laser pulse is larger than the actual plasma size, it may interact with the surgical effect of the next pulse. Moreover, if the pulse hits an existing cavitation, it does not remove tissue but increases the size of the cavitation through heat transfer to the gas. In order to avoid reheating the gas inside the cavitation, the next pulse must hit the tissue outside the bubble. Therefore in the optimum case, the cavitation diameter should approach the diameter of the plasma ball. Because the size of the cavitation bubble in the cornea decreases with decreasing pulse energies, IPRK should be performed with threshold pulse energies and optimal spot separations. Therefore threshold pulse energies (20 to 25 μJ in the human cornea), spot separations of 15 μm, and layer separations of 10 to 20 μm were chosen in this investigation based on studies using scanning electron microscopy (SEM) (T Juhasz and M Speaker: unpublished data).

Our early studies involved a cat model, which was selected for its similarities to the human cornea in

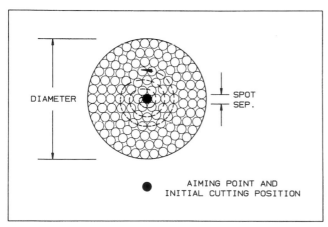

A

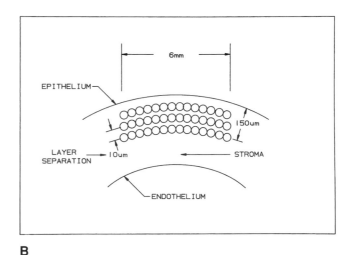

B

Figure 35–2. A. Schematic of spiral pattern configuration. Treatment begins with the deepest layer at the center of the cornea by computer-controlled galvanometers that place pulses at a preset depth and add spot separations in a spiral pattern toward the periphery, forming a preset curvature in the plane of the spiral. **B.** Schematic of laser treatment used to create spiral patterns for myopic IPRK. Parameters are as follows: layer diameter and configuration, 6-mm spiral; Z radius (curvature within the plane of each layer), 9 mm; spot separation, 15 μm; layer separation, 10 μm; energy per pulse, 25 mJ; repetition rate, 1000 Hz; number of pulses/layer, 126,340; Z-offset (initial depth), 150 μm; number of layers, 3.

thickness, curvature, and anatomic structure (the presence of a thin Bowman's layer). Intrastromal PRK was performed by layering three 6-mm spiral patterns concentrically in the central anterior cornea (Figs 35–2, 35–3). The patterns were placed in the central cornea starting with the deepest layer at 150 μm, with each subsequent layer displaced anterior to the previous one by 10 μm. Each layer was formed by computer-controlled scanning of pulses from the center of the layer toward the periphery in a spiral pattern. Each layer of a 6-mm diameter spiral pattern consists of 126,340 pulses requiring 126 seconds to be completed at 1 kHz and 63 seconds at 2 kHz. No postop medications were instilled, with the exception of Tobrex TID in both eyes for 1 week following treatment.

Postop follow-up of the cats consisted of corneal topography, ultrasonic pachymetry, and slit lamp biomicroscopy. Immediate steepening and thickening

of the central cornea were noted during the first 2 weeks postoperatively, after which gradual, progressive flattening and thinning of the central cornea were achieved (Fig 35–4). The corneas thinned by an average of 50 μm and flattened by an average of 11 D at 2 months following IPRK. Slit lamp biomicroscopy revealed moderate corneal thickening in the first few days postoperatively, which gradually resolved to reveal thinning by 3 to 4 weeks (Fig 35–3B). At the 6-month examination of the corneas, corneal topography was stable with no change from the 2-month values; slit lamp biomicroscopy was clear, with a patchy, barely detectable subepithelial haze noted (Fig 35–3C). No corneas demonstrated significant haze or scarring despite omission of treatment with an anti-inflammatory agent over the 6-month study period. Mean ultrasonic pachymetric measurements had returned to preop values by 5 months postoperatively

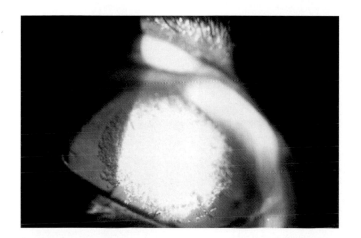

A

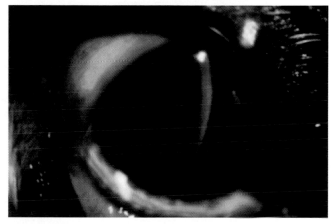

B

C

Figure 35–3. Biomicroscopic appearance of cat cornea after a three-layer myopic IPRK. **A.** Appearance 15 minutes postoperatively. The cavitation bubbles prevent visualization of the pupil, and the peripheral bubbles are already being absorbed. **B.** Appearance of cornea 24 hours following treatment shows anterior stromal haze and thickening. **C.** Appearance of cornea 6 months postoperatively without treatment with steroidal or nonsteroidal anti-inflammatory agents (NSAIDs). The broad-beam photograph was taken with maximal tangential slit illumination and shows barely detectable anterior stromal haze.

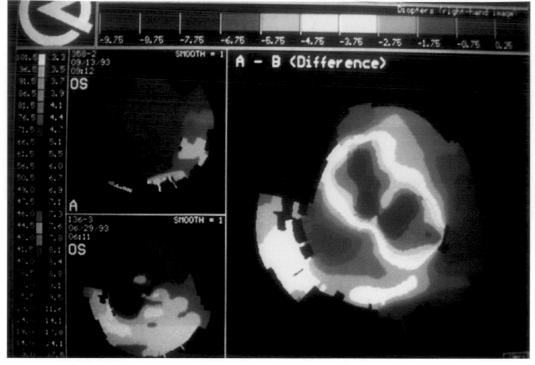

A

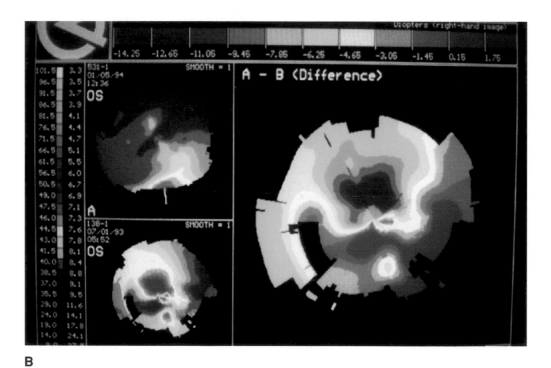

B

Figure 35–4. Topographic changes in cat corneas following three-layer myopic IPRK. Difference maps showing topographic change between preop and postop examinations at 10 weeks **(A)** and at 6 months **(B).** The color-coded dioptric power scale on the left refers to the preop *(below, left)* and postop *(above, left)* examinations, and the scale on top refers to the difference map on the right.

despite the absence of significant haze. The refractive change was stable, and slit lamp examination of the cornea did not reveal edema; the corneas appeared compact and clear.

On histologic studies, the treated corneas showed normal-appearing epithelial cells and normal epithelial thickness in all specimens (Figs 35–5, 35–6). Basement membranes were also of normal thickness without evidence of fragmentation or reactive thickening. Bowman's layer was intact in all specimens (Fig 35–6). Multiple cavitation bubbles of different sizes were present in the anterior one third of the treated zone of the corneal stroma in the acute specimens. Some bubbles coalesced to form larger spaces, while others remained small and discrete (Fig 35–7A). The presence of the gas bubbles in the anterior stroma pushed the overlying stroma, Bowman's layer, and epithelium forward (Fig 35–5). The cavities were hollow and interrupted collagen fibers were not seen within.

Stromal collagen fibers were minimally disrupted in a narrow band at the site of the laser treatment in the 1-month specimens. Mildly increased cellularity was also noted at 1 month in the immediately adjacent, intact anterior stromal lamellae. These were interpreted as reactive keratocytes (Fig 35–6A). Rare cells morphologically consistent with lymphocytes were noted. The increased cellularity was less apparent at 2 months and was absent at 6 months (Fig 35–6B).

At 6 months, the laser treatment site was not apparent histologically, except in one cornea, which was treated with five layers of IPRK. This cornea displayed a barely discernible region of scarring measuring approximately 30 μm in thickness and extending less than 1 mm laterally from the center of the application site. This cat was treated with threefold higher energy than the remaining cats at 75 μJ/pulse, and the laser patterns were applied in the midstroma rather than the anterior corneal stroma (Fig 35–6C). There was no evidence of thermal effects on the corneal stroma adjacent to the treatment site. Endothelial cells displayed normal morphology, and the monolayer was intact at all time points.

Thinning of the treated zones of the cornea was apparent in most of the cases by light microscopy, especially in the 1- and 2-month specimens.

Histology did not reveal apparent new collagen synthesis that would explain the observed thickening of the corneas at 5 to 6 months. This phenomenon cannot be explained by the experimental observations.

On SEM imaging, the acute specimens revealed multiple cavities seen in the treatment zone with del-

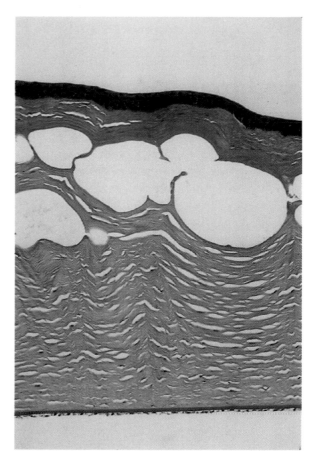

Figure 35–5. Light microscopy of an H&E stained section of a cat cornea immediately after IPRK performed at threshold energy (25 μJ/pulse). Notice the presence of multiple cavitations pushing the anterior stroma, Bowman's layer, and the epithelium forward.

icate partitions of the stroma bridging the lamellar defects. The treated zones in most specimens examined at 1 through 3 months following treatment demonstrated discernible thinning of stroma at the cut surface. The corneal stroma lamellae appeared slightly compressed at the site of laser treatment in the early specimens (1 and 2 months). Six-month specimens showed no discernible ultrastructural change. There was no evidence of thermal effects in adjacent stromal lamellae (Fig 35–7B). The corneal endothelium was intact and normocellular compared with controls (Fig 35–7C).

Further studies of wound healing after IPRK are in progress, and clinical trials of IPRK in human corneas are underway in Europe. Food and Drug Administration approval for phase I clinical trials has been obtained in the United States. This treatment has seemingly the greatest potential in creating a refractive ablation under a keratomileusis flap.

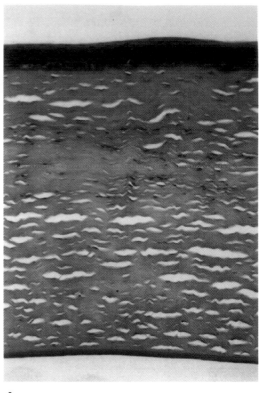

A

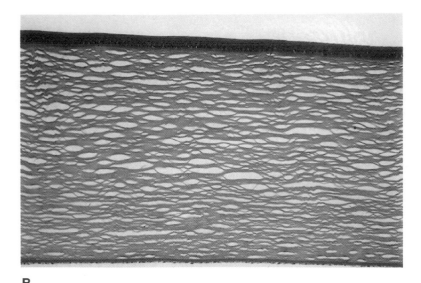

B

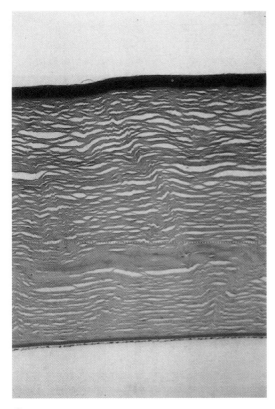

C

Figure 35–6. A. Light microscopy of an H&E stained section of a cat cornea at 1 month after IPRK with the picosecond laser. Notice the presence of compressed stroma in the area of the treatment with surrounding hypercellularity. **B.** Light microscopy of a cat cornea at 6 months after IPRK at threshold energy. The cut section of the corneas shows no hypercellularity, and the collagen lamellae are unremarkable. **C.** Light microscopy of a cat cornea at 6 months following IPRK that was treated at energies threefold above threshold (75 μJ/pulse), a five-layer pattern, and deeper placement of the laser treatment into the midstroma.

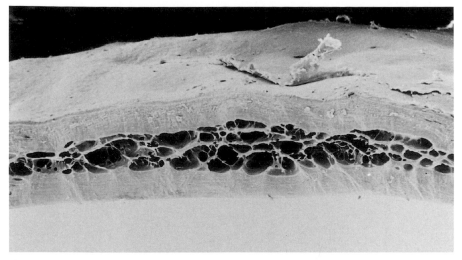

A

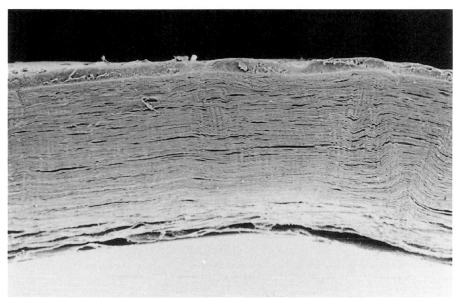

B

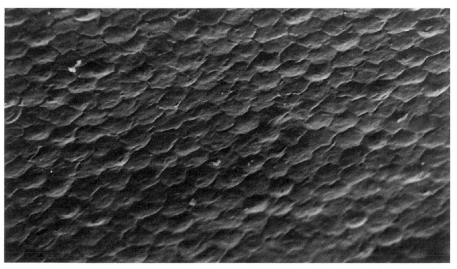

C

Figure 35–7. A. SEM of a cat cornea taken immediately after IPRK demonstrating the cavitation bubbles in the anterior stroma with gross thickening of the cornea. **B.** SEM of a cat cornea 6 months posttreatment at threshold energy. The corneal stroma is unremarkable. **C.** SEM of the endothelial cell layer of a cat cornea at 6 months after IPRK at threshold energy. The monolayer and the individual cells are normal in appearance.

REFERENCES

1. Hanna KD, Pouliquen YM, Savoldelli M, et al. Corneal wound healing in monkeys 18 months after excimer laser photorefractive keratectomy. *Refract Corneal Surg.* 1990;6: 340–345.

2. Fantes F, Hanna KD, Waring GO, Pouliquen YM, Thompson KP, Savodelli M. Wound healing after excimer laser keratomileusis (photorefractive keratectomy) in monkeys. *Arch Ophthalmol.* 1990;108:665–675.

3. Troutman RC, Veronneau-Troutman S, Jacobiec FA, Krebs W. A new laser for collagen wounding in corneal and strabismus surgery: a preliminary report. *Trans Am Ophthalmol Soc.* 1986;84:117–132.

4. Hoh H, Becker, KW. Intrastromal keratorhexis with the Nd:YAG laser—a possible method of refractive surgery? [In German.] *Klin Monatsbl Augenheilkd.* 1990;197:480–487.

5. Niemz MH, Hoppeler TP, Juhasz T, Bille JF. Intrastromal ablations for refractive corneal surgery using picosecond infrared laser pulses. *Lasers Light Ophthalmol.* 1993;5: 145–152.

6. Vogel A, Schweiger P, Freiser A, Asyo MN, Bimgruber R. Intraocular Nd:YAG laser surgery: light tissue interactions, damage range, and reduction of collateral effects. *IEEE J Quant Electron.* 1990;26:2240–2260.

7. Aron-Rosa D, Aron J, Griesemann J, Thyzel R. Use of the neodynium-YAG laser to open the posterior capsule after lens implant surgery: a preliminary report. *Am Intraoc Implant Soc J.* 1990;6:352–354.

8. Niemz MN, Klancnick EG, Bille JF. Plasma-mediated ablation of corneal tissue at 1053 nm using a ND:YLF oscillator/regenerative amplifier laser. *Lasers Surg Med.* 1991; 11:426–431.

9. Docchio F, Sacchi CA. Shielding properties of laser-produced plasmas in ocular media irradiated by single Nd:YAG pulses of different duration. *Invest Ophthalmol Vis Sci.* 1988;29:437–443.

10. Fujimoto JG, Lin WZ, Ippen EP, Puliafito CA, Steinert RF. Time resolved studies of ND:YAG laser-induced breakdown. *Invest Ophthalmol Vis Sci.* 1985;26:1771–1777.

11. Capon MRC, Mellerio J. ND:YAG lasers: plasma characteristics and damage mechanisms. *Lasers Ophthalmol.* 1986;1:95–106.

12. Zysset B, Fujimoto G, Deutsch TF. Time resolved measurements of picosecond optical breakdown. *Appl Phys B.* 1989;48:139–147.

13. Zysset B, Fujimoto JG, Puliafito CA, Birngruber R, Deutsch TF. Picosecond optical breakdown: tissue effects and reduction of collateral damage. *Lasers Surg Med.* 1989; 9:193–204.

14. Vogel A, Hentschel W, Holzfuss J, Lauterborn W. Cavitation bubble dynamics and acoustic transient generation in ocular surgery with pulsed neodymium:YAG lasers. *Ophthalmology.* 1986;93:1259–1269.

15. Mellerio J, Capon M, Docchio F. ND:YAG lasers: a potential hazard from cavitation bubble behaviour in anterior chamber procedures? *Lasers Ophthalmol.* 1987;1:190–195.

16. Doukas AG, Zweig AD, Frisoli JK, Birngruber R, Deutsch T. Non-invasive determination of shock wave pressure generated by optical breakdown. *Appl Phys B.* 1991;53: 237–245.

17. Juhasz T, Hu XH, Turi L, Bor Z. Dynamics of shock waves and cavitations generated by picosecond laser pulse in corneal tissue and water. *Lasers Surg Med.* In press.

18. Habib MS, Speaker MG, Juhasz T, Kaiser R. Acute effects of myopic intrastromal ablation of the cat cornea with the ND:YLF picosecond laser. *Invest Ophthalmol Vis Sci.* 1994; 35:2026.

19. Speaker MG, Habib MS, McCormick SA. Histopathology and corneal wound healing of the cat cornea following intrastromal ablation with the ND:YLF picosecond laser. *Invest Ophthalmol Vis Sci.* 1994;35:2026.

CHAPTER 36

193-nm Excimer Laser Treatment
of Hyperopia

David R. Hardten

INTRODUCTION

Ultraviolet radiation at a 193-nm wavelength can remove precise amounts of tissue from the anterior cornea. Early results using the excimer laser have been promising in both animal and human corneas.[1–5] The efficacy of excimer laser photorefractive keratectomy in the treatment of low, moderate, and high myopia has now been well established.[6–10] The excimer laser can also be used to remove superficial anterior corneal scars.[11–14] Hyperopic and astigmatic corrections are also possible using this technology.[15–17]

INDICATIONS

Over 20 million Americans are currently dependent on glasses or contact lenses and therefore may be potential candidates for refractive surgical procedures, with even more potential candidates worldwide.[18] Patients with anterior corneal scars whose vision is not improved by glasses or contact lenses usually require penetrating keratoplasty to achieve improved vision. Advances in technology that improve the safety and predictability

of refractive surgical procedures consequently may benefit a large number of patients.

Excimer laser photorefractive keratectomy (PRK) appears to be most reproducible for the patient within the range of −1.5 to −8.0 diopters of myopia.[6–10] Although higher degrees of myopia can also be corrected, they can be associated with higher degrees of regression or corneal haze.[8,9] Hyperopic corrections have been more elusive, but there are now some reports of success in low and moderate degrees of hyperopia.[15,16] Low and moderate degrees of astigmatism may also be corrected with the excimer laser.[15,17]

Alternatives to the use of PRK for surgical correction of hyperopia include hexagonal keratotomy, epikeratoplasty, automated lamellar keratoplasty (ALK), phakic intraocular lenses (IOLs), lens extraction with IOL implant, or holmium laser treatment.[19–30]

Several alternatives exist for the treatment of anterior corneal scars. Spectacles or contact lenses can be used to correct the refractive errors or irregular astigmatism induced by these scars. Mechanical superficial keratectomy can sometimes be used to remove corneal scars such as Salzmann's nodular dystrophy. Lamellar or penetrating keratoplasty may be useful to remove deeper scars close to the visual axis. The excimer laser

481

can be used to remove anterior corneal opacities with improved visual acuities.[11–14] This is often accompanied by a hyperopic shift in the refractive error because of corneal thinning centrally. This hyperopic shift can be reduced by removing additional tissue in the midperipheral cornea (see Chapter 38).

PREOP CONSIDERATIONS

Appropriate consideration of the risks and benefits for each individual patient should be entertained, as with all refractive surgical procedures. The vision should be assessed with a careful manifest and cycloplegic refraction, ocular dominance testing, and distance and near vision with and without correction. Anterior segment and posterior segment examinations should be carried out to screen for other conditions. Computerized topographic analysis of the corneal surface should be performed to rule out subclinical keratoconus or other corneal diseases. Appropriate reading materials should be provided to educate the patient, and the surgeon should discuss the risks and benefits of the various alternatives with the patient.

Complete anterior and posterior segment examinations are also necessary of all patients for whom excimer phototherapeutic keratectomy (PTK) with correction of hyperopia is considered. Topographic analysis using computerized topographic systems should be undertaken to better understand the abnormal anterior corneal surface. Pachymetry is helpful to ascertain that the cornea is sufficiently thick to remove the central portion of the anterior stromal scars, still preserving enough tissue to maintain the posterior corneal curvature without excessive thinning in the periphery. Analysis of the depth of the scar is important, and optical pachymetry, high-resolution anterior segment ultrasonography, or confocal microscopy can be used to determine scar depth.[31–35] Careful analysis of the refractive error with manifest and cycloplegic refractions should be carried out. The surgeon should conduct a detailed risk and benefit analysis with the patient and discuss alternative methods of treatment.

SURGICAL TECHNIQUE

Instrumentation

There are several 193-nm excimer lasers now commercially available across the world that have been used for PRK and PTK.[9,15,36,37] Some of these lasers use a large-beam diameter that ranges from 5 to 7 mm, whereas others use a scanning technique to deliver a small beam in a controlled manner across the surface of the cornea. All systems include a computer control module with an interactive menu, providing a method to develop an ablation protocol for each individual patient. Proper positioning of the eye is important, and therefore the excimer laser system should include a microscope with the ability to provide alignment in all axes. Some lasers provide a vacuum apparatus to remove particle debris from the ablation plume. Foot-pedal and fingertip controls can be used to allow the surgeon to manipulate the ablating beam. The 193-nm wavelength is totally absorbed by the cornea, breaking the molecular bonds within the cornea, which makes this wavelength uniquely applicable for corneal treatment.

Correction of Hyperopia

For PRK the patient's spectacle correction is adjusted to the corneal plane to take into account vertex distance. If astigmatism is to be treated, the astigmatism is converted into minus cylinder form. Some laser machines will treat the astigmatism first, whereas others will treat astigmatism following the spherical correction.

Preoperatively the patient should receive antibiotic, steroid, nonsteroidal, and anesthetic drops. We currently use a combination of tobramycin and dexamethasone (Tobradex, Alcon, Fort Worth, TX), diclofenac sodium (Voltaren, Ciba Vision Ophthalmics, Duluth, GA), and proparacaine. Bupivacaine can also be used as a topical anesthetic and may last longer, giving the patient some protection from the early postop pain.

The patient is positioned under the microscope, and the head position is carefully assessed to make sure that the iris plane is perpendicular to the laser beam. The eyelids are prepped with dilute betadine solution. A lid speculum is inserted to open the eyelids. Careful centration with the eye aligned in the X, Y, and Z planes is crucial. Centration on the pupil is preferred.[38,39]

The epithelium is then marked with a 7-mm optical-zone marker, again centering on the pupil. The epithelium is removed with a Tooke knife or No. 69 Bard–Parker blade. It is important to remove the epithelium totally, so that only Bowman's membrane remains. Residual epithelium will create uneven ablation.[40]

It is also possible to remove the epithelium with the excimer laser. To do this the excimer laser should be set to a depth of approximately 50 μm (200 pulses), and the beam is set to its widest aperture. The excimer laser is centered and the ablation is begun. The microscope light is dimmed so that the area of fluorescence where the epithelium is being struck by the laser beam can be seen. The ablation should be stopped when a change from a fluorescent pattern to a dark pattern is seen, indicating that the epithelium has been ablated. The epithelium may be more or less than 50 μm deep. If there is still fluorescence across the whole area after a 50-μm ablation has been performed, then an additional depth of 25 μm should be set for the laser, and the treatment is stopped when all of the epithelium has been removed.

Centration is again checked after epithelial removal. Epithelial removal should be promptly followed by the ablation to prevent drying, which can lead to increased haze and scarring.[41,42] Despite the exact epithelial removal technique, it is important to make certain that the hydration status of the corneal stroma is uniform through the duration of the procedure.[43] This can be assured by carefully applying a drop of artificial tears on the stroma. This can be dried with a Weck cell or a blade used to "squeegee" the surface to remove excess fluid.

For astigmatic corrections there must be alignment on the proper axis. This can be done by marking the patient's limbus at the 12 and 6 o'clock positions with gentian violet dye on a Sinsky hook at the slit lamp prior to the procedure. If the procedure is performed on the wrong axis, there will be a significant reduction of effect.

The ablation is then begun, centered over the pupil with the patient looking at the fixation light. Forceps fixation should be avoided to prevent globe distortion. If the patient loses fixation, it is important to stop and recenter before completing the ablation. If any excess fluid is detected at any time in the corneal stroma, the procedure should be paused and excess fluid removed by using the blade or Weck sponge to smooth the cornea. Immediately following the ablation a drop of antibiotic, steroid, and nonsteroidal medication is placed on the eye. A bandage soft contact lens should then be inserted.

Corneal Scar Removal with Correction of Hyperopia

The technique for removal of anterior corneal scars is similar to that of the photorefractive procedure,[44-47] but several other steps become important and the procedure must be carefully planned. Patient centration, preparation, and preop medications are the same as for the photorefractive technique.

It is important to remember that the excimer laser is most useful to perform a final polishing of the anterior stromal surface. If the laser alone is used to treat an irregular surface, the abnormal surface topography will be reproduced deeper in the cornea. It is therefore important first to remove large nodules mechanically. A blade or diamond burr can be used for this initial step. If only small irregularities exist and mechanical removal is not necessary, the epithelium can be left in the lower-lying areas to prevent excessive tissue removal in the depressed areas. Because the exact amount of tissue removed by the laser is more difficult to determine when using modulating fluids, after mechanical removal of tissue, or when the epithelium is left intact, the exact refractive change can be difficult to predict. Still, it is very useful to attempt to control the refractive result by using appropriately placed laser ablations. If no consideration is given to the refractive state, then a large degree of ametropia or anisometropia can occur. Following removal of a central corneal scar in a patient who had no refractive error, usually hyperopia will be induced. In this patient, it is appropriate to remove additional tissue in the midperiphery to steepen the central cornea, preventing severe hyperopic shift.

ABLATION PROFILES

Surface Ablation

Within the United States the hyperopic ablation profiles are currently carefully regulated by the companies under investigative protocols approved by the Food and Drug Administration. These ablations use a variety of masking techniques to allow more laser pulses in the midperiphery with blend zones toward the center and far periphery of the cornea. For instance, the VISX/ Taunton 2015 laser has multiple diaphragms through which the beam is passed, allowing a larger amount of ablation in the peripheral cornea than in the center (Figs 36–1, 36–2). Other systems use an expanding ring, ablatable mask, or rotating mask (Fig 36–3).[36,37] The amount of tissue that must be removed to produce a certain refractive result depends on the optical-zone size.[48,49]

Intrastromal Excimer Laser Ablation in Combination with Automated Lamellar Keratoplasty

The laser in situ keratomileusis (LASIK) procedure is currently being used for low, moderate, and high myopia.[50,51] From early results it appears that removal of stromal tissue leaving Bowman's membrane intact may induce less corneal woundhealing response. This procedure can be used for myopic corrections from −1 to −25 D. Hyperopic corrections may be possible by removing more tissue in the midperiphery than in the center under the superficial stromal flap (Figs 1–11, 1–12). Astigmatic and presbyopic corrections may also be possible. Long-term data are not available on the effectiveness and predictability of corrections using the excimer laser under a stromal flap.

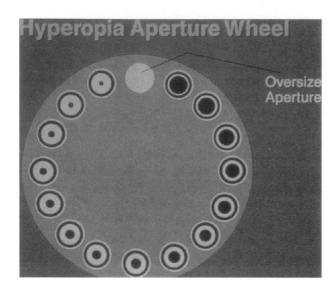

Figure 36–1. Progressively enlarging openings in the apertures allow a transition from the center, which is untreated, to the midperiphery, which receives the most treatment. Differing refractive errors are treated by adjusting the central untreated zone as well as the depth of the ablation. *(© Taunton Technologies, Inc.)*

POSTOP MEDICATIONS AND CARE

If a bandage soft contact lens is used, it is left in place for 3 to 5 days until the epithelium has healed. Antibiotic, steroid, and nonsteroidal medications should be applied QID. It is important not to use a nonsteroidal without appropriate steroid coverage and to use them only for 1 to 2 days in order to avoid inflammatory infiltrates.[52] In patients who have had ALK flaps with intrastromal excimer ablation (LASIK), no bandage contact lens is needed. These patients are comfortable with antibiotic, steroid, and nonsteroidal anti-inflammatory drops.

The antibiotic can be discontinued when the epithelium has healed. Steroid medications are used in a tapering regimen over the first 3 to 6 months. We have used mild steroids 6 times per day for the first week, QID for the first month, and BID until 3 months. Some of the corneal scars or deeper ablations may require continuation of the topical steroids for a longer period of time. If there is any increased haze, then topical steroids should be reinstituted at a higher dosage to prevent scarring. The haze in the hyperopic patients is less of a problem because of the midperipheral location. The patient should be monitored for steroid side effects such as intraocular hypertension. The corneal topography should be followed after these procedures.[53–55]

Currently the timing of the second eye is determined by the investigational protocols in the United

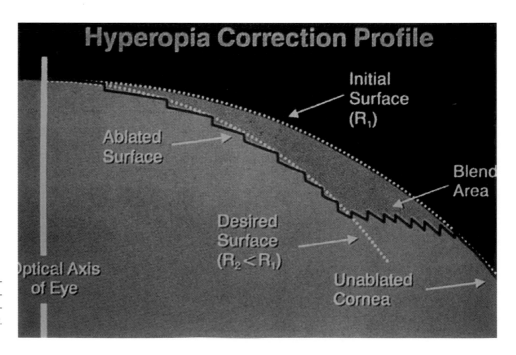

Figure 36–2. The central cornea receives no ablation, and the midperiphery is thinned the most. A peripheral blend zone is necessary. *(© Taunton Technologies, Inc.)*

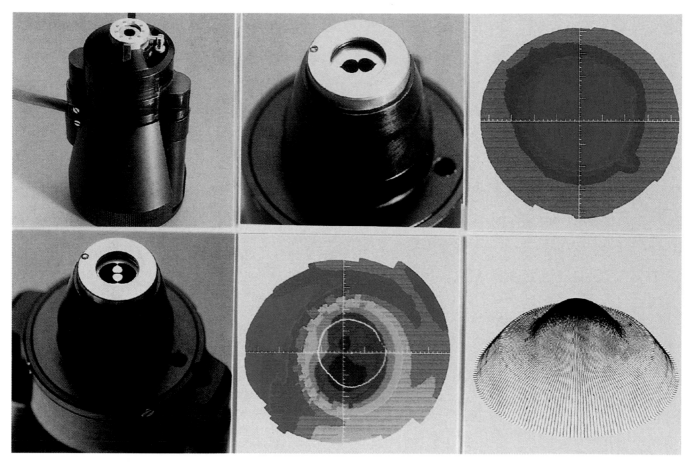

Figure 36–3. Iris mask handpiece (Aesculap-Meditec laser) for the correction of myopia and therapeutic applications *(top left)*, rotating mask for myopic corrections *(top center)*, corneal topography after correction of myopia *(top right)*, rotating mask for hyperopia and hyperopic astigmatism *(bottom left)*, corneal topography after a hyperopic correction *(bottom center)*, computer-aided design of a hyperopic correction *(bottom right)*.

States. The patient should have good function of the first eye before treatment of the second eye is performed.

RESULTS

Phillips Eye Institute—VISX/Taunton 2015 Laser

At the Phillips Eye Institute 18 eyes of 16 patients have been treated with hyperopic ablations under the phototherapeutic investigative protocol of the FDA clinical trials. These patients had other corneal disease, and the primary goal of surgery was to remove scars, with prevention or treatment of anisometropia as a secondary goal. Six eyes (33%) were of males and 12 eyes (67%) were of females. The average age of the patients was 62 ± 13 years old. The initial mean spherical equivalent was +3.6 ± 1.9 D. Follow-up is now available on 15 eyes at the 6-month examination, 14 eyes at the 12-month examination, and 11 eyes at the 24-month

examination postoperatively. Mean follow-up was 19.0 ± 8.4 months. Corneal diseases present in these eyes included anterior basement membrane dystrophy with corneal scarring, overcorrected radial keratotomy, Salzmann's nodular degeneration, or high anisometropia with amblyopia.

Treatment was performed with the VISX/Taunton 2015 excimer laser. Beam diameters between 6 and 7 mm were used for all patients. Pre- and postop management was the same as described earlier. Mechanical removal of large nodules was performed when needed. Both myopic and hyperopic recipes were used first to remove the corneal scar and then to manipulate the refractive error.

At the last follow-up, 9 eyes (50%) were within 2 D of emmetropia and 3 eyes (17%) were within 1 D (Fig 36–4). There was some regression between 3 and 12 months. Between 12 and 24 months there was minimal regression of effect in eyes that were followed up at both periods (Fig 36–5).

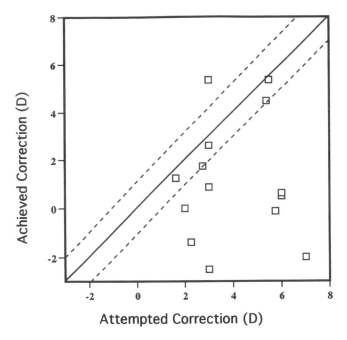

Figure 36–4. Plot of attempted versus achieved refractive error change in 14 hyperopic eyes with 12-month follow-up treated at the Phillips Eye Institute. The dashed lines represent ± 2 D of intended corrections. The dots below the line represent undercorrections and those above represent overcorrections. These eyes also had significant corneal scarring preoperatively, and the refractive outcome of the treatment is therefore less predictable.

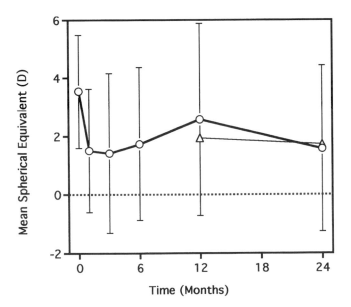

Figure 36–5. Spherical equivalent (mean ± 1 SD) following hyperopic excimer laser treatment in 18 eyes treated with hyperopic ablations at the Phillips Eye Institute. Initially more correction is obtained with some regression from 3 months to 1 year. Stability appears apparent from 12 to 24 months in the 10 eyes, with measurements at both visits represented by the triangle. These eyes also had significant corneal scarring preoperatively, and the refractive outcome of the treatment is therefore less predictable.

Three of 18 (17%) eyes had an uncorrected visual acuity (UCVA) of 20/25 or better at last follow-up. One of these eyes had a UCVA of 20/20. Most eyes had an improvement in best corrected visual acuity (BCVA) because of the reduction of corneal scarring and irregular astigmatism. Two eyes (11%) lost BCVA; both of these eyes lost two lines of BCVA. Significant topographic steepening can be seen in most patients when additional tissue has been removed in the midperipheral zones following removal of the corneal scar.

Aesculap–Meditec Laser

Dausch and coauthors have reported a series of 23 hyperopic eyes treated with the Aesculap–Meditec 193-nm excimer laser.[16] The Aesculap–Meditec laser uses a 7 × 1 mm slit profile beam moved uniformly over a mechanical mask, which for hyperopia allows treatment of the zone from 4 to 7 mm. The energy density is 250 mJ/cm^2. Dausch and colleagues followed all of these eyes for 12 months. They divided their patients into two groups. The first group consisted of 15 hyperopic eyes with preop refraction between +2.0 and +7.5 D (mean spherical equivalent +4.7 ± 1.6 D). The second group consisted of eight aphakic eyes with preop refraction between +11.0 and +16.0 D (mean spherical equivalent +13.1 ± 2.0 D).

In the low hyperopia group 12 eyes (80%) were within ± 1 D of the intended correction after 1 year. In the high hyperopia group, three eyes (37%) were within ± 1 D of the intended refraction. One eye (7%) lost two lines of BCVA in the low hyperopia group. In the high hyperopia group, two eyes (25%) lost BCVA because of decentration of the ablation zone. The Meditec laser can also be used to correct hyperopic astigmatism (Fig 36–3). FDA-sponsored studies are currently underway to evaluate the outcomes, safety, and efficacy of these treatments.

COMPLICATIONS

Complications can occur with any refractive surgical procedure. Under- and overcorrection can be seen based upon improper surgical ablation, decentration, or malfunctioning of the excimer laser, abnormal corneal hydration status, or excessive or inadequate wound-healing response. It is crucial to maintain consistent hydration of the cornea because excessive fluid on the cornea will result in an undercorrection. If desiccation of the corneal stroma is present, then overcorrection and haze can occur.[43] An enhanced wound-healing response can lead to regression, resulting in an undercorrection and possible scarring. No or minimal tissue healing can sometimes lead to an overcorrection.

The haze following hyperopic PRK is peripherally located. Bowman's membrane remains intact in the very center of the cornea, protecting this area from haze. Haze takes second place to decentration in causing a decrease in BCVA following hyperopic excimer PRK.

Infectious keratitis can result in scarring, haze, and a decrease in vision. Appropriate culture and treatment with frequent antibiotics should be used for this complication. If topical nonsteroidal anti-inflammatory drugs (NSAIDs) are used without appropriate steroid coverage, an increase in polymorphonuclear leukocyte migration into the cornea can occur, causing inflammatory infiltrates. These are best treated by discontinuing the NSAIDs and instituting frequent topical steroids.[52]

A complication unique to LASIK to correct hyperopia is displacement of the flap following the procedure (Fig 1–11). If this should occur, then the flap should be lifted, the interface cleaned of any debris, and the flap repositioned. The flap should be allowed to dry in place for 5 minutes. Taping the eye without a pressure patch can be useful to reduce the frequency of this complication. Epithelial ingrowth under the flap can also be seen if epithelium has been allowed to remain in the interface. If this is significant enough to reduce vision, the flap can be lifted at the edge and the epithelium cleaned from underneath the interface.

Decentration of the refractive cut can result in glare, irregular astigmatism, and a decrease in BCVA.[15,16,38,39] Controversy exists as to whether refractive procedures should be centered on the pupil or the corneal light reflex.[38,39,56,57] Centration on the pupil is preferred in most instances (see Chapter 9).

Treatment of hyperopia with the excimer laser is still not as reproducible as myopic treatment. Large optical zones with treatment blending into the far periphery may be important in achieving stable hyperopic corrections. A better understanding of hyperopic ablations will also help to prevent undesired hyperopic shift following excimer phototherapeutic removal of anterior corneal scars.

The excimer laser is a promising tool for refractive surgery. The techniques are still developing, and it is certain that there will be significant advances in the future. An increased understanding of the optics of refractive surgery and the corneal wound-healing response may help us to improve our results and modulate the patient's postop healing, to further our goal of predictable, safe, refractive surgery. The excimer laser is a highly complex surgical tool that requires attention to detail, an appropriate physician–patient relationship that includes careful patient counseling, and meticulous postop care to achieve high-quality results.

REFERENCES

1. Marshall J, Trokel S, Rothery S, Krueger RR. A comparative study of corneal incisions induced by diamond and steel knives and two ultraviolet radiations from an excimer laser. *Br J Ophthalmol.* 1986;70:482–501.
2. McDonald MB, Beuerman R, Falzoni W, Rivera L, Kaufman HE. Refractive surgery with the excimer laser. *Am J Ophthalmol.* 1987;103:469.
3. Puliafito CA, Steinert RF, Deutsch TF, Hillenkamp F, Dehm EJ, Adler CM. Excimer laser ablation of the cornea and lens: experimental studies. *Ophthalmology.* 1985;92:741–748.
4. Taylor DM, L'Esperance FA Jr, Del Pero RA, et al. Human excimer laser lamellar keratectomy: a clinical study. *Ophthalmology.* 1989;96:654–664.
5. Trokel SL, Srinivasan R, Braren B. Excimer laser surgery of the cornea. *Am J Ophthalmol.* 1983;96:710–715.
6. Gartry DS, Kerr Muir MG, Marshall J. Excimer laser photorefractive keratectomy: 18-month follow-up. *Ophthalmology.* 1992;99:1209–1219.
7. Sher NA, Barak M, Daya S, et al. Excimer laser photorefractive keratectomy in high myopia: a multi-center study. *Arch Ophthalmol.* 1992;110:935–943.
8. Sher NA, Chen V, Bowers RA, et al. The use of the 193-nm excimer laser for myopic photorefractive keratectomy in sighted eyes: a multi-center study. *Arch Ophthalmol.* 1991;109:1525–1530.
9. Sher NA, Hardten DR, Fundingsland B, et al. 193-nm excimer photorefractive keratectomy in high myopia. *Ophthalmology.* 1994;101:1575–1582.
10. Talley AR, Hardten DR, Sher NA, et al. Results one year after using the 193-nm excimer laser for photorefractive keratectomy in mild to moderate myopia. *Am J Ophthalmol.* 1994;118:304–311.
11. Campos M, Nielsen S, Szerenyi K, Garbus JJ, McDonnell PJ. Clinical follow-up of phototherapeutic keratectomy for treatment of corneal opacities. *Am J Ophthalmol.* 1993;115:433–440.
12. Fagerholm P, Fitzsimmons TD, Örndahl M, Öhman L, Tengroth B. Phototherapeutic keratectomy: long-term results in 166 eyes. *Refract Corneal Surg.* 1993;9(suppl):S76–S81.
13. Sher NA, Bowers RA, Zabel RW, et al. Clinical use of the 193-nm excimer laser in the treatment of corneal scars. *Arch Ophthalmol.* 1991;109:491–498.

14. Steinert RF, Puliafito CA. Excimer laser phototherapeutic keratectomy for a corneal nodule. *Refract Corneal Surg.* 1990;6:352.

15. Dausch D, Klein R, Landesz M, Schröder E. Photorefractive keratectomy to correct astigmatism with myopia or hyperopia. *J Cataract Refract Surg.* 1994;20(suppl):252S–257S.

16. Dausch D, Klein R, Schröder E. Excimer laser photorefractive keratectomy for hyperopia. *Refract Corneal Surg.* 1993;9:20–28.

17. Taylor HR, Kelly P, Alpins N. Excimer laser correction of myopic astigmatism. *J Cataract Refract Surg.* 1994;20(suppl):243–251.

18. Poggio EC, Glynn RJ, Schein OD, et al. The incidence of ulcerative keratitis among users of daily-wear and extended-wear soft contact lenses. *New Engl J Med.* 1989;321:779–783.

19. Arffa RC, Marvelli TL, Morgan KS. Long-term follow-up of refractive and keratometric results of pediatric epikeratophakia. *Arch Ophthalmol.* 1986;104:668–670.

20. Basuk WL, Zisman M, Waring GO III, et al. Complications of hexagonal keratotomy. *Am J Ophthalmol.* 1994;17:37–49.

21. Durrie DS, Schumer DJ, Cavanagh TB: Holmium: YAG laser thermokeratoplasty for hyperopia. *J Refract Corneal Surg.* 1994;10(suppl):5277–5280.

22. Ehrlich MI, Nordan LT. Epikeratophakia for the treatment of hyperopia. *J Cataract Refract Surg.* 1989;15:661–666.

23. Foss AJ, Rosen PH, Cooling RJ. Retinal detachment following anterior chamber lens implantation for the correction of ultra-high myopia in phakic eyes. *Br J Ophthalmol.* 1993;77:212–213.

24. McDonald MB, Kaufman HE, Aquavella JV, et al. The nationwide study of epikeratophakia for myopia. *Am J Ophthalmol.* 1987;103:375–383.

25. Moreira H, Campos M, Sawusch MR, McDonnell JM, Sand B, McDonnell PJ. Holmium laser thermokeratoplasty. *Ophthalmology.* 1993;100:752–761.

26. Neumann AC, McCarty GR. Hexagonal keratotomy for correction of low hyperopia: preliminary results of a prospective study. *J Cataract Refract Surg.* 1988;14:265–269.

27. Neumann AC, Sanders D, Raanan M, DeLuca M. Hyperopic thermokeratoplasty: clinical evaluation. *J Cataract Refract Surg.* 1991;17:830–838.

28. Seiler T, Matallana M, Bende T. Laser thermokeratoplasty by means of a pulsed holmium: YAG laser for hyperopic correction. *Refract Corneal Surg.* 1990;6:335–339.

29. Siganos DS, Siganos CS, Pallikaris IG. Clear lens extraction and intraocular lens implantation in normally sighted hyperopic eyes. *J Refract Corneal Surg.* 1994;10:117–124.

30. Worst JG, van der Veen G, Los LI. Refractive surgery for high myopia. The Worst-Fechner biconcave iris claw lens. *Doc Ophthalmol.* 1990;75:335–341.

31. Allemann N, Chamon W, Silverman RH, et al. High-frequency ultrasound quantitative analyses of corneal scarring following excimer laser keratectomy. *Arch Ophthalmol.* 1993;111:968–973.

32. Cavanagh HD, Petroll WM, Alizadeh H, He YG, McCulley JP, Jester JV. Clinical and diagnostic use of in vivo confocal microscopy in patients with corneal disease. *Ophthalmology.* 1993;100:1444–1454.

33. Lohmann CP, Gartry DS, Kerr MK, Timberlake GT, Fitzke FW, Marshall J. Corneal haze after excimer laser refractive surgery: objective measurements and functional implications. *Eur J Ophthalmol.* 1991;1:173–180.

34. Reinstein DZ, Silverman RH, Coleman DJ. High-frequency ultrasound measurement of the thickness of the corneal epithelium. *Refract Corneal Surg.* 1993;9:385–387.

35. Stark WJ, Gilbert ML, Gottsch JD, Munnerlyn C. Optical pachymetry in the measurement of anterior corneal disease: an evaluative tool for phototherapeutic keratectomy. *Arch Ophthalmol.* 1990;108:12–13.

36. Friedman MD, Bittenson S, Brodsky L, et al. OmniMed II: a new system for use with the emphasis rotatable mask. *J Refract Corneal Surg.* 1994;10(2 suppl):S267–S273.

37. O'Brart DP, Gartry DS, Lohmann CP, Muir MG, Marshall J. Excimer laser photorefractive keratectomy for myopia: comparison of 4.00- and 5.00-millimeter ablation zones. *J Refract Corneal Surg.* 1994;10:87–94.

38. Amano S, Tanaka S, Shimizu K. Topographical evaluation of centration of excimer laser myopic photorefractive keratectomy. *J Cataract Refract Surg.* 1993;20:616–619.

39. Uozato H, Guyton DL. Centering corneal surgical procedures. *Am J Ophthalmol.* 1987;103:264–275.

40. Campos M, Hertzog L, Wang XW, Fasano AP, McDonnell PJ. Corneal surface after de-epithelialization using a sharp and a dull instrument. *Ophthalmic Surg.* 1992;23:618–621.

41. Campos M, Trokel SL, McDonnell PJ. Surface morphology following photorefractive keratectomy. *Ophthalmic Surg.* 1993;24:822–825.

42. Maguen E, Nesburn AB, Papaioannou T, Salz JJ, Macy JI, Warren C. Effect of nitrogen flow on recovery of vision after excimer laser photorefractive keratectomy without nitrogen flow. *J Refract Corneal Surg.* 1994;10:321–326.

43. Dougherty PJ, Wellish KL, Maloney RK. Excimer laser ablation rate and corneal hydration. *Am J Ophthalmol.* 1994;118:169–176.

44. Hahn TW, Sah WJ, Kim JH. Phototherapeutic keratectomy in 9 eyes with superficial corneal diseases. *Refract Corneal Surg.* 1993;9(suppl):S115–S118.

45. Hersh PS, Spinak A, Garrana R, Mayers M. Phototherapeutic keratectomy: strategies and results in 12 eyes. *Refract Corneal Surg.* 1993;9(suppl):S90–S95.

46. Rapuano CJ, Laibson PR. Excimer laser phototherapeutic keratectomy. *CLAO J.* 1993;19:235–240.

47. Thompson V, Durrie DS, Cavanagh TB. Philosophy and technique for excimer laser phototherapeutic keratectomy. *Refract Corneal Surg.* 1993;9(suppl):S81–S85.

48. Werblin TP. Lans lecture. Lamellar refractive surgery: where have we been and where are we going? *Refract Corneal Surg.* 1989;5:167–176.

49. Munnerlyn CR, Koons SJ, Marshall J. Photorefractive keratectomy: a technique for laser refractive surgery. *J Cataract Refract Surg.* 1988;14:46–52.

50. Brint SF, Ostrick M, Fisher C, et al. 6-month results of the multi-center phase I study of excimer laser myopic keratomileusis. *J Cataract Refract Surg.* 1994;20:610–615.

51. Pallikaris IG, Siganos DS. Excimer laser in situ keratomileusis and photorefractive keratectomy for correction of high myopia. *J Refract Corneal Surg.* 1994;10:498–510.

52. Sher NA, Frantz JM, Talley A, et al. Topical diclofenac in the treatment of ocular pain after excimer photorefractive keratectomy. *Refract Corneal Surg.* 1993;9:425–436.

53. Klyce SD, Smolek MK. Corneal topography of excimer laser photorefractive keratectomy. *J Cataract Refract Surg.* 1993;19(suppl):S122–S130.

54. Lin DT. Corneal topographic analysis after excimer photorefractive keratectomy. *Ophthalmology.* 1994;101:1432–1439.

55. Moreira H, Garbus JJ, Fasano A, Lee M, Clapham TN, McDonnell PJ. Multifocal corneal topographic changes with excimer laser photorefractive keratectomy. *Arch Ophthalmol.* 1992;110:994–999.

56. Fay AM, Trokel SL, Myers JA. Pupil diameter and the principal ray. *J Cataract Refract Surg.* 1992;18:348–351.

57. Pande M, Hillman JS. Optical zone centration in keratorefractive surgery. Entrance pupil center, visual access, coaxially sighted corneal reflex, or geometric corneal center? *Ophthalmology.* 1993;100:1230–1237.

CHAPTER 37

Laser Thermokeratoplasty for Hyperopia, Astigmatism, and Myopia

Gregory S. H. Ogawa ▪ Dimitri T. Azar ▪ Douglas D. Koch

INTRODUCTION

Thermokeratoplasty is an old procedure plagued by a history of regression of effect. A better understanding of corneal and collagen response to heat, combined with state-of-the-art heat delivery systems, offers new promise for the future of thermal refractive surgery (Fig 1–10).

CLINICAL BACKGROUND

Heat has long been known to affect the curvature of the cornea. Cautery was used to treat keratoconus, beginning with Gayet in 1879 and continuing until the first penetrating keratoplasty was performed by Castroviejo in 1936.[1] In 1898 Lans first reported using cautery to decrease corneal astigmatism,[2] and in 1900 Terrien reported using cautery to correct severe astigmatism in an eye with Terrien's marginal degeneration.[3] In 1914 Wray also reported a case of astigmatism successfully treated with corneal cautery.[4] In 1933 O'Connor reported the successful, but variable, 10-year follow-up results on a patient with high myopic astigmatism whom he had treated with corneal cautery.[5]

After a hiatus, interest in thermal keratoplasty resurfaced with Stringer and Parr's 1964 report of the temperature at which corneal collagen contracts.[6] In the 1970s Gasset and colleagues worked extensively to evaluate a thermostatically controlled electric probe used at about 130°C to centrally flatten corneas with keratoconus. He demonstrated excellent 1-year results in five patients who had previously been contact lens intolerant,[6] but other investigators did not achieve such superb results. They experienced a high incidence of regression and more complications, ranging from mild surface problems to aggressive corneal melting and stromal scarring.[8,9] In one small series there was regression of effect all the way back to baseline within 1 to 6 months after the procedure.[10] Although thermal keratoplasty is no longer used in the United States as a stand-alone treatment for keratoconus, it is still used by some as a surgical adjunct that allows flattening of steep cones in order to improve the quality of the host trephination.

Rowsey and coworkers reported in 1980 their initial work with a 1.6-MHz radio-frequency probe (the Los Alamos Probe) designed to minimize the corneal surface problems of the Gasset technique of thermokeratoplasty for keratoconus.[11–13] This probe used a circulating saline electrode to deliver energy 200 to 400 μm below the surface of the probe, allowing the stroma to be heated with relative sparing of the endothelial and epithelial areas. The recurring problem of regression of effect seen with other thermal keratoplasty procedures also plagued the Los Alamos Probe, and in 1987 Rowsey formally withdrew the probe from experimentation because of the loss of clinical effect over time.[14,15]

CORNEAL COLLAGEN RESPONSE TO HEAT

Collagen can shrink down to one third of its native length upon heating. Human corneal collagen shrinks when heated to 55° to 58°C.[6] The covalent bonds of the primary collagen structure are not disturbed, but the heat provides the necessary energy to disrupt the hydrogen bonds of the tertiary collagen structure, allowing the collagen triple helix to partially unwind and form new cross-links between amino acid moieties with different collagen hydration levels.[11,16–18] The actual amount of shrinkage depends on the mechanical tensions on the collagen, and in the cornea the shrinkage is approximately 7%.[19] If collagen is heated past its shrinkage temperature into the 65° to 78°C range, then the contracted collagen relaxes as heat-labile cross-links are hydrolyzed. The aging process increases the number of thermally stable cross-links, raising the temperature required for relaxation of the collagen.[16] Further elevation of the temperatures can cause the collagen fibers to undergo necrosis.

NONREFRACTIVE CORNEAL RESPONSE TO HEAT

Heating has an impact on the various cells and structures of the cornea in addition to its effect on collagen. Very low levels of corneal heating cause either no discernible changes or only transient changes in the tissues. Higher temperatures can cause cellular destruction and disruption of structures such as Bowman's layer. The temperature elevation in the cornea varies by proximity to the heating source. Extreme heat causes significant tissue destruction near the center of the heat source, with gradually decreasing levels of tissue effect as the distance increases from the center of heating. The higher the temperature the greater the likelihood that there will be tissue destruction and an inflammatory response with subsequent wound healing and remodeling.

Histopathologic evaluation of human corneas treated with a Gasset-type thermokeratoplasty probe offers some insight into the changes the cornea undergoes with heating from a 100° to 130°C surface probe.

Bowman's layer appears to be more affected by destruction and abnormalities than would be expected with keratoconus alone.[8,20] There is also a marked loss of hemidesmosome complexes between the basement membrane and basal cells, which may be the cause of re-epithelialization problems in some thermokeratoplasty cases.[20] Other changes included corneal vascularization, epithelial thinning and irregularity, and stromal scarring.[8,20]

The Los Alamos Probe for thermokeratoplasty demonstrated similar histologic changes in a human keratoconus patient evaluated 6 months posttreatment by light and electron microscopy. Bowman's membrane was destroyed and the anterior two thirds of the stroma was scarred with contracted and folded collagen. There was no apparent effect on the endothelium.[14]

Rabbit thermokeratoplasty experiments using surface probes demonstrate less long-term histologic and refractive sequelae than are seen in humans. New Zealand albino rabbit experiments with ring thermokeratoplasty at 98°C and with Gasset-type thermal keratoplasty at 90°C show initial epithelial loss and keratocyte destruction, but by 2 weeks the corneas have either mild epithelial–anterior stromal thinning or an almost completely normal appearance to light and electron microscopy.[7,21] The keratometric changes with ring thermokeratoplasty in this rabbit model parallel the histologic changes and also revert to normal by 2 weeks' time.[21]

Normal levels of energy from the noncontact holmium : YAG laser tested in rabbits produce the expected stromal scarring, but the endothelium appears to be only minimally affected. Moreira examined the histopathologic changes in rabbit corneas produced with the MO1-1 noncontact Ho : YAG laser (Medical Optics Corporation, Carlsbad, CA) emitting 2.10-μm laser energy in 8-microsecond pulses with a per pulse energy adjustable from 4 to 5 mJ.[22] Immediately after treatment the epithelium demonstrated nuclear elongation and increased eosinophilia as indicators of thermal injury, while the stroma exhibited a decrease in the lamellar collagen pattern. At 4 weeks' time an 80% deep, epithelially based stromal wedge was evident with some overlying epithelial hyperplasia. In eyes treated with suprathreshold energies (15 J/cm^2), keratocyte nuclei became pyknotic, and at very high energies (at or exceeding 20 J/cm^2) acute endothelial injury was evident with retrocorneal membrane formation within 4 weeks of treatment. A ×400 magnification scanning electron microscope (SEM) revealed the threshold for morphologic endothelial change at the site of treatment to be 8 J/cm^2, and by 10 to 12 J/cm^2 the majority of sites demonstrated endothelial morphologic changes. Even with maximal possible endothelial injury from 32 spots treated with ≥20 J/cm^2, the total endothelial loss would be less than 1.2%.

REFRACTIVE CORNEAL RESPONSE TO HEAT

The cornea responds to heating in the 60°C range by flattening in the area of heating owing to corneal collagen contraction. If the cornea is heated centrally, then flattening occurs in the most optically active part of the cornea, and refractive power of the cornea decreases with the eye becoming relatively more hyperopic. This central flattening is the optical effect that has been sought in the treatment of centrally steep keratoconus corneas. When the cornea is heated peripherally, the contracting collagen causes peripheral flattening with a concomitant beltlike effect and resultant central steepening. The peripheral heating may be carried out in an annular pattern or in multiple radials. In general, the greater the number of peripheral burns or radials, and the smaller the optical zone, then the greater the central steepening. When the peripheral heating is brought in centrally to the range of a 4-mm–diameter optical zone, the effect begins to reverse and central flattening begins.[23–25] The optical zone diameter at which central flattening occurs seems to be pattern and modality dependent. For example, the noncontact Ho:YAG laser used in a 32-spot ring at a 3-mm optical zone produces significant central steepening on human cadaver eyes while the same laser used with 4 to 8 spots at a 3-mm optical zone causes central flattening on fresh swine eyes; a pulsed CO_2 laser used in a continuous ring pattern at a 5.5-mm optical zone causes central flattening in human cadaver eyes.[22,25,26]

An astigmatic response to heating can be achieved by treating the periphery along a single meridian. Peripheral meridional heating has a similar effect to a wedge resection, causing central steepening along the axis of treatment. If a person has a cornea steeper at 90° (axis of plus cylinder correction at 90°), then the appropriate amount of peripheral heating of the flatter 180° meridian would steepen the cornea centrally on the 180° meridian and decrease the amount of astigmatism. A treatment for hyperopia with astigmatism can be designed by treating more of the cornea or working closer to the visual axis along the flattest meridian of the cornea.[27]

In vivo human and animal models demonstrate that the effect of the corneal collagen contraction tends to decrease with time.[24,28] This regression of effect may be due to production of new collagen by corneal fibroblasts, although the actual reason for the apparent reversal of the collagen contraction is not clear.[28]

To achieve adequate refractive results with thermokeratoplasty, at least three key factors will likely play a role:

1. Collagen shrinkage temperatures
2. Collagen stability
3. Keratocyte response[25]

Because of the narrow temperature range for collagen shrinkage, thermokeratoplasty requires excellent control of corneal temperature. Normal corneal collagen appears very stable with a probable half-life of greater than 10 years.[29] We do not know as much about the stability of thermally contracted collagen. For stability of the refractive result, minimal wound healing should occur. Temperature levels probably should be minimized to reduce the potential for an inflammatory and keratocyte wound-healing response.

NONLASER TECHNIQUES OF TREATING HYPEROPIA: RADIAL THERMOKERATOPLASTY AND THE FYODOROV TECHNIQUE

The most recent and most advanced nonlaser technique of treating hyperopia and hyperopic astigmatism by thermokeratoplasty was developed by Fyodorov in Moscow and is called *radial thermokeratoplasty.* In 1981 Fyodorov began using superficial peripheral corneal thermal treatments for hyperopia, and by 1984 he and the engineers at the Moscow Research Institute for Eye Microsurgery developed a fine needle probe for deeper thermal keratoplasty.[30] It was postulated that deep treatment in the stroma would overcome the regression seen with superficial thermal treatment.[24] Fyodorov combined this depth-controlled probe with controls for energy level and duration and devised a computer program for choosing the surgical plan for each patient.[27] The first human trials using this technique in the United States began in late 1987.[31]

Radial Thermokeratoplasty: Indications and Preop Planning

Radial thermokeratoplasty indications include hyperopia, hyperopic astigmatism, presbyopia, and hyperopia resulting from overresponse to radial keratotomy.[24]

The degree of treated hyperopia generally ranges from 1 to 10 diopters, with the amount of hyperopic astigmatism limited to 5 D or less.[27] Monovision is usually the goal when treating presbyopic patients. Patients treated for overcorrection after radial keratotomy (RK) are usually not treated before 6 to 8 months after RK.[24]

The Fyodorov computer program utilizes the patient's age, sex, amount of hyperopia or hyperopic astigmatism, K's, corneal thickness, and scleral rigidity to determine treatment plans from which the surgeon can select.[30] Because of the potential for anterior-chamber–angle narrowing with peripheral corneal shrinkage, patients with narrow angles were considered for prethermokeratoplasty prophylactic laser peripheral iridectomies to reduce the chance of acute-angle–closure attacks after thermokeratoplasty.[24]

Radial Thermokeratoplasty: Surgical Technique and Postop Course

The handheld radial thermokeratoplasty probe contains a 34-gauge retractable wire heated to 600°C. A motor drives the hot, retractable wire from the probe tip for 0.3 second, extending it to a preset length of 95% of corneal pachymetry upon activation by a foot pedal.[24,27] Under topical anesthesia the peripheral cornea is treated along 6 to 16 radial rays with 2 to 4 burns per ray and an optical zone of 5 to 8 mm in diameter.[24,30] Astigmatic treatments consist of radial rays, or for more effect, limbus concave arcs enclosing rays along the flatter axis for treating hyperopic astigmatism alone, or oval optical zones when treating hyperopia with hyperopic astigmatism.[27,30] When treating RK overcorrection eyes, the burns are placed in the RK incisions.[24]

Immediately postoperatively the corneas have focal white stromal burns with loss of the overlying epithelium. Stromal edema around the burns and Descemet stress lines between the burns develop within 1 hour after the procedure.[27] Early after the procedure patients develop tearing, foreign body sensation, and redness for 24 to 72 hours until the epithelium heals. There is a subsequent decrease in measured corneal sensation after the procedure.[24,28] The scars from the burns heal from posterior to anterior, and at 1 year only the anterior stroma is still clinically scarred.[27,28]

Radial Thermokeratoplasty: Refractive Results

The results of this procedure have been variable, but in general are characterized by an initial overcorrection showing a more pronounced effect on keratometry readings than on refractive error, followed by a regression of effect with time.[24] A review of Fyodorov's cases

yielded a 53% incidence of 20/40 or better vision at 12 months, but the predictability was poor enough that none of the surgical parameters (including optical zone and number of radial rays) was found to correlate with refractive outcome in these patients. The results of this review of Fyodorov's cases is probably unreliable owing to selection bias because, of the 211 charts submitted for review, only 117 (55%) were complete enough for inclusion in the review.[32] In Neumann's series of 61 cases, the eyes were initially overcorrected with a drift to near emmetropia at 2 months. At the 2-month evaluation, the optical-zone size was the best predictor of result. By 6 months 63% of the eyes were undercorrected by at least 1 D, and by 9 to 12 months that figure rose to 83% of eyes.[27] Feldman's prospective evaluation of four eyes treated with this technique more dramatically demonstrated the regression of effect with a loss of 82% of the desired effect by the 1-year postop evaluation.[28]

Radial Thermokeratoplasty: Complications

A variety of complications have been reported with this technique, but the incidence of complications is said to be low.[24,28,30] Intraoperative complications include: improper placement of the probe/coagulations, poor heating due to corneal wetness, gaping of RK wounds if burns are not placed in the old RK incisions, microperforation by the wire probe, and malfunction of the probe heating-wire system causing excessive burning of the cornea. Early complications include: central corneal erosions, keratoconjunctivitis (probably infectious), corneal ulceration, fixed central corneal folds resulting from treatment of high astigmatism (treated by placing small burns in the periphery 90° away from the initial treatment meridian). Late complications include: overcorrection, undercorrection, induced astigmatism, peripheral corneal neovascularization in the area of thermal injury, and pterygoid growth onto the cornea.

Radial Thermokeratoplasty: Conclusion

Because of the significant regression of effect and the poor predictability of this technique, interest in it has largely died, but much of the previous excitement about it has been transferred to the newest, most controlled methods of thermokeratoplasty using lasers.

LASER THERMOKERATOPLASTY

Why should we use lasers to perform a procedure that has not worked adequately in the past? The reason is that lasers may provide an adequately controlled method to avoid heating collagen past its shrinking temperature to the relaxation and necrosis temperature ranges. More controlled heating may also minimize keratocyte injury and possibly decrease the wound-healing response with its collagen synthesis and remodeling.

Multiple types of lasers have been investigated for use in laser thermokeratoplasty (LTK), including hydrogen fluoride,[33–35] cobalt: magnesium fluoride,[36] erbium: glass,[37] carbon dioxide,[9,38] and Ho: YAG. For each of these lasers the light energy is absorbed by water in the corneal epithelium and stroma, and the heat is passively transferred to the stromal collagen. The heating allows collagen shrinkage with subsequent topographic and refractive changes in the cornea.

Carbon Dioxide Lasers

Carbon dioxide laser energy is absorbed well at the surface of the cornea, which makes it difficult to heat the deeper stroma without causing excessive surface heating. In 1980 work to heat the stroma with carbon dioxide lasers was generally unrewarding, and few changes in corneal topography were achieved.[39,40] More recently, topographic changes were achieved in a cadaver eye model, but stromal heating changes only penetrated to one third of the corneal thickness.[26] (This anterior heating may explain the flattening achieved with this laser at a 5.5-mm optical zone. The heating may have been conducted much more centrally to produce central flattening.) The carbon dioxide laser does not appear to be ideal for delivering controlled stromal heating with minimal excess tissue heating.

Holmium: YAG Lasers

There are two principal Ho: YAG laser delivery systems for LTK. The first is a contact probe type manufactured by Summit, and the second is a noncontact type manufactured by Sunrise Technologies.

Contact Holmium: YAG

Technical Description

The contact Ho: YAG laser from Summit Technology, Inc (Waltham, MA) emits infrared electromagnetic energy at the wavelength of 2.06 μm and operates with 300-microsecond pulses at a repetition frequency of 15 Hz and a pulse power of approximately 19 mJ.[41] The laser focally raises the stromal collagen temperature to approximately 60°C by delivering 25 pulses at each treatment location. The laser energy reaches the cornea through a fiber-optic hand piece with a sapphire tip that provides a cone angle of 120°. When the tip is applied to the cornea and laser energy is delivered, it creates a cone-shaped zone of collagen contraction with a base diameter at the corneal surface of 700 μm, and a depth of 450 μm.

Clinical Indications and Technique

Thus far the published trials for contact Ho: YAG LTK have been for the treatment of hyperopia and hyperopic astigmatism. For low hyperopia, eight evenly spaced treatment spots are placed in the peripheral cornea. The optical-zone size is varied with a larger ring of spots for the lower degrees of hyperopia to be treated.[42,43] For higher hyperopia the surgeon places a second ring of eight spots along the same radials as the first set of spots, but more peripheral. Topical 1% pilocarpine and anesthetic are administered preoperatively. The surgeon places an instrument similar to an RK marker on the cornea to define the locations for probe placement. The probe is manually placed in contact with cornea, and the treatment requires approximately 2 seconds at each site.[41] The epithelium generally sloughs at the treatment sights, but heals within 4 days. The patients generally have a foreign body sensation for the first 3 days after the procedure. Patients use topical antibiotics for 3 days postoperatively to help prevent infectious keratitis. For astigmatism treatment, two spots may be placed in the peripheral cornea on the flat meridian of the cornea, or for more effect spots may be placed in the periphery adjacent to the flat meridian for a total of four spots.[44]

Clinical Results

Patients treated for hyperopia with contact Ho: YAG LTK have an initial large myopic shift with gradual regression. Durrie's phase I and II US Food and Drug Administration results for patients with mild to moderate hyperopia showed an improvement in uncorrected near vision: no patients saw J2 or better preop, and 75% saw J2 or better 6 months postoperatively.[45] At 6 months postoperatively 79% of the phase II patients had refractive errors within 1 D of emmetropia. The refractive results seemed to be fairly stable between 3 and 6 months in both phase I and II studies, but the phase I patients followed for 1 year have continued to show some further regression. After 6 months of follow-up, of the 16 patients in the phase II study, 50% maintained the same best spectacle-corrected vision, while 43% lost one line and 7% lost two lines. All loss of best spectacle-corrected vision was attributed to induced irregular astigmatism.

Treatment of astigmatism with contact Ho:YAG LTK produces a flattening of the steepest meridian with a concomitant overall flattening of the cornea, causing a myopic shift in the spherical equivalent of approximately half the amount of the astigmatic correction. Thompson's 6-month results in 26 eyes with 1.5 to 4.0 -D of astigmatism treated with four spots, two on each side of the flat meridian at an 8.5-mm ablation zone (optical zone), yielded an average astigmatic correction of 1.7 D (0.4 to 4.0 D) at 6 months.[44] Uncorrected distance visual acuity improved by two or more lines in 18 eyes and remained unchanged in the other 8 eyes. Twenty-four of the 26 eyes maintained or improved their best spectacle-corrected visual acuity, and two eyes lost two lines of acuity.

Further follow-up will be needed to determine when and if refractive results will stabilize with this modality.

Complications

The number of treated patients reported is low, so the true incidence of complications is unknown. Potential complications include: irregular astigmatism, improper alignment and positioning of the probe, or lack of uniform probe pressure, which can cause inconsistent coagulation spots, persistent epithelial defects, infectious keratitis, and recurrent erosions.

Noncontact Holmium: YAG

Technical Description/Background

The noncontact Ho:YAG laser from Sunrise Technologies (Fremont, CA) functions at a 2.13-μm wavelength with a 5-Hz pulse repetition frequency and a 250-microsecond pulse duration. The system employs a compact, solid state laser with a fiber-optic noncontact delivery system mounted to a slit lamp to deliver one to eight simultaneous treatment spots, each approximately 600 μm in diameter.

Koch's in vitro studies with fresh swine eyes and this laser looked at corneal topographic changes with varying treatment zones using four to eight spots, 10 pulses per spot, and an energy density of 8 to 11 J/cm^2.[46] The topographic changes were measured with the EyeSys Corneal Analysis System (EyeSys Technologies, Inc, Houston, TX). Treatment zones of 3.0 and 3.5 mm produced central corneal flattening of up to 9 D. Treatment zones of 4.0 to 4.5 mm produced no effect, and 5.0-mm or greater treatment zones caused central

corneal steepening of over 4 D. The central steepening could be increased by using 16 treatment spots instead of 8 and by placing a second ring of 16 spots around the first. Increasing the energy density of the spots also increased the curvature changes. Astigmatic treatments were made with pairs of laser spots along the flat corneal meridian.

Moreira and colleagues treated human eye-bank eyes with the Sunrise noncontact Ho:YAG laser using a 300-μm spot size and a 9 J/cm^2 laser energy with a 32-spot treatment ring (four sets of eight spots, each set rotated by 11.25°) at 3- to 7-mm treatment zones.[22] The central cornea steepened at all of these treatment zones; less steepening occurred in a near linear fashion with enlarging treatment zones. The treatment ring produced a beltlike contraction effect in the cornea. Moreira et al also conducted rabbit histopathologic studies of the effects of noncontact Ho:YAG laser energy as described above in the section on nonrefractive corneal responses to heat. The difference in refractive results between Koch's and Moreira's work indicates that at smaller treatment zones factors like spot size, spot number, and energy density play a role in the refractive outcome.

Clinical Indications and Techniques and Results

Ongoing clinical trials with the noncontact Ho:YAG laser focus on hyperopia and astigmatism. Clinical trials for the treatment of myopia will begin after treatment patterns and techniques are developed that will not cause persistent corneal haze at the treatment locations.

Treatment trials for hyperopia began with this laser in 1993.[25,47] Eligible patients had between 1 and 5 D of hyperopia. Sixteen eyes were treated with an eight-spot pattern using 10 pulses per spot for a total treatment duration of 2 seconds. The laser used a fixation light centrally with eight peripheral helium–neon (He–Ne) target beams corresponding to the eight treatment sites. The surgeon positioned the eight He–Ne beams around the patient's entrance pupil while the patient looked at the fixation light. More recently a split He–Ne focusing beam was added to ensure focus on the anterior surface of the cornea. The treatment-zone diameters were 5.0 mm for two eyes, 5.5 mm for two eyes, and 6.0 mm for 17 eyes. Eyes treated with 5.0-mm and 5.5-mm zones did not maintain their central steepening past 1 week. The 6.0-mm group had a change in their average spherical equivalent from +2.0 D preoperatively to +1.2 D 2 years postoperatively, with a concomitant improvement in uncorrected distance visual

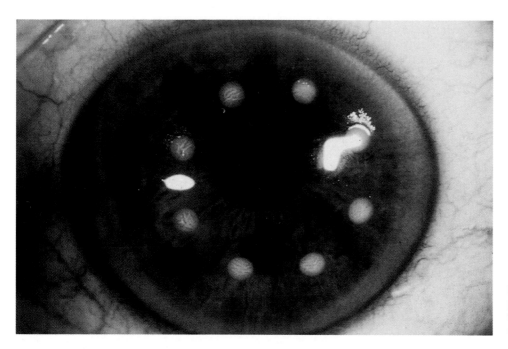

Figure 37–1. Early postoperative appearance of cornea after LTK. Note the stromal opacification in the area of treatment.

acuity from 20/125 preoperatively to 20/50 at 2 years postoperatively. Topographic changes corresponded well with the refractive changes and remained remarkably stable from 1 week to 6 months after the procedure. Postoperatively the patients had haze at all treatment sites, which was marked immediately after the procedure (Fig 37–1). The haze diminished significantly by 1 week, but it was still detectable with the slit lamp at 2 years (Fig 37–2). The mean refractive astigmatism increased by 0.2 D, and the maximum increase was 1.0 D in one patient. No patient lost two or more

lines on the Regan Contrast Acuity Charts (Paragon Services, Nova Scotia, Canada) and none of the patients lost 2 or more lines of best corrected visual acuity (BCVA) by the 1 month postop visit. Later hyperopic treatments were performed with higher energies and a greater number of spots, producing corrections of 3 D or more and good stability from 1 to 6 months after the treatment. FDA phase II studies are now underway in the United States using 8 or 16 spots with varied power settings to help further evaluate hyperopic noncontact Ho:YAG LTK.

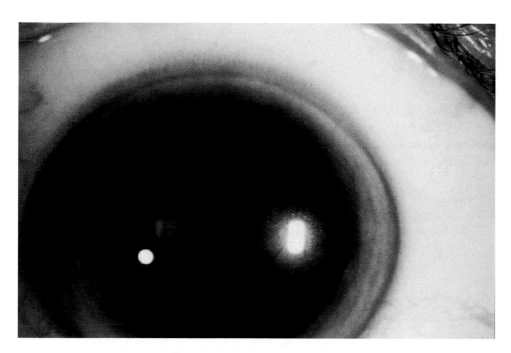

Figure 37–2. Appearance of cornea 2 years after LTK illustrated in Figure 37–1, showing barely perceptable haze.

Noncontact Ho:YAG LTK treatment for astigmatism began in trials outside the United States with a pair of treatment spots at each end of the flat meridian of the cornea at the 6- or 7-mm treatment zones. Astigmatic treatments have produced corrections of up to 4 D, with a maximum follow-up thus far in these studies of 6 months.[48]

Noncontact LTK for myopia will require having less corneal opacification than is associated with current midperipheral hyperopic and astigmatic treatments. The corneal haze in the midperiphery does not impair vision, but similar treatments for myopia closer to the center of the cornea could produce glare symptoms or decreases in contrast sensitivity. Serendipitously, myopic treatments at a 3-mm treatment zone produce twice as much flattening as the amount of steepening produced with hyperopic treatments using the same energy density.[25] The lower energies possible in myopic treatments may help decrease the amount of associated haze.

Complications

Potential complications include: irregular astigmatism, epithelial defects, infectious keratitis, and recurrent erosions. Improper focusing could lead to tissue energy delivery levels other than those desired, and improper centration or patient movement could potentially cause induced astigmatism or corneal opacity in an unwanted location. The risk of irregular astigmatism may theoretically be less with this noncontact modality because all spots are spaced by the delivery system, and the variation induced by manual alignment and applanation is not present.

Conclusions

Early studies with laser modalities of thermokeratoplasty for the treatment of low to moderate hyperopia, and possibly even myopia, appear promising. LTK appears safe and well tolerated. The lasers are generally easy to use and relatively inexpensive. The cornea is likely to tolerate repeated LTK treatments, making titration or retreatment possible. Ongoing studies to evaluate the effect of laser treatment parameters, pharmacologic modulation, and patient variables will be valuable in further refining LTK. The most important factor for LTK will be whether it can overcome the downfall of prior thermokeratoplasty techniques and achieve refractive stability.

REFERENCES

1. Gasset A. Changes in corneal curvature associated with thermokeratoplasty. In: Schachar RA, Levy NS, Schachar L, eds. *Keratorefraction*. Denison, TX: LAL Publishing; 1980;59–64.
2. Lans LJ. Experimentelle Untersuchungen uber die entstehung ver astigmatismus durch nicht-perforirende corneawunden. *Albrecht von Graefes Arch Klin Exp Ophthalmol*. 1898;45:117–152.
3. Terrien F. Dystrophie marginale symetrique des deux cornées avec astigmatisme regular consecutif et guerison par la cauterisation ignée. *Arch Ophthalmol*. 1900;20:12.
4. Wray C. Case of 6 D of hypermetropic astigmatism cured by the cautery. *Trans Ophthalmol Soc UK*. 1914;34:109–110.
5. O'Connor R. Corneal cautery for high myopic astigmatism. *Am J Ophthalmol*. 1933;16:337.
6. Stringer H, Parr J. Shrinkage temperature of eye collagen. *Nature*. 1964;204:1307.
7. Gasset AR, Shaw EL, Kaufman HE, Itoi M, Sakimoto T, Ishii Y. Thermokeratoplasty. *Trans Am Acad Ophthalmol Otolaryngol*. 1973;77:441–454.
8. Aquavella JV, Smith RS, Shaw EL. Alterations in corneal morphology following thermokeratoplasty. *Arch Ophthalmol*. 1976;94:2082–2085.
9. Kenyon KR. Histological changes in Bowman's membrane associated with thermokeratoplasty. In: Schachar RA, Levy NS, Schachar L, eds. *Keratorefraction*. Denison, TX: LAL Publishing; 1980;51–57.
10. Keates RH, Dingle J. Thermokeratoplasty for keratoconus. *Ophthalmic Surg*. 1975;6:89–92.
11. Rowsey JJ. Radiofrequency probe keratoplasty. In: Schachar RA, Levy NS, Schachar L, eds. *Keratorefraction*. Denison, TX: LAL Publishing; 1980:65–76.
12. Rowsey JJ, Gaylor JR, Dahlstrom R, et al. Los Alamos keratoplasty techniques. *Contact Intraocul Lens Med J*. 1980;6:1–12.
13. Rowsey JJ, Doss JD. Preliminary report of Los Alamos keratoplasty techniques. *Ophthalmology*. 1981;88:755–760.
14. McDonnell PJ, Garbus J, Romero JL, Rao NA, Schanzlin DJ. Electrosurgical keratoplasty: clinicopathalogic correlation. *Arch Ophthalmol*. 1988;106:235–238.
15. Rowsey JJ. Electrosurgical keratoplasty: update and retraction. *Invest Ophthalmol Vis Sci*. 1987;28:224.
16. Flory PJ, Garrett RR. Phase transitions in collagen and gelatin systems. *J Am Chem Soc*. 1958;80:4836–4845.
17. Deak G, Romhanyi G. The thermal shrinkage process of collagen fibres as revealed by polarization optical analysis of topooptical staining reactions. *Acta Morphol Acad Sci Hung*. 1967;15:195–208.
18. Verzar F, Zs-Nagy I. Elecronmicroscopic analysis of thermal collagen denaturation in rat tail tendons. *Gerontolgia*. 1970;16:77–82.

19. Allain JC, Le Lous M, Cohen-Solal, Brazin S, Maroteaux P. Isometric tensions developed during the hydrothermal swelling of rat skin. *Connect Tissue Res.* 1980;7:127–133.

20. Fogle JA, Kenyon KR, Stark WJ. Damage to epithelial basement membrane by thermokeratoplasty. *Am J Ophthalmol.* 1977;83:392–401.

21. Gruenberg P, Manning W, Miller D, Olson W. Increase in rabbit corneal curvature by heated ring application. *Ann Ophthalmol.* 1981;13:67–70.

22. Moreira H, Campos M, Sawusch MR, McDonnell JM, Sand B, McDonnell PJ. Holmium laser thermokeratoplasty. *Ophthalmology.* 1993;100:752–761.

23. Neumann AC, Sanders DR, Salz JJ, Bessinger DJ, Raanan MG, Van Der Karr M. Effect of thermokeratoplasty on corneal curvature. *J Cataract Refract Surg.* 1990;16:727–731.

24. Schachar RA. Radial thermokeratoplasty. *Int Ophthalmol Clin.* 1991;31:47–57.

25. Koch DD, Berry MJ, Vassiliadis A, Abarca AA, Villarreal R, Haft EA. Non-contact holmium:YAG laser thermal keratoplasty for treatment of hyperopia. In: Salz JJ, McDonnell PJ, McDonald MB, eds. *Corneal Laser Surgery.* St. Louis, MO: Mosby–Year Book; 1995:247–254.

26. Chandonnet A, Bazin R, Sirois C, Belanger PA. CO_2 laser annular thermokeratoplasty: a preliminary study. *Lasers Surg Med.* 1992;12:264–273.

27. Neumann AC, Sanders D, Raanan M, DeLuca M. Hyperopic thermokeratoplasty: clinical evaluation. *J Cataract Refract Surg.* 1991;17:830–838.

28. Feldman ST, William E, Frucht-Pery J, Chayet A, Brown SI. Regression of effect following radial thermokeratoplasty in humans. *Refract Corneal Surg.* 1989;5:288–291.

29. Smelser CK, Polack FM, Ozanies V. Persistence of donor collagen in corneal transplants. *Exp Eye Res.* 1965;4:349–354.

30. Caster AI. The Fyodorov technique of hyperopia correction by thermal coagulation: a preliminary report. *J Refract Surg.* 1988;4:105–108.

31. Neumann AC, Sanders DR, Salz JJ. Radial thermokeratoplasty for hyperopia: encouraging results from early laboratory and human trials. *Refract Corneal Surg.* 1989;5:52–54.

32. Neumann AC, Fyodorov S, Sanders DR. Radial thermokeratoplasty for the correction of hyperopia. *Refract Corneal Surg.* 1990;6:404–412.

33. Berry MJ, et al. Temperature distributions in laser-irradiated corneas. *Invest Ophthalmol Vis Sci.* 1991;32(1;suppl):994.

34. Koch DD, et al. HF chemical laser photothermal keratoplasty. *Invest Ophthalmol Vis Sci.* 1991;32(4;suppl):994.

35. Koch DD, et al. Laser photothermal keratoplasty: nonhuman primate results. *Invest Ophthalmol Vis Sci.* 1992;33(4;suppl):768.

36. Horn G, Spears KG, Lopez O, et al. New refractive method for laser thermal keratoplasty with the $Co:MgF_2$ laser. *J Cataract Refract Surg.* 1990;16:611–616.

37. Kanoda AN, Sorokin AS. Laser correction of hypermetropic refraction. In: Fyodorov SN, ed. *Microsurgery of the Eye: Main Aspects.* Moscow: MIR Publishers; 1987.

38. Householder J, et al. Laser induced thermal keratoplasty. *SPIE Proc.* 1994;1066:18–23.

39. Beckman H, Fuller TA, Boyman R, et al. Carbon dioxide laser surgery of the eye and adnexa. *Ophthalmology.* 1980;87:990–1000.

40. Peyman GA, Larson B, Raichand M, Andrews AH. Modification of rabbit corneal curvature with use of carbon dioxide laser burns. *Ophthalmic Surg.* 1980;11:325–329.

41. Thompson VM, Seiler T, Durrie DS, Cavanaugh TB. Holmium:YAG laser thermokeratoplasty for hyperopia and astigmatism: an overview. *Refract Corneal Surg.* 1993;9:S134–S137.

42. Seiler T, Matallara M, Bende T. Laser thermokeratoplasty by means of a pulsed Holmium:YAG laser for hyperopic correction. *Refract Corneal Surg.* 1990;6:335–339.

43. Seiler T, Matallara M, Bende T. Laser coagulation of the cornea with a holmium:YAG laser for correction of hyperopia. *Fortschr Ophthalmol.* 1991;88:121–124.

44. Thompson VM. Holmium:YAG laser thermokeratoplasty for correction of astigmatism. *J Refract Corneal Surg.* 1994;10:S293.

45. Durrie DS, Schumer DJ, Cavanaugh TB. Holmium:YAG laser thermokeratoplasty for hyperopia. *J Refract Corneal Surg.* 1994;10:S277–S280.

46. Koch DD, et al. Ho:YAG laser thermal keratoplasty: *in vitro* experiments. *Invest Ophthalmol Vis Sci.* 1993;34(4;suppl):1246.

47. Koch DD (personal communication, June 1996).

48. Koch DD, Berry MJ, Vassiliadis A, Haft EA. Laser thermal keratoplasty for correction of astigmatism and myopia. In: Salz JJ, McDonnell PJ, McDonald MB, eds. *Corneal Laser Surgery.* St. Louis, MO: Mosby–Year Book; 1995:274–276.

CHAPTER 38

Photicotherapeutic Keratectomy

Dimitri T. Azar ▪ Sandeep Jain ▪ Walter Stark

INTRODUCTION

Excimer laser phototherapeutic keratectomy (PTK) has been used in investigational protocols to treat patients with corneal pathologic conditions since 1988.[1] The high-energy ultraviolet (UV) light emitted by the excimer laser ablates corneal tissue with submicron precision and without significant injury to nonablated tissue.[1–3] It can be used for reshaping the corneal curvature, for controlled removal of corneal tissue, or in reconstructive superficial keratectomy. Excimer laser PTK has great potential to treat corneal opacities and to smooth corneal surface irregularities. The depth and shape of excimer laser ablative photodecomposition can be accurately controlled,[3–6] allowing for exact removal of the stroma and providing a relatively smooth base for better re-epithelialization.[1,3,6]

ADVANTAGES OVER MECHANICAL KERATECTOMY TECHNIQUES

The excimer laser provides corneal surgeons with an excellent cutting instrument for the management of anterior stromal opacities.[6] Unlike nonlaser corneal surgery, there is a clear boundary between the treated and untreated area at the histologic level.[7] Re-epithelialization and wound healing begin shortly after surgery and

are associated with a small degree of tissue reorganization.[7,8] Incisions made with diamond and steel blades produce relatively irregular and more diffuse tissue damage, compared to the 193-nm argon fluoride (ArF) excimer laser.[7] This is also in contrast to the 248-nm krypton excimer laser, which produces irregular and scattered areas of tissue damage (see Chapter 4).

The far UV (193-nm) laser radiation is thought to be within the limits of safety for the human eye. Adjacent tissues undergo minimal distortion and suffer no apparent thermal damage after 193-nm excimer laser PTK. The stromal lamellae show no evidence of distant disorganization.[1,3,4,6] There is evidence of endothelial cell loss after PTK when the remaining unablated stromal thickness is 40 mm or less.[6] It is not clear, however, whether similar endothelial loss would occur with equally deep mechanical lamellar dissection. Successfully treated patients can postpone or avoid more invasive surgical procedures, such as penetrating or lamellar keratoplasty.[1]

INDICATIONS FOR PHOTOTHERAPEUTIC KERATECTOMY

Opacities resulting from surgical or nonsurgical trauma, corneal inflammations, dystrophies, and degenerations limited to the anterior corneal layers have been successfully treated with PTK. Of 271 consecutive

PTK cases at 17 VISX US centers reviewed by Sanders, 55% of patients had corneal scars or leukomas, 39% had corneal dystrophies, and 5% had corneal surface irregularities.[9]

Surface irregularities resulting from epithelial dystrophies, Reis–Buckler's dystrophy, band keratopathy, peripheral corneal degenerations, and corneal surgical procedures can be improved with PTK, especially if the surface irregularities are associated with significant visual impairment. PTK is less effective in treating deep scars, nodules, and band keratopathy. Calculated posttreatment corneal thickness should not be less than 250 μm. The use of PTK to treat microbial keratitis, including infectious crystalline keratopathy,[10–13] is very limited because of the risk of spreading of microorganisms during treatment.[14]

Hyperopia may be a relative contraindication for PTK because PTK results in further flattening of the cornea. Keratoconjunctivitis is a relative contraindication. Uncontrolled uveitis, severe blepharitis, lagophthalmos, and systemic immunosuppression are contraindications under many protocols.

SURGICAL TECHNIQUE

Preop Evaluation

Under most investigational protocols, preop evaluation includes visual acuity, visual potential (evaluated with pinhole, hard contact lens, and potential acuity meter), pupil size, slit lamp biomicroscopy, and dilated fundus examination. The depth of the intended treatment is measured using an optical pachymeter.

Preop Preparation

The laser is calibrated before each treatment to ensure optimal performance. The overall operation of the laser is confirmed by ablating a standard treatment into a calibration plate made of polymethyl methacrylate (PMMA) test block or other material, depending on the laser used. The appropriate corneal ablation rate is determined using nomograms and entered into the laser computer program. Currently most procedures are performed under topical anesthesia. Before treatment, the plane of the corneal surface is determined by focusing the microscope at high magnification. Poor centration of laser treatment may result in a suboptimal outcome.

Laser Treatment

Table 38–1 summarizes the laser parameters that are ordinarily used in PTK. Nitrogen gas flow, previously used during the PMMA calibration in some lasers, is rarely used today.[15] The decision whether to ablate using the laser or to remove the epithelium manually is based on the smoothness of the epithelium relative to the envisioned smoothness of Bowman's layer. The epithelium is ablated with the laser if the anterior stromal surface is judged to be irregular. If the anterior stromal surface is judged to be smooth, the epithelium may be removed manually with a Bard–Parker blade.

A transition zone is usually created during stromal ablation. It is intended to allow smooth and uniform re-epithelialization over the ablation bed. This procedure is referred to as *standard taper* ablation. Sher et al used a "smoothing" technique in their early cases, wherein the eye was moved in a circular manner under the laser beam.[16] A similar "polish technique" was used in the Summit excimer laser clinical trials. The surgeon moved the patient's head in a controlled, circular manner under the laser beam to "polish" the corneal surface.[17,18] Stark et al described a "modified taper" technique, wherein the surgeon attempts to decrease central flattening by moving the eye under the laser in a circular fashion and treating the circumference of the ablation zone with a 20 μm–deep, 2-mm–diameter spot size.[1] This edge modification creates a ring-shaped ablation pattern at the periphery of the PTK to reduce the

TABLE 38–1. TYPICAL LASER PARAMETERS FOR PHOTOTHERAPEUTIC KERATECTOMY

	VISX Twenty/Twenty; Star	Summit ExciMed 200	Meditec LV 2000	Technolos Keracor 116
Fluence (mJ/cm²)	160 ± 10	180	250	120–200
Repetition rate (Hz)	5; 6	10	20	10
Ablation rate (μm/pulse)	0.20–0.27	0.25	0.5	—
Ablation diameter (mm)	5.5–6, including 0.5-mm transition zone	6.5	7.0	7.0

Source: Modified from Azar DT, Jain S, Woods K, et al. Phototherapeutic keratectomy: the VISX experience. In: Salz JJ, McDonnell PJ, McDonald MB, eds. *Corneal Laser Surgery.* St. Louis, MO: Mosby-Year Book; 1995:213–226.

hyperopic shift that is often seen after PTK. When corneal opacities or irregularities are associated with myopic refractive errors, a combination of PTK and PRK should be considered. By allowing for approximately 1 diopter of hyperopic shift for every 20 μm of stromal ablation, the need for PRK to correct any myopic refractive error is reduced. Talamo et al have described clinical treatment strategies for optimizing the successful application of PTK to treat superficial corneal pathology.[19] Table 38–2 summarizes this approach.

Multiple Surface Irregularities

Following epithelial removal, whether manually or using the laser, a masking fluid (1% hydroxymethylcellulose, 0.5% tetracaine, or Tears Naturale II) is usually applied to improve the smoothness of the stromal surface. The fluid in valleys prevents ablation of underlying tissue, leaving the exposed peaks to be ablated. A highly viscous fluid (2% hydroxymethylcellulose or Healon) does not cover an irregular surface uniformly and tends to partially cover peaks as well as valleys. A fluid of low viscosity tends to expose both peaks and valleys. In addition to creating a smooth corneal surface, masking agents may reduce the amount of induced hyperopia.

Elevated Central Corneal Nodules

Achievement of a smooth ablated surface and of good visual outcome in elevated corneal opacities located at the central optical zone (COZ) is difficult even when surface modulators are used. Several surgeons advocate using a blade to excise the elevated lesion prior to PTK (Figs 38–1, 38–2).[16,19]

TABLE 38–2. STRATEGIES FOR SUCCESSFUL PHOTOTHERAPEUTIC KERATECTOMY

Pathologic Lesion	Epithelial Removal	Ablation Technique	Masking Fluid
Elevated, focal	No	Small spot size	Preoperatively, to adjacent normal epithelium
Extensive, evenly distributed	No	Large spot size "Smoothing" head rotation	Intraoperatively, if irregularities are increasing
Multiple, unevenly distributed	Yes	Varying spot size	Repeated focal application

Source: Azar DT, Jain S, Woods K, et al. Phototherapeutic keratectomy: the VISX experience. In: Salz JJ, McDonnell PJ, McDonald MB, eds. *Corneal Laser Surgery.* St. Louis, MO: Mosby-Year Book; 1995:213–226.

We present a case report illustrating a surgical technique utilizing epithelial debridement to create a depression around the lesion, followed by application of surface modulators to fill the annular furrow around the lesion before laser treatment. This technique may result in removal of the elevated central corneal opacity and improve postop visual acuity.

Corneal Dystrophies

Conventional surgical methods of treating corneal dystrophies include lamellar and penetrating keratoplasty. Recurrence of the primary pathology in the corneal graft is not uncommon. Patients with superficial corneal lesions as in epithelial and basement membrane dystrophies (Schyder, Reis–Buckler, lattice, and Meesmann) may respond well to PTK, thus obviating the need for conventional invasive surgery (Fig 38–3). Patients with recurrent granular or lattice dystrophy in a graft have relatively superficial lesions. The success rate in these cases is very high and is similar to that for primary Reis–Buckler's dystrophy, in which the deposits are limited to Bowman's layer (Fig 38–4).[1] Most patients achieve a relatively smooth ablation bed by treating through the epithelium. For patients with granular dystrophy, the aim is to ablate most of the areas of diffuse haze between the granular deposits and not necessarily all the granular hyaline deposits (Fig 38–5).

Recurrent Corneal Erosions

Conventional surgical methods of treating recurrent corneal erosions include manual epithelial debridement and anterior stromal puncture. Patients suffering from recalcitrant recurrent corneal erosions (not relieved by conventional surgery) may benefit from excimer PTK. The treatment depth is relatively minimal (5 to 10 μm) and is usually limited to the Bowman's layer (Table 38–3). Accordingly, significant postop hyperopic shift is not observed and corneal wound healing is less prolonged. After epithelial debridement, a wet Weck-cell sponge can be used to sweep any residual deposits. In most cases the use of surface modulators before laser ablation is not necessary.

Corneal Scars

Treatment of corneal scars limited to the superficial stroma produces significant improvement of visual function.[1] Visual improvement with deeper postinfectious and posttraumatic scars is less likely to occur for several reasons.[16,20] The scar may ablate at a different

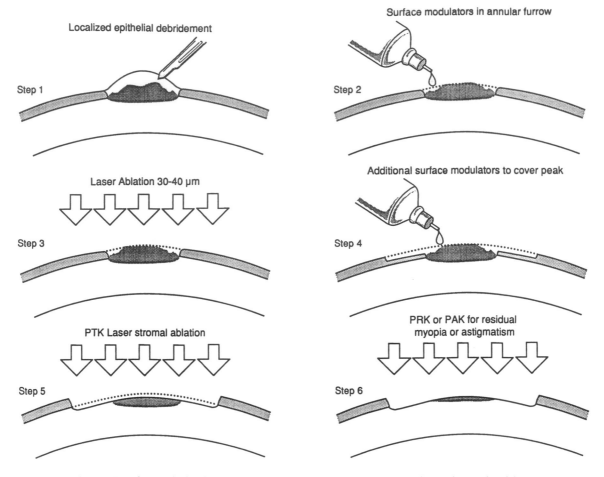

Step 1 — Localized epithelial debridement

Step 2 — Surface modulators in annular furrow

Step 3 — Laser Ablation 30-40 µm

Step 4 — Additional surface modulators to cover peak

Step 5 — PTK Laser stromal ablation

Step 6 — PRK or PAK for residual myopia or astigmatism

Figure 38–1. Schematic drawings of the surgical techniques of PTK for elevated central corneal nodules.

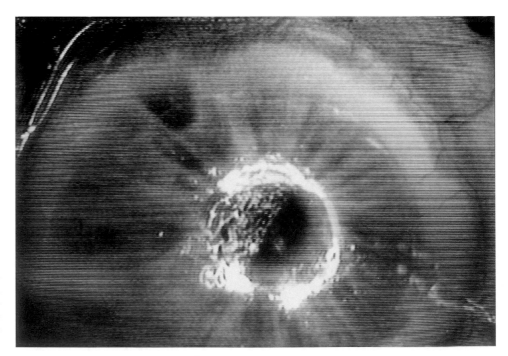

Figure 38–2. The epithelium overlying the elevated corneal nodule is scraped with blade before applying surface modulators. The postoperative outcome is shown in Figure 38–6.

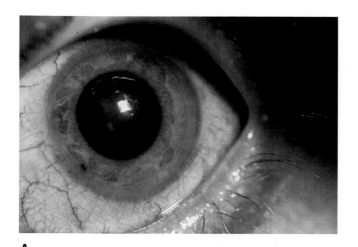

A

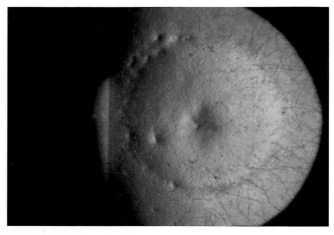

B

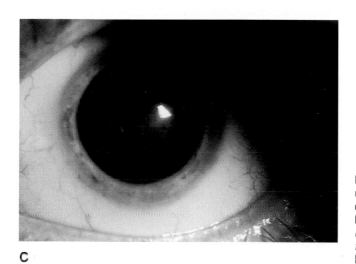

C

Figure 38–3. A 31-year-old man with a history of corneal lattice dystrophy underwent PTK. Preop BCVA was 20/200. **A.** 75-μm stromal depth after epithelial ablation. **B.** Appearance of cornea 3 months after PTK by retroillumination. **C.** Marked improvement 24 months postoperatively. *(Reproduced from Azar DT, Jain S, Woods K, et al. Phototherapeutic keratectomy: the VISX experience. In: Salz JJ, McDonnell PJ, McDonald MB, eds.* Corneal Laser Surgery. *St. Louis, MO: Mosby-Year Book; 1995:213–226.)*

TABLE 38–3. RECURRENT CORNEAL EROSIONS

Study	Laser	Eyes	Phototherapeutic Keratectomy	Follow-up (mo)	Success after Treatment	
					Initial	*Retreatment*
Ohman[32]	Summit VISX	76	1. Epithelial debridement & 3 or 5 μm PTK 2. 20 μm PTK through intact epithelium	16.3	56 (74%)	70 (92%)
Dausch[33]	Meditec (800 mJ/cm²)	74	1. 1–3 μm PTK at epithelial defect sites 2. 30–40 μm PTK at marginal epithelium	21.1	55 (74%)	—
Fagerholm[34]	Summit	37	Epithelial debridement & 3 μm PTK	11.8	31 (84%)	37 (100%)
Forster[35]	Summit	9	Epithelial debridement & 3–4 μm PTK	6.0	8 (89%)	—
Rapuano[36,37]	VISX	3	—	9.0	3 (100%)	—
John[38]	Summit	2	Epithelial debridement & 3–4 μm PTK	18.0	2 (100%)	—
Sher[16]	Taunton	1	Epithelial debridement & 30 μm PTK (simultaneous corneal scar removal)	10.0	1 (100%)	—
Hersh[39]	Summit	1	Epithelial debridement & 3.8 μm PTK	4.0	1 (100%)	—

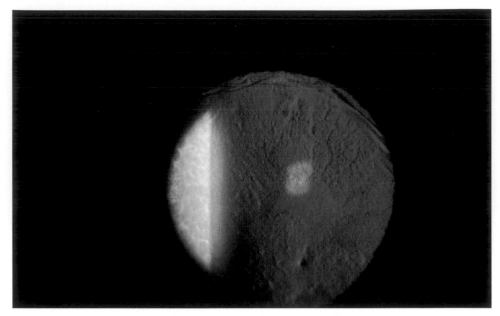

A

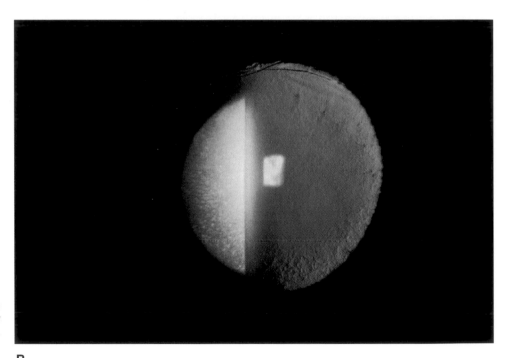

Figure 38–4. Reis–Buckler's dystrophy. **A.** Pre-PTK. **B.** Three months postoperatively. *(Reproduced from Chamon W, Azar DT, Stark WJ, Reed C, Enger C. Phototherapeutic keratectomy. Ophthalmol Clin North Am. 1993;6:399–413.)*

B

rate than the adjacent normal stroma, which may not benefit from laser ablation. This and the presence of calcified or cartilaginous tissue may result in postop irregular astigmatism. Peripheral elevated nodules may be treated with laser ablation after truncation with sharp blades. Central elevated nodules remain a major operative challenge.

Postop Management

Postop medications include prophylactic antibiotics and anti-inflammatory agents. Sub-Tenon's injection of gentamicin and dexamethasone is given immediately postoperatively. After topical application of antibiotic ointment (bacitracin and erythromycin) and instillation

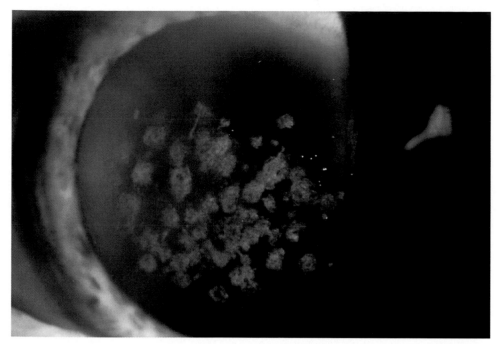

A

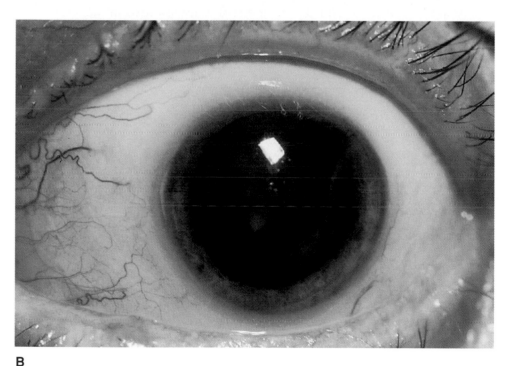

B

Figure 38–5. A 73-year-old woman with a history of granular dystrophy. The left eye was treated with 40 μm of stromal ablation combined with a modified tapering procedure. **A.** Preop clinical appearance of granular dystrophy. **B.** Nine months postoperatively. *(Reproduced from Azar DT, Jain S, Woods K, et al. Phototherapeutic keratectomy: the VISX experience. In: Salz JJ, McDonnell PJ, McDonald MB, eds. Corneal Laser Surgery. St. Louis, MO: Mosby-Year Book; 1995:213–226.)*

of a cycloplegic agent (homatropine), the eye is patched. Alternatively, a therapeutic soft contact lens is applied with frequent application of comparable medications. Since the patient may experience severe pain in the first 24 hours, topical nonsteroidal anti-inflammatory agents (NSAIDs) and systemic sedative-analgesics may be needed for the first few days. One percent (1%) prednisolone acetate or 0.1% fluoromethalone drops are used QID for 1 week and then tapered to once daily by 1 month. The benefits of continued steroid drops may be outweighed by potential side effects, such as steroid responsiveness.

Most protocols require patients to be examined every 24 to 48 hours until re-epithelialization, and then at 1 month, 3 months, 6 months, 12 months, and 24 months. Re-epithelialization occurs within 1 week in most patients. Following re-epithelialization, the post-op examination at each visit includes symptomatic evaluation, a detailed anterior segment examination, and slit lamp biomicroscopy. In addition, all measurements (visual acuity, ocular pressure, etc) taken during the preop evaluation are repeated.

Corneal haze can be graded subjectively using slit lamp biomicroscopic examination as follows: 0 = clear; 0.5 = barely detectable; 1.0 = mild, not affecting refraction; 1.5 = mildly affecting refraction; 2.0 = moderate, refraction possible but difficult; 3.0 = opacity preventing refraction, anterior chamber easily viewed; 4.0 = impaired view of anterior chamber; and 5.0 = inability to see the anterior chamber. The cornea is divided into five hypothetical layers (superficial and deep epithelium, anterior and posterior stroma, and endothelium), and each layer is graded separately. Subjective methods of grading corneal haze are not accurate and reproducible, and suffer from interobserver variability and bias. Objective methods assess the magnitude of haze by measuring corneal light scattering. In collaboration with Dr Russell McCally of the Applied Physics Laboratory at Johns Hopkins, we have developed an instrument for the objective measurement of haze. The "scatterometer" is a modified slit lamp microscope that measures back-scattered light from a defined region of the cornea under standardized illumination conditions. Corneal light scattering is related to the degree of stromal scarring following excimer laser ablations. This instrument has been tested on laboratory animals and humans and found to yield reproducible results.[21] Both objective and subjective postop corneal clarity scores are usually lower than preop scores after PTK.

CORNEAL WOUND HEALING AFTER PHOTOTHERAPEUTIC KERATECTOMY

Reformation of basement membrane complexes and reestablishment of the basement membrane usually follow epithelial scrape wounds, resulting in a smooth epithelial surface with minimal stromal scarring.[1,6,22–24] Re-epithelialization after excimer PTK usually occurs within the first week.[1–6,9,25,26] Anchorage of the epithe-

TABLE 38–4. PHOTOTHERAPEUTIC KERATECTOMY IN CORNEAL DISEASES

Pathology	Excimer Laser Used				Eyes	Follow-up (mo)	Success (%)	References
	VISX	Summit	Meditec	Taunton				
Recurrent epithelial erosions	+	+	+	+	203	16.5	77	32–39
Corneal dystrophies								
Reis–Buckler's	+	+	−	+	32	6.2	100	36, 37, 39–44
Lattice	+	+	−	−	25	11.0	92	1, 20, 39, 44
Granular	+	+	−	+	20	7.2	70	1, 16, 20, 36, 37, 42, 44
Salzmann's nodular	+	+	−	+	12	8.6	67	1, 16, 36, 37, 39
Map–dot–fingerprint	+	+	−	−	10	5.2	100	20, 44
Schnyder's	+	+	−	−	6	6.0	67	36, 37, 44
Avellino	−	−	+	−	1	12.0	100	45
Gelatinous droplike	−	+	−	−	1	4.0	100	46
Meesmann's	+	+	−	−	2	9.0	100	44
Fuch's endothelial	+	+	−	−	1	9.0	100	44
Corneal scars								
Postinfectious	+	+	−	+	12	8.5	50	16, 20, 42
Posttraumatic	+	+	−	+	23	11.1	61	16, 20, 34–37
Herpetic	+	+	−	+	24	15.0	71	16, 30, 47
Trachomatous	−	+	−	−	3	6.0	67	48
Pterygium	+	+	−	+	10	11.2	80	16, 34, 36, 37, 39, 42
Stevens–Johnson syndrome	−	+	−	−	3	11.7	67	34
Contact-lens-wear related	+	+	−	−	2	3.0	50	37, 39
Unknown etiology	+	+	−	−	12	14.6	50	1, 31, 37, 39, 49
Corneal irregularities								
Band keratopathy	+	+	−	+	136	12.3	91	16, 20, 34, 39, 50
Apical scars in keratoconus	+	+	−	−	21	9.7	81	16, 34, 36, 37, 51, 52
Corneal intraepithelial dysplasia	−	−	+	−	1	26.0	100	53

lium to the stroma is achieved 1 to 3 months later, after adequate deposition of the adhesion structures (hemidesmosomes, basal lamina, and anchoring fibrils) of the new epithelium to the underlying stroma.[3,27]

Stromal wound healing occurs after formation of new corneal epithelium and while the adhesion structures are reforming. Some reports have noted that a pseudomembrane forms almost immediately after surgery. The pseudomembrane is thought to help hyperplastic migrating epithelial cells to fill in the wound and create a smooth epithelial surface.[3,25] Epithelial hyperplasia and stromal collagen deposition help restore the original corneal surface contour of shallow wounds.[1,5,25] Generally, hyperplasia takes place in deeper ablations and when there are apparent irregularities in the stromal bed.[23,24,26]

After re-epithelialization, a hypercellular zone of keratocytes is evident at the wound margins and within the anterior stroma.[3,26] A residual depression persists after deep PTK despite deposition of newly synthesized collagen by the keratocytes.[23,24]

Following surgery the cornea may remain hazy for several months. Haze may result from the deposition of new irregular collagen fibers or from light scattering by "activated" keratocytes in the wound.[2,5,6,25] Postop treatment with steroids may reduce the thickness of the subepithelial layer of collagen and the density of subepithelial scarring.[5] Haze usually decreases after the 3- to 6-month period following surgery.[5,26]

When ablations are within 40 mm from Descemet's membrane, there is a loss of endothelial cells.[6,7] This may be related to acoustic or shock waves, and high pulse energy or resonance in the posterior cornea.[3,7,28] There is no evidence so far of endothelial cell loss or displacement if the ablations stay 40 mm above Descemet's membrane.[6,28,29]

CLINICAL OUTCOME

Clinical Study Background

To date, clinical outcomes of approximately 600 eyes, treated for various corneal diseases with excimer laser PTK, have been reported in 26 published reports (Tables 38–4 and 38–5). Four excimer lasers have been used: Twenty/Twenty (VISX Inc, Santa Clara, CA), LV 2000 (Taunton Technologies Co, Monroe, CT [now VISX 20/15]), ExciMed 200 (Summit Technologies Inc, Waltham,

TABLE 38–5. RESULTS OF MAJOR PHOTOTHERAPEUTIC KERATECTOMY STUDIES

	Sher[16] (1991)	Chamon[31] (1993)	Campos[20] (1993)	Sanders[9] (1995)	Durrie[18] (1995)
Excimer laser	Taunton LV 2000	VISX Twenty/Twenty	VISX Twenty/Twenty	VISX Twenty/Twenty	Summit ExciMed 200
Ablation technique	Myopic Combined Smoothing	Standard taper Modified taper	Uniform depth (disc ablation)	Uniform depth Standard taper Modified taper	Polish technique
Visual acuity (%)					
Better	48	74	61	80	67
Unchanged	36	16	28	10	28
Worse	15	10	11	10	11
Hyperopic shift (%)	50	Greater in standard taper	56	Greater in early treatments	20[a]
Best results >75% success	Keratoconus (apical scar)	Corneal dystrophies (lattice, granular, Reis–Buckler's) Salzmann's degeneration	Corneal dystrophies (lattice, granular, map–dot–fingerprint)	—	Corneal dystrophies (lattice, Schnyder's, Reis–Buckler's) Recurrent erosions
Moderate results 50% to 75% success	Corneal dystrophies Corneal scars Salzmann's nodule	Corneal scars Surgically induced myopia	—	—	Corneal scars Salzmann's nodule
Poor results <25% success	Band keratopathy Recurrent erosions Herpetic scars	Band keratopathy Recurrent erosions	Band keratopathy Corneal scars	—	—

[a]Data calculated from scatterplot.
Source: Modified from Azar DT, Jain S, Woods K, et al. Phototherapeutic keratectomy: the VISX experience. In: Salz JJ, McDonnell PJ, McDonald MB, eds. *Corneal Laser Surgery.* St. Louis, MO: Mosby-Year Book; 1995:213–226.

MA), and MEL 50 (Aesculap Meditec, Heroldsberg, Germany). Thirty-six percent (203) eyes were treated for recurrent corneal erosions, 20% (110) for corneal dystrophies, 16% (89) for corneal scars, 28% (157) for corneal irregularities, and 1 eye for recurrent corneal intraepithelial dysplasia. Success rates refer to the functional improvement of several parameters (visual acuity, corneal clarity, patient comfort, or cosmetic appearance) based on the goals of treatment. Because of the heterogenicity of corneal pathologies treated with PTK, no single parameter can reliably estimate the success rate.

Recurrent Epithelial Erosions and Corneal Dystrophies

Functional improvement was achieved in 77% of the 203 eyes after the initial treatment of recurrent epithelial erosions with PTK (Table 38–3). In two studies the success rate improved to 95% (107/113) with retreatment. Corneal dystrophies and degenerations that have been treated with PTK to improve visual function or comfort include: dystrophies of the epithelium and basement membrane (map–dot–fingerprint and Mees-

mann's), dystrophies of Bowman's layer (Reis–Buckler's Table 38–6), granular dystrophy (Table 38–7), lattice dystrophy (Table 38–8) and other stromal dystrophies (gelatinous droplike, macular, Schnyder), endothelial dystrophies (Fuch's), and Salzmann's nodular degeneration (Table 38–9). Greater success has been achieved in superficial corneal dystrophies like map–dot–fingerprint (100%), Meesmann's (100%), and Reis–Buckler's dystrophy (100%) than in stromal dystrophies like granular (67%), lattice (92%), and Schnyder's dystrophy (67%).

Corneal Scars

Corneal scars that have been successfully treated with PTK to improve visual function include: postinfectious (Table 38–10), posttraumatic (Table 38–11), herpetic (Table 38–12), trachomatous, and pterygium-related (Table 38–13). The success rate varies from 50% to 80%. Greater success has been achieved in superficial corneal scars such as those following pterygium surgery (80%) than in deeper postinfectious (50%) and posttraumatic scars (61%). One report has shown a high success rate

TABLE 38–6. REIS–BUCKLER'S DYSTROPHY

Study	Laser	Eyes	Phototherapeutic Keratectomy	Follow-up (mo)	Success (%)	Hyperopic Shift	
						Eyes (%)	Range (D)
Rogers[40]	Summit	11	Hydroxymethylcellulose (0.5%) Fluorescence-guided epithelial ablation PTK (19–63 μm) focal technique	6	100	100	0.25–7.0
Lawless[41]	Summit	9	Hydroxymethylcellulose (0.5%) Fluorescence-guided epithelial ablation PTK (18–60 μm) focal technique	6	100	78	0.25–8.0
Hahn[42]	Summit	2	Hydroxymethylcellulose (1.0%) Mechanical epithelial debridement PTK (50 μm) focal technique	10	100	100	0.5–1.5
Hersh[39]	Summit	2	Hydroxymethylcellulose (1.0%) Epithelial debridement/ablation PTK smoothing technique	4	100	100	up to 7.0
McDonnell[43]	Summit	1	Epithelial ablation PTK (100 μm) smoothing technique PRK −4 D	6	100	100	10.75
	VISX	1	Epithelial ablation PTK (100 μm) focal technique	6	100	100	3.8
Sher[16]	Taunton	1	Mechanical epithelial debridement PTK (50 μm) (combined "myopic & hyperopic" cut)	6	100	100	7.25
Rapuano[36,37]	VISX	1	Mechanical epithelial debridement PTK focal technique	3	100	100	1.25
Orndahl[44]	Summit VISX	2	—	9	100	—	—
Stark[1]	VISX	2	—	—	100	—	—

TABLE 38–7. GRANULAR DYSTROPHY

Study	Laser	Eyes	Photptherapeutic Keratectomy	Follow-up (mo)	Success (%)	Hyperopic Shift Eyes (%)	Hyperopic Shift Range (D)
Hahn[42]	Summit	2	Hydroxymethylcellulose (1.0%) Mechanical epithelial debridement PTK (40 μm) focal technique	8.3	66	66	Up to 2.0
Sher[16]	Taunton	2	Mechanical epithelial debridement PTK (50 μm) (Combined "myopic & hyperopic" cut)	6.0	0	100	0.3–1.1
Rapuano[36,37]	VISX	6	Epithelial debridement/ablation PTK disciform/elliptical	8.3	83	66	0.62–2.0
Orndahl[44]	Summit VISX	4	Fluorescence-guided epithelial ablation PTK (45 μm)	12.0	75	—	Up to 2.0
Stark[1]	VISX	4	PTK standard taper/modified taper	—	75	—	—
Campos[20]	VISX	1	Epithelial debridement PTK (110 μm) disciform	24.0	100		

in treating herpetic scars (80%). Despite the reported success, several investigators caution against using the excimer laser in herpetic disease because of the risk of recurrence.[1,20,24,30]

Central Elevated Corneal Nodules

We used the technique described in Figure 38–1 to treat an 87-year-old white woman with a central Salzmann's nodule and irregular astigmatism in the right eye. She had undergone cataract extraction and posterior chamber lens implantation 9 years earlier and also had received lamellar keratectomy for a Salzmann's nodular degeneration of the right cornea. At initial presentation, her best corrected visual acuity (BCVA) was 20/400 (+1.25 +3.00 × 145 correction) in the right eye and 20/20 in the left eye. Hard contact lenses improved her visual acuity to 20/50 OD. On slit lamp examination, the cornea had linear elevated subepithelial opacities 1 to 2 mm from the visual axis (Fig 38–2). Superficial

punctate keratitis was noted around the opacities. Corneal topography showed localized +5 D steepening over the opacities. Fundus examination showed age-related macular degeneration and mild epiretinal membrane. Intraocular pressure (IOP) and other ocular findings were within normal limits. PTK was performed as described above using ArF excimer (fluence: 160 mJ/cm^2; repetition rate: 5 Hz; epithelial ablation rate: 0.24 μm/pulse; stromal ablation rate: 0.27 μm/pulse) followed by photoastigmatic keratectomy (cylindrical correction). After PTK, the corneal surface appeared smooth. The central elevated opacity noted preoperatively had disappeared (Fig 38–6). Anterior stromal haze was barely detectable throughout the 12-month follow-up period.

Corneal Irregularities

Corneal scars that have been successfully treated with PTK to improve visual function include: band kerato-

TABLE 38–8. LATTICE DYSTROPHY

Study	Laser	Eyes	Phototherapeutic Keratectomy	Follow-up (mo)	Success (%)	Hyperopic Shift Eyes (%)	Hyperopic Shift Range (D)
Hersh[42]	Summit	1	Hydroxymethylcellulose (1.0%) Epithelial debridement/ablation PTK smoothing technique	4	100	0	—
Orndahl[44]	Summit VISX	11	Fluorescence-guided epithelial ablation PTK (45 μm)	12	90	—	Up to 2.0
Stark[1]	VISX	11	PTK standard/modified taper	—	90	—	—
Campos[20]	VISX	2	Mechanical epithelial debridement PTK (100–110 μm); disciform	10	100	100	3.0–8.2

TABLE 38–9. SALZMANN'S NODULAR DEGENERATION

Study	Laser	Eyes	Photocherapeutic Keratectomy	Follow-up (mo)	Success (%)	Hyperopic Shift Eyes (%)	Hyperopic Shift Range (D)
Sher[16]	Taunton	5	Epithelial debridement (1)/intact (4) PTK (40–80 μm) Combined (3)/myopic (1)/smoothing (1)	7.2	60	20	2.62
Rapuano[36,37]	VISX	3	Mechanical epithelial debridement PTK disciform/elliptical	14	66	100	1.0–5.2
Stark[1]	VISX	2	PTK standard taper/modified taper	—	100	—	—
Hersh[39]	Summit	2	Focal epithelial debridement PTK focal technique	4	100	0	—

TABLE 38–10. POSTINFECTIOUS SCAR

Study	Laser	Eyes	Photocherapeutic Keratectomy	Follow-up (mo)	Success (%)
Hahn[42]	Summit	1	Hydroxymethylcellulose (1.0%) Mechanical epithelial debridement PTK (75 μm) smoothing technique	12.0	100
Sher[16]	Taunton	5	Epithelial debridement/intact PTK (50–150 μm) combined/myopic	8.4	60
Campos[20]	VISX	6	Epithelial debridement/ablation	8.0	33

TABLE 38–11. POSTTRAUMATIC SCAR

Study	Laser	Eyes	Photocherapeutic Keratectomy	Follow-up (mo)	Success (%)
Campos[20]	VISX	4	Epithelial debridement/ablation PTK, disciform	9.0	50
Sher[16]	Taunton	8	Mechanical epithelial debridement PTK (50–220 μm) combined/myopic	6.7	62
Fagerholm[34]	Summit	9	Methylcellulose/sodium hyaluronate PTK focal technique	15.2	66
Forster[35]	Summit	1		4.0	100
Rapuano[36,37]	VISX	1		3.0	0

TABLE 38–12. HERPETIC KERATITIS

Study	Laser	Eyes	Photocherapeutic Keratectomy	Follow-up (mo)	Success (%)	Recurrences (%)
Fagerholm[34]	Summit VISX	20	Surface modulator: tetracain Epithelial debridement/ablation PTK disciform	16.8	80	25
Sher[16]	Taunton	4	Mechanical epithelial debridement PTK (50–140 μm) combined/myopic	6	25	—

TABLE 38–13. POSTPTERYGIUM SCAR

Study	Laser	Eyes	Phototherapeutic Keratectomy	Follow-up (mo)	Success (%)
Hahn[42]	Summit	1	Hydroxymethylcellulose (1.0%) Mechanical epithelial debridement PTK (80 μm) smoothing technique	7.0	100
Sher[16]	Taunton	2	Intact epithelium PTK (50 μm) smoothing technique	12.0	50
Hersh[39]	Summit	1	Hydroxymethylcellulose (1.0%) Epithelial debridement/ablation PTK smoothing technique	4.0	100
Rapuano[36,37]	VISX	1	Epithelial debridement/ablation PTK disciform/elliptical	3.0	100
Fagerholm[34]	Summit	5	Methylcellulose/sodium hyaluronate PTK focal technique	15.2	80

pathy (smooth and rough) and apical scars in keratoconus (proud nebulae). Of the 136 eyes treated for band keratopathy, 91% improved (Table 38–14), while 81% of the 21 eyes treated for apical scars in keratoconus improved. As opposed to O'Brart's high success rate (113/122) in treating band keratopathy, other investigators have had little success.[16,20] The use of EDTA is still the standard treatment for this condition.[1,16,20–24]

Results of Major Clinical Studies

Representative postop results published in the four major reports are summarized in Table 38–5. The data comparing preop to post BCVA accumulated by Sanders from 271 consecutive PTK cases at 17 VISX US centers shows that the average improvement in BCVA

was 1.8 lines ($P < .001$).[9] Ten percent (10%) of patients lost two or more lines of BCVA, while 45% gained two or more lines. Seven percent (7%) of the patients lost three or more lines, while 36% gained that much. Analysis of the reasons for decreases in BCVA showed corneal surface irregularity induced by PTK accounting for only 3% of cases. Two or more lines of improvement of uncorrected visual acuity (UCVA) were seen in 42% to 44% of patients, as opposed to reduction in 18% to 19%. Based on the dates of treatment, Sanders divided the 271 patients treated at US VISX centers into quartiles.[9,24] He found that the first quartile had an average of 5.5 D of hyperopic effect, and the last quartile had less than 2D of hyperopia. The percentages of patients in Sanders's review who experienced moderate to severe levels of pain and

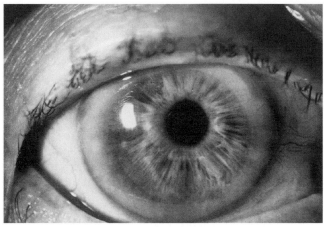

A

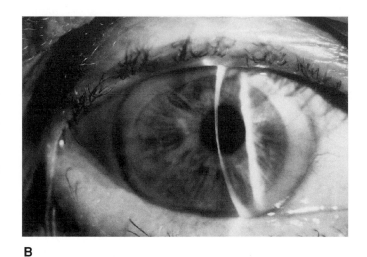

B

Figure 38–6. Postoperative appearance of patient shown in Figure 38–2. After PTK, the corneal surface appeared smooth. The linear elevated opacity noted preoperatively had disappeared by direct **(A)** and slit lamp **(B)** biomicroscopy.

TABLE 38–14. BAND KERATOPATHY

Study	Laser	Eyes	Phototherapeutic Keratectomy	Follow-up (mo)	Success (%)
O'Brart[50]	Summit	122	—	12.3	93
Hahn[42]	Summit	1	Hydroxymethylcellulose (1.0%) Mechanical epithelial debridement PTK (50 μm) focal technique	7.0	100
Hersh[39]	Summit	1	Hydroxymethylcellulose (1.0%) Epithelial debridement/ablation	4.0	100
Sher[16]	Taunton	3	Mechanical epithelial debridement PTK (50 μm) (Combined "myopic & hyperopic" cut)	6.0	7
Fagerholm[34]	Summit	8	—	18.3	87
Campos[20]	VISX	1	—	6.0	0

tearing before treatment were 10% and 8%, respectively. Of these patients, only one experienced postop tearing; the rest improved. Similarly, there was no significant worsening of photophobia, redness, or foreign body sensation. The effect of PTK on patients with moderate to severe epithelial corneal opacities shows that 86% to 88% of patients improved following treatment, and in only 1% did the condition worsen. Sixty percent (60%) to 62% of patients with anterior stromal opacities improved after treatment, and 2% worsened.[24]

Sher and colleagues reported that 15% of their patients lost two or more lines of spectacle-corrected visual acuity following PTK.[16] Chamon, Azar, Stark et al from the Wilmer Ophthalmological Institute have reported a 3% loss of one line of functional visual acuity, defined as the acuity achieved with the visual aid that a patient is wearing: either contact lenses or spectacles.[31] The mean preop visual acuity (logarithmic) was 20/92, and the mean postop visual acuity was 20/47 using manifest refraction. In 80% of patients, spectacle-corrected visual acuity had improved one line or more at the most recent follow-up visit. Four patients became contact lens tolerant after PTK.[31] Eyes treated with the standard 0.5-mm taper had an average of 5.11 and 5.28 D of induced hyperopia at 3 and 36 months, respectively. Eyes treated with the modified taper showed a trend toward a decreasing amount of induced hyperopia.[31] Chamon et al observed a positive correlation between depth of stromal ablation and amount of induced hyperopia.[31] Campos et al performed PTK on 18 eyes.[20] The follow-up ranged from 2 to 18 months, with a mean of 8 months. Corneal clarity improved in 77.7% of the patients, while 22.2% did not experience any improvement. In 61.1% of the patients, UCVA improved. An induced flattening was observed in all patients, and

a hyperopic shift was observed in 55.5%. This induced hyperopia was observed to decrease by the 6-month and 1-year follow-ups. Patients with band keratopathy and corneal calcification who underwent PTK did not experience any visual improvement.[20] Durrie et al have reported 3- to 21-month follow-up data from 67 procedures performed in phase II and phase III Summit Excimed excimer laser clinical trials for PTK.[18] BCVA improved in 67% of eyes, and 20% of eyes lost at least one line of BCVA. Hyperopic shift was noted in 19% of eyes, and there was an average reduction of corneal cylinder postoperatively.[18]

SIDE EFFECTS AND COMPLICATIONS

Delayed corneal wound healing can follow PTK.[1,2] Stark et al reported two patients in whom corneal re-epithelialization took 3 to 4 weeks, compared to 1 week or less for other patients.[1] Delayed wound healing following PTK may be associated with corneal haze, recurrent erosions, infections, corneal ulcers, and persistent epithelial defects.[1,7]

Postop pain may be severe during the first 24 to 48 hours. In some patients, moderate to severe pain may occur for several days after surgery. It is generally relieved by the time the epithelium heals. Cycloplegics, ice packs, peribulbar or retrobulbar anesthesia, narcotics, and disposable soft contact lenses may be helpful. The use of topical nonsteroidal agents like 0.1% diclofenac sodium (Voltaren Ophthalmic, CIBA Vision Ophthalmics, Atlanta, GA) in the immediate postop period has significantly reduced postop pain.

Flattening of the central cornea appears to be the principal side effect of PTK. Hyperopia is induced as a result of the corneal flattening. It may require the use of contact lenses postoperatively. Four potential mechanisms for the hyperopic shift have been hypothesized:

1. greater degrees of epithelial hyperplasia and tear film thickness at the edge of ablation;
2. greater ablation centrally if the corneal pathology thins progressively toward the visual axis;
3. greater shielding of the stroma toward the edge of the ablated zone by the ablation products ('plume'); and
4. oblique angle of incident radiation falling on more peripheral cornea, resulting in a decreased peripheral ablation[22,31,54]

The use of appropriate masking agents may minimize the hyperopic shift. Other strategies include the modified taper technique of Stark and colleagues[1] or Sher's technique of preprogramming the Taunton laser system to cut a secondary hyperopic correction ("combined" ablation).[16]

DNA damage is another potential side effect of PTK that may result from the 193-nm UV radiation or from thermal loading.[28,29,55] The shorter penetration depth of direct 193-nm excimer laser radiation, and the minimal fluorescent emission of longer UV wavelengths for energy exposures used in clinical applications, makes the potential side effects and risks of PTK very limited and remote in subablative laser energy.[56]

PTK has been less successful than initially expected in the treatment of infectious keratitis because of the possibility of spread of infectious agents during and following treatment. Reactivation of latent herpes simplex virus has been reported following excimer PTK. Involvement of the stroma in most microorganism infections extends deeper than the clinically observable lesion. As the tissue penetration depth of 193-nm radiation is no more than 1 mm, deep stromal infiltration may limit the effectiveness of treatment of infectious keratitis with the excimer laser.

Long-standing posttraumatic superficial stromal scars may prove resistant to ablation.[49] This complication may be minimized by using surface-modulating agents or by the "smoothing" technique. Gentle rotation of the head under the laser beam blends the edges of the irregularities. By maintaining the corneal surface meticulously clear of debris and cellular remnants, further irregularities may be avoided.

If there are many complications or if the eyes do not improve significantly after PTK, the patient may need to undergo more invasive treatment such as corneal transplantation.[1] Many patients who are currently treated with PTK in order to reduce the chance of needing penetrating keratoplasty (PK) end up requiring PK. With further advances in our technique and refinement of PTK indications, the need for PK after PTK will be minimized.

REFERENCES

1. Stark WJ, Chamon W, Kamp MT, Enger CL, Rencs EV, Gottsch JD. Clinical follow-up of 193-nm ArF excimer laser photokeratectomy. *Ophthalmology.* 1992;99:805–811.
2. Salz JJ, Maguen E, Macy JI, Papaioannou T, Hofbauer J, Nesburn AB. One-year results of excimer laser photorefractive keratectomy for myopia. *Refract Corneal Surg.* 1992;8:270–273.
3. Gaster RN, Binder PS, Coalwell K, Berns M, McCord RC, Burstein NL. Corneal surface ablation by 193 nm excimer laser and wound healing in rabbits. *Invest Ophthalmol Vis Sci.* 1989;30:90–97.
4. Trokel SL, Srinivasan R, Braren B. Excimer laser surgery of the cornea. *Am J Ophthalmol.* 1983;96:710–715.
5. Tuft SJ, Zabel RW, Marshall J. Corneal repair following keratectomy. *Invest Ophthalmol Vis Sci.* 1989;30:1769–1777.
6. Marshall J, Trokel S, Rothery S, Krueger RR. Photoablative reprofiling of the cornea using an excimer laser: photorefractive keratectomy. *Lasers Ophthalmol.* 1986;1:23–44.
7. Marshall J, Trokel S, Rothery S, Krueger RR. A comparative study of corneal incisions induced by diamond and steel knives and two ultraviolet radiations from an excimer laser. *Br J Ophthalmol.* 1986;70:482–500.
8. van Setten GB, Koch JW, Tervo K, et al. Expression of tenascin and fibronectin in the rabbit cornea after excimer laser surgery. *Graefe's Arch Clin Exp Ophthalmol.* 1992;230:178–182.
9. Sanders, D. Clinical evaluation of phototherapeutic keratectomy—VISX Twenty/Twenty excimer laser. Submitted to the FDA; 1994. Written communication 2/7/94.
10. Keates RH, Drago PC, Rothchild EJ. Effect of excimer laser on microbiological organisms. *Ophthalmic Surg.* 1988;19:715–718.
11. Gottsch JD, Gilbert ML, Goodman DF, Sulewski ME, Dick JD, Stark WJ. Excimer laser ablative treatment of microbial keratitis. *Ophthalmology.* 1991;98:146–149.
12. Serdarevic O, Darrell RW, Krueger RR, Trokel SL. *Am J Ophthalmol.* 1985;99:534–538.
13. Eiferman RA, Forgey DR, Cook YD. Excimer laser ablation of infectious crystalline keratopathy. *Arch Ophthalmol.* 1992;110:18.
14. Pepose JS, Laycock KA, Miller JK, et al. Reactivation of latent herpes simplex virus by excimer laser photokeratectomy. *Am J Ophthalmol.* 1992;114:45–50.
15. Krueger RR, Campos M, Wang XW, Lee M, McDonnell PJ. *Arch Ophthalmol.* 1993;111:1131–1137.

16. Sher NA, Bowers RA, Zabel RW, et al. Clinical use of 193-nm excimer laser in the treatment of corneal scars. *Arch Ophthalmol.* 1991;109:491–498.

17. Thompson V, Durrie DS, Cavanaugh TB. Philosophy and technique for excimer laser phototherapeutic keratectomy. *Refract Corneal Surg.* 1993;9(2 suppl):81–85. Review.

18. Durrie DS, Schumer JD, Cavanaugh T. Phototherapeutic keratectomy: the VISX experience. In: Salz JJ, McDonnell PJ, McDonald MB, eds. *Corneal Laser Surgery.* St. Louis, MO: Mosby-Year Book; 1995:227–235.

19. Talamo JH, Steinert RF, Puliafito CA. Clinical strategies for excimer laser therapeutic keratectomy. *Refract Corneal Surg.* 1992;8:319–324.

20. Campos M, Nielsen S, Szerenyi K, Garbus JJ, McDonnell PJ. Clinical follow-up of phototherapeutic keratectomy for treatment of corneal opacities. *Am J Ophthalmol.* 1993;115:433–440.

21. McCally RL, Hochheimer BF, Chamon W, Azar DT. A simple device for objective measurement of haze following excimer ablation of cornea. *SPIE Proc.* 1993;1877:20–25.

22. Azar DT, Chamon W, Stark WJ. Phototherapeutic keratectomy. In: Stenson S, ed. *Surgical Management in External Diseases of the Eye.* Tokyo: Igaku-Shoin. 1996:303–319.

23. Azar DT. Epithelial and stromal wound healing following excimer laser keratectomy. *Sem Ophthalmol.* 1994;9:102–105.

24. Azar DT, Jain S, Woods K, et al. Phototherapeutic keratectomy: the VISX experience. In: Salz JJ, McDonnell PJ, McDonald MB, eds. *Corneal Laser Surgery.* St. Louis, MO: Mosby-Year Book; 1995:213–226.

25. Courant D, Fritsch P, Azema A, et al. Corneal wound healing after photo-kerato-mileusis treatment on the primate eye. *Lasers Light Ophthalmol.* 1990;3:189–195.

26. Hanna KD, Pouliquen Y, Waring GO III, et al. Corneal stromal wound healing in rabbits after 193-nm excimer laser surface ablation. *Arch Ophthalmol.* 1989;107:899–900.

27. Fountain TR, De la Cruz Z, Green WR, Stark WJ, Azar DT. Reassembly of corneal epithelial adhesion structures after excimer laser keratectomy in humans. *Arch Ophthalmol.* 1994;112:967–972.

28. Bende T, Seiler T, Wollensak J. Side effects in excimer corneal surgery: corneal thermal gradients. *Graefe's Arch Clin Exp Ophthalmol.* 1988;226:277–280.

29. Ozler SA, Liaw LL, Neev J, Raney D, Berns MW. Acute ultrastructural changes of cornea after excimer laser ablation. *Invest Ophthalmol Vis Sci.* 1992;33:540.

30. Vrabec MP, Anderson JA, Rock ME, et al. Electron microscopic findings in a cornea with recurrence of herpes simplex keratitis after excimer laser phototherapeutic keratectomy. *CLAO J.* 1994;20:41–44.

31. Chamon W, Azar DT, Stark WJ, Reed C, Enger C. Phototherapeutic keratectomy. *Ophthalmol Clin North Am.* 1993;6:399–413.

32. Ohman L, Fagerholm P, Tengroth B. Treatment of recurrent corneal erosions with the excimer laser. *Acta Ophthalmologica.* 1994;72:461–463.

33. Dausch D, Landesz M, Klein R, Schroder E. Phototherapeutic keratectomy in recurrent corneal epithelial erosion. *Refract Corneal Surg.* 1993;9:419–424.

34. Fagerholm P, Fitzsimmons TD, Orndahl M, Ohman L, Tengroth B. Phototherapeutic keratectomy: long-term results in 166 eyes. *Refract Corneal Surg.* 1993;9(2 suppl):76–81.

35. Forster W, Grewe S, Atzler U, Lunecke C, Busse H. Phototherapeutic keratectomy in corneal diseases. *Refract Corneal Surg.* 1993;9(2 suppl):85–90.

36. Rapuano CJ, Laibson PR. Excimer laser phototherapeutic keratectomy. *CLAO J.* 1993;19:235–240.

37. Rapuano CJ, Laibson PR. Excimer laser phototherapeutic keratectomy for anterior corneal pathology. *CLAO J.* 1994;20:253–257.

38. John ME, et al. Excimer laser phototherapeutic keratectomy for treatment of recurrent corneal erosion. *J Cataract Refract Surg.* 1994;20:179–181.

39. Hersh PS, Spinak A, Garrana R, Mayers M. Phototherapeutic keratectomy: strategies and results in 12 eyes. *Refract Corneal Surg.* 1993;9(2 suppl):90–95.

40. Rogers C, Cohen P, Lawless M. Phototherapeutic keratectomy for Reis Buckler's corneal dystrophy. *Aust NZ J Ophthalmol.* 1993;21:247–250.

41. Lawless MA, Cohen PR, Rogers CM. Retreatment of undercorrected photorefractive keratectomy for myopia. *J Refract Corneal Surg.* 1994;10(2 suppl):174–177.

42. Hahn TW, Sah WJ, Kim JH. Phototherapeutic keratectomy in nine eyes with superficial corneal diseases. *Refract Corneal Surg.* 1993;9(2 suppl):115–118.

43. McDonnell PJ, Seiler T. Phototherapeutic keratectomy with excimer laser for Reis-Buckler's corneal dystrophy. *Refract Corneal Surg.* 1992;8:306–310.

44. Orndahl M, Fagerholm P, Fitzsimmons T, Tengroth B. Treatment of corneal dystrophies with excimer laser. *Acta Ophthalmol.* 1994;72:235–240.

45. Cennamo G, Rosa N, Rosenwasser GOD, Sebastiani A. Phototherapeutic keratectomy in the treatment of avellino dystrophy. *Ophthalmologica.* 1994;208:198–200.

46. John ME, Martines E, Cvintal T, Ballew C. Excimer laser photoablation of primary familial amyloidosis of the cornea. *Refract Corneal Surg.* 1993;9(2 suppl):138–141.

47. Fagerholm P, Ohman L, Orndahl M. Phototherapeutic keratectomy in herpes simplex keratitis: clinical results in 20 patients. *Acta Ophthalmol.* 1994;72:457–460.

48. Goldstein M, Loewenstein A, Rosner M, Lipshitz I, Lazar M. Phototherapeutic keratectomy in the treatment of corneal scarring from trachoma. *J Refract Corneal Surg.* 1994;10(2 suppl):290–292.

49. McDonnell JM, Garbus JJ, McDonnell PJ. Unsuccessful excimer laser phototherapeutic keratectomy. Clinicopathologic correlation. *Arch Ophthalmol.* 1992;110:977–979.

50. O'Brart DP, Gartry DS, Lohmann CP, et al. Treatment of band keratopathy by excimer laser phototherapeutic keratectomy: surgical techniques and long term follow up. *Br J Ophthalmol.* 1993;77:702–708.

51. Steinert RF, Puliafito CA. Excimer laser phototherapeutic keratectomy for a corneal nodule. *Refract Corneal Surg.* 1990;6:352.

52. Moodaley L, Liu C, Woodward GE, O'Brart D, Muir MK, Buckley R. Excimer laser superficial keratectomy for proud nebulae in keratoconus. *Br J Ophthalmol.* 1994;78: 454–457.

53. Dausch D, Landesz M, Schroder E. Phototherapeutic keratectomy in recurrent corneal intraepithelial dysplasia. *Arch Ophthalmol.* 1994;112:22–23.

54. Gartry D, Muir MK, Marshall J. Excimer laser treatment of corneal surface pathology: a laboratory and clinical study. *Br J Ophthalmol.* 1991;75:258–269.

55. Seiler T, Bende T, Winckler K, Wollensak J. Side effects in excimer corneal surgery: DNA damage as a result of 193 nm excimer laser radiation. *Graefe's Arch Clin Exp Ophthalmol.* 1988;226:276.

56. Krueger RR, Sliney DH, Trokel SL. Photokeratitis from subablative 193-nanometer excimer laser radiation. *Refract Corneal Surg.* 1992;8:274–279.

CHAPTER 39

Excimer Laser Prismatic Photokeratectomy

Nathalie F. Azar ▪ Dimitri T. Azar

Excimer laser photokeratectomy has been used to correct myopia and astigmatism and to smooth surface irregularities.[1] Each pulse ablates a predictable depth of tissue, resulting in controlled removal of superficial corneal stroma. Animal and human studies have demonstrated well-defined ablations with minimal damage to the adjacent tissue.[2] Complications include regression of the initial refractive effect and development of haze in the visual axis. These complications may be due in part to the postoperative wound-healing response. This study was undertaken to determine the characteristics of the wound-healing response after prismatic photokeratectomy (PPK), a new method of excimer laser ablation that may hold potential for the correction of small-angle strabismic deviations and diplopia. The excimer laser has not been previously used to treat strabismus or diplopia in primates or humans.

Diplopia results from misalignment of the visual axes. One image falls on the fovea of one eye and simultaneously on a nonfoveal point in the other eye. The same object is seen at two different locations in subjective space. In physiologic diplopia, objects outside Panum's area fall on noncorresponding points.

The angle of deviation, PD, can be calculated from the equation:

$$PD = \frac{360(n-1)}{\pi} \cdot \frac{h}{OZ}$$

where: PD is the angle of deviation (prism diopters), n is the index of refraction, h is the maximal ablation depth,

and OZ is the optical zone (diameter of laser ablation).

or PD = 42 · h/OZ

or h = PD · OZ/42

The mechanism of action and principle of prismatic keratectomy have been described. Figure 39–1 shows a schematic of PPK used to correct binocular diplopia. The prismatic correction is proportional to the depth of ablation and inversely proportional to the diameter-of-ablation zone. The healing process that follows the stromal prismatic ablation may alter the final effect depending on how well the epithelial surface conforms to the ablation bed.

Better understanding of the wound-healing response may help refine our ability to use PPK to treat patients with postsurgical and postparetic binocular diplopia. How well the epithelial surface conforms to the curvature of the underlying area of prismatic ablations will ultimately determine the success of this procedure.

EXCIMER LASER DELIVERY SYSTEM

We modified the excimer laser delivery system to achieve the desired corneal contour of prismatic abla-

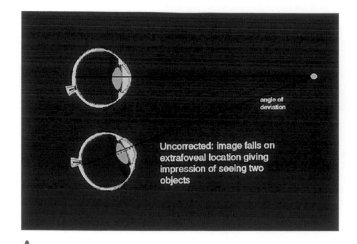

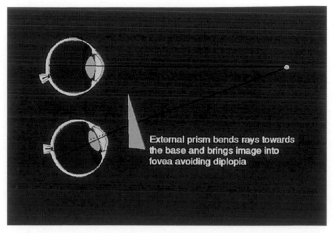

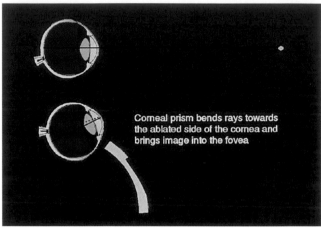

Figure 39–1. Schematic diagram of binocular diplopia **(A)**, corrected with external prism **(B)** or prismatic photokeratectomy **(C)**.

tions (Fig 39–2). We tested this method on PMMA blocks and PMMA model eyes to determine if it results in predictable degrees of prismatic effect. We used the 193-nm argon fluoride laser at fluence of 160 mJ/cm^2 and ablation rate of 5 Hz. Before the prismatic stromal ablations, we removed epithelium with the excimer laser in a 5-mm diameter zone and to a depth of 40 μm. We performed prismatic corneal ablations of 5.0 mm in diameter as follows: deep ablation: 240-μm base-up ablation; intermediate: 120-μm base-up ablation; and superficial: 60-μm base-up ablation.

PPK makes the cornea resemble a curved prism with spherical sides. Theoretical analysis of the optics of prisms with spherical sides and the relationship of the prismatic correction to the diameter of laser ablation and the maximal ablation depth have been described.[3,4] Variable degrees of "small-angle" prismatic correction may be obtained. For instance, a "deep PPK treatment"

(240 μm maximal depth and 5-mm diameter ablation) would induce 2.5 prism diopters (D).

We treated 21 pigmented rabbit eyes with PPK, photorefractive keratectomy (PRK), or phototherapeutic keratectomy (PTK). Animals were anesthetized with intramuscular injections of a 1:1 mixture of ketamine (40 mg/kg body weight) and xylazine (7 mg/kg body weight). Atropine (1%) and proparacaine eyedrops were applied preoperatively. We performed retinoscopy to determine the preoperative refractive error. Animals receiving PPK were divided into the following groups: deep PPK (n=4), intermediate PPK (n=3), and superficial PPK (n=2). Animals treated with −10 D PRK (n=5), −4 D PRK (n=4), and 100-μm PTK (n=4) served as controls. The eyes were irrigated with sterile balanced salt solution (BSS). Topical erythromycin ointment, prednisolone acetate (0.1%), and atropine (1%) were applied daily for 3 days. Animals were anesthe-

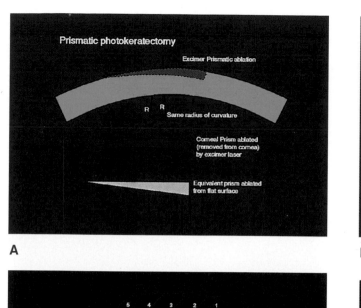

A

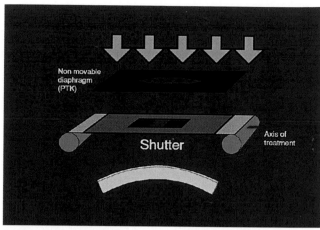

B

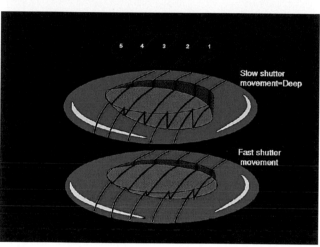

C

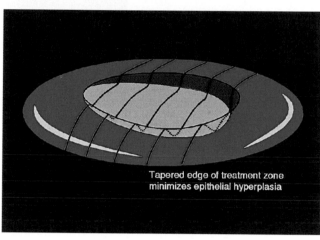

D

Figure 39–2. Prismatic photokeratectomy principle **(A)** and excimer delivery system **(B)** showing the effect of moving the shutter at various rates **(C)**. The optimal treatment **(D)** results from decentering the treatment toward the base and oscillating the circular shutter to create smooth edges.

tized with ketamine (40 mg/kg body weight) and xylazine (7 mg/kg body weight) 9 days and 3, 4, and 5 months after surgery. Atropine (1%) was given topically before biomicroscopic examination to grade corneal haze and determine the refractive error using cycloplegic retinoscopy. External or slit lamp photographs were obtained. Animals were sacrificed with an overdose of pentobarbital at the above time points and their eyes enucleated and processed for histologic examination.

RESULTS

Figure 39–3 illustrates the clinical appearance of eyes treated with the excimer laser. Epithelial wound clo-

sure was complete by 3 days in all the animals except for one animal in the intermediate PPK group (9 days) and one of the −10 D controls (4 days). Table 39–1 summarizes the histologic findings in rabbits treated with PPK and PRK. There were no significant differences in epithelial edema, which followed deeper ablations in the immediate postoperative period in the PPK and PRK groups. Stromal subepithelial haze after PPK was not as pronounced as that seen after PRK or PTK.

Epithelial hyperplasia and subepithelial scarring were seen at the deep edges and were more pronounced with 240-μm PPK treatment (Fig 39–4). Reduced epithelial thickness in the central area was observed at 9 days. At 4 and 5 months, epithelium appeared normal in the central area. The treatment ar-

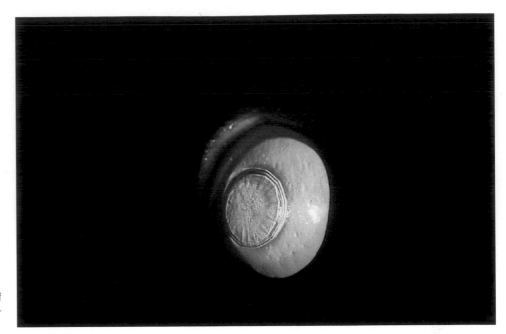

Figure 39–3. Clinical appearance of eyes treated with prismatic photokeratectomy.

TABLE 39–1. EPITHELIAL EDEMA AND STROMAL HAZE AFTER PHOTOPRISMATIC KERATECTOMY AND PHOTOREFRACTIVE KERATECTOMY

	PPK			PRK	
	60 μm	120 μm	240 μm	−4 D	−10 D
Epithelial edema					
9 days	0	0	±	0	±
121 days	0	0	0	0	0
Stromal edema					
9 days	0	1/3	1/4	+	+
121 days	0	0	0	±	+

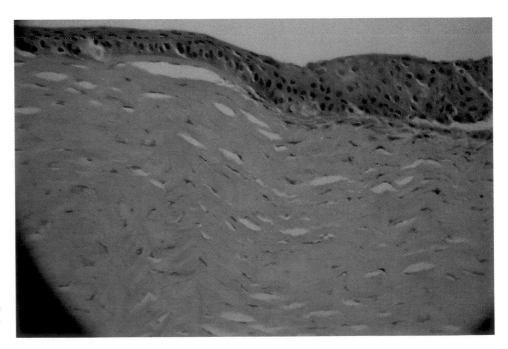

Figure 39–4. Histologic appearance of eyes treated with prismatic photokeratectomy.

eas showed absence of inflammatory cells. Evidence of keratocyte proliferation in superficial stroma was observed at day 9 but not at 5 months.

CONCLUSIONS

We achieved prismatic photoablation of PMMA blocks, lenses, and rabbit eyes. No other refractive changes accompanied the prismatic effect. We observed that re-epithelialization was complete by day 3 and that corneal haze was not evident clinically by gross and by slit lamp examination. We conclude that PPK is not only feasible in rabbit corneas but may hold important therapeutic potential for patients with binocular diplopia.

We attempted to perform topography on the PRK and PTK "controls" but were unable to obtain reproducible topographic maps preoperatively and postoperatively. We are currently investigating whether significant prismatic correction can be achieved with PPK in

monkeys, and to determine methods of optimizing epithelial conformity to the ablation bed and minimizing stromal scarring by pharmacological modulation of the epithelial and stromal wound-healing response.

REFERENCES

1. Azar DT, Jain S, Woods K, Stark W, Sanders D. Phototherapeutic keratectomy: the VISX experience. In: Salz JJ, ed. *Corneal Laser Surgery.* St. Louis, MO: Mosby-Year Book, Inc., 1995.
2. Azar DT, Hahn TW, Jain S, Yeh TC, Stetler-Stevenson W. Matrix metalloproteinases are expressed after excimer laser keratectomy. *Cornea.* In press.
3. Azar DT: A new excimer laser technique for the correction of strabismus and diplopia. SPIE Vol. 2126 *Ophthal Technol.* IV: 1994;4:40–46.
4. Azar DT: ArF excimer prismatic photokeratectomy in the treatment of consecutive small angle prismatic deviations. *Ophthalmology.* 1993;100(suppl):103.

SECTION VII

Phakic IOLs and Refractive Anterior Segment Surgery

CHAPTER 40

Refractive Cataract Surgery

Martin G. Edwards ▪ Dimitri T. Azar

The goals of cataract surgery have changed dramatically since the development of phacoemulsification and small-incision cataract surgery. The ability to create an astigmatically neutral cataract incision, accurately predict intraocular lens (IOL) power, and surgically correct preexisting astigmatism with keratorefractive techniques has resulted in higher patient and physician expectations. Today, cataract surgeons' goals include excellent uncorrected vision, rapid visual rehabilitation, and stable long-term postoperative results.

HISTORICAL PERSPECTIVE

The effect of a cataract incision on astigmatism has been known since 1864 when Donders described against-the-rule astigmatism after cataract surgery.[1] Although intracapsular cataract surgery (ICCE) leaves a significant degree of surgically induced astigmatism, it has relatively minimal refractive effect because ICCE requires aphakic spectacles or contact lenses for optical correction. After ICCE, most patients are legally blind without spectacles; with spectacles or contact lenses, astigmatism is a relatively minor component of the refractive error and has little effect on visual acuity. The development of the extracapsu-

lar cataract extraction technique (ECCE) and advancements in IOL technology reduced the need for significant spherical optical correction after cataract surgery and increased awareness of the importance of surgically induced astigmatism. As ECCE and IOL implantation became safer and corneal, vitreal, and retinal complications decreased, astigmatism became a major limiting factor in visual rehabilitation. A number of different surgical techniques were developed to reduce postoperative astigmatism, including moving the incision posteriorly, limiting the use of cautery, using an intraoperative keratometer,[2] adjusting suture tension to minimize wound gape or wound compression, selective suture removal,[3] and use of medications such as corticosteroids to alter wound healing. These techniques have allowed for better control of postoperative astigmatism; however, none allows for reproducible and consistent results. After ECCE, surgically induced astigmatism can change in direction and magnitude for at least 2 years.[4]

Phacoemulsification has allowed for the development of small-incision cataract surgery and the creation of a potentially astigmatically neutral incision with less postoperative against-the-rule shift. This technology combined with keratorefractive techniques portends today's refractive cataract surgeon.

INDIVIDUALIZED APPROACH

Successful keratorefractive procedures must be highly individualized. Individual surgeons should analyze their past 50 to 100 cases to become familiar with their degree of postoperative astigmatism induced and accuracy of IOL power calculation. Several formulas have been described for calculating the surgically induced refractive change after cataract surgery.[5–8] The techniques and general principles described here should be custom tailored to the individual surgeon. A variety of techniques, including alteration of wound construction or location, astigmatic keratotomy (AK), or use of a toric IOL, can be applied. All methods of altering postoperative astigmatism require careful consideration of preoperative astigmatism and corneal topography, which, in addition to refraction and keratometric readings, help to identify the steep axis of preoperative astigmatism.[9] Corneal topography is also useful for identifying irregular astigmatism and unsuspected keratoconus.

CALCULATION OF INTRAOCULAR LENS POWER

A number of IOL formulas have been developed, and most perform well in eyes with normal dimensions. All depend on accurate measurement of axial length and corneal power. The eye should be fixating properly and the cornea not be indented during A-scan biometry. If both eyes are not roughly equal in length or the axial length does not correlate with refraction, repeat the measurements. Posterior staphyloma can lead to erroneous measurements. Keratometry readings should likewise be accurate and consistent. Holladay and coworkers reported that 43% to 67% of large refractive surprises (more than 2 diopters [D] from predicted) using the Binkhorst or Sanders-Retslaff-Kraff (SRK) formulas were not due to formula errors but rather to inaccurate preoperative measurements.[10] Highly variable measurements coincide with less accuracy in predicting postoperative refractive results.[11] Overly long or short eyes can lead to underestimation or overestimation of the anterior chamber depth (ACD) respectively, resulting in more hyperopic correction in long eyes or more myopic correction in short eyes. The older Binkhorst formula assumes a constant ACD value and is inaccurate in overly long or short eyes. The SRKI likewise does not include ACD as part of its equation and also is less accurate in overly long or short eyes than the SRKII, in which the A constant is modified according to axial length.[12–14] The SRKT formula considers both corneal

height considerations and axial length correction factors in estimating ACD. Sanders and coworkers and Retslaff and coworkers found it to perform slightly better than the SRKII or Binkhorst formulas in long eyes.[15,16] The Holladay formula is based partly on corneal height considerations and partly on axial length correction of the assumed ACD.[17] Olsen and coworkers found the Holladay formula more accurate overall than the SRKI or SRKII formula.[12] The Olsen formula uses multiple regression equations including average corneal height, preoperative ACD, and axial length to predict postoperative ACD and is accurate in long and short eyes.[18]

A difference of 1 mm in the position of the IOL from the assumed position will result in an average of 1.3 D error in refraction. Errors in IOL power can therefore come from erroneous estimation of postoperative ACD or more anterior or posterior IOL placement than predicted with sulcus or in-the-bag fixation. Careful fixation of both haptics in the capsular bag when a continuous tear capsulorrhexis is performed will result in a more posterior position of the IOL. Armstrong compared 50 patients with a can-opener anterior capsulotomy with 50 patients with a continuous tear capsulotomy with confirmed capsular-bag lens placement. Because of the more posterior position of the IOL, the capsulorrhexis patients required a spectacle correction of 0.43 D greater than the can-opener patients when the same A constant surgeon factor was used.[19] Surgeons should individualize their own A constant using known postoperative refractive results for both techniques. When surgical techniques are used to correct preexisting astigmatism, the spherical equivalent may have to be changed by the astigmatism correction, which must be accounted for in the IOL calculation.

MOVING THE INCISION

Cataract surgical incisions centered around the 12 o'clock position usually result in some degree of against-the-rule shift. Incisions centered at the steepest meridian result in corneal flattening in that meridian. This requires one to be comfortable with operating in other than the 12 o'clock position. To predict postoperative results, the surgeon must be able to predict how much postoperative astigmatism the incision and closure techniques will induce. Wound size, construction, and location and closure technique all determine the amount of postoperative astigmatism. In general, larger incisions and clean corneal incisions result in more postoperative astigmatism. By operating on the steeper meridian, the surgeon can use these factors to reduce postoperative astigmatism.

Gayton describes a technique of using a variably sized sutureless scleral tunnel incision placed at the steep meridian of astigmatism identified by corneal topography. For against-the-rule astigmatism, a 6.0-mm incision is used for 0.75 to 1.5 D of astigmatism; a 7.0-mm incision is used for 1.75 to 2.25 D of astigmatism. For with-the-rule astigmatism a more conservative approach is recommended, with a small incision used for up to 2.0 D, a 6.0-mm incision for 2.0 to 2.25 D, and a 7.0-mm incision for 2.5 to 2.75 D of astigmatism. For lesser amounts of astigmatism use a frown-shaped incision; for greater amounts, make the wound more parallel to the limbus. Of 36 patients who underwent cataract surgery using this method, Gayton noted that 20 had their astigmatism reduced by more than 0.5 D, 14 were within ±0.5 D of the presurgical measurement, and 2 had an increased keratometric cylinder.

Rowan described a similar technique of locating the incision at the steep axis 1 mm posterior to and parallel to the surgical limbus. A 60° limbal incision is used to correct 1 D, a 90° incision is used for 2 D, and a 120° incision is used for 3 D or more of preoperative astigmatism. The incision is 75% scleral thickness and is shelved anteriorly into clear cornea. The cataract incision is completed with a 3.5-mm keratome. In 54 consecutive cases Rowan found mean keratometric cylinder was reduced from 1.51 D preoperatively to 1.10 D postoperatively. Most patients were undercorrected, and three patients shifted from against the rule to with the rule.[20]

Axt and McCaffrey observed that 6-mm phacoemulsification or 9-mm ECCE incisions located in the temporal quadrant reduced preexisting against-the-rule astigmatism. Selective suture cutting postoperatively enhanced the effect.[21] Nordan has proposed that a 6-mm incision can correct up to 3 D of astigmatism and a 10-mm incision can correct up to 8 D.[22] Poor predictability limits the usefulness of this large-incision technique. Larger amounts of astigmatism may better be corrected with an astigmatically neutral incision combined with AK.

THE ASTIGMATICALLY NEUTRAL CATARACT INCISION

It is generally accepted that smaller incisions induce less postoperative astigmatism. Several authors have found less postoperative astigmatism with a 3- to 6-mm

scleral incision than with a 10-mm ECCE corneal incision.[23,24] Hayashi and coworkers[25] used a topographic modeling system to study early postoperative changes in the corneal curvature after ECCE with an 11-mm incision and phacoemulsification with a 6-mm incision. The smaller incision resulted in less corneal steepening and stabilized more rapidly than the large wound used for ECCE.

With phacoemulsification incisions several studies have demonstrated less surgically induced astigmatism and more stable wounds with a 3- to 4-mm incision than with a 6- to 7-mm incision.[26–28] Koch and coworkers and Samuelson and coworkers found that 3-mm scleral tunnel incisions induced minimal to no astigmatism in eye bank eyes.[29,30] Increasing the incision length to 4 mm, however, resulted in an average of 0.5 D of corneal flattening. Shepherd observed that 4-mm scleral pocket incisions closed with a single horizontal suture remained stable, with an average of 0.22 D of against-the-rule shift at 3 months.[31] Other studies, however, have compared 3.5- to 4.0-mm incisions with larger (5.0- to 6.0-mm) incisions and found no difference in postoperative keratometric astigmatism between the two groups.[32–34] Martin and coworkers found no statistical difference in postoperative keratometric cylinder using no-stitch 3.2-, 5.0-, and 6.0-mm incisions; however, corneal topography showed significantly less corneal flattening with a 3.2-mm incision.

A 5-mm incision can still accommodate a rigid all-polymethyl methacrylate (PMMA) IOL, while a 3- to 4-mm incision requires insertion of a foldable IOL. Foldable IOLs have become more popular, but skeptics question their long-term safety. Freeman has described a 4.5-mm no-stitch scleral stretch incision through which a 6.0-mm rigid PMMA lens can be inserted,[35] but the astigmatic effects of this technique are not reported. Smaller incisions have been shown to result in less postoperative inflammation[28,36] and more rapid visual recovery.[24,37]

Wound architecture also plays an integral role in creating the astigmatically neutral cataract incision. Scleral tunnel incisions are less likely to induce astigmatism in part because of their posterior location. A three-step incision leads to more wound stability and consists of a scleral groove, a scleral tunnel, and a corneal lip. Ernest in a retrospective review has shown that a three-step 4-mm incision even when sutureless did not induce additional cylinder or induce against-the-rule shift.[38] Masket has found that a scleral pocket phacoemulsification incision closed with a single suture tied under keratometric control resulted in less than 1.5 D of astigmatic swing.[39] Singer described a frown incision that consistently demonstrated a lower degree of induced astigmatism than a scleral pocket incision.[40] Nielsen evaluated 40 patients with a 5- to 6-mm frown incision and found that the mean surgically induced astigmatism progressed from significant with-the-rule change on the first day to no induced astigmatism at 6 weeks to a small against-the-rule shift at 6 months.[41]

Wound-closure technique can also affect postoperative astigmatism. A single horizontal suture in 5.0-, 6.0-, and 6.5-mm scleral tunnel incisions resulted in no statistical difference between the three groups in vector astigmatic changes over a 4-week period.[42] Kondrot evaluated 100 patients in whom a 5.2-mm self-sealing no-stitch tunnel incision was used and found that although keratometry and refraction were stable at 1 month, a small degree of against-the-rule shift occured after 1 year.[43] Feil and coworkers similarly found mild against-the-rule shift 1 week postoperatively with a 3.5- to 4.0-mm no-stitch scleral tunnel with little decay at 1 month.[44] Using corneal topography Koch and coauthors reported steepening of the superior meridian 1 week postoperatively in sutured 4-mm scleral tunnel incisions that was not present in the unsutured cases. Minimal astigmatism was present in both groups 5 to 7 weeks postoperatively.[29]

Several of the above studies showed consistent results, but the study designs generally were not prospective and randomized. We have performed a multicenter prospective study of 0-, 1-, and 3-stitch closure of a 5.5-mm self-sealing scleral tunnel incision in 131 patients. Mean astigmatism was greatest in the first postoperative week in all groups and stabilized at around 1 D after 8 weeks. No-stitch and one-stitch surgery resulted in a low percentage of with-the-rule induced astigmatism 4 weeks after surgery. As opposed to no-stitch surgery, the one-stitch surgery resulted in a significantly lower against-the-rule shift. The three-stitch surgery resulted in high with-the-rule shift in the first 8 weeks after surgery, with progressive against-the-rule shift at 6 months and 1 year postoperatively.[45]

Suture tension plays a large part in surgically induced astigmatism. One tends to overtighten sutures in a soft or underinflated eye. Pacifico and Morrison describe a technique of reinflating the anterior chamber with balanced salt solution after placing and temporarily tying a nylon suture. The internal pressure from the fluid relaxed the suture, which was then permanently tied in place. The authors report a mean postoperative change in astigmatism of 0.02 ± 0.57 D at 6 weeks with this method.[46]

In summary, depending on wound size, architecture, location, and closure, cataract incisions that are constructed either to be astigmatically neutral or with significant surgically induced astigmatism appear to correct preexisting astigmatism. A 4- to 6-mm 3-step scleral tunnel or frown incision located 2 to 3 mm posterior to the limbus with appropriate suture tension will result in little to no surgically induced astigmatism. Emmetropia can be achieved with such an incision and appropriate IOL power in the spherical eye. Maloney and coauthors reviewed 4000 consecutive cataract patients and found 44% already had spherical or clinically insignificant astigmatism.[47] Forty-seven percent had 1.0 to 2.5 D of astigmatism, and 9% had 2.5 to 10.0 D of astigmatism. When an astigmatically neutral cataract incision is used, a patient with preexisting astigmatism will be left with residual postoperative astigmatism and hence will benefit from an astigmatic procedure.

ASTIGMATIC KERATOTOMY

Transverse astigmatic keratotomy (TAK) reduces astigmatism at or after cataract surgery. TAK is based on the following keratorefractive principles: (1) transverse corneal incisions flatten the adjacent cornea and steepen the cornea 90° away, (2) the flattening effect increases as the incision is moved closer to the center of the cornea, and (3) the effect increases with incision length. TAK requires accurate preoperative evaluation and identification of the steep axis of astigmatism. The surgeon should be skilled in performing small-incision cataract surgery, capsulorrhexis, hydrodissection, phacoemulsification, and small-incision IOL implantation. Necessary additional equipment includes corneal videokeratography, a corneal pachymeter, and an accurately calibrated diamond knife. TAK can be performed before or after phacoemulsification, but when it is performed before phacoemulsification, microperforations or corneal clouding may interfere with the cataract procedure. Waiting several weeks after cataract surgery has several advantages, including the ability to reevaluate postoperative astigmatism, easier localization of the visual axis with a nondilated pupil, and eliminating the effect of corticosteroids. Patients may be reluctant, however, to undergo a second procedure several weeks postoperatively. Accordingly, many surgeons perform TAK in conjunction with cataract surgery.

A number of authors have reported their results of performing TAK in conjunction with cataract surgery. Most advocate a conservative approach and a small degree of undercorrection as desirable. In various series, the incision depth, incision length, size of optical zone, and incision shape are all varied to achieve the desired effect of reducing, but not eliminating, postoperative astigmatism.[47–54]

Maloney and coworkers have described a technique of TAK used in over 600 patients immediately after phacoemulsification.[47–49] They perform intraoperative keratometry to confirm the degree and axis of astigmatism, mark the steep axis, define a 7-mm optical zone, and then mark the incision sites. They make incisions with a diamond blade set at 0.6 mm. The incision length varies with the degree of astigmatism to be corrected. The authors felt that this procedure worked better for against-the-rule astigmatism than for oblique or with-the-rule astigmatism. Davidson used a similar technique of TAK with an incision depth to 95% central pachymetry in 40 patients. Two months after surgery 74% of the patients had 20/40 or better visual acuity uncorrected. The average keratometric astigmatism was reduced from 2.6 D preoperatively to 1.5 D postoperatively in this series.[50]

Hall and coworkers[51] performed four TAK incisions before phacoemulsification in 61 eyes. They varied the optical zone depending on the degree of preoperative astigmatism. They did not perform intraoperative keratometry. They used optical zones of 7 mm for 1 to 2 D of corneal astigmatism, 6 mm for 2 to 3 D of corneal astigmatism, and 5.5 mm for more than 3 D of corneal astigmatism. All incisions were 3 mm long. Astigmatism improved in all three patients groups, but the astigmatism was undercorrected in each.

Osher used a similar technique of two 3-mm transverse incisions 0.65 mm deep perpendicular to the steepest meridian with an optical zone varying from 7 to 10 mm. The technique reduced astigmatism in 66 of 75 eyes and resulted in an oblique axis of cylinder in 9 eyes.[52] Shepherd reported 48 patients who underwent TAK immediately before cataract surgery.[53] In this series the incision was performed to 90% pachymetry in the steepest meridian using a 7-mm optical zone. Shepherd makes the incision 1 mm long for each 1 D of astigmatism. All but two patients had a decrease in corneal cylinder postoperatively, but all were undercorrected.

Thorton and Sanders found a mean decrease of 1.1 D of corneal cylinder using the Thorton nomogram[54,55] in eyes with idiopathic astigmatism. The authors propose modifying the amount of surgery for patient age, sex, and intraocular pressure. Thornton advocates performing AK at least 3 months after cataract surgery.

Arcuate keratotomy is a similar technique in which curvilinear incisions are made corresponding to the optical zone. Arcuate corneal incisions that parallel the optical zone tend to result in about 20% more corneal flattening than straight incisions. Kershner has described a technique of performing clear corneal phacoemulsification through an arcuate incision. This alone can be used to correct between 1.0 and 1.5 D of astigmatism. For more than 1.5 D of astigmatism a paired arcuate keratotomy incision is used opposite the cataract incision. The optical zone size and incision length are varied to correct increasing amounts of astigmatism.

Martin uses a similar approach and combines arcuate keratotomy with a clear corneal or scleral tunnel phacoemulsification incision.[56] For the arcuate keratotomy the blade is set at 100% pachymetric depth and arcuate incisions are made at the steepest meridian using a 7-mm optical zone. A second pair of incisions in the 8- to 9-mm optical zone gives an additional 50% more effect. The incision length is varied for increasing amounts of astigmatism, and age is factored into the nomogram. Gills advocates combining a clear corneal incision temporally for preoperative against-the-rule astigmatism and a scleral tunnel incision superiorly for with-the-rule astigmatism.[56,57] An arcuate corneal-relaxing incision is placed at the 8-mm optical zone to 100% pachymetric depth immediately anterior to the cataract incision unless there is asymmetric astigmatism. The incision is 2 mm long for each 1 D of astigmatism to be corrected.

Semilinear incisions can be combined with transverse incisions, resulting in the trapezoidal AK popularized by Ruiz. Trapezoidal AK has been shown to reduce astigmatism after penetrating keratoplasty or cataract extraction and can correct large amounts of astigmatism.[58] This method is not used currently because multiple parallel incisions are not necessary to achieve the desired effect.

Complications of TAK include undercorrection or overcorrection, creating irregular astigmatism, microperforation, macroperforation, wound dehiscence,[50] infection, prolonged instability resulting in fluctuating vision, and glare.

TORIC INTRAOCULAR LENS

Toric IOLs are currently under investigation in the United States. These investigational lenses are composed of PMMA or silicone and have a toric component on the surface of the lens with alignment markers identifying the cylinder axis. The steep axis of astigmatism should be clearly identified and marked preoperatively so that the lens can be properly oriented during surgery. Rotational stability of the IOL is required, because lens rotation after surgery may lead to increased postoperative astigmatism.

Grabow has reported preliminary results in 50 patients who received a Staar Surgical toric IOL as part of a clinical trial. The lens has about 2 D of toric correction. In 94% of patients the lenses rotated less than 30° postoperatively, and these patients' astigmatism was reduced by an average of 1.25 D. In three eyes in which the lens rotated more than 30°, the toric IOL induced an average of 0.4 D of astigmatism. Sixty-nine percent of these patients had uncorrected vision of 20/40 or better. Theoretically these lenses could also be repositioned in the early postoperative period if significant lens rotation occurs.[59]

REFERENCES

1. Donders FC. *On the Anomalies of Accommodation and Refraction of the Eye.* London: New Sydenham Society; 1864:334.
2. Lindstrom RL, Destro MA. Effect of incision size and Terry keratometer usage on postoperative astigmatism. *Am Intraocular Implant Soc J.* 1985;11:469–473.
3. Stanford MR, Fenech T, Hunter PA. Timing of removal of sutures in control of post-operative astigmatism. *Eye.* 1993;7:143–147.
4. Talamo JH, Stark WJ, Gottsch JD, et al. Natural history of corneal astigmatism after cataract surgery. *J Cataract Refract Surg.* 1991;17:313–318.
5. Holladay JT, Cravy TV, Koch DD. Calculating the surgically induced refractive change following ocular surgery. *J Cataract Refract Surg.* 1992;18:429–443.
6. Cravy TV. Calculation of the change in corneal astigmatism following cataract extraction. *Ophthalmic Surg.* 1979; 10:38–49.
7. Jaffe NS, Clayman HM. The pathophysiology of corneal astigmatism after cataract extraction. *Trans Am Acad Ophthalmol Otolaryngol.* 1975;79:615–630.
8. Olsen T. Simple method to calculate surgically induced refractive change. *J Cataract Refract Surg.* 1993;19:319.
9. Gills JP. Analysis of corneal topography in cataract surgery. *Ophthalmic Pract.* 1994;12:14–18.
10. Holladay JT, Prager TC, Ruis RS, et al. Improving the predictability of intraocular lens power calculations. *Arch Ophthalmol.* 1986;104:539–541.
11. Richards SC, Olson RJ, Richards WL. Factors associated with poor predictability by intraocular lens calculation formulas. *Arch Ophthalmol.* 1985;103:515–518.
12. Olsen T, Thim K, Corydon L. Accuracy of the newer generation intraocular lens power calculation formulas in long and short eyes. *J Cataract Refract Surg.* 1991;17:187–193.
13. Sanders DR, Retzlaff J, Kraff MC. Comparison of the SRKII formula and other second generation formulas. *J Cataract Refract Surg.* 1988;14:136–141.
14. Drews RC. Reliability of lens implant power formulas in hyperopes and myopes. *Ophthalmic Surg.* 1988;19:11–15.
15. Retzlaff JA, Sanders DR, Kraff MC. Development of the SRK/T intraocular lens implant power calculation formula. *J Cataract Refract Surg.* 1990;16:333–340.
16. Sanders DR, Retzlaff J, Kraff MC, et al. Comparison to the SRK/T formula and other theoretical and regression formulas. *J Cataract Refract Surg.* 1990;16:341–346.
17. Holladay JT, Prager TC, Chandler TY, et al. A three part system for refining intraocular lens power calculations. *J Cataract Refract Surg.* 1988;14:17–24.
18. Olsen T, Olesen H, Thim K, Corydon L. Prediction of pseudophakic anterior chamber depth with the newer IOL calculation formulas. *J Cataract Refract Surg.* 1992;18:280–285.
19. Armstrong TA. Refractive effect of capsular bag lens placement with the capsulorrhexis technique. *J Cataract Refract Surg.* 1992;18:121–124.
20. Gayton JL, Rowan P, Van Der Karr MA. Cataract incision at the steep axis. In: *Surgical Treatment of Astigmatism.* Thorofare, NJ: Slack, Inc.; 1994:129–142.
21. Axt JC, McCaffery JM. Reduction of postoperative against the rule astigmatism by lateral incision technique. *J Cataract Refract Surg.* 1993;19:380–386.
22. Nordan LT. Astigmatism control. In: Devine TM, Banko W, eds. *Phacoemulsification Surgery.* Elmsford, NY: Pergamon Press; 1991:111–118.
23. Watson A, Sunderraj P. Comparison of small-incision phacoemulsification with standard extracapsular cataract surgery: Post-operative astigmatism and visual recovery. *Eye.* 1992;6:626–629.
24. Neumann AC, McCarty GR, Sanders DR, Raanan MG. Small incisions to control astigmatism during cataract surgery. *J Cataract Refract Surg.* 1989;15:78–84.
25. Hayashi K, Nakao F, Hayashi F. Topographic analysis of early changes in corneal astigmatism after cataract surgery. *J Cataract Refract Surg.* 1993;19:43–47.
26. Steinert RF, Brint SF, White SM, Fine IH. Astigmatism after small incision cataract surgery; a prospective, randomized, multicenter comparison of 4 and 6.5 mm incisions. *Ophthalmology.* 1991;98:417–424.
27. Brint SF, Ostrick DM, Bryan JE. Keratometric cylinder and visual performance following phacoemulsification and implantation with silicone small-incision or poly (methyl methacrylate) intraocular lenses. *J Cataract Refract Surg.* 1991;17:32–36.
28. Gills JP, Sanders DR. Use of small incisions to control induced astigmatism and inflammation following cataract surgery. *J Cataract Refract Surg.* 1991;17:740–744.

29. Koch DD, Haft EA, Gay C. Computerized videokeratographic analysis of corneal topographic changes induced by sutured and unsutured 4mm scleral pocket incisions. *J Cataract Refract Surg.* 1993;19:166–169.

30. Samuelson SW, Koch DD, Kuglen CC. Determination of maximal incision length for true small-incision surgery. *Ophthalmic Surg.* 1991;22:204–207.

31. Shepherd JR. Induced astigmatism in small incision cataract surgery. *J Cataract Refract Surg.* 1989;15:85–88.

32. Martin RG, Sanders DR, Miller JD, et al. Effect of cataract wound incision size on acute changes in corneal topography. *J Cataract Refract Surg.* 1993;19:170–177.

33. Martin RG, Sanders DR, Van Der Karr MA, DeLuca M. Effect of small incision intraocular lens surgery on postoperative inflammation and astigmatism. A study of the AMO SI-18NB small incision lens. *J Cataract Refract Surg.* 1992;18:51–57.

34. Davison JA. Keratometric comparison of 4.0mm and 5.5mm scleral tunnel cataract incisions. *J Cataract Refract Surg.* 1993;19:3–8.

35. Freeman JM. Scleral stretch incision for cataract surgery. A technique for no-suture closure and control of astigmatism. *J Cataract Refract Surg.* 1991;17:696–701.

36. Sanders DR, Spigelman A, Kraff C, et al. Quantitative assessment of postsurgical breakdown of the blood-aqueous barrier. *Arch Ophthalmol.* 1983;101:131–133.

37. Uusitalo RJ, Ruusuvaara P, Jarvinen E, et al. Early rehabilitation after small incision cataract surgery. *Refract Corneal Surg.* 1993;9:67–70.

38. Ernest PH. Corneal lip tunnel incision. *J Cataract Refract Surg.* 1994;20:154–157.

39. Masket S. Keratorefractive aspects of the scleral pocket incision and closure method for cataract surgery. *J Cataract Refract Surg.* 1989;15:70–77.

40. Singer JA. Frown incision for minimizing induced astigmatism after small incision cataract surgery with rigid optic intraocular lens implantation. *J Cataract Refract Surg.* 1991;17:677–688.

41. Nielsen PJ. Induced astigmatism and its decay with a frown incision. *J Cataract Refract Surg.* 1993;19:375–379.

42. Buzzard KA, Shearing SP. Comparison of postoperative astigmatism with incisions of varying length closed with horizontal sutures and with no sutures. *J Cataract Refract Surg.* 1991;17:734–739.

43. Kondrot EC. Keratometric cylinder and visual recovery following phacoemulsification and intraocular lens implantation using a self-sealing cataract incision. *J Cataract Refract Surg.* 1991;17:731–733.

44. Feil SH, Crandall AS, Olson RJ. Astigmatic decay following small incision, self sealing cataract surgery. *J Cataract Refract Surg.* 1994;20:40–43.

45. Azar DT, Dodick J, Stark WJ, et al. Prospective, randomized, multicenter vector analysis of astigmatism after three-, one-, and no-stitch phacoemulsification cataract surgery. *Ophthalmology.* 1994;101(suppl).

46. Pacifico RL, Morrison C. Astigmatically neutral sutured small incision. *J Cataract Refract Surg.* 1991;17:710–712.

47. Maloney WF, Grindle L, Sanders D, Pearcy D. Astigmatism control for the cataract surgeon: a comprehensive review of surgically tailored astigmatism reduction (STAR). *J Cataract Refract Surg.* 1989;15:45–54.

48. Maloney WF, Sanders DR, Pearcy DE. Astigmatic keratotomy to correct preexisting astigmatism in cataract patients. *J Cataract Refract Surg.* 1990;16:297–304.

49. Maloney WF, Shapiro DR. Transverse astigmatic keratotomy. An integral part of small incision cataract surgery. *J Cataract Refract Surg.* 1992;18:190–194.

50. Davison JA. Transverse astigmatic keratotomy combined with phacoemulsification and intraocular lens implantation. *J Cataract Refract Surg.* 1989;15:38–44.

51. Hall GW, Campion M, Sorenson CM, Monthofer S. Reduction of corneal astigmatism at cataract surgery. *J Cataract Refract Surg.* 1991;17:407–414.

52. Osher RH. Paired transverse relaxing keratotomy: a combined technique for reducing astigmatism. *J Cataract Refract Surg.* 1989;15:32–37.

53. Shepherd JR. Correction of preexisting astigmatism at the time of small incision cataract surgery. *J Cataract Refract Surg.* 1989;15:55–57.

54. Thornton SP, Sanders DR. Graded nonintersecting transverse incisions for correction of idiopathic astigmatism. *J Cataract Refract Surg.* 1987;13:27–31.

55. Thornton SP. Thornton guide for radial keratotomy incisions and optical zone size. *J Refract Surg.* 1985;1:29–33.

56. Gills JP, Martin RG, Thornton SP. Astigmatic keratotomy in the cataract patient. In Gills JP.: *Surgical Treatment of Astigmatism.* Thorofare, NJ: Slack, Inc.; 1994:27–48.

57. Gills JP. Cataract surgery with a single relaxing incision at the steep meridian. *J Cataract Refract Surg.* 1994;20:368–369.

58. Lavery GW, Lindstrom RL. Clinical results of trapezoidal astigmatic keratotomy. *J Refract Surg.* 1985;1:70–74.

59. Grabow HB. Toric IOLs: another way to correct pre-op astigmatism. *Rev Ophthalmol.* 1994;1:29–31.

CHAPTER 41

Postkeratoplasty Astigmatism: Etiology and Management

Salim I. Butrus ▪ M. Farooq Ashraf ▪ Dimitri T. Azar

Corneal surgeons can achieve clear corneal grafts in most patients, especially in those who are not at high risk of allograft rejection. This is due to a remarkable improvement in modern eye banking and instrumentation, a clearer understanding of corneal wound healing, and the use of immunosuppressive agents such as corticosteroids, cyclosporine A, and others. Despite all this, a certain amount of unpredictable astigmatism follows penetrating keratoplasty (PK), sometimes frustrating surgeons and leaving patients with visual disability. Numerous studies have shown an average of 4 or more diopters (D) of astigmatism after corneal transplants.[1-10]

PATHOGENESIS OF POSTKERATOPLASTY ASTIGMATISM

Penetrating keratoplasty surgically involves resecting and suturing a donor corneal tissue to a recipient corneal bed. It requires meticulous attention to detail by the corneal surgeon. The surgeon's task begins with communication with the eye bank and ends with lengthy postoperative management of the patient. Different degrees of graft astigmatism may arise postoperatively and can be attributed to poor surgical technique. Table 41–1 enumerates factors that may contribute to postkeratoplasty astigmatism. Some are beyond the surgeon's control; others are totally or partially controlled by the surgeon.

Preoperative Factors

In general, surgeons have access to high-quality donor tissues that can be preserved and transported for days. Donors may have undetected astigmatism. Whether donor native astigmatism has any effect on final-graft astigmatism is not known.

Certainly recipient pathologic conditions can lead to astigmatism. Sectorial vascular invasion, thinning, or uneven rigidity in keratoconus will lead to uneven donor-to-recipient wound apposition, wound healing, and creation of uneven forces within the cornea. Irregular recipient corneas (scars, vessels, thinning, unequal rigidity) result in irregular opening after trephination and hence irregular astigmatism.

Operative Factors

Most donor corneal buttons today are trephined in an endothelial cell-up position in a concave Teflon block as described by Vannas.[11] This method yields a perfectly round edge graft. It is done in a more controlled fashion than when trephined epithelial cell-up in an intact

TABLE 41–1. CONTRIBUTING FACTORS TO POSTKERATOPLASTY ASTIGMATISM

Preoperative factors: recipient related
  Native astigmatism
  Topographic changes
  Recipient corneal scarring, vascularization, thinning
  Recipient uneven scleral rigidity
  Aphakia or pseudophakia (ACIOL, prior vitrectomy, or scleral fixation)

Preoperative factors: donor related
  Nonuniform peripheral changes (scarring, thinning, vascularization)
  Donor topographic variations (undetected keratoconus, high astigmatism)

Intraoperative factors: recipient related
  Effect of pressure of eyelid speculum and Flarienga ring on trephination
  Dull trephine or overused trephine blade
  Trephine tilt
  Eccentric trephination scissors
  Uneven wound architecture, poor resection
  Asymmetric wound edges

Intraoperative factors: donor related
  Inadequate punch technique
  Dull trephine or overused trephine blade
  Eccentric trephination
  Oval trephination
  Punch tilt during freehand trephination

Intraoperative donor-recipient relationship
  Donor/recipient diameter disparity
  Suture tension
  Donor/recipient torquing (improper suture orientation and location, wound override)
  Eccentric donor/recipient trephination

Postoperative factors
  Wound microdehiscense, override
  Trauma with macrodehiscence
  Timing of suture removal or adjustment
  Graft rejection, melting, necrosis, infectious keratitis
  Pharmacologic agents,
  Scleral fixated IOL, ACIOL
  Other (contact lens, IOP elevation)

Abbreviations: ACIOL, anterior chamber; IOL, intraocular lens; IOP, intraocular pressure.

globe. The donor corneoscleral rim is placed and fixated in a Teflon block to be punched with a piston-guided trephine or by a freehanded trephine. The piston-guided punch method is more precise and usually results in a circular tissue with vertical edges. If the trephine is slightly tilted, the freehanded technique may yield an oval button with shelved edges.[12–14] A dull trephine will leave irregular edges and thereby leads to irregular wound healing and astigmatism. More recent and sophisticated trephines such as the Krumeich and Hanna–Moria trephines cut donor corneas through the epithelial side, producing more reproducible results.

Although donor corneas can be correctly punched with reproducible results, recipient corneas are less likely to be trephined with the same accuracy, since more variables are involved and less predictable results are obtained. Freehand trephination is a common practice, but other trephines, such as Hessburg–Barron, are more popular despite setting a reverse shelved wound. Other, more expensive trephines such as the Krumeich cam-guided trephine, automated Hans–Gueder trephine, and mechanized Hanna–Moria trephine theoretically should give more reproducible results (Table 41–2). The Krumeich cam-guided system cuts the cornea in an applanated shape, perpendicular to the limbal plane, and theoretically produces round grafts.[15]

Many factors may affect adequate trephination in the recipient cornea. Freehanded trephination is subject to more factors that may affect the outcome such as external pressure by the eyelid speculum, Flarienga ring, or forceps stabilizing the globe.[16] Do not use dull trephines or trephines made by different manufacturers because they result in irregular edges.[17] Hold trephines perpendicular to the plane of the globe, hugging the recipient tissue 360°, because minor tilts can cause asymmetric corneal grooves and oval openings.[18,19] Eccentric trephination results in a high degree of astigmatism with an axis toward the displacement direction.[20] Finally, poor excision of the corneal tissue due to inadequate trephination or dull scissors may result in poor wound architecture, poor wound opposition and healing, and a high degree of astigmatism. Trephine tilts should be minimized during trephination of recipient corneas. This can be difficult to accomplish under the operating microscope, and a tilt more than 5° can easily occur. Olson's mathematic model has shown that buttons should be round with 0° of tilt.[21] Ovality increases with higher degrees of tilt. Cohen and associates[22] showed that maximum ovality appeared in 20° to 25° tilt; however, buttons were oval and asymmetric at 0° to 15° of tilt in eye bank eyes (Fig 41–1). They concluded that neither ovality or asymmetry correlated with degrees of tilt and factors other than tilt contribute to wound ovality and irregularity. Troutman and colleagues attempted to use intraoperative keratometry

TABLE 41–2. TYPES OF TREPHINES USED FOR PENETRATING KERATOPLASTY

Freehand: disposable, Weck, Storz, Pharmacia
Reusable: Grieshaber
Disposable suction: Hessburg–Barron
Automated: Hans–Gueder
Mechanized: Hanna–Moria
Cam guided: Krumeich, Lieberman

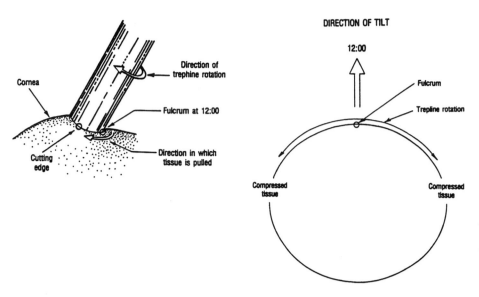

Figure 41–1. Side view of oblique trephination *(left)* showing pulling of corneal tissue. This results in oblong tissue resection in the recipient cornea *(right)*. *(From Cohen et al.* Am J Ophthalmol. *1986;101:722–725.)*

and rotate the donor button while inside the recipient wound to minimize disparity but without eliminating astigmatism.[23]

The use of oversized donor buttons is believed to reduce hyperopia and glaucoma in aphakic patients.[16] The donor button is punched from endothelial surface and hence is smaller due to retraction of the tissue. Oversized is in fact superior to undersized, and there is no difference in astigmatism, less wound leak, and less chance of collapse of the trabecular meshwork with oversized donor buttons.

Corneal wound disparity defined by mismatch between size and shape of donor button wound and its recipient wound determines degree, direction, and amount of astigmatism created. Multifactorial elements contribute to corneal wound disparity. Donor or recipient trephine, tilt, size, and eccentricity all contribute to disparity and ultimately astigmatism.

The donor button is punched from the donor endothelial side, and approximately 0.2 mm in diameter is lost in this process. Thus a 0.2-mm oversized graft is practically the same size as the recipient. The use of oversized donor over recipient (0.25 to 1 mm) gained popularity because it is believed to reduce hyperopia and the incidence of glaucoma in aphakic patients. It also has the advantages of less wound leak, easier suturing, less collapse of the trabecular meshwork, and lower incidence of glaucoma. Most studies found that oversized grafts didn't increase the incidence of astigmatism. However, the study by Perl and coworkers showed that oversized grafts compared with same-sized grafts did not affect intraocular pressure and refractive state and increased the amount of induced

astigmatism.[24] The extent of myopic error following penetrating keratoplasty in keratoconus patients can be decreased by reducing recipient-donor trephine disparity.[25]

SUTURING TECHNIQUE

Many uncontrollable factors discussed previously contribute to postkeratoplasty astigmatism; however, much attention has been focused on factors that the surgeon can manipulate operatively and postoperatively such as suture type, size, and technique. Table 41–3 summarizes different suture patterns and configurations. Different studies have shown that the final corneal astigmatism follows suture removal regardless of suture technique used. It is extremely difficult to draw conclusions from earlier studies because most studies (1) are retrospective, (2) lack controls, (3) involve different sur-

TABLE 41–3. DIFFERENT SUTURE PATTERN TECHNIQUES USED FOR PENETRATING KERATOPLASTY

Toricity	Material	Size/Pattern
Torque	Nylon (most common)	Single running (10-0):16, 24 bites
Antitorque	Mersilene	Double running (10-0 and 11-0): 12 bites each
No torque	Proline	Mixed running (10-0):16 bites and 8 interrupted
		Mixed running (10-0 or 11-0):12 bites and 12 interrupted
		Interrupted 16 bites

geons, (4) draw conclusions based on data before final suture removal, and (5) depend only on either refraction or keratometry. More recent studies, however, are prospective and employ vector analysis and computer-assisted topographic analysis. Although most established techniques to reduce postkeratoplasty astigmatism employ either selective suture removal or postoperative suture adjustment relying on keratometry or computer-assisted topographic analysis, a recent study advocated suture adjustment.[26,27] Serdarevic and coauthors observed that after suture removal, at 15 months postoperatively, astigmatism was less in the intraoperative adjustment group (1.75 ± 1.04 D) than in the postoperative adjustment group (2.23 ± 1.72 D), but this was not statistically significant.[27] The authors concluded that low astigmatism and good visual results can be obtained with either intraoperative or postoperative running suture adjustment, but intraoperative suture adjustment permits more rapid visual rehabilitation, increased safety, and increased refractive stability.

MANAGEMENT OF SIGNIFICANT POSTKERATOPLASTY ASTIGMATISM

The amount of postkeratoplasty astigmatism declines as the surgeon's experience increases. Most surgeons feel that astigmatism greater than 3 to 3.5 D is significant enough to warrant manipulation to minimize astigmatism. Table 41–4 summarizes possible ways and techniques to minimize astigmatism. The most important factor is whether the sutures have been removed. Adjusting the sutures will help reduce the amount of astigmatism and possibly the final outcome. There is no definite postoperative time period when the graft becomes "fixed," although some surgeons believe that this does not occur before 1 year. The final astigmatic stabilization occurs when all sutures are removed. For example, removing a running suture can theoretically change the amount and the axis of astigmatism up to 6 years after surgery.

Management of Astigmatism While Sutures Are In: Suture Manipulation

Surgeons try to manipulate corneal sutures to control and minimize astigmatism. To reduce suture tension at the steep meridian, sutures are adjusted either by selective removal or by adjusting the tension of single running sutures. Each approach has advantages and disadvantages. Both will reduce the amount of astigmatism for as long as the sutures are in. However, the cornea is not "fixed," and removing the running sutures any time after surgery creates large degrees of astigmatism. Because 10-0 nylon is biodegradable, it may loosen, disintegrate, and/or break, possibly leading to potentially serious problems such as microbial keratitis, epithelial breakdown, suture abscesses, graft vascularization, and rejection (Table 41–5). Both techniques only assume compression suture effects on astigmatism, ignoring wound healing or other relevant variables that may affect astigmatism.

Selective Suture Removal

This technique was popularized by Binder and colleagues,[28,29] and results of recent studies show a mean reduction of astigmatism from 2.5 to 3.0 D after selective suture removal (Table 41–6).[30] It is based on the assumption that the cornea assumes a different curvature

TABLE 41–5. COMPLICATIONS OF 10-0 NYLON PERMANENTLY LEFT IN CORNEAL GRAFT

Spontaneous breakage or degradation
Exposed knots and GPC
Suture abrasion
Suture erosion
Vascularization and fibrosis along suture tract
Infection
Inflammation graft rejection after suture removal

Abbreviation: GPC, giant papillary conjunctivitis.

TABLE 41–4. POSTOPERATIVE TECHNIQUES TO MINIMIZE POSTKERATOPLASTY ASTIGMATISM

Sutures In	Sutures Out
Suture manipulation	Relaxing incisions (<12–15 D)
Selective suture removal	Augmented relaxing incisions (12–15 D)
Suture adjustment	Corneal-wedge resections (>15 D)
Suture addition in wound	Limbal-wedge resections
Repair of wound override and	Combinations
microdehiscence	Excimer laser

TABLE 41–6. POSTKERATOPLASTY ASTIGMATISM AFTER SELECTIVE SUTURE REMOVAL

Author	No. of Eyes	Follow-up Months	Mean Astigmatic Reduction (D)
Binder[29]	56	14–16	3.7
Vanmeter[45]	31	7–12	3.2
Musch[46]	60	12	2.5
Filatov[47]	20	8	3.9

after the tight suture is selectively decompressed at a particular time. The change of astigmatism after long-term removal of the remaining sutures is less dramatic, suggesting that additional suture removal results in minimal curvature change after the corneal wound becomes "fixed."

Although it is not difficult to remove one or two 10-0 nylon sutures under a slit lamp using topical anesthesia, it does require an increased number of patient office visits. It can also be unpredictable and irreversible, and it may result in wound dehiscence, suture-induced irritation, infection, vascularization, and graft rejection. This technique also regulates the amount of astigmatism at a specific meridian of that tight suture and not the whole corneal circumference.

Suture Adjustment

A single 10-0 nylon running suture is performed and usually left on the loose side so that suture adjustment can be done 1 day and up to 6 weeks postoperatively.[31]

The technique involves rotating the suture from an area of flat meridian (cool colors) to areas of steep meridian (hot colors) (Fig 41–2). Nabors and associates took a step further by opening the anterior third of the wound along the steep meridian.[32] All studies show that a lower level of astigmatism occurs after selective removal, although it is not statistically significant in some studies (Table 41–7).

TABLE 41–7. POSTKERATOPLASTY ASTIGMATISM AFTER SUTURE ADJUSTMENT

Author	No. of Eyes	Follow-up Months	Mean Astigmatic Reduction (D)
McNeill[26]	330	19	2.87
Vanmeter[45]	26	7–12	1.50
Lin[31]	8	4	1.70
Nabors[32]	52	4	1.89
Filatov[47]	18	9	2.70

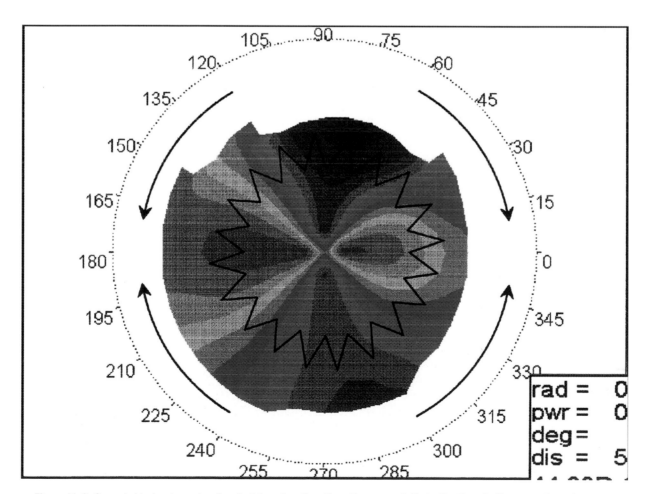

Figure 41–2. Corneal videokeratography of against-the-rule astigmatism. The arrows indicate direction of adjustment of running suture.

Suture adjustment achieves early visual rehabilitation and relatively regular keratometry mires. This is beneficial when an intraocular lens (IOL) is inserted 3 months after keratoplasty. It is a titrated procedure where adjustment is continued and stopped until stable K's are obtained. It is reversible and more predictable and results in regular astigmatism along the entire circumference of the cornea, not along one single meridian.

Suture adjustment can be performed under a slit lamp with a calm cooperative patient. The procedure must be repeated and sometimes requires a loose running suture, which may compromise the graft wound, lead to wound disruption, leak, cause infection, or recess the wound. Suture breakage occurs rarely. If it occurs, the patient usually must go to the operating room for suture placement. McNeill and Wessels encountered a broken suture in five eyes of a total of 330 eyes studied.[26]

Management of Astigmatism After Suture Removal

Relaxing Incisions

The surgical approach using relaxing incisions to minimize graft astigmatism is undertaken in cases of astigmatism high enough to cause blurring of vision with or without spectacle correction. Although the eye can often be visually rehabilitated through special contact lenses, some patients will require a surgical attempt to correct high astigmatism. Before relaxing incisions are entertained in postkeratoplasty patients, all sutures should be removed and stable refractions, keratometry, and topographic analyses observed for at least 3 months. The above three methods for evaluating postkeratoplasty astigmatism are all important and should be performed before relaxing incisions are made. In individuals with high degrees of astigmatic error (>10 D), wound overrides should be suspected, ruled out, and corrected. In patients who have significant myopia, radial keratotomy plus relaxing incisions can be performed. All incisions are made on the graft and are not extended to the host tissue.

We recommend arcuate relaxing incisions made 1 mm on the graft itself and not in the graft-host interface (Fig 41–3). Compression sutures can be placed in the orthogonal meridian to enhance the surgical effect. The technique of arcuate relaxing incisions is simple to perform, requiring office setup and topical anesthesia. The postoperative recovery period is extremely short, and visual rehabilitation is rapid and dramatic. Clinical results show 40% or greater reduction in mean astigmatism after relaxing incisions (Table 41–8).

Operative Technique

The eye is anesthetized with topical anesthetic drops. The particular meridian is marked on the slit lamp with a surgical blue marker, and the periocular skin is prepped with povidone iodine solution and draped with a plastic adhesive aperture drape. The lids are separated with a wire speculum, and the patient is asked to fixate using the surgical eye on a fixation mark built in the surgical microscope. Ultrasonic pachymetry is used to measure corneal thickness at different sites, especially at those where the cuts are planned. The Arc-T diamond knife's depth is set at less than 100% of corneal thickness. Two arcuate relaxing incisions are made at two hemimeridians that the refraction, keratometry, or topographic analysis have depicted. Most of the time the two hemimeridians are 180° apart. While using the Arc-T diamond blade, the surgeon must roll his or her fingers to achieve an arcuate incision. Some corneal surgeons tended to perform relaxing incisions of three-quarters depth in the corneal recipient-host interface with the patient situated on the slit lamp. This technique became less popular recently because of lower predictability and effectiveness and increased risk of perforations and infections. If after the first attempt astigmatism is not reduced as desired, another double arcuate incision can be performed 1 mm inside the previous ones. Alternatively, the incisions can be deepened if slit lamp evaluation shows shallow incisions. Compression sutures can be used to augment the effect of the arcuate incisions (Fig 41–4).

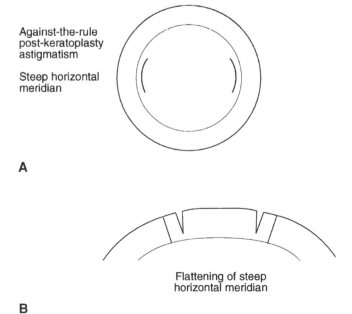

Against-the-rule post-keratoplasty astigmatism

Steep horizontal meridian

A

Flattening of steep horizontal meridian

B

Figure 41–3. Top **(A)** and side **(B)** view of arcuate keratotomy to correct steep horizontal meridian in against-the-rule postkeratoplasty astigmatism.

TABLE 41–8. MANAGEMENT OF ASTIGMATISM AFTER SUTURE REMOVAL: RELAXING INCISIONS

Study	No. of Subjects	Mean Reduction	% Reduction	Vector Correction
Troutman[36]	4	8.40	75.0	8.36
Krachmer[35]	14	4.52	48.9	7.37
Sugar[34]	17	7.53	60.0	9.51
Mandell[37]	21	6.56	67.0	8.40
Lavery[33]	12	4.70	45.7	
Cohen[48]	7	6.52	69.8	
Limberg[49]	10	4.80	48.0	No RI
Lustbader[38]	10	6.33	55.5	RI and comp. suture
Frangieh[50]	7	8.20	81.0	" "
Kirkness[51]	42	3.60	48.0	3 different techniques
Saragoussi[52]	48	4.51	50.0	
Ariffa[53]	6	7.46	77.0	Transverse, ± radial and comp.
Maxwell[54]	11	5.00	63.0	
Price[55]	58 (in graft)	2.84	54.0	
	51 (in Interface)			
Maguire[56]	6	4.22	46.0	5.99
Fronterre[39] I.	63	5.53	77.0	10.61
II.	25	9.68	77.0	9.34
III.	12	9.16	52.0	
McCartney[57]	11	7.77	66.8	

Abbreviations: RI, relaxing incision; comp, compression.

Wedge Resections

In 1967 Troutman devised the corneal wedge-resection procedure for high astigmatism.[40] Before this a repeat keratoplasty was often the procedure of choice to correct excessive graft astigmatism. Today wedge resection is reserved for cases of extremely high astigmatism and is recommended for astigmatism of 10 D or more. The procedure involves excising corneal tissue across the axis of the longer or flatter corneal meridian and suturing the two opposing ends of the resected tissue. The corneal meridian is shortened and the meridian steepened to correct the astigmatism (Fig 41–5). Although limited in numbers, previous clinical studies show an approximate 40% to 70% reduction of mean astigmatism after corneal wedge resection (Table 41–9).

Compared with relaxing incisions, wedge resections can correct large amounts of astigmatism. Moreover, the wounds are sutured, unlike the gaping wounds of relaxing incisions, and astigmatism can be customized by selective suture removal. However, it may take months for the wound to stabilize and hence for stable keratometer readings.

Operative Technique

As with relaxing incisions, all sutures should be removed and stable refractions, keratometry, and topographic analyses should be observed for at least 3 months. A retrobulbar block is used for anesthesia and akinesia. Intraoperatively the axis of the flattest meridian is identified. A keratometer-equipped surgical microscope is recommended. The surgeon should attend to intraoperative factors that may induce iatrogenic astigmatism, especially the lid speculum. Ultrasonic pachymetry is used in the axis where the resection be performed. Simultaneous partial penetrating incisions are made across the scar using a double-bladed diamond knife. The total excision area should be 90° wide and at a depth of 90% to 95%. This wedge of tissue is excised with the diamond knife or by corneal scissors by

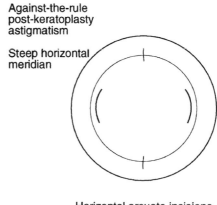

Against-the-rule
post-keratoplasty
astigmatism

Steep horizontal
meridian

Horizontal arcuate incisions
vertical compression sutures

Figure 41–4. Surgeon's view of horizontal arcuate incisions and "augmenting" vertical compression sutures.

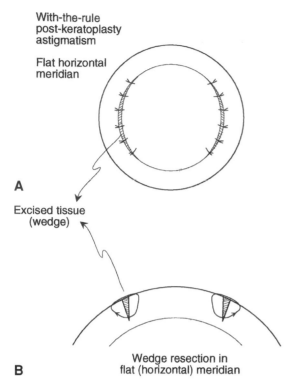

With-the-rule post-keratoplasty astigmatism

Flat horizontal meridian

A

Excised tissue (wedge)

B

Wedge resection in flat (horizontal) meridian

Figure 41–5. Top **(A)** and side **(B)** views of wedge resection to correct extreme postkeratoplasty astigmatism.

TABLE 41–9. MANAGEMENT OF ASTIGMATISM AFTER SUTURE REMOVAL: WEDGE-RESECTION STUDIES

Study	No. of Subjects	Mean Astigmatism Reduction (D)	% Reduction
Lugo[43]	14	5.09	62
Frucht-Pery[44]	11	11.04	72
Krachmer[42]	10	3.50	39

freehand dissection. For approximately every 0.1 mm of resected tissue, a 1 to 2 D correction is obtained.[41] Six to eight interrupted deep sutures are placed using 10-0 nylon. Suture loop tension is adjusted using slip knots under direct visualization of the surgical keratometer. Sutures are then tied down with square knots and buried. Tension should be placed to overcorrect the astigmatism by approximately 30% to 50%. To compensate for the astigmatic overcorrection in the meridian 90° away from the wedge resection, two compression sutures may be placed during the immediate postoperative period until the wedge-resected sutures are removed. Selective suture removal can begin 8 to 10 weeks postoperatively. Afterward, sutures can be removed every 3 to 5 weeks until a satisfactory result is obtained. Sutures may be left indefinitely if the desired

astigmatic correction occurs before all the sutures are removed.

REFERENCES

1. Jensen AD, Maumenee AE. Refractive errors following keratoplasty. *Trans Am Ophthalmol Soc.* 1974;72:123–131.
2. Perlman EM. Analysis and interpretation of refractive errors after penetrating keratoplasty. *Ophthalmology.* 1981; 88:39–45.
3. Perl T, Charlton KH, Binder PS. Disparate diameter grafting astigmatism, intraocular pressure and visual acuity. *Ophthalmology.* 1981;88:774–781.
4. Troutman RC, Swinger CA, Belmont S. Selective positioning of the donor cornea in penetrating keratoplasty for keratoconus: postoperative astigmatism. *Cornea.* 1984;3: 135–139.
5. Samples JR, Binder PS. Visual acuity, refractive error, and astigmatism following corneal transplantation for pseudophakic bullous keratoplasty. *Ophthalmology.* 1985;92: 1554–1560.
6. Meyer RF, Musch DC. Assessment of success, and complications of triple procedure surgery. *Am J Ophthalmol.* 1987; 104:233–240.
7. Swinger CA. Postoperative astigmatism. *Survey Ophthalmol.* 1987;31:219–248.
8. Troutman RC. Microsurgical control of corneal astigmatism in cataract and keratoplasty. *Trans Am Acad Ophthalmol Otolaryngol.* 1973;77:563–572.
9. Troutman RC, Gaster RN. Surgical advances and results of keratoconus. *Am J Ophthalmol.* 1980;90:131–136.
10. Raton RT. *Keratoplasty.* New York: McGraw-Hill; 1955: 146–163.
11. Vannas M. Some suggestions for improved operating technique in corneal transplantation. *Arch Ophthalmol.* 1939;140:709–794.
12. Troutman RC, Buzard K. Incisional techniques for corneal surgery. In: Troutman RC, Buzard K, eds. *Corneal Astigmatism.* St. Louis, MO: Mosby-Year Book; 1992:184–216.
13. Wright KW, Kaufman HE, Barron BA, McDonald MB, Wilson SE. *Color Atlas of Ophthalmic Surgery. Corneal and Refractive Surgery.* Philadelphia: Lippincott; 1992:15–105.
14. Abbott RL. Aphakic and pseudophakic keratoplasty. In: Brightbill FS, ed. *Corneal Surgery: Theory, Technique, and Tissue.* St. Louis, MO: Mosby-Year Book; 1993:141–157.
15. Belmont SC, Zimmerman JL, Storch RL, Anaga A, Troutman RC. Astigmatism after penetrating keratoplasty using the Krumeich guided trephine system. *Refract Corneal Surg.* 1993;9:250–254.
16. Olson R. Preventing astigmatism in penetrating keratoplasty. *Int Ophthalmol Clin.* 1988;28:37–45.
17. Perlman EM. Unusual refractive errors induced by interchanging trephines during penetrating keratoplasty. *Corneal Surg.* 1989;5:271–273.

18. VanRij G, Waring GO. Configuration of corneal trephine opening using five different trephines in human donor eyes. *Arch Ophthalmol.* 1988;106:1228–1233.

19. Mahjoub SB, Av Y-K. Astigmatism and tissue-shape disparity in penetrating keratoplasty. *Ophthalmic Surg.* 1990; 21:187–190.

20. Van Rij G, Cornell FM, Waring GO, Wilson LA, Beekhuis WH. Postoperative astigmatism after central versus eccentric penetrating keratoplasties. *Am J Ophthalmol.* 1985; 99:317–370.

21. Olson RJ. Corneal curvature changes associated with penetrating keratoplasty, a mathematical model. *Ophthalmol Surg.* 1980;11:838.

22. Cohen KL, Holman RE, Tripoli NK, Kupper LL. Effect of trephine tilt on corneal button dimensions. *Am J Ophthalmol.* 1986;101:722–725.

23. Troutman RC, Buzard K. Incisional techniques for corneal surgery. In: *Corneal Astigmatism.* St Louis, MO: Mosby–Year Book; 1992:349–404.

24. Perl T, Charlton KH, Binder PS. Disparate diameter grafting: astigmatism, intraocular pressure, and visual acuity. *Ophthalmology.* 1981;88:774–780.

25. Wilson SE, Bourne WM. Effect of recipient-donor trephine size disparity on refractive error in keratoconus. *Ophthalmology.* 1989;96:299–305.

26. McNeill JI, Wessels IF. Adjustment of single continuous suture to control astigmatism after penetrating keratoplasty. *Refract Corneal Surg.* 1989;5:216–219.

27. Serdarevic ON, Renard GJ, Pouliquen Y. Randomized clinical trial of penetrating keratoplasty—before and after suture removal comparison of intraoperative and postoperative suture adjustment. *Ophthalmology.* 1995;102:1497–1503.

28. Binder PS. Selective suture removal can reduce post keratoplasty astigmatism. *Ophthalmology.* 1985;92:1412–1416.

29. Binder PS. The effect of suture removal on post keratoplasty astigmatism. *Am J Ophthalmol.* 1988;105:637–645.

30. Burk LL, Waring GO, Radjee B, et al. The effect of selective suture removal on astigmatism following keratoplasty. *Ophthalmol Surg.* 1988;19:849–854.

31. Lin DTC, Wilson SE, Reidy JJ, Klyce SD, McDonald MB, Kaufman HE, et al. An adjustable single running suture technique to reduce post keratoplasty astigmatism. *Ophthalmology.* 1990;97:934–938.

32. Nabors G, Zwaag RV, Vanmeter WS, Wood TO. Suture adjustment for postkeratoplasty astigmatism. *Trans Am Ophthalmol Soc.* 1990;97:289–299.

33. Lavery GW, Lindstrom RL, Hofer LA, Doughman DJ. The surgical management of corneal astigmatism after penetrating keratoplasty. *Ophthalmic Surg.* 1985;16:165–169.

34. Sugar J, Kirk AK. Relaxing keratotomy for post-keratoplasty high astigmatism. *Ophthalmic Surg.* 1983;14:156–158.

35. Krachmer JH, Fenzl RE. Surgical correction of high postkeratoplasty astigmatism, relaxing incisions vs. wedge resection. *Arch Ophthalmol.* 1980;98:1400–1403.

36. Troutman RC, Swinger C. Relaxing incision for control of postoperative astigmatism following keratoplasty. *Ophthalmic Surg.* 1980;11:117–120.

37. Mandel MR, Shapiro MB, Krachmer JH. Relaxing incisions with augmentation sutures for the correction of postkeratoplasty astigmatism. *Am J Ophthalmol.* 1987;103: 441–447.

38. Lustbader JM, Lemp MA. The effect of relaxing incisions with multiple compression sutures on post-keratoplasty astigmatism. *Ophthalmic Surg.* 1990;21:416–419.

39. Fronterre A, Portesani GP. Relaxing incisions for postkeratoplasty astigmatism. *Cornea.* 10:305–11.

40. Troutman RC. Microsurgical control of corneal astigmatism in cataract and keratoplasty. *Trans Am Acad Ophthalmol Otalaryngol.* 1973;77:563–572.

41. Lindstrom RL. Surgical correction of refractive errors after penetrating keratoplasty. *Int Ophthalmol Clin.* 1994;34: 35–53.

42. Krachmer JH, Fenzl RE. Surgical correction of high postkeratoplasty astigmatism, relaxing incisions vs. wedge resection. *Arch Ophthalmol.* 1980;98:1400–1403.

43. Lugo M, Donnenfeld ED, Arentsen JJ. Corneal wedge resection for high astigmatism following penetrating keratoplasty. *Ophthalmic Surg.* 1987;18:650–653.

44. Frucht-Pery J. Wedge resection for post keratoplasty astigmatism. *Ophthalmic Surg.* 1993;24:516–518.

45. Vanmeter WS, Gussler JR, Solomon KD, Wood TO. Post keratoplasty astigmatism control. Single continuous suture adjustment versus selective interrupted suture removal. *Ophthalmology* 1991;98:177–183.

46. Musch DC, Meyer R, Sugar A, Soong HK. Corneal astigmatism after penetrating keratoplasty—the role of suture technique. *Ophthalmology.* 1989;96:698–703.

47. Filatov V, Steiner RF, Talamo JH. Post keratoplasty astigmatism with single running suture or interrupted sutures. *Am J Ophthalmol.* 1993;115:715–721.

48. Cohen KL, Tripoli NK, Noecker RJ. Prospective analysis of photokeratoplasty astigmatism. *Refract Corneal Surg.* 1989;5:388–393.

49. Limberg MB, Dingeldein SA, Green MT, Klyce SD, Insler MS, Kaufman HE. Corneal compression sutures for the reduction of astigmatism after penetrating keratoplasty. *Am J Ophthalmol.* 1989;108:36–42.

50. Frangieh GT, Kwitko S, McDonnell PJ. Prospective corneal topographic analysis in surgery for postkeratoplasty astigmatism. *Arch Ophthalmol.* 1991;109:506–510.

51. Kirkness CM, Ficker LA, Steele AD, Rice NS. Refractive surgery for graft-induced astigmatism after penetrating keratoplasty for keratoconus. *Ophthalmology.* 1991;98: 1786–1792.

52. Saragoussi JJ, Abenhaim A, Waked N, Koster HR, Pouliquen Y. Results of transverse keratotomies for astigma-

tism after penetrating keratoplasty: a retrospective study of 48 consecutive cases. *Refract Corneal Surg.* 1992;8:33–38.

53. Arffa RC. Results of a graded relaxing incision technique for postkeratoplasty astigmatism. *Ophthalmic Surg.* 1988; 19:624–628.

54. Maxwell WA, Nordan LT. Trapezoidal relaxing incision for post keratoplasty astigmatism. *Ophthalmic Surg.* 1986; 17:88–90.

55. Price FW, Whitson WE. The art of surgical correction for postkeratoplasty astigmatism. *Int Ophthal Clin.* 1994;34: 59–67.

56. Maguire LJ, Bourne WM. Corneal topography of transverse keratotomies for astigmatism after penetrating keratoplasty. *Am J Ophthalmol.* 1989;107:323–330.

57. McCartney DL, Whitney CE, Stark WJ, Wong SK, Bernitsky DA. Refractive keratoplasty for disabling astigmatism after penetrating keratoplasty. *Arch Ophthalmol.* 1987;105: 954–957.

CHAPTER 42

Phakic Intraocular Lenses

Georges Baikoff ▪ Ameed Samaha

Since the end of the 19th century different surgical procedures to correct high myopia have been advocated and tried to eliminate the need for eyeglasses or contact lenses. These surgical procedures include clear lens extraction–phakic intraocular lens (IOL) implantation[1–10] or keratorefractive surgery consisting of freeze or nonfreeze keratomileusis, epikeratoplasty, radial keratotomy, photorefractive surgery using the excimer laser, lamellar keratoplasty with the excimer laser, or intracorneal lenses or rings.

For the lower degrees of myopia up to −6 or −7 diopters (D), radial keratotomy or photorefractive keratectomy (PRK) is the procedure of choice.[1,2] The challenge is to correct severe myopia (>−8.0 D), where various alternative procedures are available. Keratorefractive surgery such as keratomileusis, epikeratophakia, and implantation of intracorneal lenses has been attempted with varying degrees of success.[3] The optical results of these surgeries are not predictable and accurate enough, and severe, sometimes irreversible complications include irregular astigmatism and corneal melting.[2,4,5]

To avoid these corneal complications, other investigators considered manipulating the lens or its total power by either clear lens extraction or phakic myopic IOL implantation.

The concept of using phakic implants to correct myopia was revived in Europe in the late 1980s and remains under clinical evaluation. It involves implanting a negative-power IOL anterior to the crystalline lens. To be recommended, the procedure should be safe, easy to perform, and provide predictable and stable optical results.

BACKGROUND

Since the evolution of IOL to correct aphakia in the 1950s, some surgeons started placing contact lenses in front of the crystalline lens in the anterior chamber (AC) to correct high myopia. The first to do so was Strampelli in 1953.[6] Later, Dannheim and Barraquer modified the design of these lenses. In 1959 Barraquer reported 239 of such implantations.[6]

The Strampelli Lens

In the Strampelli lens,[6] the radius of curvature of its nonoptical portion is 13 mm, which ensures lens separation from the iris and the corneal endothelium. The lens was thick and rigid (Fig 42–1). It was implanted in the AC using the iridocorneal angle for support. A surgical peripheral iridectomy was always performed. Difficulties were in matching AC diameter and lens length, sometimes resulting in excessive lens movement with subsequent endothelial cell damage, corneal decompo-

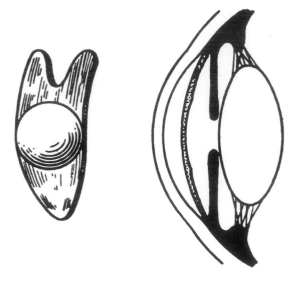

Figure 42–1. Strampelli lens of adequate length, curvature, and thickness. *(From Barraquer J. Anterior chamber plastic lenses. Results and conclusions from five years experience. Trans Ophthalmol Soc UK. 1959;79:393–424. With permission.)*

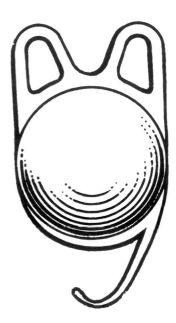

Figure 42–2. A Cogan/Boberg-Ans fenestrated lens. *(From Barraquer J. Anterior chamber plastic lenses. Results and conclusions from five years experience. Trans Ophthalmol Soc UK. 1959;79:393–424. With permission.)*

sition, iritis, and pupillary block.[6] This was more likely with smaller lens size. To avoid this pupillary block, another model was designed by Cogan and Boberg (Fig 42–2).[6] However, pupillary and peripheral iridectomy block still occurred. Hyphema, iritis, endothelial cell damage with corneal dystrophies, and increase in intraocular pressure were also common problems at that time, mainly secondary to lens thickness and rigidity.

The Dannheim Lens

The Dannheim lens[6] solved the problems of thickness, weight, and elasticity inherent in the Strampelli lens (Fig 42–3). However, it was still hard to match the lens length with the AC diameter, and the same complications remained (Fig 42–4).

The Barraquer Lens

The chief difference in the Barraquer lens is that its support is curved and maximum elasticity is in its haptics, so that it is better fitted in the AC without modifying the curvature of its optical part (Fig 42–5).[6] Despite all efforts, corneal dystrophies, hyphema, and glaucoma were still common, and many implants had to be removed later. Later Choyce[7] started to use implants with thinner haptics (0.5 mm instead of 0.911 mm) and reported a significant decrease in corneal dystrophies and other complications. However, most of his patients were uniocular aphakes except for only four high-myopic young children.[6]

For the later one third of this century, negative-power phakic myopic IOL implantation for high-myopia correction was abandoned for two reasons[8]: faulty lens design (solid lenses with thick periphery) and faulty surgical technique. When Drews[1] examined some of the explanted lenses of Barraquer, he found them to be coarse and of poor quality. Moreover, there was no concept of endothelial vitality, no viscoelastic

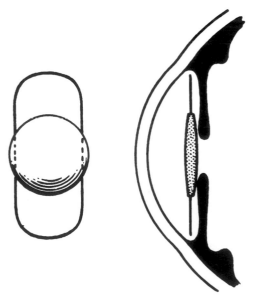

Figure 42–3. Lens slightly less long than the AC diameter as indicated by its author. *(From Barraquer J. Anterior chamber plastic lenses. Results and conclusions from five years experience. Trans Ophthalmol Soc UK. 1959; 79:393–424. With permission.)*

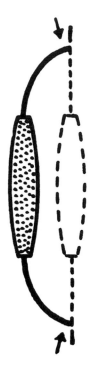

Figure 42–4. At the loop extremities the Dannheim lens curves forward toward the cornea, which it may touch. *(From Barraquer J. Anterior chamber plastic lenses. Results and conclusions from five years experience. Trans Ophthalmol Soc UK. 1959;79:393–424. With permission.)*

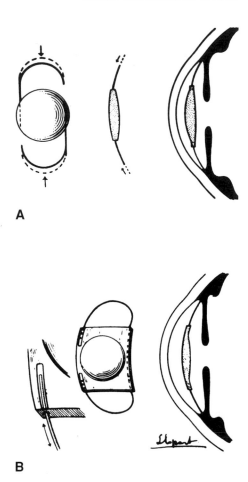

Figure 42–5. A. The Barraquer lens. The radius of curvature is not sensibly affected despite transverse pressure on the supramid (poliamida, nylon) supports. **B.** A prototype Barraquer lens. The supramid nylon loops can slide in the tunnel, thus varying its length and the diameter of the nonoptical part of the lens. The model shown in **A** is a simplified version of **B**. *(From Barraquer J. Anterior chamber plastic lenses. Results and conclusions from five years experience. Trans Ophthalmol Soc UK. 1959;79:393–424 With permission.)*

substances used to form the AC, no miotics used in many cases, and no effort to avoid traumatizing the natural crystalline lens.

There has been great progress in the design of IOLs. The surface is now well polished; the haptics are thinner and more flexible. Surgical techniques have improved markedly due to the advent of microsurgery and the invention of viscoelastic substances. As a result, the concept of minus-power IOL implantation in phakic myopes was revived in the late 1980s. Such operations were reported by Dvali[1] in 1986. Fechner, Praeger and Momose, Baikoff, and Fyodorov have all developed a mode of lens fixation. Fechner,[1,9–11] in an attempt to avoid the anterior-chamber angle for lens support, developed an iris-fixated lens derived from the Worst iris-claw lens designed in 1977[12] for aphakia correction. Baikoff[2,13–15] and Praeger-Momose[3,8,16] developed an angle-supported lens, and Fyodorov used a posterior-chamber (PC) lens supported by the anterior surface of the crystalline lens.

Few animal data on phakic IOL are available. Baikoff[13] reviewed the literature and found two animal experiments, one done on rabbits by Tchah and colleagues[4] and the other done on monkeys by Peiffer.[17] A high incidence of cataract development secondary to implant lenticular touch occured in all 12 rabbit eyes. The monkeys had a high incidence of endothelial cell loss. Peiffer reported a mean cell loss of 31% after 1 year. The consensus was against use of these implants, but Baikoff commented that in both experiments the AC IOL did not fit the different ocular anatomy of these animals compared with humans. Based on this, one must depend more on clinical investigation information to analyze and evaluate this procedure.

PATIENT SELECTION CRITERIA

Patients are selected as follows[1,2,9]:

- High myopes (>8 D) with no general health problems. No diabetes mellitus.

- Only if spectacle correction is unsatisfactory for occupational reasons or contraindicated for any important psychological reason.
- Myopia has been stable for some years.
- Patient is not a candidate for radial keratotomy (RK) or PRK (ie, low-myopic patients).
- No anterior-segment pathology, no glaucoma, no cataract, no rubeosis iridis, no uveitis or anterior synechea.
- Adequate AC depth (more than 3.5-mm depth or 3.2-mm depth according to Fechner[1] and Baikoff,[2] respectively).
- Healthy peripheral retina or retina prophylactically treated before surgery.
- Anisomyope (severe) patients.
- Patients amenable to lifelong close ophthalmologic supervision.

PREOPERATIVE EVALUATION

A full ophthalmologic examination and prophylactic treatment if necessary are needed.[1,2,9] The surgeon should measure AC depth by ultrasound and perform keratometry and careful, cycloplegic, and subjective manifest refraction. Caution is advised in subjective refractions or objective measurements of refractive errors more than −20 D. High myopes accept overcorrection easily, and automated refractometers are less accurate in myopia exceeding −20 D.[13] If difficulty is encountered, one can refer to the power of a trial contact lens to find the exact correction as suggested by Baikoff. Systematic endothelial cell count should be documented.[1,2,13]

POSTOPERATIVE FOLLOW-UP AND EXAMINATION

Postoperative examination should include visual acuity, manifest refraction, intraocular pressure, slit lamp examination to assess the AC, cornea, pupils, and IOL position and to confirm contact with the cornea or natural lens, and endothelial cell diversity at regular interals. There are three follow-up visits during the first week postoperatively, then every week for the next 3 weeks, then at week 8, week 12, in 6 months, in 12 months, and then every 6 months.[1]

SURGICAL TECHNIQUES

Different types of phakic myopic implants have been designed and tried. They include (1) the AC bioconcave iris-claw lens, iris fixation; (2) the Praeger-Momose glass optic AC lens, angle fixation; (3) the Baikoff-type lens, angle fixation; and (4) the Fyodorov phakic PC lens, anterior crystalline lens support.

The Worst-Fechner Biconcave Iris-Claw Lens

The Worst-Fechner biconcave iris-claw lens[1,9,11,12] used to correct high myopia has a posterior concave surface that provides enough space between the implant and the crystalline lens even if the latter thickens with age (Fig 42–6). It is composed of polymethylmethacrylate (PMMA) and is 0.93 mm thick for a −13.0 D lens in water.[1] The diameter of its optical part is 4.5 mm, and the refractive power of its posterior surface is −5.0 D. Additional divergent power is attained by the concave anterior surface. When more refractive power is desired, the anterior rim of the lens is ground off so that the total thickness of the lens remains 0.93 mm, but the optical part is a little smaller. Even for a −18 D lens, its optical diameter is 4 mm.[1]

Preoperative Preparation

One hour preoperatively, the pupil is constricted with 2% pilocarpine eye drops three to four times.[1] Additional steps include giving 250 ml of 20% mannitol intravenously and applying ocular compression at 40 mm Hg for 10 minutes. Systemic steroids (prednisone) used to be given, but later Fechner stopped giving them preoperatively. Finally, retrobulbar anesthesia is applied with lid akinesia or general anesthesia.

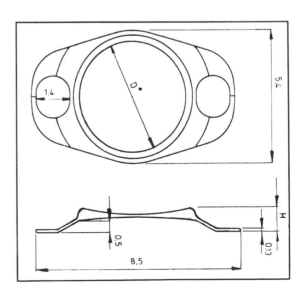

Figure 42–6. Worst-Fechner biconcave lens. *(From Fechner PU, et al. Correction of myopia by implantation of a concave Worst iris claw lens into phakic eyes.* Refract Corneal Surg. *1991;7:286–298. With permission.)*

Operative Procedure

Fornix-based conjunctival peritomy is performed between 8 over 12 to the 4 o'clock position. Then three corneoscleral incisions are made—one from 10:30 over 12 to 1:30 o'clock (the big incision), and two small (3-mm) incisions at 3 and 9 o'clock. Surgical peripheral iridectomy is done at 12 o'clock. The AC is then irrigated with acetylcholine and filled with viscoelastic substance. A Sheet's glide is placed over the pupil, and the IOL is inserted through the big incision into the AC. The big incision is partly closed with interrupted sutures to preserve the viscoelastic substance in the AC. The lens is then rotated into the horizontal position. A lens fixation forceps is introduced through one end of the big incision to hold the corresponding haptic of the lens. Then with an iris forceps introduced through the ipsilateral small incision, a 2-mm iris fold is captured and pulled through the slit in the haptic. Now the lens is fixed to the midperiphery of the iris at one side. The same procedure is applied to the other haptic, with the surgeon maintaining good centration of the IOL optic. The viscoelastic material is evacuated and replaced with balanced salt solution. All incisions are then closed with 9-0 nylon and peritomy secured to the limbus (Fig 42–7). Table 42–1 lists postoperative medications.

Intraocular Lens Calculation

Van der Heijde developed a formula and a nomogram to calculate IOL power (Table 42–2).[1] The formula is based on the following parameters:

TABLE 42–1. FECHNER PHAKIC ANTERIOR-CHAMBER INTRAOCULAR LENS PROTOCOL

1 hour preoperatively:
   2% pilocarpine eye drops
   250 ml of 20% mannitol intravenously
   100 mg of prednisone orally
   250 mg of prednisone intravenously

Postoperative day 1:
   100 mg of prednisone orally
   Prednisolone acetate 1% eyedrops hourly
   Dilation of pupil twice daily

Postoperative day 2:
   50 mg of prednisone orally
   Prednisolone acetate 1% eyedrops hourly
   Dilation of pupil twice daily

Postoperative days 3 to 14:
   Prednisolone acetate 1% eyedrops five times daily
   Pupil dilation once

Postoperative weeks 3 and 4:
   Prednisolone acetate 1% eyedrops three times daily

Modified from Fechner PU, et al. Correction of myopia by implantation of a concave Worst iris claw lens into phakic eyes. *Refract Corneal Surg.* 1991;7:286–298.

TABLE 42–2. VAN DER HEJIDE'S TABLE FOR CLAW-LENS INTRAOCULAR LENS*

K = 38	K = 43	K = 48
−5.6	−5.7	−5.9
−6.6	−6.8	−6.9
−7.6	−8.0	−8.0
−8.6	−8.8	−9.0
−9.5	−9.8	−10.0
−10.4	−10.7	−11.0
−11.3	−11.6	−11.9
−12.2	−12.5	−12.8
−13.1	−13.4	−13.7
−13.9	−14.3	−14.6
−14.7	−15.1	−15.5
−15.5	−15.9	−16.3
−16.3	−16.7	−17.1
−17.1	−17.5	−17.9
−17.8	−18.3	−18.7
−18.5	−19.0	−19.5
−19.3	−19.7	−20.2
−20.0	−20.4	−20.9
−20.6	−21.1	−21.7
−21.3	−21.8	−22.4
−21.9	−22.5	−23.0

*Assumes anterior chamber depth (distance between apex of anterior corneal surface and cardinal plane of IOL) = 3.0 mm.
Modified from Fechner PU, et al. Correction of myopia by implantation of a concave Worst iris claw lens into phakic eyes. *Refract Corneal Surg.* 1991;7:286–298.

1. The preoperative and postoperative refraction desired. Refraction is defined by the correcting glasses in the spectacle plane 12 mm in front of the cornea.
2. Refractive power of the cornea (keratometry).
3. Anterior chamber depth. This is distance between the anterior corneal surface and the cardinal plane of the IOL, which is practically identical with the anterior IOL surface. Fechner and Worst found that the anterior surface of the IOL is approximately 0.8 mm in front of the natural lens. To calculate, deduct 0.8 mm from the total AC depth as measured by ultrasound.

Praeger-Momose Glass Optic Phakic Myopic Intraocular Lens

The Praeger-Momose IOL[8,16] was first implanted by Dr Akira Momose of Japan in May 1987. This was before Fechner and Baikoff's procedures. The lens has a glass optical part with a high index of refraction—1.62. The haptics are made up of polyamide. The wetting angle is

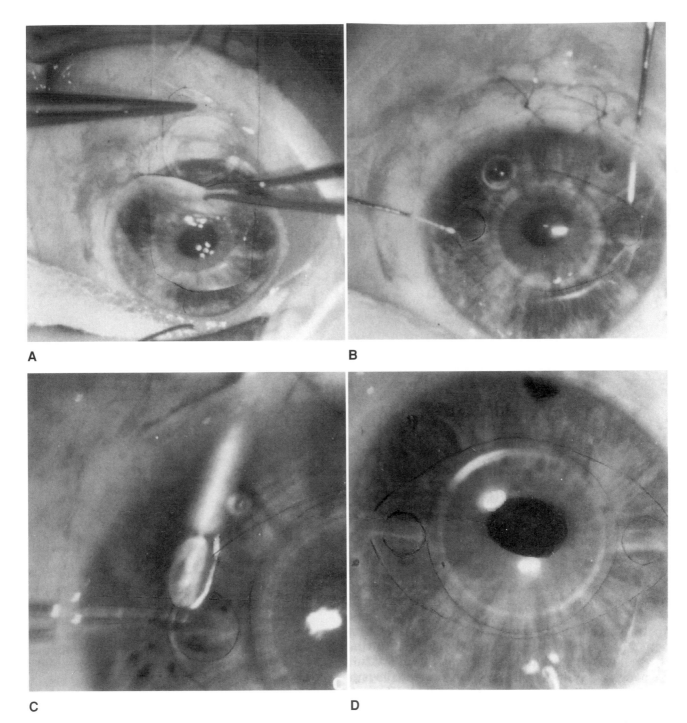

A

B

C

D

Figure 42–7. Insertion of a biconcave lens. Some contours are emphasized by retouching. **A.** The incisions at 9 and 3 o'clock and from 10:30 to 1:30 o'clock have been performed, and the anterior chamber is filled with viscous material. Presently, the IOL is being inserted over a Sheet's glide. **B.** After a peripheral iridectomy, the big incision is partly closed. The IOL is being manipulated into a horizontal position with two hooks. **C.** The haptic is grasped from above and the iris forceps has grasped iris tissue behind the IOL's haptic and presently moves through the slit in the haptic, incarcerating the iris into the claw. **D.** The end of the operation. The IOL is fixed to the iris on the contralateral side. The corneoscleral wounds are closed with 9-0 nylon sutures (not seen), and the conjunctival flap is repositioned. *(From Fechner PU, et al. Correction of myopia by implantation of a concave Worst iris claw lens into phakic eyes.* Refract Corneal Surg. *1991;7:286–298. With permission.)*

low. This AC lens uses the iridocorneal angle for support (Fig 42–8). Implantation involves one large corneoscleral incision superiorly through which the implant is introduced and fixed at the AC angle. Preoperative and intraoperative miotics are used, as is a viscoelastic substance. The incision is closed with 10-0 or 9-0 interrupted sutures.

The Baikoff Intraocular Lens

First Generation Intraocular Lens

In 1986, Baikoff presented his new angle-supported AC IOL to correct high myopia in phakic eyes. It was derived from the Kelman-type implant designed to correct aphakia (Fig 42–9).[2]

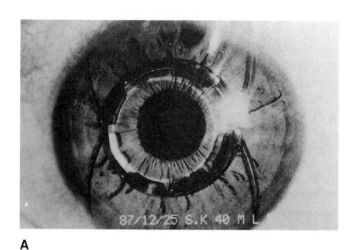

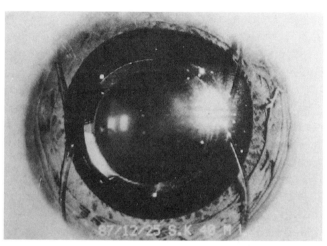

A

B

Figure 42–8. A. Phakic myopic AC IOL 5 months after surgery, undilated. *(From Baikoff G, Joly P. Comparison of minus power anterior chamber intraocular lenses and myopic epikeratoplasty in phakic eyes.* Refract Corneal Surg. 1990;6:252. *With permission.)* **B.** Same eye as in **A**, dilated. *(From Tchah H, Duffey RJ, Allarakhia L, Lindstrom RL. Intraocular lens implantation in phakic rabbit eyes.* J Cataract Refract Surg. *1989;15:554–558. With permission.)*

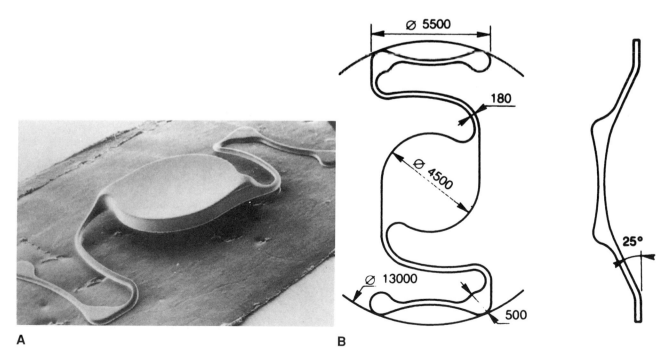

A

B

Figure 42–9. A. Minus-power AC IOL used in the study. Scanning electron micrograph shows lens with finely polished surface, concave optic, and anterior vault (× 10). **B.** Specifications for the intraocular lens. *(From Baikoff G, Joly P. Comparison of minus power anterior chamber intraocular lenses and myopic epikeratoplasty in phakic eyes.* Refract Corneal Surg. *1990;6:252. With permission.)*

The lens has a biconcave optic with an edge surface thickness of 0.7 mm for a −20 D lens. The haptic is designed to permit only localized contact with the AC angle, thus limiting the development of peripheral anterior synechiae and damage to the angle (Fig 42–10). The anterior vaulting of this model is 25°, thus placing the center of the IOL approximately 1 mm in front of the pupil and 2 mm behind the cornea. Overall diameters were 12.0, 12.50, 13.0, and 13.50 mm, with refractive power ranging from −8.0 D to −30.0 D in steps of 1.00 D. The lens has a 4.5-mm-diameter optic to provide sufficient distance between the peripheral rim of the optic and the corneal endothelium.[2,13]

Second Generation

In an attempt to limit the rate of complications associated with the first-generation Baikoff implants, Baikoff[14] modified his original design. He called the new lens ZB5M design. He lowered the angulation from 25° to 20° (Fig 42–11) and thinned out the optic edge, thereby gaining 0.6 mm in the lens-cornea spacing.[14] It is not less than 1.3 mm compared with 0.8 to 1.0 mm in the first-generation IOL. Baikoff also limited the IOL power to −18.0 D (Fig 42–12).

Implant Determination

The implant is chosen according to two parameters: lens refractive power and lens length. Rather than depending on formula calculation to determine the lens power, Baikoff applied the following rule[2]: for spectacle refraction of −10.0 D, he used a −10.0 D implant. For spectacle refraction between −11.0 and −15.0 D, he added +1.0 D to the implant power (eg, for a −13.0 D spectacle refraction, a −12.0 D implant is used). For spectacle refraction between −16 and −20.0 D, he added +2.0 D (eg, a −17.0 spectacle refraction re-

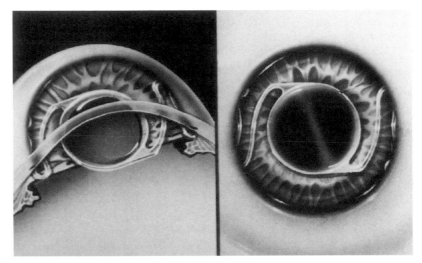

Figure 42–10. AC IOL for myopia. *(From Baikoff G, Colin J. Intraocular lenses in phakic patients. Ophthalmol Clin North Am. 1992;4:789. With permission.)*

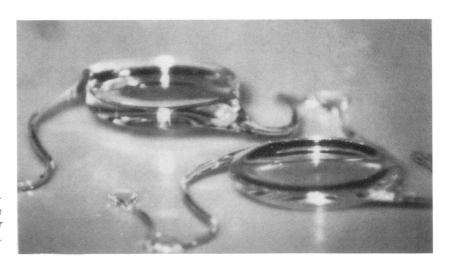

Figure 42–11. Comparison of the first and last design of the Baikoff phakic AC IOL. Both IOLs have the same power. *(From Baikoff G, Colin J. Intraocular lenses in phakic patients. Ophthalmol Clin North Am. 1992;4:789. With permission.)*

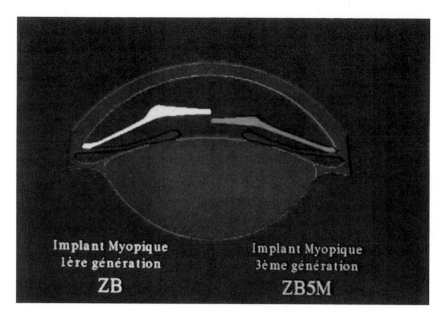

Implant Myopique
1ère génération
ZB

Implant Myopique
3ème génération
ZB5M

Figure 42–12. Schematic comparison in simulated AC of a first-generation implant and of the new design. *(From Baikoff G. The refractive IOL in a phakic eye.* Ophthalmic Pract. *1991;9:2. With permission.)*

quires a −15.0 D implant). Total diameter of the lens was determined according to the horizontal distance from white to white plus 1.0 mm.[13]

Operative Procedure

Preoperatively the pupil is constricted. The operation can be done under local or general anesthesia.[2] Baikoff used a nasal or temporal corneal incision parallel to the plane of the iris 6 to 7 mm long. This avoids the lid and the eyelid speculum if the incision is made superiorly, thus rendering the operation easier. Sodium hyaluronate was used to form the AC and coat the lens before its insertion. A Sheet's glide can be inserted above the pupil on which the implant will slide. Once the distal haptic of the implant is in the angle, the proximal haptic is introduced using a fine forceps and is secured in the opposite angle. Peripheral iridectomy is not always necessary; however, if it is to be done it should not be basal to avoid contact between the haptic and the ciliary body. After lens insertion and in the absence of pupil deformation, the proper position of IOL footplates is checked by gonioscopy. A fine probe is used to reposition the lens, if needed. Thereafter the viscoelastic substance is completely removed from the AC, which is irrigated with balanced salt solution. The corneal incision is closed using interrupted 10-0 nylon sutures. Antibiotics and corticosteroids are then injected subconjunctivally. Topical antibiotics and corticosteroids are used for 6 weeks postoperatively. If ovalization of the pupil is noted intraoperatively, the implant is changed for a smaller one. As mentioned, do not use these implants if AC depth is less than 3.2 mm.[2,15]

Since the late 1980s many investigational clinical studies have been undertaken in Europe using different implant types and surgical techniques to correct high myopia.

CLINICAL OUTCOME

Refractive and Visual Acuity Results

The optical results of phakic myopic implants seem to produce superior, more predictable, and stable results compared with other keratorefractive procedures. Fechuer, Baikoff, Colin, Mimouni, and Landesz demonstrated in their studies that emmetropia within 1 D could be achieved in 70% to 75% of eyes with preoperative mean refraction of −14.50 D. Emmetropia within 2 D was achievable in more than 90% of eyes. Fechner and colleagues had a mean deviation of 0.41 D in 123 operated eyes after an average follow-up period of 34 months (Fig 42–13). In the multicenter study done in France using Baikoff's implant, the mean deviation was −0.2 D. Taking the standard deviation into account, this study reported that 95% of eyes had a refractive error between −1.3 D and +1.3 D.

Visual acuity recovery was rapid. Preoperative visual acuity level was attained the second day postoperatively, and best corrected visual acuity (BCVA) was attained during the first postoperative month and stabilized by the sixth postoperative month (Fig 42–14). Moreover, Fechner, Baikoff, and Colin reported that in approximately 78% of eyes, BCVA has been improved by one or two Snellen lines versus 56.6% and 42% for

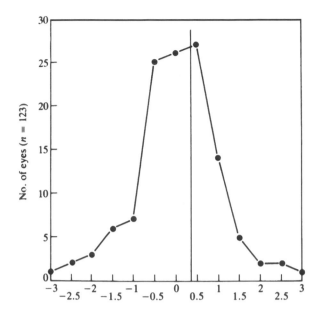

Figure 42–13. Deviation of the achieved from the calculated refraction (in diopters). Mean deviation, +0.4 D. *(From Fechner PU, et al. Correction of myopia by implantation of minus optic (Worst iris claw) lenses into the anterior chamber of phakic eyes. Eur J Implant Refract Surg. 1993;5:55. With permission.)*

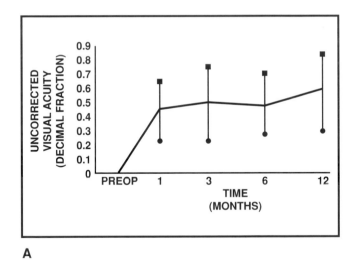

A

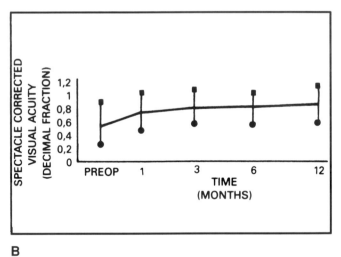

B

Figure 42–14. A. Uncorrected distance visual acuity after minus-power AC IOL implantation in phakic myopic eyes. At each time 32 to 39 eyes were examined. Line indicates mean visual acuity; error bars indicate standard deviation. **B.** Spectacle-corrected distance visual acuity after minus-power AC IOL implantation in phakic myopic eyes. There were 32 to 40 eyes examined at the postoperative time points. Line indicates mean value; error bars indicate standard deviation. *(From Baikoff G, Joly P. Comparison of minus power anterior chamber intraocular lenses and myopic epikeratoplasty in phakic eyes. Refract Corneal Surg. 1990;6:252. With permission.)*

Praeger-Momose and Mimouni in their small series, respectively. This improvement in BCVA occurs because the retinal image magnification achieved with IOL implantation eliminates the minification effect of spectacles. Accommodation was maintained, and near BCVA did not change in any patient. The mean BCVA in most of the studies was 20/40. One patient in Bai-

koff's initial series showed a decrease in BCVA from 20/20 to 20/25. Fechner had four patients who developed corneal edema with a secondary decrease in BCVA.[1]

Excellent long-term stability of postoperative refraction was noted by all the investigators. None of Fechner's patients had delayed refractive changes, and only a 0.5 D average change over a 2-year period was noted in Baikoff's series of 41 patients (Fig 42–15).

Compared with other keratorefractive procedures for high-myopia correction, namely, epikeratoplasty and keratomileusis, Baikoff[2] and Colin[5] in a retrospective study demonstrated that phakic myopic implantation provided more rapid and predictable optical correction and better BCVA results. The preoperative visual acuity level was obtained by 6M° and 12M° with epikeratoplasty and keratomileusis (nonfreeze), respectively. Results showed 27% and 33%[2,5] of cases were within 1 D of emmetropia according to the procedure versus 78% for phakic myopic implantation. Moreover, 14.3%[5] of eyes lost one to two Snellen lines of BCVA after epikeratoplasty, and many lenticules (~20%) had to be removed because of poor refractive results compared with one IOL, that had to be exchanged in Baikoff's series because of refractive error exceeding 3 D. Some 30.7% of eyes in the nonfreeze keratomileusis group lost more than two lines of BCVA. Moreover, epikeratoplasty requires donor corneal tissue and myopic keratomileusis is a difficult and nonreversible surgery. Surgical phakic myopic implantation is a relatively simple procedure and potentially easily reversible.

The above-mentioned predictability and stability of optical correction in phakic myopic implantation, improved BCVA, and the simplicity of the surgical procedure are important factors, but they are not enough to recommend this surgery. The procedure's potential complications must be carefully evaluated to ensure that the risks are less than those associated with a regular cataract surgery before the procedure can be recommended.

COMPLICATIONS

Complications can be divided into two main categories: minor and serious. Minor complications include transient iritis and uveitis, transient increase in intraocular pressure (IOP), pupillary distortion, wound dehiscence, and cataract. Serious sequelae with more vision-threatening potential include endothelial cell damage, retinal detachment, chronic uveitis, glaucoma, endophthalmitis, and expulsive choroidal hemorrhage.

Wound Dehiscence

Fechner and coworkers[1,11] reported 10 cystic wounds in 100 patients who received systemic steroids preoperatively. All underwent resuturing of the corneoscleral wound 3 to 8 weeks postoperatively with no compromise of ultimate BCVA. These wounds were not noted in patients who did not receive steroids preoperatively. Fechner and coworkers later stopped using preoperative steroids. No such complication was reported in any of the other studies.

Urrest-Zavalia Syndrome

Also known as postoperative atonic pupil, this syndrome consists of a transient increase in IOP caused by an op-, iris stromal atrophy, and irreversible paretic mydriasis. Fechner and associates[1,11,13] had two (1.6%) such cases that could have resulted from inadequate evacuation of the viscoelastic substance requiring removal within the first week after the initial operation. The pupils in these two patients were narrowed with nylon sutures, and in both cases preoperative visual acuity returned.[1]

Transient Iritis or Uveitis

Transient iritis or uveitis is usually secondary to iris trauma during surgery. Fechner reported an incidence of 6.4%, the majority of which were the first few cases that he did. Baikoff had a rate of 2%, while Mimoni in his small series of 15 patients had a rate of 13%. Praeger-Momose had no such cases in his small series. All patients responded quickly (within a week or two) to topical steroid treatment with no delayed sequelae.

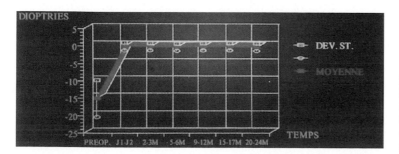

Figure 42–15. Stability of postoperative refraction after 2 years (French multicenter study). One standard deviation (DEV. ST.) above (square) and below (circle) the mean (MOYENNE) are shown. *(From Baikoff G. The refractive IOL in a phakic eye. Ophthalmic Pract. 1991;9:2. With permission.)*

Chronic Uveitis

No clinically significant or detectable ongoing inflammation has been reported in any of the studies despite the use of a flare cell meter by Fechner. However, Perez-Santonja and Benitez del Castillo using fluorophotometry were able to demonstrate the presence of prolonged (up to 14M° postoperatively) disruption of the blood-aqueous barrier (BAB) in 15 eyes with phakic iris fixation and 16 eyes with angle fixation IOLs.[18,19] Fluorophotometry is a qualitative method to assess the integrity of the BAB[19] by determining the concentration of a fluorescent tracer in the eye after intravenous injection. It is more sensitive than the flare cell meter. As proposed by Miyake, Asakura, and Kobayashi, when the IOL haptics or claws compress the uveal tissue, they may disrupt the BAB. Iris fluorescein angiography in some of Fechner's cases did not reveal any leakage from the site of lens fixation.[1] Chronic inflammation was demonstrated in recent studies by Neves and colleagues and Alio and coworkers[20,21] using cell flare photometry.

Cataract Development

Phakic AC IOL implantation is considered to be a noncataractogenic surgery.[1,2,16] There were no reports of cataract development or progression postoperatively except in one patient in Baikoff's series (0.6% incidence) who developed a cataract 1 year after surgery. According to Baikoff, it was difficult to know if this was secondary to surgical trauma to the crystalline lens or secondary to the presence of the implant in the AC. Benitez del Castillo[18] and Perez-Santonja[19] showed that there is a clinically significant decrease in lens transmittance that could be due to surgery itself or to changes in BAB permeability. However, the fact that the difference was significant 3, 6, and 14 months postoperatively but not at 1 month postoperatively indicates that BAB disruption with resultant metabolic disturbances, not surgical trauma, may decrease transmittance and speed cataract formation. However, data presented by the different studies failed to show any clinically detectable cataract formation, changes in visual acuity, or any myopic shift to suggest the possibility of early cataract formation.

Postoperative Glaucoma

There is no risk of persistent increased intraocular pressure.[1,2,13,15,16] Usually any increase is transient and may by attributed to inadequately removed viscoelastic substance, transient iritis, or steroid application regardless of the type of IOL used. The overall occurrence of transient increased IOP is 20%.[13] No cases of pupillary block glaucoma have been reported.

Intraocular Lens Instability and Decentration

IOL instability and decentration were common in the 1950s[6] with the Strampelli and the Barraquer implants, but is uncommon with the newer implants. Decentration and rotation of Baikoff's implants were observed in 2% and 4% of patients, respectively, because lens size was too small.[14,15] Baikoff reported that the lens frequently stabilizes in the new position, but if it continues to rotate or is markedly decentered, it should be replaced with a suitable size implant. Baikoff also added that lens exchange is simple and with no additional risks if done in the early postoperative period. Fechner had no such complication, although one would expect the opposite according to the Food and Drug Administration (FDA) report on IOLs published in 1983 by Stark and colleagues.[22] Moreover, Singh[1] reported his personal experience with thousands of iris-claw lens implantations in which he showed the long-lasting stability of these lenses.

Praeger, using the Momose glass optic type of AC IOLs, thought that the polyimide was too flaccid to maintain the implant in a fixed position. The weight of the glass may cause the implant to shift posteriorly. No contact was noted between the IOL and the natural lens with either a constricted or dilated pupil.

Retinal Detachment

Retinal detachment (RD) is a serious complication that can occur after any opening of an eye. It was an infrequent complication of this procedure. Both Fechner and Baikoff reported one case each in their corresponding series, accounting for an an incidence of 0.8% and 0.6%, respectively.

In two recent articles, Foss and colleagues[23] and Alio and associates[25] reported a total of six cases of retinal detachment occuring 1.5 to 13 months after phakic anterior chamber IOL implantation for high-myopia correction. The first two patients in Alio's series had RD a few weeks after Baikoff lens implantation despite preoperative prophylactic laser treatment of an area of lattice degeneration in one eye and for a horseshoe tear in the other. Both eyes were successfully treated for RD without removal of the stable AC lens. Visual results after surgery were good. Alio's third patient developed exudative and rhegmatogenous RD 8 months after phakic AC implantation. No prop retinal lesion was detected. The RD was associated with severe fibrinoid uvetis. The patient was managed with steroids, scleral buckle, and vitrectomy and had a significant loss of visual acuity. The AC was left in place.

Therefore, RD should be considered a potential serious complication of phakic AC lens implantation for myopia correction, although in many cases successful treatment with good visual acuity is possible.

Attempts recommended to decrease the risk of RD in these patients include[1]:

- Preoperative laser treatment of peripheral retinal lesions if present
- Preoperative osmotics and ocular compression
- Careful handling of the globe during surgery

Haloes and Glare

Haloes and glare are more prevalent if small diameter optical zone (OZ) IOL is used, especially at night with a mid-dilated pupil. Nocturnal haloes occured in 33% of eyes that received Baikoff's implant and in 46% of patients in the small series of Mimouni.[26] Fechner did not comment on these symptoms in his series, but Landesz and colleagues,[24] using the newly modified design of the Worst-Fechner iris-claw lens, reported the presence of haloes in 6 of 18 patients (33%) 12 months after surgery, although this modified lens had a bigger optical diameter by 0.5 mm. Landesz also found that the severity of haloes and glare seem to diminish gradually and considerably during the first 6 months postoperatively in the majority of patients.

According to Baikoff, all his patients but one tolerated these nocturnal haloes and glare with no problems. Pilocarpine 1% can be prescribed in such cases.[15]

Damage to Corneal Endothelium

Corneal endothelial cell injury remains one of the most serious complications of phakic myopic implants. Fechner in his studies used the Karickhoff method to estimate the endothelial cell density preoperatively and postoperatively at different time intervals. Results showed that the endothelial density remained good for most eyes and appeared to approximate the preoperative density.[1,11] However, in his series, Fechner had a total of 13 eyes with significant endothelial cell loss (cell count less than 300 cells/mm^2) over a mean follow-up period of 34 months postoperatively. Five were explained by operative difficulties and the other eight were of unexplained etiology, since in none of the eyes was there any detectable contact between the IOL and the endothelium.[1,16] The endothelial cell loss was progressive over the follow-up period (Fig 42–16).

The first five eyes and one of the other eight eyes developed corneal edema requiring corneal transplantation. The one with the unexplained etiology underwent a triple procedure with replacement of the iris fixation AC lens by a PC IOL. With first generation Baikoff's implants the estimated endothelial cell loss was 10% to 15% at year 1 after surgery. None of the patients had corneal decompensation after 2½ years of follow-up study of Baikoff's initial series of 41 patients.

Praeger and colleagues[8,16] showed a 5.3% endothelial cell loss postoperatively, which was not progressive after 3 years of follow-up. Mimouni and colleagues,[26] trying to find out the mechanism of damage in these patients, examined 15 patients with Baikoff's AC implants 1 year after surgery. They used specular microscopy for this purpose. There was central endothelial cell loss in 10 of 11 patients examined and paracentral cell loss in 13 of 15 patients. Four eyes (36.3%) had more than 20% central endothelial loss, and six eyes (54.5%) had less than 10% cell loss. The loss was more significant in patients who had worn contact lenses, which seem to predispose eyes to endothelial cell damage.

Mimouni in his study differentiated between chronic and acute endothelial cell loss.[26] Acute cell loss could be due to direct contact between the IOL and the cornea during surgery or during specular microscopy examination when the cornea is indented. This indentation could be equivalent to that of rubbing the eye. Mimouni also found that the greatest cell loss was in an eye with a distance less than 1 mm between the edges of the IOL and the endothelium, so he concluded that chronic damage could be the result of intermittent touch between the IOL and the endothelium.

Two and one-half years after Baikoff introduced his lens, no cases of corneal decompensation have been seen, including the French multicenter study group. Taking into account the possibility of long-term endothelial risks, a retrospective study using quantitative and topographical analysis of the corneal endothelium was undertaken by Colin, Sasagoussi, and Baikoff in different centers.[14,15] The number of examined eyes was small (29 eyes), but conclusions were firm. They found that most of the endothelial cell loss took place in the second postoperative year and later and it averaged 80% by the second year with a wide standard deviation. They also concluded that intermittent contact between the IOL and the cornea is responsible for the cell loss and probably was worse with higher implant power.

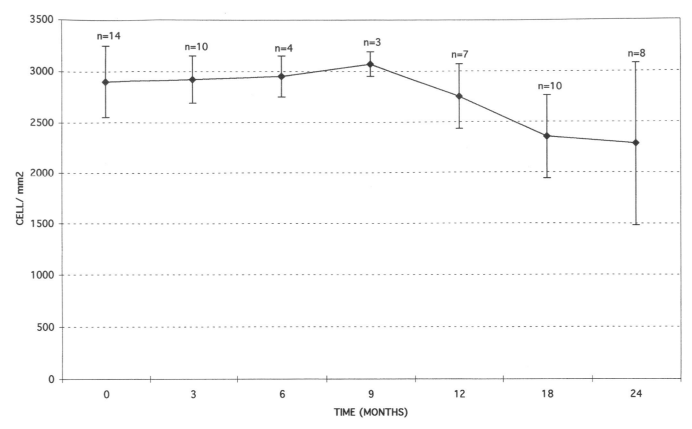

Figure 42–16. Curve of estimates of central endothelial density. *(From Baikoff G. The refractive IOL in a phakic eye. Ophthalmic Pract. 1991; 9:2. With permission.)*

These complications convinced Baikoff to modify his lens and rename it the ZB5M. A 5-year prospective study is underway to evaluate this new lens model.[13] Preliminary results after 12 months of follow-up study have been reported.[13] Sixteen eyes underwent surgery using the second-generation Baikoff AC lens. Optical results are comparable to those seen with the first-generation lens. The endothelial cell loss was measured at 3, 6, 12, and 18 months postoperatively. Results were -2.39 ± 4.87; -2.4 ± 5.0; -3.73 ± 4.53; and -4.99 ± -5.84, respectively (personal communication). There was no statistical difference between these values. The decrease in endothelial cell loss is also evident when one compares the 12-month postoperative results in the second generation and first generation lenses, although no definite conclusions can be drawn due to the small number of eyes included. Baikoff also adds that this cell loss remains inferior or equal to that seen in any cataract surgery (personal communication).

IOL was inserted and fixed horizontally to the iris through the larger superior corneoscleral incision only.

Landesz and colleagues used the noncontact and the contact specular microscope for corneal endothelial examination. The follow-up period was 6 months for 15 eyes and 12 months for 20 eyes. Preliminary refractive and visual acuity results were comparable to the previous IOL model. Haloes and glare occured in 6 of 18 patients at 12 months despite the fact that stray light measurements did not show any significant increase postoperatively. The mean endothelial cell loss was 5.3% at 6 months postoperatively in the 32 eyes and was 8.9% at 12 months postoperatively in 12 eyes. The difference between the mean cell loss at 6 and 12 months was statistically significant.[14]

To compare the endothelial cell loss in cataract surgeries with the phakic IOL implantation surgeries, Landesz and coworkers reviewed the literature. The Oxford Cataract Treatment and Evaluation team[14,27] reported a mean cell loss of 8.2% to 13.9% at 6 months and of 13.6% to 19.3% at 12 months, depending on surgical technique. Peilas and colleagues reported a mean cell loss of 26.6% at 6 months with AC IOLs and 23.8% with PC IOLs,[14] whereas Schultz and coworkers reported a mean cell loss of 7.5%.[14] Werblin,[14,28] suggesting comparison of endothelial cell loss in patients undergoing phakic IOL implantation versus phacoemulsification, found a mean cell loss of the central endothelium of

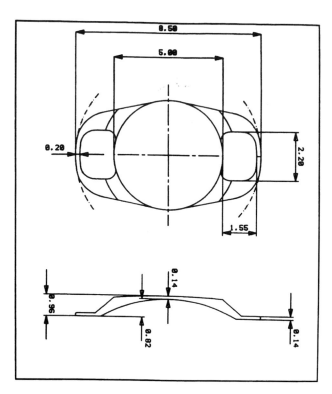

Figure 42–17. Schematic drawing of a −20.00 D convex-concave myopia claw lens. *(From Landesz M, et al. Correction of high myopia with the Worst myopic claw intraocular lens. J Refract Surg. 1995;11:16–25. With permission.)*

8.8% at 1 year after phacoemulsification, which stabilized at 11.5% after 3 years. Landesz and coauthors,[14] comparing their rate of endothelial cell loss with that of Werblin at 1 year after surgery, found no significant difference (8.9% vs. 8.8%).

Landesz mentioned that the endothelial cell count per se is not enough for complete assesment of the functional reserve of the corneal endothelium. One must also morphologically assess the endothelium in addition to cell density for better evaluation.

According to Baikoff, the AC IOL should be removed whenever the endothelial cell count is equal to or less than 50% of the normal count. The procedure of choice is lensectomy by phacoemulsification and exchange of the AC lens for a PC IOL.

Other complications such as endopthalmitis, expulsive choroidal hemorrhage, and CME occur at such an infrequent rate that they would not significantly affect the overall risk. There is one case report of ischemic optic neuropathy occurring immediately after Worst-Fechner IOL implantation to correct myopia in a phakic 33-year-old patient.[29] It was likely associated with increased IOP and systemic hypotension. Perez-Santonja and colleagues recommend the prophylactic use of carbonic anhydrase inhibitors to prevent AION.[29]

CONCLUSION

Phakic IOL implantation for myopia correction is highly predictable and reversible, is a short operation with a brief healing time, and can be performed by most opthalmologists. With phakic AC implants, refractive and visual acuity results are more stable with no fluctuations or delayed regression or progression of the refractive error. Most patients had improved BCVA. However, damage to the corneal endothelium remains the major risk factor of this procedure, and it might become evident years after the operation. Therefore, the long-term safety of this technique remains undetermined. Large-scale studies are needed to evaluate the long-term effects of this procedure before it can be unequivocally recommended.

REFERENCES

1. Fechner PU, Strobel J, Wiechmann W. Correction of myopia by implantation of a concave Worst iris claw lens into phakic eyes. *Refract Corneal Surg.* 1991;7:286–298.
2. Baikoff G, Joly P. Comparison of minus power anterior chamber intraocular lenses and myopic epikeratoplasty in phakic eyes. *Refract Corneal Surg.* 1990;6:252.
3. Praeger DL. Phakic myopic IOL—an alternative to keratolenticulorefractive procedure. *Ann Ophthalmol.* 1988;20:46.
4. Tchah H, Duffey RJ, Allarakhia L, Lindstrom RL. Intraocular lens implantation in phakic rabbit eyes. *J Cataract Refract Surg.* 1989;15:554–558.
5. Colin J, Mimouni F, Robinet A, Conrad H, Mader P. The surgical treatment of high myopia: comparison of epikeratoplasty, keratomileusis and minus power anterior chamber lenses. *Refract Corneal Surg.* 1990;6:245–251.
6. Barraquer J. Anterior chamber plastic lenses. Results and conclusions from five years experience. *Trans Ophthalmol Soc UK.* 1959;79:393–424.
7. Choyce P. Discussion to Barraquer: anterior chamber plastic lenses. Results and conclusions from five years experience. *Trans Ophthalmol Soc UK.* 1959;79:423.
8. Praeger DL. Innovations and creativity in contemporary ophthalmology: preliminary experience with the phakic myopic IOLs. *Ann Ophthalmol.* 1988;20:456–462.
9. Fechner PU, Worst JGF. A new concave intraocular lens for the correction of myopia. *Eur J Implant Refract Surg.* 1989;1:41–43.
10. Fechner PU, VanderHeijde JL, Worst JJ. The correction of myopia by lens implantation into phakic eyes. *Am J Ophthalmol.* 1989;107:659–663.
11. Fechner PU, et al. Correction of myopia by implantation of minus optic (Worst iris claw) lenses into the anterior chamber of phakic eyes. *Eur J Implant Refract Surg.* 1993;5:55.

12. Alpor JJ, Fechner PU. Intraocular lenses. In: *Intraocular Lenses.* New York: Thieme; 1986:328–335.

13. Baikoff G, Colin J. Intraocular lenses in phakic patients. *Ophthalmol Clin North Am.* 1992;4:789.

14. Baikoff G. The refractive IOL in a phakic eye. *Ophthalmic Pract.* 1991;9:2.

15. Baikoff G. Phakic anterior chamber IOL. *Int Ophthalmol Clin.* 1991;31:75.

16. Praeger DL, Mamose A, Muroff LL. Thirty-six month follow-up of a contemporary phakic intraocular lens for the surgical correction of myopia. *Ann Ophthalmol.* 1991; 23:6–10.

17. Peiffer RL, Porter DP, Eifrig DE, Boyd J. Experimental evaluation of a phakic anterior chamber implant in a primate model. I. Clinical observations. *J Cataract Refract Surg.* 1991;17:335–352.

18. Benitez del Castillo JM, Hernandez JL, Iradier MT, Del Rio MT, Garcia J. Fluorophotometry in phakic eyes with anterior chamber intraocular lens implantation to correct myopia. *J Cataract Refract Surg.* 1993;19:607–609.

19. Perez-Santonja JJ, Hernandez JL, Benitez del Castillo JM, Rodriguez C, Zato MA. Fluorophotometry in myopic phakic eyes with anterior chamber intraocular lenses to correct severe myopia. *Am J Ophthalmol.* 1994;118:316–321.

20. Neves RA, et al. Laser flare photometry in phakic myopic patients with anterior chamber lenses. *Invest Ophthalmol Vis Sci.* 1993;34:883.

21. Alio JL, de la Hoz F, Ismail M. Subclinical inflammatory reactions induced by phakic anterior chamber lenses for the correction of high myopia. *Ocular Immunol Inflam.* 1993;1:219–223.

22. Stark WJ, et al. The FDA report on intraocular lenses. *Ophthalmology.* 1983;90:311–317.

23. Foss AJE, Rosen PH, Cooling RJ. Retinal detachment following anterior chamber lens implantation for the correction of ultra-high myopia in phakic eyes. *Br J Ophthalmol.* 1993;77:212–213.

24. Landesz M, Worst JJ, Siertsema JV, van Rij G. Correction of high myopia with the Worst myopic claw intraocular lens. *J Refract Surg.* 1995;11:16–25.

25. Alio JL, Ruiz-Moreno JM, Artola A. Retinal detachment as a potential hazard in surgical correction of severe myopia with phakic anterior chamber lenses. *Am J Ophthalmol.* 1993;115:145–148.

26. Mimouni F, Colin J, Koffi V, Bonnet P. Damage to the corneal endothelium from anterior chamber intraocular lenses in phakic myopic eyes. *Refract Corneal Surg.* 1991;7: 277–281.

27. Oxford Cataract Treatment and Evaluation Team (OCTET): Longterm corneal endothelial cell loss after cataract surgery. Results of a randomised controlled trial. *Arch Ophthalmol.* 1986;104:1170–1175.

28. Werblin TF. Long term endothelial cell loss following phacoemulsification: model for evaluating endothelial damage after intraocular surgery. *J Refract Corneal Surg.* 1993; 9:29–35.

29. Perez-Santonja JJ, Bueno JL, Meza J, Garcia-Sandoval B, Serrano JM, Zato MA. Ischemic optic neuropathy after IOL implantation to correct high myopia in phakic patient. *J Cataract Refract Surg.* 1993;19:651–654.

CHAPTER 43

Refractive Aspects of Corneal Lacerations

Samuel E. Navon

Lacerating injuries of the anterior segment are a major cause of vision loss and morbidity throughout the world. Significant alterations in corneal contour may occur not only from the actual laceration, but from its surgical repair and healing as well. Therefore, it is not uncommon for vision to be limited by residual damage to the cornea, even though the visual axis is not directly involved in most cases. The importance of restoring a normal refracting surface as quickly as possible is underscored when young children are affected. In these cases the main cause of permanent vision loss is amblyopia secondary to irregular high astigmatism.

Several studies have noted a strong relationship between corneal wound length and residual astigmatism. Snell[1] found that up to 50% of patients with a small corneal laceration (1 to 4 mm) had a final visual acuity of 20/40 or better; with longer lacerations, only about 20% achieved this acuity. Similar results were obtained by Eagling,[2] who noted that lacerations involving less than one third of the corneal diameter were considerably less likely to be associated with significant astigmatism. More recently, Barr[3] reported residual astigmatism of 3 or more diopters (D) only in patients whose lacerations were longer than 4 mm. Rowsey and Hays[4] called attention to the refractive aspects of these injuries by applying basic caveats of keratorefractive surgery[5] to their management. Since then, computer-ized topography has been used to detail further the behavior of the lacerated cornea.[6,7]

In dealing with the unique characteristics of each injury, the trauma surgeon must observe carefully and apply information and techniques gleaned from the parent field of refractive surgery. This chapter presents the keratorefractive aspects of corneal lacerations with emphasis on clinical example. Familiarity with these principles often allows the surgeon to meet the challenges posed by surgical repair and visual rehabilitation.

ROLE OF COMPUTERIZED TOPOGRAPHY

Standard keratometry measures only four central points (1.5-mm radius) on the corneal surface and can therefore give misleading results for localized disturbances such as keratoconus and corneal lacerations.[8] With this technique, accurate conclusions can only be made if the surface being measured is a symmetric spherocylinder. This shortcoming was eliminated by the corneoscope, a modified Placido disk and photography system that obtains many data points out to the mid-periphery of the cornea.[9]

Computerized topography represents a further improvement on the methods described above. The instruments analyze thousands of data points over the corneal surface and readily store and retrieve data, allowing detailed comparison of serial examinations. As discussed below, these features make this technique ideally suited to study the refractive aspects of corneal lacerations.

REFRACTIVE EFFECTS OF CORNEAL LACERATIONS

As randomly oriented keratorefractive events, the effects of corneal lacerations can only be partially understood from their similarities to precise surgical incisions such as radial or astigmatic keratotomies. Nevertheless, the basic principles governing corneal mechanics still apply. For instance, wound depth, length, shape, and location can be expected to greatly influence refractive significance.

The relationship between incision depth and refractive effect is well known clinically[10] and has also been demonstrated using mathematic models of radial[11] and transverse[12] incisions. Such a model is illustrated in Figure 43–1, which shows that an incision must penetrate at least two thirds of the cornea to have a significant refractive effect; further deepening markedly increases this effect. This behavior explains why the majority of partial-thickness lacerations do not change the cornea's refractive status. In a series of 25 patients with partial-thickness lacerations, none of the eyes whose laceration was noncentral and less than 75% depth experienced a significant decrease in visual acuity or change in refraction (unpublished results). This finding supports the conventional recommendation to manage superficial corneal lacerations nonsurgically.[13]

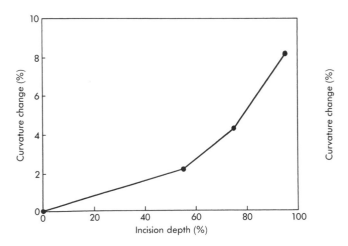

Figure 43–1. Effect of corneal incision depth on refractive change.

Deep lacerations may heal with surprisingly little astigmatism if they are shelved. This is probably because the relatively large contact area of the wound edges is less likely to deform. Figure 43–2 illustrates the topographic recovery of an extensive, but highly shelved, 95%-depth corneal laceration passing through the central zone. The two vertical branches of the laceration resemble a pair of transverse relaxing incisions. Initially, there is a great deal of surface distortion; however, tremendous flattening within the area bounded by the laceration is evident. The patient was managed with a contact lens and topical antibiotics and had a gradual but remarkable recovery. After 12 weeks visual acuity was 20/20 with −0.50 sph.

Corneal response to refractive incisions depends highly on their location. This relationship has been studied extensively and is the basis for keratotomy nomograms. Unfortunately, little is known about incisions that predominantly cross the central zone, since they have no therapeutic counterpart. The central flattening caused by radial and transverse keratotomies are distal from the actual incisions.

Mathematical models[14,15] and clinical observations[16,17] have shown steepening directly over radial and astigmatic keratotomy incisions. This phenomenon cannot be understood by considering the corneal radius to be simply expanded by the incision. Instead, a deep incision can be considered to act as a hinge that bows forward (Fig 43–3). The result is highly localized steepening across the wound. In this manner, a central laceration would act as a "reverse radial keratotomy (RK)," leading to central steepening directly across the wound and generalized flattening of the peripheral cornea (Fig 43–4).

Lacerations outside the central cornea would be expected to behave similarly to planned refractive incisions of comparable orientation. Figure 43–5 illustrates the corneal topography of a 5-mm curvilinear, full-thickness transverse corneal laceration. The wound resembles a relaxing incision used to correct steepness in the meridian perpendicular to the incision. Three diopters of central astigmatism are present, with the flat meridian perpendicular to the laceration. This astigmatism was assumed to be caused by the injury because the patient reported having equally good uncorrected vision in both eyes before the injury, and the vision in her fellow eye was 20/15 with less than 1 D of corneal astigmatism. The amount of laceration-induced astigmatism is consistent with data obtained by Lundergren and Rowsey, who found central corneal flattening of 0.58 D to 5.93 D when cir-

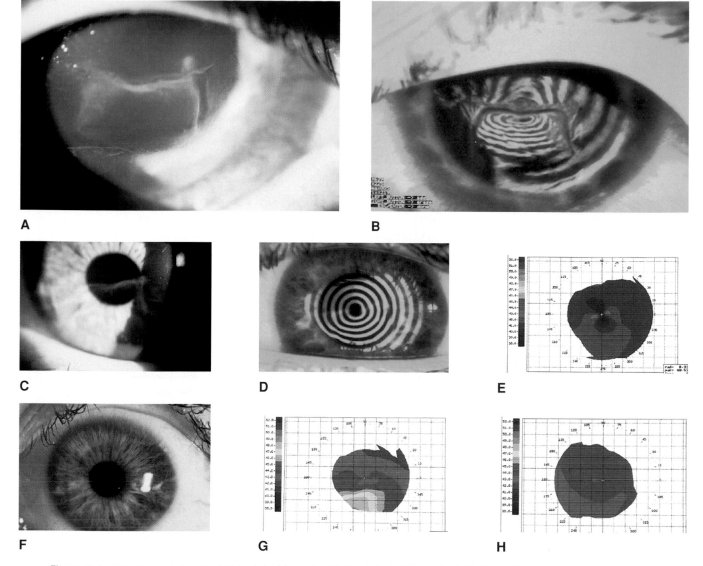

A   B

C   D   E

F   G   H

Figure 43–2. Refractive evolution of a highly shelved laceration. Highly shelved, 95% depth, 3-sided laceration passing near the visual axis. Top: **A.** Photograph and **(B)** corresponding keratoscopy. A great deal of flattening is evident between the vertical end branches. The extensive distortion did not permit computed topography. Visual acuity was 20/300 uncorrected and 20/60 with pinhole. Middle: **C.** Photograph, **(D)** the corresponding keratoscopy, and **(E)** computed topography showing marked improvement 1 month after the injury. Bottom: **F.** Photograph, **(G)** corresponding topography, and **(H)** topography of the normal fellow eye 4 months after the injury. The injured eye has less than 1 D of central astigmatism and is of similar dioptric power as the fellow eye. Visual acuity of the injured eye is 20/20 with −0.25 D sph.

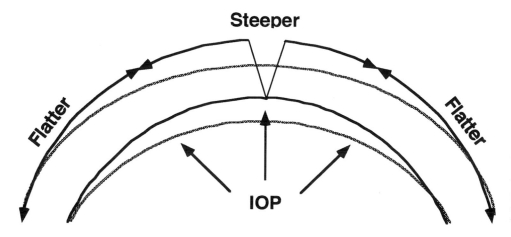

Figure 43–3. Localized steepening over a deep corneal incision. Schematic cross section of a normal (shaded) and deeply incised (solid) cornea. The stroma under the incision bulges forward to reequilibrate with the outward forces of intraocular pressure. The steepening across the cut is associated with compensatory flattening in the same meridian.

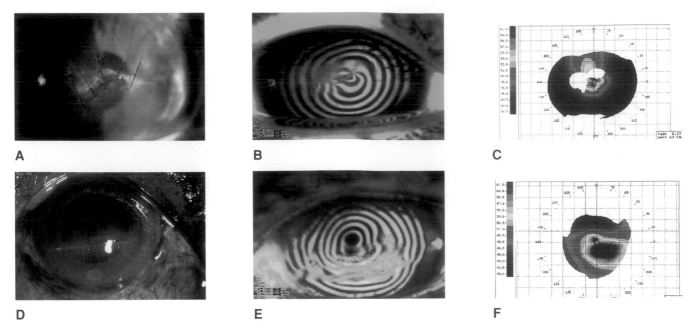

Figure 43–4. Topography of central corneal lacerations. Top: **A.** Postoperative photograph (preoperative photo was not taken), **(B)** preoperative keratoscopy, and **(C)** computed topography of an 6-mm, linear, full-thickness laceration crossing within 1 mm of the visual axis. Bottom: **D.** Preoperative photograph, **(E)** corresponding keratoscopy, and **(F)** topography of a 7-mm, linear, full-thickness laceration. Both of these wounds were sufficiently watertight to permit formed anterior chambers and intraocular pressures of about 10 mm Hg. A great deal of contour distortion is present; however, localized steepening is evident across the wounds in association with marked peripheral flattening. Note the expanded diopter range of the computed topography needed to display the distorted surfaces.

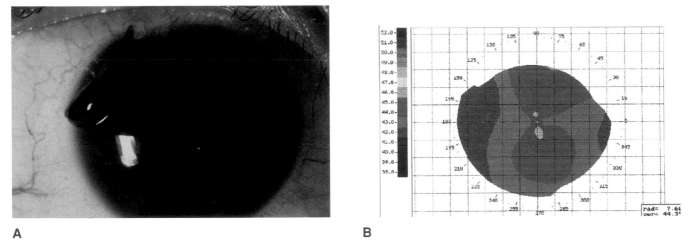

Figure 43–5. Topography of a circumferential laceration. **A.** Preoperative photograph of a 5-mm corneal laceration with iris prolapse. The patient presented about 1 hour after the injury. **B.** Corresponding corneal topography demonstrating 3 D of central astigmatism with the flattest meridian perpendicular to the laceration.

cumferential incisions of 1 to 3 o'clock were made, respectively.[18]

The above examples provide interesting information on corneal response to simple traumatic incisions; however, many lacerations have complex shapes and oblique locations that defy predetermined rules for behavior. For example, one would expect branched lacer-

ations to give rise to complex topographic patterns due to the abrupt changes in incision direction and unpredictable coupling effects between different regions of the laceration. In addition, full-thickness wounds that cause anterior chamber collapse and negligible intraocular pressure (IOP) would not be expected to yield meaningful information in the unrepaired state. This is because IOP plays a large role in shaping the contour of a deeply incised cornea by displacing the weakened area forward until a new equilibrium contour is formed.[19,20]

The above considerations argue against routinely obtaining preoperative topography of full-thickness lacerations. This is underscored by the need to manipulate these eyes as little as possible. It is, perhaps, more important to recognize whether a laceration has significant refractive implications rather than deciphering its precise topography. As discussed below, proper wound apposition at surgery followed by uneventful healing will often yield excellent refractive results regardless of the initial topography.

SURGERY

Anesthesia and Instrumentation

Corneal lacerations should be repaired using general anesthesia unless the patient is an extremely poor candidate for this approach. The increased orbital volume caused by the instillation of local anesthetic or a resultant retrobulbar hemorrhage risks collapse of the anterior chamber and a disastrous extrusion of intraocular contents. If the patient cannot tolerate general anesthesia and the injury is small and self-sealing, local anesthesia can be used with a small volume of anesthetic and constant monitoring of the eye. A recent report

demonstrating the effectiveness of low-volume (5 ml), single-site, peribulbar anesthesia for cataract surgery appears to have particular value for use with traumatized eyes under these circumstances.[21] Topical anesthesia may be appropriate for the small minority of patients with self-sealing corneal lacerations and excellent cooperation.

A Jaffe-style lid speculum is recommended because it channels the force of elastic bands toward lifting the palpebral circle off the globe. Other instruments that should be immediately available are the iris and cyclodialysis spatulas and irrigation/aspiration, phacoemulsification, and vitrectomy handpieces. A variety of corneoscleral needles are currently available, mainly in response to the exacting demands of small-incision cataract surgery. For short, deep bites a bicurve, minicurve, or compound curve needle is recommended. These needles have in common a very tight radius of curvature at their points, and they should be used to place sutures near the visual axis. For peripheral lacerations, a larger radius needle (i.e., 2 mm, 160°) works well. Finally, 11-0 sutures are occasionally useful when additional sutures are needed to form a watertight closure in a region already crowded with sutures (Fig 43-6).

Techniques

Although creativity and flexibility are the hallmarks of trauma surgery, they should complement an orderly approach to the repair of corneal lacerations. Prolapsed

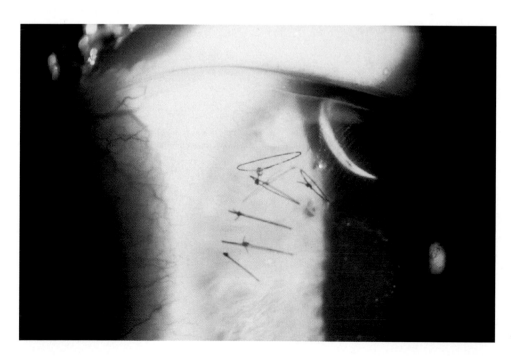

Figure 43–6. Use of 11-0 suture in an area crowded with sutures. This upright "Y"-shaped laceration was Seidel positive at its upper left arm during repair with 10-0 sutures. The fine needle and suture of 11-0 material permitted an additional suture to be placed across the leaking area, which resulted in watertight closure.

iris tissue should be examined for its viability and the presence of an epithelial membrane. In general, uveal tissue that has remained prolapsed for more than 24 hours should be excised and sent for culture and histology. Prolapsed iris can be reposited in several ways:

1. A small amount of viscoelastic or air can be used to push the iris back into the anterior chamber and tamponade it in place. If only a small amount of viscoelastic is used, it will not have to be removed at the end of the repair. Take care not to overinflate the anterior chamber, since this can paradoxically worsen the prolapse.

2. A fine spatula can be brought into the anterior chamber through a limbal paracentesis to sweep the prolapsed iris into place. This approach reduces the amount of instrument manipulation of the wound and can be performed by an assistant while the surgeon places sutures. It may also be the most effective way to avoid the development of anterior synechiae formation with wounds that extend to the limbus.[22]

3. Pharmacologic mobilization of the iris can facilitate its reposition. Centrally prolapsed iris can be brought into the anterior chamber by mydriatic contraction, and peripherally prolapsed tissue can often be effectively mobilized by miotics. Except for acetylcholine (Miochol) and carbachol (Miostat), medication should be applied at the limbus, with care not to expose it to intraocular tissues.

The wound should be gently irrigated through a fine-gauge blunt cannula. This is useful for three reasons. First, this will often result in the tactile detection (gritty sensation) of a small foreign body that was not evident by visual examination alone. Second, as with the closure of skin lacerations, irrigation may decrease any microbial load and reduce the risk of infection. Third, probing allows the surgeon to explore the anatomy of the wound accurately. This is important because the degree of shelving and the regions where a wound is full- or partial-thickness are often not evident by slit lamp examination. If excised iris tissue is not available for culture, a sterile swab can be gently passed over the wound and placed into medium. A sample of aqueous humor should be cultured and Gram stain obtained if endophthalmitis is suspected.

Meticulous attention should be given to suture technique because this will greatly influence the resulting astigmatism. Interrupted 10-0 nylon sutures usually give the best control of astigmatism and tension. In general, they should be placed 1 mm from wound edges, 1 mm apart, and deeply into the stroma—superficial placement may gape the endothelial surface. Long sutures may often be necessary (Fig 43–7). If the wound margins can provide sufficient resistance to needle passage (i.e., are not loose flaps), it is usually unnecessary to hold the wound edges with forceps. Countertraction can be obtained by grasping the limbus 180° away from the path of the needle. After the needle is passed into the tissue, the forceps can be placed just distal to the desired exit site of the needle to direct its path accurately. If at all possible, avoid suturing through the visual axis. This technique can be applied to procedures done under topical anesthesia if the limbal area to be grasped is anesthetized subconjunctivally or by direct contact with an anesthetic-soaked applicator.

It is often very difficult to predict the amount of tension initially placed sutures will finally need to appose the wound margins properly. In contrast to surgical incisions, which are precisely constructed to be watertight with minimal tension, traumatic lacerations often require large amounts of tension to achieve adequate closure. The amount of suture tension needed to close short puncture-type injuries or wounds with rough edges can be dramatic (Fig 43–8). For this reason, well-placed initial sutures are important to close the wound and relieve tension. This can be aided by closing portions of the wound with sliding knots that are initially tightened to the surgeon's best estimation and left in an adjustable state (Fig 43–9). After the wound

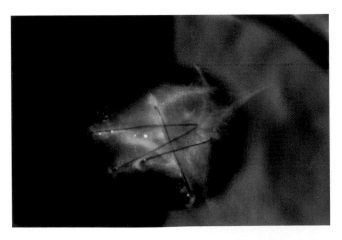

Figure 43–7. Use of long sutures to avoid crowing. This complex puncture laceration was successfully repaired with only a few long sutures. Noted the extra-long vertical suture, which sealed the apex of the "V"-shaped laceration by reaching over two sutures already in place.

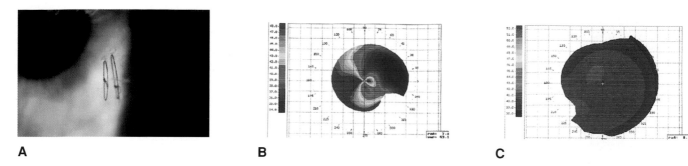

A   **B**   **C**

Figure 43–8. Distortion due to high suture tension. **A.** Postoperative photograph and **(B)** corresponding computed topography of a 2.5-mm corneal laceration due to a wood splinter. Considerable distortion is present after surgical repair. Although the wound was small, it was distinctly gaped and had rough edges. The injury was initially repaired with low suture tension and considerably less postoperative astigmatism—visual acuity on the first postoperative day was 20/30 uncorrected. A persistent wound leak was present, however, because the large gaping forces were not overcome. The second repair, shown here, was performed using enough suture tension to achieve a watertight closure. Visual acuity on the first postoperative day was 20/400. **C.** The distortion fully resolved after suture removal at 8 weeks. Final visual acuity was 20/15 uncorrected.

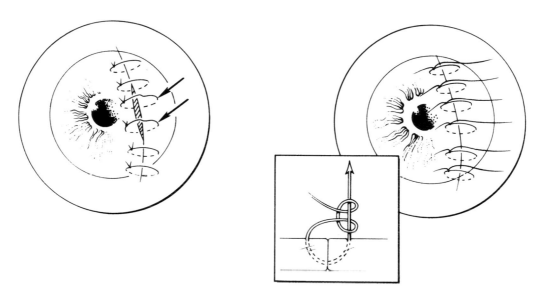

Figure 43–9. Adjustable slip knot technique for repairing corneoscleral lacerations. Left: Initial sutures tend to loosen significantly (arrows) as neighboring sutures bring the wound together and help overcome tension. Insert: Illustration of the slip knot used to approximate the wound. Right: When all sutures are placed, final adjustments in tension are made and the sutures are locked with a final throw.

margins are approximated, the sutures are readjusted to the desirable tension and locked. This method gives precise control over wound tension without the need to replace sutures.

KERATOREFRACTIVE EFFECTS OF SURGICAL REPAIR

Despite a wide variety of geometries and locations of corneal lacerations, four common patterns of behavior are evident:

1. Interrupted sutures produce localized flattening.

2. Steepening occurs distal and parallel to interrupted sutures.

3. The distortion caused by sutures is largely transient.

4. Extensively long and branched wounds may cause significant residual astigmatism.

Interrupted Sutures Produce Localized Flattening

Vertical interrupted sutures can produce significant flattening within their compression zones (Fig 43–10). This effect can be understood by considering the force vectors of sutures as detailed by Eisner[23] and de-

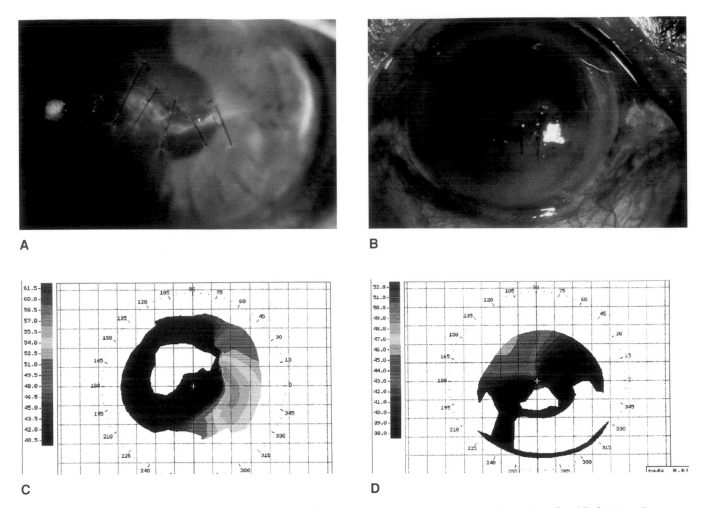

Figure 43–10. Marked flattening caused by sutures. **A** and **B.** Postoperative photographs of central corneal lacerations. **C** and **D.** Corresponding topographies showing marked flattening over the sutured cornea. Surface distortion did not permit data processing directly over the knots.

scribed by Rowsey as a basic caveat of keratorefractive surgery.[5] Although the ability to flatten increases with the length of a suture, it is a fundamental characteristic of all vertical interrupted sutures, long and short.

Rowsey and Hays[4] have suggested using sutures of varying length to repair corneal lacerations to reconstruct a physiologic corneal contour. They recommend using longer sutures in the corneal periphery to maintain its relatively flat shape and shorter sutures centrally to keep flattening to a minimum and recreate its native steeper shape. The principles behind this approach are elegant and should be thoroughly understood; however, they may not apply in several situations. First, many lacerations are not clearly oriented through both the periphery and center. Second, in many cases the shape of the laceration dictates the length of the suture needed. For instance, highly shelved lacera-

tions require longer sutures to bring the edges in contact. Often a great deal of compression is needed to make the wound watertight (Fig 43–8). A large number of shorter sutures would be needed in these situations with their attendant residual scarring. Finally, no clinical studies to date have documented the effectiveness of this approach or whether any flattening the sutures cause would be permanent. The additional flattening that occurs with longer sutures is mostly due to incorporating longer lengths of cornea into the flattened compression zone of the suture. Because this cornea is uninjured and will not be involved in scar formation or changes, do not expect the suture to cause permanent distortion. This is discussed below. We find only a minority of patients who would benefit from this type of repair and mainly use this technique on pediatric patients at risk for amblyopia. These patients require as rapid a visual recovery as possible.

Steepening Occurs Distal and Parallel to Interrupted Sutures

Steepening in the meridian parallel to, but distal from, interrupted sutures is coupled to their localized flattening effect.[5] This phenomenon is routinely observed in the with-the-rule astigmatism commonly seen with sutured cataract wounds. The mechanics that cause this effect are closely related to the flattening that is coupled to the localized steepening over a laceration. Distal steepening due to sutures is demonstrated in Figure 43–11, which shows the corneal topography of the full-thickness laceration of Figure 43–5 2 days after its repair.

The coupled flattening-steepening pattern of sutures can be quite pronounced and is most easily recognized when the sutures are radially oriented. This is because perturbations of the corneal contour tend to pass through the apex. An example of this is the bowtie pattern of normal astigmatism. Distortions that are obliquely oriented will be the origination site for a change in contour, which will then bend to make its way to the corneal apex. This phenomenon is seen in the transversely oriented sutures shown in Figure 43–6.

Distortion Caused by Sutures Is Largely Transient

The astigmatism caused by sutures can be large and can even be the main cause for decreased vision after the repair of a laceration (Fig 43–12). Thus, it is important to know whether this distortion persists after sutures are removed. The case shown in Figure 43–13 indicates that this effect may be largely transient. After removal of all sutures 8 weeks after surgery, the central cornea assumed a spherical central contour of similar dioptric power to the fellow eye. Only a small amount of localized residual flattening remained over the wound and did not appear to influence the topography of the central zone significantly. We have observed this behavior in a wide variety of corneal lacerations and consider it a universal phenomenon in all but the most extensive lacerations.

It is reasonable to expect the distortion caused by sutures to be largely transient. After sufficient tension is used to appose the wound margins, additional tension will deform the normal surrounding corneal tissue located between the suture's entrance and exit sites. The compressed tissue should resume its normal shape after the sutures are removed. This is evident from the refractive distortion caused by sutured cataract wounds, which is predictably relieved even months after surgery by selective cutting of sutures.

Figures 43–14, 43–15, and 43–16 demonstrate the keratorefractive courses of three midperipheral transverse lacerations. In each case, a substantial amount of steepening is present perpendicular to the sutured lacerations, presumably in response to localized flattening over the sutured area. The latter lacerations were large; however, after suture removal less than 1 D of astigmatism remained in each case. The eye shown in Figure 43–14 had a final dioptric power very similar to the fellow eye, while those shown in Figures 43–15 and 43–16 had about 2.5 D

(Text continued on page 574)

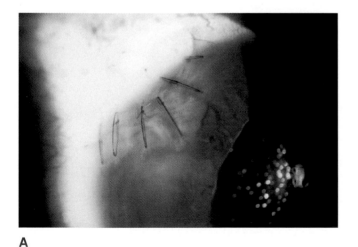

A

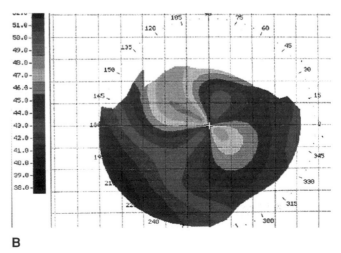

B

Figure 43–11. Compensatory corneal steepening perpendicular to a sutured wound. **A.** The circumferential laceration shown in Figure 43–5 2 days following surgical repair with interrupted 10-0 nylon sutures. **B.** Corresponding topography demonstrating 7 D of central astigmatism with the steep meridian perpendicular to the laceration.

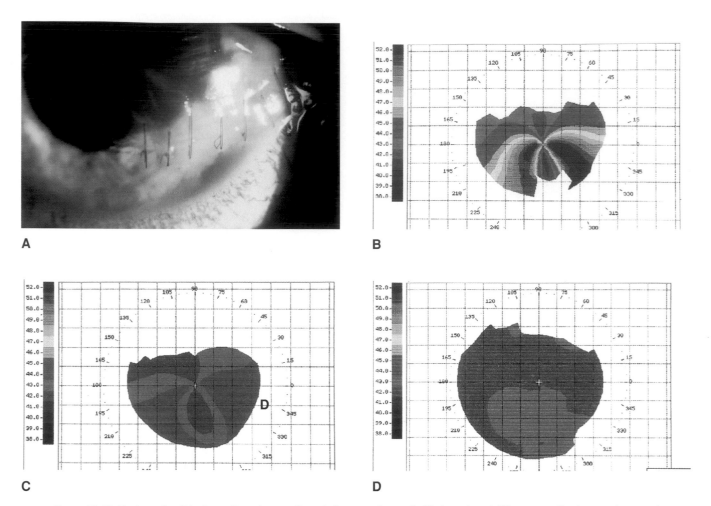

Figure 43–12. Tendency for distortion patterns to pass through the corneal apex. **A.** Photograph and **(B)** corresponding topography several days after the repair of a 7-mm oblique laceration. 16 D of central astigmatism is present in a sagging bowtie pattern. One arm of the bowtie arises adjacent and parallel to the sutures and curves centrally to pass through the corneal apex. The pattern created is highly symmetric with respect to the apex. **C.** Computed topography 8 weeks after all sutures were removed resulting in less than 1.5 D of central astigmatism and similar dioptric power as the fellow eye. **D.** Final visual acuity of the injured eye was 20/20 with −1.25 sph.

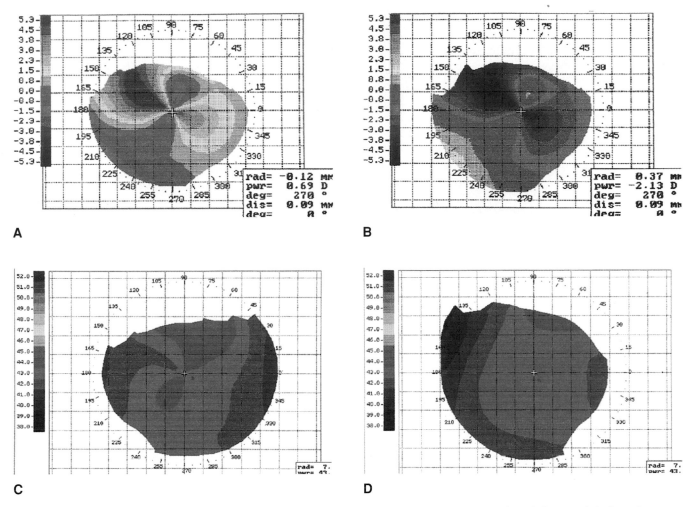

Figure 43–13. Resolution of suture- and wound-induced astigmatism after suture removal. Difference (subtraction) maps of the laceration shown in Figure 43–9 showing the change in topography from before to after surgery **(A)** and before to after suture removal **(B)**. The meridians and magnitudes of the changes are identical. Topography following removal of all sutures 10 weeks postoperatively **C.** The central cornea is essentially spherical and of similar dioptric power as the fellow eye. **D.** Final visual acuity of the injured eye was 20/15 uncorrected.

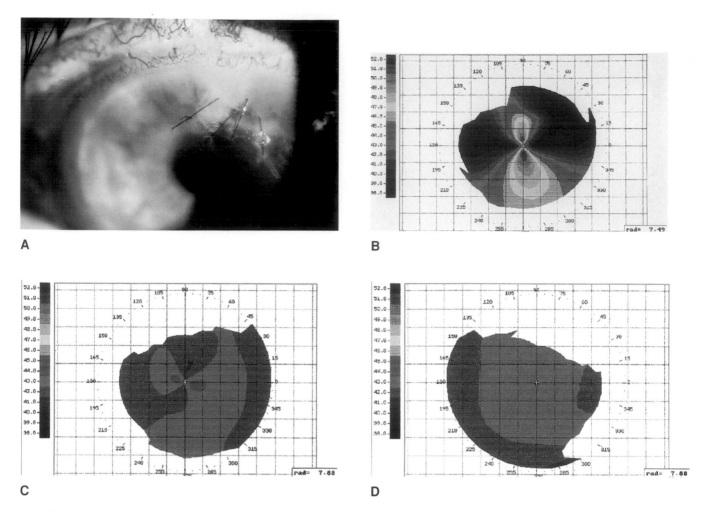

Figure 43–14. Topography after repair of a 4-mm transverse laceration. **A.** Photograph and **(B)** corresponding topography several days after the repair of a 4-mm transverse laceration. 16 D of central astigmatism is present with the steep meridian parallel to the sutures. **C.** Computed topography 8 weeks after all sutures were removed resulting in **(D)** less than 1 D of final astigmatism and similar contours between the injured and fellow eyes. Final visual acuity of the injured eye was 20/20 uncorrected.

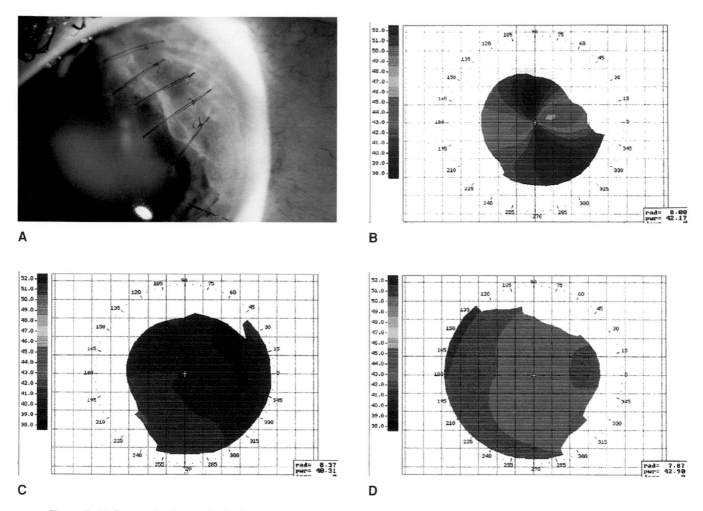

Figure 43–15. Topography after repair of a 6-mm transverse laceration. **A.** Photograph and **(B)** corresponding topography several days after the repair of a 6-mm transverse laceration. 8 D of central astigmatism is present with the steep meridian parallel to the sutures. **C.** Computed topography 8 weeks after all sutures were removed resulting in **(D)** a nearly spherical central cornea about 2.5 D flatter than the fellow eye. Final visual acuity of the injured eye was 20/25 uncorrected with an intraocular lens implanted at the time of laceration repair.

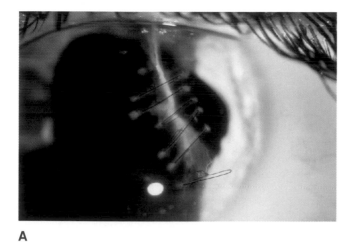

A

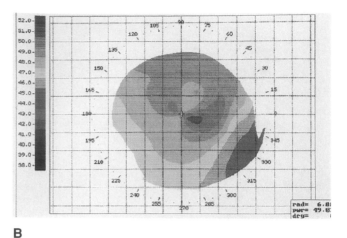

B

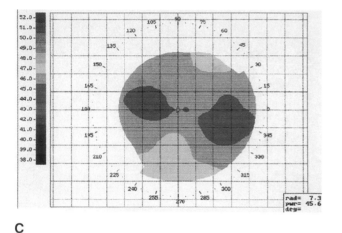

C

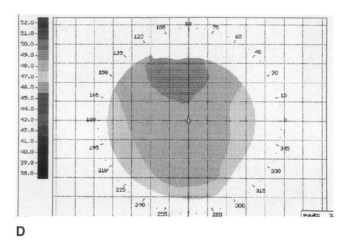

D

Figure 43–16. Topography after repair of an 8-mm transverse laceration. **A.** Photograph and **(B)** corresponding topography several days after the repair of an 8-mm transverse laceration. 8 D of central astigmatism is present with the steep meridian parallel to the sutures. **C.** Computed topography 8 weeks after all sutures were removed resulting in **(D)** a nearly spherical central cornea about 2.5 D flatter than the fellow eye. Lensectomy was performed at the time of laceration repair. Final visual acuity of the injured eye was 20/25 with a correction of +13 −1.00 × 165°.

of relative central flattening, although this was not manifested in the final refraction.

Figure 43–17 shows a radial laceration that extended from the limbus to about 4 mm from the center of the cornea, resembling a peripheral RK incision. Sutures apparently produced little distortion in this wound. The final topography showed not only less than 1 D of central astigmatism after all sutures were removed, but also less than 1 D difference in spherical power from the other eye. These results are consistent with the diminishing effect of RK incisions as they are made farther from the corneal center. The lack of any residual astigmatism is also consistent with the practice of suturing an RK to reverse the effects of the

incision in situations of overcorrection or hyperopic drift.

Extensively Long and Branched Wounds May Cause Significant Residual Astigmatism

Despite meticulous surgical repair, patients with wounds that are extensive or irregular may still end up with large amounts of residual astigmatism. We have had many examples of excellent refractive results for long wounds that are linear and nonbranching; however, it is clear that lacerations that are extensive, branched, or stellate are at greater risk of leaving the patient with high residual astigmatism (Figs 43–18, 43–19, and 43–20). A large percentage of patients with these injuries

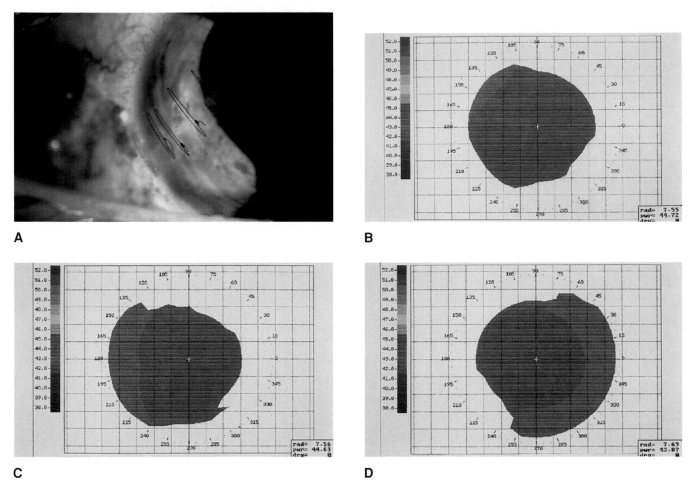

A   **B**

C   **D**

Figure 43–17. Topography after repair of a 6-mm radial laceration. **A.** Photograph and **(B)** corresponding topography several days after the repair of a 6-mm peripheral radial laceration. Less than 1 D of central astigmatism is present. This small amount of distortion is probably due to the peripheral and radial orientation of the wound. Visual acuity with sutures in place was 20/40 uncorrected. **C.** Suture removal at 8 weeks had essentially no effect on **(D)** corneal contour which had nearly identical dioptric power as the fellow eye. Final visual acuity of the injured eye was 20/20− with −0.75 × 180°.

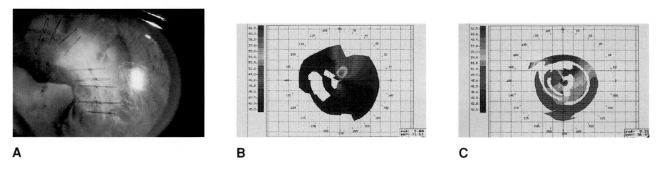

A   **B**   **C**

Figure 43–18. Topography after repair of an extensive central laceration. **A.** Photograph and **(B)** corresponding topography several days after the repair of a 10-mm central arcuate laceration which had shelved and irregular margins. Over 20 D of irregular astigmatism is present without a clear relationship to the wound. **C.** Marked distortion persisted after suture removal at 10 weeks. This patient has subsequently undergone anterior segment reconstruction with good results.

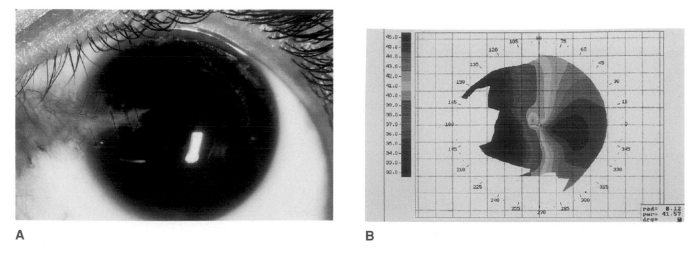

Figure 43–19. Topography after repair of an extensive V-shaped laceration. **A.** Photograph and **(B)** corresponding topography several days after the repair of an extensive V-shaped laceration. Over 20 D of irregular astigmatism is present, which did not resolve after suture removal. Visual acuity was 20/100 uncorrected and 20/30 with a hard contact lens.

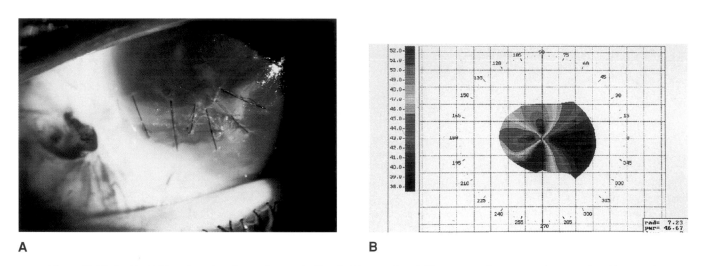

Figure 43–20. Residual high astigmatism due to aberrant healing. **A.** Photograph and **(B)** corresponding computed topography with corneal sutures in place of a 5-mm radial laceration. No reduction in the 12 D of astigmatism occurred after suture removal.

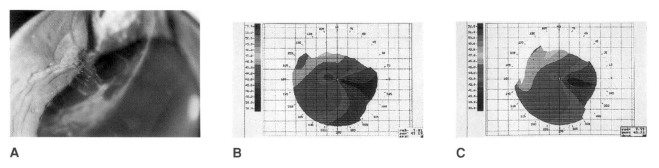

Figure 43–21. Astigmatic keratotomy to correct residual astigmatism due to a corneal laceration. **A.** Photograph and **(B.)** corresponding topography several months after the repair of an 8-mm transverse laceration. Visual acuity was 20/70 uncorrected and 20/50 with +0.75 −3.00 × 165°. The patient complained of blurry vision without correction and distorted images with correction. Astigmatic keratotomy (60° arc length at the 6-mm optical zone) was performed centered on the 250° meridian. Visual acuity at 6 weeks was 20/30 uncorrected with a manifest refraction of +0.25 −1.00 × 165° giving 20/25. The patient was very satisfied with his vision. **C.** Postkeratotomy computed topography confirms the reduction in central astigmatism.

will obtain good visual acuity only with a hard contact lens or by undergoing a surgical procedure such as astigmatic keratotomy or penetrating keratoplasty (Fig 43–21). This is in contrast to the findings of Eagling, who concluded that wound shape is not a factor in the final astigmatism produced.[2] It is clear that factors such as injury location, orientation, method of repair, and timing of suture removal must also be important in determining prognosis for a good refractive outcome.

REFERENCES

1. Snell AD. Perforating ocular injuries. *Am J Ophthalmol.* 1945;28:263–281.

2. Eagling EM. Perforating injuries of the eye. *Br J Ophthalmol.* 1976;60:732–736.

3. Barr CC. Prognostic factors in corneoscleral lacerations. *Arch Ophthalmol.* 1983;101:919–924.

4. Rowsey JJ, Hays JC. Refractive reconstruction for acute eye injuries. *Ophthalmic Surg.* 1984;15:569–574.

5. Rowsey JJ. Ten caveats in keratorefractive surgery. *Ophthalmology.* 1983;90:148–155.

6. Navon SE, Smith S. Corneal topography of a full-thickness corneal laceration. *Ophthalmic Surg.* 1994. In press.

7. Navon SE, Smith S. Residual astigmatism in corneal lacerations. In preparation.

8. Sanders DR, Gills JP, Martin RG. When keratometric measurements do not accurately reflect corneal topography. *J Cataract Refract Surg.* 1993;19:131–135.

9. Rowsey JJ, Reynolds AE, Brown R. Corneal topography: corneascope. *Arch Ophthalmol.* 1981;99:1093–1100.

10. Nordan LT. Quantifiable astigmatism correcting: concepts and suggestions. *J Cataract Refract Surg.* 1986;12:507–518.

11. Vito RP, Shin J-W. A finite element model of radial keratotomy surgery. In: Waring GO, ed. *Refractive Keratotomy for Myopia and Astigmatism.* St. Louis: Mosby; 1992.

12. Seiler T. Biomechanics of transverse incisions of the cornea. In: Waring GO, ed. *Refractive Keratotomy for Myopia and Astigmatism.* St. Louis: Mosby; 1992.

13. Hersh PS, Shingleton BJ, Kenyon KR. Management of corneoscleral lacerations. In: Shingleton BJ, Hersh PS, Kenyon KR, eds. *Eye Trauma.* St. Louis: Mosby; 1991.

14. Bryant MR, Velinsky SA, Plesha ME, Clarke GP. Computer-aided surgical design in refractive keratotomy. *CLAO J.* 1987;13:238–242.

15. Pinsky PM, Datye DV. Numerical modeling of radial, astigmatic, and hexagonal keratotomy. 1992;8:164–172.

16. Nordan LT, Grene RB. The importance of corneal asphericity and irregular astigmatism in refractive surgery. *Refract Corneal Surg.* 1990;6:200–204.

17. Henslee SL, Rowsey JJ. New corneal shapes in keratorefractive surgery. *Ophthalmology.* 1983;90:245–250.

18. Lundergren MK, Rowsey JJ. Relaxing incisions: corneal topography. *Ophthalmology.* 1985;92:1226–1236.

19. Feldman FT, Frucht-Pery J, Weinrab RN, Chaye TA, Dreher AW, Brown SI. The effect of increased intraocular pressure on visual acuity and corneal curvature after radial keratotomy. *Am J Ophthalmol.* 1989;108:126–129.

20. Maloney RK. Effect of corneal hydration and intraocular pressure on keratometric power after experimental radial keratotomy. *Ophthalmology.* 1990;97:927–933.

21. Agrawal V, Athanikar NS. Single injection, low volume periocular anesthesia in 1,000 cases. *J Cataract Refract Surg.* 1994;20:61–63.

22. Mackensen G. Microsurgery of ocular injuries. *Adv Ophthalmol.* 1970;27:115.

23. Eisner G. *Eye Surgery: An Introduction to Operative Technique.* New York: Springer-Verlag; 1990.

CHAPTER 44

Refractive Surgery in Dry Eye Syndrome

Kazuo Tsubota ▪ Ikuko Toda

While radial keratotomy (RK) is an established surgical technique to correct low to moderate myopia,[1] excimer laser photorefractive keratectomy (PRK) has the potential to correct a wider range of refractive errors.[2–4] Both approaches yield satisfactory results with few complications up to −6 diopters (D)[5] of myopia, but greater myopia is considered a relative contraindication.[6]

Because RK and PRK outcomes depend on proper wound healing of the corneal stroma and epithelium, a normal tear-film layer is necessary. Tears contain epidermal growth factor (EGF),[7] vitamin A,[8] IgA,[9] and other important proteins required to induce wound healing and prevent postoperative infection. Patients with dry eye syndrome have thus generally been considered poor candidates for PRK. Ironically, patients with dry eye syndrome and myopia of −6 D or more would benefit the most from refractive surgery. The thick eyeglasses they require are heavy and cause peripheral distortion, while contact lens (CL) wear is complicated by inadequate tear production. CL wear is also a risk factor for ulcerative keratitis,[10–12] and it is believed that patients with dry eye syndrome who wear CL are more likely to develop ulcerative keratitis.[13–16] It remains to be seen whether the benefits of eliminating CL wear in these patients outweigh the risks of refractive surgery in patients with high myopia and dry eye syndrome, and, if so, what form that surgery would take.

Recently, we proposed a subclassification of patients with dry eye syndrome into three groups[17]: Sjögren-type without reflex tearing and two non-Sjögren types with good reflex tearing but poor basic tearing.[18] Because reflex tears include essential components such as EGF and vitamin A, they may suffice for corneal wound healing, so that patients with good reflex tearing may be candidates for refractive surgery. Our experience with PRK in patients with dry eye syndrome and high myopia who had pain and recurrent ocular problems due to CL wear was generally successful.

PATIENT SELECTION

All patients had myopia of more than −6 D and astigmatism of less than 2 D. Individuals with less myopia can tolerate eyeglasses, while those with more astigmatism would still require CL even if the myopia were corrected.

We recruited 21 eyes from 13 patients with various ocular problems, ranging from discomfort to superficial punctate keratitis, associated with CL wear. In preparation for excimer laser ablation, we divided the eyes into two groups according to their refractive errors. Group A (N = 13) had myopia of > −6 D to < −10 D (mean −7.6 D), whereas group B (N = 8) had myopia of > -10 D (mean -14.5 D). All patients satisfied the following criteria: (1) presence of ocular symptoms such as fatigue, irritation, or redness,[19] (2) positive vital staining of the cornea and conjunctiva,[20] and (3) abnormal tear dynamics as determined by BUT, Schirmer test, cotton thread test,[21] or clearance test.[22]

Patients with dry eye syndrome who lacked reflex tearing were excluded from our study.[18] If the patients had decreased basic tearing, their capacity for reflex tearing was checked by the Schirmer test with nasal stimulation. The test was first performed without topical anesthesia for 5 minutes. If the result was less than 10 mm, a disposable cotton applicator was inserted into the nasal cavity toward the outlet of the ethmoid canthus and left in place for 5 minutes, during which the Schirmer test was repeated (Fig 44–1). Patients usually respond to nasal stimulation very promptly, and we often experience basic tearing of 0 mm but reflex tearing of more than 25 mm. To make sure that the reflex tears also contain the necessary components for healing, for the first three patients we confirmed the presence of EGF and vitamin A in the reflex and basic tears.

Rarely did patients not respond to nasal stimulation. Most of these patients were middle-aged women with Sjögren's syndrome. Because wounds may not heal properly without both basic and reflex tearing, these individuals were excluded from the study, as were those with keratoconus or rheumatoid arthritis.

PREOPERATIVE CARE

Our primary concern was proper corneal epithelial healing after PRK. We were thus particularly careful in evaluating the ocular surface preoperatively, since even subtle abnormalities might prevent normal wound healing.

We used a specular microscope with a special contact lens[23] to analyze the corneal epithelial morphology, including cell size and pattern. If we detected any abnormal cells such as elongated or extra large ones,[24,25] the patients did not undergo PRK. Corneal sensation was checked with a Cochet-Bonnet anesthesiometer, and patients with abnormal sensation were also excluded from the study. Permeability of the corneal epithelium was measured with a recently developed anterior fluorometer. The corneal epithelium usually has a good barrier function, yet no one was excluded based on a bad epithelial barrier function.

PRK is performed in patients with dry eye syndrome to eliminate the need for a contact lens and enable more comfortable use of eyeglasses. We thus evaluated the subjective ocular condition with a "face score" that rates patients' comfort.

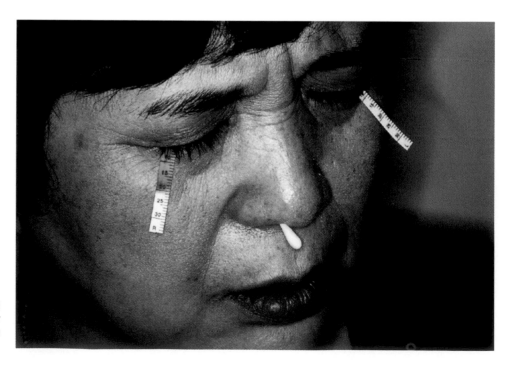

Figure 44–1. Schirmer test with nasal stimulation. A small cotton applicator is inserted into the nasal cavity to stimulate tearing.

SURGICAL TECHNIQUES

We used a Summit ExiMed UV200LA with the routine ablation parameters. The laser diameter was 4.5 mm, fluence 180 mJ/cm^2/pulse, frequency 10 Hz, and ablation rate 0.25 μm/pulse. For the patients in group A we attempted full refractive correction; for those in group B we used the laser's maximal refractive correction of 9.9 D. Because the local temperature rise during ablation may worsen complications of the procedure such as severe pain, prolonged sensory defect, and corneal haze, we kept the cornea cool by irrigating it with BSS+ (4°C) for 3 minutes[27] before and after the ablation. With this technique, the usual laser circle was not seen during the procedure. For ablations of more than 100 pulses (10 seconds), additional balanced saline solution+ was performed in the middle of the procedure.

POSTOPERATIVE CARE

Postoperative management consisted of topical antibiotics, steroids, and nonsteroidal anti-inflammatory drugs. Because dry eye itself was not treated, extensive dry eye care was given, including artificial tears and protective eyeglasses. The subjective assessments and the objective parameters were evaluated postoperatively from day 1 to day 90.

RESULTS

In all patients from groups A and B, the corneal epithelium recovered within 3 days without prolonged wound healing. Although specular microscopy revealed spindle-shaped epithelial cells at 1 week, no epithelial breakdown occurred. At 1 month, the epithelium was normal even at the cellular level.

Corneal sensation returned to normal in 69.2% of patients within 1 week and in 100% within 1 month in group A, whereas only 12.5% of these in group B recovered within 1 week and 37.5% within 1 month. The deeper the ablation, the longer the recovery for corneal sensation.

Changes in refractive error and uncorrected visual acuity are shown in Figures 44–2 and 44–3. In both groups, there was a short period of overcorrection to hyperopia followed by stabilization. We have so far followed up only to 3 months, and uncorrected visual acuity has been very stable in group A. Group B showed somewhat unpredictable results; however, refraction

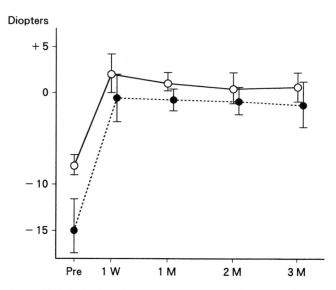

Figure 44–2. Refractive changes after PRK in patients with dry eye syndrome.

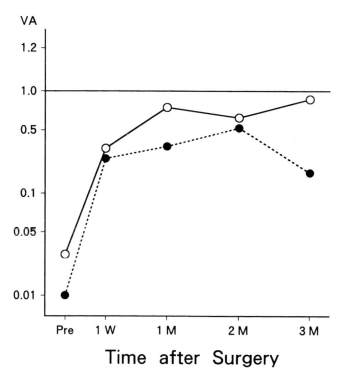

Figure 44–3. Uncorrected visual acuity after PRK in patients with dry eye syndrome.

was achieved within ±3 D of intended refraction, and uncorrected visual acuity improved in all cases. All patients could stop using CL, so that the primary objective was achieved in 100% of patients at the 3-month follow-up examination. Although some patients started to show regression after 3 months, additional PRK may help them.

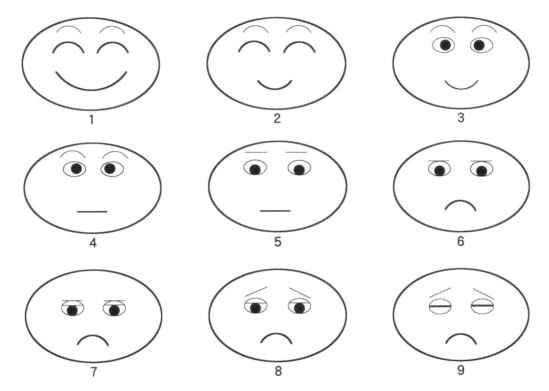

Figure 44–4. Face score for evaluation of ocular discomfort.

To evaluate subjective comfort, we used a "face score." Patients were asked before (with CL) and 3 months after PRK which depiction reflected their eye condition, ranging from very uncomfortable (number 9) to comfortable (number 1) (Fig 44–4). In all patients, the subjective complaints decreased. An additional questionnaire showed that 83.3% of patients were satisfied with the PRK results, 16.7% were neutral, and none regretted that they had undergone PRK.

COMPLICATIONS

There were no serious complications in this series. Our major concern was compromised epithelial wound healing, which may lead to persistent epithelial defect, but we experienced no such problem. As noted above, reflex tearing may be sufficient for proper wound healing after PRK.

Central subepithelial haze formation is summarized in Table 44–1. No clinically significant haze was observed, although two patients showed corneal haze of more than +2 (Fig 44–5). It may be that dry eye causes more dense subepithelial haze or that other factors (eg, racial differences) contribute to this outcome.

TABLE 44–1. HAZE SCORE OF PATIENTS WITH DRY EYE SYNDROME 3 MONTHS AFTER PHOTOREFRACTIVE KERATECTOMY

	Less than −10 D (%)	−10 D or more (%)
0	15.8	37.5
trace	15.8	25.0
1+	46.2	37.5
2+	15.3	0
3+	0	0

CASE REPORT

A 27-year-old Japanese man experienced pain and discomfort after many years of CL wear. His refractive error was −6.5 D with −0.5 D of astigmatism in the right eye and −5.5 D with −1.0 D of astigmatism in the left. The corneal and external examination revealed no abnormalities except for shortened BUT, 5 seconds in the right eye and 4 seconds in the left. The Schirmer value was 2 mm, but the reflex tearing determined by Schirmer test with nasal stimulation was more than 20 mm in both eyes. No systemic abnormalities were found. We made a diagnosis of simple dry eye with compromised basic tearing but good reflex tearing.

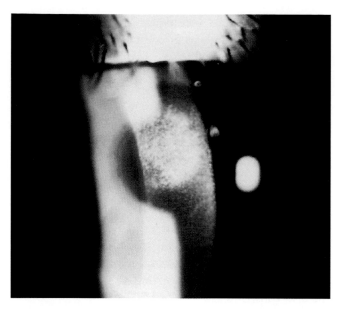

Figure 44–5. The worst corneal haze observed in patients with dry eye syndrome after PRK.

The patient underwent PRK on his right eye on July 1, 1993, and on his left eye on January 26, 1994. The corneal epithelium recovered promptly with no fluorescein staining. The visual acuity was 20/15 in both eyes on February 3, 1994. After the PRK, although the BUT remained at preoperative levels, the patient was satisfied, with a corresponding decrease in face score from 9 to 3, because he did not have to use CL anymore.

CONTACT LENS WEAR VERSUS REFRACTIVE SURGERY

Recent studies have shown that CL wear, especially use of extended-wear soft contact lenses (EWSCL), is closely associated with ulcerative keratitis.[10,12,28–30] Schein and coworkers have reported that 20 of 200,000 wearers develop the condition each year.[12] There are several ways in which CL wear may cause ulcerative keratitis. CL can (1) harbor bacteria and be a source of

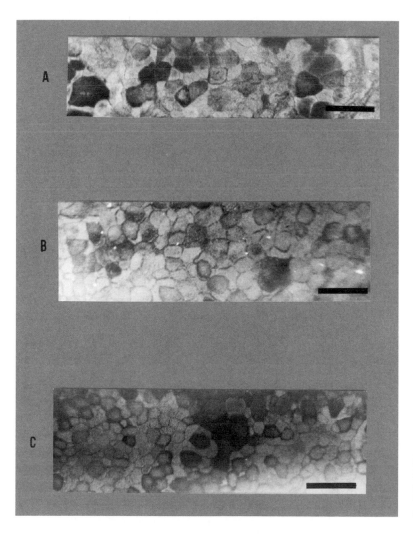

Figure 44–6. A. Specular microscopic view of the corneal epithelium in a patient who wears EWSCL. **B.** Specular microscopic view of the corneal epithelium 3 months after PRK. **C.** Specular microscopic view of normal corneal epithelium.

infection,[31,32] (2) decrease the oxygen supply and suppress epithelial metabolism,[33] (3) produce minor corneal trauma, leading to infection, and (4) suppress desquamation and interfere with normal epithelial maturation.[34] These subtle alterations are difficult to detect clinically. Specular microscopy has been successfully employed to assess subclinical epithelial abnormalities in the postoperative cornea, the diabetic cornea, in keratoconus, and after treatment with various drugs. The effect of EWSCL was also evaluated by morphometric analysis, showing the enlargement of the exposed epithelial cells.

Fig. 44–6A shows the enlarged corneal epithelial cells (mean cell area 890 μm^2) typical of EWSCL patients.[35] In contrast, the patients who underwent PRK looked normal at least 1 month postoperatively (Fig 44–6B and C). It appears that the corneal epithelium maintains the proper cell size by timely desquamation. This event may be accompanied by programmed cell death or another active mechanism rather than the shearing forces of lid movement. Although there were several reports showing epithelial hyperproliferation or other types of epithelial abnormalities after PRK, the desquamation seems to remain within normal limits. From the perspective of epithelial function, this is the most important mechanism to prevent ulcerative keratitis, because bacteria attach to the most superficial layer.

PRK may thus be preferable to chronic CL use in patients with dry eye syndrome, but this may be true only for EWSCL wearers. Preliminary data suggest that daily wear CL can maintain a healthier corneal epithelium than can EWSCL and thereby decrease the risk of ulcerative keratitis.

WHAT IS THE APPROPRIATE REFRACTIVE SURGERY FOR PATIENTS WITH DRY EYE SYNDROME?

We found normal healing of the corneal epithelium after PRK in patients with dry eye syndrome who had reflex tearing. However, ideally, refractive surgery should not depend on wound healing. PRK necessarily affects the visual axis, and these patients appeared to have more haze following PRK than most. Another consideration is that PRK, as RK, is irreversible, although repeat treatments to refine the refractive results are possible. Although no refractive surgery avoids all these issues, the intrastromal corneal ring (ICR)[36] and gel injection adjustable keratoplasty (GIAK)[37] may be alternatives to PRK and RK in patients with dry eyes (see

Chapter 27). These techniques involve inserting a (PMMA) plastic ring and gel, respectively, into the corneal stroma, both of which alter corneal curvature and decrease refractive power. Neither technique interferes with the corneal epithelium, nor do they depend on wound healing or touch the center of the cornea. Although GIAK may not be reversible, the ICR may be removed, with the restoration of preoperative forms of refractive surgery for these patients if the issues of predictability and stability can be resolved.

In addition to patients with dry eye syndrome and high myopia, those with high astigmatism or hyperopia may also find it difficult to wear eyeglasses. They are CL candidates, but because of their dry eyes may not be able to tolerate CL wear. Techniques for correcting these refractive errors are expected to be refined in the near future.

CONCLUSIONS

Dry eye is one of the most common eye diseases, affecting millions of people. The condition is a leading cause of ocular discomfort, irritation, and fatigue,[19] especially in video display terminal users[38] and CL wearers. Dry eye is also a risk factor for ulcerative keratitis in CL wearers.

Although dry eye has sometimes been considered a contraindication for refractive surgery, such patients often cannot tolerate CL wear. However, as long as patients with dry eye syndrome have reflex tearing, their wound healing is sufficient to achieve good results with PRK. The role of punctal plugs in the perioperative period in other patients with dry eyes remains to be determined.

REFERENCES

1. American Academy of Ophthalmology. Radial keratotomy for myopia. *Ophthalmology.* 1993;100:1103–1115.
2. Lohmann C, Fitzke F, O'Brart D, Muir M, Timberlake G, Marshall J. Corneal light scattering and visual performance in myopic individuals with spectacles, contact lenses, or excimer laser photorefractive keratectomy. *Am J Ophthalmol.* 1993;115:444–453.
3. Piebenga L, Matta C, Deitz M, Tauber J, Irvine J, Sabates F. Excimer photorefractive keratectomy for myopia. *Ophthalmology.* 1993;100:1335–1345.
4. Salz J, Maguen E, Nesburn A, et al. A two-year experience with excimer laser photorefractive keratectomy for myopia. *Ophthalmology.* 1993;100:873–882.

5. Seiler T, Holschbach A, Derse M, Jean B, Genth U. Complications of myopic photorefractive keratectomy with the excimer laser. *Ophthalmology.* 1994;101:153–160.

6. Heitzmann J, Binder P, Kassar B, Nordan L. The correction of high myopia using the excimer laser. *Arch Ophthalmol.* 1993;111:1627–1634.

7. Ohashi Y, Motokura M, Kinoshita Y, et al. Presence of epidermal growth factor in human tears. *Invest Ophthalmol Vis Sci.* 1989;30:1879–1887.

8. Ubels J, Loley K, Rismondo V. Retinol secretion by the lacrimal gland. *Invest Ophthalmol Vis Sci.* 1986;27:1261–1269.

9. Wiecozorek R, Jakobiec F, Sacks E, Knowles D. The immunoarchitecture of the normal human lacrimal gland. *Ophthalmology.* 1988;95:100–109.

10. Poggio E, Glynn R, Schein O, et al. The incidence of ulcerative keratitis among users of daily-wear and extended-wear soft contact lenses. *N Engl J Med.* 1989;321:779–783.

11. Poggio E, Abelson M. Complications and symptoms in disposable extended wear lenses compared with conventional soft daily wear and soft extended wear lenses. *CLAO J.* 1993;19:31–39.

12. Schein O, Glynn R, Poggio E, Seddon J, Kenyon K. The relative risk of ulcerative keratitis among users of daily-wear and extended-wear soft contact lenses: a case-control study. *N Engl J Med.* 1989;321:773–778.

13. Farris R. The dry eye: its mechanism and therapy, with evidence that contact lens is a cause. *CLAO J.* 1986;12:234–246.

14. Farris R. Contact lens wear in the management of the dry eye. *Int Ophthalmol Clin.* 1987;27:54–60.

15. Gilbard J, Gray K, Rossi S. A proposed mechanism for increased tear-film osmolarity in contact lens wearers. *Am J Ophthalmol.* 1986;102:505–507.

16. Hamano T, Hamano T, Hamano H, et al. Contact lens wear troubles and phenol red thread test. *J Jpn Contact Lens Soc.* 1986;28:104–107.

17. Tsubota K, Toda I, Yagi Y, Ogawa Y, Ono M, Yoshino K. Three different types of dry eye. *Cornea.* 1994;13:202–209.

18. Tsubota K. The importance of the Schirmer test with nasal stimulation. *Am J Ophthalmol.* 1991;111:106–108. Letter.

19. Toda I, Fujishima H, Tsubota K. Ocular fatigue is the major symptom of dry eye. *Acta Ophthalmol.* 1993;71:18–23.

20. Toda I, Tsubota K. Practical double vital staining for ocular surface evaluation. *Cornea.* 1993;12:366–367.

21. Hamano H, Hori M, Hamano T, et al. A new method for measuring tears. *CLAO J.* 1983;9:281–289.

22. Xu K, Yagi Y, Toda I, Tsubota K. Tear function index: a new measure of dry eye. *Arch Ophthalmol.* 1995;113:84–88.

23. Tsubota K. A contact lens for specular microscopic observation. *Am J Ophthalmol.* 1988;106:627–628.

24. Tsubota K, Yamada M, Naoi S. Specular microscopic observation of human corneal epithelial abnormalities. *Ophthalmology.* 1991;98:184–191.

25. Tsubota K, Yamada M, Naoi S. Specular microscopic observation of normal human corneal epithelium. *Ophthalmology.* 1992;99:89–94.

26. Tsubota K, Mashima Y, Murata H, Sato N, Ogata T. Corneal epithelium in keratoconus. *Cornea.* 1995;14:77–83.

27. Tsubota K, Toda I, Itoh S. Reduction of subepithelial haze after photorefractive keratectomy by cooling the cornea. *Am J Ophthalmol.* 1993;115:820–821.

28. Buehler P, Schein O, Stamler J, Verdier D, Katz J. The increased risk of ulcerative keratitis among disposable soft contact lens users. *Arch Ophthalmol.* 1992;110:1555–1558.

29. Matthews T, Frazer D, Minassian D, Radford C, Dart J. Risks of keratitis and patterns of use with disposable contact lenses. *Arch Ophthalmol.* 1992;110:1559–1562.

30. Alfonso E, Mandelbaum S, Fox MJ, Forster RK. Ulcerative keratitis associated with contact lens wear. *Am J Ophthalmol.* 1986;101:429–433.

31. Butrus SI, Klotz SA. Contact lens surface deposits increase the adhesion of *Pseudomonas aeruginosa. Curr Eye Res.* 1990;9:717–724.

32. Fletcher E, Fleiszig S, Brennan N. Lipopolysaccharide in adherence of *Pseudomonas aeruginosa* to the cornea and contact lens. *Invest Ophthalmol Vis Sci.* 1993;34:1930–1936.

33. Hamano H, Hori M. Effect of contact lens wear on the mitoses of corneal epithelial cells: a preliminary report. *CLAO J.* 1983;9:133–136.

34. Tsubota K, Yamada M. Corneal epithelial alterations induced by disposable contact lens wear. *Ophthalmology.* 1992;99:1193–1196.

35. Amano S, Shimizu K, Tsubota K. Corneal epithelial changes after excimer laser photorefractive keratectomy. *Am J Ophthalmol.* 1993;115:441–443.

36. Nose W, Neves R, Schanzlin D, Crockett-Billing D, Belfort R Jr. The nine-months evaluation of the intrastromal corneal ring in ten myopic eyes. *Invest Ophthalmol Vis Sci.* 1993;34:1240.

37. Simon G, Parel J, Lee W, Kervick G. Gel injection adjustable keratoplasty. *Arch Clin Exp Ophthalmol.* 1991;229:418–424.

38. Tsubota K, Nakamori K. Dry eyes and video display terminals. *N Engl J Med.* 1993;328:584.

SECTION VIII

Combined Refractive Procedures

CHAPTER 45

Combined Keratorefractive Procedures

Suhas W. Tuli ▪ Dimitri T. Azar

Refractive surgery has come a long way from procedures such as clear lens extraction and posterior corneal incisions. In the late 1930s Sato suggested using surgical incisions in the posterior cornea to treat patients with astigmatism and myopia. Cowden, Bores, and Myers began performing radial keratotomy (RK) in the United States in 1978. Since then, the procedure has improved markedly as a result of laboratory and clinical investigations and technologic innovations. However, existing keratorefractive procedures are far from perfect. The problem is compounded by variability in corneal wound healing and other individual responses to surgery. Under correction and overcorrection are frequent, and patients often undergo repeated keratorefractive procedures.

Staged procedures and combinations of two or more procedures have been used to improve visual outcome. Staged procedures have several advantages, especially for RK. Salz and colleagues[1] argued that a four-incision RK followed by four more incisions helps reduce undercorrection and allows staging of the surgery based on observing the eyes' response to the first four incisions. The authors cite the additional advantages of decreased risk of perforation and infection and decreased endothelial cell loss. A marked reduction in the percentage of overcorrections was reported in their study. However, the disadvantages of such a procedure include the risks inherent to multiple operations, an increase in scarring, and an increase in the amount of time required to achieve the final outcome.

Two or more keratorefractive procedures can be combined when one procedure is not ideal. This allows the surgeon to minimize the disadvantages of one procedure while exploiting its advantages. There are few laboratory or clinical data on combination procedures. Such combination procedures can be performed for (1) unplanned undercorrections, (2) unplanned overcorrections, (3) disabling complications produced by the first procedure, or (4) to achieve optimal effect (as a planned operation).

COMBINATION PROCEDURES FOR UNPLANNED UNDERCORRECTION

Undercorrection After Radial Keratotomy

Although not as undesirable a complication as overcorrection, undercorrection after RK is more common. Patients with undercorrection after RK have traditionally been treated with reoperations that involve adding, lengthening, or deepening incisions or decreasing the optical zone. These procedures are discussed in Chapter 20. Briefly, if an aspect of the RK procedure that explains the undercorrection can be identified, it is logical to repeat the surgery. When such explanatory factors cannot be identified, however, minimal benefit can be achieved by reoperation.[2] Furthermore, reoperations are more difficult and less predictable. When reoperations are not feasible options, the alternatives include nonsurgical techniques or different keratorefractive procedures.

Keratomileusis

RK can correct myopia to a limit of 4-6 diopters (D). Keratomileusis can correct moderate to high myopia.[3] Thus patients with residual high myopia after RK may benefit from keratomileusis. Swinger and colleagues rehabilitated two patients who had residual myopia of −16 D and −5.75 D after RK by performing keratomileusis.[4] The authors used post-RK keratometry readings to calculate the lathing parameters. Both autoplastic and homoplastic myopic keratomileusis (MKM) were performed. They found that autoplastic MKM was more accurate, simpler, and less time-consuming than homoplastic surgery. However, autoplastic surgery cannot remove the anterior radial scars, which, with poor surgical technique, may come closer to the visual axis.

Nordan and associates[5] have also performed myopic keratomileusis on patients undercorrected by RK. The authors used pre-RK keratometry data to calculate lathing parameters. They argued that the biomechanical properties of the cornea change after RK. Hence, the keratometry readings after RK may not be reliable for calculating the lathing parameters for myopic keratomileusis, because the nomograms are made for a normal cornea. Thus, in addition to the problems associated with determining the appropriate lathing parameters after RK, the complexities of instrumentation restrict the use of this procedure to those experienced in it. The use of LASIK to correct residual high myopia after RK seems to be promising. The ideal interval between RK and LASIK remains to be determined (see Chapters 26 and 34).

Epikeratoplasty

Epikeratoplasty is a potential surgical modality for selected patients with pediatric and adult aphakia, keratoconus, and high myopia. In epikeratoplasty, a donor lamellar specimen is frozen and carved on a cryolathe, then preserved by lyophilization for storage until surgery. During surgery the lamellar specimen is rehydrated and sutured into an annular keratectomy in the recipient cornea after the host epithelium is removed (see Chapter 29). This procedure is used to correct moderate to high myopia in patients with keratoconus. There are very little published data on the use of epikeratophakia to treat patients with undercorrection after RK. As opposed to keratomileusis, epikeratophakia offers a technique where calculations need not be altered by previous manipulation of the recipient corneal bed. Another potential advantage of epikeratophakia is the addition of mass to a potentially compromised tissue in a reversible manner. Keates and coworkers[6] successfully rehabilitated a patient presenting with high residual myopia of −6.4 D using epikeratophakia. This patient had a poor response to an eight-incision RK (Fig 45–1). No splitting of the RK incisions was observed intraoperatively, and the sutures were placed in between the RK incisions. McDonald and colleagues have treated as many as 20 patients with epikeratoplasty after RK.[7] With the advent of LASIK and PRK, the use

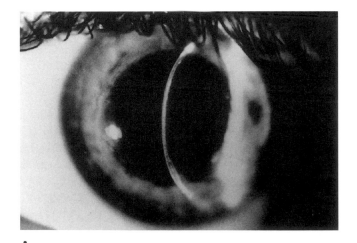

A

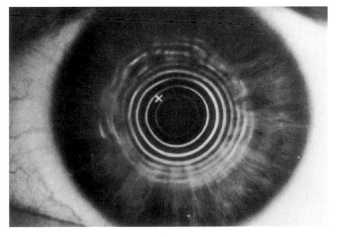

B

Figure 45–1. A. Slit lamp photograph 22 months after RK and 4 months after myopic epikeratophakia. Note absence of scarring between previous RK wounds and lenticule. **B.** Photokeratoscopic appearance of the same patient 21 months after radial keratotomy and 3 months after myopic epikeratophakia. Note central flattening with lack of significant astigmatism. *(From Keates RH, Watson SA, Levy SN. Epikeratophakia following previous refractive surgery: two case reports.* J Cataract Refract Surg. *1986;12:536–540. With permission.)*

of epikeratoplasty after RK has diminished significantly.

Photorefractive Keratectomy

RK is currently the most widely used surgical technique to correct myopia.[8] In the recently reported results of the multicenter PERK study, 43% of patients had experienced a hyperopic shift of ≥1 D by 10 years after treatment.[9] As a safeguard against the development of hyperopia, several investigators advocate "conservative RK," which leaves the patient with intentional undercorrection. However, significant undercorrection may occur in some patients even without a conservative approach.

RK acts indirectly through peripheral radial incisions that flatten the central cornea. There is a limit, however, to the amount of central corneal flattening one can achieve in this way.[10,11] Photorefractive keratectomy (PRK), on the other hand, acts by ablating tissue directly from the central cornea.[12,13] Thus, performing PRK after RK has the theoretical advantage of having additive effects, and it may be possible to combine the advantages of the two procedures. Several authors have reported good results with this procedure.[14–19] We analyzed the visual outcomes of 55 eyes of 45 patients (unpublished data) that had undergone PRK for residual myopia after RK (Fig 45–2); 18.9% of eyes lost 2 or more lines of best-corrected visual acuity (BCVA) at 1 month, and the percentage declined to 11.1% at 12 months. A BCVA of 20/40 or better was achieved in most eyes at 6 months and by all patients at 12 months. Three eyes actually showed improvement in BCVA compared with pre-PRK status. The percentage of eyes with 20/40 or

better uncorrected visual acuity increased from none (0%) preoperatively to 76% at 12 months. The refraction data revealed an initial mean overcorrection, which gradually regressed toward emmetropia. The percentage of eyes within ± 1 D of intended correction increased from 44.4% at 1 month to 65% at 12 months. We analyzed the outcomes of patients after PRK based on their pre-RK and pre-PRK refraction. Patients with smaller refractive errors tended to have more predictable and stable outcomes after the procedure compared with those with higher refractive errors (Table 45–1 and Fig 45–3). A definite correlation between the RK response and the PRK response was not evident. The long-term outcome of the procedure is yet to be determined.

Undercorrection After Photorefractive Keratectomy

With the increased use of PRK, the incidence of residual myopia after PRK is also increasing. The standard method of correcting PRK undercorrections is retreatment with the excimer laser (see Chapters 31 and 33). In the VISX FDA study, retreatment was performed in approximately 4% of eyes. Radial keratotomy may play an important role in correcting low residual myopia after PRK. The advantages of this latter approach include: four or less "mini-RK" incisions may be sufficient; the optical zone is usually large; and subepithelial scarring is not increased. The role of RK for the correction of large (>2.500) degrees of residual myopia after PRK remains to be determined.

Undercorrection After Epikeratophakia

With small undercorrections after epikeratophakia, stability of refraction can be achieved by removing sutures earlier or using intensive steroid treatment. For large undercorrections in myopic epikeratophakias, a suggested technique involves the retrephination of the len-

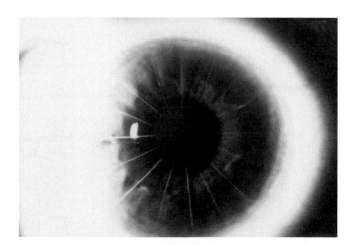

Figure 45–2. Postoperative clinical appearance of a patient who underwent PRK for residual myopia of −6 D after 16-incision RK.

TABLE 45–1. PERCENTAGE OF PATIENTS WITH 20/40 OR BETTER UNCORRECTED VISUAL ACUITY BASED ON PREPHOTOREFRACTIVE KERATECTOMY REFRACTION

Follow-up (mo)	Based on Prephotorefractive Keratectomy Refraction		
	0 D to −2.5 D (%)	−2.62 D to −5 D (%)	> −5 D (%)
1	75	46.0	22.2
3	75	61.5	29.4
6	75	63.6	29.4
12	100	77.8	40.0

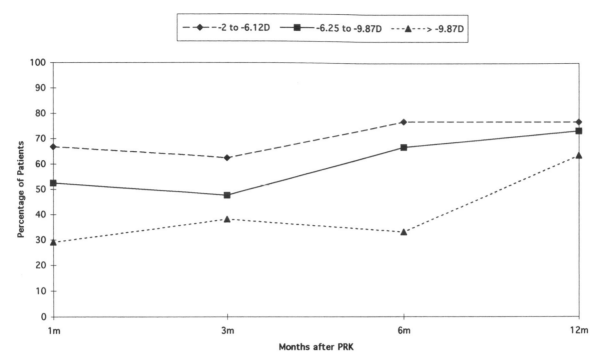

Figure 45–3. Percentage of patients within ±1 D of intended correction based on pre-RK (original) refraction at various time points after PRK.

TABLE 45–2. PREDICTABILITY OF TWO PROCEDURES VERSUS A SINGLE PROCEDURE

Emmetropia	After Myopic Keratomileusis (%)	After Myopic Keratomileusis and a Secondary Procedure (%)
±1 D	45	55
±2 D	69	81
±3 D	85	91

Modified from Maxwell WA. Myopic keratomileusis: initial results and myopic keratomileusis combined with other procedures. *J. Cataract Refract Surg* 1987;13:518–524.

ticule, careful dissection of the lenticule away from the keratectomy bed, and placement of loose cardinal sutures to stabilize the lenticule. The cardinal sutures are removed 1 week postoperatively. Another modality of treatment is RK, where great care must be taken to ensure proper depth, since corneal thickness changes significantly due to the shape of the epikeratophakia lenticule. If there is persistent significant undercorrection, despite the above measures, the lenticule must be replaced.[20]

Undercorrection After Keratomileusis

Maxwell[21] and Bas[22] reported on patients who, originally having undergone keratomileusis, remained undercorrected, for which they underwent RK and astigmatic keratotomy (AK). Maxwell reported that the percentage of patients within ±1 D of emmetropia increased from 45% to 55% if they underwent a secondary procedure following MKM (Table 45–2). One can make the RK and AK calculations for a patient who has undergone keratomileusis as if no previous surgery were performed. Careful pachymetry measurements are essential because corneal thickness varies in previously lathed tissue.

COMBINATION PROCEDURES FOR UNPLANNED OVERCORRECTION

Overcorrection After Radial Keratotomy

Overcorrection after RK is a major complication with passing years. Procedures to rectify this complication are discussed in Chapter 25, and are covered only briefly here. Noninvasive techniques include glasses and contact lenses. The post-RK cornea is thought to be less than ideal for contact lens fitting because of its topographic changes and the potential for corneal infections and vascularization. Other treatments for unplanned overcorrection include purse-string sutures, hexagonal keratotomy, hyperopic keratomileusis, PRK, thermokeratoplasty, and epikeratoplasty.

The disadvantage of hexagonal keratotomy is the need to cut across previous incisions, which further weakens them, rendering this an unacceptable option. Hyperopic keratomileusis is a more realistic possibility, but it requires a homoplastic donor and is unpredictable. PRK is an attractive alternative but has not yet been proven to be uniformly successful (see Chapter 36). Epikeratoplasty can add mass to a potentially compromised cornea. Carlson and colleagues performed epikeratoplasty in four eyes of three patients who were overcorrected after RK.[23] Intraoperatively there was gaping of the RK incisions despite their being sutured. Postoperatively the authors found that contact lens fitting was facilitated by the improved corneal topography after epikeratoplasty. The best approach for overcorrection after RK, however, is to suture the wounds with pursestring sutures.

Pursestring Sutures

The pursestring suture both sterilizes the ocular surface by correcting excessive wound gape and promotes wound healing, which corrects hyperopia.

In this procedure the incisions are split open with a blunt instrument such as a Sinskey hook. Epithelial plugs are removed by irrigating the cornea with balanced salt solution. Each incision is then sutured by either interrupted or circular pursestring sutures. The sutures are placed at a diameter (optical zone, OZ) of 7 mm, tied with a slip knot, adjusted with intraoperative quantitative keratometric control, and then tied with a square knot and buried. If more effect is required, additional sutures can be placed at the 5-mm OZ.[24] Alió and colleagues[25] (Fig 45–4) described a combined technique of interrupted sutures across the RK incision with a single pursestring suture to manage overcorrections. Damiano and associates[26] successfully used a double pursestring suture for the same purpose.

Radial Thermokeratoplasty

Radial thermokeratoplasty seems to be a viable modality to treat patients with overcorrection after RK. Fyodorov's technique includes a thermal microprobe that applies intense heat directly to the corneal stroma in the periphery. The device consists of a handpiece containing a thermal needle composed of a loop of 34-guage wire that is electrically heated to 600°C. The thermal needle, driven by an electric motor through a guard, penetrates 85% to 95% of the corneal stroma. The intense heat that is applied to the cornea causes the collagen surrounding the burn to shrink completely and tightens the peripheral cornea. This causes the central cornea to bulge (Fig 45–5). The procedure, which can correct from 1 to 5 D of hyperopia, can be used to reverse RK overcorrection. When used to treat overcorrection due to RK, the burns

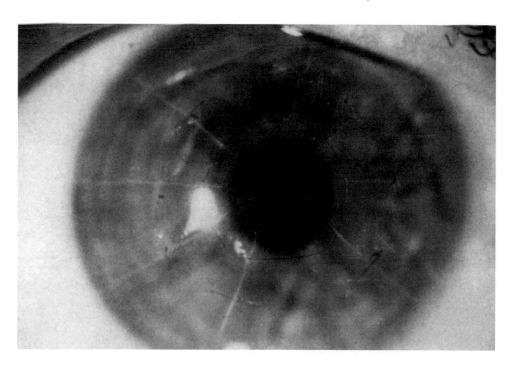

Figure 45–4. Slit lamp photograph of pursestring and radial incision sutures. *(From Alió J, Ismail M. Management of radial keratotomy overcorrections by corneal sutures. J Cataract Refract Surg. 1993;19: 595–599. With permission.)*

should be placed in the previous incision sites. This technique should not be used until the RK incisions have stabilized (ie, after at least 6 to 8 months). Conversely, patients with thermokeratoplasty overcorrections can be treated with RK incisions.[27] The potential danger with this technique is a shallowing of the angle, which can occur as the peripheral cornea shrinks; therefore, a preoperative prophylactic laser peripheral iridectomy is advisable.

An alternative to thermokeratoplasty is the use of an intrastromal pulsed holmium:YAG laser, which works on a principle similar to that of thermokeratoplasty.[28] Thermokeratoplasty is known to cause recurrent erosions, corneal scars, and necrosis. Intrastromal lasers are less invasive and cause no surface defects. Also, their focused laser beam causes a cone-shaped coagulation, which leads to a more pronounced shrinkage of the collagen fibrils. This property of intrastromal lasers results in a greater refractive effect and increased stability. Thus the intrastromal laser can be used within the RK incisions to shrink collagen and reverse overcorrection.

Overcorrection After Epikeratophakia and Keratomileusis

Overcorrection after epikeratophakia and keratomileusis is best treated by resuturing or by replacing the lenticules.[20,29] Other options include selective suture removal and contact lenses.

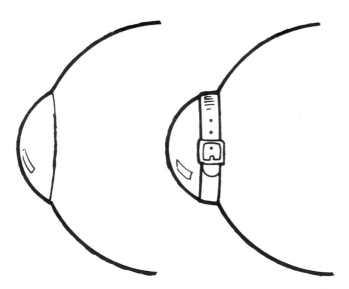

Figure 45–5. Mechanism of action of radial thermokeratoplasty. Shrinking of the peripheral cornea causes the central cornea to bulge forward as if a belt were placed around the peripheral cornea and tightened. *(From Schachar RA. Radial thermokeratoplasty.* Int Ophthalmol Clin. *1991;31:47–57.)*

SECONDARY SURGERY FOR DISABLING SIDE EFFECTS OF RADIAL KERATOTOMY

Penetrating keratoplasty (PK) following RK is indicated when persistent glare exists because of incisions that were made too close to, or within, the visual axis; corneal ulceration; or irregular astigmatism or bullous keratopathy.[30] A possible intraoperative complication that can occur during PK is the disruption of the RK incisions and inadequate wound closure,[31] which can cause irregular astigmatism postoperatively. Leakage of aqueous can occur at the RK incision/circumferential keratoplasty wound junction. Beatty and colleagues[32] performed penetrating keratoplasty after RK on whole human frozen eyes. The authors tried a variety of techniques to determine the most effective method for PK wound closure. They found that meticulous closure of the RK/circumferential corneal wound junctions with either a criss-crossed interrupted or a double-running antitorque suturing technique to be the most effective (Figs 45–6 to 45–8). They recommend (1) paracentesis of the anterior chamber, (2) reinforcement of the cornea using an aqueous humor–Healon exchange, (3) preplacement of transverse 10-0 nylon sutures across each RK incision, 0.5 mm peripheral to the planned corneal button wound, (4) partial-thickness corneal trephination with a sharp disposable or nondisposable corneal trephine, (5) microsurgical dissection of a vertically oriented circumferential wound, (6) radial cardinal suture placement with at least one 10-0 interrupted nylon suture between each radial incision, (7) meticulous closure of the RK-circumferential corneal wound junctions with either a criss-crossed interrupted or a double-running antitorque suturing technique, and (8) peripheral placement of a second transverse 10-0 nylon suture 1.0 mm from the corneal limbus. McNeill and colleagues[33] have used a simple corneal pursestring suture to stabilize the peripheral host cornea during PK (Fig 45–9).

PLANNED COMBINATION REFRACTIVE SURGICAL PROCEDURES

Radial Keratotomy and Photorefractive Keratectomy

The corneal biomechanics are altered during RK, the most widely used technique to reduce myopia, by deep peripheral incisions, which induce indirect flattening of the center. The nonlinear characteristics of corneal bio-

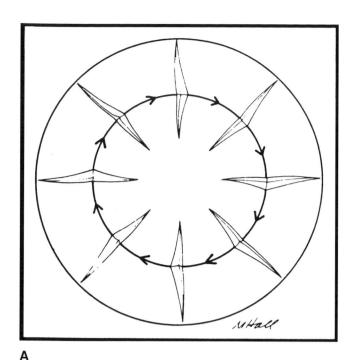

A

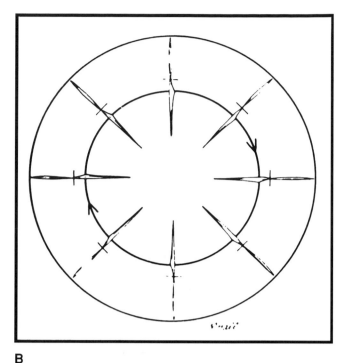

B

Figure 45–6. A. Clockwise trephine rotation in unsutured corneal tissue. RK wound separation and torque occur in the same clockwise direction. Note separation of RK incisions along their entire length. Wound dehiscence occurs central and peripheral to trephine groove. **B.** Clockwise trephine rotation in corneal tissue with preplaced transverse sutures across radial keratotomy incisions 0.5 mm peripheral to trephine groove. Separation of the radial incisions is markedly reduced during trephination of the cornea. *(From Beatty RF, Robin JB, Schanzlin DJ. Penetrating keratoplasty after radial keratotomy. J Refract Surg. 1986;2:207–214. With permission.)*

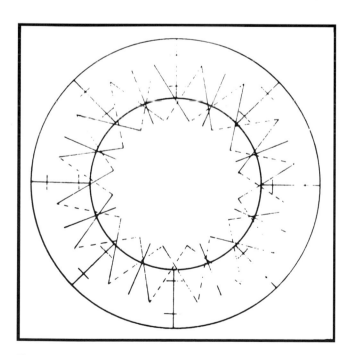

Figure 45–7. Eight-bite double-running antitorque suture technique. Both sutures run clockwise, staggered by 22.5°. At the RK incision and circumferential wound intersection, one suture is placed deeply through tissue and the other suture overlies the intersection point. Radial sutures and transverse sutures are left in place to be selectively removed postoperatively. *(From Beatty RF, Robin JB, Schanzlin DJ. Penetrating keratoplasty after radial keratotomy. J Refract Surg. 1986;2:207–214. With permission.)*

mechanics often limit the amount of central flattening that can be achieved. PRK is an alternative technique to flatten the central cornea. PRK removes tissue directly from the center of the cornea and reprofiles its anterior surface, thereby imparting a new refractive surface. If used alone in patients with high myopia, PRK may cause increased scarring in the visual axis due to removal of excessive tissue. Additionally, hyperplasia of the epithelium may cause regression, thus negating the effect of treatment.

The use of RK alone in high myopia may not be sufficient to correct such a high refractive error. It may theoretically be possible to combine RK and PRK to maximize their refractive effect and offset their disadvantages. There are no published laboratory or clinical data regarding the intentional combination of these two procedures. The questions that must be answered are the efficacy of the combined procedure, the time interval between the two procedures, and the sequence of operation. The increased haze that might develop after PRK due to activation of keratocytes in the RK incision sites is the issue of prime concern with such a combination procedure.

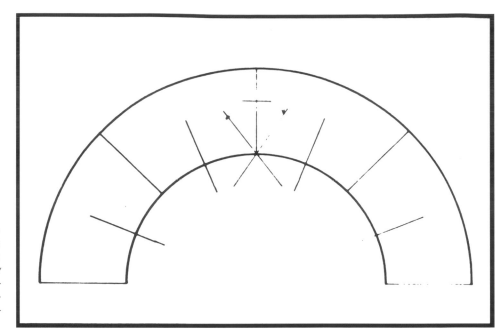

Figure 45–8. The criss-crossed interrupted suture technique combines intrastromal wound splinting with wound compression. *(From Beatty RF, Robin JB, Schanzlin DJ. Penetrating keratoplasty after radial keratotomy. J Refract Surg. 1986;2:207–214. With permission.)*

LASIK—Automated Lamellar Keratectomy and Photorefractive Keratectomy

Laser in situ keratomileusis, or LASIK, is another interesting surgical combination—automated lamellar keratectomy (ALK) and PRK. It is increasingly being used to treat patients with myopia (see Chapter 34). ALK, although not very accurate, has been used to treat patients with high myopia (see Chapter 26). It consists of a second shaping resection of the cornea after a pri-

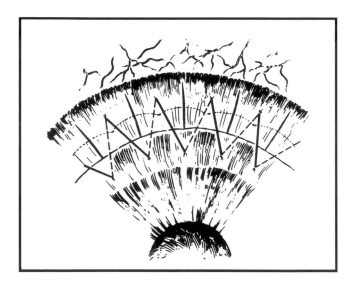

Figure 45–9. The pursestring suture (fine dashed line) runs just outside the corneal trephine mark. The running keratoplasty suture (solid and dashed lines) passes over the pursestring suture and completes the stabilization of the peripheral cornea. *(From McNeill JI, Wilkins DL. A pursestring suture for penetrating keratoplasty following radial keratotomy. Refract Corneal Surg. 1991;7:392–394. With permission.)*

mary cap is resected. The flap or first disc, when replaced, conforms to the shape of the resected bed, thus altering corneal anterior curvature. The thickness of the second resection determines the power of the correction. The keratome depends on the speed of the pass to give the proper thickness of the resection.

An alternative way to make a second refractive cut is to use the 193-nm excimer laser. With this, the corneal tissue can be removed with precision, a lenticular cut can be made, and astigmatism can be corrected at the same sitting. The disadvantages that surgeons face with surface excimer ablations, especially in high myopes, are scarring and regression of refractive effect. The epithelial healing response may play an important role in the refractive outcome. An exuberant response can cause undercorrection; conversely, a thin atrophic layer of epithelium causes an overcorrection. Making excimer ablations deep in the stroma circumvents the epithelial healing process and thus improves its predictability and decreases scarring. A large series of patients undergoing this procedure was first reported by Lucio Burrato.[34] The issue of whether the ablation should be on the cap or on the bed has been resolved in favor of treating the stromal bed under a flap. The advantages cited for cap ablation are perfect centration and the possibility of replacing the cap with homoplastic tissue in case the ablation is unsatisfactory. With the flap technique the major advantage is the ease of surgery, ease of apposition of the flap, and reduced postoperative astigmatism. It is not entirely clear whether the endothelium may be damaged because the ablations are closer to Descemet's membrane.

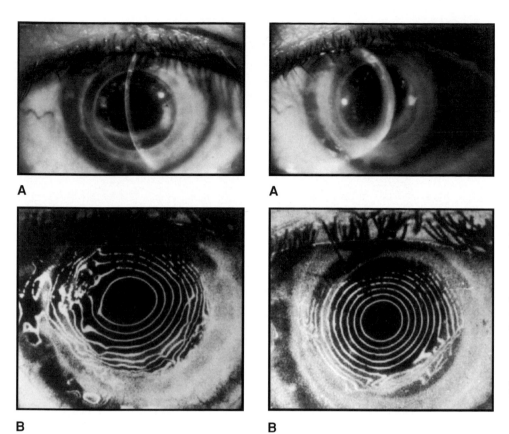

A

A

B

B

Figure 45–10. A and **B**, left. Clinical and photokeratoscopic appearance of a 51-year-old aphakic patient with high-degree postkeratoplasty astigmatism. **A** and **B**, right. Clinical and photokeratoscopic appearance of the same patient 2 years after a combined procedure using corneal relaxing incisions and epikeratophakia. *(From Busin M, Spitsnaz M. Combined relaxing incisions and epikeratophakia for the correction of aphakia and high postkeratoplasty degree astigmatism. Ophthalmic Surg. 1991;22:137–141. With permission.)*

Epikeratophakia and Astigmatic Keratotomy

The management of patients with postkeratoplasty astigmatism combined with aphakia remains a nightmare for the keratorefractive surgeon. Such management routinely includes implanting an intraocular lens (IOL) during or after penetrating keratoplasty followed by AK to correct astigmatism. In cases where an IOL cannot be implanted due to anatomic unsuitability, an epikeratophakia alone can treat the aphakia if the astigmatism is minimal. If the astigmatism is high, an AK can be performed, followed later by epikeratophakia. This procedure would, however, delay visual rehabilitation because the surgeon must wait for the corneal curvature to stabilize after AK before proceeding with epikeratophakia. Another possibility is to combine the two procedures in one sitting,[35] the distinct advantage of this being faster visual rehabilitation (Fig 45–10). The other advantage cited by Busin and colleagues is that epithelial plugs are prevented from entering the incisions due to presence of the epilens. This may help maintain corneal stability.

Casebeer and colleagues[36] reported a patient with keratoconus who underwent epikeratophakia followed by RK and AK. RK cannot be performed in patients

with keratoconus; however, improving the structural integrity of the cornea with epikeratophakia can make RK possible in such patients.

Other Combination Procedures

There are isolated reports of combination procedures like removal of a clear crystalline lens combined with keratomileusis and RK, or a synthetic intracorneal implant and RK either on the corneal surface or within the keratomileusis bed.[37] Goosey and coauthors[38] reported an interesting case of a 3-year-old child who had unilateral posttraumatic corneal scar with aphakia. He underwent rotational autokeratoplasty so that the scar no longer obscured the visual axis. This was followed later by epikeratophakia to correct aphakia (Fig 45–11). Choyce successfully implanted Baikoff ZB5M IOLs in both eyes of a 35-year-old high myope (−11.0D, OU) for residual myopia of −4.5 D and −5.0 D in the right and left eye, respectively, after RK[39] (Fig 45–12). Another interesting combination of keratorefractive procedures has been suggested by Hjortdal and colleagues: the epi lens can be attached to the surface of the cornea to obtain a curvature change, after which the corneal surface can be finely tuned by excimer laser ablation to obtain the exact desired shape.[40]

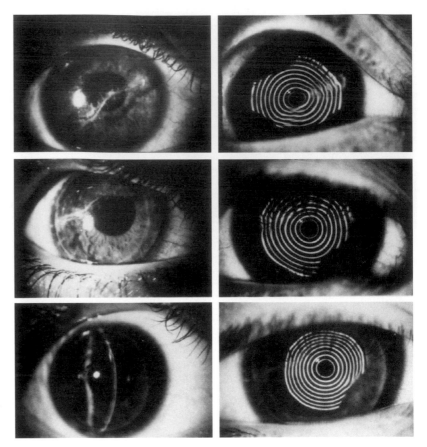

Figure 45–11. Slit lamp and corneascope appearance of a 3-year-old child with unilateral posttraumatic central corneal scar and aphakia. Top left and right. Preoperative appearance. Middle left and right. Two months after rotational epikeratoplasty. Bottom left and right. 1 year after epikeratophakia. *(From Goosey JD, Vila-Coro AA. Epikeratophakia following rotational autokeratoplasty in a child. Cornea. 1987; 6:140–143. With permission.)*

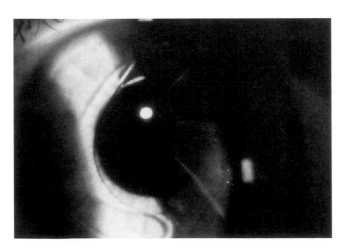

Figure 45–12. Slit lamp photomicrograph shows radial keratotomy scars and the Baikoff ZB5M minus power IOL. The distance between the IOL and the corneal endothelium is 2.0 mm. *(From Choyce DP. Residual myopia after radial keratotomy successfully treated with Baikoff ZB5M IOLs. Refract Corneal Surg. 1993;9:475. With permission.)*

High myopia and astigmatism often complicate penetrating keratoplasty, making it difficult to rehabilitate the eye. Treatment options include RK, epikeratoplasty, keratomileusis, PRK, and minus-power anterior-chamber (AC) lenses. RK has been used to treat patients with intolerable myopia after penetrating keratoplasty[41–43] (Fig 45–13). The authors found a high amount of variability, and the predictability was limited by the complex topographic changes occuring in corneal transplants. They also believe that complex corneal biomechanical changes may predispose these eyes to develop irregular astigmatism. The potential complications that can occur after RK in the keratoplasty patient are vascularization, weakening of structural integrity of the graft, and epithelial erosions. Young and colleagues[43] have reported vascularization of the radial incisions, which can trigger an acute allograft rejection in the keratoplasty patient. Keates and coworkers[6] performed epikeratophakia on a patient with postkeratoplasty myopia (Fig 45–14). The disadvantage of this procedure is the delayed regression of its effect that can occur in high myopia. There are reports of successful rehabilitation after keratomileusis performed in postkeratoplasty patients.[44] The implantation of minus-power

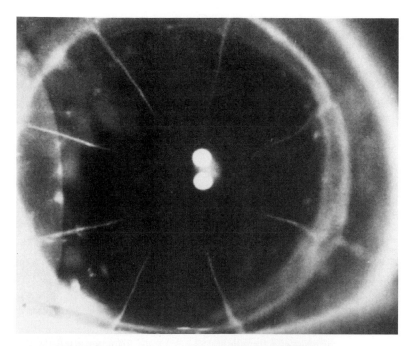

Figure 45–13. Clinical photograph of a 71-year-old woman 1 year after RK for high myopia. The patient had previously undergone penetrating keratoplasty after corneal ulceration. *(From Shapiro MB, Harrison DA. Radial keratotomy for intolerable myopia after penetrating keratoplasty.* Am J Ophthalmol. *1993;115:327–331. With permission.)*

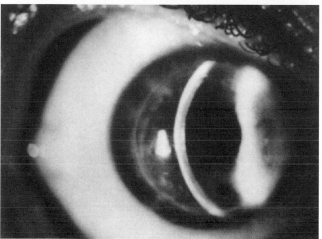

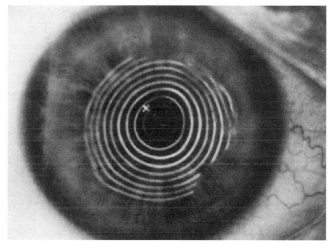

A

B

Figure 45–14. Clinical photograph **(A)** and photokeratoscopic appearance **(B)** 12 years after penetrating keratoplasty and 5 months after keratoconic epikeratophakia. *(From Keates RH, Watson SA, Levy SN. Epikeratophakia following previous refractive surgery: two case reports.* J Cataract Refract Surg. *1986;12:536–540. With permission.)*

AC lenses as a secondary procedure after penetrating keratoplasty may increase the risk of graft endothelial damage, postoperative intraocular infection, and possible graft rejection. PRK holds promise in this situation but has not yet been performed and reported.

REFERENCES

1. Salz JJ, Villasenor RA, Elander R, Reader AL, Swinger C, Buchbinder M. Four-incision radial keratotomy for low to moderate myopia. Ophthalmology. 1986;93:727–738.

2. Villasenor RA, Cox KO. Radial keratotomy: reoperations. *J Refract Surg.* 1985;1:34–37.

3. Swinger CA, Barker BA. Prospective evaluation of myopic keratomileusis. *Ophthalmology.* 1984;91:785–792.

4. Swinger CA, Barker BA. Myopic keratomileusis following radial keratotomy. *J Refract Surg.* 1985;1:53–55.

5. Nordan LT, Havins WE: Undercorrected radial keratotomy treated with myopic keratomileusis. *J Refract Surg.* 1985;1:56–58.

6. Keates RH, Watson SA, Levy SN: Epikeratophakia following previous refractive surgery: two case reports. *J Cataract Refract Surg.* 1986;12:536–540.

7. Waring GO. Radial keratotomy. In: Kaufman HE, et al, eds. *The Cornea.* New York: Churchill Livingstone; 1988: 849–896.

8. Waring GO. *Refractive Keratotomy for Myopia and Astigmatism.* St. Louis, MO: Mosby–Year Book; 1992.

9. Waring GO, Lynn MJ, McDonnell PJ, and the PERK Study Group. Results of the prospective evaluation of radial keratotomy (PERK) study 10 years after surgery. *Arch Ophthalmol.* 1994;112:1298–1308.

10. Villasenor RA, Cox KO. Radial keratotomy: reoperations. *J Refract Surg.* 1985;1:34–37.

11. Salz JJ. Radial keratotomy. In: Thompson FB, ed. *Myopia Surgery. Anterior and Posterior Segments.* New York: Macmillan; 1990:31–65.

12. Marshall J, Trokel S, Rothery S, Krueger RR. Photoablative reprofiling of the cornea using an excimer laser: photorefractive keratectomy. *Lasers Ophthalmol.* 1986;1:21–48.

13. Taylor DM, L'Esperance FA, Del Pero RA, et al. Human excimer lamellar keratectomy. *Ophthalmology.* 1989;96: 654–664.

14. Meza J, Perez-Santonja JJ, Morena E, Zato MA. Photorefractive keratectomy after radial keratotomy. *J Cataract Refract Surg.* 1994;20:485–489.

15. Ribeiro JC, McDonald MB, Klyce SD. Photorefractive keratectomy after radial keratotomy in a patient with severe myopia. *Am J Ophthalmol.* 1994;118:106–108.

16. McDonnell PJ, Garbus JJ, Salz JJ. Excimer laser myopic photorefractive keratectomy after undercorrected radial keratotomy. *Refract Corneal Surg.* 1991;7:146–150.

17. Frangie JP, Park SB, Kim J, Aquavella JV. Excimer laser keratectomy after radial keratotomy. *Am J Ophthalmol.* 1993; 115:634–639.

18. Durrie DS, Schumer DJ, Cavanaugh TB. Photorefractive keratectomy for residual myopia after previous refractive keratotomy. *Refract Corneal Surg.* 1994;10(suppl 2):S235–S238.

19. Seiler T, Jean B. Photorefractive keratectomy as a second attempt to correct myopia after radial keratotomy. *Refract Corneal Surg.* 1992;8:211–214.

20. Lindstrom R, ed. Consultations in refractive surgery. *J Refract Surg.* 1988;4:194–195.

21. Maxwell WA. Myopic keratomileusis: initial results and myopic keratomileusis combined with other procedures. *J Cataract Refract Surg.* 1987;13:518–524.

22. Bas AM, Nano HD. In situ myopic keratomileusis results in 30 eyes at 15 months. *Refract Corneal Surg.* 1991;7:223–231.

23. Carlson KA, Goosey JD. Epikeratoplasty following overcorrected radial keratotomy. *Investigative Ophthalmol Vis Sci* suppl 1988;29:390.

24. Lindquist TD, Rubenstein JB, Lindstrom RL. Correction of hyperopia following radial keratotomy: quantification in human cadaver eyes. *Ophthalmic Surg.* 1987;10:432–437.

25. Alió J, Ismail M. Management of radial keratotomy overcorrections by corneal sutures. *J Cataract Refract Surg.* 1993;19:595–599.

26. Damiano RE, Forstot SL, Dukes DK. Surgical correction of hyperopia following radial keratotomy. *Refract Corneal Surg.* 1992;8:75–79.

27. Schachar RA. Radial thermokeratoplasty. *Int Ophthalmol Clin.* 1991;31:47–57.

28. Seiler T, Matallana M, Bende T. Laser thermokeratoplasty by means of a pulsed Holmium:YAG laser for hyperopic correction. *Refract Corneal Surg.* 1990;6:335–339.

29. Nichols BD, Lindstrom RL, Spigelman AV. The surgical management of overcorrection in myopic epikeratophakia. *Am J Ophthalmol.* 1988;105:354–356.

30. Robin JB, Beatty RF, Dunn S, et al: *Mycobacterium chelonei* keratitis following radial keratotomy. *Am J Ophthalmol.* 1986;102:72–79.

31. McNeill JI. Corneal incision dehiscence during penetrating keratoplasty nine years after radial keratotomy. *J Cataract Refract Surg.* 1993;19:542–543.

32. Beatty RF, Robion JB, Schanzlin DJ. Penetrating keratoplasty after radial keratotomy. *J Refract Surg.* 1986;2: 207–214.

33. McNeill JI, Wilkins DL. A purse-string suture for penetrating keratoplasty following radial keratotomy. *Refract Corneal Surg.* 1991;7:392–394.

34. Burrato L, Ferrari M. Retrospective comparison of freeze and non-freeze myopic epikeratophakia. *Refract Corneal Surg.* 1989;5:94–97.

35. Busin M, Spitsnaz M. Combined relaxing incisions and epikeratophakia for the correction of aphakia and high postkeratoplasty degree astigmatism. *Ophthalmic Surg.* 1991;22:137–141.

36. Casebeer JC, Shapiro DR. Radial keratotomy in intact keratoplasty graft. *Refract Corneal Surg.* 1993;9:133–135.

37. Woo GC, Wilson MA. Current methods of treating and preventing myopia. *Optometry Vision Sci.* 1990;67: 719–727.

38. Goosey JD, Vila-Coro AA. Epikeratophakia following rotational autokeratoplasty in a child. *Cornea.* 1987;6: 140–143.

39. Choyce DP. Residual myopia after radial keratotomy successfully treated with Baikoff ZB5M IOLs. *Refract Corneal Surg.* 1993;9:475.

40. Hjortdal JO, Ehlers N. Epikeratophakia for high myopia. *Acta Ophthalmol.* 1991;69:754–760.

41. Gothard TW, Agapitos PJ, Bowers RA, Mma S, Chen H, Lindstrom RL. Four incision radial keratotomy for high myopia after penetrating keratoplasty. *Refract Corneal Surg.* 1993;9:51–57.

42. Shapiro MB, Harrison DA. Radial keratotomy for intolerable myopia after penetrating keratoplasty. *Am J Ophthalmol.* 1993;115:327–331.

43. Young SR, Lundergan MK, Olson RJ. Late complications of combined radial and transverse keratotomy after penetrating keratoplasty associated with atopic keratoconjunctivitis. *Refract Corneal Surg.* 1989;5:194–197.

44. Kremer F, Kremer I. Postkeratoplasty myopia treated by keratomileusis. *Ann Ophthalmol.* 1993;25:370–372.

CHAPTER 46

Combined Radial and Astigmatic Keratotomy

J. B. Stevens ▪ Kenneth R. Kenyon ▪ Peter A. Rapoza ▪ David Miller ▪ R. Bruce Grene

The cornea has been referred to as an "anatomically eccentric, radially asymmetric, aspheric optical surface."[1] Hence, the incisional surgical correction of combined myopic astigmatism, although technically feasible and visually satisfactory, nonetheless is several times more complex than simple radial keratotomy (RK) or astigmatic keratotomy (AK). Despite this challenge, given advances in instrumentation, technique, and experience, it is possible to combine RK and AK procedures successfully.

PATIENT SELECTION

Combining RK and AK is essentially equal to the sum of its component parts, but given the increased difficulty of predicting outcome, careful patient selection is all the more mandatory. The patient's refractive error must fall within the range of compound myopic astigmatism for which surgical nomograms are applicable, and the patient must have a realistic appreciation of the somewhat decreased predictability of possible refractive outcomes. The patient should have a stable cycloplegic refraction (0.50 diopters [D] or less change per year over the previous 2 years). Although it is not mandatory that patients discontinue contact lens wear before preliminary evaluation for refractive surgery, patients wearing PMMA and RGP contact lenses should discontinue them for 3 weeks, while soft contact lens wearers should remove them 1 week before cycloplegic refraction and manual keratometry, since these measurements are critical to surgical planning. If irregular astigmatism is present as detected by manual keratometry or computerized topography, then the patient should remain without contact lenses and be reevaluated weekly until the corneal surface configuration has stabilized. This permits differentiation of contact-lens-related corneal warpage (which should diminish, or at least stabilize) from keratoconus (which is a contraindication to incisional keratotomy).

CONTRAINDICATIONS

Ophthalmic and systemic conditions generally considered contraindications to incisional refractive surgery include severe connective tissue disorders or history of abnormal wound healing, chronic steroid use, poorly controlled diabetes mellitus, major psychiatric disorders, uncontrolled glaucoma, recurrent herpes simplex keratitis, and vitreoretinal disorders that might require future major surgical intervention. Significant ocular surface disease should be diagnosed and optimally managed. Although patients with severe dry eyes, blepharitis, or meibomian gland dysfunction may be initially inappropriate for refractive surgery, attentive management may render them suitable candidates[2] or may facilitate their tolerance of contact lenses.

PREOPERATIVE EVALUATION

Preoperative evaluation includes testing of uncorrected and best corrected visual acuity (BCVA) (both dry and cycloplegic), manual keratometry, slit lamp biomicroscopy (with special attention to the possible presence of epithelial basement membrane disease, stromal scarring or vascularization, keratoconus, or guttatae), intraocular pressure measurement, dilated ophthalmoscopy (especially to identify myopic macular degeneration or peripheral retinal breaks or detachments), and determination of ocular dominance. (For reasons discussed elsewhere, refractive surgery is usually first performed on the nondominant eye.) Preoperative preparation also includes patient education regarding postoperative discomfort, photophobia, glare, starburst, fluctuating vision, irregular astigmatism, the potential complications of perforation and of infection, and the possible necessity of reoperation (enhancement[s]).

On the day of surgery, patients should eat minimally, refrain from wearing eye make-up, and arrange for transportation home. Following a written or video presentation of the surgery and its potential risks, benefits, and alternatives, and after discussion with the surgeon, patients are asked to sign an informed consent document.

SIMULTANEOUS RADIAL KERATOTOMY AND ASTIGMATIC KERATOTOMY

From both the patient's and the surgeon's viewpoint, there are several obvious advantages to performing RK and AK as a single, combined procedure. The one-stage approach is both efficient and economical while also speeding visual recovery. Hence, in all but the most complex of cases, we prefer simultaneous RK and AK. However, should considerations of high astigmatism combined with low myopia or hyperopia, patient age greater than 50 years, or unpredicted prior refractive

surgical outcome supervene, it may be prudent to perform deliberately staged surgical procedures.

In the performance of simultaneous RK-AK there are three potentially confounding elements: pattern and placement of incisions, structural integrity of the cornea, and predictability of the nomograms.

Pattern and Placement of Incisions

In RK for simple myopia, the actual orientation of the radial incisions need only be symmetric (ie, equally spaced). In combined RK-AK, however, the appropriate and accurate placement of the radial incisions is far more critical. For low levels of astigmatism (less than 1 D of cylinder), some astigmatic correction can be achieved by orienting one pair of radial incisions to coincide with the meridian of the plus cylinder axis. Additional astigmatic effect (up to 1 D of cylinder) can be accomplished by lengthening this same pair of radial incisions by approximately 0.25 to 0.50 mm. Thus, for astigmatism of less than 1.25 D, no additional astigmatic incisions per se should be required. When indicated for myopic astigmatism of greater than 1.25 D, there are currently three basic patterns of combined RK and AK: (1) transverse incisions (straight or arcuate, single or multiple, symmetric or asymmetric) between radials (Fig 46–1), (2) nonintersecting, interrupted transverse incisions that "jump" the radials ("jump-T") (Fig 46–2A), or (3) radials that are interrupted to "jump" the transverse incisions placed in the steep meridian ("jump-radial") (Fig 46–2B).

Structural Integrity

If radial incisions are performed first, the effect of both incision and manipulation is to weaken the cornea. Although this is usually of no significant concern when only a single astigmatic incision is to be performed, it can create technical difficulties for placing either straight or arcuate incisions at precise length, depth, and consistent configuration. For this reason, and especially when two or more astigmatic incisions are required, the transverse incisions should precede the radial incisions.

Predictability

As is detailed elsewhere, the effect of flattening (reduced curvature) in a given corneal meridian, induced by either a radial or transverse incision, is "coupled" with approximately equal steepening (increased curvature) in the orthogonal meridian (90°

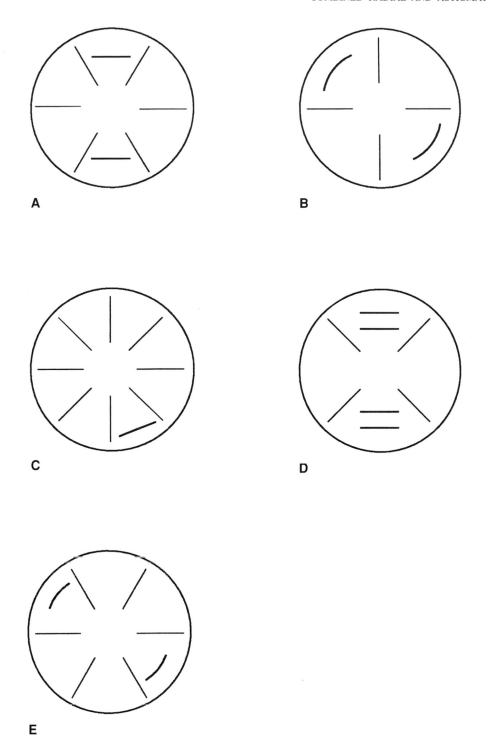

Figure 46–1. Transverse incisions between radials. **A.** Straight. **B.** Arcuate. **C.** Single. **D.** Multiple. **E.** Asymmetrically placed.

away).[3] Theoretically, if AK alone is performed, the spherical equivalent of the cornea remains unchanged. This is not always the case, however, especially when AK is combined with RK.[4–10] Although the astigmatic reduction clinical trial (ARC-T)[10] results did

show roughly 1:1 correspondence in 100 eyes each of straight-T versus arcuate AKs, they also showed very high variability. Recent clinical experience suggests that the relationship is nonlinear and that the coupling ratio is 2:1 for the flattening of the steep merid-

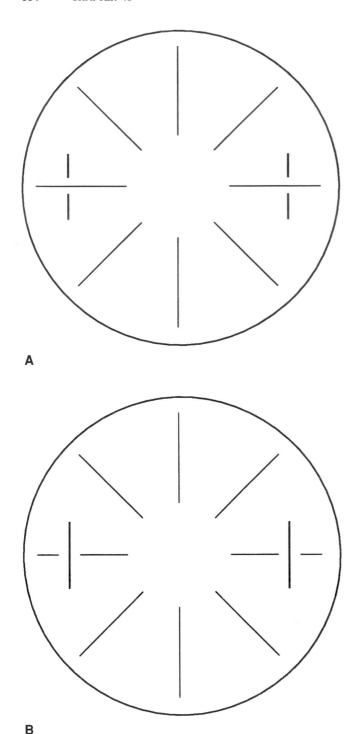

A

B

Figure 46–2. A. Nonintersecting interrupted T incisions. **B.** Nonintersecting interrupted radial incisions.

ian versus the "coupled" steepening of the flat meridian (ie, for every 2 D of flattening, only 1 D of steepening is produced, with a resultant decrease in the spherical equivalent). Other recent clinical experience appears to demonstrate a consistent finding

of up to 2.0 D of additional decrease in cylinder when arcuate transverse incisions are combined with simultaneous RK than when the identical AK is performed alone.[11] Of interest in this regard is the ARC-T. As detailed below, one segment of this study entailed performing (1 month after initial AK) either RK alone or RK plus simultaneous AK as indicated by refraction at that time. The authors found that the group having solely RK as the second-stage surgery had a greater magnitude of change of all three refractive parameters (sphere, cylinder, and spherical equivalent) than the group having simultaneous RK plus AK enhancement.[12] Could this even imply an inhibitory effect of AK on RK if performed simultaneously?

From a practical surgical planning standpoint, we assume that the effects of simultaneous RK and AK are, in fact, simply additive. Thus, we use an RK nomogram and spherical equivalent myopia for planning radial incisions, in conjunction with an AK nomogram for determining the transverse incisions. With the rather rare aforementioned exceptions, for which we deliberately stage these procedures, we have enjoyed clinically excellent results with this exceedingly straightforward approach. Furthermore, and most important, we have encountered several instances when in using the staged approach, a seemingly stable AK result was subsequently destabilized by the later RK procedure, thereby necessitating further intervention to produce an acceptable outcome. This was especially encountered when arcuate incisions of greater than 60° were performed. Hence we no longer use 90° arcuate incisions, and alternatively we employ a modified Ruiz procedure to correct higher astigmatism. Lesson: less is more, and more is too much!

STAGED RK AND AK

Despite the foregoing caveats, the combination of RK and AK can be effectively accomplished as a "staged" procedure; in fact, there may even be some advantage to doing so. Ibrahim and colleagues[13] found relative stabilization of any significant AK undercorrection or overcorrection after approximately 3 months. Such stabilization may make two-stage procedures more predictable than those in which RK and AK are performed simultaneously. In the more recent ARC-T,[10] good results were obtained when the AK component preceded the RK component of a two-stage procedure by 1 month. In this prospective clinical trial of arcuate keratotomy, a modification of the nomogram derived by Lindstrom[14] was used, and a group of nine surgeons initially performed AK on 160 eyes of 95 patients. Based on the refraction at 1 month postoperatively, 41% of these eyes required either no additional surgery or AK enhancement alone. Of the remainder, at 1 month postoperatively 75 eyes underwent RK as a second surgery and 19 underwent simultaneous RK plus AK enhancement. As shown in Tables 46–1 and 46–2, there was a significant change in both cylinder and spherical equivalent in all patients undergoing RK in the second stage but, as mentioned above, even more for those having RK alone than for those having RK plus AK enhancement. The true reason for this is not yet known and definitely bears further study. Any consistently contributing parameters can then be titrated to provide ever-more-predictable results.

RK itself can induce astigmatism, as demonstrated by the prospective evaluation of radial keratotomy (PERK) study: 14% of eyes undergoing the standardized eight-incision RK experienced an increased astigmatism of more than 1 D. The reason for this was presumably a difference in precision of individual incisions or variable wound healing. A greater increase in astigmatism was associated with a smaller diameter optical zone.[15,16] Hence there is a rationale for initially performing RK, waiting 1 month or more to assess the residual myopia and astigmatism, and then proceeding with simultaneous AK and, as required, RK enhancement.

Despite improved nomograms and "cookbook" methodologies, all incisional refractive surgery remains substantially individualized and individually variable. Hence, to help the refractive surgeon of moderate experience decide whether to perform either staged or combined RK-AK, it may be advisable to review one's own results to ascertain consistent patterns of results that would indicate an outcome bias. The data can then be used to advantage in subsequent surgical planning and performance.

VARIABLES

Variables affecting outcome of combined RK-AK (either simultaneous or staged) are similar to those affecting each procedure individually. They include:

TABLE 46–1. 6-MONTH RESULTS OF STAGED ASTIGMATIC KERATOTOMY–RADIAL KERATOTOMY FROM THE ARC-T STUDY.*

	RK[†]	RK + AK[†]
Number of patients	75	19
Percentage of total	47%	12%
Total decrease in SE	4.5 ± 1.6(−0.4 − 7.9)	3.6 ± 1.2(0.9 − 5.3)
Total decrease in cylinder	2.9 ± 1.6(0.3 − 9.4)	2.5 ± 1.0(0.3 − 3.7)

*Results at 6 months for patients undergoing either RK or RK plus AK enhancement. Data refer to second-stage (enhancement) surgery, compared with initial presentation. All patients underwent AK alone as first-stage surgery.[9]
[†]Values are expressed as the mean number of diopters, plus or minus the standard deviation. Numbers in parentheses represent the range of values in diopters.
Abbreviation: SE = spherical equivalent.

TABLE 46–2. INCREMENTAL RESULTS OF SECOND-STAGE SURGERY FROM THE ARC-T STUDY*

	RK[†]	RK + AK[†]
Number of patients	67	18
Percentage of total	42%	11%
Incremental decrease in SE	4.5 ± 1.6(−1.0 − 8.6)	3.8 ± 1.3(0.9 − 5.5)
Incremental decrease in cylinder	1.5 ± 1.1(0.3 − 5.6)	1.3 ± 0.6(0.3 − 2.5)

*Results of second surgery (measured 6 months later) minus the results of initial AK alone, as measured 1 month after initial AK.[9]
[†]Values are expressed as the mean number of diopters, plus or minus one standard deviation. Numbers in parentheses represent the range of values in diopters.
Abbreviation: SE = spherical equivalent.

1. Distance of incisions from the visual axis. The closer the incisions, the more effect, up to about 2 mm from the center for transverse incisions. We typically use a 6-mm optical zone for transverse incisions and do not go below a 3-mm optical zone for radial incisions.
2. Length of incisions. The longer the incisions, the greater the effect, for the length typically used in combined surgeries (30° to 60° of arc for the transverse component).
3. Depth of incision. There is an increased effect with deeper incisions (80% to 95% depth recommended).
4. Number of incisions. After one pair of transverse incisions, or four radial incisions, additional incisions provide disproportionately less additional result. Hence we never use more than eight radial or four transverse incisions.
5. Patient's age. For a given incision, the older the patient, the greater the effect.

Recent data from the ARC-T group indicate no statistical difference between the results of arcuate and straight transverse incisions in that study population, since both and straight T incisions brought 58% of patients to 1 D or less residual refractive astigmatism.[17] Although others[11] have found up to 30% more effect from arcuate than from straight incisions, in our practice we also have found no significant difference. Again, it may be useful to review one's own cases, looking particularly for a consistent pattern of outcome, and then plan accordingly.

OTHER RELEVANT STUDIES

A number of relevant studies appear in the literature. The study by Neumann and associates[18] seems to answer best the question regarding interrupted T versus interrupted radial incisions. They evaluated three different patterns of combined RK-AK. Two of these patterns were composed of radial incisions with interrupted T incisions and T incisions with interrupted radials. They found that the latter (47 patients) corrected 93.1% of preoperative cylinder, with 89% of patients experiencing less than 20° of postoperative axis deviation compared with preoperative axis. By comparison, the 47 patients with interrupted T incisions had 82.3% of preoperative cylinder corrected, with 77% of them experiencing postoperative axis deviation of less than 20°. Because of the scatter of the data with both techniques, there is probably no statistically significant difference.

As part of a larger study, Agapitos and colleagues[19] studied 20 eyes with idiopathic astigmatism, of which 10 were corrected with transverse incisions between radial incisions and 8 were corrected with radial incisions with interrupted T incisions. All were performed as "simultaneous" combined procedures. Again, the authors found a high degree of variability coupled with poor predictability, but this study did demonstrate that two currently acceptable methods of RK-AK could produce large shifts in corneal astigmatism along with significant shifts of spherical equivalent in the hyperopic direction.

Thornton and Sanders[20] also found, incidental to their other conclusions, that astigmatism correction could effectively be combined with simultaneous myopia correction. They used eight-incision radial keratotomies with one pair of straight T incisions (between the radial incisions) whose lengths were titrated per the Thornton nomogram,

according to the magnitude of result desired. Preoperative idiopathic refractive astigmatism of 1.00 to 2.25 D was reduced to less than 1.00 D at 3-month follow-up examination in 85% of treated eyes. Most results were within 20° of the intended axis.

More recently, Thornton[21] has suggested treating a highly astigmatic patient (eg, plano −4.00 D) with a single pair of *inverse* arcuate incisions in lieu of the more common alternative of concentric arcuate transverse incisions. Such concentric incisions would, of necessity, be combined with RK to treat the 2.00 D of myopia that—because of the coupling effect—would result from standard AK alone. He suggests that the termini of an inverse arcuate incision, having radial as well as transverse components, may obviate the need for separate radial incisions. Using this technique on a patient with initial refraction of plano −2.50 × 100°, his patient's resultant refraction was −0.50 −0.50 × 110, with uncorrected visual acuity of 20/25.

Lipshitz and colleagues[22] reported on their use of straight transverse incisions with interrupted radial incisions (using centrifugal technique) in 32 eyes of 22 patients to correct compound myopic astigmatism. With up to 18 months' follow-up study, the mean residual astigmatism was 0.1 D of cylinder (preoperative mean was 1.6 D cylindric refractive error). The mean preoperative spherical refractive error was −5.25 D (range −2.25 to −9.50), decreasing to a mean postoperative value of 0.60 (range 0.00 to −4.50 in the patient whose preoperative myopia was −9.50 D). Their results support the finding of Neumann and colleagues that correcting compound myopic astigmatism by simultaneous straight transverse and jump-radial incisions is both effective and accurate.

Regarding change over ensuing years, the retrospective study by Salz and coworkers[23] is of note. In that study, of 225 eyes of 135 patients undergoing RK-AK by a single surgeon, 100 eyes were followed for 2 to 10 years and analyzed for stability of result. With a conservative approach to both patient selection and surgical planning, 69% of eyes achieved postoperative uncorrected visual acuity of greater than or equal to 20/40 (100% for preoperative levels of less than or equal to −3.00 D, 47% for −6.00 to −11.60 D preoperatively). Of the 100 eyes followed for 2 years or greater, 77% changed by less than 1.00 D from the result at 1 year, with 17% experiencing a hyperopic shift of greater than or equal to 1.0 D, and 6% regressing by greater than or equal to 1.0 D. This study reinforces the advisability of aiming for undercorrection rather than emmetropia.

Comparable results were later found by Schneider and coauthors,[24] who performed combined RK-AK on 350 eyes (with 93% better than or equal to 20/40 at the last follow-up visit). Their results appeared stable up to 5 years postoperatively in 80% of the cases documented. In the remaining 20%, they noted a tendency toward increasing effect, especially of the transverse incisions.

Another study in support of undercorrection, and therefore freedom to enhance, is that of Werblin and Stafford.[25] They reported considerable success with a relatively conservative approach to combined myopic astigmatism, using the Casebeer system for keratorefractive surgery in 205 consecutive eyes. Their goal was slight residual myopia. Paired transverse T incisions were performed, along with four- or eight-incision RK, as the primary procedures. Enhancements were performed in 33% of the eyes studied, with up to a total of 16 radial incisions (initial surgery plus enhancement) deemed acceptable. All radial incisions were performed centripetally. With 100% follow-up study of patients at 1 year, they found uncorrected visual acuity of 20/40 or better in 99% of patients and of 20/25 or better in 96%.

Reasons for a lack of perfectly predictable outcome in any study, or in any individual patient, include variations in individual surgical technique, the difficulty in repetitively performing manual microsurgery to submicrosurgical tolerances, idiosyncracies of individual patients' wound healing, and, despite remarkable technologic progress in less than a decade, the lack of instrumentation to reproduce reliably precise incisions. Indeed, among the greatest contributors to variability are incision depth, perpendicularity, and length, which may even vary within a single incision. Yet it remains a poor carpenter who blames his tools.

SURGICAL PLAN AND PROCEDURE

Surgical calculations should be based on the cycloplegic refraction and should be verified (but not modified) in accordance with manual keratometry, the latter to be repeated by the surgeon immediately before surgery in patients with high astigmatism, where the precise orientation of AK incision placement is even more critical. It is important to avoid the potentially major error introduced by the cyclotorsional rotation of the globe when the patient is supine. Thus, at this same time, with the patient seated upright at the keratometer or slit lamp, either the vertical or horizontal meridian can be marked with a marking pen or other instrument at the limbus. Other anatomic landmarks (eg, conjunctival vascular frond, pingueculum) can also be precisely localized at this time, to provide intraoperative cues as to ocular orientation.

All data are recorded on a "Planning and Procedure Report" before surgery. After consulting the appropriate nomograms, plan and record on this sheet the number, length and orientation (surgeon's view) of incisions to be used. We currently prefer the Genesis (two-pass) technique (which uses the goal of 0.75 D of residual myopia), and we favor the number of incisions that will provide the desired correction while preserving the largest possible optical zone. Especially for combined RK-AK, the six-incision RK technique, when appropriate, is most attractive. It permits a higher degree of myopic correction than does the four-incision technique, while leaving greater arcs (60° versus 45°) of unoperated cornea than does the eight-incision technique, to be used for AK incision without the necessity of incision interruption, or "jumping."

After routine sedation (5 or 10 mg of diazepam) plus topical anesthesia (lidocaine 4% or proparacaine 1% plus tetracaine 0.5%), the patient is positioned on the operating table. Before prepping and draping of the eye, and with the minimal illumination level of the operating microscope, the surgeon views the patient's eye monocularly and marks the visual axis. This is performed with a blunt visual axis marker or Sinskey hook, while the patient fixates on a spot marked at the center of the microscope's objective lens through which the surgeon is sighting.[26] The 3.0-mm optical zone (OZ) marker is imprinted concentric to the visual axis mark to provide a guide for pachymetry measurements in the major corneal hemimeridians. Using the previously specified anatomic or marking pen landmarks, and with the aid of the Mendez protractor or microscope reticule, the surgeon imprints the AK marker at the axis and OZ appropriate for the astigmatic incision(s).

Real-time pachymetry is performed first for the RK, at the 3.0-mm OZ imprint, in at least the four prime quadrants, as well as at the site(s) of the intended AK incisions. Using these measurements, and with the aid of the calibrating microscope, the surgeon sets the Genesis RK knife for 100% of thinnest stromal depth at the 3.0-mm OZ mark (plus or minus personal bias factor of up to 10 μm). In concert with the Genesis RK blade, we use a double-edged AK blade with a 15° angle for transverse incisions, set at 100% of pachymetry minus 20 μm. For surgeons who use a different RK technique (centripetal or centrifugal alone), it is possible to use one single-edged knife (preferably front-cutting for easier visualization), simply resetting the blade under the microscope for the subsequent incisions.

While the surgeon is calibrating the diamond knives, the surgical assistant preps the patient's eyelids, orbit, and brow with a povidone-iodine 10% swab, placing a small amount directly on the globe as well. The patient is then instructed to rest comfortably with eyes closed, so as to prevent dehydration (and thinning) of the cornea before the surgical procedure starts. A fenestrated plastic drape is positioned, a closed-blade spring speculum is inserted, and an additional round of anesthetic drops is instilled. The patient is instructed to keep the uninvolved eye gently closed to avoid inducing lid spasm and Bell's phenomenon of the operated eye.

If the corneal surface indentations previously used for pachymetry have diminished, the AK impressions can be repeated and the OZ marker of correct diameter for the myopic correction imprinted. Using the appropriate RK incision marker, these imprints should then be added with precision, since the radial marks should either flank the astigmatic marks (for a four- or six-incision RK) or bisect them (for an eight-incision RK with interrupted "jump" incisions).

While making the AK incisions, we fixate the globe gently with Bores forceps to prevent torsional or saccadic movement. During RK incisions, only a cellulose surgical sponge (Weck-cel) is necessary for fixation; this will substantially diminish patients' postoperative discomfort and eliminate subconjunctival hemorrhage from forceps fixation. Care is taken not to apply pressure to the globe, since increased intraocular pressure (IOP) may lead to spreading of the incisions, deeper incisions, or perforations. The corneal surface must remain dry during surgery, and such dehydration may induce thinning. The thinnest quadrant (usually the inferotemporal) is therefore incised first, since it is the most likely site for a perforation to occur. Note that in accordance with standard Genesis technique, only one blade depth is permitted for all RK incisions and no peripheral deepening is required. However, and as is common, should the pachymetry of the AK incision sites vary by more than 20 μm, the blade length is adjusted accordingly.

Should a corneal microperforation occur in the course of an RK incision, it is almost invariably at the central extent of the incision where the cornea is thinnest; it should be managed in accordance with the extent of aqueous leakage. Usually, minute punctures are self-sealing and require neither interruption of the case nor suture closure. Microperforation occurring while performing an AK incision is potentially more significant. The stromal thickness along the course of an astigmatic incision, especially an arcuate one, is relatively uniform. Thus the extent of anterior-chamber (AC) entry may be more lengthy, and more serious AC shallowing might develop. Furthermore, the possibility of postoperative wound gape or override (and attendant overcorrection) is somewhat likely, especially for longer-arc-length incisions. Hence it is sometimes necessary to use one or two interrupted sutures of 10-0 nylon intraoperatively to stabilize an AK-related corneal perforation.

POSTOPERATIVE CARE

Immediately postoperatively, instill both topical antibiotic and steroid drops (a combination drop can be both convenient and cost-effective). A nonsteroidal anti-inflammatory drop may be of benefit for pain prophylaxis. No eye patch is applied except if there is a significant epithelial defect, and neither eye patch, soft contact lens, nor collagen shield is appropriate for microperforations. Patients then immediately commence application of combined antibiotic-steroid drops four times daily. Patients rarely require any additional pain medications other than acetaminophen or aspirin. Patients should be instructed to continue abstinence from eye make-up for 1 week, to avoid particularly dusty environments and potentially contaminated water (pond, pool, hot tub) for 1 week, and to refrain from reading the night of surgery.

Patients are examined on the first postoperative day, at which time uncorrected visual acuity, wound depth and integrity (with Seidel test), and tactile IOP are assessed. Reaffirm the limited restrictions, and remind patients to use protective eyewear for sports. Antibiotic and steroid drops are continued. Patients next return in 1 to 2 weeks for reexamination plus refraction. At this time, a cycloplegic refraction, performed late in the day, can be the best approximation of final outcome. Patients then return in 4 to 6 weeks, at which time either the satisfactory visual outcome or the potential need for enhancement can usually be ascertained.

We have devised a rapid pictorial method for demonstrating the magnitude of the patient's residual refractive error and comparing it to the preoperative refractive error. This involves a circular, clear plastic template with orthogonal slits for tracing, marked with a measuring grid, and stamped with protractor-type degree measurements around the perimeter (Fig 46–3). Using this, the principal meridians are easily marked, as is the magnitude of refractive error along them. In essence, this represents a cross section through the conoid of Sturm. Although such a cross section would in actuality form an ellipse, a simple but adequate approximation can be achieved by connecting with straight lines the terminus of one principal meridian to the terminus of the next (Fig 46–4). This technique facilitates the patient's as well as the surgeons's ability to quantify the amount of correction achieved versus the amount of residual refractive error and helps the patient to participate in an active and informed manner in decisions regarding the need for enhancements.

ENHANCEMENTS

If the cycloplegic refraction 2 weeks postoperatively demonstrates more than 0.50 D of residual myopia, continue steroid drops to slow wound healing and prescribe intermittent compression of the globe four times a day, using gentle pressure from the "heel" (base of the palm) of the hand or from the fingertip. Alternatively, pressure patching at night might also compress the central cornea and thereby augment the desired flattening. Any or all of these measures are continued for up to 6 weeks after surgery, at which time the uncorrected visual acuity and cycloplegic refraction are rechecked and an enhancement performed if indicated.

Remember that surgical enhancement should be attempted only if the patient is unhappy with the result, rather than for any arbitrary residual refractive error. If indicated, it would be based on biomicroscopic examination of incision depth, length, and regularity

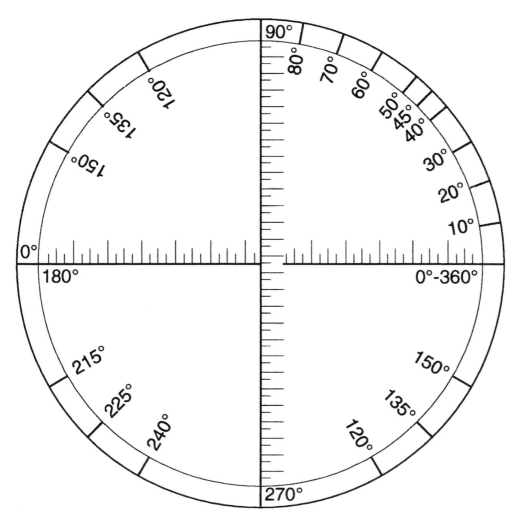

Figure 46–3. Template for pictorial representation of refractive error.

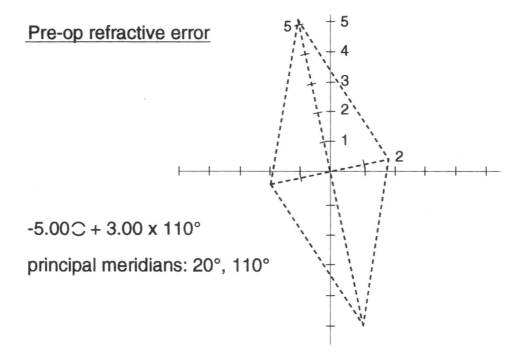

Pre-op refractive error

-5.00○ + 3.00 x 110°

principal meridians: 20°, 110°

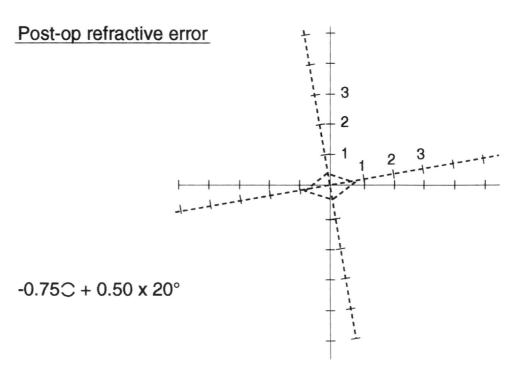

Post-op refractive error

-0.75○ + 0.50 x 20°

Figure 46–4. Pictorial representation of refractive error: preoperative and postoperative comparison.

and carried out in the manner prescribed for enhancing RK or AK alone. In brief, after the axis of the residual astigmatism is identified in the manner previously detailed, the existing incisions are opened with a Sinskey hook and are deepened or extended as is appropriate to the magnitude of refractive error and axis of astigmatism. It is almost never appropriate to perform enhancement more than twice, since it may increase the risk of destabilizing the cornea.

COMPLICATIONS

As with RK or AK individually, unacceptable refractive errors comprise the most frequent problems in a com-

bination procedure. Enhancements for undercorrection have been reviewed above. For overcorrections, our best results have been obtained using one or more 10-0 nylon interrupted compression sutures placed perpendicular to the wound at the 6-mm OZ, under light tension. We have found sutures of 10-0 Prolene or Mersilene to be less effective than nylon for this purpose, since the former tend to erode, expose, and irritate and require premature removal. Another example of compression sutures used to repair an AK overcorrection, with simultaneous placement of RK incisions (all as a second-stage procedure), is shown in Figure 46–5.

A problem can occur from the intersection of incisions, which may lead to wound gape, increased glare, recurrent epithelial erosion, microbial keratitis, and de-

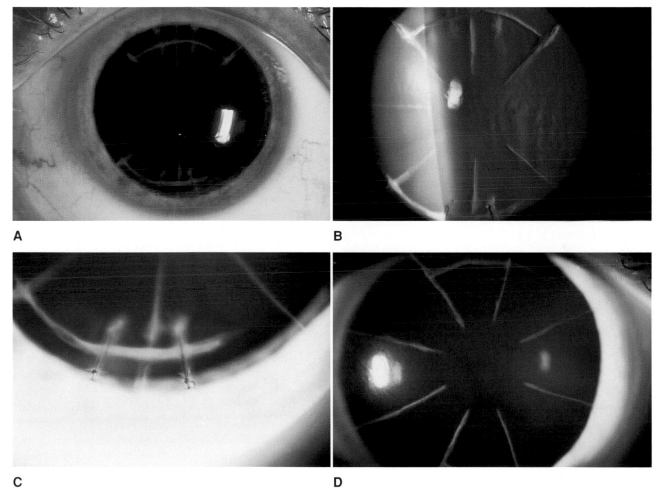

A **B** **C** **D**

Figure 46–5. A 45-year-old patient with refractive error −7.00 −4.50 × 180 in each eye. **A** to **C.** In the left eye, two 90° AK incisions were performed at axis 70° and 270° with a resultant refractive error of −10.25 −0.50 × 90. One month later, an eight-incision RK with a 3.0-mm OZ was performed because the radial incisions "jumped" the previous AK incisions, which resulted in a marked astigmatic overcorrection (−0.75 −6.0 × 90). Four weeks later, two compression sutures of 10-0 nylon were inserted in each of the AK incisions and the refractive error stabilized at −2.00 −1.50 × 180 for 1 year. In the right eye, an eight-incision RK at the 3.0-mm OZ with a refraction of +0.50 −4.50 × 190 at 3 months postoperatively. **D.** AK with 60° arcuate incision at 90° that jumped the 1 o'clock RK incision and a 45° arcuate incision at axis 270° that did not intersect the 5 or 7 o'clock RK incisions. The postoperative refraction remained stable for 6 months at −1.25 −0.75 × 45°.

creased predictability of the refractive result. For this reason, one must be particularly careful to avoid intersecting either fresh or prior incisions when performing either simultaneous or staged RK-AK procedures. Because incisions previously placed may, as the wound heals, become less visible, the risk of inadvertent intersection can actually increase. Such intersections are readily managed by a single 10-0 nylon suture.

Despite the theoretical risks of additional surgery, including the possibilities of inadvertently intersecting incisions, the ARC-T group found few such complications. In the 94 eyes that had received astigmatic correction alone as a first stage, and then either RK alone (75 eyes) or simultaneous RK and AK enhancement (19 eyes) as a second-stage procedure, there were 14 complications, specifically 1 case of conjunctivitis, 11 eyes with wound gape, and 2 with wound gape requiring resuturing. Because AK wound gape occurred primarily with 90° arc incisions, as stated previously, we therefore currently do not create arcs greater than 60°. Although overcorrection and undercorrection remain common, AK combined with RK was demonstrated to be a safe procedure whose "complications are outweighed by significant functional improvement in most eyes."[10]

Microperforations, as indicated previously, are almost invariably self-sealing and require no particular treatment. If persistent at the 24-hour postoperative check, we either decrease or discontinue topical steroids to facilitate wound healing while continuing antibiotics. We attempt to avoid this difficulty by working on a dry field, so that an aqueous leak is immediately appreciated and reliably managed. As with any ocular surgery, the possibility for additional complications (including iridocyclitis, microbial keratitis, and endophthalmitis) exists but is exceedingly and increasingly rare.

SUMMARY AND FUTURE DIRECTIONS

To improve predictability of either simultaneous or sequential RK and AK, surgeons require better control over the known nondemographic variables affecting outcome, including stromal wound healing, corneal surface topography, and ocular rigidity. Finite-element modeling and computer simulation[27] may hold great promise for increasing predictability by elucidating the multivariate stress relationships within the cornea. Meanwhile, prospective studies remain to be done to determine differences in outcome between the various patterns of combined RK-AK, as well as long-term

studies to determine any significant differences for staged versus simultaneous procedures. Because there is not yet a single "universal" standard protocol or nomogram, every surgeon must critically evaluate and decide on a strategy that can with practical experience be critically reassessed and modified to suit the individual variations of both patient and surgeon. Despite the inevitable questions to be answered and problems to be solved in this decade of rapid advancement in incisional refractive surgical techniques, the combination of RK and AK has taken the correction of refractive errors truly "a cut above" that of RK alone.

REFERENCES

1. Holliday JT, Waring GO. Optics and topography of radial keratotomy. In Waring GO, ed. *Refractive Keratotomy for Myopia and Astigmatism*. St. Louis: Mosby-Year Book; 1992:136.
2. Rapoza PA, Kenyon KR, Assil KK. Myopia Astigmatism. In: Roy FH, ed. *Master Techniques in Ophthalmic Surgery*. Baltimore: Williams & Wilkins; 1995:983–993.
3. Lans LJ. Experimentelle Untersuchungen über Entstehung von Astigmatismus durch nicht-perforirend Corneawunden. *Arch Ophthalmol.* 1898;45:117–152.
4. Thornton SP. Astigmatic keratotomy: a review of basic concepts with case reports. *J Cataract Refract Surg.* 1990;16: 430–435.
5. Lundergan MK, Rowsey JJ. Relaxing incisions. Corneal topography. *Ophthalmology.* 1985;92:1222–1236.
6. Hoffmann RF. The surgical correction of idiopathic astigmatism. In Sanders DR, Hoffmann RF, Salz JJ, eds. *Refractive Corneal Surgery.* Thorofare, NJ: Slack; 1986:241–290.
7. Lavery GW, Lindstrom RL. Clinical results of trapezoidal astigmatic keratotomy. *J Refract Surg.* 1985;1:70–74.
8. Tchah H, Hoffmann R, Duffey R, Vivanti J, Lindstrom R. Delimited peripheral arcuate keratotomy for astigmatism: "bowtie configuration". *J Refract Surg.* 1988;5: 183–190.
9. Price FW, Grene RB, Marks RG, et al. Astigmatism reduction clinical trial: A multi-center prospective evaluation of the predictability of arcuate keratotomy: evaluation of surgical nomogram predictability. *Arch Ophthalmol.* 1995; 113:277–282.
10. Grene R, Kenyon K, Durrie D, et al. Astigmatism reduction clinical trial (ARC-T): The ARC-T study, A multi-center prospective evaluation of the surgical results of arcuate keratotomy for the reduction of astigmatism. Submitted.
11. Friedlander MH. Presented at "Radial and Astigmatic Keratotomy: A Practical Course," Boston, MA: The Massachusetts Eye and Ear Infirmary, 1994.

12. Price FW, Grene RB, Marks, RG, et al. Arcuate transverse keratotomy for astigmatism followed by subsequent radial or transverse keratotomy. *J. Refract Surg.* 1996:68–76.

13. Ibrahim O, Hussein H, El-Sahn M, El-Nawawy S, Kassem A, Waring G. Trapezoidal keratotomy for the correction of naturally occurring astigmatism. *Arch Ophthalmol.* 1991; 109:1374–1381.

14. Lindstrom RL. The surgical correction of astigmatism: a clinician's perspective. *Refract Corneal Surg.* 1990;6: 441–454.

15. Waring GO, Lynn MJ, Nizam A, et al. Results of the prospective evaluation of radial keratotomy (PERK) study five years after surgery. *Ophthalmology.* 1991;98:1164–1176.

16. Lynn MJ, Waring III GO, Sperduto RD, and the PERK study group. Factors affecting the outcome and predictability of radial keratotomy in the PERK study. *Arch Ophthalmol.* 1987;105:42–51.

17. Grene RB. ARC-T vs. STRAIGHT-T: A Clinical Comparison. ASICO Newsletter, 1994.

18. Neumann AC, McCarty GR, Sanders DR, Raanan MG. Refractive evaluation of astigmatic keratotomy procedures. *J Cataract Refract Surg.* 1989;15:25–31.

19. Agapitos PJ, Lindstrom RL, Williams PA, Sanders DR. Analysis of astigmatic keratotomy. *J Cataract Refract Surg.* 1989;15:13–18.

20. Thornton SP, Sanders DR. Graded non-intersecting transverse incisions for correction of idiopathic astigmatism. *J Cataract Refract Surg.* 1987;13:27–31.

21. Thornton SP. Inverse arcuate incision: a new approach to the correction of astigmatism. *Refract Corneal Surg.* 1994; 10:27–30.

22. Lipshitz I, Mayron Y, Loewenstein A. Combined transverse and interrupted radial keratotomy for compound myopic astigmatism. *Refract Corneal Surg.* 1992;8:280–285.

23. Salz JJ, Salz JM, Salz M, Jones D. Ten years' experience with a conservative approach to radial keratotomy. *Refract Corneal Surg.* 1991;7:12–22.

24. Schneider DM, Draghic T, Murphy RK. Combined myopia and astigmatism surgery. A review of 350 cases. *J Cataract Refract Surg.* 1992;18:370–374.

25. Werblin TP, Stafford GM. The Casebeer system for predictable keratorefractive surgery: one-year evaluation of 205 consecutive cases. *Ophthalmology.* 1993;100:1095–1102.

26. Uozato H, Guyton DL. Centering corneal surgical procedures. *Am J Ophthalmol.* 1987;103:264–275.

27. Pinsky PM, Datye D-V. Numerical modeling of radial, astigmatic, and hexagonal keratotomy. *Refract Corneal Surg.* 1992;8:164–172.

SECTION IX

Contact Lenses

CHAPTER 47

Orthokeratology

Joseph Pasternak

It has long been known that the use of contact lenses can induce corneal topographic changes and cause dramatic visual changes after lens removal.[1] The most commonly recognized change is "spectacle blur"—a transient myopic shift induced by epithelial edema.[2] Many studies suggest that corneal topographic changes induced by lens wear are variable and unpredictable,[3-16] while others indicate that the base curve of the contact lens fitted correlates with the corneal topographic change induced.[17] Recent computer-assisted topography studies demonstrate that although rigid and soft lenses can induce variable amounts of topographic change,[18] both flattening and steepening the cornea, a correlation between the resting position of the lens and the change induced does exist[19] (Fig 47-1).

For more than 30 years, some contact lens practitioners have attempted to put this information to use, believing that contact lenses can purposely flatten the cornea to modify the eye's refractive state. The field of orthokeratology, "the reduction or elimination of refractive anomalies through programmed applications of contact lenses,"[20] was introduced to the United States by Grant and May in 1963.[21] By 1987, over 100,000 orthokeratology procedures had been performed in North America.[22]

Orthokeratology has gained in popularity as patient awareness and the desire to eliminate glasses or contact lenses has increased. Advocates contend that the use of rigid contact lenses to change the curvature of the cornea is safe—much less invasive than refractive surgical procedures—and that myopia and astigmatism can be substantially reduced. Opponents argue that this technique is unpredictable and that the time and expense involved are disproportionate to the rare and unpredictable freedom from optical devices that is achieved.

PROCEDURES

The initial description of Grant and May's orthokeratology technique[23] involved fitting a rigid PMMA lens 0.37 diopters (D) flatter than the patient's flattest corneal meridian, with emphasis on the center thickness of the lens. Treatments were done in two stages: the adaptive phase and the retainer phase. The lenses were worn 12 to 15 hours daily, and patients were followed at regular intervals. As the cornea flattened, new lenses were applied, again 0.37 D flatter than the flattest meridian. An average of 3½ pairs of lenses were prescribed over the first year, and an additional 2½ pairs of lenses over the second year. After an average period of 18 to 24 months, the orthokeratologists would determine that the second phase—the "retainer lens" phase—had been reached

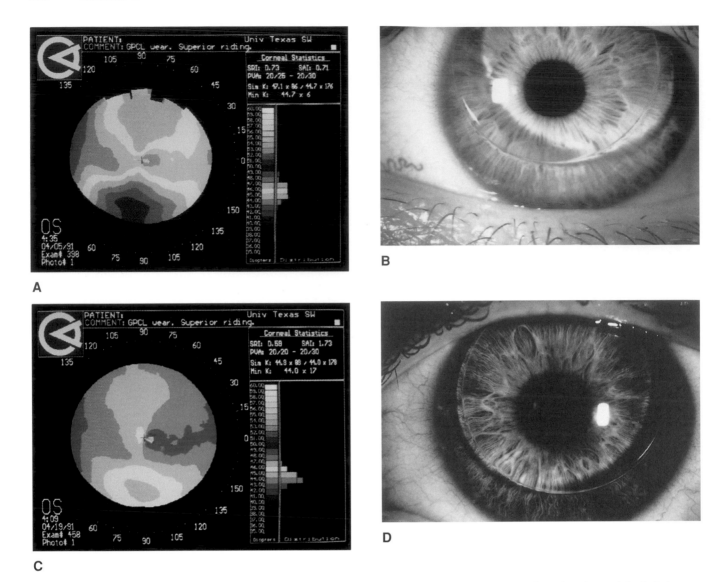

Figure 47–1. A. Cornea that wore a superior-riding rigid gas-permeable contact lens that had central irregular astigmatism and the typical pattern of relative flattening beneath the decentered contact lens and relative steepening inferiorly outside of the resting position of the lens. The topographic pattern simulates early keratoconus. **B.** Superior resting position of the gas-permeable contact lens worn on the cornea in **A. C.** Cornea that wore a superior-riding rigid gas-permeable contact lens that had central irregular astigmatism and the typical pattern of relative flattening beneath the decentered contact lens and relative steepening inferiorly outside of the resting position of the lens. The topographic pattern simulates early keratoconus. **D.** Superior resting position of the gas-permeable contact lens worn on the cornea in **C.** *(From Ruiz-Montenegro, et al. Ophthalmology. 1993;100:130. With permission.)*

when unaided vision reached 20/20, or refraction stabilized to plano ± 0.50 D. Hyperopic eyes could be treated in a similar fashion, but the contact lens was made to fit more steeply than the steepest corneal meridian.

A number of orthokeratology techniques have been published,[20,22,24–29] and all involve fitting a series of loose, flat lenses with larger diameters, flatter base curves, and deeper sagital depths for a given corneal base curve than a standard cosmetic contact lens. Lenses are fit from 0.5 to 2.75 D flatter than the flattest

corneal meridian,[27] and peripheral curvature and edge contour are modified.[30,31] In all cases, the power of the lens is modified to compensate for the base curve changes and to yield the best corrected visual acuity. The adaptive phase, during which the corneal curvature is in a state of flux, can last from 2 months[26] to 3 years,[22] with an average of 18 months. The number of lens changes required during the adaptive phase varies in different series from 2 to 11.[22,25,27] When a stable corneal curvature and refractive error have been reached, the retainer lens stage begins.

PREDICTABILITY OF REFRACTIVE CORRECTIONS

Orthokeratologists claim that their success rate is high and that patients of all ages can experience a lessening of myopia, hyperopia, and astigmatism.[26,31] The optometric literature abounds with claims of success, but the majority of reports are uncontrolled and anecdotal. Very few scientific studies have been performed and reported in the medical literature. In 1980, Binder[27] undertook to evaluate the orthokeratology procedure as performed by Grant and May, experts in the field who introduced the procedure, which they helped popularize. In their study of 20 orthokeratology patients, the majority of refractive changes took place in the first 9 months, and the majority of corneas reached their best level of uncorrected vision between 11 and 18 months. The patients with initial refractive errors of more than 2.5 D had an average 1.52 D reduction in myopia and improved sixfold (five lines) in uncorrected vision. Patients with less than 2.5 D of myopia had a mean decrease of 0.38 D of myopia, and a threefold (five lines) improvement in uncorrected visual acuity. Twenty-five percent (5/20) had no response. Disconcertingly, 7 of 25 eyes in the greater-than-2.50 D group experienced an increase in myopia during the study, and sudden changes in visual acuity and refractive error occurred while the patients were wearing the same lens.

Polse[25] evaluated two randomized groups in the more recent Berkeley Orthokeratology Study, a randomized, controlled clinical trial. Eyes were treated for an average of 14 months, and 36% of the orthokeratology treatment group experienced greater than 1.0 D of reduction in myopia at the end of the treatment period, compared with 12% of those eyes fitted with cosmetic contact lenses. This corresponded with an improvement in uncorrected visual acuity of 0.3 logmar (an improvement from 20/100 to 20/50) in 36.6% of the treatment group compared with 20.8% of cosmetic lens wearers who improved the same amount. Thirteen percent (4/30) of treated patients had more than 2.0 D reduction in myopia (Table 47–1).

REFRACTIVE FLUCTUATION

In Binder's study, the average uncorrected visual acuity was 20/120 before treatment, which improved to a mean of 20/40 throughout the 24 months of the study. However, there was great deal of variability as to when the best uncorrected vision was achieved. Not only did the best vision vary on a month-to-month basis, but there was no predictability as to how long after lens removal the best vision would be experienced. Some patients experienced their best vision immediately after lens removal, others experienced it on awakening, and still others experienced it up to 12 to 24 hours later. Patients with a refractive error less than 4.00 D had a 50% probability of achieving 20/25 uncorrected visual acuity and a 70% probability of 20/40 at some time during the study period, but not necessarily at the end of the study, nor at any predictable time after lens removal. Binder concluded that orthokeratology responses were uncontrollable, unpredictable, and unstable. Even as practiced by experts, the chance of obtaining 20/40 uncorrected visual acuity through orthokeratology was small.

STABILITY AND TREATMENT PERMANENCE

Several orthokeratology studies showed that corneal curvature fluctuated throughout the study periods and could not demonstrate any predictability, stability, or permanence of treatment effect.[25,27,32] The lack of persistence of effect has remained a controversial area in orthokeratology treatment regimens. Early orthokeratologists felt that their treatment effects would be permanent, but they promptly observed that the cornea demonstrated memory and elasticity, and corneal molding tended to regress after discontinuation of con-

TABLE 47–1. MEAN CHANGE IN REFRACTIVE ERROR DURING ORTHOKERATOLOGIC INTERVENTION

		Mean Initial Refractive Error (D)	Mean Change in Refractive Error (D)	Statistical Significance
Binder (1983)	Treatment Groups	>2.50 (−3.25 ± 1.02)	1.52	$P < .01$
		<2.50 (−1.87 + 0.40)	0.38	$.1 < P < .2$
Polse (1980)	Treatment Group	—	0.97	$P < .01$
	Control Group	—	0.49	$P < .01$
Kerns (1976)	Treatment Group	—	0.87	
	Control Group	—	—	

tact lens wear. A cornea will return to its initial topographic configuration from 3 to 8 weeks after lens removal.[21] Some corneal topographic changes induced by contact lenses have been shown to be present for years,[6,10,33] but the majority of evidence supports the tendency of the cornea to return to its original topography. Although this tissue property is advantageous for reversal of unwanted contact lens–induced changes, in orthokeratology it harkens the return of myopia and the loss of many months of programmed corneal shaping.

Kerns[32] undertook one of the earliest orthokeratology studies in which 26 cosmetic contact lens and 36 orthokeratology patients were fit and followed for 1000 days. The orthokeratology group had an average of 0.87 D reduction of myopia. After this period, lens use was discontinued, and within 100 days there was a complete regression of effect and return to prefit levels of refractive error. Binder's[27] group discontinued contact lens wear after reaching a stable period—the "retainer lens" stage—or after 18 to 24 months, whichever came first. In 75% of patients who reached retainer lens stage, uncorrected visual acuity immediately deteriorated toward prefit levels. In all patients, horizontal and vertical corneal meridians returned toward their prefit topography. Only 3 of 75 patients retained a greater than 0.7 D reduction in myopia after 3 months.

There is general agreement that the cornea has a strong tendency to return to its original topography, and the concept of retainer lenses is an integral part of orthokeratology. Analogous to retainer wear in orthodontics, the retainer lens is worn after the desired endpoint has been reached to maintain the permanence of the effect. There is much disagreement among orthokeratologists about the appropriate lens to use as a retainer and how often the retainer should be worn. Recommendations vary for modifying the base curve of the last adaptive orthokeratology lens, and wear time can vary from a few hours a day to not at all.[28,34,35] Some reports indicate that patients can go months to years without loss of effect.[22] One technique even advocates the use of a nighttime retainer cellulose acetyl butyrate (CAB) lens.[36]

MECHANISMS OF CORNEAL SHAPING

Several physiologic explanations for the effect of contact lenses on corneal topography have been proffered. Most orthokeratology lenses are designed to be larger, thicker, and flatter than cosmetic lenses, suggesting that mechanical pressure of the lens on the cornea modifies corneal curvature.[37] However, topographic changes have been noted after use of cosmetic lenses, including soft lenses,[17–19] suggesting other factors may also play a role. The action of the eyelids may convey a transfer of pressure through the lens and massage the corneal contour into the conformation of the lens. Others have suggested that tear volume underneath the contact lens creates a hydraulic pressure gradient against the cornea, exerting a dynamic force very dependent on lens positioning.[38] This mechanism could account for the observation of correlation between lens position and induced topographic changes.

Metabolic effects such as low transmissibility of oxygen through PMMA lenses may be variables in the orthokeratologic effect. Ocular rigidity has also been postulated as a factor in the variability of treatment results.[39] Patients with low ocular rigidity have been reported to have greater amounts of induced corneal astigmatism, but the imprecision in measuring ocular rigidity calls any correlation into question.[40]

The curvature of the peripheral cornea may significantly affect the potential for orthokeratologic corneal remodeling. Early orthokeratologists made use of a nine-ring photoelectric keratoscope (PEK) that could evaluate 42% of the corneal surface. By assessing the curvature of the mid-peripheral cornea, orthokeratolo-

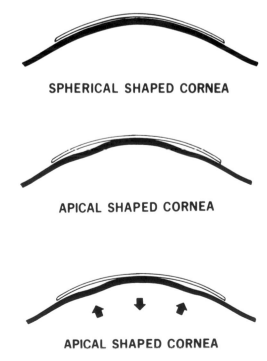

SPHERICAL SHAPED CORNEA

APICAL SHAPED CORNEA

APICAL SHAPED CORNEA

Figure 47–2. Curvature of cornea.

gists attempted to estimate the potential for refractive error modification. They observed that some corneas were not spherical but had a paracentral invagination. Application of a contact lens not only flattened the central cornea but also induced a peripheral corneal steepening, making an aspheric eye more spherical. These aspheric eyes were seen to have a greater treatment effect[32] (Fig 47–2).

LIMITATIONS AND ADVERSE EFFECTS

A major limitation of orthokeratology is the inability to predict the refractive outcome in myopia during the study period.[27] This poor predictability necessitates frequent and continued monitoring and repeated evaluation. Significant adverse effects of orthokeratology are uncommon, and contact lens complications such as infection, ulceration, and inducement of astigmatism compare with cosmetic rigid contact lens use.[33] Nonetheless, orthokeratology has not seen a widespread practice in the ophthalmologic community. The lack of predictability of induced myopic reduction, the variability and transience of the efficacy, and the length of time and expense involved in achieving the potential benefits have led many to dismiss orthokeratology as being of little clinical value. For many patients who do experience an improvement in unaided vision, the quality of vision has been described as less than that with their refractive correction. For the same given level of visual acuity, they described their vision as irregular and variable, like "looking through a fishbowl" or "looking through a dirty windshield".[27]

CONTACT LENSES AFTER KERATOREFRACTIVE SURGERY

The relatively large number of patients who are undercorrected or overcorrected after radial keratotomy (RK) necessitates a sound approach to contact lens fitting in these individuals. Unfortunately, very little information is available on the potential effects of contact lens–induced corneal topographic changes in eyes that have undergone RK.

The usual ametropic cornea being fit with a contact lens is aspheric—most steep centrally, with gradual flattening toward the periphery.[41] Accordingly, most contact lens fitting sets are designed with curvatures that gradually flatten toward the edges. In contrast, post-RK eyes have a central plateau shape and steepen from the center toward the periphery, often with a midperipheral "knee." The difference in central and mid-peripheral corneal power can reach up to 5 D.[42] Lenses fit to match the central corneal topography will be quite flat and will tend to be unstable due to bridging over the mid-peripheral knee, with potential for movement, rocking, decentration, and variable vision.

Many skilled practitioners have described methods for fitting lenses on eyes that have undergone RK, a task that is very challenging. Some advocate fitting soft lenses, which give better comfort and centration and are easier to adapt to a potentially irregularly shaped cornea.[43,44] However, both daily and extended wear soft contact lenses have been associated with the rapid development of superficial neovascularization along keratotomy incisions, as well as inclusion cysts, deposits of debris, and focal thickening of Descemet's membrane.[45] Most experts agree that gas-permeable lens material is the lens of choice after RK,[42,46–48] with a large diameter to allow good tear flow and base curves to match the mid-peripheral contour to avoid rocking and decrease undue pressure on the periphery.

El Hage[48] advocated the use of a rigid gas-permeable lens to reform the cornea with a special design using a flat central curve and steep peripheral curvatures to apply pressure to the mid-periphery. Theoretically this lens could alter the mid-peripheral contour to induce a myopic shift and neutralize excessive hyperopia. Astin[38] examined changes in corneal curvature resulting from the use of regularly fit contact lenses in patients who had undergone RK. The lenses were fit to allow good tear flow and provide good lens movement, and the eyes were all at least 1 year out from surgery and felt to be stabilized. Corneal pachymetry, keratometry, and refraction were evaluated before and after varying periods of hard and soft contact lens wear in different individuals. Although pachymetry remained stable, myopia and astigmatism tended to decrease after lens wear and central corneal curvature flattened. Individual variability was high, but changes tended to be greater in those patients wearing soft lenses, particularly soft lenses with low water content and high center thickness.

Diurnal variation in refraction and corneal curvature is seen in many RK patients, even years after surgery.[49] Vision is clearest in the morning after lid pressure during sleep induces corneal flattening. As the cornea deturgesces throughout the day, refraction progresses toward myopia. The adjunctive use of afternoon contact lens wear for a number of hours after unaided vision in the morning could potentially counteract the diurnal myopic shift and improve unaided vision during the evening.[38]

Contact lens wear after RK causes an increased risk of irregular astigmatism, neovascularization, epithelial erosions, and potential for infection; however, with proper handling techniques and correct fitting, some post-RK patients might gain the additional benefit of contact lens–induced myopia reduction.

SUMMARY

Orthokeratology is defined as the programmed application of contact lenses to reduce or eliminate refractive anomalies, primarily myopia. Many different techniques of orthokeratology have been described, all consisting of two phases of therapy: an adaptive phase and a retainer lens phase. An orthokeratology lens tends to be fit flatter, looser, and larger than a conventional lens and mechanically alters the central corneal contour over time. The corneal flattening effect induced by an orthokeratology lens will tend to regress unless a retainer contact lens is used to maintain the effect. Many anecdotal reports laud the potential myopia-reducing benefits of orthokeratology, but controlled scientific studies are limited, and all demonstrate a high degree of variability, instability, and lack of predictability of the orthokeratology technique. It appears that 1 D of myopia is the maximum reduction achievable with any degree of predictability. Orthokeratology proponents contend that initial corneal responses can be used to predict and maximize outcomes and that treatment goals are aimed at decreasing dependence on optical aids.

No scientific studies are available to support the claims that newer modifications of orthokeratology techniques are viable alternatives to keratorefractive surgery. Judicial patient selection and careful contact lens fitting in patients who have undergone keratorefractive surgery may afford a potentially beneficial adjunct in limiting visual fluctuation.

REFERENCES

1. Woo GC, Wilson MA. Current methods of treating and preventing myopia. *Optom Vision Sci.* 1990;679:719–727.
2. Tredici T. Orthokeratology—help or hindrance. *Trans Am Acad Ophthalmol Otolaryngol.* 1974;78:425.
3. Pratt-Johnson JA, Warner DM. Contact lenses and corneal curvature changes. *Am J Ophthalmol.* 1965;60:852–855.
4. Morrison RJ, Kaufman KJ, Cerulli E. Effect of contact lenses on the cornea after various periods of wear. *Am J Optom.* 1967;41:688–690.
5. Sarver MD, Harris MG. Corneal lenses and "spectacle blur." *Am J Optom.* 1967;44:502–504.
6. Hartstein J. Corneal warping due to wearing of corneal contact lenses. *Am J Ophthalmol.* 1965;60:1103–1104.
7. Mobilia EF, Kenyon KR. Contact lens induced corneal warpage. *Int Ophthalmol Clin.* 1986;26:43–53.
8. Miller D. Contact lens induced corneal curvature and thickness changes. *Arch Ophthalmol.* 1968;80:430–432.
9. Riegstorff RH. Corneal curvature and astigmatic changes subsequent to contact lens wear. *J Am Optom Assoc.* 1965; 36:996–1000.
10. Rubin ML. The tale of the warped cornea: a real life melodrama. *Arch Ophthalmol.* 1967;77:711–712. Letter.
11. Levenson DS. Changes in corneal curvature with long term PMMA contact lens wear. *CLAO J.* 1983;9:121–125.
12. Levenson DS, Berry CV. Findings on follow-up of corneal warpage patients. *CLAO J.* 1983;9:126–129.
13. Hovding G. Variations of central corneal curvature during the first year of contact lens wear. *Acta Ophthalmol.* 1983; 61:17–28.
14. Koetting RA, Castellano CF, Keating MJ. PMMA lenses worn for twenty years. *J Am Optom Assoc.* 1986;57: 459–461.
15. Rengstorff RH. The relationship between contact lens base curve and corneal curvature. *J Am Optom Assoc.* 1973; 44:291–293.
16. Hill JF, Rengstorff RH. Relationship between steeply fitted contact lens base curve and corneal curvature changes. *Am J Optom Physiol Opt.* 1974;51:340–342.
17. Bailey H, Carney LG. A survey of corneal changes from corneal lens wear. *Contact Lens J.* 1977;6:3–13.
18. Wilson TE, Lin DTC, Klyce SD, Reidy JJ, Insler MS. Topographic changes in contact lens–induced corneal warpage. *Ophthalmology.* 1990;97:734–744.
19. Ruiz-Montenegro J, Mafra CH, Wilson SE, Jumper JM, Klyce SD, Mendelson EN. Corneal topographic alterations in normal contact lens wearers. *Ophthalmology.* 1993;100: 128–134.
20. Tredici T. Role of orthokeratology: a perspective. *Ophthalmology.* 1979;86:698–705.
21. Grant SC, May CH. Orthokeratology—control of refractive errors through contact lenses. *J Am Opt Assoc.* 1971; 42:1277–1283.
22. King P. Orthokeratology: seeing is believing. *Sci Technol Dimen.* 1987;1:21–*Orthokeratology, a Synopsis of Techniques.* San Diego: International Society of Orthokeratology; 1972.
23. May CH, Grant SC, Norlan J. *Orthokeratogy, a Synopsis of Techniques.* San Diego: International Society of Orthokeratology; 1972.
24. Ziff SL. Orthokeratology. *J Am Optom Assoc.* 1971;42: 231–234.

25. Polse KA. Corneal changes accompanying orthokeratology. *Arch Ophthalmol.* 1984;101:1873–1878.
26. Paige N, Mustaler KL. Orthokeratology: a retrospective study. *Contact Lens Spect.* 1986;1:24–28.
27. Binder P, May CH, Grant SC. An evaluation of orthokeratology. *Ophthalmology.* 1980;87:729–744.
28. Heikkela THC. Orthokeratology: the case analysis concept. *J Orthokeratol.* 1976;2:29–39.
29. Bier N, Lowther GE. Myopia control study: effect of different contact lens refractive corrections on progression of myopia. *AOA Proc.* 1985.
30. Wygloda RJ. Personal communication, 1994.
31. Buffington RD, Lilley JY. A predictable approach to orthokeratology. *Contact Lens Spect.* 1986;1:24–28.
32. Kerns RL. Research in orthokeratology. *J Am Optom Assoc.* 1977;48:345–359.
33. Hartstein JH. Keratoconus that developed in patients wearing corneal contact lenses. *Am J Ophthalmol.* 1968;60:1103–1105.
34. Kirscher DW. Orthokeratology: reduction of refractive error with contact lenses. *J Orthokeratol.* 1976;2:47.
35. Grant SC, May CH. Effects of corneal change on the visual system. *Contacto.* 1972;16:65–69.
36. Nolan JA. Night retainers. *Optom Weekly.* 1977;68:42–44.
37. Watkins JR. The one commonality among various fitting techniques that make orthokeratology work. *Contacto.* 1977;21:26–31.
38. Astin CLK. Kerotoreformation by contact lenses after radial keratotomy. *Ophthal Physiol Opt.* 1991;11:156–162.
39. Hartstein J, Becker B. Research into the pathogenesis of keratoconus. *Arch Ophthalmol.* 1970;84:728–729.
40. Friedman DM. Ocular rigidity and corneal astigmatism; are they related? *Rev Optom.* 1978;115:65–67.
41. Rowsey JJ, Balyeat HD, Monlux R, et al. Prospective evaluation of radial keratotomy; photokeratoscopic corneal topography. *Ophthalmology.* 1988;95:322–334.
42. McDonnell P, Garbus J, Caroline P, Yoshinaga P. Computerized analysis of corneal topography as an aid in fitting contact lenses after radial keratotomy. *Ophthalmology Surg.* 1992;23:55–59.
43. Shivitz TA, Russell BM, Arrowsmith PN, Marks RG. Optical correction of postoperative radial keratotomy patients with contact lenses. *Contact Lens Assoc Ophthalmol.* 1986;12:1244–1248.
44. Vickery JA. Post RK and the soft lens. *Contact Lens Forum.* 1986;Oct:34–35.
45. Bores LD, Myers W, Cowden J. Radial keratotomy; an analysis of the American experience. *Ann Ophthalmol.* 1981;13:941–948.
46. Janes J, Reichie RN. Refractive surgery and contact lenses. *Contact Lens Forum.* 1986;28–32.
47. Greco A. Fitting the postoperative keratotomy patient. *Int Eyecare.* 1986;2:188–190.
48. El Hage S, Baker R. Controlled keratoreformation for postoperative radial keratotomy patients. *Int Eyecare.* 1986;2:490–530.
49. Wyszinski P, O'Dell L. Diurnal cycle of refraction after radial keratotomy. *Ophthalmology.* 1987;94:120–124.

SECTION X

Systemic Associations

CHAPTER 48

Ocular and Systemic Associations with Ametropia

Jeffrey C. Lamkin

Excluding presbyopia, approximately 35% to 40% of the general population (of North America) suffers from a visually significant refractive error.[1,2] The majority of these patients require only a reliable refractive correction, since there are no associated ocular or systemic disorders mandating intervention. Still, a significant minority of patients with refractive error will suffer morbidity or even mortality from related disorders affecting the eye or other organ systems. The purpose of this chapter is not to catalogue exhaustively each and every syndrome that has been passingly associated with a certain refractive state. Rather, it is to review briefly those disorders, both systemic and ocular, that have been clearly associated with either myopia or hyperopia and that are of day-to-day relevance to the practicing ophthalmologist. The refractive surgeon should be aware of these associations to facilitate timely diagnosis and therapy.

GLAUCOMA

Ocular Hypertension and Primary Open-Angle Glaucoma

Myopia is one of several ocular risk factors for the development of ocular hypertension and subsequent glaucomatous optic nerve damage.[3] Tomlinson and Phillips[4] found that intraocular pressure (IOP) tended to vary directly with the axial length. They found an average IOP in myopes of 15.5 mm Hg, compared with 13.9 mm Hg in the hyperopic group. Podos measured IOP in 17 myopes with no evidence of primary open-angle glaucoma (POAG) and found that 3 of 32 (9%) had pressures exceeding 21 mm Hg (5% of normal eyes will have IOP greater than 21 mm Hg).[5]

Daubs and Crick[6] performed a case-control study of the relationship between myopia, ocular hypertension, and POAG, assessing relative risks. Their definition of POAG was quite simple—characteristic visual field loss. The "characteristics" of the definitive field patterns were not included, however. Interestingly, they found no increased risk of ocular hypertension among myopes, regardless of the degree of myopia. On the other hand, they found a significant progressive trend toward POAG as the spherical equivalent became more myopic. Additionally, the combined effect of myopia and marked elevations in IOP (31 to 80 mm Hg) produced a synergistic effect on visual field loss; that is, myopes seemed more susceptible to comparable levels of ocular hypertension than emmetropes and hyperopes. This finding was corroborated by Perkins and Phelps,[7] who found that one in three myopes with IOP

627

greater than 21 mm Hg went on to develop glaucomatous field defects, compared with one in 20 emmetropes and one in 40 hyperopes. This latter study also showed that myopes were more likely to develop visual field loss at IOP less than 21 mm Hg (normal tension glaucoma).

Numerous studies have focused on the prevalence of myopia among patients with glaucoma and that of glaucoma among patients with myopia. Estimates of the frequency of myopia among patients with glaucoma range from 6.6% to 37.8% (compared with 3% to 25% of the general population).[8] Approximately 9% to 28% of myopic patients also carry the diagnosis of POAG. Wilson and associates[9] performed a case-control study investigating the relationship between POAG and various personal characteristics and exposures. Using multiple logistic regression for simultaneous evaluation of numerous factors, they found that black race and untreated systolic hypertension were the most important independent risks. Myopia was a "suggestive association," both for patients with overt POAG as well as for individuals suspected of having glaucoma.

Mastropasqua and associates[8] compared the refractive errors in patients with open-angle glaucoma to those of nonglaucomatous myopic eyes and found a significantly higher frequency of high myopia in patients with POAG.

Patients with coincident myopia and POAG present unique diagnostic and therapeutic challenges. The myopic optic disc is typically larger with a larger central cup, and early glaucomatous changes may be difficult to recognize. Myopic tilting of optic discs and peripapillary atrophy can further obscure analysis of optic nerve topography (Fig 48–1). Furthermore, myopes are significantly more likely to develop nonglaucomatous atypical nerve fiber bundle defects on perimetry, complicating the interpretation of serial visual fields.[10]

At least one report provides evidence that myopes respond more favorably to medical treatment of POAG.[11] Phelps found a significantly lower rate of progression of glaucomatous visual field defects among a myopic subgroup. In addition, his patients with POAG plus myopia were significantly more likely to show improvement in visual field testing after 1 year. The author concluded that myopia facilitates the optic neuropathy induced by elevated IOP without contributing an independent pathophysiologic insult.

Clearly, all myopes should undergo routine tonometry. Visual field testing is indicated if IOP is clearly elevated or if morphologic abnormalities of the optic nerve suggest glaucoma.

Pigment Dispersion Syndrome and Pigmentary Glaucoma

In 1940, Sugar[12] described a 29-year-old man with glaucoma characterized by particularly heavy pigment deposition in the anterior segment. In 1949, Sugar and Barbour[13] more completely defined the syndrome, including an association with myopia. Subsequently numerous additional series have confirmed these landmark observations.[14]

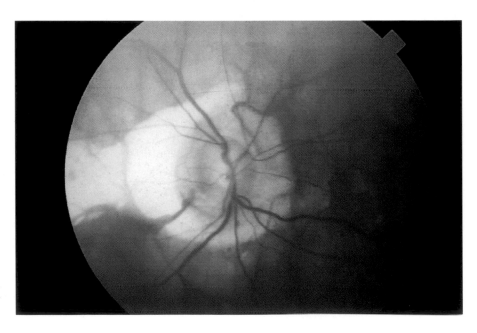

Figure 48–1. Optic nerve of axial myope. Note the vertical elongation, peripapillary atrophy, and relatively large cup.

The majority of patients with pigmentary dispersion, with or without glaucoma, are young myopic men with particularly deep anterior chambers (ACs). These findings are believed to be important in the pathophysiology of the disorders.[13] Based on the classic pattern of radial midperipheral transillumination defects of the iris, the excessive pigment is felt to be liberated by abnormal contact between the pigment epithelium of the iris and the zonules of the lens. This iris-zonule contact is not seen in the normal-sized eye. Only in eyes with particularly deep ACs and concave irides does this contact occur. The myopic eye is, on average, longer than the emmetropic or hyperopic eye and predisposed to develop a deeper AC. As the myopic eye continues to lengthen in the second and third decades, the ciliary ring may enlarge faster than the lens-zonule diaphragm, resulting in iridozonular contact. Male eyes are, on average, longer than female eyes, thus explaining the sex predilection as well.

The hallmarks of pigmentary dispersion syndrome must be sought out in the young myope, particularly men. These include a pigment spindle on the corneal endothelium, radial midperipheral transillumination defects of the iris, pigment on the anterior lens capsule, and heavy pigment in the trabecular meshwork and on Schwalbe's line. Once IOP is found to be elevated, or glaucomatous optic nerve or visual field changes are noted, the diagnosis of pigmentary glaucoma is generally made. Wide fluctuations in IOP are another of the syndrome's hallmarks. These are believed to be secondary to "showers" of liberated pigment accumulating in the trabecular meshwork after significant pupillary movement or vigorous exercise.[15] Management of patients with pigmentary glaucoma is not unlike that for patients with POAG, except the patients are typically younger and tolerate miotic therapy poorly. Laser trabeculoplasty often lowers IOP temporarily (weeks or months), typically for a shorter period than in POAG. Standard filtration surgery is successful.

Steroid-Induced Glaucoma

Elevated IOP in response to topical corticosteroid therapy was initially reported by Francois in 1954.[16] Subsequent studies employing steroid challenges established that older patients, as well as those with previously diagnosed POAG, were particularly susceptible.[17] Three decades of clinical research have established that approximately one third of the general (nonglaucomatous) population will develop a moderate rise in IOP after 4 to 6 weeks of topical corticosteroid administration. The pressure response is significant or marked (greater than 31 mm Hg) in only 5% to 6% of the population, however.

The response to chronic therapy among patients with definite glaucoma is clearly different. Virtually every such patient will suffer a measurable pressure increase. Patients with a family history of glaucoma are also at very high risk for this so-called steroid response. Diabetics and patients with collagen vascular diseases are more likely to respond to steroids as well, albeit not as often or dramatically, as patients with glaucoma or a family history of glaucoma.

In 1966, Podos and colleagues[5] noted that high myopes seemed vulnerable to steroid-induced pressure rises as well. In their series of myopes with no evidence of glaucoma, 15 (88%) responded to a topical steroid challenge with a significant increase in IOP. A subsequent study confirmed that over 85% of high myopes will suffer a significant increase in response to a topical steroid challenge.[18]

The pressure rise seen in this condition is typically delayed 10 to 14 days after initiation of therapy. In some cases, however, the response may be much faster (hours to days) or strikingly delayed (months or years). This medication effect should always be suspected as a contributing factor in any recent rise of IOP encountered during steroid therapy, regardless of the timing of onset. Note that corticosteroids may exert this untoward effect with any route of exposure, including systemic treatment or endogenous hypercortisol states (eg, Cushing's syndrome).

Pathogenesis is believed to be related to abnormal accumulation of glycosaminoglycans within the trabecular meshwork in susceptible individuals. Following cessation of exposure, IOP tends to return toward normal within days to weeks, although rare cases take significantly longer. In very rare cases the glaucoma may be permanent, although many of these cases may represent previously undiagnosed or latent POAG. Some myopes at higher risk of developing POAG may fall into this category.

The obvious caveat is that steroids should be used with great caution and careful follow-up examination in all patients, particularly those most likely to have a steroid response. This group clearly includes myopes, particularly high myopes. No patient should be treated indefinitely with these agents, and "steroid sparing" medications, both topical and systemic, are clearly preferable. (Topical nonsteroidal agents have never been associated with rises in IOP.) Depot periocular steroid injections should be avoided at all costs, since steroid response in this case is often long lasting and refractory to treatment. If topical steroids are clearly indicated, fluorometholone or medrysone are known to elicit the least effect.

Pediatric Glaucomas

The eye of the infant and young child is more distensible and elastic than that of the adult. For this reason, significant rises in IOP can cause lengthening of the globe in young children, particularly those less than 2 years of age.

During adolescence, elevated IOP can induce myopia by a different mechanism. Cherny and associates[19] have reported a case of chronic angle closure glaucoma in a 19-year-old girl with a previously documented hyperopic refractive error. She developed progressive unilateral myopia (−6 diopter [D] versus −1D), gross cupping, and field loss associated with elevated IOP. The axial length of the affected eye remained within 0.4 mm of the fellow eye, and the lens was measured as only 0.4 mm more anterior than the contralateral lens. Keratometry revealed 5 D of additional corneal power in the affected eye relative to the fellow eye. The authors concluded that elevated IOP had induced changes in the corneal curvature, rather than an increase in the overall axial length, to account for the myopic shift.

Congenital Glaucoma

B-scan ultrasonography of an eye with congenital glaucoma will typically show significant globe lengthening. Obviously, the more severe the glaucoma, the greater the degree of enlargement. Eyes with significant secondary axial myopia will probably have suffered optic nerve damage from the glaucoma. This, plus secondary amblyopia, renders the myopia more an epiphenomenon than a management issue. Obviously, eyes with useful vision should receive full correction, if possible, to minimize ongoing amblyopia.

Because of preexistent structural abnormalities in the corneas of patients with congenital glaucoma, as well as the preexistent limitations on visual acuity due to the underlying disease processes, patients with moderate or severe disease may not be suitable candidates for refractive surgery.

Juvenile Glaucoma

Juvenile open-angle glaucoma (JOAG) is defined as primary open-angle glaucoma in young adults up to 30 years of age. There is generally a family history of POAG, and it is often transmitted on an autosomal dominant basis.[20] Like pigment dispersion syndrome, there is a male preponderance, and myopia is a frequent association.[21] In fact, one series reported that as many as 50% of patients with true JOAG are also myopic.[22]

Gonioscopy may reveal subtle abnormalities in the angle, including abnormal width and prominence of the trabecular meshwork, absence of the angle recess, and mesodermal remnants. JOAG is often resistant to traditional medical therapy. Trabeculoplasty, as used in POAG, typically fails as well. Patients with JOAG can respond significantly to YAG laser trabeculopuncture,[20] a procedure using the cutting action of the YAG laser to incise trabecular tissue. This is usually attempted before traditional surgical intervention. Trabeculotomy remains the surgical procedure of choice. Traditional filtration surgery frequently fails due to the exuberant wound healing process of young adults, and filtration with antimetabolites may result in a better success rate.

Several forms of secondary glaucoma are seen in young adults (eg, Sturge-Weber syndrome, Axenfelds's anomaly, Peter's anomaly, aniridia, traumatic). Only pigmentary glaucoma carries a clear association with myopia (see above).

Early-Onset POAG

Some investigators consider early-onset POAG to be synonymous with JOAG, while others recognize this as a distinct entity of open-angle glaucoma with no recognizable pattern of inheritance and normal AC angles.[20] Any association with myopia probably resembles that for POAG.

Myopia and Filtration Surgery

One of the well-known complications of glaucoma filtration surgery is hypotony. It is typically due to overfiltration but can also arise secondary to persistent choroidal effusions, aqueous hyposecretion, or cyclodialysis. In the setting of hypotony, the posterior choroid becomes thickened with resulting macular wrinkling, thickening, and striae formation. Optic disc edema is also seen (Fig 48–2). Central acuity is generally diminished, sometimes permanently, due to chronic cystoid macular edema. Postoperative hypotony may be more common with the use of antimetabolites in the early postoperative period.

In 1992, Stamper and colleagues[23] reported on 15 patients with significant hypotony after trabeculectomy with postoperative antimetabolite therapy, in-

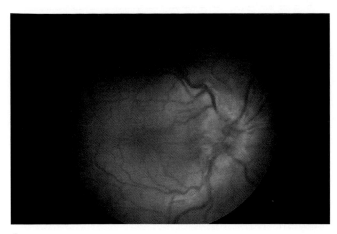

A

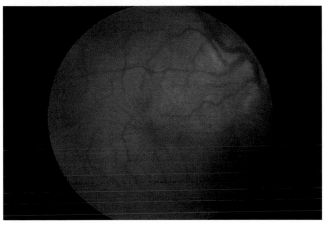

B

Figure 48–2. Hypotonous maculopathy. A 37-year-old myopic man 3 weeks after filtration surgery with mitomycin C for traumatic glaucoma. **A.** Nerve fiber layer edema around optic nerve head, extending into the macula. **B.** Macular edema with striae account for visual acuity of 20/200.

cluding eight in whom maculopathy and visual loss developed. Patients who developed maculopathy were significantly younger (46 versus 73 years old) and significantly more myopic (−7.5 D versus −1.11 D). Perioperative management of the myope undergoing filtration surgery should include safeguards against overfiltration (thicker trabeculectomy flaps with more sutures, delayed suture lysis, cautious use of antimetabolites, etc).

Primary Angle-Closure Glaucoma

The possible mechanisms leading to secondary closure of the AC angle are numerous, including anterior segment inflammation, neovascularization of the anterior segment, lens dislocation, and intraocular cysts and tumors. The most common cause, primary angle closure,

is without a clear precipitating factor or event. The underlying factors leading to primary angle closure are multiple. Different patients represent varying combinations of anatomic and physiologic factors that, in sum, lead to physical obstruction of the trabecular meshwork by iris stroma, with subsequent elevation in IOP.

Relative pupillary block refers to the resistance to flow of aqueous humor from the posterior chamber (PC) into the AC. The resistance, which is present in every eye, is created by the normal contact between iris and lens. In most eyes, the resistance is minimal and fluid moves easily into the AC, although a small pressure gradient does persist. In anatomically predisposed eyes, the resistance is significantly higher. This results in a larger pressure gradient (higher pressure in the PC) and anterior bowing of the midperipheral iris (Fig 48–3). If the bowing is sufficient, iris stroma can physically obstruct the access of aqueous humor to the trabecular meshwork, with subsequent elevation in IOP.

Eyes predisposed to primary angle closure have a disparity between the size or position of the crystalline lens and the size of the remainder of the anterior segment (and the eye itself). Thus, eyes that are too small or have lenses that are inappropriately large are at risk.[24] Lowe[25,26] has shown that eyes that are 1 mm shorter than average are at increased risk, and other investigators have substantiated the importance of short axial length.[27] Shorter eyes have smaller corneas with shallower ACs, making relative pupillary block more likely to lead to trabecular obstruction.[24] In general, shorter eyes are hyperopic, and the syndrome of primary angle closure is less common among myopes, who tend to have larger, deeper ACs. The one exception to this rule is the patient whose myopia is lenticular, either due to spherophakia (eg, Weill-Marchesani syndrome) or ectopia lentis. In these cases, the amount of iris-lens contact is increased, and angle closure develops in normally sized ACs.

It is important to be aware of the possibility of classic primary angle-closure glaucoma presenting in a gradual or insidious fashion (subacute and chronic angle closure). The syndrome of sudden painful visual loss associated with nausea and vomiting is well recognized as acute glaucoma and is the most common presentation for primary angle-closure glaucoma, but many eyes have become irreversibly blind as the trabecular meshwork becomes silently, but visibly, occluded by the same mechanism.[28]

Treatment of patients with angle-closure glaucoma generally consists of a medical regimen appropriate for

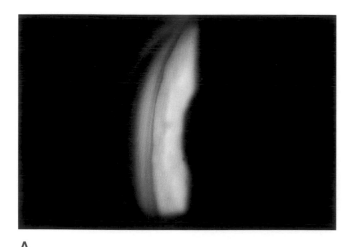
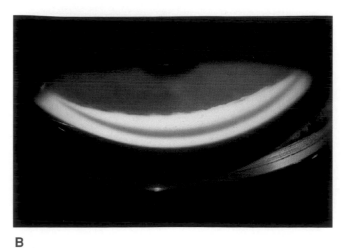

A   B

Figure 48–3. Primary angle-closure glaucoma. **A.** Three-mirror gonioscopy of a normal angle shows an easily visible trabecular meshwork and scleral spur. **B.** In a narrow angle of a +4.00 D hyperope, only the anterior meshwork is (barely) visible. The iris contour is markedly convex, reflecting an inappropriately large lens with increased relative pupillary block.

the IOP, followed by laser iridotomy. Rarely, surgical iridectomy is required, should laser treatment fail due to corneal edema or hyphema. Failure to relieve angle closure with iridotomy or iridectomy rules out the relative pupillary block as the causative mechanism. Malignant glaucoma and other causes of secondary angle closure (eg, rubeosis) should then be aggressively sought. Because of the strong tendency for bilateral symmetry in anterior segment morphology, a case of acute angle-closure glaucoma is unlikely to be primary if the fellow AC is deep, with a wide-open angle. For the same reason, the patient who has suffered unilateral primary angle-closure glaucoma is at significant risk for contralateral involvement in the future and is generally considered a candidate for prophylactic laser iridotomy.

CHORIORETINAL DISORDERS

Myopic Macular Degeneration

The classic findings of the myopic fundus are a direct result of the pathophysiology of the abnormally elongated globe. Thus, this form of macular degeneration occurs in patients whose myopia is mostly axial. This is generally the high myope (> -6 D).

Anywhere from 11% to 36% of the general population is myopic, with 1.7% to 2.1% highly myopic.[29] This prevalence of high myopia depends strongly on ethnic origin and is particularly low among Egyptians (0.2%) and high among Spaniards (9.6%).[30] Roughly 2.1% of American 21-year-olds are highly myopic.

Women are more frequently affected and seem more susceptible to developing associated macular degeneration.[31]

The clinical findings of myopic macular degeneration are probably a direct result of axial elongation with progressive distension of the posterior globe leading to thinning of the sclera, choroid, and retina. The optic nerve is usually elongated vertically and may appear tilted, raised nasally, and flattened temporally. With sufficient stretching temporally, the sclera adjacent to the optic nerve may become visible as a temporal crescent (myopic conus; Figs 48–1 and 48–4). In 10% of cases, the scleral exposure entirely surrounds the disc.

If the posterior distension is exaggerated in a circumscribed area of the fundus, a staphyloma develops. If the localized outpouching spares the fovea, the staphyloma may be silent. If the fovea is involved, central acuity is affected.[32]

Diffuse distension with thinning of the retinal pigment epithelium (RPE) and choroid makes the larger vessels of the choroid quite prominent, resulting in the so-called tigroid fundus seen clinically but most dramatically on fluorescein angiography (Fig 48–5). Because (normal) late scleral fluorescence is more visible, the contrast of the myopic angiogram is lessened. Profound atrophy of the RPE and choroid may occur in focal patches resembling the geographic atrophy seen in age-related macular degeneration. These patches tend to enlarge and coalesce with time.

The finding considered pathognomonic of myopic macular degeneration is the lacquer crack (Fig 48–5).

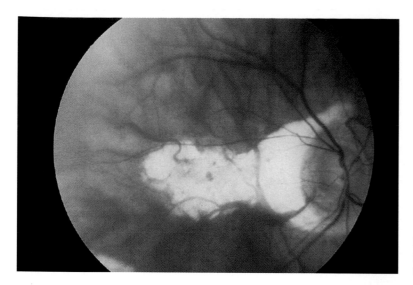

Figure 48–4. Myopic conus. Note the tilted optic nerve and peripapillary atrophy extending into the macula (same eye as Fig 48–1).

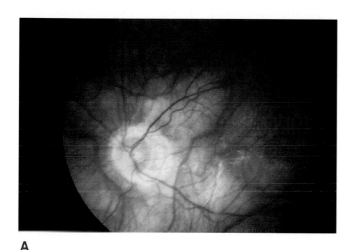

A

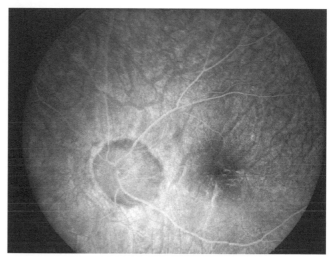

B

Figure 48–5. Myopic fundus. Diffuse atrophy of the RPE renders the larger choroidal vessels easily visible against the sclera. **A.** The vessels stand out on color photography. The linear hypopigmented streaks inferior and temporal to the macula are lacquer cracks, a form of dry macular degeneration. **B.** On fluorescein angiography, the choroidal vessels are even more striking. The lacquer cracks appear as window defects (early hyperfluorescence that fades in late views).

These linear or stellate lesions are macroscopic ruptures in Bruch's membrane and RPE. They tend to reflect more severe mechanical and anatomic disruption of the myopic fundus. In one study of 22 eyes with lacquer cracks, only one eye maintained 20/20, with the remainder in the 20/50 to 20/100 range.

The lesions are generally narrow (50 to 200 μm) but may be wider and expose choroidal vessels. Their distribution is random but typically confined to the posterior pole, with 17% in continuity with a temporal crescent.[33] Smaller cracks can be quite subtle on biomicroscopy or ophthalmoscopy but are readily distinguished on fluorescein angiography.

Subretinal hemorrhage is frequently associated with new or enlarging lacquer cracks. Their presence thus does not necessarily indicate concomitant choroidal neovascularization. The classic appearance of such a hemorrhage is round, focal, deep, and dense. The center of the fovea may be involved. The hemorrhage is usually along the course of the crack, although it may be just adjacent to it. Less than 5% of these hemorrhages arise in the absence of a definable lacquer crack. Not infrequently, hemorrhages recur in the same location months or years later. They typically resorb completely over weeks to months, with little long-term impact on vision (apart from the underlying disease process).

The most feared complication of myopic macular degeneration is choroidal neovascularization (CNV). Foerster was the first to describe hemorrhagic degeneration of the myopic macula in the 1860s. In 1901, Ernst Fuchs[34] described a dark lesion in the fovea of a high myope complaining of sudden loss of vision, attributing the color of the lesion to hyperplasia of the RPE. With the advent of fluorescein angiography, it has become clear that CNV is associated with these dark lesions. Thus, the "Fuchs' spot" is a different manifestation of the same process (CNV) originally described by Foerster. As discussed above, the appearance of a simple subretinal hemorrhage is not firm evidence of CNV. If associated with subretinal fluid or fibrosis, then CNV is almost certainly present.

Some 5% to 10% of the myopic population will develop CNV, with high myopes disproportionately affected. One series reported a 40% prevalence of CNV in high myopia,[35] although most other series report a significantly lower rate. In this same series, 12% of patients developed bilateral CNV. In a study with a longer follow-up period, the rate of bilaterality was 41%.[36]

Clinically, the development of CNV is heralded by painless loss of vision or metamorphopsia. The findings on biomicroscopy are often different from CNV of other etiologies (Figs 48–6 and 48–7). Myopic membranes are distinguished by a tendency to become hyperpigmented and to be clinically indolent, with scanty hemorrhage and fluid leakage. Subretinal lipid exudate is uncommon, particularly relative to its prominence in CNV associated with age-related macular degeneration (AMD). Fluorescein angiography confirms early hyperfluorescence, which increases in size and intensity in late views. The clinical indolence is also quite apparent on angiography, since the leakage is not pronounced. In fact, in some cases, the hyperfluorescence does not appear to enlarge significantly with time but instead remains confined to the borders of the clinically visible lesion. These findings are in contrast to those of CNV due to AMD. In the latter case, the leakage tends to be dramatic and obvious, with definite enlargement of late hyperfluorescence.

CNV often develops in direct continuity with lacquer cracks, with estimates ranging from 57% to 82% of all myopic CNV.[37,38] The membranes are usually quite close to center of the fovea, with the majority involving the fovea center at the time of examination.

The natural history of myopic CNV is clearly different from that of the most common cause of CNV, AMD. One report has claimed a relatively benign prognosis, with stabilization of useful acuity in 63% of un-treated patients.[35] Avila reported that 96% of myopic CNV stabilized spontaneously, with stable or improved vision in 54% (Fig 48–6).[37] Subsequent studies with better documentation of disease activity have not substantiated such a favorable picture. Over 50% of affected eyes will deteriorate to 20/200 or worse (Fig 48–7) and up to one third of affected patients will become legally blind.[39,40]

Because of the controversy regarding the natural history of the disorder, the role of laser photocoagulation in treatment has been uncertain as well. Only one randomized controlled trial has been performed to date.[41] This study investigated the value of krypton red laser photocoagulation in preventing visual loss in patients with CNV outside the fovea center due to myopia. Patients over 55 years of age and in whom the fovea center could not be reliably located were excluded. The study, limited by small patient numbers and limited follow-up study (1 to 2 years), documented significantly higher rates of improvement of visual acuity in treated eyes. Untreated eyes were significantly more likely to lose visual acuity. Some 31.4% of treated patients developed recurrences, but only 9% developed subfoveal recurrences.

Several factors hinder treatment of patients with myopic CNV. First, as discussed above, the anatomic derangements of the myopic fundus can make localization of the fovea center an educated guess, at best, in some cases. Because most of the membranes are close to the fovea, this is vital in discussing therapy with the patient. Second, lacquer cracks have been reported to extend after laser treatment. Thirdly, in myopic maculae, the atrophy caused by the laser itself may enlarge considerably over time, resulting in unplanned loss of foveal photoreceptors (and vision) months or years later.[36,40,42] This risk seems to be greater with argon green than krypton red laser.

In summary, laser treatment for CNV outside the fovea center is probably justified, if the patient understands most of the important issues. Treatment of subfoveal disease in myopia has not been specifically studied. Results from the macular photocoagulation study[43] of subfoveal CNV in AMD are sometimes cautiously extrapolated for less common causes of CNV. Ultimately, the decision to treat must be undertaken with the complete education and understanding of the patient.

Lattice Degeneration of the Retina

Lattice degeneration, along with peripheral cystoid and cobblestone degeneration, is one of the three most com-

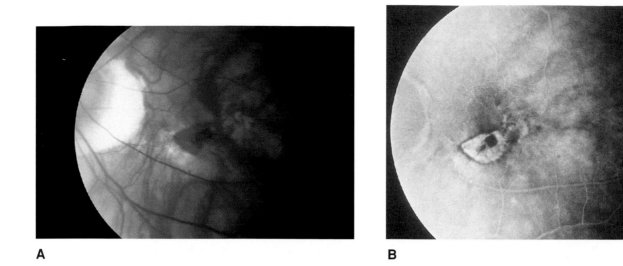

A

B

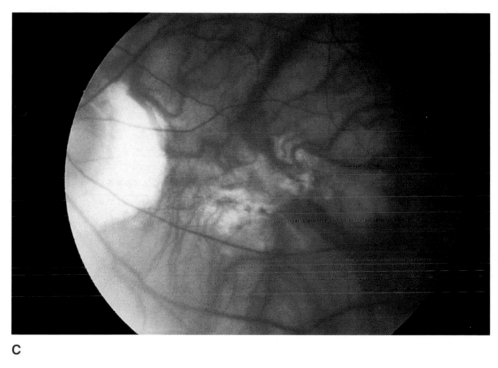

C

Figure 48–6. Myopic choroidal neovascularization (CNV). The 48-year-old highly myopic man presented with a 2-week history of mild metamorphopsia in his left eye. Visual acuity is 20/60. **A.** The appearance of the membrane clinically is typical for myopic CNV—a relatively flat, hyperpigmented lesion with scant overlying fluid and no hemorrhage. **B.** The fluorescein angiogram at presentation confirms classic CNV with little leakage. **C.** Six months later, the lesion, left untreated, has undergone spontaneous fibrous involution, with visual acuity stable at 20/60.

mon degenerations of the peripheral retina. Like cobblestone degeneration, lattice degeneration bears a clear association with increased axial length. Lattice degeneration is the only one of the three to be associated with primary retinal detachment (although cobblestones can lead to secondary retinal tears).

The condition was originally described by Gonin in 1920.[44] It was originally considered to be identical

histopathologically to typical peripheral cystoid degeneration (TPCD), but in 1937 Linder described the three histologic hallmarks distinct from TPCD.[45] These include localized retinal thinning, overlying vitreous liquefaction, and enhanced vitreoretinal adhesion at the lesions' borders due to glial proliferation. Many other morphologic terms have been used to describe the condition (pigmentary degeneration, equatorial degenera-

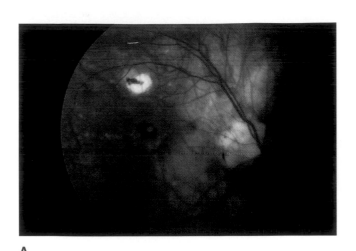

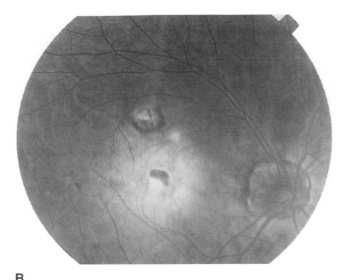

A   B

Figure 48–7. Myopic CNV. This 32-year-old woman presented with a 1-week history of decreased reading vision and purple chromatopsia. Visual acuity is 20/100. **A.** Note the classic hyperpigmented plaque just superior to the foveal center with a rim of surrounding atrophy of the RPE. The lesion in the superior macula probably represents scarring from previous CNV that spontaneously involuted. **B.** Angiography discloses a classic membrane with surrounding blocked fluorescence, mostly due to hyperpigmentation. Note relative lack of fluorescein leakage. This lesion was also left untreated, due to its proximity to the fovea. Acuity subsequently dropped to 20/200 after 3 months of observation.

tion, galaxy bands), but the term *lattice degeneration* has come to be the most widely accepted since Schepens introduced it in 1952.[46]

Lattice degeneration is found in anywhere from 6% to 11% of the general population,[47] with peak prevalence in young adults (histopathologic changes have been detected in a 17-month-old child).[45] There is no predilection for gender, right versus left eye, or race. Involvement is bilateral in up to 40% of patients studied clinically (nearly 50% in autopsy reviews).

The association of lattice degeneration with myopia has been demonstrated by numerous investigators.[47] Seventy-five percent of eyes with lattice degeneration are myopic to some degree.[48] With myopia of 1 D or greater, the incidence of lattice degeneration is 15%, twice that of the general population.[49] The incidence of lattice degeneration has also been shown to increase with increasing axial length in two independent studies.[46]

The primary clinical features of lattice degeneration are well described, including latticelike sclerotic vascular changes, multiple tiny yellow-white flecks on the inner retinal surface, hyperplasia or atrophy of the RPE, and oval or linear erosions of the retinal surface. When the yellowish flecks are extensive and coalescent, the retina appears shiny and wet, and the term "snail-track degeneration" is applied.

The clinical importance of lattice degeneration is its clear association with rhegmatogenous retinal detachment. Atrophic holes within lattice degeneration form in up to 1% to 2% of the general population and in 25% of patients known to have the disorder. The prevalence of atrophic breaks increases with age and is twice as common in the inferior quadrants, most often the inferotemporal.[46] Interestingly, the risk of progressive detachment due to atrophic holes clearly diminishes with age. This risk is small, as less than 1% of eyes with atrophic holes and lattice degeneration will develop retinal detachment. When it does occur and progress, however, the typical patient is an asymptomatic young myope. It is important to be aware of this small subset of patients.

The risk of progressive retinal detachment is much greater when a retinal break forms secondary to vitreous traction. Because of the abnormally strong vitreoretinal adhesion at the borders of lattice lesions, there is significant risk of retinal break formation at the time of acute posterior vitreous separation. Byer[50] followed 204 eyes with lattice degeneration over 3 to 10 years and found that 1.5% developed tears at the margin of lattice lesions. It is important to bear in mind that retinal breaks can also form in regions that appear unaffected by the degeneration. Some studies have asserted that posterior vitreous detachment occurs earlier in eyes with lattice degeneration, but other data contradict this.[47]

Retinal detachment, the most feared complication of lattice degeneration, is relatively uncommon, although more common than in the general population. The risk of detachment in all patients with lattice degeneration is estimated at 0.3% to 0.5%, while 20% to 32% of all rhegmatogenous retinal detachments are associated with lattice degeneration.[46,49] The greatest risk is undoubtedly in the older patient, at the time of vitreous detachment, but young myopes with asymptomatic inferior atrophic holes and an intact posterior hyaloid must be watched carefully.

The importance of lattice degeneration in the myopic patient is obvious. All myopes should undergo dilated retinal examination as a part of their initial comprehensive examination. If no lattice degeneration is discovered by the end of the third decade, it is unlikely to develop subsequently. If there is active lattice degeneration, the patient should undergo routine dilated examination, perhaps every 1 to 2 years.

Prophylactic retinopexy (laser or cryotherapy) of lattice degeneration may be of value in certain cases. Atrophic holes are of low risk but must be followed carefully in the young myope. Atrophic holes detected after vitreous separation are generally treated only if there is evidence of ongoing vitreous traction. Other lattice lesions (ie, without retinal breaks) may also be followed without treatment, even when accompanied by symptoms of vitreoretinal traction (flashes and floaters), provided there is no history of detachment in the fellow eye. With such a history, the standard of care is generally to treat prophylactically, especially in the setting of symptoms of vitreoretinal traction. In the absence of vitreoretinal symptoms (flashes, floaters), candidates for prophylactic treatment of lattice degeneration in the fellow eye include those with a poor functional outcome after repair of the contralateral retinal detachment and patients less able to detect or attend to acute posterior vitreous separation (retarded or homebound patients). Lattice degeneration associated with retinal breaks and subretinal fluid (localized or subclinical retinal detachment) or new symptomatic retinal breaks are also generally treated.

Retinal Detachment

The risk of rhegmatogenous retinal detachment clearly increases with increasing axial length. Depending on the series, between 40% and 80% of retinal detachments

occur in eyes with axial myopia.[47] Ogawa[51] compared the refractive errors among 1166 Japanese eyes with retinal detachment to those of 11671 eyes without it. He found that among patients with retinal detachment, 8.58% were hyperopic (> +0.75 D) and 82.16% were myopic (> −0.50 D). Among the controls, 24.29% were hyperopic and 34.41% myopic. During the first 60 years of life the risk of retinal detachment in patients with at least 5 D of myopia has been estimated to be approximately 2.4%, compared with 0.06% for emmetropic patients.[52]

The axially myopic eye has abnormally low levels of hyaluronic acid within the vitreous gel. This leads to premature liquefaction of the gel, which increases the incidence of posterior vitreous separation at earlier ages than in emmetropic eyes. This in turn increases the incidence of new retinal break formation. The liquefaction also increases the likelihood of subsequent retinal detachment after a retinal break. Thus, vitreous liquefaction, together with the increased incidence of lattice degeneration, increases the incidence of retinal detachment(Fig 48–8). These factors also increase the risk of retinal detachment after cataract extraction and laser capsulotomy.[53]

Repair of myopic retinal detachment is not significantly different than for other eyes, except that intraoperative and postoperative complications are more frequent. These include inadvertent perforation due to thin sclera, excessive fluid drainage with hypotony, retinal incarceration, choroidal effusion and hemorrhage, and postoperative glaucoma (including steroid induced).

Highly myopic eyes are also at risk for progressive retinal detachment after idiopathic macular hole formation. This is distinctly uncommon in emmetropic or hyperopic eyes.[54] Pars plana vitrectomy with gasfluid exchange and prone positioning is necessary for repair.

Other Peripheral Retinal Degenerations

White Without Pressure

This not uncommon but poorly understood peripheral retinal change occurs most commonly in the young black myopic eye. Thirty-five percent of myopic eyes under 40 years of age show some white without pressure, but this rate falls to 9.5% of patients over 40 years old.[55] Virtually all patients with axial lengths greater than 33 mm show some white without pressure, as do 50% of those with lengths of 26 to 33 mm. The con-

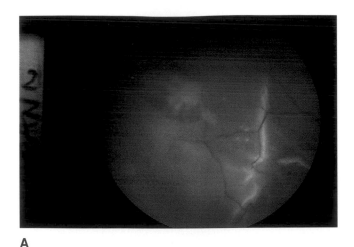

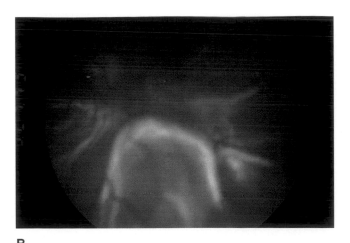

A   **B**

Figure 48–8. Retinal detachment in a 48-year-old −4.50 D myope with sudden visual loss. **A.** A large flap tear in the superonasal quadrant accounts for the extensive detachment. **B.** Macular detachment is the most important negative prognostic factor in rhegmatogenous retinal detachment.

dition is 9 to 10 times more common in blacks than whites.[47]

The changes appear as an unusual whitish sheen to the inner retinal surface. If the change is only seen on depressed examination, it is referred to as white with pressure. The cause of the appearance is not known but is believed to be due to an abnormality in the vitreoretinal interface. Affected areas are generally geographic with irregular borders and may change with time.

The condition does not seem to constitute any risk for primary retinal detachment but does carry an important implication for patients with a history of a giant tear in the fellow eye. In some of these patients, the white without pressure progresses with subsequent formation of retinal breaks, often giant tears. Freeman[56] has advocated prophylactic encircling buckles in these patients before break formation.

Cobblestone Degeneration

Cobblestone degeneration (also known as pavingstone degeneration) is a common peripheral retinal disorder characterized by round or oval punched-out regions of peripheral chorioretinal atrophy, most commonly inferiorly. The disorder is probably secondary to choroidal vascular insufficiency affecting localized areas of the choriocapillaris. The local ischemia leads to focal atrophy of the RPE and outer retina.

The disorder affects 17% to 22% of autopsy eyes. More extensive disease is usually bilateral.[47] The incidence increases with age and axial length, occurring in over 50% of myopes.[55]

The disorder is not associated with the formation of primary retinal breaks but can be the source of secondary breaks in an eye with a progressive retinal detachment. When subretinal fluid reaches an atrophic patch, the retina can tear at its margin due to the enhanced chorioretinal adherence within the patch itself.

Peripheral Pigmentary Degeneration

The peripheral retina of axially elongated eyes often shows significant variation in outer retinal and subretinal pigmentation. It may be diffusely darkened and show discrete focal hyperpigmentation or even a pseudo–retinitis pigmentosa appearance. The pigmentary "degeneration" is strongly associated with increasing axial length and age.[47,55] It is nearly always bilateral, with no sex predilection. The cause is not understood but is probably a reaction of the RPE to globe elongation and aging.

The peripheral pigmentary changes of the axially myopic eye do not constitute any independent risk for retinal breaks or detachments beyond that of the myopia itself.

Idiopathic Multifocal Choroiditis

In 1973, Nozik and Dorsch described a "new chorioretinopathy" characterized by multiple, small, yellow-white lesions of the RPE and inner choroid that appeared similar to those seen in the presumed ocular histoplasmosis syndrome (POHS).[57] Two features have come to distinguish the syndrome from POHS. First, there is usually little or no peripapillary scarring; more important, there is often AC or vitreous inflammation, which is not seen in POHS.

Several other reports have subsequently defined the syndrome more fully.[58] The disorder tends to affect otherwise healthy younger people (generally less than 45 years of age), with a female:male ratio of up to 3:1. The majority of cases, perhaps higher than 80%, will become bilateral. Recurrent episodes of choroiditis and panuveitis occur, which are often asymptomatic. Any initial symptoms relate to vitreous floaters, since most involved eyes are white and quiet. The choroiditis typically involves the postequatorial fundus, with numerous 100- to 300-μm lesions. Occasionally, active choroiditis near the center of the macula can result in a scotoma or metamorphopsia. Many patients (between 25% and 50%) will develop choroidal neovascularization (CNV) with loss of central acuity. A smaller subset develops progressive subretinal fibrosis, with no angiographic evidence of CNV. Angiographic distinction between active choroiditis and CNV may be difficult. Both are hyperfluorescent early, with leakage in late views. Typically, the leakage associated with CNV is more pronounced, with greater enlargement in late images. Treatment of active choroiditis is generally reserved for lesions threatening the center of the macula. Oral corticosteroids are sometimes successful in this situation. Any patient with active CNV is generally treated promptly, most often with laser photocoagulation strategies guided by those used for more common causes of CNV. Some reports have suggested that steroids can quiet CNV,[59] but this is not widely accepted.

In 1982, Doran and Hamilton[60] added a series of four patients with multifocal choroiditis and macular degeneration to Nozik's original two patients. They noted that two of their four patients were myopic. In two subsequently published series, 20 of 22 affected patients were mildly myopic.[59,61] Scheider[62] has proposed an interesting hypothesis for the preponderance of myopic females. Probably because of menstruation, younger women are significantly more likely to develop asymptomatic bacteremia than younger men or older women. Myopic eyes tend to have more attenuated choroidal vasculature, increasing the chance for infectious thrombosis during bacteremic episodes. The combination of these risk factors, Scheider reasons, may result in the significantly higher incidence of the disorder among young myopic women. However, the myopia in multifocal choroiditis is generally mild or moderate, where there is less likely to be pathologic thinning or attenuation of ocular structure.

It is important to note that the term *multifocal choroiditis* is purely descriptive and can apply to a variety of etiologies and syndromes with systemic manifestations. The most common uveitic disorders associated with secondary multifocal choroiditis include sarcoidosis, tuberculosis, and syphilis.[63] Less common causes include *Pneumocystis carinii* (in immunosuppressed patients), herpes family viruses (usually herpes zoster), atypical mycobacteria, and fungi. The association with mild to moderate myopia has only been demonstrated in idiopathic cases.

Choroidal Hemorrhages/Effusions

Fluid may collect in the potential space between the choroid and sclera, the suprachoroidal space, after any type of intraocular surgical procedure or trauma. If the fluid represents a transudate or exudate—that is, the noncellular components of blood—the collection is referred to as a choroidal effusion. A critical pathophysiologic factor in the development of choroidal effusions is hypotony. A drop in hydrostatic pressure surrounding the branches of the posterior ciliary arteries passing between sclera and choroid can tip the scales, which normally balance fluid flux in the suprachoroidal space and keep it dry. The result is a progressive collection, either rapid (seconds to minutes) or slow (hours to days), of a transudate, with secondary retinal and choroidal elevation. The elevation is typically dome shaped, solid, and smooth. A true effusion, or transudate, will transilluminate.

Any procedure than can cause significant hypotony, particularly a sudden drop from high pressure to low, can lead to choroidal effusion. One such circumstance is drainage of bullous subretinal fluid during scleral buckling. Scleral buckling elements themselves can impede the normal evacuation of fluid from the suprachoroidal space through the vortex veins, causing or aggravating the effusions. Any anterior segment procedure that leads to hypotony can result in the same end, but the most common scenario is a slow leak from a filtering bleb, either intentional (glaucoma surgery) or inadvertent (cataract surgery). Choroidal inflammation of any cause can lead to fluid transudation into the suprachoroidal space. Infectious, postoperative, or idiopathic inflammation can lead to the same endpoint. Heavy scatter laser treatment of neovascular retinopathies can trigger effusions as well (Fig 48–9).

If the branches of the posterior ciliary artery are ruptured or sheared open by significant mechanical de-

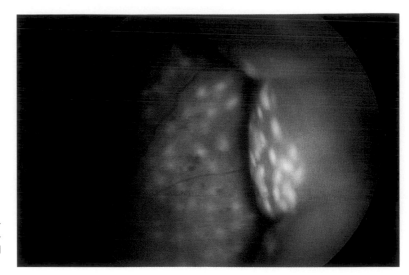

Figure 48–9. Choroidal effusions. Intense scatter laser treatment in this patient with ischemic central retinal vein occlusion with rubeosis has resulted in moderate choroidal effusion.

formation of the globe, whole blood can accumulate in the suprachoroidal space. Disruption of larger-caliber vessels will result in more rapid accumulation of larger choroidal hemorrhages than if the smallest vessels are involved. If the hemorrhage develops extremely rapidly, typically during a surgical procedure, intraocular contents may be significantly displaced through the open wound (suprachoroidal expulsive hemorrhage). Like effusions, choroidal hemorrhages are smooth and dome shaped but are dark and do not transilluminate. An interesting sign of choroidal hemorrhage is unilateral scleral icterus.[64]

Axial myopia has been associated with both choroidal effusions and hemorrhages by several investigators.[65] In 1966, Hawkins and Schepens[66] reviewed a series of 1500 patients undergoing retinal detachment repair. Choroidal effusion developed in 23 percent of cases, while hemorrhage occurred in 1 percent. Effusions were more common among high myopes and the elderly. Numerous studies have evaluated risk factors in suprachoroidal expulsive hemorrhage. In the most statistically rigorous review, several risk factors for expulsive hemorrhage emerged from age-adjusted bivariate analysis: increased axial length, glaucoma, elevated IOP, systemic atherosclerosis, and intraoperative tachycardia >85 bpm.[67]

Most effusions and delayed hemorrhages can be observed for spontaneous resolution. Indications for intervention include significant AC shallowing (causing lens/implant-corneal touch, persistent angle closure), severe secondary glaucoma, or prolonged contact of extremely large bullous detachments ("kissing choroidals"). Oral corticosteroids have been used in an attempt to stabilize hemorrhages, although there is no firm evidence of their efficacy. Surgical drainage is the definitive treatment.[65]

Recognition of risk factors is important for prevention. In eyes with axial myopia, a Flieringa ring can reduce the amount of mechanical distortion the globe undergoes during anterior segment procedures. Preoperative lowering of IOP, medically, surgically (paracentesis), or both, can reduce the magnitude of any pressure drop. Safety sutures permit rapid wound closure in the event of an expulsive hemorrhage. During scleral buckling, tension on harness sutures should be minimized immediately before drainage, which should be performed in the most controlled manner possible. Intraoperative hypertension and tachycardia should be minimized.

Retinopathy of Prematurity

Each year brings significant new advances in neonatology and care of the premature infant. With increasing survival rates among very low birthweight children, the visual impact of retinopathy of prematurity is increasing. The cryoretinopathy of prematurity (ROP) natural history study estimates that more than 65% of children weighing less than 1251 g at birth will develop some degree of ROP, with over 80% of children less than 1000 g being affected.[68] Obviously, a comprehensive discussion of the disorder is beyond the scope of this chapter. ROP results from exposure of immature retinal vasculature to vaso-obliteration if it is profound and long lasting. Normalization of arterial oxygen content results in vasoproliferation that can become uncontrolled, leading to neovascularization, vitreous hemorrhage, cicatrization, and retinal detachment.

High myopia can complicate any stage of ROP, although it is more common with more advanced disease. Several reports have placed its prevalence between 17% and 87%, reflecting the varying severity of the underlying ROP.[69] The myopia tends to progress during the first year or two of life and subsequently stabilizes. It does not regress as part of the hyperopic shift seen in normal children. (Premature infants without ROP are slightly myopic due to increased corneal and lenticular curvature. This myopia is temporary because normal eye growth leads to anterior segment flattening.) The nature of the myopia in infants with ROP has been disputed in the literature, with one report ascribing it to increased axial length and another suggesting a permanent augmentation of lenticular refractive power (Fig 48–10).[70]

Exudative Age-Related Macular Degeneration

As the leading cause of legal blindness in Americans over age 60, AMD has been extensively studied for risk factors associated with the more aggressive, wet form. It is clear that increasing age is the primary risk factor.[71] Women seem to be at increased risk for visual loss.[72] Between 10% and 20% of patients with profound visual loss have a family history of severe macular degeneration.[73] Severe disease in one eye constitutes a risk for severe disease contralaterally.[74] The effect of light ocular pigmentation is felt to be reflected in the notable rarity of exudative AMD in blacks and Orientals.[75]

Several reports have indicated that AMD is more common in hyperopic patients than in emmetropes and myopes.[76] In 1993, Sandberg and colleagues[77] compared refractive errors of 198 patients with unilateral exudative AMD with refractive errors of 129 patients with bilateral dry disease. The groups were otherwise matched according to sex, age, and acuity in the better-seeing eye. They found that patients with unilateral exudative disease were, on average, +1 D more hyperopic (in their better eyes) than the group with bilaterally dry disease. Furthermore, patients with +0.75 D or more of hyperopia were at significantly higher risk of having neovascular disease than other patients (odds ratio, 2.40). The association held up regardless of the definition of AMD or the eye used for analysis. The authors concluded that hyperopia was associated with neovascularization among patients referred with AMD (Fig 48–11).

Hyperopia has not been shown to be a risk factor for recurrence of choroidal neovascularization after laser treatment. For a more complete discussion of the treatment of patients with AMD, the MPS reports offer an outstanding review.

Central Serous Chorioretinopathy

One of the common caricatures in clinical ophthalmology is the young type A man with recent onset of monocular metamorphopsia and slightly blurred vision. Many times, the ophthalmologist can make a provi-

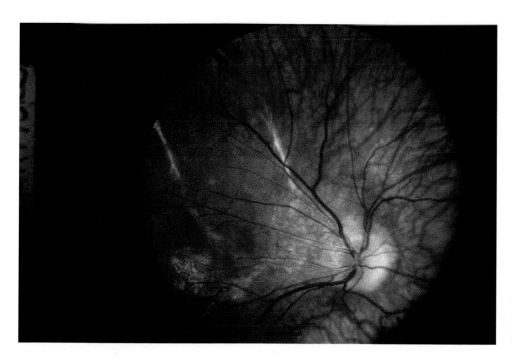

Figure 48–10. Retinopathy of prematurity. This 17-year-old patient presented with 20/400 acuity in the right eye secondary to cicatricial macular ectopia. Refractive error in her worse eye was −12.50 D.

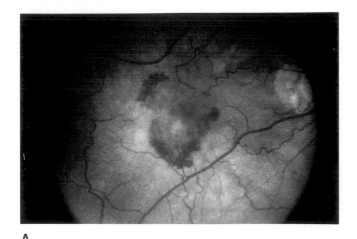
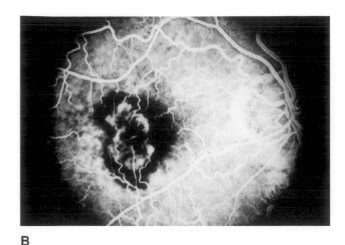

A   **B**

Figure 48–11. Exudative age-related macular degeneration. **A.** Extensive subfoveal CNV has dropped visual acuity to counting fingers. Refractive error is +1.25 D. **B.** Mid-phase angiogram confirms classic CNV with surrounding hypofluorescence corresponding to subretinal hemorrhage.

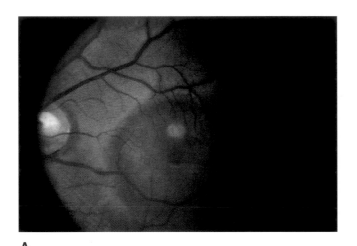
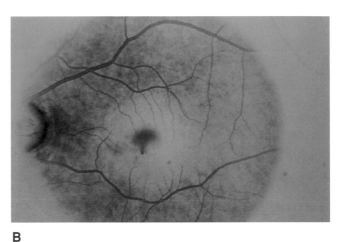

A   **B**

Figure 48–12. Central serous chorioretinopathy. **A.** A 2500-μm disciform detachment of the macula in a 34-year-old male engineer. Distance acuity is 20/30. Overcorrection of +1.50 D improves acuity to 20/25. **B.** Angiogram reveals the classic but uncommon smokestack pattern of dye leakage (seen in less than 20% of cases).

sional diagnosis of central serous chorioretinopathy before performing a dilated macular examination.

The syndrome is yet another example of a well-recognized yet incompletely understood condition. Increasing evidence suggests that choroidal hyperperfusion may be the primary pathogenic event. At any rate, the RPE develops one or more focal regions of altered permeability and faulty adherence to Bruch's membrane, with secondary serous detachment of the macula and, in one third of patients, detachment of the RPE itself (Fig 48–12).

One of the interesting features of the reduced central acuity is that it is often improved with low hyperopic correction. This is because the serous elevation of the macula shortens the effective axial length. Weak plus lenses add the additional convergence necessary for proper image placement. Many of these patients are quite capable of adding their own low hyperopic correction through accommodation, masking the effect of additional plus lenses.

Because of accommodation, as well as the generally self-limited course of the disease (95% recover at least 20/30 acuity spontaneously), hyperopic correction is rarely prescribed. Laser treatment has been shown to shorten the course of an individual attack without affecting the final visual acuity. One study of krypton red laser treatment suggested that treatment with this longer wavelength, with better penetration to the level of the RPE, may in fact reduce the recurrence rate.[78] Treatment is generally deferred for 3 to 4 months to allow spontaneous remission. In cases where prompt visual recovery is important, laser treatment may be considered earlier.

There is no definite association of this disorder with any premorbid refractive error. There is one report of the condition arising in a young boy with Haller-mann-Streiff syndrome and +13 D refractive error.[79] The authors reviewed their 247 cases of central serous chorioretinopathy and found only six with hyperopia greater than +4 D. They concluded that there was no significant association with premorbid hyperopia, although the number of patients with low hyperopia or myopia were not included.

Best Disease

This uncommon macular dystrophy/degeneration is seen primarily in persons of European, African, and Hispanic descent.[80] It is inherited on an autosomal dominant basis with variable expressivity. Presenting findings typically include bilateral, but asymmetric, loss of central acuity and metamorphopsia. The fundus findings evolve from a seemingly normal appearance (with an abnormal electrooculogram [EOG]) to a round atrophic scar, with several stages in between. These intermediate stages include a tiny yellow dot in the fovea (previtelliform), a fried-egg yolk lesion (vitelliform [Fig 48–13]), cyst formation with or without the classic pseudohypopyon, and severe pigment disruption with yellow flecks throughout the macula (scrambled egg). Ultimately, the lesion becomes a punched-out atrophic scar.

The classic yellow deposits represent lipofuscin accumulation, initially at the level of the pigment epithe-lium. The overlying retina remains healthy until later in the disease. Up through the vitelliform and cyst stages, the acuity is near normal as the lipofuscin granules remain entirely within the RPE. For this reason, new cases are rarely diagnosed at these stages. Once "scrambling" occurs, lipofuscin is liberated into the subretinal space, with secondary RPE disruption and damage to the overlying photoreceptors. At this point, acuity begins to diminish, and affected patients report to the ophthalmologist. At its worst, acuity reaches the 20/200 to 20/400 range. In roughly 10% of affected patients, the characteristic lesions are multiple and extrafoveal.[81]

The EOG is characteristically depressed (light-peak to dark-trough ratio of less than 1.5), even in seemingly unaffected carriers. The full-field ERG remains normal. Fortunately, over 85% of affected patients retain at least 20/40 vision in one eye; less than 5% will become legally blind.[82] There is no treatment that successfully halts or reverses visual loss.

An association with hyperopia has been established for many years. Tasman[83] found that 44% of affected patients had hyperopia of at least +3 D. Astigmatism is common as well.[84]

Choroidal Folds

Choroidal folds are a direct manifestation of mechanical distortion of the choroid and overlying Bruch's membrane-RPE complex. They can arise from a variety of conditions and do not represent a specific disorder. The entities commonly associated with choroidal folds include postoperative or posttraumatic hypotony, posterior scleritis, tumors of the choroid or orbit, thyroid

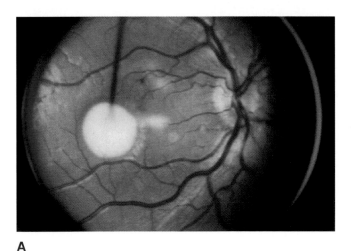

A

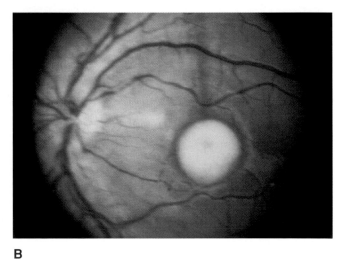

B

Figure 48–13. Best disease. **A.** The vitelliform stage of the disease is the most striking and pathognomonic but is uncommonly seen. **B.** Findings in each eye generally parallel one another, although acuity is typically well preserved in at least one eye.

eye disease, vein occlusions, uveal effusion, scleral buckling surgery, optic disc edema of any etiology, optic disc drusen, choroiditis, and choroidal neovascularization. Each of these diverse disorders causes biomechanical stress within the choroid, resulting in choroidal folds.[85]

The clinical appearance varies from dramatic to quite subtle. Focal lesions (tumors) cause only limited focal folds, while more diffuse processes (posterior scleritis) cause more widespread changes. In the troughs of the folds, the RPE is crowded together, whereas on the crests of the folds, the RPE is stretched thin. This leads to the characteristic alternating dark and light striae seen clinically and angiographically (Fig 48–14). In general, acuity is not affected by choroidal folds, unless folds involve the macula itself. In this case, there may be sufficient distortion of photoreceptors to drop central acuity measurably. Most cases are asymptomatic.

Kalina and Mills[86] originally described the syndrome of acquired hyperopia associated with choroidal folds and no other discernible ocular abnormality. Dailey and associates[87] subsequently defined the syndrome more fully. They reported seven healthy adults with hyperopic shifts in refraction associated with new choroidal folds. CT scanning or B-scan ultrasound testing documented flattening of the posterior sclera, thickening of the choroid, and mild to moderate optic nerve enlargement. Five of 11 also had

a space visible between the optic nerve and its sheath. The authors considered these features characteristic of the syndrome. They reviewed the literature and found that of the 15 patients reported with the syndrome, 14 were men. The only affected woman had primary amenorrhea and was found to have severely atrophic ovaries. Interesting associated findings include mild disc edema, vertical strabismus, focal RPE mottling, and angiographic changes similar to central serous chorioretinopathy. None of the reported patients have developed choroidal neovascularization. The authors found that refractive correction restored excellent acuity, which tended to remain stable over time (although one patient spontaneously remitted after several years, and a second went from unilateral to bilateral involvement).

Acquired Retinoschisis

This interesting degeneration of the peripheral retina has been reported to affect up to 22% of patients over age 40 years.[88] Most autopsy series suggest a lower prevalence, probably between 1% and 5%.[47] Although the term *senile retinoschisis* has been applied in the past (to differentiate the disorder from the juvenile form), true schisis cavities can be seen in patients in their third and fourth decades.[89] Thus, the term *acquired retinoschisis* is probably preferable. Still, the incidence and severity of this condition clearly increase with age.

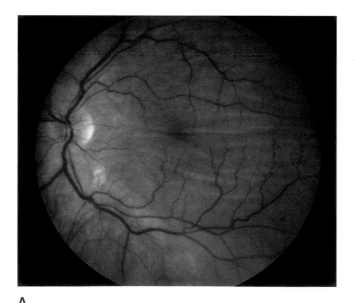

A

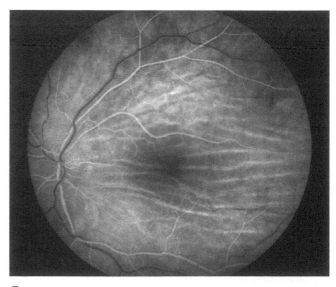

B

Figure 48–14. Idiopathic choroidal folds in a 42-year-old man with an otherwise normal eye examination and newly diagnosed choroidal folds. Visual acuity can be improved from 20/80 to 20/20 with +1.75 D overcorrection. **A.** Note the alternating light and dark striae passing through the macula. **B.** Angiography makes the folds particularly striking.

Retinoschisis means, literally, a splitting of the neural retina. In juvenile retinoschisis, a distinct disorder, the splitting occurs within the nerve fiber layer. In the reticular form, distinguished clinically (in some cases) by fine white lines corresponding to retinal blood vessels and by a particularly transparent inner layer, the schisis cavity is within the nerve fiber layer, similar to juvenile schisis. Most experts agree that the reticular form is more frequently associated with retinal detachment. Both forms are closely associated with peripheral cystoid degeneration of the retina and probably represent the severe end of a common disease spectrum.

Retinoschisis manifests itself clinically as retinal elevation, similar to true retinal detachment (in which there is a physical separation between the RPE and photoreceptors). Unlike retinal detachment, the inner layer of a schisis cavity is quite transparent (particularly in the bullous, reticular type) and immobile (Fig 48–15). Unlike many detachments, the shape and location of a schisis cavity will not change with head movements, and its inner surface is very smooth.

Still, chronic retinal detachment may be quite difficult to distinguish from schisis. Clinical tests to separate the two include perimetry and laser photocoagulation. Because of the electrical discontinuity created within the retina by a schisis cavity, the visual field defect is absolute and has abrupt borders. In retinal detachment, the field defect is relative (because the neural connections to the central nervous system are not broken) with less distinct borders. Laser burns to the outer layer of a schisis cavity should produce a white spot. Laser energy applied to bare RPE through a true detachment will elicit a weak gray burn or no response at all.

There are two important complications of retinoschisis. The first is posterior progression of the schisis cavity with a symptomatic visual field defect. Byer[90] reported that, over 9 years, 3.2% of his patients with retinoschisis experienced posterior progress, 74% of which extended posterior to the equator. Interestingly, none were symptomatic. Hirose and associates[91] followed 696 eyes, with follow-up study ranging from 1 month to 15 years, and found that 14% showed some extension. Macular involvement, greatly feared, is actually quite uncommon. Brockhurst[92] documented only two cases among more than 22,000 patient visits to a tertiary retinal specialty service. Thus, prophylactic laser treatment to prevent posterior progression is probably not indicated.

The second, and more important, complication of retinoschisis is true retinal detachment. Both Byer's[90] and Hirose's[91] surveys reflect that approximately 6% of patients with retinoschisis develop retinal breaks. Unlike true retinal detachment, these breaks are not full thickness but rather are limited to either the outer (3.7%) or inner (1.6%) layer.[91] Rarely (0.8% of affected patients), breaks develop in both outer and inner layers. Both types of breaks may be quite difficult to find clinically. An isolated inner layer break (usually small) leads to communication of the vitreous and schisis cavities but not to true detachment. For detachment to oc-

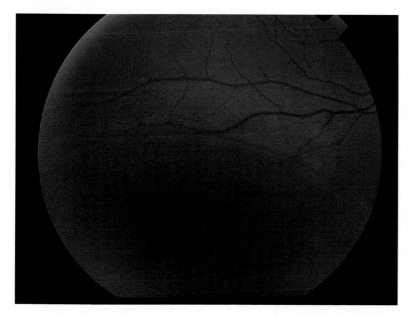

Figure 48–15. Acquired peripheral retinoschisis in a 63-year-old asymptomatic man with +1.75 D refractive error. The smooth, domelike elevation of the retina inferotemporally is characteristic of the disorder.

cur, there must be a break in the outer layer that allows fluid to gain access to the subretinal space. Isolated outer layer breaks (usually larger) allow schisis cavity fluid, generated by the cellular elements of the retina, to leak under the retina and create localized retinal detachments. In this setting, the detachment is generally slow or nonprogressive, with little visual significance.[46,47] In the setting of combined inner and outer layer breaks, however, vitreous fluid can leak through each break into the subretinal space. These detachments may or may not be progressive but are more likely to be so than those associated only with outer layer breaks. Breaks in retinoschisis are responsible for 2% to 3% of progressive retinal detachments,[47,93] while the incidence of progressive detachment in patients with retinoschisis is very low (0.5%).[91]

Many investigators have confirmed that retinoschisis is more common in hyperopes.[47] Hagler and Woldoff[93] reported their experience with 82 phakic eyes with retinoschisis. Sixty-six percent of the eyes were hyperopic, while only 7% were myopic and 27% emmetropic.[93] In another series, the refractive errors ranged from −15 D to +7.25 D, but 83% were in the hyperopic range (0 to +7.25 D).[94]

Because the risk of visual loss due to posterior progression is small, treatment is generally reserved for cases of true retinal detachment. Laser barriers may also be used in the setting of combined inner and outer layer breaks without subretinal fluid, since the risk of progressive detachment is higher. In the setting of a small detachment, laser retinopexy circumscribing the entire area of schisis can prevent spread of subretinal fluid and visual loss. Scleral buckling surgery is required if the area of schisis or detachment is extensive. Extensive detachments with numerous breaks, as well as the rare case of progressive macular schisis, may require vitrectomy with gas-fluid exchange. This surgery will not restore vision in regions of schisis, however, because the neural connections of the retina have been irreversibly interrupted.

Asteroid Hyalosis

In 1894, Benson[95] differentiated asteroid hyalosis from synchysis scintillans, likening the appearance of the vitreous particles to "stars on a clear night." The particles, spherical bodies consisting of calcium soaps and insoluble lipids, are yellow-white and highly refractile. They are generally suspended throughout the vitreous gel, which is otherwise structurally normal.[96] Although they may be somewhat more dense in the inferior vit-

reous cavity, they are largely unaffected by gravity and do not pool inferiorly when the eye is at rest (unlike synchysis scintillans). If sufficiently dense, they may entirely obscure the fundus. Even in these cases, patients are surprisingly undisturbed. It is with great rarity that an affected patient complains of floaters or reduced vision.

The condition is unilateral in 75% of patients, and there is no racial or sexual predilection. The incidence clearly increases with increasing age. Numerous reports have linked the disorder with various metabolic disorders, most notably diabetes and hypercholesterolemia. A controlled study showed that affected patients generally have normal serum calcium levels.[97] Bergen and associates[98] performed a cross-sectional study of over 12,000 patients undergoing examinations in a general eye clinic, identifying 101 (0.83%) with asteroid hyalosis. They found a 29% prevalence of diabetes in affected patients compared with 10% of age-matched controls. Additional significant associations with asteroid hyalosis included arterial hypertension and atherosclerotic heart disease.

In 1987, Weiter and Albert[96] reviewed findings in 30 patients with asteroid hyalosis. Fifteen were hyperopic to some degree (50%), with 12 emmetropes and only 3 myopes. They also found a significantly lower rate of vitreous liquefaction and posterior vitreous separation among affected patients, implying the presence of a particularly solid vitreous gel with firm retinal adhesion. Retinal detachment was particularly uncommon. In Bergen's[98] series of 101 patients, the average refractive error among affected patients was +1.10 D, compared to +0.19 D among the controls. Over 75% were hyperopic to some degree.

Fluorescein angiography is of great help in visualizing fundus details in severe cases, since the barrier and exciter filters optically eliminate the particles. Treatment is rarely indicated, since most patients are blithely unaware of their condition. In severe cases, pars plana vitrectomy can be effective. Vitrectomy is sometimes required to allow adequate laser treatment of diabetic retinopathy as well. The lower incidence of posterior vitreous separation and increased vitreoretinal adherence may increase the risk of postvitrectomy retinal detachment, however.

Nanophthalmos and Uveal Effusions

Nanos is the Greek root, meaning dwarf; thus, nanophthalmos means, literally, dwarf's eye. There is no strict cutoff of axial length defining the syndrome, but eyes that are 21 mm or shorter are generally considered nanophthalmic.[99] The condition may be sporadic or familial (either dominant or recessive). There is no sex predilection (unlike the idiopathic uveal effusion syndrome, which is more common in men).

Because of the short axial length, these eyes are always highly hyperopic (at least +8 D). Every feature of the eye is smaller than normal, with the notable exception of the lens, which is of normal size but much too large for the small AC. Normally, the lens occupies less than 5% of the internal volume of the eye. In nanophthalmos, the lens may represent 11% to 32% of the space,[100] with a significant incidence of pupillary block and angle-closure glaucoma.

It has long been recognized that cataract and filtration procedures on nanopthalmic eyes result in a significant rate of vision-threatening choroidal (uveal) effusions.[101] Effusions can also develop spontaneously. This is because the sclera in patients with this condition is markedly thickened and disorganized histologically.[102] These changes result in significantly increased resistance to vascular flow through the vortex venous system. Osmotically active serum proteins tend to accumulate in the suprachoroidal space as well. These proteins normally exit the eye transsclerally (since there are no lymphatic channels); thicker sclera presents a relative barrier to their diffusion. As they build up in the suprachoroidal space, they create a hydrostatic imbalance and predispose to the formation of effusions, either spontaneous or after trauma (surgical or otherwise).

In 1980, Brockhurst reported on 10 patients with nanophthalmos who had undergone decompression of the vortex veins along with drainage sclerotomics for uveal effusion.[103] Eight cases resulted in complete reattachment. Ten years later he reported on the successful use of vortex vein decompression before planned cataract extraction in patients with nanophthalmos, with a lower rate of postoperative effusion and angle closure.[104]

It is important to realize that some emmetropic or myopic patients can suffer from a similar syndrome that is due to abnormally thick sclera, but without associated nanophthalmos, shortened axial length, and hyperopia. This has been referred to by Gass and Jallow[105] as the idiopathic uveal effusion syndrome. Its implications and treatment strategies are similar to those for patients with nanophthalmos.

Inherited Retinal Degenerations

Myopia is far more commonly associated with inherited retinal degenerations than hyperopia. Conversely, virtually every class of retinal degeneration has been reported in association with myopia, including congenital achromatopsia, congenital stationary night blindness, classic retinitis pigmentosa (Fig 48–16), choroideremia, and gyrate atrophy (see below). In Sieving and Fishman's review[106] of 268 eyes with inherited retinal degenerations, 201 were myopic (75%). The association with myopia may be strongest for congenital stationary night blindness.[107]

The two main exceptions to this rule are Leber's congenital amaurosis and so-called preserved para-arteriolar RPE. Both are autosomal recessive forms of RP and are characterized by moderate to high hyperopia.[108,109] Isolated pedigrees of early-onset autosomal dominant RP[110] and X-linked congenital stationary night blindness,[69] each associated with hyperopia, have been reported as new exceptions to the myopia-RP association.

OPTIC NERVE DISORDERS

A normal retina contains approximately 1 million ganglion cells, each one of which sends a cellular process through the nerve fiber layer into the optic nerve. These fibers all exit the eye through the lamina cribrosa at the optic nerve head. In eyes with abnormally small lamina, the normal complement of nerve fibers will be crowded. The physical crowding of the small optic nerve head predisposes to a variety of alterations in normal axonal function. These so-called discs-at-risk are more likely to be found in eyes with other abnormally small dimensions, including axial length. Thus, axial hyperopes may be at increased risk for two important disorders of small optic nerve heads.

Optic Disc Drusen

Optic disc drusen represent hyaline, calcific deposits within the prelaminar portion of the optic nerve head. They may be buried within its substance (early in life) or exposed at the surface of the disc (as time passes). Like astrocytic hamartomas of the optic nerve head, optic disc drusen may autofluoresce (Fig 48–17). They may be inherited in a dominant fashion. They are associated with retinitis pigmentosa as well. They commonly cause asymptomatic visual field loss, but unless they are associated with vascular occlusion (usually venous) or choroidal neovascularization, they do not threaten central acuity.

It is accepted that they are more common in small, crowded optic nerve heads.[111,112] This is believed to be due to relative impairment of axoplasmic transport by

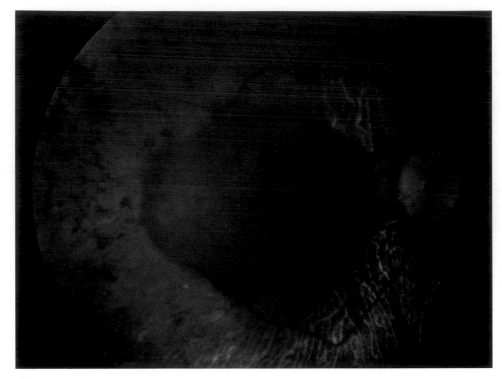

A

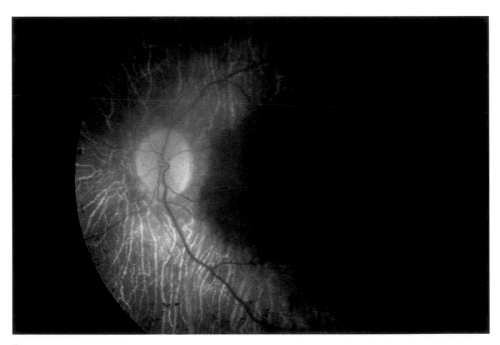

B

Figure 48–16. Retinitis pigmentosa (RP) in a 48-year-old man with recessive RP. **A.** Right eye. **B.** Left eye. Visual acuity is LP OU; manifest retinoscopy is −4.75 D.

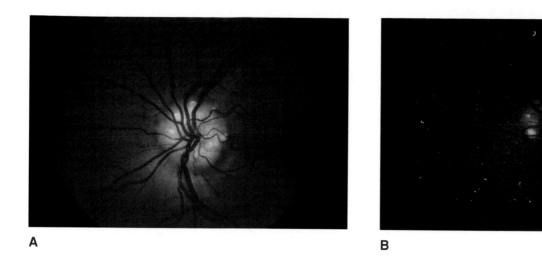

Figure 48–17. Optic disc drusen. **A.** The "rock-candy" appearance of the optic disc makes the presence of disc drusen obvious. **B.** Optic disc drusen may autofluoresce if they are not buried deep within the nerve head. That is, they will "light up" with both barrier and exciter filters in place before fluorescein injection.

the congestion of the crowded nerve head. The connection between hyperopia and disc drusen is disputed, however. Although historically an association has been assumed, more recently, this has been questioned.[113] Strassman and associates[114] reported a case of bilateral disc drusen in a high hyperope and suggested that future studies of refractive error and disc drusen focus on high hyperopes.

Nonarteritic Anterior Ischemic Optic Neuropathy

As with optic disc drusen, patients with a small crowded optic nerve head seem to be at risk for developing a common cause of significant visual loss, nonarteritic anterior ischemic optic neuropathy (AION). This syndrome is well recognized as a leading cause of sudden, painless, monocular visual loss in older adults. Although the peak incidence is in the seventh and eighth decades, it can occur in patients in their late 40s.[115] Acuity can range from normal to NLP, although severe visual losses (LP or NLP) are more common with the arteritic variety. The sine qua non is disc edema (at least for the nonarteritic type); the classic visual field defect is altitudinal. Same-eye recurrences are rare, but 40% of cases become bilateral with time.

The pathogenesis is believed to be related to insufficiency of the posterior ciliary supply to the prelaminar portion of the optic nerve. Systemic associations with AION, including diabetes, hypertension, and atherosclerotic vascular disease, may merely represent the coincidence of various disorders of aging. On the other hand, they may provide important pathogenetic clues.

Small optic nerve size has come to be accepted as important in the pathogenesis of this disorder (Fig 48–18). Beck and colleagues[116] found that the optic cup of the fellow eye is smaller or absent in a significantly higher number of patients with nonarteritic AION than control eyes (or those with arteritic AION). Subsequently, disc area and diameter have been shown to be smaller in nonarteritic AION as well.[117] Thus, in the patient with AION, if the fellow optic nerve is large, with a large cup, nonarteritic disease is less likely and the index of suspicion for giant cell arteritis is higher. With a small fellow optic nerve, nonarteritic disease is possible, but, because giant cell arteritis affects optic nerves of any size, it must still be aggressively ruled out. Thus, the clinical use of this sign is somewhat questionable.

Katz and Spencer[118] have addressed the question of refractive error and nonarteritic AION. They compared the refractive errors of 50 patients with nonarteritic AION and an age- and eye-matched control group. The mean refractive error for the AION patients was +0.26 D, while that of the controls was −0.86 D. The difference of +1.12 D was significant (P = .027). The authors did not conclude if myopia was a protective or hyperopia a predisposing factor. Still, they concluded that eyes with nonarteritic AION tended to be slightly hyperopic.

Idiopathic Intracranial Hypertension (Pseudotumor Cerebri)

This condition is also misleadingly referred to as benign intracranial hypertension. There is little that is be-

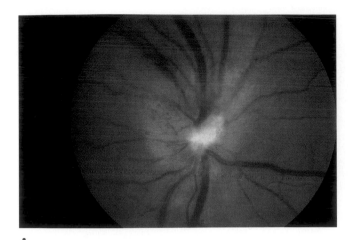

A

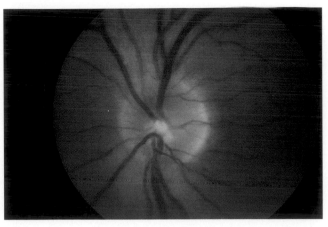

B

Figure 48–18. Nonarteritic anterior ischemic optic neuropathy (AION). This 72-year-old healthy man presented with a 48-hour history of blurred vision in the right eye. Acuity is 20/80, and visual field testing reveals an inferior altitudinal field defect. **A.** Note the (relatively mild) segmental optic disc edema. **B.** Careful examination of the fellow optic nerve head may help differentiate between arteritic and nonarteritic disease. In this case, the fellow nerve is small and crowded, with a glial plug occupying its central portion.

nign about the condition, including its symptoms (disabling headaches and visual loss, including blindness), diagnosis (lumbar puncture), and treatment (carbonic anhydrase inhibitors, lumboperitoneal shunt, or optic nerve sheath fenestration). The disorder affects 1 in 100,000 of the general population and nearly 20 of every 100,000 obese women.[119] An idiopathic disorder that leads to elevated intracranial pressure, it has been associated with the use of numerous medications and the withdrawal of others (corticosteroids). The major symptoms are headache, transient visual observations, horizontal diplopia, pulsatile tinnitus, and neck and back pain. Papilledema is the hallmark (Fig 48–19), although it may be quite asymmetric or even unilateral.

The important permanent sequela of the disease is visual loss. In the neurologic literature, 25% of affected patients suffer some degree of visual loss. Careful ophthalmologic studies have documented a higher rate of visual compromise—as high as 49%, with severe loss in 6% (field constriction to less than the central 10°, or acuity less than 20/200).[120] Orcutt found that high-grade and atrophic papilledema were significant risk factors for visual loss in this condition. Of note, high myopia, along with anemia and older age, were also significant predictors for visual loss. Four of the 135 eyes in the study had myopia greater than −10 D. Three of these had visual field deterioration, and one lost acuity to the 20/200 level. Thus, more aggressive treatment of

pseudotumor cerebri should be considered in the high myope.

SYSTEMIC ASSOCIATIONS

Diabetes Mellitus

Patients with both newly diagnosed and chronic diabetes are subject to unpredictable refractive changes with fluctuations in blood sugar levels. This well-recognized phenomenon, described over 120 years ago,[121] is not completely understood. Since Elschnig's original observations that a myopic shift with acute hyperglycemia is seen only in phakic eyes, it has become widely accepted that the site of diabetic refractive shifts is in the lens, rather than the cornea or axial length. Most reports have dealt with the short-term variations in poorly controlled or recently diagnosed diabetes. More recently, interest has been dedicated to chronic diabetes and permanent refractive changes.

Transient Refractive Shifts

Myopic Shifts

Conventional teaching holds that acute elevation in blood sugar causes a myopic shift with a gradual hyperopic shift back toward the baseline refraction as blood sugar comes under control. This is what Elschnig originally reported and Duke-Elder[121] undertook to ex-

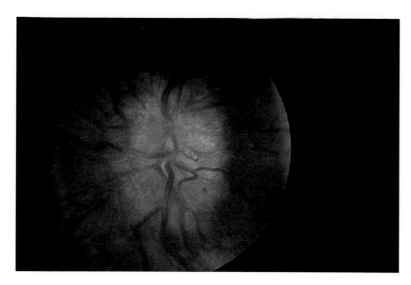

Figure 48–19. True papilledema. This 34-year-old woman presented to her obstetrician complaining of new-onset headaches. A neurologic evaluation was normal, as was CT scanning of the brain. Lumbar puncture documented normal fluid with an opening pressure of 280 mm.

plain. He hypothesized an osmotic imbalance between the lens and aqueous humor, with hyperglycemia leading to lens hydration, decreased radius of curvature, and increased lenticular power.

In its normal state, the lens is in "glucose balance," absorbing glucose from the aqueous at a rate equal to its consumption. In hyperglycemia, lens fibers take on more glucose than is required metabolically, leading to intracellular accumulation of glucose and its metabolic by-products, sorbitol and fructose. Lens fiber membranes are far less permeable to these latter two than glucose, making them more important osmotically.

Osmotic swelling can have varying effects on the refractive power of the lens. In animal studies, intravenously induced hyperglycemia causes a hyperopic shift, and this has become increasingly recognized in humans as well (see below). Most reports of refractive shifts in humans deal with myopic shifts in hyperglycemia. In 1933, Granstrom[122] suggested that newly diagnosed diabetics are more likely to suffer a myopic shift with acute hyperglycemia, while chronic diabetics were more likely to suffer hyperopic variations. He found no changes in corneal curvature, AC depth, or macular changes and ascribed refractive variations to the lens. Other reports have corroborated the myopic shift of hyperglycemia.[123] Gwinup and Villareal[124] induced hyperglycemia intravenously in six phakic type II diabetics and found low-grade myopic shifts in each of the 12 eyes, with a return to baseline 45 minutes after the injection. They estimated that a rise in blood glucose of 100 mg/dl typically caused a −0.5 D shift in refrac-

tive error. Interestingly, the eight aphakic eyes tested became more hyperopic, for unclear reasons (possibly on the basis of microscopic reductions in axial length due to mild retinal swelling).

When hyperglycemia induces myopia, it is believed to be a result of a geometric change in the lens, namely, decreased radii of curvature of the anterior and posterior lens capsules. This shift may be perceived as blurry vision by the young emmetrope or improved reading vision by the presbyope.

Hyperopic Shifts

Although clinical experience has emphasized this tendency for a myopic shift with hyperglycemia, there are several reports of hyperopic shifts that regressed gradually in association with the achievement of long-term euglycemia.

In 1944, Bellows[125] was the first to suggest that hyperopia was the more common direction for diabetic refractive shifts. In 1956, Rosen[126] reported on a single patient with a documented hyperopic shift due to hyperglycemia, and Planten[127] subsequently reported that 21 of 23 hyperglycemic patients became transiently hyperopic. Two additional studies have added 22 additional patients with hyperglycemic hyperopia to this group.[128,129] Even though some of the patients have clearly had a hyperopic shift during untreated hyperglycemia, most of the reports document new symptomatic hyperopia commensurate with the onset of therapy, usually insulin.[130] Even in these cases, however, the hyperopia regressed (ie, the eyes became more myopic) as blood sugar normalized over days to weeks.

In the most recent series, Saito and associates[129] documented increased lens thickness and decreased AC depth during the hyperopic period, supporting the proposed mechanism of hyperglycemic refractive shifts—that is, osmotic lens swelling.

But if osmotic lens swelling acts to decrease the crystalline lens' radius of curvature, thus increasing its refractive power, how can a larger lens create a hyperopic shift? To answer this apparent paradox, it is important to realize that the refractive power of any lens is a combination of its radius of curvature and its index of refraction. Obviously, imbibition of water by the crystalline lens will lead to a reduction in its refractive index. This will decrease the lens power, resulting in a hyperopic shift. If the curvature change associated with oxmotic swelling outweighs the drop in refractive index, the net result will be a hyperglycemic myopic shift. If, on the other hand, the change in refractive index outweighs that of curvature, then hyperglycemia will result in new, transient hyperopia.

Which factor predominates varies among patients, partly explaining the discrepancy in the literature. Obviously, any type of refractive shift, including astigmatic changes, can occur with disturbances in blood glucose. New onset of blurry vision due to refractive error in a known diabetic should imply instability in blood sugar levels. Prescription of refractive correction or refractive surgery is clearly unwise during a period of known or anticipated blood sugar swings. Likewise, this discussion should also serve to underline the importance of suspecting new-onset diabetes in any patient suffering an abrupt change in refractive error, regardless of its direction.

One other, less common mechanism for a hyperopic shift in newly diagnosed diabetics is accommodative paresis. It has been reported to affect as many as 19% of all new diabetics and 77% of diabetic patients less than 30 years of age with refractive changes.[131] Usually the change occurs when insulin therapy is started and disappears over 2 to 6 weeks. In this setting, not only is additional hyperopic correction needed for best vision, but accommodative amplitudes are clearly decreased, as is uncorrected near vision. It is important to realize that scatter laser treatment for proliferative diabetic retinopathy can cause transient accommodative paresis as well, with an accompanying transient hyperopic shift.

As discussed above, acute iatrogenic hyperglycemia has been shown to induce hyperopia in aphakic eyes.[124] The mechanism is unclear.

Permanent Myopia

Only more recently has the increased incidence of permanent myopia among diabetics been recognized. Fledelius[132] was the first to demonstrate this. His review of 2832 eyes included 762 diabetic eyes. With age-matched controls, diabetics were significantly more likely to have a myopic refractive error than nondiabetics (37.9% versus 27.5%). Of note, the myopia was nearly always mild (less than −2.0 D). A second study by the same author showed that this permanent diabetic myopia was more often of adult onset (after 20 years of age) than myopia in nondiabetics.[133] With subsequent ultrasound information, Fledelius showed that, when compared with nondiabetics with similar refractive errors, the lenses of diabetics were significantly thicker (mean difference, 0.2 mm).[134] Lens thickness correlated positively with duration of diabetes. He ascribed the low-grade, adult-onset myopia of diabetes to this lens thickening.

Myopia and Diabetic Retinopathy

In 1967, Jain and associates[135] were the first to suggest that myopia may be associated with less progressive diabetic retinopathy. In their study, myopes of greater than −5 D were less likely to develop retinopathy. In 1985, Rand[136] demonstrated an increased risk of proliferative retinopathy in association with HLA-DR phenotypes 3/0, 4/0, and x/s (non 3 or 4). Interestingly the risk was negated by myopia as low as −2 D.[136] This relationship was shown to be important for nonproliferative disease as well, in a second study.[137] Of further interest, myopia did not lessen severity of retinopathy among patients with the nonsusceptible HLA phenotype. The authors invoked possible ocular (reduced retinal perfusion in myopes) and nonocular causes for myopia's effect on the natural history of diabetic retinopathy in genetically susceptible individuals.

Acquired Immunodeficiency Syndrome

Blurred vision and photophobia are among the most common ocular complaints of patients with acquired immunodeficiency syndrome (AIDS). New-onset and rapidly progressive myopia have been reported in patients with human immunodeficiency virus (HIV) infection.[138] Associated infections and the use of multiple potent medications may be important, but the exact incidence and etiology of the myopia seen in patients with AIDS is unclear.

Albinism

Albinism is a inherited disorder of melanin synthesis that causes hypopigmentation systemically. When eyes, skin, and hair seem equally affected, the disorder is referred to as oculocutaneous albinism. When the eyes are significantly more affected than skin and hair (which may appear normal), it is referred to as ocular albinism. Both disorders are inherited on an autosomal recessive basis, except for the Nettleship-Falls variety of ocular albinism, which is X-lined recessive. Estimates of prevalence range from 1 in 5000 to 1 in 100,000, depending on the variant. For a comprehensive discussion of the disorder, excellent reviews are available.[139]

Ocular findings include moderately or severely reduced vision, nystagmus, hypopigmented irides with prominent transillumination, and sometimes foveal hypoplasia. The fundus is usually strikingly blond with visible choroidal vessels and sclera. Visual pathway alterations include excessive chiasmal decussation of temporal retinal ganglion cell axons, lateral geniculate disorganization, and optic tract changes.

Carriers of the recessive conditions (most often female carriers of the X-linked variety) may show partial iris transillumination and unusual areas of RPE hypopigmentation.

Systemic findings in oculocutaneous albinism include deafness, progressive neurologic dysfunction, and mental retardation.[69] Two forms of albinism are potentially lethal. The Hermansky-Pudlak variant includes a coagulopathy with bleeding diatheses and easy bruisability. In Chediak-Higashi syndrome, there is granulocyte dysfunction with recurrent sinopulmonary infections and high incidence of various refractive errors in albinism. In one review, five of 16 albino patients were myopic (31%), two of whom were highly myopic (> -12 D).[140]

Pierre Robin Syndrome

This is a well-recognized branchial arch malformation syndrome. Incomplete development of the first branchial arch causes mandibular hypoplasia, with secondary glossoptosis and cleft palate. Ears are typically low set, and congenital heart and neurologic disease are common.

Ophthalmic abnormalities include megalocornea, cataract, and vitreoretinal degeneration with retinal detachment.[69] Congenital glaucoma is quite common. Al-

though high myopia has been reported,[141] it may be a secondary manifestation of the glaucoma rather than a primary part of the malformation sequence.

Wagner's and Stickler's Syndromes

Historically, these entities have generally been considered as part of the same disease spectrum.[142] However, there are two important differences between the disorders that clearly distinguish them from one another. First, although ocular findings in each may be quite similar, the risk of retinal detachment for patients with Wagner's syndrome is not higher than that of the general population, while patients with Stickler's syndrome have a 50% lifetime risk. Second, in Wagner's syndrome, the findings are limited to the eye; in Stickler's syndrome, there are prominent abnormalities of the musculoskeletal system, reflecting a systemic abnormality in collagen synthesis.

The features common to the two disorders include a high incidence of myopia (greater than 50%), posterior subcapsular cataract, and the hallmark of the disorders—so-called optically empty vitreous degeneration with epiretinal membranes and latticelike changes.[47] The retina undergoes progressive pigmentary degeneration with loss of ERG waveforms and vascular sheathing, while there is also progressive choroidal atrophy. The myopia of these disorders is often severe (> -6 D). Both are inherited in an autosomal dominant pattern.

In Stickler's syndrome (also known as hereditary artho-ophthalmopathy), the preretinal vitreous membranes contract and create irregular, often posterior, retinal breaks, which typically progress to retinal detachment. Giant retinal tears are more common in this disorder as well. Nonocular findings include facial malformations identical to Pierre Robin syndrome, cleft palate, hearing loss, and skeletal abnormalities—loose joints, marfanoid habitus, arachnodactyly, and kyphoscoliosis. The disorder is inherited on an autosomal dominant basis, with extremely variable expressivity and nearly complete penetrance. It is hypothesized that the abnormalities are due to aberrant synthesis of type II collagen.[143]

Other entities that could be confused with these vitreoretinal degenerations include juvenile retinoschisis (usually hyperopic or emmetropic), Marfan syndrome (ectopia lentis), and Ehlers-Danlos syndrome (retinal detachment only seen in type VI). Generally, the systemic manifestations will distinguish each. Note

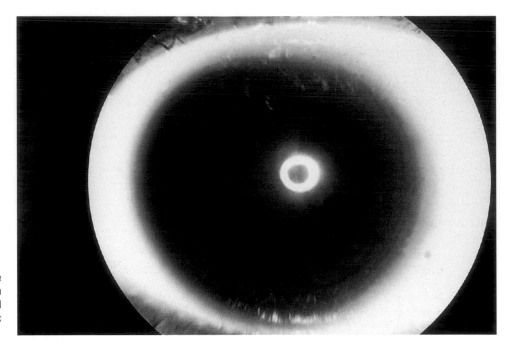

Figure 48–20. Marfan syndrome. The lens in this high myope (axial length 27 mm) dislocated temporally and posteriorly. Acuity with an aphakic contact lens is 20/20.

that life expectancy in patients with Wagner's and Stickler's syndromes is normal.

Marfan Syndrome

This is another autosomal dominant disorder of the eyes and musculoskeletal system associated with myopia and retinal detachment. The condition is named for a French pediatrician who described it in 1896, but an earlier report documented what is probably the same condition.[47] Although there is some overlap of Stickler's and Marfan syndromes (tall slender habitus with long limbs and arachnodactyly), characteristic radiologic findings distinguish the former, while the latter is associated with serious, often fatal, cardiovascular problems. Furthermore, ectopia lentis is not normally seen as part of Stickler's syndrome but is one of the hallmarks of Marfan syndrome (Fig 48–20). The most typical direction for lens dislocation in this syndrome is superotemporally.

Axial myopia is very common in patients with Marfan syndrome, often apparent by age 5 years. Over 20% of patients are highly myopic. The findings of ectopia lentis and retinal detachment are positively correlated with increasing axial length. The incidence of retinal detachment is also increased by ectopia lentis or cataract extraction. This probably reflects increased vitreous liquefaction due to disruption of the posterior capsule–zonular barrier. In Maumenee's[144] series of 160 affected patients, no patient with normal axial length

developed a retinal detachment. Furthermore, each of the 16 eyes that did develop retinal detachment had ectopia lentis.

The cardiovascular complications of the disorder may overshadow any ocular findings. Abnormal dilatation of the aortic root can lead to aortic valvular insufficiency and dissecting thoracic aortic aneurysm, which may be suddenly fatal. The life expectancy of patients with Marfan syndrome is greatly reduced, with 50% of male patients dead by age 41 and 50% of women by age 49.[145] Mitral valve disease, although less dramatic and severe than aortic valve disease, may be more common.

The newly diagnosed high myope with any marfanoid changes must undergo a comprehensive family history and medical evaluation to rule out significant cardiovascular disease.

Weill-Marchesani Syndrome

Patients with Weill-Marchesani syndrome, another inherited cause of ectopia lentis, are easily differentiated from those with Marfan syndrome. First, the inheritance is autosomal recessive. More obviously, these patients are usually short, with abnormally stiff limbs.

There are ocular differences as well. The myopia in this condition is not axial, as in Marfan syndrome. Rather, it is purely a curvature myopia, due to microspherophakia and increased lenticular refractive power.[69] The severity of myopia varies from moderate to extremely high (−20 D). Microspherophakia should be suspected if the equator of the lens can be seen through a dilated pupil. With ectopia lentis, the risk of retinal detachment and acute angle-closure glaucoma rises.

Down Syndrome

This well-known inherited complex is the most common chromosomal syndrome. Its incidence strongly depends on maternal age. With advancing age, nondisjunction of the 21st chromosome becomes more likely, resulting in Down syndrome. Five percent of cases are due to an inherited translocation between chromosome 21 and either chromosome 15 or 22 and are independent of maternal age. This subset of Down syndrome can subsequently be inherited on a dominant basis. Thus, karyotyping is important in genetic counseling.

The systemic findings are well recognized. They include short stature, flattened occiput with low-set ears, and a small nose. The tongue is large and fissured with glossoptosis. Feet are short, and the hands show an exaggerated simian crease. Abdominal protuberance may be associated with umbilical hernia. Hypotonia and seizures are common. Congenital heart disease and cryptorchidism are common associated problems as well.[69]

Ocular findings are also well known. Epicanthal folds are seen in a minority of affected patients, but the "mongoloid" slant (upwardly displaced lateral canthi) and hypertelorism are quite characteristic. Blepharitis and ectropion complicate external disease. Esotropia is common. Keratoconus can be seen in patients with Down syndrome, possibly related to eye rubbing. Brushfield spots are whitish yellow nodules at the junction of the outer third of the iris. They can be seen, generally in small numbers, in 15% to 20% of the normal population. In patients with Down syndrome, the lesions are numerous, arranged concentric with the pupil. Histologically, they represent focal accumulations of extracellular matrix material within the iris stroma.

Myopia is significantly more common in patients with Down syndrome. One review cited a 50% prevalence of myopia (15% of hyperopia).[146] Another reported that 35% of Down syndrome patients were highly myopic, although the definition of high myopia was not stated.[147] More recently, Shapiro and France[148] reported that 27% of patients had myopia of −5 D or greater.

Alport's Syndrome

This inherited oculorenal syndrome is part of the differential for bilateral congenital cataract. The most common pattern of inheritance is autosomal dominant, but recessive pedigrees, both autosomal and X-linked, have been described.[69] Synthesis of certain basement membranes, particularly glomerular, is impaired. The lenticular basement membrane may also be involved, leading to anterior lenticonus (Fig 48–21A) and anterior polar cataract (Fig 48–21B). Systemic manifestations include asymmetric hearing loss and chronic renal failure with hematuria, proteinuria, and uremia by early to mid-adulthood.

Ocular manifestations include the characteristic lens changes, along with calcium crystalline deposits in the conjunctiva and retina (Figs 48–21C and D). Juvenile corneal arcus, pigment dispersion, and angle-closure glaucoma may also be seen. Along with crystals, there is a nonprogressive pigmentary retinopathy. Optic nerve drusen can be seen as well.

The lens changes induce a curvature type of myopia.[69] The retinal findings do not increase the risk of rhegmatogenous retinal detachment. As with other types of lenticular myopia, the best refractive surgery may be lens extraction.

Fetal Alcohol Syndrome

This is another not uncommon but poorly understood congenital complex that has been linked to excessive maternal consumption of alcohol during pregnancy. Incidence is from 1 to 5 per 1000 live births.[149] Systemic features include mental retardation, low birth weight, short stature, cardiovascular and skeletal anomalies, behavioral instability, and thin vermillion borders. Ophthalmic findings include blepharophimosis, telecanthus, strabismus, anterior segment dysgenesis, and optic nerve hypoplasia.

One study has reported eight of nine fetal alcohol syndrome patients with myopia as high as −18 D. The type of myopia or associated fundus findings were not described.[150]

Congenital Rubella

This potentially devastating congenital infection has become significantly less common with routine vaccination for the rubella virus.[151] Still, maternal infection with the virus during pregnancy, particularly during the first trimester, can result in fetal transmission with significant morbidity or even fetal death. Systemic

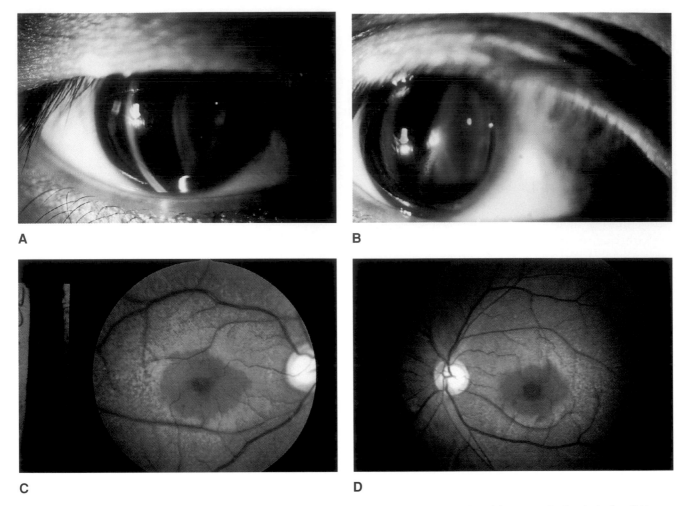

Figure 48–21. Alport's syndrome. **A.** The excessive curvature of the anterior lens capsule may be subtle on examination (note the slight forward bowing of the slit beam) but obvious as a curvature myopia. **B.** The anterior polar cataract is often unimportant visually. **C.** The crystalline retinopathy is not significant visually and does not increase the risk of retinal detachment. **D.** The crystals impart a fine sheen to the retina, sparing the macula in this patient.

manifestations include hearing loss, retardation, congenital heart disease, anemia, hepatitis, pneumonitis, and diabetes.

The ocular findings are numerous, including microphthalmia, corneal leukoma, chronic uveitis, cataracts, and "salt and pepper" retinopathy. Glaucoma is uncommon, except in association with microphthalmia.

The myopia in patients with congenital rubella is usually moderate or high. Myopia of −6 D or greater, seen in 1.9% of healthy newborns,[152] is found in more than 4% of patients with congenital rubella.[153]

Gyrate Atrophy

Although this disorder is caused by a systemic deficiency of a mitochondrial enzyme (ornithine-oxalate-aminotransferase), the ocular findings greatly over-shadow the impact of the systemic findings (alopecia and muscle weakness). The autosomal recessive inborn error of metabolism leads to hyperornithinemia. The ocular manifestations consist of a relentlessly progressive tapetoretinal degeneration (rod and cone loss) and cataract (posterior sutural). The geographic areas of progressive RPE atrophy are strikingly characteristic of the disorder, but electroretinography is required to confirm the diagnosis.

Myopia is seen in the majority of affected patients, with one review claiming a 90% prevalence.[30] The degree of myopia is usually moderate or high.

Cerebral Palsy

This is a heterogeneous group of disorders characterized by motor and cognitive impairment that can be congenital or acquired early in childhood. The simple name belies the diversity of etiologies and is somewhat misleading but firmly entrenched.[154] Different classification schema have been offered. The simplest is by the date of onset—that is, congenital versus acquired. A more common one is by pattern of motor involvement: paraplegic (legs only), diplegic (legs greater than arms), and generalized (including cranial nerves). In their studies of the prevalence of various refractive errors in cerebral palsy (CP), Fantl and Perlstein[155] have divided the disorders into three groups based on the most prominent type of motor abnormality: spastic, dyskinetic, and ataxic. The spastic pattern, accounting for 60% of affected children, is characterized by increased stretch reflexes compatible with an upper motor neuron lesion within the pyramidal tract. The dyskinetic pattern, seen in 35%, is dominated by abnormal amounts and types of spontaneous movements (choreoathetoid, rigidity, tremor), probably secondary to lesions in the extrapyramidal systems (basal ganglia). Ataxic CP is the rarest, affecting only 5% of children with CP. It is characterized by signs of cerebellar involvement.

Each of the various classes of CP share a basic pathophysiology. Intrauterine, peripartum, or postnatal hypoxia leads to ischemic necrosis of a portion of the central nervous system, resulting in the typical patterns of motor involvement, with or without significant cognitive loss. The list of maternal, fetal, and neonatal disorders that can lead to hypoxic insult is very long but includes preeclampsia and eclampsia, dystocia of any cause, prematurity, neonatal infections, and neonatal jaundice. In many cases, no clear precipitant can be identified.

Fantl and Perlstein performed a preliminary study in 1961[153] that was subsequently corroborated by a larger, more definitive one in 1967.[1] They performed cycloplegic refractions on 417 affected children and found that higher degrees of hyperopia were more common in children with CP than in healthy children; 27.3% of their cases were +2.0 D or greater, compared with 2% to 15% of a group of healthy children. Low hyperopia was less common in CP—49.7% versus 64% to 88% of healthy children. High myopia was also slightly more common in affected children—3.8% versus 0.5% to 1.0%. They analyzed the refractions with regard to the type of CP and the underlying etiology. Confirming theories previously formulated, they found that the tendency for high hyperopia was greatest in the dyskinetic type of cerebral palsy, typically associated with neonatal causes of hypoxia. Conversely, the tendency toward high myopia seemed to be associated with the spastic pattern of CP, which usually devel-

TABLE 48–1. MEDICAMENTOSA: SOME MEDICATIONS ASSOCIATED WITH TEMPORARY MYOPIA

ACTH
Acetazolamide
Aconitine
Arsenicals
Aspirin
Chlorthalidone (Hygroton)
Dichlorphenamide
Digitalis and derivatives
Ethoxzolamide
Hexamethonium
Hydralazine
Hydrochlorothiazide
Isosorbide (Isordil)
Isotretinoin (Accutane)
Methylene blue
Morphine
Penicillamine
Phenothiazines
Prednisone
Prochlorperazine (Compazine)
Promethazine hydrochloride (Phenergan)
Spironolactone
Sulfonamides
Tetracyclines
Trichlormethiazide

Abbreviation: ACTH = adrenocorticotropic hormone.

oped following a prenatal insult (toxemia, dystocia, prematurity). Not surprisingly, insults occurring well after childbirth did not seem to have any effect on the development of refraction. That is, on the basis of refraction, children with acquired CP are indistinguishable from normal children.

Reversible Myopia and Pseudomyopia

Many medications have been reported to cause reversible myopia.[30] Table 48–1 includes a partial list. Mechanisms include ciliary body edema with anterior displacement of the lens and ciliary spasm.

Systemic illness can induce ciliary spasm,[69] most commonly syphilis, encephalitis, and myasthenia gravis. Severe metabolic akalosis (diarrhea), diphtheria and influenza infections, jaundice, labyrinthitis, and severe systemic edema have also been associated with a reversible (pseudo) myopia.

REFERENCES

1. Fantl EW, Perlstein MA. Refractive errors in cerebral palsy. Their relationship to the causes of brain damage. *Am J Ophthalmol.* 1967;63:857.

2. Framingham Eye Study. VII Visual acuity. *Surv Ophthalmol.* 1980;24:472.

3. Thomas JV. Primary open angle glaucoma. In: Albert DM, Jakobiec FA, eds. *Principles and Practice of Ophthalmology.* Philadelphia: Saunders; 1993:1342–1345.

4. Tomlinson A, Phillips CJ. Applanation tension and axial length of the eyeball. *Br J Ophthalmol.* 1970;54:548.

5. Podos SM, Becker B, Morton WR. High myopia and primary open angle glaucoma. *Am J Ophthalmol.* 1966;62:1039.

6. Daubs JG, Crick RP. Effect of refractive error on the risk of ocular hypertension and open angle glaucoma. *Trans Ophthal Soc UK.* 1981;101:121.

7. Perkins ES, Phelps CD. Open angle glaucoma, ocular hypertension, low-tension glaucoma, and refraction. *Arch Ophthalmol.* 1982;100:1464.

8. Mastropasqua L, Lobefalo L, Mancini A, Ciancaglini M, Palma S. Prevalence of myopia in open angle glaucoma. *Eur J Ophthalmol.* 1992;2:33.

9. Wilson MR, Hertzmark E, Walker AM, Childs-Shaw K, Epstein DL. A case-control study of risk factors in open angle glaucoma. *Arch Ophthalmol.* 1987;105:1066.

10. Greve EL, Furuno F. Myopia and glaucoma. *Arch Exp Ophthalmol.* 1980;213:33.

11. Phelps CD. Effect of myopia on prognosis in treated primary open-angle glaucoma. *Am J Ophthalmol.* 1982;93:622.

12. Sugar HS. Concerning the chamber angle. I. Gonioscopy. *Am J Ophthalmol.* 1940;23:853.

13. Sugar HS, Barbour FA. Pigmentary glaucoma: a rare clinical entity. *Am J Ophthalmol.* 1949;32:90.

14. Richardson TM. Pigmentary dispersion syndrome and glaucoma. In: Albert DM, Jakobiec FA, eds. *Principles and Practice of Ophthalmology.* Philadelphia: Saunders; 1993:1414–1426.

15. Linner E. The association of ocular hypertension with the exfoliation syndrome, the pigmentary dispersion syndrome and myopia. *Surv Ophthalmol.* 1980;25:145.

16. Francois J. Cortisone et tension oculaire. *Ann Ocul.* 1954;187:805.

17. Arrigg CA. Corticosteroid-induced glaucoma. In: Albert DM, Jakobiec FA, eds. *Principles and Practice of Ophthalmology.* Philadelphia: Saunders; 1993:1462–1467.

18. Wang RF, Guo BK. Steroid-induced ocular hypertension in high myopia. *China Med J.* 1984;97:24.

19. Cherny M, Brooks AMV, Gillies WE. Progressive myopia in early onset chronic angle closure glaucoma. *Br J Ophthalmol.* 1992;76:758.

20. Melamed S, Ashkenazi I. Juvenile-onset open-angle glaucoma. In: Albert DM, Jakobiec FA, eds. *Principles and Practice of Ophthalmology.* Philadelphia: Saunders; 1993:1345–1350.

21. Goldwyn R, Waltman SR, Becker B. Primary open angle glaucoma in adolescents and young adults. *Arch Ophthalmol.* 1970;84:579.

22. Melamed S, Latina MA, Epstein DL. Neodymium-YAG laser trabeculopuncture in juvenile open-angle glaucoma. *Ophthalmology.* 1987;94:163.

23. Stamper RL, McMenemy MG, Lieberman MF. Hypotonus maculopathy after trabeculectomy with subconjunctival 5-fluorouracil. *Am J Ophthalmol.* 1992;

24. Campbell DG. Primary angle-closure glaucoma. In: Albert DM, Jakobiec FA, eds. *Principles and Practice of Ophthalmology.* Philadelphia: Saunders; 1993:1365–1368.

25. Lowe R. Causes of shallow anterior chamber in primary angle-closure glaucoma: ultrasonic biometry of normal and angle-closure glaucoma eyes. *Am J Ophthalmol.* 1969;67:87.

26. Campbell DG. Primary angle-closure glaucoma. In: Albert DM, Jakobiec FA, eds. *Principles and Practice of Ophthalmology.* Philadelphia: Saunders; 1993:1372.

27. Storey J, Phillips CI. Ocular dimensions in angle-closure glaucoma. *Br J Physiol Opt.* 1971;26:228.

28. Epstein DL. Angle-closure glaucoma. In: Epstein DL, ed. *Chandler and Grant's Glaucoma.* Philadelphia: Lea & Febiger; 1986:249.

29. Soubrane G, Coscas G. Choroidal neovascular membrane in degenerative myopia. In: Ryan SJ, ed. *Retina,* vol. 2. St. Louis, MO: Mosby; 1989:201–217.

30. Curtin BJ. *The Myopias: Basic Science and Clinical Management.* Philadelphia: Harper & Row; 1985.

31. Green JL, Rabb MF. Degeneration of Bruch's membrane and retinal pigment epithelium. *Int Ophthalmol Clin.* 1981;21:27.

32. Noble KG, Carr RE. Pathologic myopia. *Ophthalmology.* 1982;89:1099.

33. Pruett RC, Weiter JJ, Goldstein RB. Myopic cracks, angioid streaks, and traumatic tears in Bruch's membrane. *Am J Ophthalmol.* 1987;103:537.

34. Fuchs E. Der centrale schwarze Fleck bei Myopie. *Z Augenheilkd.* 1901;5:171.

35. Hotchkiss ML, Fine SL. Pathologic myopia and choroidal neovascularization. *Am J Ophthalmol.* 1981;91:177.

36. Fried M, Siebert A, Meyer-Schwickerath G, Wessing A. Natural history of Fuchs' spot: a long-term follow-up study. *Doc Ophthalmol Proc Series.* 1981;28:215.

37. Avila MP, Weiter JJ, Jalkh AE, Trempe CL, Pruett RC, Schepens CL. Natural history of choroidal neovascularization in degenerative myopia. *Ophthalmology.* 1984;91:1573.

38. Klein RM, Curtin BJ. Lacquer crack lesions in pathologic myopia. *Am J Ophthalmol.* 1975;79:386.

39. Hampton GR, Kohn D, Bird AC. Visual prognosis of disciform degeneration in myopia. *Ophthalmology.* 1983;90:923.

40. Curtin BJ. The posterior staphyloma of pathologic myopia. *Trans Am Ophthalmol Soc.* 1977;75:67.

41. Soubrane G, Pison J, Bornert P, Perrenoud F, Coscas G. Neo-vaisseux sous-retiniens de la myopie degenerative:

resultats de la photocoagulation. *Bull Soc Ophthalmol Fr.* 1986;86:269.

42. Jalkh AE, Weiter JJ, Trempe CL, Pruett RC, Schepens CL. Choroidal neovascularization in degenerative myopia: role of laser photocoagulation. *Ophthalmic Surg.* 1987; 18:721.

43. Macular Photocoagulation Study Group. Visual outcome after laser photocoagulation for subfoveal choroidal neovascularization secondary to age-related macular degeneration. The influence of initial lesion size and initial visual acuity. *Arch Ophthalmol.* 1994; 112:480.

44. Gonin J. Pathogenie et anatomie pathologique dues decollements retiniens. *Bull Mem Soc d'Ophtalmol.* 1920;33:1.

45. Lindner K. Zur Klinik des Glaskorpers III, Glaskorper und Nezhautabhebung. *Arch Ophthalmol.* 1937;137:157.

46. Byer NE. Lattice degeneration of the retina. *Surv Ophthalmol.* 1979;23:213.

47. Michels RG, Wilkinson CP, Rice TA. *Retinal Detachment.* St. Louis, MO: Mosby; 1990:49–76, 104–117, 137–139.

48. Byer NE. Clinical study of lattice degeneration of the retina. *Trans Am Acad Ophthalmol Otolaryngol.* 1965;69: 1064.

49. Hyams SW, Neumann E. Peripheral retina in myopia; with particular reference to retinal breaks. *Br J Ophthalmol.* 1969;53:300.

50. Byer NE. Changes in and prognosis of lattice degeneration of the retina. *Trans Am Acad Ophthalmol Otolaryngol.* 1974;78:114.

51. Ogawa A, Tanaka M. The relationship between refractive errors and retinal detachment—analysis of 1166 retinal detachment cases. *Jpn J Ophthalmol.* 1988;32:310.

52. Bohringer HR. Statistische zu Haufigkeit und Risiko der Netzhautablosung. *Ophthalmologica.* 1956;131:331.

53. Koch DD, Liu JF, Gill EP, Parke DW. Axial myopia increases the risk of retinal complications after neodymium-YAG laser posterior capsulotomy. *Arch Ophthalmol.* 1989;107:986.

54. Morita H, Ideta H, Ito K, Yonemoto J, Sasaki K, Tanaka S. Causative factors of retinal detachment in macular holes. *Retina.* 1991;11:281.

55. Karlin DB, Curtin BJ. Axial length measurements and peripheral fundus changes in the myopic eye. In: Pruett RC, Regan CDJ, eds. *Retina Congress.* New York: Appleton-Century-Crofts; 1974.

56. Freeman HM. Fellow eyes of giant retinal breaks. *Trans Am Ophthalmol Soc.* 1978;76:343.

57. Nozik RA, Dorsch W. A new chorioretinopathy associated with anterior uveitis. *Am J Ophthalmol.* 1973; 76:758.

58. Singerman LJ. Discussion of Morgan CM, Schatz H. Recurrent multifocal choroiditis. *Ophthalmology.* 1986;93: 1138.

59. Morgan CM, Schatz H. Recurrent multifocal choroiditis. *Ophthalmology.* 1986;93:1138.

60. Doran RML, Hamilton AM. Disciform macular degeneration in young adults. *Trans Ophthalmol Soc UK.* 1982; 102:471.

61. Watzke RC, Packer AJ, Folk JC, et al. Punctate inner choroidopathy. *Am J Ophthalmol.* 1984;98:572.

62. Scheider A. Multifocal inner choroiditis. *Ger J Ophthalmol.* 1993;2:1.

63. Deutsch TA, Tessler HH. Inflammatory pseudohistoplasmosis. *Ann Ophthalmol.* 1985;17:461.

64. Tolentino FI, Brockhurst RJ. Unilateral scleral icterus due to choroidal hemorrhage. *Arch Ophthalmol.* 1963;70:358.

65. McMeel WJ. Uveal circulatory problems. In: Albert DM, Jakobiec FA, eds. *Principles and Practice of Ophthalmology.* Philadelphia: Saunders; 1993:379–386.

66. Hawkins WR, Schepens CL. Choroidal detachment and retinal surgery: a clinical and experimental study. *Am J Ophthalmol.* 1966;62:812.

67. Speaker MD, Guerriero PN, Met JA, et al. A case-control study of risk factors for intraoperative suprachoroidal expulsive hemorrhage. *Ophthalmology.* 1991;98:202.

68. Palmer EA, Flynn JT, Hardy RJ, et al. Incidence and early course of retinopathy of prematurity. *Ophthalmology.* 1991;98:1628.

69. Fong DS, Pruett RC. Systemic associations with myopia. In: Albert DM, Jakobiec FA, eds. *Principles and Practice of Ophthalmology.* Philadelphia: Saunders; 1993:3142–3151.

70. Gordon RA, Donzis PB. Myopia associated with retinopathy of prematurity. *Ophthalmology.* 1986;93:1953.

71. Sarks SH, Sarks JP. Age-related macular degeneration: atrophic form. In Ryan SJ, ed. *Retina.* St. Louis, MO: Mosby; 1989:149–173.

72. Marshall J. The aging retina: physiology or pathology. *Eye.* 1987;1:282.

73. Gass JD. Drusen and disciform macular detachment and degeneration. *Arch Ophthalmol.* 1973;90:206.

74. Elman MJ, Fine SL. Exudative age-related macular degeneration. In: Ryan SJ, ed. *Retina.* St. Louis, MO: Mosby; 1989:175–200.

75. Weiter JJ, Delori FC, Wing GL, Fitch KA. Relationship of senile macular degeneration to ocular pigmentation. *Am J Ophthalmol.* 1985;99:285.

76. The Eye Disease Case-Control Study Group: Risk factors for neovascular age-related macular degeneration. *Arch Ophthalmol.* 1992;10:1701.

77. Sandberg MA, Tolentino MJ, Miller S, Berson E, Gaudio AR. Hyperopia and neovascularization in age-related macular degeneration. *Ophthalmology.* 1993;100:1009.

78. Novak MA, Singerman LJ, Rice TA. Krypton and argon laser photocoagulation for central serous chorioretinopathy. *Retina.* 1987;7:162.

79. Blair NP, Brockhurst RJ, Lee W. Central serous choroidopathy in the Hallermann-Streiff syndrome. *Ann Ophthalmol.* 1981;13:987.

80. Reichel E, Sandberg MA. Hereditary macular degenerations. In: Albert DM, Jakobiec FA, eds. *Principles and Prac-*

tice of Ophthalmology. Philadelphia: Saunders; 1993:1250–1252.

81. Baird LA, Cross HE. Genetic counseling of families with Best macular dystrophy. *Trans Am Acad Ophthalmol Otolaryngol.* 1975;79:865.

82. Mohler CW, Fine SL. Long-term evaluation of patients with Best's vitelliform dystrophy. *Ophthalmology.* 1981; 88:688.

83. Tasman W. Variations of vitelliform macular degeneration. *Dev Ophthalmol.* 1981;2:121.

84. Deutman AF. Macular dystrophies. In: Ryan SJ, ed. *Retina.* St. Louis, MO: Mosby; 1989:264–268.

85. Friberg TR. Choroidal and retinal folds. In: Albert DM, Jakobiec FA, eds. *Principles and Practice of Ophthalmology.* Philadelphia: Saunders; 1993:889–996.

86. Kalina RE, Mills RP. Acquired hyperopia with choroidal folds. *Ophthalmology.* 1980;87:44.

87. Dailey RA, Mills RP, Stimac GK, Shults WT, Kalina RE. The natural history and CT appearance of acquired hyperopia with choroidal folds. *Ophthalmology.* 1986;93:1336.

88. Rutnin U, Schepens CL. Fundus appearance in normal eyes. III. Peripheral degenerations. *Am J Ophthalmol.* 1967;64:1040.

89. Hirose T. Retinoschisis. In Albert DM, Jakobiec FA, eds. *Principles and Practice of Ophthalmology.* Philadelphia: Saunders; 1993:1070–1078.

90. Byer NE. A long term natural history of senile retinoschisis with implications for management. *Ophthalmology.* 1986;93:1127.

91. Hirose T, Marcil G, Schepens CL, Freeman HM. Acquired retinoschisis: observations and treatment. In: Pruett RC, Regan CDJ, eds. *Retina Congress.* New York: Appleton-Century-Crofts; 1974:489.

92. Brockhurst RJ. Discussion of Dobbie JG. Cryotherapy in the management of senile retinoschisis. *Trans Am Acad Ophthalmol Otolaryngol.* 1969;73:1060.

93. Hagler S, Woldoff HS. Retinal detachment in relation to senile retinoschisis. *Trans Am Acad Ophthalmol Otolaryngol.* 1973;773:99.

94. Byer NE. Clinical study of senile retinoschisis. *Arch Ophthalmol.* 1968;79:36.

95. Benson AH. Diseases of the vitreous. *Trans Ophthalmol Soc UK.* 1894;14:101.

96. Weiter JJ, Albert DM. Degenerative conditions of the vitreous. *Bull Soc Belge Ophthalmol.* 1987;223:115.

97. Jervey ED, Anderson WB. Asteroid hyalitis: a study of serum calcium levels in affected patients. *South Med J.* 1965;58:191.

98. Bergen RL, Brown GC, Duker JS. Prevalence and association of asteroid hyalosis with systemic diseases. *Am J Ophthalmol.* 1991;111:289.

99. Brockhurst RJ. Uveal effusion. In: Albert DM, Jakobiec FA, eds. *Principles and Practice of Ophthalmology.* Philadelphia: Saunders; 1993:548–559.

100. Kimbrough RL, Trempe CL, Brockhurst RJ, et al. Angle-closure glaucoma in nanophthalmos. *Am J Ophthalmol.* 1979;88:572.

101. Brockhurst RJ. Nanophthalmos with uveal effusion: a new clinical entity. *Trans Am Ophthalmol Soc.* 1974; 72:371.

102. Trelstad RL, Silbermann NN, Brockhurst RJ. Nanophthalmic sclera: ultrastructural, histological, and biochemical observations. *Arch Ophthalmol.* 1982;100:1935.

103. Brockhurst RJ. Vortex vein decompression for nanophthalmic uveal effusion. *Arch Ophthalmol.* 1980;98:1987.

104. Brockhurst RJ. Cataract surgery in nanophthalmic eyes. *Arch Ophthalmol.* 1990;108:965.

105. Gass JDM, Jallow S. Idiopathic serous detachment of the choroid, ciliary body, and retina (uveal effusion syndrome). *Ophthalmology.* 1982;89:1018.

106. Sieving PA, Fishman GA. Refractive errors of retinitis pigmentosa patients. *Br J Ophthalmol.* 1978;62:163.

107. Khouri G, Mets MB, Smith VC, Wendell M, Pass AS. X-linked congenital stationary night blindness. Review and report of a family with hyperopia. *Arch Ophthalmol.* 1988;106:1417.

108. Wagner RS, Caputa AR, Nelson LB, Zanoni D. High hyperopia in Leber's congenital amaurosis. *Arch Ophthalmol.* 1985;103:1507.

109. Heckenlively JR. Preserved para-arteriole retinal pigment epithelium in retinitis pigmentosa. *Br J Ophthalmol.* 1982;66:26.

110. Lam BL, Judisch GF. Early-onset autosomal dominant retinitis pigmentosa with severe hyperopia. *Am J Ophthalmol.* 1991;111:454.

111. Mullie MA, Sanders MD. Scleral canal size and optic nerve head drusen. *Am J Ophthalmol.* 1985;99:356.

112. Cogan DG. Pathology of the optic nerve. In: Albert DM, Jakobiec FA, eds. *Principles and Practice of Ophthalmology.* Philadelphia: Saunders; 1993:2361.

113. Walsh FB, Hoyt WF. *Clinical Neuro-Ophthalmology,* 4th ed. Baltimore: William & Wilkins; 1982:355–365.

114. Strassman I, Silverston B, Seelenfreund M, Landau L, Scher A, Berson D. Optic disc drusen and hypermetropia. *Metab Ped Sys Ophthalmol.* 1991;14:37.

115. Glaser JS. The ischemic optic neuropathies. In Albert DM, Jakobiec FA, eds. *Principles and Practice of Ophthalmology.* Philadelphia: Saunders; 1993:2568–2578.

116. Beck RW, Servais GE, Hayreh SS. Anterior ischemic optic neuropathy. IX. Cup-to-disc ratio and its role in pathogenesis. *Ophthalmology.* 1987;94:1503.

117. Mansour AM, Shoch D, Logani S. Optic disk size in ischemic optic neuropathy. *Am J Ophthalmol.* 1988;106:587.

118. Katz B, Spencer WH. Hyperopia as a risk factor for nonarteritic anterior ischemic optic neuropathy. *Am J Ophthalmol.* 1993;116:754.

119. Corbett JJ. Idiopathic intracranial hypertension (pseudotumor cerebri). In: Albert DM, Jakobiec FA, eds. *Principles*

and Practice of Ophthalmology. Philadelphia: Saunders; 1993:2698–2706.

120. Orcutt JC, Page NGR, Sanders MD. Factors affecting visual loss in benign intracranial hypertension. *Ophthalmology.* 1984;91:1303.

121. Duke-Elder S, Abrams D. Ophthalmic optics and refraction. In: Duke-Elder S, ed. *System of Ophthalmology,* vol. V. London: Henry Kimpton; 1970:368–370.

122. Granstrom KO. Refraktionsveraderungen bei Diabetes Mellitus. *Acta Ophthalmol.* 1933;1:1.

123. Mantyjarvi M. Myopia and diabetes, a review. *Acta Ophthalmol.* 185:82.

124. Gwinup G, Villareal A. Relationship of serum glucose concentration to changes in refraction. *Diabetes.* 1976; 25:29.

125. Bellow JG. The crystalline lens in diabetes mellitus. 1944; 32:498.

126. Rosen M. Diabetes mellitus with relative hyperopia. *Am J Ophthalmol.* 1956;41:680.

127. Planten J Th. Physiologic optic approach of lens and cataract. *Ophthalmologica.* 1975;171:249.

128. Eva PR, Pascoe PT, Vaughan DG. Refractive change in hyperglycemia: hyperopia, not myopia. *Br J Ophthalmol.* 1982;66:500.

129. Saito Y, Ohmi G, Kinoshita S, et al. Transient hyperopia with lens swelling at initial therapy in diabetes. *Br J Ophthalmol.* 1993;77:145.

130. Caird FL, Pirie A, Ramsell TG. *Diabetes and the Eye.* Oxford: Blackwell; 1969:122–126.

131. Marmor MF. Transient accommodative paralysis and hyperopia in diabetes. *Arch Ophthalmol.* 1973;89:419.

132. Fledelius HC. Is myopia getting more frequent? A cross-sectional study of 1416 Danes aged 16 years. *Acta Ophthalmol.* 1983;61:545.

133. Fledelius HC. Myopia and diabetes mellitus with special reference to adult-onset myopia. *Acta Ophthalmol.* 64:33.

134. Fledelius HC, Miyamoto K. Diabetic myopia—is it lens-induced? An oculometric study comprising ultrasound measurements. *Acta Ophthalmol.* 1987;65:469.

135. Jain IS, Luthra CL, Das T. Diabetic retinopathy and its relation to errors of refraction. *Arch Ophthalmol.* 1967;77:59.

136. Rand LJ, Krolewski AS, Aiello LM, Warram JH, Baker RS, Maki T. Multiple factors in the prediction of risk of proliferative retinopathy. *N Engl J Med.* 1985;313:1433.

137. Baker RS, Rand LJ, Krolewski AS, Maki T, Warram JH, Aiello LM. Influence of HLA-DR phenotype and myopia on the risk of nonproliferative and proliferative diabetic retinopathy. *Am J Ophthalmol.* 1986;102:693.

138. McMullen WW, D'Amico DJ. AIDS and its ophthalmic manifestations. In Albert DM, Jakobiec FA, eds. *Principles*

139. Witkop CJ Jr, Quevedo WC Jr, Fitzpatrick TB. Albinism and other disorders of pigment metabolism. In: Stanbury JB, Wyngaarden JB, Frederickson DS, et al, eds. *The Metabolic Basis of Inherited Disease,* 5th ed. New York: McGraw-Hill; 1985:301.

140. Edmunds RT. Vision of albinos. *Arch Ophthalmol.* 1949; 42:775.

141. Crandall A. Developmental ocular abnormalities and glaucoma. *Int Ophthalmol.* 1984;24:73.

142. Godel V, Nemet P, Lazar M. The Wagner-Stickler syndrome complex. *Doc Ophthalmol.* 1981;52:179.

143. Robertson JE, Meyer SM. Hereditary vitreoretinal degenerations. In Ryan SJ, ed. *The Retina,* vol. 1. St. Louis, MO: Mosby; 1979:474–476.

144. Maumenee IH. The eye in the Marfan syndrome. *Trans Am Ophthalmol Soc.* 1981;79:684.

145. Murdoch JL, Walker BA, Halpern BL, et al. Life expectancy and causes of death in the Marfan syndrome. *N Engl J Med.* 1972;286:804.

146. Gardiner PA. Visual defects in cases of Down's syndrome and in other mentally handicapped children. *Br J Ophthalmol.* 1967;51:469.

147. Lowe RF. The eyes in mongolism. *Br J Ophthalmol.* 1949; 33:131.

148. Shapiro MB, France TD. The ocular features of Down's syndrome. *Am J Ophthalmol.* 1985;99:659.

149. Clarren SK, Smith DW. The fetal alcohol syndrome. *N Engl J Med.* 1978;298:1063.

150. Miller M, Israel J, Cuttone J. The fetal alcohol syndrome. *J Pediatr Ophthalmol.* 1981;18:6.

151. Kieval SJ. Viral infections of the retina in the pediatric patient. In: Albert DM, Jakobiec FA, eds. *Principles and Practice of Ophthalmology.* Philadelphia: Saunders; 1993: 962–963.

152. Goldschmidt E. Refraction in the newborn. *Acta Ophthalmol.* 1969;47:370.

153. Wolff SM. The ocular manifestations of congenital rubella. A prospective study of 328 cases of congenital rubella. *J Pediatr Ophthalmol.* 1973;10:101.

154. Adams RD, DeLong GR. Developmental and other congenital abnormalities of the nervous system. In: Petersdorf et al, eds. *Harrison's Principles of Internal Medicine,* 10th ed. New York: McGraw-Hill; 1983:2137–2138.

155. Fantl EW, Perlstein MA. Ocular refractive characteristics in cerebral palsy. *Am J Dis Child.* 1961;102:36.

INDEX

A

Ablative photodecompensation, 417
Ablative photodecomposition, 49
Acanthamoeba
  keratitis, 79
  postoperative infection, 322
Accommodation
  age-related values for, 309, 310*t*
  equal amplitude, postoperative
    considerations, 123
  and hyperopia, in young person,
    309
  preoperative evaluation, 119
  spasm of
    causes, 122
    postoperative considerations, 122–
      123
    signs and symptoms, 122
  unequal amplitude, postoperative
    considerations, 123
Achromatopsia, congenital, 647
Acne rosacea, ocular manifestations, 77
Acquired immunodeficiency syndrome
  HIV-related diffuse infiltrative
    lymphadenopathy in, tear film
    deficiency in, 82
  myopia in, 652
Acquired retinoschisis, 644–646, 645*f*
α-Actin, in corneal wound healing, 24–
  25
Acular. *See* Ketorolac
Adenovirus conjunctivitis, 79–80, 80*f*
Adie syndrome, tear film deficiency in,
  82
β-Adrenergic blockers, tear film
    deficiency caused by, 82
Aelotropic materials, 197
Age
  astigmatism reduction using arcuate
    keratome and, 237

as contraindication to refractive
    surgery, 102–103, 259
  exudative macular degeneration
    related to, 641, 642*f*
  refractive correction with radial
    keratotomy and, 261, 274–
    275
Airborne contamination, precautions
    against, 211
Air purification, 211
Airy, George Biddell, 157
AK. *See* Astigmatic keratotomy
AKC. *See* Atopic keratoconjunctivitis
Albinism
  Chediak-Higashi syndrome, 653
  genetics of, 653
  Hermansky-Pudliak variant, 653
  ocular, 653
  oculocutaneous, 653
Alcon EyeMap EH290 Corneal
    Topographer, 162
ALK. *See* Automated lamellar
    keratoplasty
Alkali injury, corneal, wound healing
    in, 25–26
Allergan Medical Optics, 385–386,
    404
Allergic conjunctivitis, 84–85
Alloplastic keratophakia, advantages
    of, 373
Alloplastic lenticular implants,
    advantages and
    disadvantages of, 373
Alport's syndrome, 655, 656*f*
Ametropia, 3–4
  ocular and systemic associations
    with, 627–661
Amikacin, for postoperative ocular
    infections, 322
Aminoglycosides, for postoperative
    ocular infections, 322

Amiodarone, ocular effects, 95
Amphotericin-B, for postoperative
    ocular infections, 322
Amyloidosis, ocular manifestations, 96
Analgesia, topical, postoperative
    therapy, 65
Analgesic(s). *See also* Nonsteroidal anti-
    inflammatory drugs
  tear film deficiency caused by, 82
Ancef, for postoperative infections, 337
Anesthesia
  for laser in situ keratomileusis, 458
  for surgical repair of corneal
    lacerations, 565
Anesthesiometer, 225
Angle kappa, 127–128
Angle lambda, 127–128, 128*f*, 130, 154*f*
Angle of deviation, in diplopia, 519
Angle of incidence, 113, 114*f*
Angle of refraction, 113, 114*f*
Anhidrotic ectodermal dysplasia, tear
    film deficiency in, 82
Animal model(s)
  of corneal wound healing, 29, 31–32,
    34, 35*f*, 35–36, 37*f*, 257–258
  for myopic intrastromal
    photorefractive keratectomy,
    474–477, 475*f*–477*f*
  for prismatic photokeratectomy, 520–
    521
  for synthetic epikeratoplasty, 408*f*,
    408–412, 409*t*, 410*f*–411*f*
Aniridia, keratoconus and, 93
Aniseikonia, 118
Anisometric blur suppression, with
    monovision, 138–139
Anisometropia
  correction of, 116
  postkeratotomy, 287
  postoperative considerations, 122
  preoperative evaluation, 117–118

EAST GLAMORGAN GENERAL HOSPITAL
CHURCH VILLAGE, near PONTYPRIDD

EAST GLAMORGAN GENERAL HOSPITAL
CHURCH VILLAGE. near PONTYPRIDD

EAST GLAMORGAN GENERAL HOSPITAL
CHURCH VILLAGE. near PONTYPRIDD

This is not the end. It is not
even the beginning of the end. But it
is, perhaps, the end of the beginning.

Winston Churchill
The ''Victory of Egypt'' speech at
Mansion House, London, 10 November 1942